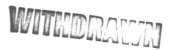

HANDBOOK OF COMPETENCE AND MOTIVATION

Handbook of
Competence and Motivation

SECOND EDITION

Theory and Application

Edited by

Andrew J. Elliot
Carol S. Dweck
David S. Yeager

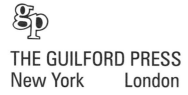

THE GUILFORD PRESS
New York   London

Copyright © 2017 The Guilford Press
A Division of Guilford Publications, Inc.
370 Seventh Avenue, Suite 1200, New York, NY 10001
www.guilford.com

Printed in the United States of America

This book is printed on acid-free paper.

Last digit is print number: 9 8 7 6 5 4 3 2 1

Library of Congress Cataloging-in-Publication Data

Names: Elliot, Andrew J., editor. | Dweck, Carol S., 1946– editor. | Yeager, David S., editor.
Title: Handbook of competence and motivation : theory and application / edited by Andrew J. Elliot, Carol S. Dweck, David S. Yeager.
Description: Second edition. | New York : Guilford Press, [2017] | Includes bibliographical references and index.
Identifiers: LCCN 2016036820 | ISBN 9781462529605 (hardcover)
Subjects: LCSH: Achievement motivation.
Classification: LCC BF504 .H36 2017 | DDC 153.8—dc23
LC record available at https://lccn.loc.gov/2016036820

About the Editors

Andrew J. Elliot, PhD, is Professor of Psychology at the University of Rochester. He has been a visiting professor at Cambridge University and Oxford University, United Kingdom; King Abdulaziz University, Saudi Arabia; and the University of Munich, Germany; and a Visiting Fellow at Churchill College (Cambridge) and Jesus College (Oxford). Dr. Elliot's research focuses on achievement motivation and approach–avoidance motivation. He is editor of *Advances in Motivation Science* and author of approximately 200 scholarly publications. The recipient of multiple awards for his teaching and research contributions to educational and social/personality psychology, Dr. Elliot has given keynote or university addresses in more than 20 countries, and his lab regularly hosts professors, postdocs, and graduate students from around the globe.

Carol S. Dweck, PhD, is the Lewis and Virginia Eaton Professor of Psychology at Stanford University. Her research focuses on the critical role of mindsets in students' achievement and has led to successful intervention to foster student learning. She is a member of the American Academy of Arts and Sciences and the U.S. National Academy of Sciences, and is the recipient of nine different lifetime achievement awards for her research. Dr. Dweck addressed the United Nations at the beginning of its new global development agenda and has advised governments on educational and economic policies. Her bestselling book *Mindset: The New Psychology of Success* brought her research to the wider public.

David S. Yeager, PhD, is Assistant Professor of Psychology at the University of Texas at Austin. His research focuses on motivation and adolescent development and on the use of behavioral science to make improvements toward pressing social issues. Dr. Yeager is co-chair of the Mindset Scholars Network, an interdisciplinary network devoted to improving the science of learning mindsets and expanding educational opportunity. He holds appointments at the Carnegie Foundation for the Advancement of Teaching, the Population Research Center and the Charles A. Dana Center at the University of Texas at Austin, and the Center for Advanced Study in the Behavioral Sciences. Dr. Yeager is the recipient of more than 15 awards in social, developmental, and educational psychology.

Contributors

Katherine A. Adams, PhD,
Department of Applied Psychology,
New York University, New York, New York

Eric M. Anderman, PhD,
Department of Educational Studies,
The Ohio State University, Columbus, Ohio

Sian L. Beilock, PhD, Department of Psychology
and Committee on Education,
University of Chicago, Chicago, Illinois

Rebecca S. Bigler, PhD,
Department of Psychology,
University of Texas at Austin, Austin, Texas

Clancy Blair, PhD,
Department of Applied Psychology,
New York University, New York, New York

Kathryn L. Boucher, PhD,
School of Psychological Sciences,
University of Indianapolis, Indianapolis, Indiana

Shannon T. Brady, MS,
Graduate School of Education,
Stanford University, Stanford, California

Fabrizio Butera, PhD, Institute of Psychology,
University of Lausanne, Lausanne, Switzerland

Ruth Butler, PhD, School of Education,
Hebrew University of Jerusalem,
Jerusalem, Israel

Andrei Cimpian, PhD,
Department of Psychology,
New York University, New York, New York

Geoffrey L. Cohen, PhD,
Department of Psychology
and Graduate School of Education,
Stanford University, Stanford, California

David E. Conroy, PhD,
Department of Kinesiology,
The Pennsylvania State University,
University Park, Pennsylvania;
Department of Preventive Medicine,
Northwestern University, Chicago, Illinois

Rhonda G. Craven, PhD,
Institute of Positive Psychology and Education,
Australian Catholic University,
Sydney, Australia

Ronald E. Dahl, MD,
Community Health Sciences Division,
School of Public Health,
University of California, Berkeley,
Berkeley, California

Céline Darnon, PhD,
Social and Cognitive Psychology Laboratory,
Clermont Auvergne University,
Clermont-Ferrand, France

Carsten K. W. De Dreu, PhD,
Institute of Psychology,
Social and Organizational Psychology,
Leiden University, Leiden, The Netherlands;
Center for Experimental Economics
and Political Decision Making,
University of Amsterdam,
Amsterdam, The Netherlands

Maria K. DiBenedetto, PhD,
Bishop McGuinness Catholic High School,
Kernersville, North Carolina

Andrea G. Dittmann, BA,
Kellogg School of Management,
Northwestern University, Evanston, Illinois

Carol S. Dweck, PhD,
Department of Psychology, Stanford University,
Stanford, California

Jacquelynne S. Eccles, PhD,
School of Education,
University of California, Irvine,
Irvine, California

Andrew J. Elliot, PhD,
Department of Clinical and Social Sciences
in Psychology, University of Rochester,
Rochester, New York

Meiyu Fang, PhD, Graduate Institute
of Human Resource Management,
National Central University,
Jhongli City, Taiwan

Julio Garcia, PhD,
Department of Psychology
and Graduate School of Education,
Stanford University, Stanford, California

Barry Gerhart, PhD,
Department of Management
and Human Resources,
University of Wisconsin–Madison,
Madison, Wisconsin

J. Parker Goyer, PhD,
Department of Psychology
and Graduate School of Education,
Stanford University, Stanford, California

DeLeon L. Gray, PhD,
Department of Teacher Education
and Learning Sciences, College of Education,
North Carolina State University,
Raleigh, North Carolina

Wendy S. Grolnick, PhD,
Department of Psychology, Clark University,
Worcester, Massachusetts

Jeremy M. Hamm, PhD,
Department of Psychology and Social Behavior,
University of California, Irvine,
Irvine, California

Judith M. Harackiewicz, PhD,
Department of Psychology,
University of Wisconsin–Madison,
Madison, Wisconsin

Liat Hasenfratz, PhD,
Martin Buber Society of Fellows,
Hebrew University of Jerusalem,
Jerusalem, Israel

Amy Roberson Hayes, PhD,
Department of Psychology,
University of Texas at Tyler, Tyler, Texas

Jutta Heckhausen, PhD,
Department of Psychology and Social Behavior,
University of California, Irvine,
Irvine, California

Chris S. Hulleman, PhD,
Center for the Advanced Study
of Teaching and Learning,
University of Virginia, Charlottesville, Virginia

Jeremy P. Jamieson, PhD,
Department of Clinical and Social Sciences
in Psychology, University of Rochester,
Rochester, New York

Ruth Kanfer, PhD,
Department of Psychology,
Georgia Institute of Technology,
Atlanta, Georgia

Maximilian Knogler, PhD,
School of Education,
Technical University of Munich,
Munich, Germany

Beth E. Kurtz-Costes, PhD,
Department of Psychology and Neuroscience,
University of North Carolina at Chapel Hill,
Chapel Hill, North Carolina

Hae Yeon Lee, MA,
Department of Psychology,
University of Texas at Austin, Austin, Texas

Michael P. Leiter, PhD,
School of Psychology, Deakin University,
Geelong, Victoria, Australia

Herbert W. Marsh, PhD, DSc,
Institute of Positive Psychology and Education,
Australian Catholic University,
Sydney, Australia

Andrew J. Martin, PhD,
School of Education,
University of New South Wales,
Sydney, Australia

Christina Maslach, PhD,
Department of Psychology,
University of California, Berkeley,
Berkeley, California

Daniel C. Molden, PhD,
Department of Psychology,
Northwestern University, Evanston, Illinois

Arlen C. Moller, PhD,
Department of Psychology,
Illinois Institute of Technology, Chicago, Illinois

Bernard A. Nijstad, PhD,
Department of Organizational Behavior
and Human Decision Making,
University of Groningen,
Groningen, The Netherlands

Meagan M. Patterson, PhD,
Department of Educational Psychology,
University of Kansas, Lawrence, Kansas

Reinhard Pekrun, PhD,
Department of Psychology,
University of Munich, Munich, Germany;
Institute for Positive Psychology
and Education, Australian Catholic University,
Sydney, Australia

Raymond P. Perry, PhD,
Department of Psychology,
University of Manitoba, Winnipeg,
Manitoba, Canada

Eva M. Pomerantz, PhD,
Department of Psychology,
University of Illinois at Urbana–Champaign,
Champaign, Illinois

C. Cybele Raver, PhD,
Department of Applied Psychology,
New York University, New York, New York

Christopher S. Rozek, PhD,
Department of Psychology,
University of Chicago, Chicago, Illinois

Emily Q. Rozenzweig, PhD,
Department of Human Development
and Quantitative Methodology,
University of Maryland, College Park, Maryland

Richard M. Ryan, PhD,
Institute for Positive Psychology and Education,
Australian Catholic University,
Sydney, Australia;
Department of Clinical and Social Sciences
in Psychology, University of Rochester,
Rochester, New York

Robert J. Rydell, PhD,
Department of Psychological and Brain Sciences,
Indiana University Bloomington, Indiana

Marjorie W. Schaeffer, MA,
Department of Psychology,
University of Chicago, Chicago, Illinois

Dale H. Schunk, PhD,
Department of Teacher Education
and Higher Education,
University of North Carolina at Greensboro,
Greensboro, North Carolina

Jacob Shane, PhD,
Department of Psychology, Brooklyn College,
City University of New York,
Brooklyn, New York

Christopher M. Spray, PhD,
School of Sport, Exercise and Health Sciences,
Loughborough University,
Loughborough, United Kingdom

Nicole M. Stephens, PhD,
Kellogg School of Management,
Northwestern University, Evanston, Illinois

Robert J. Sternberg, PhD,
Department of Human Development,
Cornell University, Ithaca, New York

Sarah S. M. Townsend, PhD,
Marshall School of Business,
University of Southern California,
Los Angeles, California

Elliot M. Tucker-Drob, PhD,
Department of Psychology,
University of Texas at Austin, Austin, Texas

Katie J. Van Loo, PhD,
Department of Psychological and Brain Sciences,
Indiana University Bloomington, Indiana

Nico W. Van Yperen, PhD,
Department of Psychology,
University of Groningen,
Groningen, The Netherlands

Gregory M. Walton, PhD,
Department of Psychology, Stanford University,
Stanford, California

Kathryn R. Wentzel, PhD,
Department of Human Development
and Quantitative Methodology,
University of Maryland,
College Park, Maryland

Allan Wigfield, PhD,
Department of Human Development
and Quantitative Methodology,
University of Maryland,
College Park, Maryland

Taniesha A. Woods, PhD,
independent consultant, New York, New York

David S. Yeager, PhD,
Department of Psychology,
University of Texas at Austin, Austin, Texas

Alexander Seeshing Yeung, PhD,
Institute of Positive Psychology and Education,
Australian Catholic University,
Sydney, Australia

Barry J. Zimmerman, PhD,
Doctoral Program in Educational Psychology,
Graduate Center, City University of New York,
New York, New York

Contents

PART III. RELEVANT PROCESSES

PART IV. DEVELOPMENT

PART V. SOCIAL GROUPS AND SOCIAL INFLUENCES

PART VI. PSYCHOLOGICAL INTERVENTIONS

Purchasers of this handbook can visit *www.guilford.com/elliot3-materials*
to download a free supplemental e-book featuring several notable, highly
cited chapters from the first edition.

A Conceptual History of the Achievement Goal Construct
ANDREW J. ELLIOT

Motivation from an Attribution Perspective
and the Social Psychology of Perceived Competence
BERNARD WEINER

Self-Theories: Their Impact on Competence Motivation
and Acquisition
CAROL S. DWECK and DANIEL C. MOLDEN

Competence Motivation in the Classroom
TIM URDAN and JULIANNE C. TURNER

Cultural Competence: Dynamic Processes
CHI-YUE CHIU and YING-YI HONG

PART I

INTRODUCTION

CHAPTER 1

Competence and Motivation

Theory and Application

ANDREW J. ELLIOT
CAROL S. DWECK
DAVID S. YEAGER

A dozen years ago, the *Handbook of Competence and Motivation* (Elliot & Dweck, 2005) was published. The *Handbook* consisted of 35 chapters written by well-known scholars across diverse disciplines, and it had an ambitious aim—to refocus the achievement motivation literature using the concept of competence. Specifically, we (Elliot and Dweck) sought to establish competence as the conceptual core of the achievement motivation literature, and proposed that this conceptual shift be accompanied by a shift in terminology from *achievement motivation* to *competence motivation*.

Why did we ground the achievement motivation literature in the concept of competence? We did so because we saw two primary weaknesses in this literature: (1) The literature lacked coherence and a clear set of structural parameters on which to base theory and guide operationalization (in short, there was no obvious, consensual answer to the question "What should and should not be included within a literature on achievement motivation?"), and (2) the literature was too narrowly focused and limited in scope, especially relative to its potential. As a function of these weaknesses, the literature that had developed represented a collection of loosely related conceptual ideas and empirical findings based on a colloquial, primarily Western notion of the term *achievement*.

We sought to provide a North Star for this literature by establishing competence as its conceptual core. We chose competence as the conceptual core because doing so addressed both of the weaknesses we had identified. First, *competence* may be precisely and clearly defined as a condition or quality of effectiveness, ability, sufficiency, or success. Therefore, *competence motivation* encompasses the appetitive energization and direction of behavior with regard to effectiveness, ability, sufficiency, or success (as well as the aversive energization and direction of behavior with regard to ineffectiveness, inability, insufficiency, or failure). Second, competence motivation is broadly and deeply applicable to psychological functioning: It is ubiquitous in everyday life, it has an important influence on emotion and well-being, it is operative and integral throughout the lifespan, and it is relevant to individuals across cultures. In short, we believed that competence had great potential as a precise, broadly applicable concept that could help integrate and provide guidance for a literature that was failing to reach its full potential.

We (and The Guilford Press) were extremely pleased with the reception that the *Handbook* received. This was subjectively represented by the many positive comments we received from scholars in the field, and objectively represented by the large number of citations of the chapters in the volume and the large number of copies sold. Given this positive reception, Guilford approached us to request that we edit a second edition of the *Handbook*. We agreed and (slightly) expanded our editorial team.

We (Elliot, Dweck, and Yeager) were not interested in a second edition that merely rehashed the material from the initial edition; instead, we wanted new, fresh chapters. Indeed, this is what we both solicited and received from our authors. Structurally, whereas some of the sections of the *Handbook* are the same as the original, others are different. Likewise, some of the chapter topics are the same, while others are different. Many of the authors are the same, but again, many are different. What is, emphatically, the same across the two editions of the *Handbook* is the caliber of the authors and the chapters that they have provided. As in the initial volume, we have received chapters from well-known researchers in their areas of expertise and they have, without exception, delivered excellent, authoritative, state-of-the-science reviews of their focal topic. What is decidedly new in this edition of the *Handbook* is a focus on application.

Since the first edition of the *Handbook* was published, the field has entered a new and exciting phase in which there has been a burgeoning interest in applying basic motivational theory, concepts, and ideas to real-world contexts. Most notably, there has been an influx of research on the implementation and testing of motivational interventions in schools (especially), the workplace, and the ballfield (for reviews, see Karabenick & Urdan, 2014; Lazowski & Hulleman, 2016; Lin-Siegler, Dweck, & Cohen, 2016; Spitzer & Aronson, 2015; Wilson & Buttrick, 2016; Yeager & Walton, 2011). This and related work holds considerable promise for both "giving away" knowledge gleaned in the ivory tower and feeding back important information from the "front lines" that can aid in theory refinement and development. For this reason, in this second edition

of the *Handbook,* we changed the charge to our authors, explicitly asking them to include coverage of the link between theory and application. This extended focus may be concretely seen in the new title: *Handbook of Competence and Motivation, Second Edition: Theory and Application.* It is our hope that this extended focus of the *Handbook* will broaden and deepen our coverage of this important area of inquiry, and prompt new insights from the theory-to-practice interface.

The *Handbook* reflects and celebrates the renaissance of motivation as a field, not just the field of competence motivation, but the field of motivation more generally. After the "cognitive revolution," the field fell into disarray, and research on motivation slowed to a trickle. In fact, in the 1980s, the esteemed series, the *Nebraska Symposium on Motivation,* even considered dropping the term *motivation* from its title (it did not do so for fear of losing name recognition and, accordingly, library subscriptions). How far the field has come since then is manifest in informative, programmatic research and applications grounded in attribution theories, goal theories, approach–avoidance theories, expectancy–value theories, need theories, implicit theories, cultural theories, identity theories, and more. We believe that there has never been a more exciting time in the field of motivation in general and competence motivation in particular. We hope the present excitement is only exceeded by the era to come (which will be, we anticipate, covered in the future editions of the *Handbook*).

This volume comprises six sections. Part I is simply an introduction to the volume, and it leads into Part II, which focuses on the constructs that are central to the competence motivation literature. These constructs are intelligence and ability (i.e., competence per se), the motives that energize competence-relevant behavior, the goals that direct competence-relevant behavior, the attributions used to explain competence and incompetence, the perceptions that one has of one's competence, the ways in which one values competence, implicit theories about competence, and anxiety regarding incompetence.

Part III focuses on processes that are relevant to competence motivation. In these chapters, competence is not the central focus, but it is nevertheless integrally implicated in the processes under consideration. These processes are challenge and threat appraisals, social comparison, autonomy, performance incentives, emotions, belonging, stereotype threat, self-regulated learning, intrinsic motivation, creativity, and burnout. These chapters nicely illustrate the broad reach of competence motivation across a diverse set of important psychological processes.

Part IV shifts from constructs and processes to issues regarding the development of competence motivation. Here the coverage encompasses mental representations in early childhood, self-regulation in early childhood, competence motivation in adolescence, competence motivation in the aging process, and gene–environment interactions in the emergence of competence motivation.

Following development, the focus in Part V is on demographic categories and socialization contexts that have a critical, pervasive influence on competence motivation. The roles of gender, social class, race, and social identity are addressed, as are the influences of parents, peers, teachers and schools, coaches, and employers and the workplace. Finally, Part VI provides a general primer on the intervention approach to application that is having a major impact on contemporary theory and research.

We believe that this second edition of the *Handbook* nicely builds on the foundation laid by the initial edition. The chapters herein clearly demonstrate that research on competence and motivation is continuing apace, with much fruit emerging on both the theoretical and applied fronts. We trust that, like ourselves, you will learn much from and be inspired by what you read in the pages that follow.

REFERENCES

Elliot, A. J., & Dweck, C. S. (Eds.). (2005). *Handbook of competence and motivation.* New York: Guilford Press.

Karabenick, S. A., & Urdan, T. C. (Eds.). (2014). *Advances in motivation and achievement: Vol. 18. Motivational interventions.* Bingley, UK: Emerald.

Lazowski, R. A., & Hulleman, C. S. (2016). Motivation interventions in education: A meta-analytic review. *Review of Educational Research, 86,* 602–640.

Lin-Siegler, X., Dweck, C. S., & Cohen, G. L. (2016). Instructional interventions that motivate classroom learning. *Journal of Educational Psychology, 108,* 295–299.

Spitzer, B., & Aronson, J. (2015). Minding and mending the gap: Social psychological interventions to reduce educational disparities. *British Journal of Educational Psychology, 85,* 1–18.

Wilson, T. D., & Buttrick, N. R. (2016). New directions in social psychological interventions to improve academic achievement. *Journal of Educational Psychology, 108,* 392–396.

Yeager, D. S., & Walton, G. (2011). Social-psychological interventions in education: They're not magic. *Review of Educational Research, 81,* 267–301.

PART II

CENTRAL CONSTRUCTS

CHAPTER 2

Intelligence and Competence in Theory and Practice

ROBERT J. STERNBERG

Intelligence tests are supposed to measure a construct that is (1) unified (so-called "general intelligence"), (2) relatively fixed by genetic endowment, and (3) distinct from and precedent to the competencies that schools develop (see, e.g., Carroll, 1993; Hunt, 2010; Mackintosh, 2011). All three of these assumptions are open to question.

A major goal of work here is to integrate the study of intelligence and related skills (see reviews in Sternberg, 1990; Sternberg, Jarvin, & Grigorenko, 2011; Sternberg & Kaufman, 2011) with the study of competence (Cianciolo, Matthew, Wagner, & Sternberg, 2006; Sternberg, 2014). Intelligence tests measure achieved skills or competencies. Even abstract reasoning tests measure achievement in dealing with geometric symbols, skills taught in Western schools (see Ang, Van Dyne, & Tan, 2011; Niu & Brass, 2011).

HOW INDIVIDUALS TRANSLATE SKILLS INTO ACHIEVEMENT

Achievement does not just depend on abilities, of course. It depends on the interaction of abilities with other key attributes of the person. Consider a model for how basic skills or abilities are translated into achievement.

Elements of the Model

The model of developing competencies has five key elements (although certainly they do not constitute an exhaustive list of elements in the ultimate development of competencies from precursor abilities): metacognitive skills, learning skills, thinking skills, knowledge, and motivation (Dai & Sternberg, 2004). Although it is convenient to separate these five elements, they are fully interactive. They influence each other, both directly and indirectly. For example, learning leads to knowledge, but knowledge facilitates further learning.

These elements are, to some extent, domain specific. The development of competencies in one area does not necessarily lead to the development of competencies in another area, although there may be some transfer, depending on the relationship of the areas, a point that has been made with regard to intelligence by others as well (e.g., Gardner, 2011; Sternberg, 2002, 2003; Sternberg & Grigorenko, 2007).

In the augmented theory of successful intelligence (Sternberg, 1984, 1985, 1999, 2003), intelligence is viewed as having four aspects: analytical, creative, practical, and wisdom-based skills. These aspects can be somewhat domain specific. For example, our research suggests that the development of competencies in one creative domain (Sternberg & Lubart, 1995, 1996) or in one practical domain (Hedlund et al., 2003; Sternberg, Wagner, & Okagaki, 1993; Sternberg, Wagner, Williams, & Horvath, 1995) shows modest-to-moderate correlations with the development of competencies in other such domains. However, psychometric research suggests more domain generality for the analytical domain (Jensen, 1998; Sternberg & Grigorenko, 2002). Moreover, people can show analytical, creative, practical, or wisdom-based competence in one domain without showing all three of these kinds of competencies, or even two of the three.

1. *Metacognitive skills.* Metacognitive skills (or metacomponents; Sternberg, 1985) refer to people's understanding and control of their own cognition. Seven metacognitive skills are particularly important: problem recognition, problem definition, problem representation, strategy formulation, resource allocation, monitoring of problem solving, and evaluation of problem solving (Sternberg, 1985). All of these skills are modifiable (Sternberg & Grigorenko, 2007; Sternberg, Kaufman, & Grigorenko, 2008).

2. *Learning skills.* Learning skills (knowledge-acquisition components) are essential to the model (Sternberg, 1985; Sternberg et al., 2008), although they are certainly not the only learning skills that individuals use. Examples of learning skills are selective encoding, which involves distinguishing relevant from irrelevant information; selective combination, which involves putting together the relevant information; and selective comparison, which involves relating new information to information already stored in memory (Sternberg, 1985).

3. *Thinking skills.* There are four main kinds of thinking skills (or performance components) that individuals need to master (Sternberg, 1985, 1994; Sternberg et al., 2008; Sternberg & Weil, 1980). It is important to note that these are sets of, rather than individual, thinking skills. Critical (analytical) thinking skills include analyzing, critiquing, judging, evaluating, comparing and contrasting, and assessing. Creative thinking skills include creating,

discovering, inventing, imagining, supposing, and hypothesizing. Practical thinking skills include applying, using, utilizing, and practicing (Sternberg et al., 2000; Sternberg & Hedlund, 2002). Wisdom-based skills include utilizing knowledge toward a common good and balancing one's own interests with others (Sternberg, 2013). These various skills are the first step in the translation of thought into real-world action.

4. *Knowledge.* There are two main kinds of knowledge that are relevant in academic situations. Declarative knowledge is of facts, concepts, principles, laws, and the like. It is "knowing that." Procedural knowledge is of procedures and strategies. It is "knowing how."

5. *Motivation.* One can distinguish among several different kinds of motivation. A first kind of motivation is achievement motivation (McClelland, 1985; McClelland, Atkinson, Clark, & Lowell, 1976). People who are high in achievement motivation seek moderate challenges and risks. They are attracted to tasks that are neither very easy nor very hard. They are strivers—constantly trying to better themselves and their accomplishments. A second kind of motivation, competence (self-efficacy) motivation, refers to persons' beliefs in their own ability to solve the problem at hand (Bandura, 1996). This kind of self-efficacy can result both from intrinsic and extrinsic rewards (Amabile, 1996; Sternberg, 1996). Of course, other kinds of motivation are important, too. Indeed, motivation is perhaps the indispensable element needed for school success. Without it, the student never even tries to learn. And, of course, if a test is not important to the examinee, he or she may do poorly simply through a lack of effort to perform well.

Dweck (1999, 2002, 2007; Dweck & Elliott, 1983) has shown that one of the most important sources of motivation is individuals' motivation to enhance their intellectual skills (also see essays in Aarts & Elliot, 2011). What Dweck and her colleagues have shown is that some individuals are entity theorists with respect to intelligence: They believe that to be smart is to show oneself to be smart, and that means not making mistakes or otherwise showing intellectual weakness. Incremental theorists, in contrast, believe that to be smart is to learn and to increase one's intellectual skills. These individuals are not afraid to make mistakes, and even believe that making a mistake can be useful because it is a way to learn. Dweck and her colleagues' research suggests that, under normal conditions, entity and incremental theorists perform about the same in school. But under conditions of challenge, incremental theorists do better because they are more willing to undertake difficult challenges and to seek mastery of new, difficult material.

6. *Context.* All of the elements discussed earlier are characteristics of the learner. Returning to the issues raised at the beginning of this chapter, a problem with conventional tests is that they assume that individuals operate in a more or less decontextualized environment (see Grigorenko & Sternberg, 2001b; Sternberg, 1985, 1997 ; Sternberg & Grigorenko, 2001). A test score is interpreted largely in terms of the individual's internal attributes. But a test measures much more, and the assumption of a fixed or uniform context across test-takers is not realistic. Contextual factors that can affect test performance include native language, family background, emphasis of test on speedy performance, and familiarity with the kinds of material on the test, among many other things.

Interactions of Elements

The novice works toward competence (and then expertise) through deliberate practice (Ericsson, 1996; Ericsson, Krampe, & Tesch-Römer, 1993). But this practice requires an interaction of all five of the key elements. At the center, driving the elements, is motivation. Without it, the elements remain inert. Eventually, one reaches a kind of expertise, at which one becomes a reflective practitioner of a certain set of skills. But expertise occurs at many levels. The expert first-year graduate or law student, for example, is still a far cry from the expert professional. People therefore cycle through many times, on the way to successively higher levels of expertise.

Motivation drives metacognitive skills, which in turn activate learning and thinking

skills, which then provide feedback to the metacognitive skills, enabling one's level of expertise to increase (see Sternberg, 1985). The declarative and procedural knowledge acquired through the extension of the thinking and learning skills also results in these skills being used more effectively in the future.

How does this model relate to the construct of intelligence?

LIMITATIONS ON THE *g* FACTOR

Some intelligence theorists point to the stability of the alleged general (*g*) factor of human intelligence as evidence for the existence of some kind of stable and overriding structure of human intelligence (e.g., Bouchard, 1998; Hunt, 2010; Kyllonen, 2002).

In a collaborative study among children near Kisumu, Kenya (Sternberg, 2007; Sternberg et al., 2001), we devised a test of practical intelligence that measures informal knowledge for an important aspect of adaptation to the environment in rural Kenya, namely, knowledge of the identities and use of natural herbal medicines that may be used to combat illnesses. The children use this informal knowledge on average once a week in treating themselves or suggesting treatments to other children, so this knowledge is a routine part of their everyday existence. By "informal knowledge," I refer to kinds of knowledge not taught in schools and not assessed on tests given in the schools.

The idea of this research was that children who knew what these medicines were, what they were used for, and how they should be dosed would be in a position better to adapt to their environments than would children without this informal knowledge. We do not know how many, if any, of these medicines actually work, but from the standpoint of measuring practical intelligence in a given culture, the important thing is that the people in Kenya believe that the medicines work. For that matter, it is not always clear how effective are the medicines used in the Western world.

We found substantial individual differences in the tacit knowledge of children of like age and schooling relative to these natural herbal medicines. More important, however, was the correlation between scores on this test and scores on an English language vocabulary test (the Mill Hill), a Dholuo equivalent (Dholuo is the community and home language), and the Raven Coloured Progressive Matrices. We found significantly *negative* correlations between our test and the English language vocabulary test. Correlations of our test with the other tests were trivial. The better children did on the test of indigenous tacit knowledge, the worse they did on the test of vocabulary used in school, and vice versa. Why might we have obtained such a finding?

Based on ethnographic observation, we believe a possible reason is that parents in the village may emphasize either a more indigenous or a more Western education. Some parents (and their children) see little value to school. They do not see how success in school connects with the future of children who will spend their whole lives in a village, where they do not believe they need the kinds of competencies the school teaches. Other parents and children seem to see Western schooling as valuable in itself or potentially as a ticket out of the confines of the village. The parents therefore tend to emphasize one type of education or the other for their children, with corresponding results. The kinds of competencies the families value differ, and so therefore do scores on the tests. From this point of view, the intercorrelational structure of tests tells us nothing intrinsic about the structure of intelligence per se, but something about the way abilities as developing forms of competencies structure themselves in interaction with the demands of the environment.

In another study (Grigorenko et al., 2004), we examined the academic and practical skills of Yup'ik Eskimo children who live in the Southwestern portion of Alaska. The Yup'ik generally live in geographically isolated villages along water that are accessible primarily by air. Most of us would have no choice in traveling from one village to another because we would be unable to navigate the terrain using, say, a dogsled. These villages are embedded in mile after mile of frozen tundra that, to us, would all look relatively the same. The Yup'ik, however, can navigate this terrain because they learn to find landmarks that most of us would

never see. They also have extremely impressive hunting and gathering skills that almost none of us would have. Yet most of the children do quite poorly in school. Their teachers often think that they are rather hopeless students. The children therefore have developed extremely impressive competencies for surviving in a difficult environment, but because these skills often are not ones teachers (who typically are not from the Yup'ik community) have, the children are viewed as not very competent.

Nuñes (1994) has reported related findings based on a series of studies she conducted in Brazil (see also Ceci & Roazzi, 1994). Street children's adaptive intelligence is tested to the limit by their ability to form and successfully run a street business. If they fail to run such a business successfully, they risk either starvation or death at the hands of death squads should they resort to stealing. Nuñes and her collaborators have found that the same children who are doing the mathematics needed for running a successful street business cannot do well the same types of mathematics problems presented in an abstract, paper-and-pencil format.

If the situations were reversed, and privileged children who do well on conventional ability tests or in school were forced out on the street, many of them would not survive long. Indeed, in the ghettoes of urban America, many children and adults who, for one reason or another end up on the street, in fact barely survive or do not make it at all.

Jean Lave (1989) has reported similar findings with Berkeley housewives shopping in supermarkets. There just is no correlation between their ability to do the mathematics needed for comparison shopping and their scores on conventional paper-and-pencil tests of comparable mathematical skills. Similarly, Ceci and Liker (1986) found that expert handicappers at race tracks generally had only average IQs. There was no correlation between the complexity of the mathematical model they used in handicapping and their scores on conventional tests. In each case, important kinds of developing competencies for life were not adequately reflected by the kinds of competencies measured by the conventional ability tests.

The problems with the conventional model of abilities do not just apply in what to us are exotic cultures or exotic occupations. In one study (Sternberg, Ferrari, Clinkenbeard, & Grigorenko, 1996; Sternberg, Grigorenko, Ferrari, & Clinkbeard, 1999), high school students were tested for their analytical, creative, and practical abilities via multiple-choice and essay items. The multiple-choice items were divided into three content domains: verbal, quantitative, and figural pictures. Students' scores were factor-analyzed, then later correlated with their performance in a college-level introductory psychology course.

We found that when students were tested for not only analytical abilities but also creative and practical abilities (as follows from the model of successful intelligence; Sternberg, 1985, 1997a, 1997b), the strong general factor that tends to result from multiple-ability tests becomes much weaker. Of course, there is always some general factor when one factor-analyzes but does not rotate the factor solution, but the general factor was weak and, of course, disappeared with a varimax rotation. We also found that all of analytical, creative, and practical abilities predicted performance in the introductory psychology course (which itself was taught analytically, creatively, or practically, with assessments to match). Moreover, although the students identified as highly analytical were the traditional population—primarily white, middle- to upper-middle-class, and well educated—the students who were identified as highly creative or highly practical were much more diverse in all of these attributes. Most importantly, students whose instruction better matched their triarchic pattern of abilities outperformed those students whose instruction more poorly matched their triarchic pattern of abilities.

Thus, conventional tests may unduly favor a small segment of the population by virtue of the narrow kind of competencies they measure. When one measures a broader range of competencies, the results look quite different. Moreover, the broader range of competencies includes kinds of skills that will be important in the worlds of work and the family.

Even in developed countries, practical competencies probably matter as much or more than do academic ones for many aspects of life success. Goleman (2005), for example, has claimed that emotional competencies are more important than academic ones, although he has offered no direct evidence (see also Boyatzis, Gaskin, & Wei, 2015; Mayer, Salovey, Caruso, & Cherkasskiy, 2011; Sternberg, 2015). In a study we did in Russia (Grigorenko & Sternberg, 2001a), although both academic and practical intelligence predicted measures of adult physical and mental health, the measures of practical intelligence were the better predictors.

Analytical, creative, and practical abilities, as measured by our own or anyone else's tests, are simply forms of developing competencies. All are useful in various kinds of life tasks. But conventional tests may unfairly disadvantage those students who do not do well in a fairly narrow range of kinds of competencies. By expanding the range of competencies we measure, we discover that many children not now identified as able have, in fact, developed important kinds of competence. The abilities that conventional tests measure are important for school and life performance, but they are not the only abilities that are important.

Teaching in a way that departs from notions of abilities based on a general factor also pays dividends. In a recent set of studies, we have shown that generally lower socioeconomic class third-grade and generally middle-class eighth-grade students who are taught social studies (a unit in communities) or science (a unit on psychology) for successful intelligence (analytically, creative, and practically, as well as for memory) outperform students who are taught just for analytical (critical) thinking or just for memory (Sternberg, Torff, & Grigorenko, 1998). The students taught "triarchically" outperform the other students not only on performance assessments that look at analytical, creative, and practical kinds of achievements, but even on tests that measure straight memory (multiple-choice tests already being used in the courses). None of this is to say that analytical abilities are not important in school and life—obviously, they are. Rather, what our data suggest is that other types of abilities—creative and practical ones—are important as well, and that students need to learn how to use all three kinds of abilities together. However, in practice, teachers are used to teaching in conventional ways and attaining improvements can be challenging (Sternberg et al., 2014).

Thus, teaching students in a way that takes into account their more highly developed competencies and also enables them to develop other kinds of competence results in superior learning outcomes, regardless of how these learning outcomes are measured. The children taught in a way that enables them to use kinds of skills other than memory actually remember better, on average, than do children taught for memory.

We have also done studies in which we measured informal procedural knowledge in children and adults. We have done such studies with business managers, college professors, elementary school students, sales people, college students, and general populations. This important aspect of practical intelligence, in study after study, has been found to be uncorrelated with academic intelligence, as measured by conventional tests, in a variety of populations, occupations, and at a variety of age levels (Sternberg et al., 2000). Moreover, the tests predict job performance as well as or better than do tests of IQ. The lack of correlation of the two kinds of ability tests suggests that the best prediction of job performance will result when both academic and practical intelligence tests are used as predictors.

Although the kind of informal procedural competence we measure in these tests does not correlate with academic competence, it does correlate across work domains. For example, we found that subscores (for managing oneself, managing others, and managing tasks) on measures of informal procedural knowledge are correlated with each other, and that scores on the test for academic psychology are moderately correlated with scores on the test for business managers (Sternberg et al., 2000). So the kinds of developing competencies that matter in the world of work may show certain correlations with each other that are not shown with the kinds of skills that matter in the world of the school.

It is even possible to use these kinds of tests to predict effectiveness in leadership. Studies of military leaders showed that tests of informal knowledge for military leaders predicted the effectiveness of these leaders,

whereas conventional tests of intelligence did not. We also found that although the test for managers was significantly correlated with the test for military leaders, only the latter test predicted superiors' ratings of leadership effectiveness (Sternberg et al., 2000).

Both conventional academic tests and our tests of practical intelligence measure forms of developing competencies that matter in school and on the job. The two kinds of tests are not qualitatively distinct. The reason the correlations are essentially null is that the kinds of skills they measure are quite different. The people who are good at abstract, academic kinds of skills are often people who have not emphasized learning practical, everyday kinds of skills, and vice versa, as we found in our Kenya study. Indeed, children who grow up in challenging environments such as the inner city may need to develop practical over academic skills as a matter of survival. As in Kenya, practical skills may better predict their survival than do more academic kinds of skills. The same applies in business, where tacit knowledge about how to perform on the job is as likely or more likely to lead to job success than is the academic skills set that in school seems so important.

PUTTING THEORY INTO PRACTICE

My colleagues and I put these ideas into practice in a series of studies and implementations concerning college admissions.

The Rainbow Project

The Rainbow Project (for details, see Sternberg, 2010; Sternberg, Bonney, Gabora, & Merrifield, 2012; Sternberg & the Rainbow Project Collaborators, 2006) was the first project designed to enhance university admissions procedures at the undergraduate level. The Rainbow measures were intended, in the United States, to supplement the Standard Achievement Test (SAT) or American College Tests (ACT), but they may supplement any conventional standardized test of abilities or achievement.

A collaborative team of investigators sought to study how successful such an augmentation could be. Even if we did not use the SAT or ACT, in particular, we still would need some kind of assessment of the memory and analytical abilities the tests assess.

Methodological Considerations

In the Rainbow Project (Sternberg, 2010; Sternberg & the Rainbow Project Collaborators, 2006), data were collected at 15 schools across the United States, including eight 4-year undergraduate institutions, five community colleges, and two high schools.

The participants were 1,013 students predominantly in their first year as undergraduates or their final year of high school. Analyses are described here only for undergraduate students because they were the only ones for whom the authors had data available regarding undergraduate academic performance. The final number of participants included in these analyses was 793.

Baseline measures of standardized test scores and high school grade-point averages were collected to evaluate the predictive validity of current tools used for undergraduate admission criteria, and to provide a contrast for the current measures. Students' scores on standardized university entrance exams were obtained from the College Board.

The measure of analytical skills was provided by the SAT plus multiple-choice analytical items we added, measuring inference of meanings of words from context, number series completions, and figural matrix completions.

Creative skills were measured by multiple-choice items and by performance-based items. The multiple-choice items were of three kinds. In one, students are presented with verbal analogies preceded by counterfactual premises (e.g., "Money falls off trees"). They have to solve the analogies as though the counterfactual premises were true. In a second, students are presented with rules for novel number operations, for example, "flix," which involves numerical manipulations that differ as a function of whether the first of two operands is greater than, equal to, or less than the second. Participants have to use the novel number operations to solve presented math problems. In a third, participants are first presented with a figural series that involves one or more

transformations; they then have to apply the rule of the series to a new figure with a different appearance, and complete the new series. These are not typical of assessments of creativity and were included to measure relative quickness of participants' responses and for relative ease of scoring.

Creative skills also were measured using open-ended measures. One measure required writing two short stories with a selection from among unusual titles, such as "The Octopus's Sneakers"; another required orally telling two stories based on choices of picture collages; and still another required captioning cartoons from among various options. Open-ended performance-based answers were rated by trained raters for novelty, quality, and task appropriateness. Multiple judges were used for each task, and satisfactory reliability was achieved.

Multiple-choice measures of practical skills were of three kinds. In the first, students are presented with a set of everyday problems in the life of an adolescent and have to select the option that best solves each problem. In the second, students are presented with scenarios requiring the use of math in everyday life (e.g., buying tickets for a ballgame), and have to solve math problems based on the scenarios. In the third, students are presented with a map of an area (e.g., an entertainment park) and have to answer questions about navigating effectively through the area depicted by the map.

Practical skills also were assessed using three situational judgment inventories: the Everyday Situational Judgment Inventory (Movies), the Common Sense Questionnaire, and the College Life Questionnaire, each of which tap different types of tacit knowledge. The general format of tacit knowledge inventories has been described in Sternberg and colleagues (2000), so only the content of the inventories used in this study are described here. The movies presented everyday situations that confront undergraduate students, such as asking for a letter of recommendation from a professor who shows, through nonverbal cues, that he or she does not recognize the student very well. One then has to rate various options for how well he or she would work in response to each situation. The Common Sense Questionnaire provided everyday business problems, such as being assigned to work with a coworker whom one cannot stand, and the College Life Questionnaire provided everyday university situations for which a solution was required.

Unlike the creativity performance tasks, the practical performance tasks did not give participants a choice of situations to rate. For each task, participants were told that there was no "right" answer, and that the options described in each situation represented variations on how different people approach different situations.

Consider examples of the kinds of items one might find on the Rainbow Assessment. One example of a creative item might be to write a story using the title "3516" or "It's Moving Backward." Another example might show a collage of pictures in which people are engaged in a wide variety of activities helping other people. One would then orally tell a story that takes off from the collage. An example of a practical item might show a movie in which a student has just received a poor grade on a test. His roommate had a health crisis the night before, and he had been up all night helping his roommate. His professor hands him back the test paper, with a disappointed look on her face, and suggests to the student that he study harder next time. The movie then stops. The student then has to describe how he would handle the situation. Or the student might receive a written problem describing a conflict with another individual with whom she is working on a group project. The project is getting mired down in the interpersonal conflict. The student has to indicate how she would resolve the situation to get the project done. All materials were administered in either of two formats. A total of 325 of the university students took the test in paper-and-pencil format, whereas a total of 468 students took the test on the computer via the World Wide Web.

No strict time limits were set for completing the tests, although the instructors were given rough guidelines of about 70 minutes per session. The time taken to complete the battery of tests ranged from 2 to 4 hours.

As a result of the lengthy nature of the complete battery of assessments, participants were administered parts of the battery using an intentional incomplete overlapping design. The participants were randomly assigned to the test sections they were to complete.

Creativity in this (and the subsequent Kaleidoscope Project) was assessed on the basis of the novelty and quality of responses. Practicality was assessed on the basis of the feasibility of the products with respect to human and material resources.

The Data

The conservative analysis described below does not correct for differences in the selectivity of the institutions at which the study took place. In a study across so many undergraduate institutions differing in selectivity, validity coefficients will seem to be lower than are typical because an A at a less selective institution counts the same as an A at a more selective institution. When the authors corrected for institutional selectivity, the results described below became stronger. But correcting for selectivity has its own problems (e.g., on what basis does one evaluate selectivity?), so uncorrected data are used in this report. The authors also did not control for university major: Different universities may have different majors, and the exact course offerings, grading, and populations of students entering different majors may vary from one university to another, rendering control difficult.

When examining undergraduate students alone, the sample showed a slightly higher mean level of SAT scores than those found in undergraduate institutions across the United States. The standard deviation was above the normal 100-point standard deviation, which means that the authors did not suffer from restriction of range. The means, although slightly higher than typical, are within the range of average undergraduate students.

Another potential concern is pooling data from different institutions. Data were pooled because in some institutions the authors simply did not have large enough numbers of cases for the data to be meaningful.

Three meaningful factors were extracted from the data: practical performance tests, creative performance tests, and multiple-choice tests (including analytical, creative, and practical). In other words, multiple-choice tests, regardless of what they were supposed to measure, clustered together. Thus, method variance proved to be very important. The results show the importance of measuring skills using multiple formats, precisely because method is so important in determining factorial structure. The results show the limitations of exploratory factor analysis in analyzing such data, and also of dependence on multiple-choice items outside the analytical domain. In the ideal, one wishes to ensure that one controls for method of testing in designing aptitude and other test batteries.

Undergraduate admissions offices are not interested, exactly, in whether these tests predict undergraduate academic success. Rather, they are interested in the extent to which these tests predict school success *beyond* those measures currently in use, such as the SAT and high school grade-point average (GPA). In order to test the incremental validity provided by Rainbow measures above and beyond the SAT in predicting GPA, a series of statistical analyses (called *hierarchical regressions*) was conducted that included the items analyzed earlier in the analytical, creative, and practical assessments.

If one looks at the simple correlations, the SAT-V (Verbal), SAT-M (Math), high school GPA, and the Rainbow measures all predict first-year GPA. But how do the Rainbow measures fare on incremental validity? In one set of analyses, the SAT-V, SAT-M, and high school GPA were included in the first step of the prediction equation because these are the standard measures used today to predict undergraduate performance. Only high school GPA contributed uniquely to prediction of undergraduate GPA. Inclusion of the Rainbow measures roughly doubled prediction (percentage of variance accounted for in the criterion) versus the SAT alone.

These results suggest that the Rainbow tests add considerably to the prediction achieved by SATs alone. They also suggest the power of high school GPA in prediction, particularly because it is an atheoretical composite that includes within it many variables, including motivation and conscientiousness.

Although one important goal of this study was to predict success in the undergraduate years, another important goal involved developing measures that reduce ethnic-group differences in mean levels. There are a number of ways one can test for group differences in these measures, each of which involves a test of the size of the effect of ethnic group. Two different measures were chosen: ω^2 (omega squared) and Cohen's *d*.

There were two general findings. First, in terms of overall differences, the Rainbow tests appeared to reduce ethnic-group differences relative to traditional assessments of abilities such as the SAT. Second, in terms of specific differences, it appears that Latino students benefited the most from the reduction of group differences. The black students, too, seemed to show a reduction in difference from the white students' mean for most of the Rainbow tests, although a substantial difference appeared to be maintained with the practical performance measures.

Although the group differences are not perfectly reduced, these findings suggest that measures can be designed that reduce ethnic- and racial-group differences on standardized tests, particularly for historically disadvantaged groups such as black and Latino students. These findings have important implications for reducing adverse impact in undergraduate admissions.

The SAT is based on a conventional psychometric notion of cognitive skills. Using this notion, it has had substantial success in predicting undergraduate academic performance. The Rainbow measures alone roughly doubled the predictive power of undergraduate GPA when compared to the SAT alone. Additionally, the Rainbow measures predict substantially beyond the contributions of the SAT and high school GPA. These findings, combined with encouraging results regarding the reduction of between-ethnicity differences, make a compelling case for furthering the study of the measurement of analytic, creative, and practical skills for predicting success in the university.

One important goal for the current study, and future studies, is the creation of standardized assessments that reduce the different outcomes between different groups as much as possible to maintain test validity. The measures described here suggest results toward this end. Although the group differences in the tests were not reduced to zero, the tests did substantially attenuate group differences relative to other measures such as the SAT. This finding could be an important step toward ultimately ensuring fair and equal treatment for members of diverse groups in the academic domain.

The principles behind the Rainbow Project apply at other levels of admissions as well. Consider two examples.

The Advanced Placement Project

Stemler, Grigorenko, Jarvin, and Sternberg (2006) and Stemler, Sternberg, Grigorenko, Jarvin, and Sharpes (2009) placed creative and practical items on advanced placement tests of psychology, statistics, and physics. These tests are used for college admissions. Here is an example for psychology:

> A variety of explanations have been proposed to account for why people sleep.
>
> a) Describe the Restorative Theory of sleep (*memory*).
> b) An alternative theory is an evolutionary theory of sleep, sometimes referred to as the "Preservation and Protection" theory. Describe this theory and compare and contrast it with the Restorative Theory. State what you see as the two strong points and two weak points of this theory compared to the Restorative Theory (*analytical*).
> c) How might you design an experiment to test the Restorative Theory of sleep? Briefly describe the experiment, including the participants, materials, procedures, and design (*creative).
> d) A friend informs you that she is having trouble sleeping. Based on your knowledge of sleep, what kinds of helpful (and health-promoting) suggestions might you give her to help her fall asleep at night (*practical*)?

The authors found that by asking such questions, as they did in the other studies, they were able both to increase the range of skills tested and substantially reduce ethnic-group differences in test scores. Thus, it is possible to reduce group differences in not only tests of aptitude but also tests of achievement.

The University of Michigan Business School Project

Hedlund, Wilt, Nebel, Ashford, and Sternberg (2006) devised a test that could be used to supplement the Graduate Management Admissions Test (GMAT) for graduate business school admissions. The idea of the test was to create scenarios actually likely to be encountered in business, encompassing a variety of business challenges, including a personnel shortage, strategic decision making, a problem subordinate, a consulting challenge, interdepartmental negotiations, and project management. There were two versions of the test. One had long and involved scenarios providing relatively comprehensive information about the problem, including graphs and charts. The other version presented relatively short vignettes, such as the one below:

Scenario 1: Personnel Shortage

1a. You are a senior-level manager in the human resources department of a medium-size manufacturing plant (2,500 employees). Your primary responsibility is to oversee employee selection and staffing. The plant has found itself in a unique situation in which product demand has been high but unemployment levels are low. This situation has resulted in a personnel shortage in key areas of the plant (20 % in production, 15% in maintenance, and 25% in engineering). To avoid layoffs and reduce overhead costs, the company has previously used temporary laborers to compensate for fluctuations in product demand. For the past 6 months, product demand has been very high, and future projections continue to be positive for the next 3–6 months. In the short term (3 months or less), temporary workers are more cost-effective; however, their commitment to the job and work quality is less than that of full-time employees. In the long term (6 months or more), hiring full-time employees is more cost-effective. However, if production demands drop, as they often do, the plant would have to lay off employees, which it has never done in its entire 25-year history. The plant was faced with the following options:

_____ Hire temporary employees to compensate for the immediate shortage and reassess the situation in 3 months.

_____ Hire full-time employees, but let them know that if production demands decrease, you will have to let them go.

_____ Hire a few full-time employees to fill some of the positions and fill the rest with temporary employees to minimize layoffs should production demand diminish.

_____ Ask members of each department to evaluate their own personnel needs and recommend the best approach for their own department.

_____ Research the situation in more detail to get a better indication of future product demand and of the relative costs and benefits of various staffing options before making any final decisions.

_____ Present the available information to members of top management and have them make a final decision on how to best handle the personnel shortage.

_____ Offer overtime hours for existing employees, to see if they would like the opportunity to make more money, before hiring temporary laborers or full-time employees.

Each of the options was rated on a 1 (low) to 7 (high) scale for how effective it would be as a solution to the problem. The answers were compared with those of experts.

The longer versions did not include response options, but it did include a set of questions to be addressed, based on the detailed scenarios the students read:

• *Problem identification and rationale.* "What do you see as the main problem in this situation?"; "Why do you consider it to be the main problem?"; "What additional problems need to be addressed?"

• *Solution generation and rationale.* "What would you do to address the main problem you have identified?"; "What alternative courses of action did you consider?"; "Why did you choose your particular course of action?"

• *Information processing.* "What information did you focus on in developing a response to the situation?"; "How did you use the information to arrive at a response to the situation?" "Did you draw on any personal experiences in developing a response to the situation?"; "If so, please explain. What additional information/resources would you need to address this problem?"

• *Outcome monitoring and obstacle recognition.* "What outcome do you hope will result from the course of action you have chosen?"; "What obstacles, if any, do you anticipate to obtaining this outcome?"

We found, first, that both measures significantly predicted academic success as measured by first-year grades. Second, we found that when our measures were used as supplements to the GMAT, they increased predictive validity of first-year grades by roughly 3–4% (i.e., .03 to .04 incremental R^2). Third, we found that our measures significantly predicted quality of performance on an independent project (whereas the GMAT did not). Fourth, we found that our measure positively correlated with participation in extracurricular and leadership activities (whereas the GMAT correlated negatively). Finally, we found that our measures substantially reduced (but did not eliminate) ethnic-group differences relative to the GMAT.

The Kaleidoscope Project

It is one thing to have a successful research project, and another actually to implement the procedures in a high-stakes situation. My colleagues and I have had the opportunity to do so. The results of a second project, Project Kaleidoscope, are reviewed here (Sternberg, 2009; Sternberg, Bonney, Gabora, Karelitz, & Coffin, 2010; Sternberg & Coffin, 2010).

Tufts University in Medford, Massachusetts, has strongly emphasized the role of active citizenship in education. It has put into practice some of the ideas from the Rainbow Project. In collaboration with Dean of Admissions Lee Coffin, we instituted Project Kaleidoscope, which represents an implementation of the ideas of Rainbow but goes beyond that project to include in its assessment the construct of wisdom (see also Karelitz, Jarvin, & Sternberg, 2010; Sternberg, 2009, 2010; Sternberg et al., 2010).

On the application for all of the over 15,000 students applying annually to Arts, Sciences, and Engineering at Tufts, we placed questions designed to assess wisdom, analytical and practical intelligence, and creativity synthesized (WICS), an extension of the theory of successful intelligence (Sternberg, 2003). The program is still in use, but the data reported here are for the first year of implementation.

The questions were optional. Whereas the Rainbow Project was a separate high-stakes test administered with a proctor, the Kaleidoscope Project was a section of the Tufts-specific supplement to the Common Application. It just was not practical to administer a separate high-stakes test such as the Rainbow assessment for admission to one university. Moreover, the advantage of Kaleidoscope is that it got us away from the high-stakes testing situation in which students must answer complex questions in very short amounts of time under incredible pressure.

Students were encouraged to answer just a single question so as not overburden them. Tufts University competes for applications with many other universities, and if our application was substantially more burdensome than those of our competitor schools, it would put us at a real-world disadvantage in attracting applicants. In the theory of successful intelligence, successful intelligent individuals capitalize on strengths and compensate for or correct weaknesses. Our format gave students a chance to capitalize on a strength.

As examples of items, a creative question asked students to write stories with titles such as "The End of MTV" or "Confessions of a Middle School Bully." Another creative question asked students what the world would be like if some historical event had come out differently, for example, if Rosa Parks had given up her seat on the bus. Yet another creative question, a nonverbal one, gave students an opportunity to design a new product or an advertisement for a new product. A practical question queried how students had persuaded friends of an unpopular idea they held. A wisdom question asked students how a passion they had could be applied toward a common good.

Creativity and practicality were assessed in the same way as in the Rainbow Project. Analytical quality was assessed by the organization, logic, and balance of the essay. Wisdom was assessed by the extent to which the response represented the use of abilities and knowledge for a common good by balancing one's own, others', and institutional interests over the long and short term, through the infusion of positive ethical values.

Note that the goal is not to replace SAT and other traditional admissions measurements such as GPAs and class rank with some new test. Rather, it is to reconceptualize

applicants in terms of academic/analytical, creative, practical, and wisdom-based abilities, using the essays as one but not the only source of information. For example, highly creative work submitted in a portfolio also could be entered into the creativity rating, or evidence of creativity through winning of prizes or awards. The essays were major sources of information, but if other information was available, the trained admissions officers used it.

Applicants were evaluated for creative, practical, and wisdom-based skills, if sufficient evidence was available, as well as for academic (analytical) and personal qualities in general.

Among the applicants who were evaluated as being academically qualified for admission, approximately half completed an optional essay. Doing these essays had no meaningful effect on chances of admissions. However, *quality* of essays or other evidence of creative, practical, or wisdom-based abilities did have an effect. For those rated as an A (top rating) by a trained admission officer in any of these three categories, average rates of acceptance were roughly double those for applicants not getting an A. Because of the large number of essays (over 8,000), only one rater rated applicants except for a sample to ensure that interrater reliability was sufficient, which it was.

Many measures do not look like conventional standardized tests, but they have statistical properties that mimic them. We were therefore interested in convergent–discriminant validation of our measures. The correlation of our measures with a rated academic composite that included SAT scores and high school GPA were modest but significant for creative, practical, and wise thinking. The correlations with a rating of quality of extracurricular participation and leadership were moderate for creative, practical, and wise thinking. Thus, the pattern of convergent–discriminant validation was what we had hoped it would be.

The average academic quality of applicants in Arts and Sciences for whom we had data rose in the first year of the implementation, in terms of both SAT and high school GPA. In addition, there were notably fewer students in what before had been the bottom one-third of the pool in terms of academic quality. Many of those students, seeing the new application, seem to have decided not to bother to apply. Many stronger applicants applied.

Thus, adopting these new methods does not result in less qualified applicants applying to the institution and being admitted. Rather, the applicants who are admitted are *more* qualified, but in a broader way. Perhaps most rewarding were the positive comments from a large number of applicants who felt our application gave them a chance to show themselves for who they are. Of course, many factors are involved in admissions decisions, and Kaleidoscope ratings were only one small part of the overall picture.

We did not get meaningful differences across ethnic groups, a result that surprised us, given that the earlier Rainbow Project reduced but did not eliminate differences. And after a number of years in which applications by underrepresented minorities were relatively flat in terms of numbers, this year, they went up substantially. In the end, applications from African Americans and Hispanic Americans increased significantly, and admissions of African Americans were up 30%, and those of Hispanic Americans, 15%. These results suggest that ethnic/race differences that sometimes are taken for granted are actually dependent on the kinds of material being tested (Sternberg, Grigorenko, & Kidd, 2005). So our results, like those of the Rainbow Project, showed that it is possible to increase academic quality and diversity simultaneously, and to do so in for an entire undergraduate class at a major university, not just for small samples of students at some scattered schools. Most importantly, we sent a message to students, parents, high school guidance counselors, and others, that we believe there is more to a person than the narrow spectrum of skills assessed by standardized tests, and that these broader skills can be assessed in a quantifiable way.

The Panorama Project

During my years as Provost at Oklahoma State University, the Panorama Project, a project similar to Kaleidoscope, was implemented, but tailored to the needs of a large and diverse land-grant institution. The results had not yet been formally analyzed when I left Oklahoma State, but the admissions office and others in the administration were happy with the results.

CONCLUSION

Conventional tests of abilities have tended to value the kinds of skills most valued by Western schools. This system of valuing is understandable given that Binet and Simon (1905) first developed intelligence tests for the purpose of predicting school performance. Moreover, these skills are important in school and in life. But in the modern world, the conception of abilities as fixed or even as predetermined is an anachronism. Moreover, our research and that of others (reviewed more extensively in Sternberg, 2003; Sternberg et al., 2011) shows that the set of abilities assessed by conventional tests measures only a small portion of the kinds of competencies relevant for life success. It is for this reason that conventional tests predict only about 10% of individual-difference variation in various measures of success in adult life (Herrnstein & Murray, 1994).

Not all cultures value equally the kinds of expertise measured by these tests. In a study comparing Latino, Asian, and Anglo subcultures in California, for example, we found that Latino parents valued social kinds of competence as more important to intelligence than did Asian and Anglo parents, who placed more value on cognitive kinds of competence (Okagaki & Sternberg, 1993). Predictably, teachers also placed more value on cognitive kinds of competence, with the result that the Anglo and Asian children would be expected to do better in school, and they did. Of course, cognitive skills matter in school and in life, but so do social skills. Both need to be taught in the school and the home to all children. This latter kind of competence may become even more important in the workplace. Until we expand our notions of abilities and recognize that when we measure them, we are measuring highly diverse competencies, we risk consigning many potentially excellent contributors to our society to bleak futures. We may also be potentially overvaluing students with skills for success in a certain kind of schooling, but not necessarily with equal skills for success later in life.

REFERENCES

Aarts, H., & Elliot, A. (Eds.). (2011). *Goal-directed behavior*. New York: Ballantine.

Amabile, T. M. (1996). *Creativity in context*. Boulder, CO: Westview Press.

Ang, S., Van Dyne, L. V., & Tan, M. L. (2011). Cultural intelligence. In R. J. Sternberg & S. B. Kaufman (Eds.), *Cambridge handbook of intelligence* (pp. 582–602). New York: Cambridge University Press.

Bandura, A. (1996). *Self-efficacy: The exercise of control*. New York: Freeman.

Binet, A., & Simon, T. (1905). Méthodes nouvelles pour le diagnostic du niveau intellectuel des anormaux [New methods for the diagnosis of the intellectual level of abnormal children]. *L'Année Psychologique, 11*, 191–336.

Bouchard, T. J., Jr. (1998). Genetic and environmental influences on adult intelligence and special mental abilities. *Human Biology, 70*, 257–279.

Boyatzis, R. E., Gaskin, J., & Wei, H. (2015). Emotional and social intelligence and behavior. In S. Goldstein, D. Princiotta, & J. A. Naglieri (Eds.), *Handbook of intelligence* (pp. 243–262). New York: Springer.

Carroll, J. B. (1993). *Human cognitive abilities: A survey of factor-analytic studies*. New York: Cambridge University Press.

Ceci, S. J., & Liker, J. (1986). Academic and nonacademic intelligence: An experimental separation. In R. J. Sternberg & R. K. Wagner (Eds.), *Practical intelligence: Nature and origins of competence in the everyday world* (pp. 119–142). New York: Cambridge University Press.

Ceci, S. J., & Roazzi, A. (1994). The effects of context on cognition: Postcards from Brazil. In R. J. Sternberg & R. K. Wagner (Eds.), *Mind in context: Interactionist perspectives on human intelligence* (pp. 74–101). New York: Cambridge University Press.

Cianciolo, A. T., Matthew, C. T., Wagner, R. A., & Sternberg, R. J. (2006). Tacit knowledge, practical intelligence, and expertise. In N. Charness, K. A. Ericsson, P. Feltovich, & R. Hoffman (Eds.), *Cambridge handbook of expertise and expert performance* (pp. 613–632). New York: Cambridge University Press.

Dai, D. Y., & Sternberg, R. J. (Eds.). (2004). *Motivation, emotion, and cognition: Integrative perspectives on intellectual functioning and development*. Mahwah, NJ: Erlbaum.

Dweck, C. S. (1999). *Self-theories: Their role in motivation, personality, and development*. Philadelphia: Psychology Press/Taylor & Francis.

Dweck, C. S. (2002). Messages that motivate: How praise molds students' beliefs, motivation, and performance (in surprising ways). In J. Aronson (Ed.), *Improving academic achievement: Impact of psychological factors on education* (pp. 37–60). San Diego, CA: Academic Press.

Dweck, C. S. (2007). *Mindset: The new psychology of success*. New York: Ballantine.

Dweck, C. S., & Elliott, E. S. (1983). Achievement motivation. In P. H. Mussen (General Ed.) & E. M. Hetherington (Vol. Ed.), *Handbook of child psychology: Socialization, personality, and social development* (4th ed., Vol. 4, pp. 644–691). New York: Wiley.

Ericsson, K. A. (Ed.). (1996). *The road to excellence: The acquisition of expert performance in the arts and sciences, sports and games*. Hillsdale, NJ: Erlbaum.

Ericsson, K. A., Krampe, R. T., & Tesch-Römer, C. (1993). The role of deliberate practice in the acquisition of expert performance. *Psychological Review, 100*, 363–406.

Gardner, H. (2011). *Frames of mind: The theory of multiple intelligences* (3rd ed.). New York: Basic Books.

Goleman, D. (2005). *Emotional intelligence*. New York: Bantam Books.

Grigorenko, E. L., Meier, E., Lipka, J., Mohatt, G., Yanez, E., & Sternberg, R. J. (2004). Academic and practical intelligence: A case study of the Yup'ik in Alaska. *Learning and Individual Differences, 14*, 183–207.

Grigorenko, E. L., & Sternberg, R. J. (2001a). Analytical, creative, and practical intelligence as predictors of self-reported adaptive functioning: A case study in Russia. *Intelligence, 29*, 57–73.

Grigorenko, E. L., & Sternberg, R. J. (Eds.). (2001b). *Family environment and intellectual functioning: A life-span perspective*. Mahwah, NJ: Erlbaum.

Hedlund, J., Forsythe, G. B., Horvath, J. A., Williams, W. M., Snook, S., & Sternberg, R. J. (2003). Identifying and assessing tacit knowledge: Understanding the practical intelligence of military leaders. *Leadership Quarterly, 14*, 117–140.

Hedlund, J., Wilt, J. M., Nebel, K. R., Ashford, S. J., & Sternberg, R. J. (2006). Assessing practical intelligence in business school admissions: A supplement to the Graduate Management Admissions Test. *Learning and Individual Differences, 16*, 101–127.

Herrnstein, R. J., & Murray, C. (1994). *The bell curve*. New York: Free Press.

Hunt, E. B. (2010). *Human intelligence.* New York: Cambridge University Press.

Jensen, A. R. (1998). *The g factor: The science of mental ability.* Westport, CT: Praeger/Greenwood.

Karelitz, T. M., Jarvin, L., & Sternberg, R. J. (2010). The meaning of wisdom and its development throughout life. In W. Overton (Ed.), *Handbook of lifespan human development* (pp. 837–881). New York: Wiley.

Kyllonen, P. C. (2002). *g*: Knowledge, speed, strategies, or working-memory capacity?: A systems perspective. In R. J. Sternberg & E. L. Grigorenko (Eds.), *The general factor of intelligence: How general is it?* (pp. 415–445). Mahwah, NJ: Erlbaum.

Lave, J. (1989). *Cognition in practice.* New York: Cambridge University Press.

Mackintosh, N. J. (2011). *IQ and human intelligence* (2nd ed.). New York: Oxford University Press.

Mayer, J. D., Salovey, P., Caruso, D. R., & Cherkasskiy, L. (2011). Emotional intelligence. In R. J. Sternberg & S. B. Kaufman (Eds.), *Cambridge handbook of intelligence* (pp. 528–549). New York: Cambridge University Press.

McClelland, D. C. (1985). *Human motivation.* New York: Scott, Foresman.

McClelland, D. C., Atkinson, J. W., Clark, R. A., & Lowell, E. L. (1976). *The achievement motive.* New York: Irvington.

Niu, W., & Brass, J. (2011). Intelligence in worldwide perspective. In R. J. Sternberg & S. B. Kaufman (Eds.), *Cambridge handbook of intelligence* (pp. 623–646). New York: Cambridge University Press.

Nuñes, T. (1994). Street intelligence. In R. J. Sternberg (Ed.), *Encyclopedia of human intelligence* (Vol. 2, pp. 1045–1049). New York: Macmillan.

Okagaki, L., & Sternberg, R. J. (1993). Parental beliefs and children's school performance. *Child Development, 64,* 36–56.

Stemler, S., Sternberg, R. J., Grigorenko, E. L., Jarvin, L., & Sharpes, D. K. (2009). Using the theory of successful intelligence as a framework for developing assessments in AP Physics. *Contemporary Educational Psychology, 34,* 195–209.

Stemler, S. E., Grigorenko, E. L., Jarvin, L., & Sternberg, R. J. (2006). Using the theory of successful intelligence as a basis for augmenting AP exams in psychology and statistics. *Contemporary Educational Psychology, 31*(2), 344–376.

Sternberg, R. J. (1984). What should intelligence tests test?: Implications of a triarchic theory of intelligence for intelligence testing. *Educational Researcher, 13,* 5–15.

Sternberg, R. J. (1985). *Beyond IQ: A triarchic theory of human intelligence.* New York: Cambridge University Press.

Sternberg, R. J. (1990). *Metaphors of mind.* New York: Cambridge University Press.

Sternberg, R. J. (1994). Cognitive conceptions of expertise. *International Journal of Expert Systems: Research and Application, 7,* 1–12.

Sternberg, R. J. (1996). What should we ask about intelligence? *American Scholar, 65*(2), 205–217.

Sternberg, R. J. (1997a). *Successful intelligence.* New York: Plenum Press.

Sternberg, R. J. (1997b). What does it mean to be smart? *Educational Leadership, 54*(6), 20–24.

Sternberg, R. J. (1999). Intelligence as developing expertise. *Contemporary Educational Psychology, 24,* 359–375.

Sternberg, R. J. (Ed.). (2002). *Why smart people can be so stupid.* New Haven, CT: Yale University Press.

Sternberg, R. J. (2003). *Wisdom, intelligence, and creativity synthesized.* New York: Cambridge University Press.

Sternberg, R. J. (2007). Intelligence and culture. In S. Kitayama & D. Cohen (Eds.), *Handbook of cultural psychology* (pp. 547–568). New York: Guilford Press.

Sternberg, R. J. (2009). The Rainbow and Kaleidoscope Projects: A new psychological approach to undergraduate admissions. *European Psychologist, 14,* 279–287.

Sternberg, R. J. (2010). *College admissions for the 21st century.* Cambridge, MA: Harvard University Press.

Sternberg, R. J. (2013). Personal wisdom in the balance. In M. Ferrari & N. Weststrate (Eds.), *The scientific study of personal wisdom: From contemplative traditions to neuroscience* (pp. 53–74). New York: Springer.

Sternberg, R. J. (2014). The development of adaptive competence. *Developmental Review, 34,* 208–224.

Sternberg, R. J. (2015). Multiple intelligences in the new age of thinking. In S. Goldstein, D. Princiotta, & J. A. Naglieri (Eds.), *Handbook of intelligence* (pp. 229–242). New York: Springer.

Sternberg, R. J., Bonney, C. R., Gabora, L., Karelitz, T., & Coffin, L. (2010). Broadening the spectrum of undergraduate admissions. *College and University, 86*(1), 2–17.

Sternberg, R. J., Bonney, C. R., Gabora, L., & Merrifield, M. (2012). WICS: A model for college and university admissions. *Educational Psychologist, 47*(1), 30–41.

Sternberg, R. J., & Coffin, L. A. (2010). Kaleidoscope: Admitting and developing "new leaders for a changing world." *New England Journal of Higher Education, 24,* 12–13.

Sternberg, R. J., Ferrari, M., Clinkenbeard, P. R., & Grigorenko, E. L. (1996). Identification, instruction, and assessment of gifted children: A construct validation of a triarchic model. *Gifted Child Quarterly, 40,* 129–137.

Sternberg, R. J., Forsythe, G. B., Hedlund, J., Horvath, J., Snook, S., Williams, W. M., et al. (2000). *Practical intelligence in everyday life.* New York: Cambridge University Press.

Sternberg, R. J., & Grigorenko, E. L. (Eds.). (2001). *Environmental effects on cognitive abilities.* Mahwah, NJ: Erlbaum.

Sternberg, R. J., & Grigorenko, E. L. (Eds.). (2002). *The general factor of intelligence: How general is it?* Mahwah, NJ: Erlbaum.

Sternberg, R. J., & Grigorenko, E. L. (2007). *Teaching for successful intelligence* (2nd ed.). Arlington Heights, IL: Skylight Training and Publishing.

Sternberg, R. J., Grigorenko, E. L., Ferrari, M., & Clinkenbeard, P. (1999). A triarchic analysis of an aptitude–treatment interaction. *European Journal of Psychological Assessment, 15*(1), 1–11.

Sternberg, R. J., Grigorenko, E. L., & Kidd, K. K. (2005). Intelligence, race, and genetics. *American Psychologist, 60*(1), 46–59.

Sternberg, R. J., & Hedlund, J. (2002). Practical intelligence, *g,* and work psychology. *Human Performance, 15*(1/2), 143–160.

Sternberg, R. J., Jarvin, L., Birney, D., Naples, A., Stemler, S., Newman, T., et al. (2014). Testing the theory of successful intelligence in teaching grade 4 language arts, mathematics, and science. *Journal of Educational Psychology, 106,* 881–899.

Sternberg, R. J., Jarvin, L., & Grigorenko, E. L. (2011). *Explorations of the nature of giftedness.* New York: Cambridge University Press.

Sternberg, R. J., & Kaufman, S. B. (Eds.). (2011). *Cambridge handbook of intelligence.* New York: Cambridge University Press.

Sternberg, R. J., Kaufman, J. C., & Grigorenko, E. L. (2008). *Applied intelligence.* New York: Cambridge University Press.

Sternberg, R. J., & Lubart, T. I. (1995). *Defying the crowd: Cultivating creativity in a culture of conformity.* New York: Free Press.

Sternberg, R. J., & Lubart, T. I. (1996). Investing in creativity. *American Psychologist, 51,* 677–688.

Sternberg, R. J., Nokes, K., Geissler, P. W., Prince, R., Okatcha, F., Bundy, D. A., et al. (2001). The relationship between academic and practical intelligence: A case study in Kenya. *Intelligence, 29,* 401–418.

Sternberg, R. J., & The Rainbow Project Collaborators (2006). The Rainbow Project: Enhancing the SAT through assessments of analytical, practical and creative skills. *Intelligence, 34*(4), 321–350.

Sternberg, R. J., Torff, B., & Grigorenko, E. L. (1998). Teaching triarchically improves school achievement. *Journal of Educational Psychology, 90,* 1–11.

Sternberg, R. J., Wagner, R. K., & Okagaki, L. (1993). Practical intelligence: The nature and role of tacit knowledge in work and at school. In H. Reese & J. Puckett (Eds.), *Advances in lifespan development* (pp. 205–227). Hillsdale, NJ: Erlbaum.

Sternberg, R. J., Wagner, R. K., Williams, W. M., & Horvath, J. A. (1995). Testing common sense. *American Psychologist, 50,* 912–927.

Sternberg, R. J., & Weil, E. M. (1980). An aptitude–strategy interaction in linear syllogistic reasoning. *Journal of Educational Psychology, 72,* 226–234.

CHAPTER 3

Achievement Motives

DAVID E. CONROY

The thrill of victory and agony of defeat are well known to anybody who has pursued competence. Images of the victorious and vanquished are characterized by facial expressions, gestures, and postures that suggest a highly emotional experience. These emotional experiences are powerful because they reflect how people interpret the meaning of an outcome in relation to their broader self-concept. Competence is a psychological motive that both organizes daily experience and shapes our self-concept. Over time, self-conscious emotions typically experienced as a result of competence pursuits may be evoked by the mere thought of pursuing competence. These anticipatory self-conscious emotional experiences provide an early stimulus around which achievement strivings are organized. Achievement motives were conceived to describe these anticipatory affective experiences and explain how they organize achievement pursuits.

Achievement motives have been reviewed in a number of chapters and review articles over the years (e.g., Conroy, Elliot, & Thrash, 2009; Elliot, Conroy, Barron, & Murayama, 2010; Pang, 2010; Schultheiss & Brunstein, 2005). For this volume, the goal is to develop an integrative perspective on how these motives organize affective, cognitive, and behavioral experiences

during competence pursuits. Research on achievement motives has slowed since its peak in the mid- to late 20th century, so recent developments in psychological theorizing and assessment are integrated to highlight the enduring scientific and practical value of achievement motives. Special attention is given to developments in dual-process models of motivation and behavior, with an aim of simultaneously differentiating and integrating these motivational systems. Following this theoretical review, this chapter addresses applications—both established and potential—of these motives in a number of the specific contexts in which people pursue competence most frequently.

THEORY

To understand the conceptual origins of the achievement motive construct, it is useful to return to White's (1959) theorizing about effectance motivation and competence. Limitations of theories based on primary drives, particularly for "explaining exploratory behavior, manipulation, and general activity" (p. 328), led White to propose a novel effectance motive. Many of these unexplained, often playful behaviors exist both selectively and persistently from infancy onward, without any proximal survival function (unlike needs). They are not aroused by deficits but instead appear to arise organically and generate satisfaction from growing intrinsic feelings of efficacy. Functionally, this motive appears to facilitate the exploratory behaviors that support long-term growth and mastery in the absence of short-term instrumental value. In that sense, the competence motive is an essential wellspring and organizer of human experience.

Although White (1959) posited an undifferentiated competence motive, he noted that "the motives of later childhood and of adult life are no longer simple and can almost never be referred to a single root" (p. 323). He left open the possibility of phenotypic differentiation because of the variety of experiences that people obtain from interacting with their environments. A fundamental differentiation involves splitting this undifferentiated motive into separate appetitive and aversive achievement motives (Elliot, 1999). Approach versions of the achievement motive involve striving for success. Avoidance versions of the motive involve striving to avoid failure. This idea was formalized in the classic achievement motivation theory by Atkinson, McClelland, and their colleagues (Atkinson, 1957; McClelland, Atkinson, Clark, & Lowell, 1953) when they differentiated between a motive to approach success and a motive to avoid failure. These approach and avoidance achievement motives recalled early theorizing by Murray (1938) about a need for achievement ("to do things as rapidly and/ or as well as possible" [p. 164]) and a need for infavoidance ("to avoid humiliation, to quit embarrassing situations or to avoid conditions which may lead to belittlement: the scorn, derision or indifference of others, to refrain from action because of fear of failure" [p. 192]).

These deficit-based needs were translated into motives by grounding them in anticipatory self-conscious emotions (Atkinson, 1957; McClelland et al., 1953). The motive to approach success, often described as a need for achievement or a hope for success, involves an anticipatory pride evoked by a competence-relevant situation. The motive to avoid failure, or fear of failure, involves an anticipatory shame evoked by a competence-relevant situation. Pride and shame are central to achievement motives because they reflect common consequences of competence and incompetence, respectively, in relation to the self. This connection to the self is critical because it accounts for the exploratory, often playful activities that cannot be explained by deficit-based needs but serve long-term development—an issue at the heart of the critique by White (1959). Furthermore, these emotions evoke distinct approach and avoidance motivational tendencies via characteristic action tendencies (or thought–action repertoires; Barrett & Campos, 1987; Fredrickson, 1998; Frijda, 2007; Lazarus, 1991). Pride heightens expressiveness as people seek to draw attention to their accomplishments and enhanced status; pride produces approach motivational tendencies. In contrast, shame catalyzes withdrawal as people seek to hide from attention drawn to their perceived defects or shortcomings; shame produces avoidance motivational tendencies.

As people interact with their environments and experience these emotions more consistently, they begin to form associations between the prospect of pursuing competence and experienced pride or shame. Over time, operant motivation emerges as anticipatory pride or shame, evoked by the prospect of competence evaluation, function to organize strivings (see Staddon & Cerutti, 2003). This notion of anticipatory emotion is critical and represents a special case of future-oriented emotions. It does not rely on affective forecasting but instead involves an evoked emotional experience in anticipation of a competence-related possibility (Baumgartner, Pieters, & Bagozzi, 2008).

Of course, emotions are transient states that vary over time and across situations, whereas motives are conceived as relatively stable individual differences. Recent developments in personality research can bridge this gap (Fleeson, 2001). As seen in Figure 3.1, momentary experiences of anticipatory pride (or shame) accumulate over time and across contexts, and produce a distribution, and distributions for different people can be compared. In Figure 3.1, Person B's

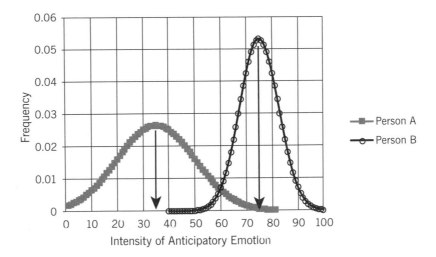

FIGURE 3.1. Simulated density distributions of anticipatory pride reveal individual differences in an appetitive achievement motive. Based on the central tendencies of each distribution (marked with an arrow), Person B has a greater estimated achievement motive than Person A.

level of anticipatory pride is typically—but not always—stronger than that of Person A. Each person's distribution can be summarized as a central tendency (e.g., as a mean, median, or mode). Such summary statistics can be used to compare individual differences. For example, contrasting the central tendency of the two distributions leads to the inference that Person B has a stronger motive to approach success than Person A.[1] Thus, it is possible to link transient self-conscious emotional experiences with more stable individual differences provided that one conceptualizes emotions as intensive longitudinal data that generate a distribution. In practice, this type of intensive longitudinal data on anticipatory self-conscious emotions has never been collected to assess achievement motives. Instead, single-occasion assessments are typically used as a shorthand for these distributions.

Two primary approaches have been used to assess motives. Early efforts involved fantasy-based, projective assessments (Murray, 1938), and scoring systems were developed to code narratives for achievement-related imagery (Birney, Burdick, & Teevan, 1969; Heckhausen, 1963; McClelland, Atkinson, Clark, & Lowell, 1976; Winter, 1994, 1999). Others developed self-report

measures that were more efficient and aligned more closely with contemporary psychometric approaches (Conroy, Willow, & Metzler, 2002; Herman, 1990; Jackson, 1974; Schultheiss, Yankova, Dirlikov, & Schad, 2009; Spence & Helmreich, 1983). When used together, these methods yielded scores that were effectively independent (Köllner & Schultheiss, 2014; Spangler, 1992). Initially, these findings stimulated debate about the validity of the two assessment methods, and camps coalesced around their preferred method. Ultimately, this failure in convergent validity led to a transformative new insight into achievement motives: These two assessment approaches for motives were actually assessing parallel motive systems (McClelland, Koestner, & Weinberger, 1989).

Dual-Process Models of Achievement Motives

Dual-process models have seen widespread application in different areas of psychology (Bargh & Chartrand, 1999; Chaiken & Trope, 1999; Kahneman, 2011; Smith & DeCoster, 2000; Strack & Deutsch, 2004). These theories posit parallel memory systems that organize human affect, behavior, and cognition (Smith & DeCoster, 2000).

The first, System 1, represents a fast and effortless system based on associative networks that are acquired slowly through accumulating experience over time. In the case of achievement motives, these associative networks reflect the probability that competence-based incentives (e.g., success or failure) will evoke anticipatory self-conscious emotions (e.g., pride or shame). This system largely operates outside of awareness. In contrast, the second, System 2, represents a slow and effortful system that draws on rule-based networks that form and adapt in response to novel or otherwise salient experiences. In the case of achievement motives, rules-based networks represent recalled episodic affective experiences or the semantic characteristics of prior competence pursuits. This system operates largely within the scope of conscious awareness. These two systems overlap with the different methods used to assess motives. For many years, the terms *implicit* and *explicit* (or *self-attributed*) were used as modifiers to describe the system under consideration. For clarity, the nature of the system should be differentiated from the method of measurement so the explicit–implicit distinction is discouraged when referring to the systems in dual-process models (Fazio & Olson, 2003).

As shown in Figure 3.2, both motivational systems have the potential to influence affective, behavioral, and cognitive dynamics as competence pursuits unfold over time. These systems can also influence each other. The associative networks that provide the basis for System 1 create a template within which rules-based processing occurs. This system biases information processing and provides default affective, behavioral, and cognitive responses to changing contextual conditions. The volitional nature of System 2 relative to System 1 provides an opportunity for agency, values, and beliefs about the self (and task) to intervene on affective, behavioral, and cognitive responses. As experience interacting with the environment accumulates, System 2 gradually uploads changes in rules-based processing to (incrementally) shape the associative networks underlying System 1. Research on self-regulation indicates that System 2 processes can easily override System 1 processes to determine a response if the individual is willing to exert the effort required to engage and sustain activity by System 2.

Both systems are critical for regulating affect, behavior, and cognition during competence pursuits; however, their relative influence can wax and wane as a function of situational incentives and other factors (McClelland et al., 1989). It is even possible that they may interact to amplify or dampen the influence of the complementary system, although this proposition has received little attention in the achievement motive domain. This general model has been applied in a variety of contexts, but research on competence and achievement motivation was arguably one of the early proving grounds for dual-process models of motivation.

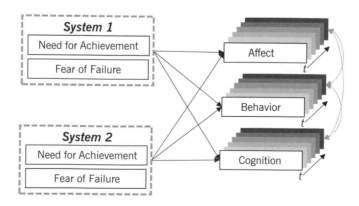

FIGURE 3.2. Dual-process model of achievement motives influencing affective, behavioral, and cognitive outcomes over time in dynamic contextual conditions.

System 1 Achievement Motives: Automatic/Impulsive

The earliest efforts to measure achievement motives derived from the Thematic Apperception Test (TAT; Murray, 1943), which test involves presenting a series of cards with images and providing instructions to write a separate story about each image. Narratives written about each story are then coded for achievement imagery, and inferences are made about motive strength. Murray (1938) wrote that latent needs—such as achievement or infavoidance—will manifest in the content of these narratives. This approach was extended by McClelland and colleagues using some of the original TAT cards and some novel images (Atkinson, 1950, p. 19; McClelland et al., 1976; McClelland, Clark, Roby, & Atkinson, 1949). The standard prompts for generating narratives based on these images were as follows:

1. What is happening? Who are the persons?
2. What has led up to this situation? That is, what has happened in the past?
3. What is being thought? What is wanted? By whom?
4. What will happen? What will be done? (McClelland et al., 1976, p. 98)

The coding systems at the core of this enterprise are summarized in Tables 3.1 and 3.2 to illustrate the evolution of content codes for appetitive and aversive

achievement motives over time. McClelland and colleagues (1976) used an empirical approach to identify scoring categories that differentiated high need achievers from low need achievers, but this approach led to some counterintuitive categories in the coding system (e.g., negative affect is coded as an indicator of an appetitive achievement motive). Heckhausen (1963) developed a streamlined scoring system that was theoretically consistent with appetitive motivational strivings; however, it was nearly four decades before that was translated into English, so it has received limited attention to date (Schultheiss, 2001). An effort to code the aversive achievement motive, fear of failure, was undertaken by Birney and colleagues (1969). Most recently, best practices for assessing motives from narratives were formalized as the Picture Story Exercise (Schultheiss & Pang, 2007). These procedures address administration methods, coder training, and scoring (including options for adjusting motive scores for word counts in narratives).

There have been concerns that the requirement to produce elaborate narrative responses to Picture Story Exercise stimuli may present too great a time demand or induce self-presentational processes that obscure motives. Two measures address this concern. First, the Operant Motive Test involves presenting respondents with 15 somewhat ambiguous line drawings and elaborating on the needs of a protagonist

TABLE 3.1. The Evolution of Content Coded for the Appetitive Achievement Motive

McClelland et al. (1953)	Heckhausen (1963; translated by Schultheiss, 2001)	Winter (1994)
• Achievement imagery	• Need for achievement and success	• Adjectives that positively evaluate performances
• Stated need for achievement	• Instrumental activity to achieve success	• Goals or performances that are described in ways that suggest positive evaluation
• Instrumental activity (successful, doubtful, or unsuccessful)	• Expectation of success	• Mention of winning or competing with others
• Anticipatory goal states (positive or negative)	• Praise	• Failure, doing badly, or other lack of excellence
• Obstacles or blocks (personal or environmental)	• Positive affect	• Unique accomplishments
• Nurturant press	• Success theme	
• Affective states (positive or negative)		
• Achievement thema		

TABLE 3.2. Evolution of Content Coded for the Aversive Achievement Motive

Heckhausen (1963; translated by Schultheiss, 2001)	Birney, Burdick, & Teevan (1969)
• Need to avoid failure • Instrumental activity to avoid failure • Expectation of failure • Criticism • Negative affect • Failure • Failure theme	• Hostile Press imagery • Need press relief • Successful/unsuccessful instrumental activity • Goal anticipation • Affective reactions to press • Blocks • Press thema

in the image (Bauman, Kazén, & Kuhl, 2010; Kuhl & Scheffer, 1999). Instead of producing detailed stories, respondents are encouraged to provide their first thoughts or spontaneous associations (even if only a few words). The other key difference with this measure is that content is scored for both motive and volitional content; that is, scores indicate both *what* a person seeks to achieve and *how* he or she seeks to achieve it. Five levels of achievement motives can be scored. Two are based on positive affect (i.e., flow, inner standards), and three are based on negative affect (i.e., coping with failure, pressure to achieve, and failure). Scores from these five levels of motives can be combined to compare approach versus avoidance, positive affect versus negative affect, or self-determined versus incentive-focused motivation.

The second approach that circumvents the long narratives in the Picture Story Exercise was initially developed as the Achievement-Motive Grid for children and later expanded to a Multi-Motive Grid for adults (Schmalt, 1999, 2005; Sokolowski, Schmalt, Langens, & Puca, 2000). These measures assess motives by presenting ambiguous stimuli to arouse the achievement motive and providing statements that participants can select to describe what they spontaneously think the protagonist in the stimulus image is thinking or feeling. The Achievement-Motive Grid yields scores for an appetitive achievement motive and two aversive achievement motives (one active, one passive). The Multi-Motive Grid yields six scores: one for approach and another for avoidance versions of each motive. This approach has been described as "semi-projective" (Schmalt, 1999, p. 111). Of course, the risk inherent in combining selected features from

theoretically distinct approaches, such as projective and self-report assessments, is that scores may capture blends of System 1 and System 2 motives and be unsuitable as a pure measure of motives in either system.

Winter (1994) adapted the classic TAT-based approach into a system for coding running text generated in a less structured fashion. The strength of this approach is its potential applications "in the wild" for studying motivational processes in the context of everyday life without interruption (or even awareness). A key limitation of the approach is its failure to differentiate between appetitive and aversive motives. Nevertheless, it has been applied profitably to study differences in achievement, affiliation, and power motives in contexts that would otherwise be inaccessible to researchers (e.g., Presidential behavior; for a review, see Winter, 2005). Schultheiss (2013) has explored a method to automate this coding using Linguistic Inquiry and Word Count software. Results were promising and suggest that automated coding of running text may be able to provide valid estimates of undifferentiated motives. Whether this method is sensitive to differences between appetitive and aversive motives remains to be seen. One interesting possibility for future work involves applying the logic of the Implicit Association Test (IAT; Greenwald, McGhee, & Schwartz, 1998; Greenwald, Nosek, & Banaji, 2003) to characterize the associative networks associated with success and failure. The IAT is a timed sorting task in which choice reaction times are measured with different category–attribute pairings. In this case, one might use failure and success as categories, and pride and shame as attributes. In the first block of trials, each category is paired with a different attribute and, in the second block of trials, those pairings are reversed. The difference in response times between compatible and incompatible category–attribute pairings provides an indirect (implicit) measure of the relative strength of the category–attribute pairings. Brunstein and Schmitt (2004) applied a similar approach with self- versus other-related category labels and successful versus nonsuccessful attributes. They found that implicit motive scores positively predicted performance on a separate reaction time test when participants were informed that they would receive feedback if they had a top performance (but did not predict performance if participants were not notified of upcoming feedback). One limitation of their approach is that the category–attribute exemplars may confound anticipatory affective responses with self-concept (a threat akin to including perceived competence items in a motive questionnaire). Future research will need to evaluate the impact of these exemplars on predictive validity of the resulting scores.

To provide more nuanced assessment, a Single-Category IAT (Karpinski & Steinman, 2006) may be implemented by pairing a single category (e.g., success) with one of two attributes (e.g., pride, shame). Again, the difference in response times between compatible (e.g., success–pride) and incompatible (e.g., success–shame) trials can be used to estimate an indirect measure of, in this example, the appetitive achievement motive. The aversive achievement motive could be assessed similarly by replacing success as a category exemplar with failure.

In summary, the literature has a rich history of assessing System 1 achievement motives by content coding narratives generated after viewing ambiguous images. Coding systems for approach and avoidance motives have been developed and refined (see Tables 3.1 and 3.2). At this point, the Heckhausen (1963; Schultheiss, 2001) coding system provides the most conceptually coherent categories and is recommended for future work in this area. Emerging alternatives capitalize on narratives from unstructured prompts and reaction time tests. Regardless of the method, a consistent set of findings have linked System 1 achievement motives with procedural or nondeclarative outcomes.

One of the early, attention-grabbing theoretical predictions attempted to address the limitations of expected utility predictions of behavioral choice. So-called "departures" from rationality have attracted tremendous interest in the flourishing behavioral economics literature, so it is worth reviewing the role of motives in these unexpected decisions. In this case, each motive was hypothesized to interact with the expected utility (cost) of succeeding (or failing) to produce separate tendencies to approach success (T_{AS}) or avoid failure (T_{AF}) (Atkinson, 1957). Equations (3.1) and (3.2) represent these tendencies as functions of the motives to approach success (M_{AS}) or avoid failure (M_{AF}), the subjective probability of success (P_S) or failure (P_F), or incentive value of success (IV_S) or failure (IV_F).

$$T_{AS} = M_{AS} \times P_S \times IV_S \qquad (3.1)$$

$$T_{AF} = M_{AF} \times P_F \times IV_F \qquad (3.2)$$

If one assumes that the probabilities of success and failure are inverse values (i.e., $P_F = 1 - P_S$), and that the incentive values for success and failure are inverse functions of the probabilities of success and failure, respectively (i.e., $IV_S = 1 - P_S$; $IV_F = 1 - P_F$), the previous equations can be reduced from six to three unknowns: MA_S, MA_F, and P_S. As shown in Equation (3.3), the difference between these tendencies yields the resultant motivational (RM) tendency, which decides whether an individual is likely to choose an action or not.

$$RM = T_{AS} - T_{AF} \qquad (3.3)$$
$$= (M_{AS} \times P_S \times (1 - P_S))$$
$$- (M_{AF} \times (1 - P_S) \times (1 - (1 - P_S)))$$

This model leads to predictions that (1) people with a strong motivation to approach success (driven by M_{AS}) will tend to select moderately difficult tasks where their effort will likely determine their success, and (2) people with a strong motivation to avoid failure (driven by M_{AF}) will tend to select extremely easy or extremely difficult tasks to protect their sense of self (see Figure 3.3). In this theory, motives serve to explain individual differences in violated expectancy–value predictions.

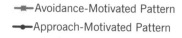

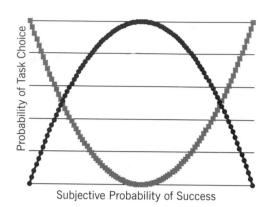

FIGURE 3.3. Theoretically predicted relations between the subjective probability of success and task choice for approach- and avoidance-motivated individuals.

Many other predictions have been made about the effects of implicit achievement motives on affective, behavioral, and cognitive outcomes during competence pursuits. A full review is beyond the scope of this chapter, but a number of reviews and collections are available elsewhere for interested readers (Atkinson, 1974; Birney et al., 1969; Heckhausen, 1967; McClelland, 1980; McClelland et al., 1976; Pang, 2010; Schultheiss & Brunstein, 2005). Consistent with the memory system underlying System 1 motives, McClelland (1980) concluded that implicit motives predict spontaneous behavioral outcomes rather than planned or declarative outcomes. This literature has been strongly weighted toward the appetitive achievement motive. Given the assessment challenges reviewed earlier, findings have been somewhat mixed. Those assessment challenges may also help to explain why research in this area has not sustained its initial momentum.

System 2 Achievement Motives: Controlled/Reflective

As an alternative to the time-consuming methods used to assess System 1 achievement motives, researchers developed a variety of questionnaire-based measures of motives. Although originally (and controversially) hypothesized to exhibit strong convergent validity with implicit measures, this hypothesis has been refuted repeatedly. As discussed earlier, self-report measures that draw on declarative memory are now presumed to assess System 2 motives. Ray (1986) catalogued and briefly critiqued over 70 scales that have been developed or applied to measure either achievement motives or closely related constructs.

Two of the most popular measures of the approach-valenced achievement motive are from the Personality Research Form (PRF) and the Work and Family Orientation Scale (Jackson, 1974; Spence & Helmreich, 1983). The 16-item achievement scale of the PRF was based on the taxonomy of needs proposed by Murray (1938). Questions have been raised and never fully resolved about the dimensionality of this scale (Jackson, Ahmed, & Heapy, 1976; Jackson, Paunonen, Fraboni, & Goffin, 1996). A second measure, the Work–Family Orientation Questionnaire, was developed to measure individual differences in work, mastery, competitiveness, and personal unconcern with achievement (Spence & Helmreich, 1983). Similar to the PRF achievement scale, the items are "relatively free of references to specific situational contexts" (p. 41) so they are assumed to represent a transcontextual motive disposition. The work and mastery items resemble the appetitive achievement motive because of their links with self-referenced definitions of competence, preference for challenge, and positive attitudes toward effort. Competitiveness items include content focused on normative definitions of competence (e.g., "I try harder when I'm in competition with other people"), and personal unconcern items are almost antithetical to an approach-based achievement motive. The work and mastery scales are often combined to form a single score for the appetitive achievement motive; however, the competitiveness scale also represents an appetitive motive, albeit one that often blends achievement and social incentives. These scores have been linked with a variety of achievement outcomes (Spence & Helmreich, 1983).

Some of the most common measures of aversive achievement motives, historically, have drawn from the anxiety literature, especially when couched in terms of evaluation-related anxiety (e.g., test anxiety; Alpert & Haber, 1960; Sarason & Mandler, 1952). These measures were not developed to measure an aversive achievement motive, so scores often included content-irrelevant variance. Consequently, a mixed picture of convergent and discriminant validity has emerged from one measure to another (Gelbort & Winer, 1985; Jackaway & Teevan, 1976; Macdonald & Hyde, 1980; Mulig, Haggerty, Carballosa, Cinnick, & Madden, 1985).

More recently, measures have been developed to assess fear of failure directly via beliefs in the aversive consequences of failing that might evoke avoidance strivings (Conroy et al., 2002). These beliefs were identified from an inductive content analysis of interviews with athletes and performing artists. These interviews produced a transcontextual model of aversive consequences of failing, and items were written to measure the strength of beliefs that each consequence is likely (Conroy, 2001). A series of factor analyses on samples of young adults informed the removal of items with irrelevant variance and other model modifications, culminating in a robust measurement model of fear of failure (Conroy, Metzler, & Hofer, 2003; Conroy et al., 2002). This model has a hierarchical structure with first-order factors representing beliefs in five different aversive consequences of failing, and a second-order factor representing a general fear of failure. The five aversive consequences that emerged included experiencing shame and embarrassment, devaluing one's self-estimate, having an uncertain future, having important others lose interest, and upsetting important others. Beliefs about experiencing shame and embarrassment consistently exhibit strong associations with the higher-order factor and also show the strongest associations with variables theorized to be linked with fear of failure (Conroy, 2004; Conroy et al., 2003; Sagar & Stoeber, 2009). It is clear that shame is at the core of this higher-order fear of failure construct. A five-item short form of this measure is available. It has strong psychometric properties and is recommended for use in assessing the aversive achievement motive (Conroy et al., 2003, 2002).

Whereas most research on competence motivation focuses on task-related outcomes such as level of aspiration, persistence, and effort, two exciting recent lines of work on System 2 achievement motives are highlighted below. These studies were selected to illustrate (1) the potential for stable individual differences in System 2 motives to predict context-sensitive within-person fluctuations in affect, behavior, and cognition, and (2) the relevance of these motives for explaining social behavior that is not task-relevant per se.

First, although most research on motives has focused on correlations with static outcomes, these motives have been linked with context-sensitive *changes* in competence-relevant outcomes. For example, golfers with a strong appetitive achievement motive decreased their level of dysfunctional performance-avoidance achievement goal pursuit more rapidly over the course of a round than did golfers with a weak motive (Schantz & Conroy, 2009). Golfers with a strong aversive achievement motive also reported sharper increases in affective arousal after performing poorly on a hole. Thus, the appetitive achievement motive is linked to improved regulation over time, and the aversive achievement motive is linked with somatic responses that characterize threat.

In another study, college students used diaries to record the qualities of interpersonal interactions for 14 days, as well as their end-of-day experience of various emotions, including hubristic pride (Conroy et al., 2015). On days when participants reported generally more communal interactions, a strong aversive achievement motive buffered against experiencing hubristic pride. In contrast, people with a weak aversive achievement motive were significantly more likely to experience hubristic pride at the end of days when people treated them with more warmth. In this case, the aversive achievement motive has roots in relational insecurity (Elliot & Reis, 2003), which appears to buffer against overreacting to social warmth with a maladaptive social emotion. Taken together, these findings illustrate that time-invariant motives can play a role in regulating the ebb and flow of time-varying outcomes in response to changing contextual conditions.

In another line of work, my colleagues and I have found that System 2 achievement motives are linked with systematic differences in interpersonal behavior. At a dispositional level, the appetitive achievement motive supports flexible interpersonal behavior and agency; however, deficits in this motive were linked with perceived problem of being overly submissive (Conroy, Elliot, & Pincus, 2009). This problem is subtle because it only emerges from self-reports and not from the reports of well-acquainted peers. Additionally, the appetitive achievement motive does not appear to bias perceptions of others' interpersonal problems. In contrast, the aversive achievement motive is associated with generalized interpersonal distress in self- and peer reports. When people with a strong aversive achievement motive are scrutinized, they exhibit one of two prototypical patterns of problems: either excessive nonassertiveness or excessive vindictiveness. This pattern aligns with expectations based on the motive's grounding in shame (Gilbert & McGuire, 1998; Lewis, 1971). Specifically, nonassertiveness corresponds with the action tendency to withdraw, appease others, and not draw attention to oneself, whereas vindictiveness corresponds with the strategy of reattributing blame externally to down-regulate shame by up-regulating anger. By connecting achievement motives with social behavior, these findings reveal that competence is a relevant motive across many contexts of daily life, and its influence transcends formal achievement settings and processes. As White (1959) wrote, "Effectance motivation is persistent in the sense that it regularly occupies the spare waking time between episodes of homeostatic crisis" (p. 321).

In follow-up studies, System 2 achievement motives were linked with interpersonal impacts during a cooperative dyadic competence pursuit (Conroy & Pincus, 2011). Participants were paired in low-acquaintance dyads to compete against other teams in a puzzle-solving competition. When participants were not informed that feedback on their performance would be provided publicly, the appetitive achievement motive was completely unassociated with interpersonal behavior, but the aversive achievement motive was associated with the established pattern of appeasement or aggression. When participants were informed ahead of time that feedback on their performance would be provided publicly, stronger effects appeared. Participants with a strong appetitive achievement motive were perceived by their partners as more distant, possibly due to their increased absorption in the task and detachment from social interaction. Notwithstanding their apparent detachment to their partners, they perceived themselves as more friendly and engaged. In contrast, participants with a strong aversive achievement motive were no longer perceived as appeasing or aggressive but instead became highly sensitive to rejection. They perceived their partners as cold–submissive, cold, cold–dominant, and dominant. Over time, this pattern is likely to cause interpersonal difficulties because people are more likely to undermine their relationships out of insecurity about their status. Taken as a whole, these studies reveal the appetitive achievement motive as a source of flexible and secure interpersonal behavior, whereas the aversive achievement motive bastardizes competence strivings with relational insecurities—an extension of important early findings by Elliot and Reis (2003).

Congruence of Motivational Systems

The two memory systems from which these motives spring are conceived as distinct because fitness increases when people are capable of slow and rapid learning from their experience (Smith & DeCoster, 2000). Research on motives specifically has supported the independence of these systems and, as noted earlier, meta-analyses have revealed small correlations between corresponding motive measures from the two systems, ranging from an average of .09 to .14 (Köllner & Schultheiss, 2014; Spangler, 1992). These averages represent a summary across people, and some people are likely to experience greater concordance than others. Such concordance is generally thought to be beneficial because the two motivational systems will be aligned and people's spontaneous behavior will match their planned behavior (Thrash, Cassidy, Maruskin, & Elliot, 2010). In cases where System 1 and System 2 motives are discordant, people may experience frustration with their efforts or decreased satisfaction with the product of their work. Some have even hypothesized that motive discordance reduces global well-being as people pursue goals with one system that do not align with the other system (Brunstein, 2010).

Factors that influence congruence have been well developed elsewhere and are not reviewed here (see Thrash et al., 2010). For the purposes of this chapter, the important point is that motives do not always converge, so it is important not to treat System 1 and System 2 motives as isomorphic or interchangeable. It is even possible that these systems may interact to amplify or dampen their respective effects on affect, behavior, and cognition. Ideally, future work will aspire to comprehensive assessments of appetitive and aversive achievement motives in both systems, but this is an expensive and time-consuming proposition. Practically, a more reasonable compromise may be for researchers to be clear about the system they are assessing, to develop hypotheses sensitive to the limited scope of their measures, and to model appetitive and aversive motives simultaneously. Even this modest recommendation would advance the literature, which too frequently has relied on bivariate comparisons of either an appetitive or an aversive motive with an antecedent or consequence.

Developmental Origins of Achievement Motives

Socialization is one of the primary theoretical influences on the development of achievement motives (McClelland, 1985; McClelland et al., 1989), but developmental trajectories have not been well characterized for either System 1 or System 2 motives. To the extent that data are available, they suggest tremendous variation and no clear age-related pattern in the System 1 appetitive achievement motive (Jenkins, 1987; Veroff, Depner, Kulka, & Douvan, 1980); there are no known data on the age-related differences in the corresponding aversive achievement motive. Data on System 2 motives are equally sparse. The norms for the PRF do not indicate any age-related differences in achievement scale scores (Jackson, 1999). The only other known study of lifespan differences in something resembling System 2 achievement motives comes from measures of imaginal processes related to achievement and fear of failure, both of which decrease with age (Giambra, 1974). These processes may overlap somewhat with motives as conceptualized here, but they are not identical constructs, so it is unclear how well the observed age-related differences will generalize. To date, all of the available data on developmental differences in achievement motives has been based on cross-sectional data which is vulnerable to age × cohort confounds that can mask intraindividual developmental processes. It is very difficult to draw strong conclusions about the functional form of developmental trajectories for System 1 and System 2 achievement motives based on the available evidence.

Notwithstanding the lack of clear developmental trajectories for motives, it is possible to implicate critical factors in the development of achievement motives. Early childhood is likely to provide the seminal experiences that provide a template for interpreting the meaning of momentary competence and incompetence in relation to the self (McClelland, 1958). Children's earliest autonomous experiences with competence occur in the context of self-care such as eating, toilet training, and getting dressed. Parents of children with strong System 1 appetitive achievement motives have exhibited warm and supportive styles with age-appropriate, if perhaps somewhat demanding, expectations for early mastery and independence (McClelland & Pilon, 1983; Rosen & D'Andrade, 1959; Winterbottom, 1958). In contrast, children with strong System 1 aversive achievement motives grow up with more affectional deprivation and parents who respond to their failures in a more neutral or critical manner (Greenfeld & Teevan, 1986; Singh, 1992; Teevan, 1983; Teevan & McGhee, 1972). Children with strong aversive motives appear to learn that competence is a route to a relational incentive, namely, parental approval and affection. Most of this work is based on samples of boys older than 5 years, so caution should be used when generalizing conclusions.

Early childhood experiences have also been implicated in the development of System 2 achievement motives. In this system, the appetitive achievement motive has been linked with high parental expectations for children's performance and a readiness to assist children with difficulties (Hermans, ter Laak, & Maes, 1972). Interestingly, parents of children with a strong appetitive achievement motive tend to offer more specific help but less nonspecific help. Their children also refuse help more frequently, and it is unclear whether the help offering drives the refusals or vice versa. This finding reveals a key limitation of this literature: Observational studies of parenting interactions are needed to unpack emergent *sequences* of parent–child behaviors that influence motive development. Parents of children with strong appetitive achievement motives also tend to be highly responsive to children's successes but less responsive to off-task expressions of insecurity.

Parents of children with strong System 2 avoidance achievement motives have lower expectations and offer less help and task-oriented reinforcement (Hermans et al., 1972). Adolescents and young adults with strong System 2 avoidance achievement motives report that their parents use more love withdrawal (Elliot & Thrash, 2004). From a mechanistic perspective, children appear to internalize the way their parents and other important figures treat them after failing or succeeding, and mimic that behavior in how they treat themselves (Conroy, 2003; Conroy & Coatsworth, 2007; Conroy & Pincus, 2006). The characteristic pattern is that others criticize them when they fail, and they subsequently self-criticize when failing. Overall, these findings are too limited to draw strong conclusions, but they are consistent with findings that the appetitive achievement motive is linked with attachment security, whereas the aversive achievement motive is characterized by insecurity (Elliot & Reis, 2003). This insecurity appears to be rooted in competence being a contingency for self-worth (Elliot et al., 2010).

This portrait of the developmental antecedents of achievement motives can be fleshed out by incorporating work on the socialization of self-conscious emotion propensities. From that work, three likely influences have been identified (Elliot et al., 2010). First, a *mutually responsive orientation* in the parent–child relationship is likely to play a role in internalizing the rules, standards, and goals that are prerequisites of self-conscious emotions. This orientation is characterized by sensitivity, acceptance, cooperation, committed compliance with rules, responsiveness to needs, and shared positive affect (Kochanska, 1997; Kochanska & Murray, 2000). This orientation may have its most direct influence on the development of pride propensities, but it is possible that it may amplify the influence of other parenting practices on shame propensities. Second, *criticism and love withdrawal* (mentioned earlier) fit within a broader class of critical/rejecting parenting practices that contribute to shame propensities (Alessandri & Lewis, 1993, 1996; Mills, 2003; Stuewig & McCloskey, 2005; Sullivan, Bennett, & Lewis, 2003). When coupled with incompetence, these practices create self-worth contingencies and internal attribution patterns that make shame for failing more likely (Lewis & Sullivan, 2005; McGregor & Elliot, 2005). Finally, parents' use of *generic (person-focused) and nongeneric (specific; behavior-focused) praise* shapes attributional patterns linked with self-conscious emotions and motivation (Cimpian, Arce, Markman, & Dweck, 2007). Nongeneric praise for success orients children toward specific, unstable, and controllable attributions that evoke pride. On the other hand, generic praise orients children toward global, stable, and uncontrollable attributions. By itself, generic praise does not evoke shame but it does create an attributional framework that can evoke shame if applied to explain future failures. Praise appears to be most potent when competence-based outcomes are ill-defined and feedback provides information that can inform self-evaluations.

In summary, the limited literature suggests that children acquire achievement motives at the knees of their parents and other important figures through the evaluative styles and self-conscious emotional propensities that are modeled and conditioned, respectively.

The specifics of this socialization process need to be characterized better, and special attention should be paid to disentangling the reciprocal effects of parents and children on each other. Although the pattern of findings appears to be reasonably similar for corresponding motives in System 1 and System 2, the interplay of these systems in motive formation is presently unknown.

APPLICATIONS

Achievement motives have been incorporated into (or have at least informed) a number of applications to address social problems over the past half century. The most notable of these were aimed at improving educational and occupational outcomes (McClelland, 1978). These projects grew from work linking the appetitive achievement motive with entrepreneurial success, economic growth, and upward mobility (McClelland, 1961). Unfortunately, despite some intriguing successes, few of these efforts have been sustained or had the transformative impact that was envisioned. Rather than revisiting these applications, this chapter provides an opportunity to look ahead to ways in which our new understanding of achievement motives can be applied to improve well-being and productivity in a contemporary context.

Drawing from evidence that motives are socialized, a suite of developmentally focused applications can be envisioned. These applications are social in nature and necessarily involve figures such as family members and educators (a term used in its broadest sense to include teachers, coaches, and others who supervise, guide, and provide feedback during children's voluntary structured activities). Key developmental milestones around which interventions could be staged include early experiences with autonomous competence (e.g., toilet training, eating, learning to speak, read, and write), the emergence of self-conscious emotions, and transitions into increasingly autonomous competence pursuits. Training could be designed to increase awareness of the implications of different behaviors on children's motivation (e.g., how they provide praise) and to promote strategies for increasing the use of a desired behavioral repertoire.

One of the key challenges in this work will involve identifying the key moments when families or educators will be most receptive to new information and strategies for supporting their children. The milestones identified earlier provide a starting point for such decisions, but the people who can use this behavioral technology profitably often have many competing demands for their attention and little bandwidth to spare as a result. Creative strategies for integrating training with existing commitments (e.g., well-baby visits, parent–teacher conferences, inservice trainings) may help in this regard. This work will require interdisciplinary collaborations to create positive mesosystem influences on children's development.

One example of this kind of work can be found in youth sport research aimed at training coaches to increase their use of a prosocial behavioral repertoire. The vast majority of youth sport coaches are well-intentioned volunteers, without formal training in developmental psychology or coaching. In practice, these coaches have been amenable to behavioral training that will help them provide a more optimal experience for participating youth, but the added time commitment for training is a common and understandable barrier. Integrating the training with organizational meetings hosted by league administrators is one strategy that has been used to overcome that barrier without compromising the coaches' autonomy and engendering resentment. Coaches who complete training have been responsive, as indicated by greater levels of reinforcements/rewards and lower levels of punitive behaviors (Conroy & Coatsworth, 2004). Unfortunately, these behavioral differences were either not strong enough or were not timed with critical moments sufficiently to reduce System 2 aversive achievement motives in a sample of 7- to 18-year-old youth. A follow-up study elaborated that coaching behaviors are associated with changes in self-blame which, in turn, are associated with changes in System 2 aversive achievement motives (Conroy & Coatsworth, 2007). Perceived criticism and self-criticism following failure were especially prominent in this process. Punitive behaviors tend to be rare in youth sport settings, so it may be necessary to raise awareness about how biased person perception can lead well-intended feedback to be perceived as critical.

Similar efforts could be developed as a part of inservice training for educators. Early childhood education seems like an especially promising time for this training because many of the developmental antecedents associated with motive development should already be familiar parts of training. Scaffolding new knowledge and strategies on established developmental sensitivities will reduce the burden of training and should increase uptake and facilitate implementation. Reaching children during their earliest experiences with autonomous competence pursuits also decreases the likelihood that an aversive motive will need to be retrained. The lack of a deeply ingrained emotional foundation may also accelerate changes in the slow-learning System 1. In contrast, intervening at later ages may require (1) that suboptimal emotional associations with competence incentives be weakened before forming a new motive, and (2) longer time for System 2 changes to exert an influence on System 1 motives. Consequently, more intense training may be required for later intervention, and the cost and burden of such training presents a significant barrier to widespread implementation and adoption.

Beyond these types of (early) developmental applications, some of the recent work linking achievement motives with interpersonal behavior seems ripe for application in industry. Complex tasks, demanding group members, and poor interpersonal processes can undermine group productivity (Forsyth, 2009). Most readers will have some experience working with difficult individuals—group members who have been either overly engaged and dominated the task without consideration of others or insufficiently engaged and not contributing to the group. System 2 achievement motives can contribute to these patterns. In high-stakes personnel selection processes, it may be advantageous to screen and identify excesses in System 2 aversive achievement motives—either from self-reports on a questionnaire or passively, using archives of running text on social media or other digital forms. Additionally, leaders may benefit from training on how to manage these often highly motivated but occasionally difficult employees. Some excellent (and best-selling) books have been written to fill this need (e.g., Sutton, 2010); however, none appear to capitalize on our new understanding of how achievement motives contribute to these challenges.

CONCLUSION

In closing, this chapter has summarized over half a century of research on achievement motives, with an emphasis on their grounding in anticipatory pride and shame. The nature of these self-conscious emotions is critical for understanding the motives' automatic and deliberate, approach and avoidance influences on affect, behavior, and cognition during competence strivings. Although research on motives has slowed in recent years, the theoretical and technological advances reviewed earlier invite us to reinvigorate this corner of the competence motivation literature. This work is needed to shed light on the dynamics of the self and its regulatory influences under conditions of competence and incompetence.

NOTE

1. For this illustration, the distribution was assumed to be Gaussian (normal). This assumption is reasonable for pride based on its adaptive nature but shame is more likely to have a skewed, and possibly zero-inflated, distribution (Conroy, Ram, Pincus, & Rebar, 2015). The appropriate summary statistic may vary for distributions with different forms.

REFERENCES

Alessandri, S. M., & Lewis, M. (1993). Parental evaluation and its relation to shame and pride in young children. *Sex Roles, 29*(5–6), 335–343.

Alessandri, S. M., & Lewis, M. (1996). Differences in pride and shame in maltreated and nonmaltreated preschoolers. *Child Development, 67*(4), 1857–1869.

Alpert, R., & Haber, R. N. (1960). Anxiety in academic achievement situations. *Journal of Abnormal and Social Psychology, 61*(2), 207–215.

Atkinson, J. W. (1950). Studies in projective

measurement of achievement motivation (*Abstract in University Microfilms, 10*(4), Publication No. 1945). Ann Arbor: University of Michigan.

Atkinson, J. W. (1957). Motivational determinants of risk-taking behavior. *Psychological Review, 64,* 359–372.

Atkinson, J. W. (1974). *Motivation and achievement.* Washington, DC: Winston.

Bargh, J. A., & Chartrand, T. L. (1999). The unbearable automaticity of being. *American Psychologist, 54,* 462–479.

Barrett, K. C., & Campos, J. J. (1987). Perspectives on emotional development: II. A functionalist approach to emotions. In J. D. Osofsky (Ed.), *Handbook of infant development* (2nd ed., pp. 555–578). Oxford, UK: Wiley.

Bauman, N., Kazén, M., & Kuhl, J. (2010). Implicit motives: A look from personality systems interaction theory. In O. C. Schultheiss & J. C. Brunstein (Eds.), *Implicit motives* (pp. 375–403). New York: Oxford University Press.

Baumgartner, H., Pieters, R., & Bagozzi, R. P. (2008). Future-oriented emotions: Conceptualization and behavioral effects. *European Journal of Social Psychology, 38*(4), 685–696.

Birney, R. C., Burdick, H., & Teevan, R. C. (1969). *Fear of failure.* New York: Van Nostrand Reinhold.

Brunstein, J. C. (2010). Implicit motives and explicit goals: The role of motivational congruence in emotional well-being. In O. C. Schultheiss & J. C. Brunstein (Eds.), *Implicit motives* (pp. 347–374). New York: Oxford University Press.

Brunstein, J. C., & Schmitt, C. H. (2004). Assessing individual differences in achievement motivation with the Implicit Association Test. *Journal of Research in Personality, 38*(6), 536–555.

Chaiken, S., & Trope, Y. (1999). *Dual-process theories in social psychology.* New York: Guilford Press.

Cimpian, A., Arce, H.-M. C., Markman, E. M., & Dweck, C. S. (2007). Subtle linguistic cues affect children's motivation. *Psychological Science, 18*(4), 314–316.

Conroy, D. E. (2001). Progress in the development of a multidimensional measure of fear of failure: The Performance Failure Appraisal Inventory (PFAI). *Anxiety, Stress, and Coping, 14*(4), 431–452.

Conroy, D. E. (2003). Representational models associated with fear of failure in adolescents and young adults. *Journal of Personality, 71,* 757–783.

Conroy, D. E. (2004). The unique psychological meanings of multidimensional fears of failing.

Journal of Sport and Exercise Psychology, 26(3), 484–491.

Conroy, D. E., & Coatsworth, J. D. (2004). The effects of coach training on fear of failure in youth swimmers: A latent growth curve analysis from a randomized, controlled trial. *Journal of Applied Developmental Psychology, 25*(2), 193–214.

Conroy, D. E., & Coatsworth, J. D. (2007). Coaching behaviors associated with changes in fear of failure: Changes in self-talk and need satisfaction as potential mechanisms. *Journal of Personality, 75*(2), 383–419.

Conroy, D. E., Elliot, A. J., & Pincus, A. L. (2009). The expression of achievement motives in interpersonal problems. *Journal of Personality, 77*(2), 495–526.

Conroy, D. E., Elliot, A. J., & Thrash, T. M. (2009). Achievement motivation. In M. R. Leary & R. H. Hoyle (Eds.), *Handbook of individual differences in social behavior* (pp. 382–399). New York: Guilford Press.

Conroy, D. E., Metzler, J. N., & Hofer, S. M. (2003). Factorial invariance and latent mean stability of performance failure appraisals. *Structural Equation Modeling, 10*(3), 401–422.

Conroy, D. E., & Pincus, A. L. (2006). A comparison of mean partialing and dual-hypothesis testing to evaluate stereotype effects when assessing profile similarity. *Journal of Personality Assessment, 86*(2), 142–149.

Conroy, D. E., & Pincus, A. L. (2011). Interpersonal impact messages associated with different forms of achievement motivation. *Journal of Personality, 79,* 675–706.

Conroy, D. E., Ram, N., Pincus, A. L., & Rebar, A. L. (2015). Bursts of self-conscious emotions in the daily lives of emerging adults. *Self and Identity, 14*(3), 290–313.

Conroy, D. E., Willow, J. P., & Metzler, J. N. (2002). Multidimensional fear of failure measurement: The Performance Failure Appraisal Inventory. *Journal of Applied Sport Psychology, 14*(2), 76–90.

Elliot, A. J. (1999). Approach and avoidance motivation and achievement goals. *Educational Psychologist, 34*(3), 169–189.

Elliot, A. J., Conroy, D. E., Barron, K. E., & Murayama, K. (2010). Achievement motives and goals: A developmental analysis. In R. M. Lerner, M. E. Lamb, & A. M. Freund (Eds.), *Handbook of lifespan development: Vol. 2. Social and emotional development* (pp. 474–510). New York: Wiley.

Elliot, A. J., & Reis, H. T. (2003). Attachment and exploration in adulthood. *Journal of Personality and Social Psychology, 85*(2), 317–331.

Elliot, A. J., & Thrash, T. M. (2004). The intergenerational transmission of fear of failure. *Personality and Social Psychology Bulletin, 30*(8), 957–971.

Fazio, R. H., & Olson, M. A. (2003). Implicit measures in social cognition research: Their meaning and use. *Annual Review of Psychology, 54*(1), 297–327.

Fleeson, W. (2001). Toward a structure- and process-integrated view of personality: Traits as density distributions of states. *Journal of Personality and Social Psychology, 80,* 1011–1027.

Forsyth, D. (2009). *Group dynamics* (5th ed.). Pacific Grove, CA: Brooks/Cole.

Fredrickson, B. L. (1998). What good are positive emotions? *Review of General Psychology, 2*(3), 300–319.

Frijda, N. (2007). *The laws of emotion.* Mahwah, NJ: Erlbaum.

Gelbort, K. R., & Winer, J. L. (1985). Fear of success and fear of failure: A multitrait–multimethod validation study. *Journal of Personality and Social Psychology, 48*(4), 1009–1014.

Giambra, L. M. (1974). Daydreaming across the life span: Late adolescent to senior citizen. *International Journal of Aging and Human Development, 5*(2), 115–140.

Gilbert, P., & McGuire, M. T. (1998). Shame, status, and social roles: Psychobiology and evolution. In P. Gilbert & B. Andrews (Eds.), *Shame: Interpersonal behavior, psychopathology, and culture* (pp. 99–125). New York: Oxford University Press.

Greenfeld, N., & Teevan, R. C. (1986). Fear of failure in families without fathers. *Psychological Reports, 59*(2, Pt. 1), 571–574.

Greenwald, A. G., McGhee, D. E., & Schwartz, J. L. (1998). Measuring individual differences in implicit cognition: The implicit association test. *Journal of Personality and Social Psychology, 74*(6), 1464–1480.

Greenwald, A. G., Nosek, B. A., & Banaji, M. R. (2003). Understanding and using the implicit association test: I. An improved scoring algorithm. *Journal of Personality and Social Psychology, 85*(2), 197–216.

Heckhausen, H. (1963). *Hoffnung und Furcht in der Leistungsmotivation* [Hope and fear components of achievement motivation]. Meisenheim am Glan, Germany: Anton Hain.

Heckhausen, H. (1967). *The anatomy of achievement motivation.* New York: Academic Press.

Herman, W. (1990). Fear of failure as a distinctive personality treait measure of test anxiety. *Journal of Research and Development in Education, 23,* 180–185.

Hermans, H. J., ter Laak, J. J., & Maes, P. C. (1972). Achievement motivation and fear of failure in family and school. *Developmental Psychology, 6*(3), 520–528.

Jackaway, R., & Teevan, R. (1976). Fear of failure and fear of success: Two dimensions of the same motive. *Sex Roles, 2*(3), 283–293.

Jackson, D. N. (1974). *Manual for the Personality Research Form.* Goshen, NY: Research Psychology Press.

Jackson, D. N. (1999). *Personality Research Form manual* (3rd ed.). Port Huron, MI: Sigma Assessment Systems.

Jackson, D. N., Ahmed, S. A., & Heapy, N. A. (1976). Is achievement a unitary construct? *Journal of Research in Personality, 10*(1), 1–21.

Jackson, D. N., Paunonen, S. V., Fraboni, M., & Goffin, R. D. (1996). A five-factor versus six-factor model of personality structure. *Personality and Individual Differences, 20*(1), 33–45.

Jenkins, S. R. (1987). Need for achievement and women's careers over 14 years: Evidence for occupational structure effects. *Journal of Personality and Social Psychology, 53*(5), 922–932.

Kahneman, D. (2011). *Thinking fast and slow.* New York: Farrar, Straus & Giroux.

Karpinski, A., & Steinman, R. B. (2006). The single category implicit association test as a measure of implicit social cognition. *Journal of Personality and Social Psychology, 91*(1), 16–32.

Kochanska, G. (1997). Mutually responsive orientation between mothers and their young children: implications for early socialization. *Child Development, 68*(1), 94–112.

Kochanska, G., & Murray, K. T. (2000). Mother–child mutually responsive orientation and conscience development: From toddler to early school age. *Child Development, 71*(2), 417–431.

Köllner, M. G., & Schultheiss, O. C. (2014). Meta-analytic evidence of low convergence between implicit and explicit measures of the needs for achievement, affiliation, and power. *Frontiers in Psychology, 5,* 826.

Kuhl, J., & Scheffer, D. (1999). *Der operante Multi-Motiv-Test (OMT): Manual* [Scoring manual for the Operant Multi-Motive Test (OMT)]. Osnabrück, Germany: University of Osnabrück.

Lazarus, R. S. (1991). *Emotion and adaptation.* New York: Oxford University Press.

Lewis, H. B. (1971). *Shame and guilt in neurosis.* New York: International Universities Press.

Lewis, M., & Sullivan, M. W. (2005). The development of self-conscious emotions. In A. J. Elliot & C. S. Dweck (Eds.), *Handbook of competence and motivation* (pp. 185–201). New York: Guilford Press.

Macdonald, N. E., & Hyde, J. S. (1980). Fear of success, need achievement, and fear of failure: A factor analytic study. *Sex Roles, 6*(5), 695–711.

McClelland, D. C. (1958). Methods of measuring human motivation. In J. W. Atkinson (Ed.), *Motives in fantasy, action, and society* (pp. 7–42). Princeton, NJ: Van Nostrand.

McClelland, D. C. (1961). *The achieving society.* New York: Van Nostrand.

McClelland, D. C. (1978). Managing motivation to expand human freedom. *American Psychologist, 33*(3), 201–210.

McClelland, D. C. (1980). Motive dispositions: The merits of operant and respondent measures. In L. Wheeler (Ed.), *Review of personality and social psychology* (Vol. 1, pp. 10–41). Beverly Hills, CA: Sage.

McClelland, D. C. (1985). *Human motivation* (2nd ed.). Glenview, IL: Scott, Foresman.

McClelland, D. C., Atkinson, J. W., Clark, R. A., & Lowell, E. L. (1953). *The achievement motive.* New York: Appleton-Century-Crofts.

McClelland, D. C., Atkinson, J. W., Clark, R. A., & Lowell, E. L. (1976). *The achievement motive.* Oxford, UK: Irvington.

McClelland, D. C., Clark, R. A., Roby, T. B., & Atkinson, J. W. (1949). The projective expression of needs: IV. The effect of the need for achievement on thematic apperception. *Journal of Experimental Psychology, 39*(2), 242–255.

McClelland, D. C., Koestner, R., & Weinberger, J. (1989). How do self-attributed and implicit motives differ? *Psychological Review, 96*(4), 690–702.

McClelland, D. C., & Pilon, D. A. (1983). Sources of adult motives in patterns of parent behavior in early childhood. *Journal of Personality and Social Psychology, 44*(3), 564–574.

McGregor, H. A., & Elliot, A. J. (2005). The shame of failure: Examining the link between fear of failure and shame. *Personality and Social Psychology Bulletin, 31,* 218–231.

Mills, R. S. L. (2003). Possible antecedents and developmental implications of shame in young girls. *Infant and Child Development, 12*(4), 329–349.

Mulig, J. C., Haggerty, M. E., Carballosa, A. B., Cinnick, W. J., & Madden, J. M. (1985). Relationships among fear of success, fear of failure, and androgyny. *Psychology of Women Quarterly, 9*(2), 284–287.

Murray, H. A. (1938). *Explorations in personality.* Oxford, UK: Oxford University Press.

Murray, H. A. (1943). *Thematic Apperception Test.* Cambridge, MA: Harvard University Press.

Pang, J. S. (2010). The achievement motive: A review of theory and assessment of N achievement, hope of success, and fear of failure. In O. C. Schultheiss & J. C. Brunstein (Eds.), *Implicit motives* (pp. 30–70). New York: Oxford University Press.

Ray, J. J. (1986). Measuring achievement motivation by self-reports. *Psychological Reports, 58*(2), 525–526.

Rosen, B. C., & D'Andrade, R. (1959). The psychosocial origins of achievement motivation. *Sociometry, 22*(3), 185–218.

Sagar, S. S., & Stoeber, J. (2009). Perfectionism, fear of failure, and affective responses to success and failure: The central role of fear of experiencing shame and embarrassment. *Journal of Sport and Exercise Psychology, 31*(5), 602–627.

Sarason, S. B., & Mandler, G. (1952). Some correlates of test anxiety. *Journal of Abnormal Psychology, 47*(4), 810–817.

Schantz, L. H., & Conroy, D. E. (2009). Achievement motivation and intraindividual affective variability during competence pursuits: A round of golf as a multilevel data structure. *Journal of Research in Personality, 43*(3), 472–481.

Schmalt, H.-D. (1999). Assessing the achievement motive using the grid technique. *Journal of Research in Personality, 33*(2), 109–130.

Schmalt, H.-D. (2005). Validity of a short form of the Achievement-Motive Grid (AMG-S): Evidence for the three-factor structure emphasizing active and passive forms of fear of failure. *Journal of Personality Assessment, 84*(2), 172–184.

Schultheiss, O. C. (Trans.). (2001). *Manual for the assessment of hope of success and fear of failure* [English translation of Heckhausen's need achievement measure]. Unpublished manuscript, University of Michigan, Ann Arbor, MI.

Schultheiss, O. C. (2013). Are implicit motives revealed in mere words?: Testing the marker-word hypothesis with computer-based text analysis. *Frontiers in Psychology, 4,* 748.

Schultheiss, O. C., & Brunstein, J. C. (2005). An implicit motive approach to competence. In A. J. Elliot & C. S. Dweck (Eds.), *Handbook of competence and motivation* (pp. 31–51). New York: Guilford Press.

Schultheiss, O. C., & Pang, J. S. (2007). Measuring implicit motives. In R. W. Robins, R. C. Fraley, & R. Krueger (Eds.), *Handbook of research methods in personality psychology* (pp. 322–344). New York: Guilford Press.

Schultheiss, O. C., Yankova, D., Dirlikov, B., & Schad, D. J. (2009). Are implicit and explicit motive measures statistically independent?: A fair and balanced test using the picture story exercise and a cue- and response-matched questionnaire measure. *Journal of Personality Assessment, 91*(1), 72–81.

Singh, S. (1992). Hostile press measure of fear of failure and its relation to child-rearing attitudes and behavior problems. *Journal of Social Psychology, 132*(3), 397–399.

Smith, E. R., & DeCoster, J. (2000). Dual-process models in social and cognitive psychology: Conceptual integration and links to underlying memory systems. *Personality and Social Psychology Review, 4,* 108–131.

Sokolowski, K., Schmalt, H. D., Langens, T. A., & Puca, R. M. (2000). Assessing achievement, affiliation, and power motives all at once: The Multi-Motive Grid (MMG). *Journal of Personality Assessment, 74*(1), 126–145.

Spangler, W. D. (1992). Validity of questionnaire and TAT measures of need for achievement: Two meta-analyses. *Psychological Bulletin, 112*(1), 140–154.

Spence, J. T., & Helmreich, R. L. (1983). Achievement-related motives and behaviors. In J. T. Spence (Ed.), *Achievement and achievement motives: Psychological and sociological approaches* (pp. 7–74). San Francisco: Freeman.

Staddon, J. E. R., & Cerutti, D. T. (2003). Operant conditioning. *Annual Review of Psychology, 54,* 115–144.

Strack, F., & Deutsch, R. (2004). Reflective and impulsive determinants of social behavior. *Personality and Social Psychology Review, 8*(3), 220–247.

Stuewig, J., & McCloskey, L. A. (2005). The relation of child maltreatment to shame and guilt among adolescents: Psychological routes to depression and delinquency. *Child Maltreatment, 10*(4), 324–336.

Sullivan, M. W., Bennett, D. S., & Lewis, M. (2003). Darwin's view: Self-evaluative emotions as context-specific emotions. *Annals of the New York Academy of Sciences, 1000,* 304–308.

Sutton, R. I. (2010). *The no asshole rule.* New York: Business Plus.

Teevan, R. C. (1983). Childhood development of fear of failure motivation: A replication. *Psychological Reports, 53*(2), 506.

Teevan, R. C., & McGhee, P. E. (1972). Childhood development of fear of failure motivation. *Journal of Personality and Social Psychology, 21*(3), 345–348.

Thrash, T. M., Cassidy, S. E., Maruskin, L. A., & Elliot, A. J. (2010). Factors that influence the relation between implicit and explicit motives: A general implicit–explicit congruence framework. In O. C. Schultheiss & J. C. Brunstein (Eds.), *Implicit motives* (pp. 308–346). New York: Oxford University Press.

Veroff, J., Depner, C., Kulka, R., & Douvan, E. (1980). Comparison of American motives: 1957 versus 1976. *Journal of Personality and Social Psychology, 39*(6), 1249–1262.

White, R. W. (1959). Motivation reconsidered: The concept of competence. *Psychological Review, 66,* 297–333.

Winter, D. G. (1994). *Manual for scoring motive imagery in running text* (4th ed.). Unpublished manuscript, University of Michigan, Ann Arbor, MI.

Winter, D. G. (1999). Linking personality and "scientific" psychology: The development of empirically derived Thematic Apperception Test measures. In L. Gieser & M. I. Stein (Eds.), *Evocative images: The Thematic Apperception Test and the art of projection* (pp. 107–124). Washington, DC: American Psychological Association.

Winter, D. G. (2005). Things I've learned about personality from studying political leaders at a distance. *Journal of Personality, 73*(3), 557–584; discussion 553–555.

Winterbottom, M. R. (1958). The relation of need for achievement to learning experiences in independence and mastery. In J. W. Atkinson (Ed.), *Motives in fantasy, action, and society* (pp. 453–478). Princeton, NJ: Van Nostrand.

CHAPTER 4

Achievement Goals

ANDREW J. ELLIOT
CHRIS S. HULLEMAN

The achievement goal construct has been central to the study of achievement motivation for many decades. Theoretical and empirical work on achievement goals first appeared in the 1980s, gained considerable momentum in the 1990s, and has become truly voluminous in the new millennium. In any social scientific literature, as ideas and findings accumulate, the literature becomes increasingly complex, and there is a danger of losing sight of the forest in the midst of the ever-expanding bounty of trees. The achievement goal literature is no exception, and our primary aim in this chapter is to provide the forest view for this literature. Specifically, in this chapter, we overview and organize various conceptual models of achievement goals that have been proffered and studied over the last four decades within the achievement goal literature. In addition, we overview the field-based intervention work conducted on the basis of these models, highlighting the need for additional empirical effort in this largely overlooked area of application.

THE ACHIEVEMENT GOAL CONSTRUCT

Before discussing models of achievement goals, we provide a conceptual definition of the achievement goal construct. In doing so,

we address the terms *achievement* and *goal* separately, then combine them in a full conceptual definition.

Achievement may be defined in a variety of different ways, but achievement goal theorists widely agree that the conceptual centerpiece of achievement is competence (Elliot & Dweck, 2005). *Competence* may be technically defined as a condition or quality of effectiveness, ability, sufficiency, or success (see *Webster's Revised Unabridged Dictionary* and the *Oxford English Dictionary*). Colloquially, competence, and therefore achievement, represents whether one is doing well or poorly at a task or activity.

Goal may also be defined in a variety of different ways, but here, achievement goal theorists diverge in their opinion of what is best. There is agreement that goal represents the purpose of behavior (Dweck, 1996; Maehr, 1989), but *purpose* may be conceptualized in two distinct ways. One conceptualization of purpose is that of the *aim* or end state that guides an individual's behavior; the other conceptualization is that of the underlying *reason* that an individual engages in behavior (Elliot & Thrash, 2001). Some achievement goals theorists view a goal as aim, others view it as reason, and still others view it as a combination of both aim and reason (Dweck, 1986; Elliot, 2005; Kaplan

& Maehr, 2007; Nicholls, 1989; Urdan & Maehr, 1995).[1] As we present our overview, we make note of these different viewpoints and their implications.

Putting "achievement" and "goal" together, *achievement goal* may be defined as the purpose for engaging in competence-relevant behavior. This definition is embraced by all, or nearly all, achievement goal theorists, although the specific emphasis on purpose as aim, reason, or a combination of both, differs across theorists. Achievement goals are posited to create a framework for how individuals interpret, experience, and select themselves into and out of achievement situations (Dweck, 1986; Nicholls, 1984).

THE DICHOTOMOUS ACHIEVEMENT GOAL MODEL

The initial model of achievement goals was grounded in a dichotomous distinction between mastery goals and performance goals (Dweck, 1986; Maehr & Nicholls, 1980; Nicholls, 1984).[2] These two goals varied with regard to their *focus of competence*: A mastery goal focuses on the development of competence and task mastery, whereas a performance goal focuses on the demonstration of competence relative to others. Both mastery and performance goals were construed as approach goals, in that both focused on success (Ames, 1992; Dweck & Leggett, 1988; Meece, Blumenfeld, & Hoyle, 1988; Nicholls, Patashnick, Cheung, Thorkildsen, & Lauer, 1989). Mastery and performance goals were presumed to be applicable across competence-relevant domains such as school, sports, work, avocational pursuits, and so on.

The distinct foci of mastery and performance goals were posited to lead to different patterns of affect, cognition, and behavior (i.e., to different nomological networks). Mastery goals were posited to give rise to a positive, adaptive set of affective, cognitive, and behavioral processes and outcomes, whereas performance goals were posited to lead to a negative, maladaptive set of processes and outcomes (Dweck, 1986; Nicholls, 1984). Perceived competence was considered an important moderator of these patterns (Elliott & Dweck, 1988; Nicholls,

1989); mastery goals were expected to lead to a positive pattern regardless of whether one had high or low perceived ability, whereas performance goals were expected to lead to a particularly negative pattern when one had low perceived ability.

Although mastery and performance goals were explicitly differentiated with regard to their focus of competence only, subsequent theorists have noted that it is possible to identify two distinct subcomponents of the focus of competence within each of the two goals (Elliot, 1999; Urdan & Mestas, 2006). Mastery goals focus on developing competence and on mastering a task, whereas performance goals focus on demonstrating competence and on outperforming others. As such, one subcomponent of the focus of competence that may be identified is one's standpoint on competence—whether one is viewing competence from the standpoint of developing it (mastery goal) or demonstrating it (performance goal; Korn & Elliot, 2016). Another subcomponent of the focus of competence that may be identified is the standard of competence—whether one is using a task/self-based standard (mastery goal) or an other-based standard (performance goal) in evaluating one's competence (Elliot & McGregor, 2001). In conceptualizing mastery and performance goals, some theorists emphasized the standpoint of competence (develop vs. demonstrate) more than the standard of competence (task/self-based vs. other-based), or vice versa, but in the main, mastery and performance goals were construed as a combination of both of these subcomponents (Grant & Dweck, 2003; Hulleman, Schrager, Bodman, & Harackiewicz, 2010).

Related to this issue of standpoint and standard is the issue of reason and aim. Mastery goals were conceptualized in terms of trying to master a task or improve over time (aim), in order to develop one's ability (reason), whereas performance goals were conceptualized in terms of trying to do better than others (aim), in order to demonstrate one's ability (reason). In other words, the standard of competence served as the aim, and the standpoint on competence served as the reason within each of the two goals. Consistent with the aforementioned point regarding standpoint and standard, theorists vary in the degree to which they emphasize reason, aim, or both, in their achievement goal conceptualizations.

Operationally, researchers have used many different measures and manipulations of mastery and performance goals. Whereas some of these measures and manipulations have emphasized the standpoint on competence, others have emphasized the standard of competence, and still others have emphasized both (see Bouffard, Boisvert, Vezeau, & Larouche, 1995; Butler, 1987; Button, Mathieu, & Zajac, 1996; Duda & Nicholls, 1992; Elliott & Dweck, 1988; Harackiewicz & Elliot, 1993; Nicholls, Patchnick, & Nolen, 1985; Poortvliet, Janssen, Van Yperen, & Van de Vliert, 2007; Roberts & Treasure, 1995; Roedel, Schraw, & Plake, 1994; Stipek & Gralinski, 1996). The empirical yield from research on the dichotomous model provided relatively strong support for the positive implications of mastery goals for a host of processes and outcomes (Elliot, 2005; Pintrich & Schunk, 1996; Senko, Hulleman, & Harackiewicz, 2011). Performance goals, on the other hand, produced a decidedly mixed empirical yield: Some research linked these goals to negative processes and outcomes; other research linked them to positive processes and outcomes; and still other work did not reveal any clear pattern (for reviews, see Harackiewicz, Barron, & Elliot, 1998; Urdan, 1997; Wolters, Yu, & Pintrich, 1996). There is some evidence that performance goals emphasizing the demonstration of ability fare worse than those emphasizing normative comparison (Edwards, 2014; Grant & Dweck, 2003; Hulleman et al., 2010; Senko & Tropiano, in press; Wartburton & Spray, 2014), but more research is needed to systematically test this possibility. Research testing perceived competence as a moderator of mastery and performance goals tended not to yield the anticipated interactions (for reviews, see Hong, Chiu, Dweck, Lin, & Wan, 1999; Kaplan & Midgley, 1997).

THE TRICHOTOMOUS ACHIEVEMENT GOAL MODEL

Conceptually, the dichotomous model overlooked an important distinction with a long and rich history in the achievement motivation literature—the distinction between approach and avoidance motivation (see Elliot & Covington, 2001, for a review). With regard to competence motivation, the approach–avoidance distinction identifies two different types of goal pursuit— striving to approach success and striving to avoid failure. As noted earlier, both mastery and performance goals were construed as approach goals in the dichotomous approach to achievement goals; avoidance goals were not explicitly represented. This approach–avoidance distinction represents a second component of competence, beyond the focus of competence, namely, the valence of competence.

The trichotomous model of achievement goals (Elliot & Harackiewicz, 1996) extended the dichotomous model by integrating the approach–avoidance distinction within performance goals. Rather than positing a single, omnibus performance goal, the trichotomous model bifurcated performance goals into separate performance-approach and performance-avoidance goals. Performance-approach goals were conceptualized in terms of striving to demonstrate competence relative to others, whereas performance-avoidance goals were conceptualized in terms of striving to avoid demonstrating incompetence relative to others. Mastery goals remained unchanged from the dichotomous model, as they continued to be conceptualized in terms of striving to develop competence and task mastery.

Incorporation of the approach–avoidance distinction was not just conceptually important, it was also important because it offered an explanation for why performance goals in the dichotomous model produced a relatively sporadic empirical yield. Performance-avoidance goals, with their use of a negative outcome (incompetence) as the hub of regulation, were posited to give rise to a negative, maladaptive pattern of affective, cognitive, and behavioral processes and outcomes. Performance-approach goals are more complex forms of regulation, in that they use a positive outcome (competence) as the hub of regulation, which should facilitate positive processes and outcomes, but they also focus on showing or demonstrating competence, which often has detrimental implications for processes and outcomes. Furthermore, performance-approach goals can emerge from appetitively based dispositions (e.g., need for achievement, approach temperament) and aversively based dispositions (e.g., fear of failure, avoidance temperament) (Elliot & Church, 1997; Elliot & Thrash, 2002). Thus, performance-approach goals were posited to be positive predictors of some outcomes but negative or null predictors of others. This bifurcation of omnibus performance goals into separate approach and avoidance forms of regulation helps provide additional precision regarding the implications of performance-based goal pursuit. Predictions for mastery goals remained the same as those articulated in the dichotomous model: They were posited to lead to a host of positive processes and outcomes. In the trichotomous model, perceived competence was construed as an antecedent rather than a moderator of achievement goal adoption. High perceptions of ability were posited to predict approach goals (mastery and performance-approach alike) and low perceptions of ability were positive to predict performance-avoidance goals. Other antecedent of the trichotomous achievement goals were also posited, such as entity and incremental theories of ability (Cury, Da Fonséca, Rufo, & Sarrazin, 2002), and the aforementioned achievement motives (need for achievement, fear of failure; Elliot & Church, 1997) and temperaments (approach temperament, avoidance temperament; Elliot & Thrash, 2002).

With regard to both the standpoint/standard issue and the reason/aim issue, the trichotomous model continued in the tradition of the dichotomous model. This is the case for the way achievement goals were both conceptualized and operationalized. Researchers have used many different measures and manipulations of the goals in the trichotomous model, with variation in the emphasis on standpoint on competence, standard of competence, or both (see Cury, Da Fonséca, Rufo, Peres, & Sarrazin, 2003; Elliot & Church, 1997; Elliot & Harackiewicz, 1996; Kavussanu, Morris, & Ring, 2009; Middleton & Midgely, 1997; Skaalvik, 1997; Vandewalle, 1997; Zweig & Webster, 2004). The empirical yield from research on the trichotomous model has highlighted the predictive utility of separating performance-approach and performance-avoidance goals into separate forms of self-regulation. Performance-avoidance goals have been linked to a wide array of negative processes and outcomes (e.g., threat appraisal, less self-regulated learning, procrastination, help avoidance, worry, low intrinsic motivation, low performance), whereas performance-approach goals have been linked to some positive processes and outcomes (e.g., challenge appraisal, effort, persistence, high performance) and a few negative processes and outcomes (e.g., emotionality, unwillingness to seek help) (for reviews, see Elliot, 1999; Midgley, Kaplan, & Middleton, 2001; Smith, Duda, Allen, & Hall, 2002). Several studies have supported perceived competence as an antecedent of the three goals of the trichotomous model (Elliot & Church, 1997; Leondari & Gialamas, 2002; Lopez, 1999; Pajares, Britner, & Valiante, 2000; Skaalvik, 2007; Tanaka, Takehara, & Yamauchi, 2006; cf. Spray & Warburton, 2011).

THE 2 × 2 ACHIEVEMENT GOAL MODEL

Although the trichotomous model integrated the approach–avoidance distinction into performance goals, it left mastery goals intact. This raised the question of whether the definition and valence components of competence could be fully crossed to create a 2 × 2 model of achievement goals. Such a model would comprise the three goals of the trichotomous model (with mastery goals taking on an approach label, mastery-approach) plus a fourth, mastery-avoidance goal. This fully crossed 2 × 2 model is precisely what was proposed to extend the trichotomous model (Elliot, 1999; Elliot & McGregor, 2001; Pintrich, 2000).

Many achievement goals researchers and theorists initially had difficulty conceiving of a goal that combined mastery and avoidance, most likely because mastery goals had been portrayed in a purely positive light since the inception of the achievement goal approach. Conceptually, however, combining mastery and avoidance is straightforward, as mastery-based goals simply focus on a particular definition of competence, and a particular valence of competence, and these two components can easily be integrated. The 2 × 2 model made an explicit shift to defining competence entirely in terms of standards of competence; standpoints on competence were construed as more relevant to the reason than the aim of competence-based goal pursuit. Thus, for mastery-avoidance goals, competence was defined in terms of a task-based reference or a person's own intrapersonal trajectory, and competence was valenced in terms of incompetence. So, mastery-avoidance goals entail striving to avoid task-based or intrapersonal incompetence.

Pragmatically, it is easy to imagine examples of mastery-avoidance goal pursuit in everyday life: trying not to forget what one has learned in math class, trying not to miss a soccer penalty kick, and trying not to make fewer sales than one made last year. Perfectionism (i.e., trying not to do anything incorrectly) is a prototypical case of mastery-avoidance regulation; athletes toward the end of their career undoubtedly focus on mastery-avoidance goals as their performance trajectory asymptotes or heads downward, and mastery-avoidance goals may be particularly salient as individuals age and begin to notice a decline in their cognitive and motor skills (Elliot & McGregor, 2001; Pintrich, 2000).

Precise empirical predictions regarding the consequences of mastery-avoidance goals are not easy to proffer. Like performance-approach goals, mastery-avoidance goals are complex forms of regulation in that they represent a hybrid combination of both positive and negative components; that is, the focus on task-based and intrapersonal competence is commonly thought to promote processes that facilitate optimal functioning, and the focus on incompetence is commonly thought to prompt aversive and self-protective processes. In any given achievement situation, the mastery component of the goal may be more salient than the avoidance component of the goal, thereby promoting more positive regulatory processes. However, the opposite may be the case in other achievement settings, leading to more negative regulatory processes. Given this variation, it is best to offer a more general predictive pattern: The pattern for mastery-avoidance goals is likely to be more positive than that for performance-avoidance goals, and more negative than that for mastery-approach goals. Predictions for the other three goals of the 2 × 2 model—mastery-approach, performance-approach, and performance-avoidance—are comparable to those offered

for these goals in the trichotomous model. The pattern for performance-based goals may be somewhat different given that these goals do not explicitly include a demonstration of competence component; a focus on demonstration is thought to have largely negative implications (Dykman, 1998; Hulleman et al., 2010). Therefore, performance-approach goals may be somewhat more beneficial and performance-avoidance goals may be somewhat less deleterious in the 2 × 2 model, relative to the trichotomous model (to the extent that operationalization follows conceptualization). In keeping with the trichotomous model, perceived competence was construed as an antecedent of achievement goal adoption in the 2 × 2 model; the precise nature of the link between perceived competence and mastery-avoidance goal adoption would likely depend on the salience of the mastery- and avoidance-based components of the goal (as described earlier).

As with the prior models, researchers have used a number of different measures and manipulations of the goals of the 2 × 2 model. These operationalizations vary in the degree to which they emphasize the standard of competence alone or also include the standpoint on competence (Baranik, Barron, & Finney, 2007; Conroy, Elliot, & Hofer, 2003; Elliot & McGregor, 2001; Ferron, Le Bars, & Gernigon, 2005; Guan, McBride, & Xiang, 2007; Riou et al., 2012; Schiano-Lomoriello, Cury, & Da Fonséca, 2005; Van Yperen, 2006). Although, as noted earlier, findings for performance-approach goals may vary depending on whether their operationalization focuses on standards, standpoints, or both, systematic empirical work on this operationalization issue focused across the 2 × 2 achievement goals has yet to be conducted. The empirical pattern for mastery-avoidance goals tends to be negative, as they have been found to be positive predictors of anxiety, procrastination, and maladaptive forms of perfectionism, and negative predictors of performance (for reviews, see Baranik, Stanley, Bynum, & Lance, 2010; Hulleman et al., 2010; Senko & Freund, 2015; Van Yperen & Orehek, 2013). However, the findings are mixed for some variables, such as help seeking, intrinsic motivation, and broad affective experience (Baranik et al., 2010; Karabenick, 2003; Madjar, Kaplan, & Weinstock,

2011; Wang, Biddle, & Elliot, 2007), and mastery-avoidance goals have been shown to be effective forms of regulation for older adults (Senko & Freund, 2015). The findings are also mixed for perceived competence as a predictor of mastery-avoidance goals (Chiang, Yeh, Lin, & Hwang, 2011; Van Yperen, 2006; Wang et al., 2007). These mixed findings for mastery-avoidance goals are to be anticipated given their hybrid nature (they represent a combination of mastery and avoidance).

THE 3 × 2 ACHIEVEMENT GOAL MODEL

In explicitly defining achievement goals entirely in terms of standards of competence, the 2 × 2 achievement goal model made salient the dual nature of mastery-based goals. These goals focus on both an absolute standard of competence and on an intrapersonal standard of competence. Although absolute and intrapersonal standards often go together in goal pursuit (e.g., trying to do a task as well as it can be done, and trying to do better than one's prior performance in a mastery-approach goal), this need not be the case. Task-based goals can be pursued independently of self-based goals, and vice versa. For example, one can try to get a lot of math problems correct (a task-approach goal) without trying to do better than one has done before on math problems (a self-approach goal). Likewise, one can try to avoid performing worse on a math exam than one has performed before (a self-avoidance goal) without trying to avoid getting a lot of math problems wrong (a task-avoidance goal). As such, task-based goals focused on an absolute standard can be separated from self-based goals focused on an intrapersonal standard, and both of these can be differentiated from other-based goals focused on an interpersonal standard. Crossing each of these standards (the definition component of competence)—task, self, others—with approach–avoidance (the valence component of competence) yields a 3 × 2 achievement goal model, a model proposed by Elliot, Murayama, and Pekrun (2011).

Six separate goals comprise the 3 × 2 model: a *task-approach* goal focused on approaching task-based competence, a *task-avoidance* goal focusing on avoiding task-based incompetence, a *self-approach* goal focusing on approaching self-based competence, a *self-avoidance* goal focusing on avoiding self-based incompetence, an *other-approach* goal focusing on approaching other-based competence, and an *other-avoidance* goal focusing on avoiding other-based incompetence. Other-approach and other-avoidance goals are identical to performance-approach and performance-avoidance goals, respectively, in the 2 × 2 model. The new ("other") label is simply used in the 3 × 2 model in order to fit with the "task" and "self" labels that must be used to bifurcate the mastery-based goal construct. Task-based goals define competence in terms of the absolute demands of the task, such as getting a problem correct, understanding a concept, or trying to hit a ball. Examples of task-approach goals are trying to get a problem correct, trying to understand a concept, or trying to hit a ball, whereas examples of task-avoidance goals are trying to avoid getting a problem incorrect, trying to avoid misunderstanding a concept, or trying to avoid missing a ball. Self-based goals define competence in terms of one's own intrapersonal trajectory, such as how one has done in the past. Examples of a self-approach goal are trying to get more problems correct than before, trying to understand a concept more quickly than before, and trying to hit a ball further than before.

Contrasting task-based and self-based standards of competence evaluation, task-based standards are more closely integrated with the task itself, and at least, under some circumstances, one can receive immediate and ongoing feedback directly from the task as one is working on it. That is, determining success or failure using a task-based standard can be simple, direct, and require minimal cognitive processing.[3] Self-based standards, on the other hand, are more separable from task engagement, in that one must compare one's current competence to a mental representation of one's competence at another point in time, such as the past. Thus, although self-based standards are inherently and ideographically optimally challenging (each person is his or her own baseline), their use in regulation is more complex and requires more cognitive capacity. Based on these differences, one could posit that task-approach goals are optimally suited to facilitate absorption in the task (i.e., "flow") and intrinsic motivation, whereas self-approach goals may be best suited to facilitate persistence and eagerness through optimal challenge. Task-avoidance and self-avoidance goals represent hybrid combinations of positive and negative components and, as with mastery-avoidance goals, it is difficult to anticipate their predictive pattern network accordingly (other than the broad statement of being more positive than other-avoidance goals and more negative than task-approach and self-approach goals). As noted earlier, performance-based and other-based goals are equivalent, so predictions for performance-approach and performance-avoidance goals in the 2 × 2 model would hold for other-approach and other-avoidance goals in the 3 × 2 model; likewise, perceived competence would be construed as an antecedent of achievement goal adoption in the 3 × 2 model, and the nature of the link between perceived competence and the hybrid goal constructs would depend on the salience of the definition and valence components of the goal (as described earlier regarding mastery-avoidance goals).

Researchers have used a number of different measures of the 3 × 2 achievement goals; all of these operationalizations focus specifically on the standards of competence alone (Elliot et al., 2011; Gillet, Lafrenière, Huyghebaert, & Fouquereau, 2015; Mascret, Elliot, & Cury, 2015a; Méndez-Giménez & Fernández-Río, 2014). The full set of six goals has yet to be instantiated via experimental manipulation. Much of the existing empirical work on the 3 × 2 model has tested whether this model is a better fit to the data than a variety of alternative models such as the 2 × 2 and trichotomous models. The data are clearly and consistently supportive of the 3 × 2 model over all possible alternatives, a finding observed across several different countries and languages (English, French, Spanish, Mandarin, Hungarian, Norwegian; Diseth, 2015; Elliot et al., 2011; Gillet et al., 2015; Mascret et al., 2015a, 2015b; Méndez-Giménez & Fernández-Río, 2014; Urbán, Orosz, Kerepes, & Jánvári, 2014; Wu, 2012). Only a small number of studies

to date have tested links between the goals of the 3 × 2 model and various processes and outcomes. The findings that have emerged across multiple research teams are as follows: Task-approach goals are a positive predictor of task interest and satisfaction (Elliot et al., 2001; Gillet et al., 2015; Mascret et al., 2015a, 2015b) and task absorption (Elliot et al., 2011; Flanagan, Putwain, & Caltabiano, 2015), and are positively associated with perceived competence (Diseth, 2015; Elliot et al., 2011; García-Romero, 2015; Mascret et al., 2015a); self-approach goals are a positive predictor of task interest and satisfaction (Gillet et al., 2015; Mascret et al., 2015a, 2015b), other-approach goals are a positive predictor of performance attainment (Diseth, 2015; Elliot et al., 2011) and are positively associated with perceived competence (Diseth, 2015; Elliot et al., 2011; García-Romero, 2015; Mascret et al., 2015a), and other-avoidance goals are a positive predictor of worry (Elliot et al., 2011; Flanagan et al., 2015) and a negative predictor of performance attainment (Elliot et al., 2011; Johnson & Kestler, 2013). These findings are consistent with predictions from the 3 × 2 model and provide further support for the need to attend to the task–self distinction.

Although the aforementioned findings on model fit and nomological network clearly support the 3 × 2 model, other aspects of the existing data point to issues in need of attention. First, in a number of studies, all six of the 3 × 2 goals are positively correlated, many to a moderate or strong degree; in no study are any of the goals significantly negatively correlated. This would not be expected from the perspective of the 3 × 2 model, especially for goals differing on both the definition and valence of competence distinctions (e.g., task-approach goals and other-avoidance goals). Second, the predictive patterns that have been observed are weaker than in research with other achievement goal models, and many relations that would be anticipated have not materialized. This is even the case with other-approach and other-avoidance goals, the two constructs that are unchanged from the trichotomous and 2 × 2 models.

We think it likely that the high intercorrelations among the goals and the weak predictive patterns are interrelated problems, and that both emerge from commonly known limitations of self-report measures. When respondents are presented with a large pool of items that all share common features and that seem reasonable or even socially desirable, they tend to "satisfice" (i.e., put in minimal effort and engage in minimal discrimination; Krosnick, 2000). Satisficing leads to reduced variance, inflated intercorrelations, and reduced predictive power (Krosnick, 1991; Podsakoff, MacKenzie, Lee, & Podsakoff, 2003). Particularly when presented as standards alone, the common features of achievement goals (they share definitions and valences of competence; they all represent commitments to competence) are highly salient, and all items sound reasonable or even socially desirable (given that they represent commitments to competence). As such, we think that the 3 × 2 measure is prone to satisficing by respondents, producing the observed empirical difficulties. These empirical difficulties have been seen, albeit to a lesser degree, in the 2 × 2 model with regard to performance-approach and performance-avoidance goals (Law, Elliot, & Murayama, 2012; Linnenbrink-Garcia et al., 2012), but the expansion of items and inclusion of an additional and more nuanced distinction between task- and self-based goals appears to have exacerbated these difficulties. We think the solution is twofold. First, achievement goal researchers would do well to implement recommendations from the satisficing literature for how to structure measures and items to combat this problem; possible foci in this regard are the instructions for the measure, the formatting of the items and/or response options, and the interspacing of the items. Second, until this problem is addressed, achievement goal researchers may do well to opt for assessing a subset of the 3 × 2 goals in any given investigation. For example, researchers can focus on studying the ways in which task-approach and self-approach goals have both similar and different implications for achievement-relevant processes and outcomes. Another possibility would be to assess the 2 × 2 goals, but to use either task-based or self-based goals as indicators of the mastery-based goal constructs in the interest of conceptual and operational clarity.

OTHER IMPORTANT TOPICS AND DIRECTIONS

The dichotomous, trichotomous, 2 × 2, and 3 × 2 models have been developed programmatically, with one model emerging as an extension and/or revision of the prior model. However, by no means is a later model meant to make obsolete a former model; a researcher's specific question of interest should dictate the goal model on which he or she focuses. Likewise, and as illustrated earlier, using a subset of the goals from a particular model that match one's research question is a sensible empirical strategy. What is of critical importance is the use of clear and consistent terminology in labeling the goals that one selects, and ensuring clear and rigorous operationalization that maps onto the labels that one is using. Careful attention to these terminological and methodological issues is essential for clarity of interpretation and the development of a cumulative body of work that has direct implications for application.

Our review of achievement goal models and constructs is not exhaustive. Other models and constructs of note include the following: the social achievement goal model (Ryan & Shim, 2006), work avoidance goals (Nicholls, 1989; Nolen, 1988), extrinsic goals (Maehr, 1983; Pintrich & Garcia, 1991), socially based goals (including social approval goals, social responsibility goals, social status goals, and prosocial goals; Urdan & Maehr, 1995), and outcome goals (Grant & Dweck, 2003). Furthermore, our aim has been to provide a "forest" view of achievement goal models without delving into the many important ideas and insights that have contributed to and are emerging within this literature. Noteworthy examples include the following: achievement goal structures (Ames, 1992; James & Yates, 2007; Maehr & Midgley, 1996), multiple goal adoption (Barron & Harackiewicz, 2001; DeShon, Kozlowski, Schmidt, Milner, & Wiechmann, 2004), achievement goal complexes (Elliot & Thrash, 2001; Senko & Tropiano, in press; Urdan & Mestas, 2006), achievement goal fit (Jackson, Harwood, & Grove, 2010; Kristof-Brown & Stevens, 2001), dominant achievement goals (Van Yperen, 2006); cultural influences on achievement goal adoption and pursuit (McInerney,

McInerney, & Marsh, 1997; Zusho & Clayton, 2011), multiple domains of achievement goals (Duda & Nicholls, 1992; Van Yperen, Blaga, & Postmes, 2014), achievement goals and interpersonal behavior (Darnon, Muller, Schrager, Pannuzzo, & Butera, 2006; Pooertvliet et al., 2007), achievement goals and moral behavior (Mouratidou, Barkoukis, & Rizos, 2012; Van Yperen, Hamstra, & van der Klauw, 2011), achievement subgoals (e.g., target goals: Harackiewicz & Sansone, 1991; boundary goals: Corker & Donnellan, 2012), achievement goal difficulty (Senko & Hulleman, 2013), subsets of achievement goal types (e.g., personal best goals: Martin, 2006; potential-based goals: Elliot, Murayama, Kobeisy, & Lichtenfeld, 2015), achievement goal contagion (Eren, 2009), achievement goals within goal systems (Bodmann, Hulleman, & Harackiewicz, 2008), and integration of the achievement goal approach with other major contemporary theories of motivation (Ciani, Middleton, Summers, & Sheldon, 2010; Hulleman, Durik, Schweigert, & Harackiewicz, 2008; Johnson, Shull, & Wallace, 2011). As clearly seen in these necessarily selective listings, the achievement goal literature is broad and generative, and continues to develop apace.

Notably, up to this point, our chapter has emphasized personal achievement goals. However, achievement goals can also be operationalized in terms of environmental emphasis. From this perspective, elements of the context in which the individual engages in achievement-relevant behavior can shape an individual's achievement goal adoption. Consideration of environmental influence naturally leads to the development and testing of interventions designed to impact achievement goal adoption. Unfortunately, intervention work on achievement goals is an area that has not received as much theoretical and empirical attention as we think it deserves, and it is to this topic we now turn.

ACHIEVEMENT GOAL INTERVENTIONS

A review of achievement goal interventions within applied contexts—educational, sports/exercise, work—reveals that two basic types of interventions have been utilized: one focused on structural aspects of the achievement context (structure-focused), and the other focused directly on student's personal achievement goal adoption (person-focused). We now describe each type of intervention, provide a few examples of each, and discuss the need for and promise of interventions in this literature.

First, some interventions have focused on structural aspects of the achievement context that are presumed to influence personal achievement goal adoption. Research using this type of intervention is usually grounded in the TARGET framework (Ames, 1992; Epstein, 1989) that highlights six aspects of achievement contexts that influence students' adoption of achievement goals: the *Tasks* in which students engage, the level of *Authority* given to students to guide their own learning, how students receive *Recognition* for their efforts, how students are *Grouped* while learning, how students are *Evaluated*, and the amount and flexibility of *Time* given to students to learn. Variation in each of these aspects of the achievement environment is posited to influence whether students adopt mastery-based or performance-based achievement goals. For example, regarding tasks, teachers may give students moderately challenging and intrinsically interesting tasks that would be posited to promote mastery-based goal adoption, or they may give students rote, repetitive tasks that would be posited to promote performance-based goal adoption. A study by Linnenbrink (2005) illustrates this approach. She first classified teachers as being more mastery-focused, performance-focused, or both-goal-focused in their teaching practices. She next provided materials to teachers that described their classroom emphasis and offered suggestions for teaching practices that focused on the evaluation and recognition aspects of the TARGET model. Finally, she structured small-group activities in each classroom to be consistent with the teacher's observed achievement goal profile and that focused on the evaluation and recognition aspects of the TARGET model. The results revealed that students whose teachers and small groups emphasized learning strategies consistent with both mastery-based and performance-based goals had the best outcomes (e.g., self-efficacy, interest, grades). In another study in a sport context, Wadsworth, Robinson, Rudisill, and Gell (2013) randomly assigned elementary physical education students to be taught using either mastery-based or performance-based instruction, defined according to TARGET emphases. Each instructor taught half of their classes with each climate: The mastery-based climate focused on private recognition for individual progress, task-focused evaluation, and opportunity for choice. The performance-based climate focused on public displays of progress and other-referenced criteria for judging student ability, and offered limited choice. The results revealed that regardless of teacher, students in the mastery-based climate were more physically active during class than students in the performance-based climate. The TARGET approach is not just applicable to teachers and students; it may also be applied to other achievement contexts and relationships as well (e.g., employers and employees, coaches and players). Additional examples of this type of intervention can be found in the sports context (e.g., Boone, 1995; Lloyd & Fox, 1992; Solmon, 1996; Treasure, 1993; Todorovich & Curtner-Smith, 2001, 2002) and the education context (e.g., Anderman, Maehr, & Midgley, 1999; Guthrie, Wigfield, & VonSecker, 2000; Maehr & Midgley, 1996; Miller & Meece, 1997; O'Keefe, Ben-Eliyahu, & Linnenbrink-Garcia, 2013; Peng, Cherng, & Chen, 2013).

Second, some interventions have focused specifically on the reasons for and aims of individuals' personal achievement goals. Research using this type of intervention is usually grounded in either the dichotomous or the trichotomous achievement goal model, and the emphasis is on directly and explicitly trying to guide individuals toward mastery-based rather than performance-based goal pursuit. A study in the work context by Noordzij, Van Hooft, Mierlo, Dam, and Born (2013) illustrates this approach. They developed a mastery-based goal intervention for unemployed Dutch job seekers. The mastery-based goal intervention (labeled "learning goal orientation") defined learning goals as focused on improvement and skills development, and encouraged participants to adopt these goals, and reflect on their learning and progress. Participants were given feedback on learning-goal progress,

and possible obstacles for goal achievement were discussed. The results revealed that job seekers in the learning-goal intervention had higher levels of learning goals and lower levels of avoidance-based goals than those in the control condition. These differences in goal adoption led to higher rates of employment. In an education context, Smeding, Darnon, Souchal, Toczek-Capelle, and Butera (2013) developed a mastery-based goal intervention for French college students. The intervention reframed examinations as an opportunity to learn and helped students connect exams to their own learning goals, as opposed to the standard perception that exams are an opportunity to demonstrate one's competence compared to others. Across three randomized field experiments, the results indicated that the intervention boosted exam performance for poorer undergraduate students, and reduced the achievement gap typically seen in these courses. A second example, this time in an education context, is provided by Martin (2005, 2008), who developed an intervention that addressed a variety of constructs related to student motivation. One aspect of the intervention involved having students work individually through modules that directly encouraged the adoption and pursuit of mastery-based goals (other aspects of the intervention focused on self-regulated learning and utility value). The results indicated that high school students in the intervention group increased in their valuing of school, task management, and persistence, whereas control students decreased in all three variables over the year. In addition, intervention students decreased in their anxiety, failure avoidance, and lack of control, whereas control students increased in these variables over the year. Additional examples of this type of intervention can be found in the work context (e.g., Van Hooft & Noordzij, 2009) and the education context (e.g., Bernacki, Nokes-Malach, Richey, & Belenky, 2016; Hoyert & O'Dell, 2006; Martin, 2005, 2008; Muis, Ranellucci, Franco, & Crippen, 2013; Quintanilla, 2007; Ranellucci, Hall, Muis, & Lajoie, in press).

Overall, the results of this brief review are encouraging in that interventions inspired by the achievement goal approach appear to be effective in improving student motivation and learning. Of course, the literature is at a nascent stage of development, and much more empirical work is needed before strong statements can be made about the effectiveness of these types of interventions. However, the findings published to date echo reviews of interventions based on other motivation constructs in social and educational psychology that have found positive effects (Lazowski & Hulleman, 2016; Yeager & Walton, 2011). For example, in their meta-analysis of 92 intervention studies designed to boost motivation in education settings, Lazowski and Hulleman (2016) found the interventions had an average effect size of $d = 0.49$ across behavioral, performance, and self-report measures.

The field of motivation research in general, and that of achievement goals in particular, has been incredibly productive over the last several decades, producing theories, constructs, and tests thereof. However, some have argued that this theoretical and empirical productivity has not resulted in a commensurate benefit to practice (Berliner, 2006; Kaplan, Katz, & Flum, 2012). Within the achievement goal literature, there are numerous meta-analyses of self-reported goals and their relationships with other motivational constructs and outcomes (Baranik et al., 2010; Burnette, O'Boyle, VanEpps, Pollack, & Finkel, 2013; Cellar et al., 2011; Huang, 2011, 2012; Hulleman et al., 2010; Lochbaum & Gottardy, 2015; Lochbaum, Jean-Noel, Pinar, & Gilson, in press; Payne, Youngcourt, & Beaubien, 2007; Richardson, Abraham, & Bond, 2012; Van Yperen et al., 2014; Wirthwein, Sparfeldt, Pinquart, Wegerer, & Steinmayr, 2013). There are also as few meta-analyses of laboratory manipulations of achievement goals and their relation to outcomes (Rawsthorne & Elliot, 1999; Utman, 1997; Van Yperen et al., 2014). However, there are no meta-analyses of field studies of achievement goal interventions. Although, as noted earlier, such intervention research is at an early stage of development, a meta-analysis may nevertheless be of benefit. Specifically, even a small-scale meta-analysis may (1) clearly document the relatively small number of published studies in this area, (2) provide tentative empirical confirmation (or not) of our conclusions from our narrative review, and (3) identify strengths and weaknesses in the existing work, and perhaps detect moderators worthy of study.

In short, we hope that our overview of the relative paucity of research in the area, coupled with the promise of the existing work, will encourage achievement goal researchers to consider stepping out into "real-world" achievement contexts to conduct intervention work. There is much to be learned from intervention studies that cannot be learned from correlational studies, observational studies, and laboratory experiments (see Hulleman & Barron, 2016; Lazowski & Hulleman, 2016). It is only through intervention work that we can examine whether changes in practice inspired by theoretical insight can lead to actual benefits in the classroom, in the boardroom, and on the ballfield.

CLOSING REMARKS

In this chapter, we have taken the broad, "forest" view of the achievement goal literature. We have covered the models and constructs used in achievement goal research, as well as the issue of field-based achievement goal interventions. What we find in such an overview is a research tradition that has developed in programmatic fashion on both the theoretical and empirical fronts but has yet to fulfill its potential on the applied front. It is our hope that as this literature progresses, moving through its fourth decade, achievement goal researchers will not only continue to strive for theoretical clarity and empirical precision but also work toward forging a stronger theory–application interface.

NOTES

1. In addition, some achievement goal theorists not only combine aim and reason together, but also include other concepts (e.g., emotions, attributional tendencies, effort) within a general, omnibus goal orientation construct (see Ames, 1992).

2. A variety of different terms have been used in the literature for each of these two goals. Mastery goals have also been labeled task goals, task involvement, and learning goals, and performance goals have also been labeled

ego goals, ego involvement, and ability goals (see Ames, 1992, for an overview).

3. Although feedback can be immediate and direct with a task-based standard, it is certainly not so in all instances. For example, in situations where the task is difficult and a correct or incorrect answer is not known by the individual him- or herself, feedback must be obtained from an external source.

REFERENCES

Ames, C. (1992). Classrooms: Goals, structures, and student motivation. *Journal of Educational Psychology, 84*, 261–271.

Anderman, E. M., Maehr, M. L., & Midgley, C. (1999). Declining motivation after the transition to middle school: Schools can make a difference. *Journal of Research and Development in Education, 32*, 131–147.

Baranik, L. E., Barron, K. E., & Finney, S. J. (2007). Measuring goal orientation in a work domain: Construct validity evidence for the 2 × 2 framework. *Educational and Psychological Measurement, 67*, 697–718.

Baranik, L. E., Stanley, L. J., Bynum, B. H., & Lance, C. E. (2010). Examining the construct validity of mastery-avoidance achievement goals: A meta-analysis. *Human Performance, 23*, 265–282.

Barron, K. E., & Harackiewicz, J. M. (2001). Achievement goals and optimal motivation: Testing multiple goal models. *Journal of Personality and Social Psychology, 80*, 706–722.

Berliner, D. C. (2006). Educational psychology: Searching for essence throughout a century of influence. In P. A. Alexander & P. H. Winne (Eds.), *Handbook of educational psychology* (2nd ed., pp. 3–42). Hove, UK: Psychology Press.

Bernacki, M., Nokes-Malach, T., Richey, J. E., & Belenky, D. M. (2016). Science diaries: A brief writing intervention to improve motivation to learn science. *Educational Psychology, 26*, 26–46.

Bodmann, S. M., Hulleman, C. S., & Harackiewicz, J. M. (2008). Achievement goal systems: An application of goal systems theory to achievement goal research. *International Review of Social Psychology, 21*, 71–96.

Boone, J. W. (1995). *Achievement goals and motivational climates for physical education.* Unpublished doctoral dissertation, Louisiana State University, Baton Rouge, LA.

Bouffard, T., Boisvert, J., Vezeau, C., & Larouche, C. (1995), The impact of goal orientation on self-regulation and performance among college students. *British Journal of Educational Psychology, 65*, 317–329.

Burnette, J. L., O'Boyle, E. H., VanEpps, E. M., Pollack, J. M., & Finkel, E. J. (2013). Mindsets matter: A meta-analysis of implicit theories and self-regulation. *Psychological Bulletin, 139*, 655–701.

Butler, R. (1987). Task-involving and ego-involving properties of evaluation: Effects of different feedback conditions on motivational perceptions, interest, and performance. *Journal of Educational Psychology, 79*, 474–482.

Button, S. B., Mathieu, J. E., & Zajac, D. M. (1996). Goal orientation in organizational research: A conceptual and empirical foundation. *Organizational Behavior and Human Decision Processes, 67*, 26–48.

Cellar, D. F., Stuhlmacher, A. F., Young, S. K., Fisher, D. M., Adair, C. K., et al. (2011). Trait goal orientation, self-regulation, and performance: A meta-analysis. *Journal of Business Psychology, 26*, 467–483.

Chiang, Y., Yeh, Y., Lin, S., & Hwang, F. (2011). Factor structure and predictive utility of the 2 × 2 achievement goal model in a sample of Taiwan students. *Learning and Individual Differences, 21*, 432–437.

Ciani, K. D., Middleton, M. J., Summers, J. J., & Sheldon, K. M. (2010). Buffering against performance classroom goal structures: The importance of autonomy support and classroom community. *Contemporary Educational Psychology, 35*, 88–99.

Conroy, D. E., Elliot, A. J., & Hofer, S. M. (2003). A 2 × 2 achievement goals questionnaire for sport. *Journal of Sport and Exercise Psychology, 25*, 456–476.

Corker, K. S., & Donnellan, M. B. (2012). Setting lower limits high: The role of boundary goals in achievement motivation. *Journal of Educational Psychology, 104*, 138–149.

Cury, F., Da Fonséca, D., Rufo, M., Peres, C., & Sarrazin, P. (2003). The trichotomous model and investment in learning to prepare for a sport test: A mediational analysis. *British Journal of Educational Psychology, 73*, 529–543.

Cury, F., Da Fonséca, D., Rufo, M., & Sarrazin, P. (2002). Perceptions of competence, implicit theory of ability, perception of motivational climate, and achievement goals: A test of trichotomous conceptualization of endorsement of achievement motivational in the physical education setting. *Perceptual and Motor Skills, 95*, 233–244.

Darnon, C., Muller, D., Schrager, S. M., Pannuzzo, N., & Butera, F. (2006). Achievement goal promotion at university: Social desirability and social utility of mastery and performance goals. *Journal of Educational Psychology, 98,* 766–776.

Deshon, R. P., Kozlowski, S. W. J., Schmidt, A. M., Milner, K. R., & Wiechmann, D. (2004). A multiple goal, multilevel model of feedback effects on the regulation of individual and team performance. *Journal of Applied Psychology, 89,* 1035–1056.

Diseth, Å. (2015). The advantages of task-based and other-based achievement goals as standards of competence. *International Journal of Educational Research, 72,* 59–69.

Duda, J. L., & Nicholls, J. (1992). Dimensions of achievement motivation in schoolwork and sport. *Journal of Educational Psychology, 84,* 1–10.

Dweck, C. S. (1986). Motivational processes affecting learning. *American Psychologist, 41,* 1040–1048.

Dweck, C. S. (1996). Implicit theories as organizers of goals and behavior. In P. M. Gollwitzer & J. A. Bargh (Eds.), *The psychology of action: Linking cognition and motivation to action* (pp. 69–90). New York: Guilford Press.

Dweck, C. S., & Leggett, E. L. (1988). A social cognitive approach to motivation and personality. *Psychological Review, 95,* 256–273.

Dykman, B. (1998). Integrating cognitive and motivational factors in depression: Initial tests of a goal-orientation approach. *Journal of Personality and Social Psychology, 74,* 139–158.

Edwards, O. V. (2014). Differentiating performance approach goals and their unique effects. *Universal Journal of Educational Research, 2,* 134–145.

Elliot, A. J. (1999). Approach and avoidance motivation and achievement goals. *Educational Psychologist, 34,* 149–169.

Elliot, A. J. (2005). A conceptual history of the achievement goal construct. In A. J. Elliot & C. S. Dweck (Eds.), *Handbook of competence and motivation* (pp. 52–72). New York: Guilford Press.

Elliot, A. J., & Church, M. A. (1997). A hierarchical model of approach and avoidance achievement motivation. *Journal of Personality and Social Psychology, 72,* 218–232.

Elliot, A. J., & Covington, M. V. (2001). Approach and avoidance motivation. *Educational Psychology Review, 13,* 73–92.

Elliot, A. J., & Dweck, C. S. (2005). Competence as the core of achievement motivation. In A. J. Elliot & C. S. Dweck (Eds.), *Handbook of competence and motivation* (pp. 3–12). New York: Guilford Press.

Elliot, A. J., & Harackiewicz, J. M. (1996). Approach and avoidance achievement goals and intrinsic motivation: A mediational analysis. *Journal of Personality and Social Psychology, 70,* 461–475.

Elliot, A. J., & McGregor, H. A. (2001). A 2 × 2 achievement goal framework. *Journal of Personality and Social Psychology, 80,* 501–519.

Elliot, A. J., Murayama, K., Kobeisy, A., & Lichtenfeld, S. (2015). Potential-based achievement goals. *British Journal of Educational Psychology, 85,* 192–206.

Elliot, A. J., Murayama, K., & Pekrun, R. (2011). A 3 × 2 achievement goal model. *Journal of Educational Psychology, 103,* 632–648.

Elliot, A. J., & Thrash, T. M. (2001). Achievement goals and the hierarchical model of achievement motivation. *Educational Psychology Review, 13,* 139–156.

Elliot, A. J., & Thrash, T. M. (2002). Approach–avoidance motivation in personality: Approach and avoidance temperaments and goals. *Journal of Personality and Social Psychology, 82,* 804–818.

Elliott, E. S., & Dweck, C. S. (1988). Goals: An approach to motivation and achievement. *Journal of Personality and Social Psychology, 54,* 5–12.

Epstein, J. L. (1989). Family structures and student motivation. In R. E. Ames & C. Ames (Eds.), *Research on motivation in education: Vol. 3. Goals and cognitions* (pp. 259–295). New York: Academic Press.

Eren, A. (2009). Examining the teacher efficacy and achievement goals as predictors of Turkish student teachers' conceptions about teaching and learning. *Australian Journal of Teacher Education, 34,* 69–87.

Ferron, F., Le Bars, H., & Gernigon, C. (2005). Development and validation of a 2 × 2 goal involvement states questionnaire for sport. *Journal of Sport and Exercise Psychology, 27,* S64–S65.

Flanagan, M. J., Putwain, D. W., & Caltabiano, M. L. (2015). The relationship between goal setting and students' experience of academic test anxiety. *International Journal of School and Educational Psychology, 3,* 189–201.

García-Romero, C. (2015). Relationship between the 3 × 2 achievement goals and perceived competence in physical education students. *Sportis: Scientific Journal of School Sport, Physical Education and Psychometricity, 1,* 293–310.

Gillet, N., Lafrenière, M., Huyghebaert, T., & Fouquereau, E. (2015). Autonomous and controlled reasons underlying achievement goals: Implications for the 3 × 2 achievement goal model in educational and work settings. *Motivation and Emotion, 39,* 853–858.

Grant, H., & Dweck, C. S. (2003). Clarifying achievement goals and their impact. *Journal of Personality and Social Psychology, 85,* 541–553.

Guan, J., McBride, R., & Xiang, P. (2007) A comparison of the trichotomous and 2 × 2 achievement goal models in high school physical education settings. *Measurement in Physical Education, and Exercise Science, 11,* 109–129.

Guthrie, J. T., Wigfield, A., & VonSecker, C. (2000). Effects of integrated instruction on motivation and strategy use in reading. *Journal of Educational Psychology, 92,* 331–341.

Harackiewicz, J. M., Barron, K. E., & Elliot, A. J. (1998). Rethinking achievement goals: When are they adaptive for college students and why? *Educational Psychologist, 33,* 1–21.

Harackiewicz, J. M., & Elliot, A. J. (1993). Achievement goals and intrinsic motivation. *Journal of Personality and Social Psychology, 65,* 904–915.

Harackiewicz, J. M., & Sansone, C. (1991). Goals and intrinsic motivation: You *can* get there from here. In M. Maehr & P. Pintrich (Eds.), *Advances in motivation and achievement* (Vol. 7, pp. 21–49). Greenwich, CT: JAI Press.

Hong, Y. Y., Chiu, C. Y., Dweck, C. S., Lin, D. M., & Wan, W. (1999). Implicit theories, attributions, and coping: A meaning system approach. *Journal of Personality and Social Psychology, 77,* 588–599.

Hoyert, M. S., & O'Dell, C. D. (2006). A brief intervention to aid struggling students: A case of too much motivation? *Journal of Scholarship of Teaching and Learning, 6*(1), 1–13.

Huang, C. (2011). Achievement goals and achievement emotions: A meta-analysis. *Educational Psychology Review, 23,* 359–388.

Huang, C. (2012). Discriminant and criterion-related validity of achievement goals in predicting academic achievement: A meta-analysis. *Journal of Educational Psychology, 104,* 48–73.

Hulleman, C. S., & Barron, K. E. (2016). Motivation interventions in education: Bridging theory, research, and practice. In L. Corno & E. M. Anderman (Eds.), *Handbook of educational psychology* (3rd ed., pp. 160–171). New York: Routledge/Taylor & Francis.

Hulleman, C. S., Durik, A. M., Schweigert, S. B., & Harackiewicz, J. M. (2008). Task values, achievement goals, and interest: An integrative analysis. *Journal of Educational Psychology, 100,* 398–416.

Hulleman, C. S., Schrager, S. M., Bodmann, S. M., & Harackiewicz, J. M. (2010). A meta-analytic review of achievement goal measures: Different labels for the same constructs or different constructs with similar labels? *Psychological Bulletin, 136,* 422–449.

Jackson, B., Harwood, C. G., & Grove, J. R. (2010). On the same page in sporting dyads: Does dissimilarity on 2 by 2 achievement goal constructs impair relationship functioning? *Journal of Sport and Exercise Psychology, 32,* 805–827.

James, V. H., & Yates, S. M. (2007). Extending the multiple-goal perspective to tertiary classroom goal structures. *International Education Journal, 8,* 68–80.

Johnson, M. L., & Kestler, J. L. (2013). Achievement goals of traditional and nontraditional aged college students: Using the 3 × 2 achievement goal framework. *International Journal of Educational Research, 61,* 48–59.

Johnson, P. D., Shull, A., & Wallace, J. C. (2011). Regulatory focus as a mediator in goal orientation and performance relationships. *Journal of Organizational Behavior, 32,* 751–766.

Kaplan, A., Katz, I., & Flum, H. (2012). Motivation theory in educational practice: Knowledge claims, challenges, and future directions. In K. Harris, S. Graham, & T. Urdan (Eds.), *Educational psychology handbook: Vol. 2. Individual differences and cultural and contextual factors* (pp. 165–194). Washington, DC: American Psychological Association.

Kaplan, A., & Maehr, M. L. (2007). The contributions and prospects of goal orientation theory. *Educational Psychology Review, 19,* 141–184.

Kaplan, A., & Midgley, C. (1997). The effect of achievement goals: Does level of academic efficacy make a difference? *Contemporary Educational Psychology, 22,* 415–435.

Karabenick, S. A. (2003). Seeking help in large college classes: A person-centered approach. *Contemporary Educational Psychology, 28,* 37–58.

Kavussanu, M., Morris, R. L., & Ring, C. (2009). The effects of achievement goals on performance, enjoyment, and practice of a novel motor task. *Journal of Sports Sciences, 27,* 1281–1292.

Korn, R. M., & Elliot, A. J. (2016). The 2 × 2 standpoints model of achievement goals. *Frontiers in Psychology.* Retrieved from *https://doi.org/10.3389/fpsyg.2016.00742.*

Kristof-Brown, A. L., & Stevens, C. K. (2001). Goal congruence in project teams: Does the fit between members' personal mastery and performance goals matter? *Journal of Applied Psychology, 86,* 1083–1095.

Krosnick, J. A. (1991). Response strategies for coping with the cognitive demands of attitude measures in surveys. *Applied Cognitive Psychology, 5,* 213–236.

Krosnick, J. A. (2000). The threat of satisficing in surveys: The shortcuts respondents take in answering questions. *Survey Methods Newsletter, 20,* 4–8.

Law, W., Elliot, A. J., & Murayama, K. (2012). Perceived competence moderates the relation between performance-approach and performance-avoidance goals. *Journal of Educational Psychology, 104,* 806–819.

Lazowski, R. A., & Hulleman, C. S. (2016). Motivation interventions in education: A meta-analytic review. *Review of Educational Research, 86,* 602–640.

Leondari, A., & Gialamas, V. (2002). Implicit theories, goal orientations, and perceived competence: Impact on students' achievement behavior. *Psychology in the Schools, 39,* 279–291.

Linnenbrink, E. A. (2005). The dilemma of performance-approach goals: The use of multiple goal contexts to promote students' motivation and learning. *Journal of Educational Psychology, 97,* 197–213.

Linnenbrink-Garcia, L., Middleton, M. J., Ciani, K. D., Easter, M. A., O'Keefe, P. A., & Zusho, A. (2012). The strength of the relation between performance-approach and performance-avoidance goal orientations: Theoretical, methodological, and instructional implications. *Educational Psychologist, 47,* 281–301.

Lloyd, J., & Fox, K. (1992). Achievement goals and motivation to exercise in adolescent girls: A preliminary intervention study. *British Journal of Physical Education Research Supplement, 11,* 12–16.

Lochbaum, M., & Gottardy, J. (2015). A meta-analytic review of the approach–avoidance achievement goals and performance relationships in the sport psychology literature. *Journal of Sport and Health Science, 4,* 164–173.

Lochbaum, M., Jean-Noel, J., Pinar, C., & Gilson, T. (in press). A meta-analytic review of Elliot's (1999) *Hierarchical Model of Approach and Avoidance Motivation* in the sport, physical activity, and physical education literature. *Journal of Sport and Health Science.*

Lopez, D. F. (1999). Social cognitive influences on self-regulated learning: The impact of action-control beliefs and academic goals on achievement-related outcomes. *Learning and Individual Differences, 11,* 301–319.

Madjar, N., Kaplan, A., & Weinstock, M. P. (2011). Clarifying mastery-avoidance goals in high school: Distinguishing between intrapersonal and task-based standards of competence. *Contemporary Educational Psychology, 36,* 268–279.

Maehr, M. L. (1983). On doing well in science: Why Johnny no longer excels, why Sarah never did. In S. Paris, G. Olson, & H. Stevenson (Eds.), *Learning and motivation in the classroom* (pp. 179–210). Hillsdale, NJ: Erlbaum.

Maehr, M. L. (1989). Thoughts about motivation. In C. Ames & R. Ames (Eds.), *Research on motivation in education: Goals and cognitions* (Vol. 3, pp. 299–315). New York: Academic Press.

Maehr, M. L., & Midgley, C. (1996). *Transforming school cultures.* Boulder, CO: Westview Press.

Maehr, M. L., & Nicholls, J. G. (1980). Culture and achievement motivation: A second look. In N. Warren (Ed.), *Studies in cross cultural psychology* (Vol. 3, pp. 221–267). New York: Academic Press.

Martin, A. J. (2005). Exploring the effects of a youth enrichment program on academic motivation and engagement. *Social Psychology of Education, 8,* 179–206.

Martin, A. J. (2006). Personal bests (PBs): A proposed multidimensional model and empirical analysis. *British Journal of Educational Psychology, 76,* 803–825.

Martin, A. J. (2008). Enhancing student motivation and engagement: The effects of a multidimensional intervention. *Contemporary Educational Psychology, 33,* 239–269.

Mascret, N., Elliot, A. J., & Cury, F. (2015a). Extending the 3 × 2 achievement goal model to the sport domain: The 3 × 2 Achievement Goal Questionnaire for Sport. *Psychology of Sport and Exercise, 17,* 7–14.

Mascret, N., Elliot, A. J., & Cury, F. (2015b). The 3 × 2 achievement goal questionnaire for teachers. *Educational Psychology.* [Epub ahead of print]

McInerney, V., McInerney, D. M., & Marsh, H. W. (1997). Effects of metacognitive strategy training within a cooperative group learning context on computer achievement and anxiety: An aptitude–treatment interaction study. *Journal of Educational Psychology, 89,* 686–695.

Meece, J. L., Blumenfeld, P. C., & Hoyle, R. H. (1988). Students' goal orientations and cognitive engagement in classroom activities. *Journal of Educational Psychology, 80,* 514–523.

Mèndez-Giménez, A., & Fernández-Río, J. (2014). Examining the 3 × 2 achievement goal model in the physical education context. *Cuadernos de Psicología del Deporte, 14,* 157–168.

Middleton, M., & Midgley, C. (1997). Avoiding the demonstration of lack of ability: An underexplored aspect of goal theory. *Journal of Educational Psychology, 89,* 710–718.

Midgley, C., Kaplan, A., & Middleton, M. (2001). Performance approach goals: Good for what, for whom, under what circumstances, and at what cost? *Journal of Educational Psychology, 93,* 77–86.

Miller, S. D., & Meece, J. L. (1997). Enhancing elementary students' motivation to read and write: A classroom intervention study. *Journal of Educational Research, 90,* 286–299.

Mouratidou, K., Barkoukis, V., & Rizos, S. (2012). Achievement goals and moral competence in sport: Examining the moderating role of demographic characteristics. *European Psychologist, 17,* 34–43.

Muis, K. R., Ranellucci, J., Franco, G. M., & Crippen, K. J. (2013). The interactive effects of personal achievement goals and performance feedback in an undergraduate science class. *Journal of Experimental Education, 81,* 556–578.

Nicholls, J. G. (1984). Achievement motivation: Conceptions of ability, subjective experience, task choice, and performance. *Psychological Review, 91,* 328–346.

Nicholls, J. G. (1989). *The competitive ethos and democratic education.* Cambridge, MA: Harvard University Press.

Nicholls, J. G., Patashnick, M., Cheung, P., Thorkildsen, T., & Lauer, J. (1989). Can achievement motivation succeed with only one conception of success? In F. Halisch & J. Van den Beroken (Eds.), *Competence considered* (pp. 190–204). Lisse, The Netherlands: Swets & Zeitlinger.

Nicholls, J. G., Patashnick, M., & Nolen, S. (1985). Adolescents' theories of education. *Journal of Educational Psychology, 77,* 683–692.

Nolen, S. B. (1988). Reasons for studying: Motivational orientations and study strategies. *Cognition and Instruction, 5,* 269–287.

Noordzij, G., Van Hooft, E. A., Mierlo, H., Dam, A., & Born, M. P. (2013). The effects of a learning-goal orientation training on self-regulation: A field experiment among unemployed job seekers. *Personnel Psychology, 66,* 73–755.

O'Keefe, P., Ben-Eliyahu, A., & Linnenbrink-Garcia, L. (2013). Shaping achievement goal orientations in a mastery-structured environment and concomitant changes in related contingencies of self-worth. *Motivation and Emotion, 37,* 50–64.

Pajares, F., Britner, S. L., & Valiante, G. (2000). Relation between achievement goals and self-beliefs of middle school students in writing and science. *Contemporary Educational Psychology, 25,* 406–422.

Payne, S. C., Youngcourt, S. S., & Beaubien, J. M. (2007). A meta-analytic examination of the goal orientation nomological net. *Journal of Applied Psychology, 92,* 128–150.

Peng, S. L., Cherng, B. L., & Chen, H. C. (2013). The effects of classroom goal structures on the creativity of junior high school students. *Educational Psychology, 33,* 540–560.

Pintrich, P. R. (2000). Multiple goals, multiple pathways: The role of goal orientation in learning and achievement. *Journal of Educational Psychology, 92,* 544–555.

Pintrich, P., & Garcia, T. (1991). Student goal orientation and self-regulation in the college classroom. In M. Maehr & P. Pintrich (Eds.), *Advances in motivation and achievement* (Vol. 7, pp. 371–402). Greenwich, CT: JAI Press.

Pintrich, P. R., & Schunk, D. H. (1996). *Motivation in education: Theory, research, and applications.* Englewood Cliffs, NJ: Prentice Hall.

Podsakoff, P. M., MacKenzie, S. M., Lee, J., & Podsakoff, N. P. (2003). Common method variance in behavioral research: A critical review of the literature and recommended remedies. *Journal of Applied Psychology, 88,* 879–903.

Poortvliet, P. M., Janssen, O., Van Yperen, N. W., & Van de Vliert, E. (2007). Achievement goals and interpersonal behavior: How mastery and performance goals shape information exchange. *Personality and Social Psychology Bulletin, 33,* 1435–1447.

Quintanilla, Y. T. (2007). *Achievement motivation strategies: An integrative achievement motivation program with first year seminar students.* Unpublished doctoral dissertation, Texas A & M University, Corpus Christi, TX.

Ranellucci, J., Hall, N. C., Muis, K. R., & Lajoie, S. P. (in press). Mastery, maladaptive learning behavior, and academic achievement: An intervention approach. *Journal of Experimental Education.*

Rawsthorne, L. J., & Elliot, A. J. (1999). Achievement goals and intrinsic motivation: A meta-analytic review. *Personality and Social Psychology Review, 3,* 326–344.

Richardson, M., Abraham, C., & Bond, R. (2012). Psychological correlates of university students' academic performance: A systematic review and meta-analysis. *Psychological Bulletin, 138,* 353–387.

Riou, F., Boiché, J., Doron, J., Romain, A., Corrion, K., Ninot, G., et al. (2012). Development and validation of the French Achievement Goals Questionnaire for Sport and Exercise (FAGQSE). *European Journal of Psychological Assessment, 28,* 313–320.

Roberts, G. C., & Treasure, D. C. (1995). Achievement goals, motivational climate, and achievement strategies and behaviors in sport. *International Journal of Sport Psychology, 26,* 64–80.

Roedel, T. D., Schraw, G., & Plake, B. S. (1994). Validation of a measure of learning and performance goal orientations. *Educational and Psychological Measurement, 54,* 1013–1021.

Ryan, A. M., & Shim, S. S. (2006). Social achievement goals: The nature and consequences of different orientations toward social competence. *Personality and Social Psychology Bulletin, 32,* 1246–1263.

Schiano-Lomoriello, S., Cury, F., & Da Fonséca, D. (2005). Development and validation of the Approach and Avoidance Questionnaire for Sport and Physical Education Setting (AAQSPE). *European Revue of Applied Psychology, 55,* 85–98.

Senko, C., & Freund, A. M. (2015). Are mastery-avoidance goals always detrimental?: An adult development perspective. *Motivation and Emotion, 39,* 477–488.

Senko, C., & Hulleman, C. S. (2013). The role of goal attainment expectancies in achievement goal pursuit. *Journal of Educational Psychology, 105,* 504–521.

Senko, C., Hulleman, C. S., & Harackiewicz, J. M. (2011). Achievement goal theory at the crossroads: Old controversies, current challenges, and new directions. *Educational Psychologist, 46,* 26–47.

Senko, C., & Tropiano, K. L. (in press). Comparing three models of achievement goals: Goal orientations, goal standards, and goal complexes. *Journal of Educational Psychology.*

Skaalvik, E. M. (1997). Self-enhancing and self-defeating ego orientation: Relations with task and avoidance orientation, achievement, self-perceptions, and anxiety. *Journal of Educational Psychology, 89,* 71–81.

Smeding, A., Darnon, C., Souchal, C., Toczek-Capelle, M. C., & Butera, F. (2013). Reducing the socio-economic status achievement gap at university by promoting mastery-oriented assessment. *PLoS ONE, 8,* e71678.

Smith, M., Duda, J., Allen, J., & Hall, H. (2002). Contemporary measures of approach and avoidance orientations: Similarities and differences. *British Journal of Educational Psychology, 72,* 155–190.

Solmon, M. A. (1996). Impact of motivational climate on students' behaviors and perceptions in a physical education setting. *Journal of Educational Psychology, 88,* 731–738.

Spray, C. M., & Warburton, V. E. (2011). Temporal relations among mulitdimensational perceptions of competence and trichotomous achievement goals in physical education. *Psychology of Sport and Exercise, 12,* 515–524.

Stipek, D. J., & Gralinski, J. H. (1996). Children's beliefs about intelligence and school performance. *Journal of Educational Psychology, 88,* 397–407.

Tanaka, A., Takehara, T., & Yamauchi, H. (2006). Achievement goals in a presentation task: Performance expectancy, achievement goals, state anxiety, and task performance. *Learning and Individual Differences, 16,* 93–99.

Todorovich, J. R., & Curtner-Smith, M. D. (2001). Influence of the motivational climate in physical education on third grade pupils' goal orientations. *Research Quarterly for Exercise and Sport, 72*(Suppl. 1), 82.

Todorovich, J. R., & Curtner-Smith, M. D. (2002). Influence of the motivational climate in physical education on sixth grade pupils goal orientations. *European Physical Education Review, 8,* 119–138.

Treasure, D. (1993). *A social-cognitive approach to understanding children's achievement behavior, cognitions, and affect in competitive sport.* Unpublished doctoral dissertation, University of Illinois at Urbana–Champaign, IL.

Urbán, G., Orosz, G., Kerepes, L., & Jánvári, M. I. (2014). Hungarian adaptation of the 3 × 2 Achievement Goal Questionnaire. *Pszichológia, 34,* 73–97.

Urdan, T., & Maehr, M. (1995). Beyond a two-goal theory of motivation and achievement: A case for social goals. *Review of Educational Research, 65,* 213–243.

Urdan, T., & Mestas, M. (2006). The goals behind performance goals. *Journal of Educational Psychology, 98,* 354–365.

Urdan, T. C. (1997). Achievement goal theory: Past results, future directions. In M. Maehr & P. Pintrich (Eds.), *Advances in motivation and achievement* (Vol. 10, pp. 243–269). Greenwich, CT: JAI Press.

Utman, C. (1997). Performance effects of motivational state: A meta-analysis. *Personality and Social Psychology Review, 1,* 170–182.

Vandewalle, D. (1997). Development and validation of a work domain goal orientation instrument. *Educational and Psychological Measurement, 57,* 995–1015.

Van Hooft, E. A. J., & Noordzij, G. (2009). The effects of goal orientation on job search and reemployment: A field experiment among unemployed job seekers. *Journal of Applied Psychology, 94,* 1581–1590.

Van Yperen, N. W. (2006). A novel approach to assessing achievement goals in the context of the 2 × 2 framework: Identifying distinct profiles of individuals with different dominant achievement goals. *Personality and Social Psychology Bulletin, 32,* 1432–1445.

Van Yperen, N. W., Blaga, M., & Postmes, T. (2014). A meta-analysis of self-reported achievement goals and non-self-report performance across three achievement domains (work, sports, and education). *PLoS ONE, 9,* 1–16.

Van Yperen, N. W., Hamstra, M. R. W., & Van der Klauw, M. (2011). To win, or not to lose, at any cost: The impact of achievement goals on cheating. *British Journal of Management, 22,* S5–S15.

Van Yperen, N. W., & Orehek, E. (2013). Achievement goals in the workplace: Conceptualization, prevalence, profiles, and outcomes. *Journal of Economic Psychology, 38,* 71–79.

Wadsworth, D. D., Robinson, L. E., Rudisill, M. E., & Gell, N. (2013). The effect of physical education climates on elementary students' physical activity behaviors. *Journal of School Health, 83,* 306–313.

Wang, C. K. J., Biddle, S. J. H., & Elliot, A. (2007). The 2 × 2 achievement goals framework in a physical education context. *Psychology of Sport and Exercise, 8,* 147–168.

Warburton, V., & Spray, C. (2014). Appearance- and competition-focused performance goals: Examining their links with performance in physical education. *European Physical Education Review, 20,* 305–318.

Wirthwein, L., Sparfeldt, J. R., Pinquart, M.,

Wegerer, J., & Steinmayr, R. (2013). Achievement goals and academic achievement: A closer look at moderating factors. *Educational Research Review, 10,* 66–89.

Wolters, C. A., Yu, S. L., & Pintrich, P. R. (1996). The relation between goal orientation and students' motivational beliefs and self-regulated learning. *Learning and Individual Differences, 8,* 211–238.

Wu, C. (2012). The cross-cultural examination of 3 × 2 achievement goal model in Taiwan. *Procedia: Social and Behavioral Sciences, 69,* 422–427.

Yeager, D. S., & Walton, G. M. (2011). Social-psychological interventions in education: They're not magic. *Review of Educational Research, 81,* 267–301.

Zusho, A., & Clayton, K. (2011). Culturalizing achievement goal theory and research. *Educational Psychologist, 46,* 239–260.

Zweig, D., & Webster, J. (2004). Validation of a multidimensional measure of goal orientation. *Canadian Journal of Behavioural Science, 36,* 232–248.

CHAPTER 5

An Attribution Perspective on Competence and Motivation
Theory and Treatment Interventions

RAYMOND P. PERRY
JEREMY M. HAMM

Attribution theories encompass a collection of social cognition perspectives concerning the psychological construal of life events. Their early development began with Heider's (1944, 1958) seminal discourse on perceived causes of behavior, followed by Rotter (1954), de Charms (1968), Jones and Davis (1965), Kelley (1967), and Weiner (1970), among others (see Jones et al., 1971). This chapter examines competence as a psychological construct based on Weiner's (1986, 1995, 2006, 2012) attribution theory that links causal attributions, cognitions, emotions, motivation, and behavior. His theory provides two attribution accounts of competence that focus on an individual's own (intrapersonal) and others' (interpersonal) life experiences.

Within this perspective, we extend Weiner's (2005) attributional analysis of competence to include cognitive treatments that can modify competence appraisals responsible for adverse motivational states. After discussing Weiner's theory and competence as an attribution construct, we describe cognitive treatments that change attribution → motivation → performance paths from maladaptive to adaptive. Integral to this perspective is the premise that competence can arise from causal ascriptions and that attribution-based cognitive treatments can alter competence appraisals and maladaptive motivational states.

AN ATTRIBUTION PERSPECTIVE ON COMPETENCE AND MOTIVATION

As a motivational construct, *competence* is viewed as a psychological entity instrumental to human adaptation in diverse settings (see Elliot & Dweck, 2005). It is thought to evolve from exogenous (e.g., socioeconomic status [SES], peer group status) and endogenous (e.g., IQ, gender) factors that prescribed its prominence, stability, and generalizability. Research attests to its versatility and utility as a construct, spawning a variety of definitions linked to ability, intelligence, self-worth, self-concept, self-efficacy, mastery, perceived control, and goal pursuit. Beginning with White's (1959) early construal of competence that focused on an organism's capacity to influence the environment (p. 297), later conceptions portray competence as personality-related inferences having ability-like qualities, being relatively stable, and serving a basic psychological need (e.g., Baumeister & Leary, 1995; Deci & Ryan, 1990).

In Weiner's (2005) analysis, a competence appraisal originates from an unexpected or negative event that instigates a causal search process to identify an explanation of the event. The ascription that results from causal thinking (e.g., low ability, disorganized) triggers a competence appraisal (e.g., incompetent) analogous to *attribution-based personality inferences* such as arrogance and modesty (e.g., Hareli & Weiner, 2000, 2002b). After a notable success (outcome), for example, if an actor tells an observer that it was due to high ability (causal attribution), the observer may infer that the actor is arrogant (personality inference). In contrast, if the actor implies that the success was a result of tenacious effort (causal attribution), the observer may regard the actor as modest (personality inference).

Personality inferences arising from causal thinking can be portrayed in attribution path sequences as follows: outcome (event) → causal attribution → cognition (*personality inference*) → affect → motivation → behavior. Assuming that attribution-based competence appraisals are personality-like inferences, they can be depicted within an attribution path sequence: outcome (event) → causal attribution → cognition (*competence appraisals*) → affect → motivation → behavior. This logic implies that competence appraisals are rooted in causal thinking, and that they have consequences for adaptive and maladaptive affect → motivation → performance path sequences. Hence, it is conceivable that attribution-based cognitive treatments that reliably change causal ascriptions will also modify competence appraisals that produce maladaptive attribution → motivation → performance path sequences.

Weiner's Attribution Theory of Emotion and Motivation

Janus: A Roman deity whose two faces simultaneously perceive the past and future

Weiner contends that causal thinking arises from attribution processes common to human nature, regardless of cultures,

civilizations, and periods in history (1972, 1985a, 1986, 2006, 2012). Studies conducted over decades attest to the prevalence of attribution processes in achievement and social settings. In accounting for attribution processes, Weiner posits that life experiences initiate "why" questions that trigger *causal search* processes to identify the causes of events. These causal ascriptions are phenomenological in their subjective construal and do not necessarily correspond to reality. In turn, the causes cue cognitions (e.g., expectations, responsibility appraisals, personality inferences) and emotions (e.g., hope, pride, guilt, gratitude) that regulate subsequent motivation, goal striving, and performance outcomes. Like Janus, epilogue is prologue: Perceptions of past experiences are integral to future events.

Weiner proposes that attributions resulting from causal search have three properties or dimensions: *Locus of causality* refers to a cause residing within or outside the person (e.g., aptitude vs. chance); *stability* implies that the cause changes or endures over time (e.g., fatigue vs. industriousness); *controllability* suggests that the cause can or cannot be altered by either oneself or another person (e.g., laziness vs. the weather). In a simple illustration, each dimension is viewed as a dichotomy that forms a locus (internal, external) by stability (stable, unstable) by controllability (controllable, uncontrollable) 2 × 2 × 2 attribution taxonomy. Since every cause has these three properties, all causes can be placed in one of the eight cells of this matrix (Figure 5.1).

These three attributional dimensions regulate cognitions and emotions, which determine subsequent motivation and behavior. For example, an internal attribution for success (e.g., high ability) activates pride stemming from the locus dimension, but an external attribution (e.g., teaching quality) does not. The stability dimension prompts expectations about future successes and failures, whereby stable (vs. unstable) causes relate to whether such outcomes will recur. Following failure, an unstable cause (e.g., low effort) triggers feelings of hope because the cause can change; a stable cause (e.g., low aptitude) elicits hopelessness because the cause will not change. The controllability dimension cues responsibility appraisals

	Internal		External	
	Stable	**Unstable**	**Stable**	**Unstable**
Controllable	Never studies	Didn't study for this test	Instructor is biased	Friends failed to help
Uncontrollable	Low aptitude	Sick day of test	School has high standards	Bad luck

FIGURE 5.1. Examples of ascriptions following failure in a $2 \times 2 \times 2$ attribution matrix based on the three causal dimensions underpinning all causal attributions in Weiner's (1985a, 2012) theory.

concerning the outcome, as well as feelings of guilt or shame following failure. Thus, the locus, stability, and controllability of causal attributions can have direct implications for motivation and behavior (see Figure 5.2).

Consider a student who fails an important course test and attributes the failure to a lack of aptitude. If the student perceives aptitude as an *internal, stable, uncontrollable* cause, then low expectations of future success and hopelessness are linked to the stability dimension, along with low self-esteem and shame arising from the locus and controllability dimensions. Uncontrollable causes also reduce personal responsibility for an outcome and motivation to change future circumstances. Expectations of future failure, paired with negative emotions and less self-responsibility, in turn, deplete motivation and erode performance, making persistence in the course much less likely.

In contrast, when the student ascribes failure to *internal, unstable, controllable* causes, very different consequences arise for motivation and performance. Controllable causes (e.g., low effort) increase perceived responsibility for an outcome, as well as guilt, which together initiate actions to rectify the situation. Guilt is a motivating emotion and is less psychologically debilitating than shame or hopelessness. Expectations about future performance will be positive because lack of effort is an unstable and controllable cause that can change. Students who ascribe internal, controllable causes to their performance will work harder, feel better about their studies, be more persistent, and obtain higher grades. Simply put, two students of equal intelligence may perform very differently depending on how they

explain their academic successes and failures.

Differences between ability and effort attributions in stability and controllability lie at the heart of many motivation and performance outcomes in achievement situations. Although both causes are internal, ascribing poor performance to low ability (stable, uncontrollable) decreases motivation, whereas low effort (unstable, controllable) increases motivation. Lack of effort, bad strategy, or poor note taking are controllable causes often ascribed for failure, but because they can be altered by trying harder, using a better strategy, or taking clearer notes, they can increase motivation and performance. External (uncontrollable) causes, such as bad luck, poor teaching, or test difficulty, may create less negative affect and are less harmful to pride and self-esteem, but they are likely to impair motivation nonetheless. From Weiner's (2005) perspective, ability and effort ascriptions can also play a pivotal role in contributing to competence appraisals.

Intrapersonal and Interpersonal Attributional Processes

Two perspectives on attribution processes have developed from Weiner's (1970, 1972, 1985a, 1985b) original theory that focus on either an individual's self-perceptions (*intrapersonal*) or an individual's perceptions of others' actions (*interpersonal*). Weiner's (1985a, 1986, 2012) intrapersonal theory deals with the causal analysis of one's own experiences involving *self-focused* attribution → cognition → affect → motivation → behavior path sequences. For example,

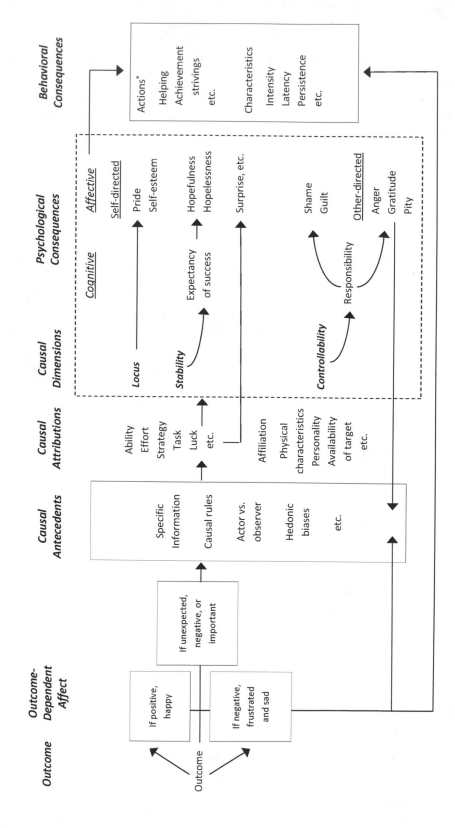

FIGURE 5.2. Weiner's attribution theory (1985a, 2012) of motivation and emotion. *Actions, interpersonal (helping) and intrapersonal (achievement strivings) domains. From Weiner (1985a, p. 565). Copyright © 1985 American Psychological Association. Adapted by permission.

consider a student who fails a test and identifies the cause as low ability; such an attribution triggers low expectations about future performance, appraisals of not being responsible for the failure, shame, little motivation to rectify the failure, and poor performance next time.

Weiner's (1995, 2006) interpersonal theory deals with an observer's causal analysis of others' experiences, which produces *others-focused* attribution → cognition → affect → motivation → behavior path sequences. For example, if after seeing a person (actor) fail a test, an observer identifies the cause of failure as low ability (causal search), the observer will develop low expectations about the person's future performance, judge the individual as not responsible for the failure, express sympathy for the person, be motivated to help, and likely assist the individual.

Thus far, we have described Weiner's theory in the context of achievement settings, but both intrapersonal and interpersonal theories apply to social settings as well. After being refused for a date, for example, an individual may ascribe the rejection to bad timing (unstable, controllable), which sustains motivation to try again from an intrapersonal perspective. Alternatively, attributing the rejection to being unattractive (stable, uncontrollable) inhibits motivation to ask again.

From its expectancy × value origins over 45 years ago, Weiner's (1970, 1972, 1979) theory has evolved in conceptual complexity, coherence, and fidelity, standing the test of time. Its structural framework includes key cognitive and affective processes, multiple determinants of motivation, assorted psychological and behavioral outcomes, and generalizability across motivation domains. Although Weiner's theory is recognized for its stature, elegance, and logical precision (e.g., Fiske & Taylor, 1991), it is not without flaws or critics whose conceptual and empirical scrutiny bettered the study of human motivation. For example, Weiner's debate with M. Covington in the *Journal of Educational Psychology* (ability vs. effort) advanced our understanding of attribution processes and motivation (Brown & Weiner, 1984; Covington & Omelich, 1984; Weiner & Brown, 1984), as did Weiner's responses to critics (e.g., 1983, 1985b).

Attribution Theory and Competence

Weiner's (2005) attribution approach to competence as a psychological entity focuses on how causal properties (locus, stability, controllability) relate to appraisals of competence. Weiner contends that laypeople and psychologists alike view competence as an enduring quality that regulates the pursuit of goals in mathematics, music, athletics, and so on. People are appraised as competent (incompetent) in these activities because they possess (lack) mathematics aptitude, musical talent, or athletic ability (internal, stable, uncontrollable causes). For example, high ability (*uncontrollable,* stable) is an internal, enduring cause that can lead to high competence appraisals when ascribed to success. Following success, competence can also be perceived as a *controllable* entity (e.g., industrious) that varies (unstable) through practice, learning, or experience. Other controllable, unstable causes such as "reflective thinker" or "organized" may also imply high competence (see Figure 5.1).

Following failure, however, uncontrollable and stable causes (e.g., low aptitude, lethargy) can trigger low competence appraisals. From an attributional perspective, these conceptions of competence can be depicted as theoretical path sequences that account for competence as a psychological entity. Hence, competence appraisals (competent, incompetent) result from causes ascribed to failure and success outcomes as follows: outcome → causal attribution → cognition (*competence appraisal*) → affect → motivation → performance (Figure 5.3a).

In Weiner's taxonomy (Figure 5.1), causal ascriptions activate both adaptive (controllable cause) and maladaptive (uncontrollable cause) motivation path sequences that include competence appraisals. Each sequence features uncontrollable (Path 1) or controllable (Path 2) causes that lead to low or high (maladaptive or adaptive) competence appraisals, depending on failure or success outcomes. Following failure, a *Path 1* (*uncontrollable* cause) sequence is depicted as low ability → cognition (*low competence appraisal*) → negative affect → low motivation → failure. Following success, Path 1 is represented as high ability → cognition (*high competence appraisal*) → positive affect →

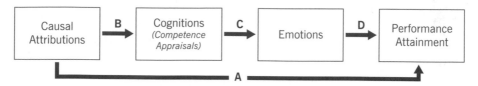

FIGURE 5.3a. Attribution–cognition–emotion–performance sequence. From Perry, Chipperfield, Hladkyj, Pekrun, and Hamm (2014, p. 6). Copyright © 2014 Emerald Group Publishing Limited. Adapted by permission.

high motivation → success. Following failure, a *Path 2* (*controllable* cause) sequence is portrayed as bad strategy → cognition (*moderate competence appraisal*) → affect → moderate motivation → improved performance. Following success, a Path 2 sequence is expressed as good strategy → cognition (*high competence appraisal*) → affect → high motivation → success. Thus, Path 1 and 2 sequences incorporate attribution-linked competence appraisals (competent, incompetent) that can impact motivation and performance as follows: outcome → attribution → cognition (*competence appraisal*) → affect → motivation → performance (see Table 5.1 on page 71).

These attribution path sequences provide a conceptual framework that accounts for competence appraisals, similar to how attributional processes relate to personality inferences (Hareli & Weiner, 2002a, 2002b). This premise rests on empirical evidence and logical argumentation. Evidence supporting this logic comes from studies of Weiner's interpersonal (others-focused) attribution theory that accounts for attribution-mediated personality inferences. Weiner (1995, 2012) argues that an observer infers personality qualities of an actor when the actor conveys high ability ("I guess I'm just brilliant") or intense effort ("I tried so hard it just about killed me") following a success outcome. In the ability scenario, the observer infers that the actor is arrogant and in the effort scenario, the observer concludes that the actor is modest. Thus, competence appraisals may be akin to personality-like inferences activated by attributions described by Weiner in path sequences like those discussed earlier.

Weiner's attribution perspective does not imply that competence is uniformly stable or unstable, but depending on its attribution origins as subjectively determined by the individual, competence is situation-specific and fleeting, or stable and generalizes across domains. Weiner accounts for the specificity–generality of competence appraisals in relation to the stability dimension, which is not focused on having more or less of an entity, as is the case from a structural (trait) perspective, but rather on the attributional properties that contribute to competence appraisals. If a competence appraisal arises from controllable and unstable causes, then it will vary with circumstances and be more amenable to change. A key issue in this attributional approach to competence concerns whether attribution-based treatments can alter maladaptive attribution → motivation → performance paths to boost low competence appraisals.

COMPETENCE AND ATTRIBUTIONAL RETRAINING TREATMENTS

Questions instigated by the assorted approaches to competence in this handbook and elsewhere include the following: What are the origins of competence? What defines its nature and structure? How can it be measured? Does competence have a developmental trajectory? Can it be changed? An affirmative response to the last question implies that change is wanted and that methods exist to effect change. If maladaptive motivational states arising from competence appraisals imply that change is needed, attribution-based motivation treatments may provide the means to do so. With Weiner's (2005) attributional account of competence in mind, we now consider how to modify competence appraisals when change is desired.

Weiner's (1972, 1985a, 2012) theory has guided the development of attribution-based treatment interventions, referred to as *attributional retraining* (AR), that seek to alter causal ascriptions in maladaptive attribution → motivation → performance path sequences. Essentially, AR reframes individuals' accounts of life experiences by shifting causal thinking from maladaptive to adaptive. In fostering adaptive causal attributions in achievement settings, AR consistently boosts persistence and performance by facilitating motivation, task engagement, and goal striving (Perry, Chipperfield, Hladkyj, Pekrun, & Hamm, 2014; Perry, Hall, & Ruthig, 2005). Adaptive causes create motivational states that enhance task completion and goal attainment; maladaptive causes create motivational states that erode task persistence and achievement. Following failure, if AR replaces lack of ability with low effort, a maladaptive path (low ability → low motivation → poor performance) changes to an adaptive path (insufficient effort → increased motivation → better performance).

The AR studies in this chapter concern young adults in achievement settings who face challenging and adverse learning conditions that create maladaptive motivational states. These conditions are exacerbated by transitions in K–16 education settings that typify developmental shifts at semistructured intervals over the life course that include new jobs, new partners, a first child, and retirement (e.g., Erikson, 1963; Heckhausen, Wrosch, & Schulz, 2010). For example, school-to-college transitions are imbued with many novel challenges, such as pressure to excel, frequent failure, unstable social networks, new living arrangements, critical career choices, and financial struggles (Perry, 2003; Perry, Stupnisky, Daniels, & Haynes, 2008). A survey of 28,000 college students reveals that 45% felt "things were hopeless," 50% experienced "overwhelming anxiety," 85% were "overwhelmed by all [they] had to do," and 30% reported being so depressed that they had difficulty functioning at least once in the last year (American College Health Association, 2012). Estimates by the U.S. Department of Education suggest that the challenges in this transition also have negative consequences for persistence and goal attainment: Nearly 30% of freshman students enrolled in 4-year programs withdraw from their institutions

within their first year, and only 57% graduate after 6 years (Snyder & Dillow, 2013).

Attributional Retraining and Competence Appraisals

From an attributional perspective, changing competence appraisals rests on three assertions. First, competence appraisals are activated by causal attributions, a premise stemming from Weiner's (2005) contention that attributional processes trigger competence appraisals similar to personality inferences. Empirical evidence supports this premise in that attributional processes can activate personality inferences (e.g., modest, arrogant) in social encounters (Hareli & Weiner, 2002a, 2002b). Second, attribution-based motivation treatments can change causal ascriptions that are theoretically linked to motivation and performance. Thus, AR treatments mitigate motivation and performance deficits by altering causes from maladaptive to adaptive (Weiner, 1986, 1988). Supporting this premise is compelling evidence that AR consistently impacts attributions, cognitions, affects, motivation, and performance in accordance with Weiner's theory (e.g., Perry, Chipperfield, et al., 2014; Perry, Hechter, Menec, & Weinberg, 1993; Perry et al., 2005).

Finally, AR treatments can alter competence appraisals given that AR treatments change causal attributions. Whether causal attributions are linked to competence appraisals is an open question since this has not been studied from an attributional perspective. Unpublished evidence from two samples of students (ages 17–20; ns = 884, 263) shows two internal causes that vary in controllability (ability, effort) predict competence appraisals consistent with Weiner's (2005) assertions (Perry & Hamm, 2015). Low ability (uncontrollable) attributed to failure related *positively* to incompetence appraisals (rs = .25, .33), whereas low effort (controllable) related *negatively* to incompetence appraisals (rs = −.11, −.16).

Thus, given such attribution–competence appraisal associations, AR treatments could change competence appraisals by modifying the associated causal ascriptions (see Figure 5.3b). Based on this logic, four AR treatment protocols can be used to change competence

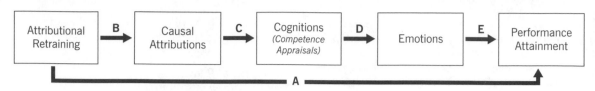

FIGURE 5.3b. Paths underpinning attributional retraining effects on performance. From Perry, Chipperfield, Hladkyj, Pekrun, and Hamm (2014, p. 6). Copyright © 2014 Emerald Group Publishing Limited. Adapted by permission.

appraisals (see Table 5.1 later in this chapter) and classified according to their attribution content within the context of Weiner's taxonomy: AR Protocol 1 treatments introduce or emphasize controllable causes (e.g., Perry, Schönwetter, Magnusson, & Struthers, 1994); Protocol 2 AR treatments curtail uncontrollable causes (e.g., Wilson & Linville, 1982); Protocol 3 AR treatments do both (e.g., Perry, Stupnisky, Hall, Chipperfield, & Weiner, 2010); and Protocol 4 AR treatments alter the dimensional properties of causes (locus, stability, controllability; e.g., Perry & Penner, 1990).

For example, Protocol 1 can change a maladaptive path (*lack of ability* → low competence → low motivation → poor performance) to an adaptive path (*insufficient effort* → adequate competence → higher motivation → improved performance), whereby insufficient effort, a controllable cause, can be replaced with greater effort in order to foster competence and motivation. Protocol 2 and Protocol 3 AR treatments are designed to accomplish similar theoretical changes. Protocol 4 AR treatments alter causal dimensions from stable to unstable by implying that causes change with time (e.g., low ability increases with experience; Wilson & Linville, 1982), or from internal to external (e.g., Storms & Nisbitt, 1970). Thus, when AR protocols alter the attribution properties of a cause from uncontrollable (or stable) to controllable (or unstable), they also produce adaptive path changes that can have positive implications for attribution → motivation → performance sequences (e.g., Perry & Penner, 1990; Weiner, 1988).

Because AR studies have not examined competence specifically, only indirect evidence is available concerning whether AR treatments can change competence

appraisals. This limits our analysis of motivation treatments to AR presented in achievement settings and our arguments to extrapolations of those studies. Excluded also from this chapter are treatment studies: that involve social cognition theories other than Weiner's; that are not attribution-based, such as goal setting, skill development, or knowledge acquisition; that do not concern motivation or performance (e.g., psychotherapy); or, that focus on very young or very old populations (e.g., Chapin & Dyck, 1976; Sarkisian, Prohaska, Davis, & Weiner, 2007). Before examining the potential of AR to change competence appraisals, we introduce three criteria that can be used to assess the quality of motivation treatments: the theoretical basis of the motivation treatment, the experimental design of the treatment study, and the fidelity of the empirical evidence supporting treatment efficacy.

Motivation Treatments and Theoretical Perspective

For motivation treatments to be considered high quality, they should be conceptually coherent and underpinned by a strong theory. This echoes Kurt Lewin's (1951) admonition, summarized as "there is nothing so practical as a good theory." Strong theories afford testable predictions of psychological processes that govern behavioral outcomes (Heckhausen et al., 2010) and enable "prediction across an array of areas with a parsimonious construct system" (Weiner, 2006, p. xvi). The principles comprising strong theories are supported by laboratory and field studies that stress internal and external validity and that can be replicated across diverse motivation domains. In addition to cross-domain replication, strong theories are bolstered by converging evidence that encompasses multiple indicators within domains. For instance, in achievement settings this may involve theoretically consistent effects on critical self-report measures (e.g., perceptions of competence) in conjunction with pertinent objective measures (e.g., test performance).

Beyond these attributes, strong theories specify *how* psychological processes interrelate via a process approach that focuses on mechanisms by which key theoretical variables influence motivation (Hayes, 2013). Such theories develop over extended periods of time and include a range of critical processes (cognitive, affective) that account for motivated behavior. Strong theories address questions concerning *when* and *under what conditions* the specified processes influence behavior (Cohen, Cohen, West, & Aiken, 2003; Hayes, 2013). Although strong theories predict motivational phenomena across domains, their utility in a given situation can depend on the context. Thus, to inform high-quality motivation treatments, strong theories include contextual variables that specify circumstances in which fundamental tenets hold true and when they do not.

Motivation Treatments and Experimental Design

High-quality motivation treatments are based on experimental designs that minimize threats to internal and external validity (Cohen et al., 2003; Cook & Campbell, 1979; Shadish, Cook, & Campbell, 2002). Internal validity concerns inferences about cause-effect linkages based on several criteria: the predictor (independent variable) precedes the outcome (dependent variable) in time; the predictor covaries with (causes) the outcome; and, alternative explanations for the predictor-outcome effect are improbable. Randomized treatment studies within laboratory settings provide ideal conditions to assess internal validity since they afford strong experimental control over extraneous influences on treatment effects (see Perry & Penner, 1990; Perry et al., 1994, 2010).

The external validity of motivation treatments concerns the generalizability of the cause (treatment)–effect relationship (Campbell & Stanley, 1963; Rosenthal & Rosnow, 2008). The assessment of external validity requires well-designed, randomized field trials that show treatment effects despite variation in settings, populations, and treatment iterations (e.g., Perry, Chipperfield, et al., 2014). Establishing internal validity (emphasizing experimental control) and external validity (emphasizing generalizability) is a process that unfolds over time and entails sustained programs of research that produce consistent findings (Shadish et al., 2002).

Whether focusing on internal or external validity, random assignment of participants to treatment conditions can establish unbiased estimates of treatment effects (Maxwell & Delaney, 2004). Doing so ensures that experimental treatment groups have equivalent expected values on relevant pretreatment variables (Rosenthal & Rosnow, 2008; Shadish et al., 2002). Sound experimental designs involve random assignment to treatment conditions and suitable comparison conditions that entail some combination of (1) no treatment, (2) an unrelated filler task, or (3) a conceptually relevant alternative treatment. Well-designed treatment studies assess multiple outcomes over time and include at least one pretest and posttest measure with which to examine selection biases and subject attrition in longitudinal field research.

Experimental design is improved when motivation protocols take into account treatment activation, content, delivery method, consolidation, boosters, and setting (see Haynes, Perry, Stupnisky, & Daniels, 2009; Perry, Chipperfield, et al., 2014). *Pretreatment activation tasks* entail procedures that initiate cognitive processes to heighten participant receptiveness and engagement with treatment content. *Treatment content* refers to the material (message) conveyed in the treatment designed to modify motivational states consistent with theory principles (e.g., adopting academic goals can increase performance). *Delivery method* pertains to procedures that are used to impart treatment content (e.g., text-based documents, audio or video formats, *in vivo* social exchanges). *Consolidation* involves posttreatment tasks that facilitate deep processing of treatment content through such procedures as group discussions, achievement tests, or writing assignments.

Boosters are posttreatment protocols that reintroduce aspects of the original treatment content after the initial administration. *Setting* refers to the context in which the treatment is presented to participants (e.g., individually, one-on-one, small groups, online distribution). Regardless of setting, high-quality treatment delivery procedures are standardized to ensure consistency within conditions (see Campbell & Stanley, 1963; Shadish et al., 2002). Hence, participants who receive a treatment in one session experience the same experimental procedures as those who receive them in another session (i.e., uniform administration of treatments).

Motivation Treatment Efficacy

The efficacy of motivation treatments rests on the reliability and magnitude of effects observed in laboratory and field trials. Reliability is inferred from evidence that shows the treatments consistently affect theoretically or logically derived outcomes. Reliability is supported by multiple studies demonstrating that treatment effects on such outcomes can be reproduced and are therefore robust. Magnitude verification implies that the *size* of these effects are important based on established criteria (Shadish et al., 2002). Cohen (1988) has proposed that $d = 0.20$ be considered a small effect; $d = 0.50$, a medium effect; and, $d = 0.80$ or higher, a large effect (p. 40).

Three types of empirical evidence may be used to verify that motivation treatment effects are reliable and substantial (Haynes et al., 2009; Shadish et al., 2002; Weiner, 2006). Type I empirical fidelity requires evidence that motivation treatments impact theory-related psychological process variables underpinning the treatment. Treatments informed by substantive conceptual frameworks include a broad range of psychological variables and demonstrate that the intervention impacts these outcomes in line with theoretical propositions. Thus, an emotion-based treatment designed to facilitate motivation should foster positive posttreatment emotions that contribute to adaptive motivational states (Pekrun, Chapter 14, this volume).

Type II empirical fidelity concerns evidence that a motivation treatment influences objective outcomes in relevant motivation domains. For instance, a control-enhancing treatment designed to increase motivation in an achievement setting should facilitate performance and persistence on theoretically or logically derived objective measures (e.g., final course grades). Establishing Type I and Type II treatment efficacy may involve (1) outcome changes over time (e.g., within-group Time 1 to Time 2 changes) and (2) posttreatment differences between experimental groups (e.g., treatment vs. no-treatment differences). The use of objective ("gold standard") outcomes can provide the most compelling evidence of Type II empirical fidelity.

Type III empirical fidelity combines Type I and Type II evidence and provides the strongest support for treatment efficacy whereby motivation interventions impact objective ("gold standard") measures via theoretically derived psychological processes. As such, Type III evidence entails a mediation approach that examines *how* treatments exert their influence. Field studies that include multiple posttreatment measurements are well suited to assess this form of fidelity in that they can examine longitudinal mediation models (path sequences) involving psychological variables that account for treatment effects on objective outcomes. Thus, an attribution-based treatment may influence long-term motivation and performance via a cascade of cognitive and affective changes (mediators) implied by theory, such as, attribution-based treatment → increased emphasis on adaptive attributions (e.g., effort) → high expectancy of future success → feelings of hope → enhanced motivation → improved performance.

Type III empirical fidelity is strengthened by designs that incorporate a pretreatment assessment of motivation and examine which individuals benefit from a treatment (moderation). Aptitude × Treatment Interaction (ATI) approaches, for example, imply that some treatments are more (less) effective for individuals who differ in critical qualities (cf. Cronbach & Snow, 1977; Perry et al., 2005). Qualities are aptitudes that vary between individuals and moderate treatment efficacy, such as age, personality, or gender. Field studies that assess treatment effects using moderation and mediation (conditional process modeling) are compelling in terms of empirical fidelity because they simultaneously test *how* and *under what conditions* the treatment has benefits (see Hayes, 2013). Thus, conditional process models test whether aptitude variables moderate (weaken, strengthen) a treatment's effects on theory-driven, mediated path sequences. See Table 5.1 for a summary of attribution path sequences, AR protocols, and the treatment evidence typology.

RESEARCH ON ATTRIBUTIONAL RETRAINING TREATMENTS

Attribution-based motivation treatments, referred to as AR, are designed to change maladaptive causal ascriptions and related motivation and performance outcomes (Perry, Chipperfield, et al., 2014). Based on Weiner (1970, 1985a, 2012), AR Treatment Protocols 1, 2, 3, and 4 foster internal (vs. external), unstable (vs. stable), and controllable (vs. uncontrollable) causes that are expected to influence cognitions, emotions, motivation, and performance. AR treatments are motivation interventions that are derived from an established social cognition theory, supported by a solid body of research, and readily adapted to diverse achievement and affiliative settings. They involve multicomponent treatment protocols that entail empirically supported theoretical propositions, presentation of context-relevant attribution information, structured delivery formats, and evidence-based consolidation procedures.

AR effects have been assessed in laboratory experiments and quasi-experimental

---

TABLE 5.1. Attribution-Based Paths Underpinning Competence Appraisals, AR Treatment Protocols, and AR Treatment Evidence Typology

Attribution-based paths contributing to maladaptive and adaptive competence appraisals

Path 1 (uncontrollable cause): Failure → low ability → cognition (*low competence appraisal*) → affect → low motivation → failure

Path 2 (controllable cause): Failure → bad strategy → cognition (*moderate competence appraisal*) → affect → moderate motivation → potential success

Attribution-based treatment protocols

Protocol 1: emphasize controllable causes (e.g., adaptive to attribute poor performance to insufficient effort, poor study strategy, lack of attention)

Protocol 2: deemphasize uncontrollable causes (e.g., maladaptive to attribute poor performance to lack of ability, teaching quality, test difficulty)

Protocol 3: do both (e.g., adaptive to focus on insufficient effort and poor strategy as causes of poor performance and to downplay ability, test difficulty)

Protocol 4: alter dimensional properties of causes (e.g., ability is unstable and can increase through persistent effort)

Attribution-based treatment evidence typology

Type I: psychological evidence (e.g., treatment has effects on cognitive, emotion, and motivation process variables consistent with theory)

Type II: achievement performance evidence (e.g., treatment has effects on objective performance outcomes, such as test grades, GPA, course withdrawals)

Type III: mediated and moderated performance evidence (e.g., treatment increases performance for failure-prone students via theory-derived process variables)

field trials using pre-post randomized treatment designs. Perry and colleagues (2010) conducted a prototypical longitudinal, quasi-experimental, randomized field study that examined AR treatment (vs. no treatment) efficacy for first-year students whose performance differed on an initial test in a two-semester course (low, average, high). A Protocol 3 AR treatment was presented early in the first semester in 1-hour laboratory sessions. The *causal search activation* stage required students to rate the contribution of several causes to previous academic failures only after they received feedback on their first course test.

Immediately thereafter, the *attribution induction* stage involved a video of two students who discussed how they improved their grades over time by changing their attributions for poor performance from uncontrollable (e.g., test difficulty) to controllable (e.g., insufficient effort). The *consolidation* stage required students to process treatment content deeply via (1) group discussion led by a trained research assistant or (2) writing an aptitude test that resulted in failure so students could apply the AR message by ascribing their poor performance to controllable causes. Data on theory-related attributions, emotions, and performance indicators were collected over an academic year.

Students who received AR (vs. no treatment) endorsed a controllable cause (bad strategy) and downplayed an uncontrollable cause (poor teaching) for failure 5 months posttreatment (Type I psychological evidence). For low- and average-initial-performance students, AR effects on performance (Type II evidence) were noteworthy: AR students did better than their no-AR peers by approximately one letter grade on classroom tests, final grades, and overall first-year grade point averages (GPAs). In the next sections, we review the theoretical underpinnings of AR treatments, the research design and methodology of AR studies, and the evidence informing AR treatment efficacy.

Attributional Retraining Treatments and Theoretical Fidelity

Given the merits of strong theory for designing high-quality motivation interventions,

Weiner's (1972, 1985a, 1986, 1995, 2006, 2012) attribution theory provides a substantive conceptual framework for the development of attribution-based treatment interventions. The fundamental principles are clear, specific, testable, and supported by over 45 years of empirical evidence from replicated laboratory and field studies. His theory describes a rich array of psychological processes (e.g., cognitions, emotions) that stem from the causal dimensions that govern motivated behavior (Figure 5.2). The theory is context-specific in stipulating that negative, important, and unexpected events elicit attribution → cognition → affect → motivation → behavior path sequences (e.g., failing a midterm examination after expecting to excel; Stupnisky, Stewart, Daniels, & Perry, 2011; Wong & Weiner, 1981). Based on this conceptual framework, high-quality attribution-based motivation treatments (1) modify key psychological processes that influence motivated behavior (e.g., causal ascriptions), (2) specify when recipients are amenable to treatment (e.g., following failure experiences), (3) prime recipients to receive treatment content (e.g., initiate causal search), and (4) identify high-risk (e.g., failure-prone) individuals who can benefit from treatment.

Fidelity of Experimental Designs Underpinning Attributional Retraining Studies

Attribution-based treatment studies conducted in achievement settings establish internal validity with experimental, randomized, laboratory designs and external validity with quasi-experimental, randomized, field designs. Common to each AR study in the next sections is the random assignment of participants to treatment conditions, which produces unbiased estimates of treatment effects (Maxwell & Delaney, 2004; Shadish et al., 2002). Each study design is also alike in that AR efficacy is based on posttreatment differences between an AR condition and relevant comparison condition (typically no treatment; i.e., AR vs. no-AR).

Early AR treatment studies stressed internal validity through well-controlled laboratory settings that simulated classroom analogue conditions. These include five classroom analogue studies that used common core experimental designs in which attribution-based treatments informed recipients that their performance on a test was due to effort (vs. ability or test difficulty; Perry et al., 1994; Perry & Magnusson, 1989), or that urged recipients to adopt controllable attributions for poor performance (vs. no treatment: Menec et al., 1994, Studies 1 and 2; Perry & Penner, 1990). The results of these laboratory-based AR Protocol 1 and Protocol 4 treatment studies were consistent in that AR recipients outperformed their peers in the no-treatment comparison conditions (Menec et al., 1994; Perry et al., 1994; Perry & Menec, 1989; Perry & Penner, 1990).

Twenty-two field studies used quasi-experimental, randomized treatment designs to assess the external validity of attribution-based treatment effects (Perry, Chipperfield, et al., 2014). The studies had similar quasi-experimental designs but varied in pre- and posttreatment assessments, time spans, and treatment comparison conditions. Sixteen AR Protocol 1, 2, and 3 studies showed that students who received AR did better than their no-AR peers on class tests, final grades, and year-end GPAs assessed up to 6 months posttreatment. Details on the treatment effects are provided below in the section "Empirical Fidelity of AR Efficacy" (Boese, Stewart, Perry, & Hamm, 2013; Hall et al., 2007; Hall, Hladkyj, Perry, & Ruthig, 2004; Hall, Perry, Chipperfield, Clifton, & Haynes, 2006; Hamm, Perry, Chipperfield, et al., 2014; Hamm, Perry, Clifton, Chipperfield, & Boese, 2014; Haynes-Stewart et al., 2011; Jesse & Gregory, 1986–1987; Noel, Forsyth, & Kelley, 1987; Parker et al., 2016; Perry & Struthers, 1994; Perry et al., 2010, 2015; Ruthig, Perry, Hall, & Hladkyj, 2004; Van Overwalle & de Matsenaere, 1990; Van Overwalle, Segebarth, & Goldchstein, 1989).

Further to randomly assigning students to treatment conditions, these AR field studies controlled critical confounds integral to competitive achievement settings by using covariance procedures (see Richardson, Abraham, & Bond, 2012). The majority controlled students' actual or self-reported high school grades (HSGs) in core disciplines (e.g., English, mathematics, chemistry, physics) given their notable influence on university GPA (*r* = .40; see the meta-analysis by Richardson et al., 2012). Several other studies controlled academic year, course load, faculty, registration status, age, or gender in demonstrating that attribution-based treatments promote achievement outcomes (e.g., Hall et al., 2004, 2007; Haynes-Stewart et al., 2011). Van Overwalle and colleagues (1989; Van Overwalle & de Metsenaere, 1990) adjusted for students' pretreatment (baseline) test performance and found that AR recipients outperformed their no-AR peers on a subsequent test and were less likely to fail their final examinations. Hall and colleagues (2004, 2006) replicated and extended these results whereby, controlling for pretreatment differences in motivation (e.g., perceived control, learning emotions), AR (vs. no-AR) recipients had higher scores on motivation measures 5 months posttreatment.

Five AR Protocol 1, 2, and 3 field studies assessed pre-post treatment changes in motivation and performance over extended time periods. Using a pre-post, quasi-experimental, randomized treatment design, Wilson and Linville (1982) found that AR (vs. no-AR) increased performance over a 12-month period. Several pre-post treatment field studies replicated and extended these results by showing that AR (vs. no-AR) improved performance and motivation outcomes up to 5 months posttreatment (Haynes, Daniels, Stupnisky, Perry, & Haldkyj, 2008; Haynes, Ruthig, Perry, Stupnisky, & Hall, 2006; Struthers & Perry, 1996; Wilson & Linville, 1985).

Moreover, AR Protocol 1, 2, 3, and 4 studies have consistently found effects on theory-related outcomes despite variability in treatment components (Perry, Chipperfield, et al., 2014). Activation (priming) procedures include (1) introducing AR only after students receive feedback on their first class test (e.g., Hamm, Perry, Clifton, et al., 2014), (2) asking students to rate the influence of causal attributions as a result of poor performance prior to AR (e.g., Perry et al., 2010), and (3) providing students with false failure feedback prior to AR (e.g., Menec et al., 1994). AR studies have varied in causal induction content, but typically they indicate that poor performance attributed to insufficient effort increases success (Protocol

1; e.g., Menec et al., 1994); performance improves over time (Protocol 2; e.g., Noel et al., 1987; Wilson & Linville, 1982); shifting emphasis from uncontrollable to controllable causes facilitates performance (Protocol 3; e.g., Perry et al., 2010); or persistent effort may increase ability (Protocol 4; Perry & Penner, 1990). AR treatment content has also contrasted adaptive and maladaptive attributions for poor test performance by emphasizing the benefits of adaptive causes (Protocol 3; e.g., Hall et al., 2006).

AR delivery methods used to present attribution-based treatment content have included student testimonials (e.g., Wilson & Linville, 1985), professor testimonials (e.g., Perry & Penner, 1990), and student social exchanges (e.g., Hamm, Perry, Clifton, et al., 2014). AR delivery methods also include live presentations by research assistants (e.g., Perry et al., 1994; Perry & Magnusson, 1989), text-based handouts (e.g., Hall et al., 2006), and narrated, text-based videos (e.g., Hamm, Perry, Chipperfield, et al., 2014; Parker et al., 2016). Contextual settings in which AR has been administered typically involve small groups of 10–50 students in a classroom environment (e.g., Perry et al., 2010; Wilson & Linville, 1982).

Recent studies have focused on mass delivery of attribution-based treatment content by developing scalable AR treatments for online achievement settings as part of blended learning courses that enable 2,500+ students to receive AR at times and locations of their choosing (e.g., Parker et al., 2016). Some AR studies standardized treatment delivery using scripted messages (e.g., Perry & Magnusson, 1989; Perry et al., 1994). Other studies standardized delivery with large-screen projectors that presented prerecorded (scripted) videos to groups of students (e.g., Perry & Penner, 1990) or with personal computers that employed automated software to enable online distribution (e.g., Hamm, Perry, Chipperfield, et al., 2014).

Four treatment consolidation procedures used in past studies include group discussion, aptitude tests, written elaboration of attribution content, and personalized causal attribution mapping. Group discussion promotes consolidation by having students describe the causes of their academic experiences with a group coordinator after AR content is presented (e.g., Struthers & Perry, 1996). Aptitude tests foster consolidation in presenting falsified failure feedback, so that students practice the AR treatment content by ascribing controllable or unstable attributions to the failure (e.g., Hall et al., 2004; Menec et al., 1994; Perry & Penner, 1990; Perry et al., 2010). The writing procedure promotes deep processing of attribution content whereby students summarize the AR content, then list reasons why they may not do well in their courses and how the AR treatment content applies to them (Hall et al., 2004, 2006). Variants of this procedure require students to summarize the AR content and discuss their conclusions with others (Van Overwalle & De Metsenaere, 1990; Van Overwalle et al., 1989).

Perry and colleagues (2013, 2015) have developed online causal attribution mapping (CAM) technology to personalize consolidation. Following AR treatment, the CAM procedure presents an online visual matrix (radar plot) of participants' pretreatment causal thinking using a four-cell attribution matrix. This attribution matrix combines the locus (internal, external) and controllability (controllable, uncontrollable) dimensions orthogonally and shows which quadrant depicts the student's causal thinking profile with a radar plot. Students whose causal thinking profile is portrayed by the external or uncontrollable quadrants receive immediate feedback that they should adopt internal–controllable attributions to maximize future performance. This personalized consolidation procedure seeks to foster deeper processing of AR treatment content and to promote its long-term retention (see Figure 5.4).

Few AR treatment protocols have used boosters to reinstate AR treatment content. An early laboratory study gave a booster 1 week after AR but found no evidence that treatment efficacy increased (Menec et al., 1994); a recent longitudinal, randomized treatment field trial provides more promising results (Perry, 2015). Longitudinal field studies are needed to clarify whether boosters can increase AR efficacy when administered on more than one occasion and over extended time intervals (e.g., every 2 months during the academic year).

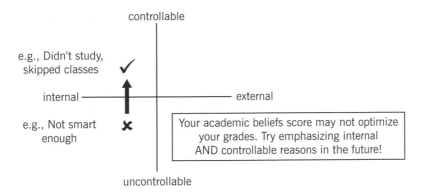

FIGURE 5.4. Online causal attribution mapping radar plot depicting an individual's causal thinking profile. From Perry et al. (2013). Copyright © 2013 by the authors. Adapted by permission.

Empirical Fidelity of Attributional Retraining Efficacy

Psychological Evidence (Type I)

Attribution-based treatment efficacy is supported by over 30 years of empirical evidence in achievement settings (Forsterling, 1985; Haynes et al., 2009; Perry et al., 2005; Perry, Chipperfield, et al., 2014). Type I (psychological) evidence concerns theory-related cognitions and emotions and consistently shows that AR can impact attribution-related outcomes. Causal attributions are proximal, theory-based psychological outcomes that AR treatments should change, as revealed by recipients endorsing internal, unstable, and controllable causes for poor performance, and/or disavowing uncontrollable causes (whether internal–external or stable–unstable).

Field studies show that AR recipients emphasize internal, unstable, controllable attributions for failure (e.g., poor strategy, low effort) posttreatment relative to their no-AR peers (e.g., Hamm, Perry, Clifton, et al., 2014; Haynes et al., 2006; Perry et al., 2010). Results support the efficacy of AR Protocol 1 treatments that instill controllable and unstable causes for achievement failure. These AR effects have implications for self-directed competence appraisals based on Weiner's (2005) propositions, whereby failure attributed to insufficient effort engenders a belief that future performance can improve (unstable) and is subject to personal modification (controllable). Ascribing poor

performance to insufficient effort or to poor study strategy (unstable, controllable causes) may preserve or improve perceived competence because one can always try harder or adopt a better study strategy in the future.

AR (vs. no-AR) treatments also alter uncontrollable attributions for failure that are *internal* and stable (e.g., low ability); *external* and stable (e.g., poor teaching); and external and *unstable* (e.g., test difficulty) (Hall et al., 2006; Hamm, Perry, Chipperfield, et al., 2014; Menec et al., 1994; Perry et al., 2010). Results support the efficacy of AR Protocol 2 treatments in modifying causal thinking by deemphasizing uncontrollable and/or stable causes for failure. AR effects on uncontrollable and stable attributions have implications for *self-directed* competence appraisals. Without treatment, such maladaptive attributions are theorized to result in beliefs that future failure is probable (stable cause) and cannot be avoided through personal action (uncontrollable cause).

Particularly detrimental to attribution-based competence appraisals are internal, stable, and uncontrollable causes, such as low ability. An emphasis on this attribution not only implies that nothing can be done to succeed in the future (stable, uncontrollable), but also that the cause of poor performance is directly due to personal qualities (internal). In other words, a low-ability attributions means that future failure is only inevitable for oneself. Thus, the capacity of AR treatments to curtail internal, stable, uncontrollable attributions following failure in achievement settings may reduce perceptions of personal incompetence appreciably.

Extending the research beyond single attributions (e.g., Haynes et al., 2006; Stewart, Chipperfield, Perry, & Weiner, 2012), Perry and colleagues (2010) and Hamm, Perry, Clifton, and colleagues (2014) used multivariate analyses of covariance (MANCOVA) and discriminant function analyses (DFA) to assess AR effects on multiple causal attributions. Perry and colleagues used this MANCOVA–DFA approach to examine posttreatment AR effects on complex causal thinking by assessing students' endorsement of multiple causes (e.g., effort, strategy, teaching quality, test difficulty). Their 6-month field study revealed DFA results (weightings) whereby AR (vs. no-AR) students jointly endorsed a controllable cause (bad strategy) and downplayed an uncontrollable cause (poor teaching) posttreatment. Hamm, Perry, Clifton, and colleagues replicated and extended these DFA results in showing that AR (vs. no-AR) recipients simultaneously favored strategy and disavowed poor teaching as causes of poor performance 5 months posttreatment. These effects on complex causal thinking (d = 0.56) underscore the capability of AR Protocol 3 treatments to both inculcate adaptive (controllable) and weaken maladaptive (uncontrollable) attributions.

Taken together, empirical evidence supports the efficacy of Protocol 1, 2, and 3 AR treatments to curb uncontrollable attributions (whether internal–external or stable–unstable) and to increase internal, unstable, and controllable attributions for poor performance. Based on the conceptual model in Figure 5.3b, such changes in causal thinking could boost attribution-based competence appraisals and subsequent motivational states by altering attribution path sequences following failure from maladaptive (e.g., low ability $\rightarrow$ low competence appraisal $\rightarrow$ low motivation $\rightarrow$ poor performance) to adaptive (e.g., low effort $\rightarrow$ higher competence appraisal $\rightarrow$ higher motivation $\rightarrow$ improved performance).

Some empirical evidence also indicates that AR Protocol 1 and AR Protocol 3 treatments influence other theory-related motivation outcomes. Laboratory and field studies show AR (vs. no-AR) positively influences students' beliefs about success, expectancies of future performance, and perceptions of control (Boese et al., 2013; Hall et al., 2004; Haynes et al., 2006; Menec et al., 1994). Field studies also reveal that AR recipients rate themselves as more responsible for their academic outcomes and report higher intrinsic and mastery motivation than their no-AR peers 5 months posttreatment (Boese et al., 2013; Hamm, Perry, Clifton, et al., 2014; Haynes et al., 2008).

These findings point to the potential of AR treatments to increase attribution-based competence motivation in keeping with Elliot and Dweck's (2005) observations in the first edition of this handbook. They argued that shifting the conceptual focus from *achievement* to *competence* motivation is advantageous because the latter represents a basic human need for competence or mastery (Deci & Ryan, 1990; Skinner, 1995; White, 1959). Fulfilling this psychological need may depend, in part, on maintaining perceptions of personal control (belief in one's capacity to influence events; see Skinner, 1996). Given that enhancing perceived (personal) control contributes to the need for competence/mastery, AR treatments may foster competence motivation in that students who receive AR (vs. no-AR) experience higher perceptions of control posttreatment (Hall et al., 2004) and increased perceived control over time (Haynes et al., 2006).

Finally, some research suggests AR Protocol 1 and AR Protocol 3 treatments enhance positive and diminish negative learning-related emotions. One field study showed that AR impacts two key emotions in achievement settings based on Pekrun's (2006; Chapter 14, this volume) control–value theory of emotion, in that AR (vs. no-AR) students reported more enjoyment and less boredom 5 months posttreatment (Hamm, Perry, Chipperfield, Clifton, & Dubberley, 2012). Several field studies point to AR's effects on attribution-related emotions consistent with Weiner's (1985a, 1995, 2012) theory. AR (vs. no-AR) students reported more hope and pride and less helplessness, shame, and anger posttreatment (Hall et al., 2004, 2007; Hamm, Perry, Chipperfield, et al., 2014; Hamm, Perry, Clifton, et al., 2014). As shown by Hamm, Perry, Clifton, and colleagues (2014), for failure prone students, AR effects on motivation and emotion (ds = 0.72, 0.57) were moderate and relatively consistent with those found for causal attributions (d = 0.56).

Achievement Performance Evidence (Type II)

Type II (achievement) evidence has received the most attention and is briefly summarized here, since our focus is on AR treatments and attribution-based competence appraisals (Type I evidence). See Perry, Chipperfield, and colleagues (2014) for a more comprehensive account of AR effects on performance. Five laboratory-based AR Protocol 1 and AR Protocol 4 studies show that AR recipients outperform their no-treatment peers on tests based on Graduate Record Exam (GRE)-like items, lecture material, and homework assignments given immediately following or 1 week posttreatment (Menec et al., 1994, Studies 1 and 2; Perry & Magnusson, 1989; Perry & Penner, 1990; Perry et al., 1994). Quasi-experimental AR Protocol 1, 2, and 3 field studies reveal that AR (vs. no-AR) facilitates performance on class tests, final course grades, and year-end GPAs up to 12 months posttreatment (e.g., Boese et al., 2013; Hall et al., 2004; Haynes et al., 2006; Perry et al., 2010; Wilson & Linville, 1982).

Other AR Protocol 1 and AR Protocol 3 field studies show that AR (vs. no-AR) recipients are less likely to fail year-end final exams and two-semester courses (Haynes-Stewart et al., 2011; Van Overwalle & De Metsenaere, 1990). Perry and colleagues (2010) found medium to large AR effects on performance: AR students whose initial test performance in a course was average did better than their no-AR peers by nearly a full standard deviation on a later class test (d = 0.92; Ms = 77 vs. 64%), a half standard deviation in final course grades (d = 0.43; Ms = 66 vs. 72%), and a half standard deviation on first-year cumulative GPAs (d = 0.51; Ms = 3.05 vs. 2.57). These means depict substantial effect sizes that translate into almost a one and a half letter grade advantage on a later test, and roughly a one letter grade gain on final course grades and cumulative GPAs.

Several AR Protocol 1 and AR Protocol 3 field studies show that AR treatments also impact *persistence* in achievement settings. Relative to their no-AR peers, AR recipients were less likely to withdraw from their courses over a 6-month period (Hamm, Perry, Clifton, et al., 2014; Parker et al., 2016) and more likely to graduate from university over a 5-year period (Perry, Hamm, et al., 2014). These studies highlight the magnitude of AR effects on "gold standard" persistence outcomes. Failure-prone students who received AR (vs. no-AR) were 61% less likely to withdraw from a course in their first year of university (26 vs. 48%) and more than twice as likely to graduate after 5 years in comparison to their no-AR counterparts (57 vs. 35%).

Mediated (and Moderated) Performance Evidence (Type III)

Type III evidence concerns AR effects on performance via theory-linked (mediated) psychological processes. AR Protocol 1 and AR Protocol 3 treatment studies have used mediation models and path analyses to test whether AR–performance links are due to changes in attributions, cognitions, emotions, and motivation consistent with Weiner's (1985a, 2012) theory. Hall and colleagues (2007) found that achievement emotions (i.e., happiness, pride, hope) mediated the influence of AR on course grades, and Haynes and colleagues (2008) showed that AR effects on students' GPAs were mediated by mastery motivation. Perry and colleagues (2012) extended these results by testing whether AR (vs. no-AR) influenced performance via a theoretical sequence of processes involving emotions and cognitions. AR impacted enjoyment and boredom 5 months posttreatment, which in turn affected cognitive elaboration and intrinsic motivation, and these predicted final course grades 6 months posttreatment.

These studies provide preliminary support for the premise that AR–performance effects are mediated by theory-derived psychological variables. However, a critical qualification is that attribution-based treatments primarily increase performance for failure-prone individuals who have motivation deficits, and hence experience difficulty adapting to novel or competitive achievement settings (Haynes et al., 2009; Perry, 2003). Research also indicates that AR benefits other motivationally at-risk individuals who have an external locus of control (Perry & Penner, 1990), are low in perceived success (Perry & Struthers, 1994), have objective failure experiences (Menec et al., 1994), are overly optimistic (Haynes et al., 2006), are high in failure-avoidance (Boese et al., 2013), or low in elaborative learning (Hall et al., 2004, 2007).

Given that AR treatments should indirectly improve the performance of failure-prone students, Hamm, Perry, Chipperfield, and colleagues (2014) simultaneously assessed *how* (mediators) and *under what conditions* (moderators) AR improves academic performance. Path analysis coupled with moderated mediation showed that for high-risk students with low levels of cognitive elaboration, an AR (vs. stress reduction) treatment reduced endorsements of uncontrollable causes for failure 5 months posttreatment (partially standardized β (beta) = −.33). In turn, deemphasizing uncontrollable attributions contributed to higher perceived academic control (β = .35) which predicted more positive (β = .24) and less negative (β = −.37) attribution-related emotions. Finally, perceived control (β = .08) and the positive (β = .35) and negative (β = −.12) emotions predicted overall course performance 6 months posttreatment.

Hamm, Perry, Chipperfield, and colleagues' (2014) study points to specific psychological processes by which AR treatments may foster adaptive attribution-based competence appraisals and motivation. Their findings suggest that AR effects on perceived control are mediated by attribution processes wherein AR enhances perceptions of control over time by reducing the endorsement of stable and uncontrollable causes (e.g., ability). These results provide indirect evidence that adaptive changes in causal thinking following AR may have positive consequences for long-term perceptions of personal competence. However, further research is needed to evaluate the impact of AR on competence using more direct measures of the construct.

ATTRIBUTIONAL RETRAINING AND CHANGING COMPETENCE APPRAISALS

Based on Weiner's (2005) theory, this chapter delineates how AR Protocol 1, 2, 3, and 4 treatments impact cognitive, affective, and motivation outcomes in achievement settings and, by implication, in competence appraisals. If *intrapersonal* ascriptions trigger competence appraisals in a manner similar to *interpersonal* personality inferences such as modesty and arrogance (Hareli & Weiner, 2000, 2002b), then AR can change these appraisals. Whether this logic accounts for competence appraisals and maladaptive motivational states depends on three assertions. First, Weiner's (1985a, 1986, 2012) theory provides an empirically validated framework for studying competence, assuming that competence appraisals arise from causal ascriptions. This analysis is depicted by Path 1 and Path 2 attribution sequences that portray competence appraisals arising from uncontrollable and controllable causes: *Path 1* = outcome → *uncontrollable* attribution → cognition (competence appraisal) → affect → motivation → performance; *Path 2* = outcome → *controllable* attribution → cognition (competence appraisal) → affect → motivation → performance.

Second, AR treatments are capable of changing competence appraisals given consistent research showing that AR modifies attribution processes and motivation outcomes (Perry, 2003; Perry et al., 2005; Perry, Chipperfield, et al., 2014). Informing this premise is that many AR studies exhibit best-evidence practices integral to the scientific method that include established theory; experimental designs having internal and external validity; replication of findings; and Type I (psychological), Type II (performance), and Type III (moderated mediation) effects that are moderate to large in size. Third, changing competence appraisals arising from Path 1 and Path 2 attribution sequences rests on four treatment alternatives: AR *Protocol 1* introduces or strengthens controllable causes; AR *Protocol 2* weakens uncontrollable causes; AR *Protocol 3* strengthens controllable causes *and* weakens uncontrollable causes; AR *Protocol 4* changes dimensional properties of maladaptive causes from uncontrollable to controllable or stable to unstable (e.g., low ability as unstable rather than stable).

Future research is needed to address the efficacy of the AR protocols to change competence appraisals with respect to Path 1 and Path 2 attribution sequences. For example, AR Protocol 2 may change a Path 1 (uncontrollable cause) competence appraisal, but it may not be required to change a Path 2 (controllable cause) competence appraisal that is adaptive. Though AR Protocols 1, 2, 3, and 4 offer opportunities to change competence appraisals, research is lacking on AR Protocol 4 efficacy with respect to Type I (psychological), Type II (performance), and Type III (moderated mediation) outcomes. Also unresolved is the efficacy of AR Protocols 1, 2, 3, and 4 when compared to each other. Beyond these questions, several issues bear further attention given that AR's benefits for young adults in achievement settings is both persuasive and encouraging (see Perry, Chipperfield, et al., 2014).

Attributional Retraining Self-Regulation and Competence Appraisals

New technologies offer opportunities to individualize AR treatments using self-regulation processes that require active (vs. passive) cognitive engagement. One possibility entails personalized attributional information, whereby AR recipients view their pretreatment attributions as a causal search activation or consolidation procedure. AR that involves such active engagement procedures may facilitate deeper processing of content tailored to each recipient. For example, Perry and colleagues (2013) introduced an online, personalized, attribution-based treatment that can be delivered to recipients from any location with Internet access. The consolidation procedure gave students a visual illustration of their ascriptions for performance using causal attribution mapping (CAM) technology (see Figure 5.4).

CAM technology actively engages deep cognitive processing of attribution content by having students reflect on and respond to their pretreatment attribution thinking patterns depicted by the four-cell (internal vs. external, controllable vs. uncontrollable) radar plot described earlier. Students who endorsed external or uncontrollable causes for poor performance pretreatment received a message encouraging them to adopt internal–controllable attributions. The CAM procedure had recipients describe how they could apply this personalized attribution feedback to their daily lives. The cognitive elaboration of the individualized attribution feedback was expected to promote deep processing of treatment material, improve content retention, and increase AR treatment efficacy.

As noted by Hamm, Perry, Chipperfield, and colleagues (2014), Weiner's (1985a, 2012) construal of causal search suggests conceptual parallels to cognitive elaboration. Weiner posits causal search involves an appraisal process to specify the causes of success or failure. Not unlike cognitive elaboration, causal search involves attending to circumstances that led to the outcome, integrating pertinent situational information, and analyzing and specifying factors that contributed to the outcome. This implies causal search and cognitive elaboration may share similarities concerning the appraisal of context-relevant information and a metacognitive synthesis of existing and new knowledge to adapt to novel learning conditions inherent in the transition to college. For instance, effective causal search depends on (1) being aware of relevant, possible determinants of an outcome and (2) deeply reflecting on this information so as to come to a functional attribution that facilitates adaptation. Similarly, effective cognitive elaboration requires (1) being aware of relevant, existing knowledge and (2) reflecting deeply on how such knowledge relates to new information so as to understand and apply novel material that fosters adaptation. Thus, these constructs may share common roots in information processing, and both may be motivated by a need for mastery.

Attributional Retraining and Competence Appraisals across the Lifespan

AR treatments that alter competence appraisals are relevant across the lifespan, particularly so for life-course transitions that erode appraisals of personal competence.

School-to-college transitions, for example, are imbued with pressures to excel, novel tasks, difficult course content, frequent failures, financial demands, and unstable social networks that can have detrimental effects on perceptions of personal competence (cf. Perry, 1991, 2003; Perry et al., 2005). Perry and colleagues' (2008) comprehensive field study of five separate 1-year cohorts (*n* > 3,000) reveals that nearly half of first-year students exhibit maladaptive causal thinking during such transitions, characterized by uncontrollable factors deemed to be major determinants of performance. The efficacy of attribution-based treatments to reduce uncontrollable attributions in these *devalued control* and *relinquish control* students holds promise for other demanding periods in the life course when AR may be an effective motivation treatment.

Few studies, however, have administered AR treatments to other vulnerable populations striving for important goals in which competence also features prominently. For example, the number of U.S. adults aged 65+ will double from 2010 to 2050, and though people now live longer, old age is accompanied by increasing dependence that undermines perceptions of competence (Centers for Disease Control and Prevention, 2013). From an attribution theory perspective, these developments might be ameliorated through the development of AR treatments that delay the onset of functional dependence. Internal, stable, and uncontrollable causal ascriptions arising from negative outcomes inherent in the aging process may be important in this regard. Such maladaptive causes weaken perceptions of competence in both early (e.g., test failure ascribed to low ability) and late adulthood (e.g., falling ascribed to old age) because they imply that the event will likely recur (stable) and cannot be avoided through personal action (uncontrollable).

Research on older adults is consistent with this logic and the detriments of attributing negative life events to low ability in young adults (e.g., Perry et al., 2008). Stewart, Chipperfield, Perry, and Hamm (2016) found that endorsing old age as a cause of heart attack or stroke negatively predicted lifestyle behavior change, and positively predicted frequency of physician visits and likelihood of hospitalization over 3 years. Underscoring the harmful consequences of this internal, stable, and uncontrollable cause is evidence that older adults who attribute health problems to old age (vs. those who did not) experienced more health symptoms, engaged in fewer health-promoting behaviors, and were more than twice as likely to die over a 2-year follow-up (36 vs. 14%; Stewart et al., 2012).

Thus, AR treatments may have benefits for older adults in terms of health and dependence outcomes (see Sarkisian et al., 2007). Similar to attribution-based treatments for young adults, AR could reshape older adults' causal thinking by replacing stable–uncontrollable attributions for health problems (old age) with adaptive causes that are unstable–controllable (insufficient activity). Such adaptive changes in causal thinking may reduce attribution-based appraisals of personal incompetence and sustain health engagement, functional independence, and autonomy at a critical juncture in the lifespan.

Whether causal thinking gives rise to competence appraisals, as Weiner (2005) proposes, or whether attribution-based treatments can change maladaptive competence appraisals are open questions subject to empirical verification. This chapter provides the logical argumentation and preliminary empirical evidence that support affirmative responses to both questions under certain conditions. Just as causal ascriptions can be a source of personality inferences, such as modesty and arrogance, they may contribute in a similar manner to competence appraisals. If so, then AR treatments may replace maladaptive with adaptive competence appraisals given that they can change causal attributions, such as low ability, that trigger low competence appraisals. With this in mind, four AR protocols can change maladaptive (Path 1) to adaptive (Path 2) attribution sequences (see Table 5.1 and Figure 5.3b). Although research is lacking that shows AR alters competence appraisals, abundant evidence supports the efficacy of AR in changing causal attributions; thus, it seems plausible that AR can modify competence appraisals arising from such ascriptions.

ACKNOWLEDGMENTS

This research was supported by grants awarded to Raymond P. Perry from the Royal Society of Canada, the Social Sciences and Humanities Research Council of Canada (435–2012–1143), and the Alexander von Humboldt Foundation (Germany), and a Social Sciences and Humanities Research Council of Canada Postdoctoral Fellowship to Jeremy M. Hamm. We are indebted to Bernard Weiner (UCLA) and Judith G. Chipperfield (University of Manitoba) for their insightful and informative comments on previous drafts of the chapter.

REFERENCES

American College Health Association. (2012). *American College Health Association National College Health Assessment II: Reference group executive summary fall 2012.* Hanover, MD: Author.

Baumeister, R. F., & Leary, M. (1995). The need to belong: Desire for interpersonal attachments as a fundamental human motivation. *Psychological Bulletin, 117*(3), 497–529.

Boese, G. D., Stewart, T. L., Perry, R. P., & Hamm, J. M. (2013). Assisting failure prone individuals to navigate achievement transitions using a cognitive motivation treatment (attributional retraining). *Journal of Applied Social Psychology, 43*(9), 1946–1955.

Brown, J., & Weiner, B. (1984). Affective consequences of ability and effort ascriptions: Controversies, resolutions, and quandaries. *Journal of Educational Psychology, 76,* 146–158.

Campbell, D. T., & Stanley, J. C. (1963). *Experimental and quasi-experimental designs for research.* Boston: Houghton Mifflin.

Centers for Disease Control and Prevention. (2013). *The state of aging and health in America 2013.* Atlanta, GA: U.S. Department of Health and Human Services

Chapin, M., & Dyck, D. (1976). Persistence in children's reading behavior as a function of *N* length and attributional retraining. *Journal of Abnormal Psychology, 85,* 511–515.

Cohen, J. (1988). *Statistical power analysis for the behavioral sciences.* Hillsdale, NJ: Erlbaum.

Cohen, J., Cohen, P., West, S. G., & Aiken, L. S. (2003). *Applied multiple regression/correlation analysis for the behavioral sciences* (3rd ed.). London: Erlbaum.

Cook, T. D., & Campbell, D. T. (1979). *Quasi-experimentation: Design and analysis issues for field settings.* Boston: Houghton Mifflin.

Covington, M. V., & Omelich, C. L. (1984). Controversies or consistencies?: A reply to Brown and Weiner. *Journal of Educational Psychology, 76,* 159–168.

Cronbach, L. J., & Snow, R. E. (1977). *Aptitudes and instructional methods: A handbook for research on interactions.* Oxford, UK: Irvington.

de Charms, R. (1968). *Personal causation: The internal affective determinants of behavior.* New York: Plenum Press.

Deci, E. L., & Ryan, R. M. (1990). A motivational approach to the self: Integration in personality. In R. Dienstbier (Ed.), *Nebraska Symposium on Motivation* (Vol. 38, pp. 237–288). Lincoln: University of Nebraska Press.

Elliot, A. J., & Dweck, C. S. (2005). Competence and motivation: Competence as the core of achievement motivation. In A. J. Elliot & C. S. Dweck (Eds.), *Handbook of competence and motivation* (pp. 3–14). New York: Guilford Press.

Erikson, E. H. (1963). *Childhood and society* (2nd ed.). New York: Norton.

Fiske, S. T., & Taylor, S. E. (1991). *Social cognition* (2nd ed.). New York: McGraw-Hill.

Forsterling, F. (1985). Attributional retraining: A review. *Psychological Bulletin, 98,* 495–512.

Hall, N. C., Hladkyj, S., Perry, R. P., & Ruthig, J. C. (2004). The role of attributional retraining and elaborative learning in college students' academic development. *Journal of Social Psychology, 144,* 591–612.

Hall, N. C., Perry, R. P., Chipperfield, J. G., Clifton, R. A. & Haynes, T. L. (2006). Enhancing primary and secondary control in achievement settings through writing-based attributional retraining. *Journal of Social and Clinical Psychology, 25,* 361–391.

Hall, N. C., Perry, R. P., Goetz, T., Ruthig, J. C., Stupnisky, R. H. & Newall, N. E. (2007). Attributional retraining and elaborative learning: Improving academic development through writing-based interventions. *Learning and Individual Differences, 17,* 280–290.

Hamm, J. M., Perry, R. P., Chipperfield, J. G., Clifton, R. A., & Dubberley, K. M. A. (2012, April). *Attributional Retraining: Facilitating emotional stability in vulnerable young adults in transition.* Paper presented at the annual meeting of the Western Psychological Association, San Francisco, CA.

Hamm, J. M., Perry, R. P., Chipperfield, J. G., Parker, P. C., Murayama, K., & Weiner, B. (2014, February). *Facilitating adaptive explanatory thinking among vulnerable young adults using attributional retraining: Long-term effects on cognition, emotion, and performance.* Paper presented at the annual meeting of the Society for Personality and Social Psychology, Austin, TX.

Hamm, J. M., Perry, R. P., Clifton, R. A., Chipperfield, J. G., & Boese, G. (2014). Attributional retraining: A motivation treatment with differential psychosocial and performance benefits for failure prone individuals in competitive achievement settings. *Basic and Applied Social Psychology, 36,* 221–237.

Hareli, S., & Weiner, B. (2000). Accounts for success as determinants of perceived arrogance and modesty. *Motivation and Emotion, 24*(3), 215–236.

Hareli, S., & Weiner, B. (2002a). Dislike and envy as antecedents of pleasure at another's misfortune. *Motivation and Emotion, 26*(4), 257–277.

Hareli, S., & Weiner, B. (2002b). Social emotions and personality inferences: A scaffold for a new direction in the study of motivation. *Educational Psychologist, 37*(3), 183–193.

Hayes, A. F. (2013). *Introduction to mediation, moderation, and conditional process analysis: A regression-based approach.* New York: Guilford Press.

Haynes, T. L., Daniels, L. M., Stupnisky, R. H., Perry, R. P., & Hladkyj, S. (2008). The effect of attributional retraining on mastery and performance motivation among first-year college students. *Basic and Applied Social Psychology, 30,* 198–207.

Haynes, T. L., Perry, R. P., Stupnisky, R. H., & Daniels, L. M. (2009). A review of attributional retraining treatments: Fostering engagement in college students. In J. Smart (Ed.), *Higher education: Handbook of theory and research* (Vol. 24, pp. 227–272). New York: Springer.

Haynes, T. L., Ruthig, J. C., Perry, R. P., Stupnisky, R. H., & Hall, N. C. (2006). Reducing the academic risks of over-optimism: The longitudinal effects of attributional retraining on cognition and achievement. *Research in Higher Education, 47,* 755–779.

Haynes-Stewart, T. H., Clifton, R. A., Daniels, L., M., Perry, R., P., Chipperfield, J., G., & Ruthig, J., C. (2011). Attributional retraining: Reducing the likelihood of failure. *Social Psychology of Education, 14,* 75–92.

Heckhausen, J., Wrosch, C., & Schulz, R. (2010). A motivational theory of life-span development. *Psychological Review, 117*(1), 32–60.

Heider, F. (1944). Social perception and phenomenal causality. *Psychological Review, 51,* 358–374.

Heider, F. (1958). *The psychology of interpersonal relations.* New York: Wiley.

Jesse, D. M., & Gregory, W. L. (1986–1987). A comparison of three attributional approaches to maintaining first year college GPA. *Educational Research Quarterly, 11,* 12–25.

Jones, E. E., & Davis, K. E. (1965). From acts to dispositions: The attribution process in person perception. In L. Berkowitz (Ed.), *Advances in experimental social psychology* (Vol. 2, pp. 219–266). New York: Academic Press.

Jones, E. E., Kanouse, D. E., Kelley, H. H., Nisbett, R. E., Valins, S., & Weiner, B. (1971). *Attribution: Perceiving the causes of behavior.* Morristown, NJ: General Learning Press.

Kelley, H. H. (1967). *Attribution theory in social psychology.* In D. Levine (Ed.), *Nebraska Symposium on Motivation* (Vol. 15, pp. 129–238). Lincoln: University of Nebraska Press.

Lewin, K. (1951). *Field theory in social science: Selected theoretical papers* (D. Cartwright, Ed.). New York: Harper & Row.

Maxwell, S. E., & Delaney, H. D. (2004). *Designing experiments and analyzing data: A model Comparison perspective* (2nd ed.). Mahwah, NJ: Erlbaum.

Menec, V. H., Perry, R. P., Struthers, C. W., Schönwetter, D. J., Hechter, F. J., & Eichholz, B. L. (1994). Assisting at-risk college students with attributional retraining and effective teaching. *Journal of Applied Social Psychology, 24,* 675–701.

Noel, J. G., Forsyth, D. R., & Kelley, K. (1987). Improving performance of failing students by overcoming self-serving attributional biases. *Basic and Applied Psychology, 8,* 151–162.

Parker, P. C., Perry, R. P., Hamm, J. M., Chipperfield, J. G., & Hladkyj, S. (2016). Enhancing the academic success of high-risk competitive student athletes using a motivation treatment intervention (attributional retraining). *Psychology of Sport and Exercise, 26,* 113–122.

Pekrun, R. (2006). The control–value theory of achievement emotions: Assumptions, corollaries, and implications for educational research. *Educational Psychology Review, 18,* 315–341.

Perry, R. P. (1991). Perceived control in college students: Implications for instruction in higher education. In J. Smart (Ed.), *Higher education: Handbook of theory and research* (Vol. 7, pp. 1–56). New York: Agathon Press.

Perry, R. P. (2003). Perceived (academic) control and causal thinking in achievement settings: Markers and mediators. *Canadian Psychologist, 44,* 312–331.

Perry, R. P. (2015). *Motivation boosters to enhance AR treatment efficacy.* Unpublished data analysis, Department of Psychology, University of Manitoba, Winnipeg, Canada.

Perry, R. P., Chipperfield, J. G., Hladkyj, S.,

Pekrun, R., & Hamm, J. M. (2014). Attribution-based treatment interventions in some achievement settings. In S. Karabenick & T. Urdan (Eds.), *Advances in motivation and achievement* (Vol. 18, pp. 1–35). Bingley, UK: Emerald.

Perry, R. P., Chipperfield, J. G., Pekrun, R., Chuchmach, L., Stewart, T. L., & Murayama, K. (2012, January). *Attributional retraining in achievement settings: Longitudinal effects of a motivation treatment on cognition, emotion, and performance.* Paper presented at the Hawaii International Conference on Education, Honolulu, HI.

Perry, R. P., Hall, N. C., & Ruthig, J. C. (2005). Perceived (academic) control and scholastic attainment in higher education. In J. C. Smart (Ed.), *Higher education: Handbook of theory and research* (Vol. 20, pp. 363–436). Dordrecht, The Netherlands: Springer.

Perry, R. P., & Hamm, J. M. (2015). *Attributions and competence.* Unpublished data analysis, Department of Psychology, University of Manitoba, Winnipeg, Manitoba, Canada.

Perry, R. P., Hamm, J. M., Chipperfield, J. C., Hladkyj, S., Parker, P. C., & Pekrun, R. (2014, February). *Long-term benefits of an attribution-based treatment intervention in competitive achievement settings: Five-year graduation rates.* Paper presented at the annual meeting of the Society for Personality and Social Psychology, Austin, TX.

Perry, R. P., Hamm, J. M., Chipperfield, J. G., Hladkyj, S., Parker, P. C., & Pekrun, R. (2015, February). *An attribution-based treatment intervention in competitive achievement settings.* Paper presented at the annual meeting of the Society for Personality and Social Psychology, Long Beach, CA.

Perry, R. P., Hechter, F. J., Menec, V. H., & Weinberg, L. E. (1993). Enhancing achievement motivation and performance in college students: An attributional retraining perspective. *Research in Higher Education, 34,* 687–723.

Perry, R. P., Hladkyj, S, Wiebe, K., Chipperfield, J. G., Hamm, J. M., & Parker, P. C. (2013, January). *A cognitive (motivation) treatment intervention to facilitate the transition from high school to college.* Paper presented at the Hawaii International Conference on Education, Oahau, HI.

Perry, R. P., & Magnusson, J. (1989). Causal attributions and perceived performance: Consequences for college students' achievement and perceived control in different instructional conditions. *Journal of Educational Psychology, 81,* 164–172.

Perry, R. P., & Penner, K. S. (1990). Enhancing academic achievement in college students through attributional retraining. *Journal of Educational Psychology, 82,* 262–271.

Perry, R. P., Schönwetter, D. J., Magnusson, J. L., & Struthers, C. W. (1994). Students' explanatory schemas and the quality of college instruction: Some evidence for buffer and compensation effects. *Research in Higher Education, 35,* 349–371.

Perry, R. P., & Struthers, C. W. (1994, April). *Attributional retraining in the college classroom: Some causes for optimism.* Paper presented at the annual meeting of the American Educational Research Association, New Orleans, LA.

Perry, R. P., Stupnisky, R. H., Daniels, L. M., & Haynes, T. L. (2008). Attributional (explanatory) thinking about failure in new achievement settings. *European Journal of Psychology of Education, 23*(4), 459–475.

Perry, R. P., Stupnisky, R. H., Hall, N. C., Chipperfield, J. G., & Weiner, B. (2010). Bad starts and better finishes: Attributional retraining and initial performance in competitive achievement settings. *Journal of Social and Clinical Psychology, 29*(6), 668–700.

Richardson, M., Abraham, C., & Bond, R. (2012). Psychological correlates of university students' academic performance: A systematic review and meta-analysis. *Psychological Bulletin, 138*(2), 353–387.

Rosenthal, R., & Rosnow, R. L. (2008). *Essentials of behavioral research: Methods and data analysis* (3rd ed.). New York: McGraw-Hill.

Rotter, J. B. (1954). *Social learning and clinical psychology.* New York: Prentice-Hall.

Ruthig, J. C., Perry, R. P., Hall, N., & Hladkyj, S. (2004). Optimism and attributional retraining: Longitudinal effects on academic achievement, test anxiety, and voluntary course withdrawal in college students. *Journal of Applied Social Psychology, 34,* 709–730.

Sarkisian, C. A., Prohaska, T. R., Davis, C., & Weiner, B. (2007). Pilot test of an attribution retraining intervention to raise walking levels in sedentary older adults. *Journal of the American Geriatrics Society, 55,* 1842–1846.

Shadish, W. R., Cook, T. D., & Campbell, D. T. (2002). *Experimental and quasi-experimental designs for generalized causal inference.* Boston: Houghton Mifflin.

Skinner, E. A. (1995). *Perceived control, motivation, and coping.* Thousand Oaks, CA: Sage.

Skinner, E. A. (1996). A guide to constructs of control. *Journal of Personality and Social Psychology, 71*(3), 549–570.

Snyder, T. D., & Dillow, S. A. (2013). *Digest of Education Statistics 2012* (NCES 2014-015). Washington, DC: National Center for

Education Statistics, Institute of Education Sciences, U.S. Department of Education.

Stewart, T. L., Chipperfield, J. G., Perry, R. P., & Hamm, J. M. (2016). Attributing heart attack and stroke to "old age": Implications for subsequent health outcomes among older adults. *Journal of Health Psychology, 21*(1), 40–49.

Stewart, T. L., Chipperfield, J. G., Perry, R. P., & Weiner, B. (2012). Attributing illness to "old age": Consequences of a self-directed stereotype for health and mortality. *Psychology and Health, 27,* 881–897.

Storms, M. D., & Nisbett, R. E. (1970). Insomnia and the attribution process. *Journal of Personality and Social Psychology, 16,* 319–328.

Struthers, C. W., & Perry, R. P. (1996). Attributional style, attributional retraining, and inoculation against motivational deficits. *Social Psychology of Education, 1,* 171–187.

Stupnisky, R. H., Stewart, T. L., Daniels, L. M., & Perry, R. P. (2011). When do students ask why?: Examining the precursors and outcomes of causal search among first-year college students. *Contemporary Educational Psychology, 36*(3), 201–211.

Van Overwalle, F., & de Metsenaere, M. (1990). The effects of attribution-based intervention and study strategy training on academic achievement in college freshmen. *British Journal of Educational Psychology, 60,* 299–311.

Van Overwalle, F., Segebarth, K., & Goldchstein, M. (1989). Improving performance of freshmen through attributional testimonies from fellow students. *British Journal of Educational Psychology, 59,* 75–85.

Weiner, B. (1970). New conceptions in the study of achievement motivation. *Progress in Experimental Personality Research, 5,* 67–109.

Weiner, B. (1972). *Theories of motivation: From mechanism to cognition.* Chicago: Markham.

Weiner, B. (1979). A theory of motivation for some classroom experiences. *Journal of Educational Psychology, 71,* 3–25.

Weiner, B. (1983). Some methodological pitfalls in attributional research. *Journal of Educational Psychology, 75*(4), 530–543.

Weiner, B. (1985a). An attributional theory of achievement motivation and emotion. *Psychological Review, 92,* 548–573.

Weiner, B. (1985b). "Spontaneous" causal thinking. *Psychological Bulletin, 97,* 74–84.

Weiner, B. (1986). *An attributional theory of achievement motivation and emotion.* New York: Springer-Verlag.

Weiner, B. (1988). Attribution theory and attributional therapy: Some theoretical observations and suggestions. *British Journal of Clinical Psychology, 27,* 93–104.

Weiner, B. (1995). *Judgments of responsibility: A foundation for a theory of social conduct.* New York: Guilford Press.

Weiner, B. (2005). Motivation from an attribution perspective and the social psychology of perceived competence. In A. J. Elliot & C. S. Dweck (Eds.), *Handbook of competence and motivation* (pp. 73–84). New York: Guilford Press.

Weiner, B. (2006). *Social motivation, justice, and the moral emotions: An attributional approach.* Mahwah, NJ: Erlbaum.

Weiner, B. (2012). An attribution theory of motivation. In P. A. M. Van Lange, A. W. Kruglanski, & E. T. Higgins (Eds.), *Handbook of theories of social psychology* (Vol. 1, pp. 135–155). Thousand Oaks, CA: Sage.

Weiner, B., & Brown, J. (1984). All's well that ends. *Journal of Educational Psychology, 76,* 169–171.

White, R. W. (1959). Motivation reconsidered: The concept of competence. *Psychological Review, 66*(5), 297–333.

Wilson, T. D., & Linville, P. W. (1982). Improving the academic performance of college freshmen: Attribution therapy revisited. *Journal of Personality and Social Psychology, 42,* 367–376.

Wilson, T. D., & Linville, P. W. (1985). Improving the performance of college freshmen with attributional techniques. *Journal of Personality and Social Psychology, 49,* 287–293.

Wong, P. T., & Weiner, B. (1981). When people ask "why" questions, and the heuristics of attributional search. *Journal of Personality and Social Psychology, 40*(4), 650–663.

CHAPTER 6

Competence Self-Perceptions

HERBERT W. MARSH
ANDREW J. MARTIN
ALEXANDER SEESHING YEUNG
RHONDA G. CRAVEN

More than a decade ago, Elliot and Dweck (2005) concluded that competency self-perceptions are all-pervasive and powerful, "a basic psychological need that has a pervasive impact on daily life, cognition and behavior, across age and culture . . . an ideal cornerstone on which to rest the achievement motivation literature but also a foundational building block for any theory of personality, development and well-being" (p. 8). Perceived competencies are a key construct in most theoretical models of achievement motivation, and have been widely studied since the beginning of psychological research. The popularity of research into competence self-perceptions and associated positive self-belief constructs stems from their universal importance and multidisciplinary appeal. The importance of these constructs is highlighted by the frequency with which their enhancement is identified as a major focus of concern in diverse settings, including education, child development, mental and physical health, social services, industry, and sports/exercise. For many developmental researchers and early childhood programs (e.g., Fantuzzo, McDermott, Manz, Hampton, & Burdick,

1996), self-concept and competence perceptions more generally have been a "cornerstone of both social and emotional development" (Kagen, Moore, & Bredekamp, 1995, p. 18; also see Davis-Kean & Sandler, 2001; Marsh, Ellis, & Craven, 2002). Similarly, the importance of a person's sense of competence has been widely accepted as a critical psychological construct that leads to success in educational settings (Chen, Yeh, Hwang, & Lin, 2013; Marsh & Craven, 2006; Marsh & Yeung, 1997a, 1977b), social and emotional situations (Donahue, Robins, Roberts, & John, 1993; Harter, 2012; Marsh, Parada, Craven, & Finger, 2004), and daily life more generally (Elliot & Dweck, 2005). However, given the plethora of ways to conceptualize competence self-perceptions, in this chapter we discuss the different operationalizations of competence self-perceptions and the implications for advancing theory, research, and practice.

Indeed, there is a revolution sweeping psychology (e.g., Seligman & Csikszentmihalyi, 2000) that emphasizes a positive psychology, focusing on how healthy, normal, and exceptional individuals can get the most from life. Self-perceptions of competence and associated positive self-beliefs, as emphasized in this chapter, are at the heart of this revolution (Bandura, 2008a, 2008b; Bruner, 1996; Hunter & Csikszentmihalyi, 2003; Marsh & Craven, 2006). More generally, the phenomena of perceived competence and associated self-beliefs are widely accepted as a universal aspect of being human and as central to understanding the quality of human existence (Bandura, 2008a, 2008b; Bruner, 1996; Harter, 1986, 1998; Marsh & Craven, 2006; Schunk & Pajares, 2005). Thus, an individual's sense of competence has become central to the field of positive psychology (Marsh & Craven, 2006; Seligman & Csikszentmihalyi, 2000). Furthermore, a person's sense of competence in a specific domain not only leads to a range of positive outcomes in that domain but may also influence his or her competence perceptions in other domains and modify how that person acts, feels, and adjusts to a changing environment.

DIFFERENT THEORETICAL CONCEPTUALIZATIONS OF COMPETENCE PERCEPTIONS

Researchers have conceptualized competence self-beliefs in different ways and from a variety of theoretical perspectives (e.g., self-concept, self-esteem, self-efficacy, expectations of success, confidence, competency). In the social sciences, particularly in the motivation and self-belief areas, researchers tend to focus on their preferred constructs, paying relatively little attention to testing how (or whether) they differ from other constructs. This leads to jingle-jangle fallacies (Marsh, 1994; Marsh, Craven, Hinkley, & Debus, 2003), in which two scales with similar names might measure different constructs while two scales with apparently dissimilar labels might measure similar constructs. In this chapter we operationalize competence perceptions as the competence component of self-concept, but we also juxtapose the different terms used to represent competency self-perceptions, in an attempt to clarify some of the prevalent areas of confusion (also see Schunk & Pajares [2005], which is organized around self-efficacy).

Definition of Self-Concept

The construct of self-concept has had a long and illustrious history, dating back to Socrates and Plato (see Hattie, 1992); Marsh (2007) has argued that current self-concept theories can be traced back to William James. In his seminal work, *The Principles of Psychology* (1890/1963), James proposed that the self is both multifaceted and hierarchical, "with the bodily Self at the bottom, the spiritual Self at the top, and the extracorporeal material selves and the various social selves between" (p. 313). This assertion, along with James's distinction between the self-as-knower, the I, and the self-as-known, the Me, played an important role in developing self-concept theory. However, despite the rich beginning provided by James, advances in theory, research, and measurement of self-concept were slow, particularly during the heyday of behaviorism. Researchers in that era (e.g., Shavelson, Hubner, & Stanton, 1976; Wells & Marwell, 1976; Wylie, 1979) noted the poor quality of the theoretical models and self-concept measurement instruments, leading Shavelson and colleagues (1976) to conclude, "it appears that self-concept research has addressed itself to substantive problems before problems of definition, measurement, and interpretation have been resolved" (p. 410). Similarly, Hattie (1992) described this period as one of "dustbowl empiricism," in which the predominant research design in self-concept studies was "throw it in and see what happens." Thus, in her review of self-concept research, Byrne (2002) concluded, "Without question, the most profound happening in self-concept research during the past century was the wake-up call sounded regarding the sorry state of its reported findings, which was followed by a conscious effort on the part of methodologically oriented researchers to rectify the situation" (p. 898).

In the period since the 1980s, self-concept research has seen a renaissance, characterized by growth in the quality and sophistication of the theoretical models, quantitative methodology, measurement instruments, and research design. This was stimulated in part by Shavelson and colleagues' (1976) seminal review article, which reviewed existing self-concept research and instruments, proposed a new theoretical model of self-concept, and provided a blueprint for the development of a whole new generation of multidimensional self-concept instruments (see review by Marsh & Hattie, 1996). Integrating key features from 17 different conceptual definitions of self-concept identified in their review, Shavelson and colleagues broadly defined *self-concept* as a person's self-perceptions formed through experience with and interpretations of his or her environment. This included feelings of self-confidence, self-worth, self-acceptance, competence, and ability. They noted that self-concept is influenced especially by the evaluations of significant others, by reinforcements, and by attributions for one's behavior. Furthermore, self-concept was seen to be multifaceted and hierarchically organized, with perceptions of personal behavior in specific situations at the base of the hierarchy, inferences about self in broader domains (e.g., social, physical, and academic) in the middle of the hierarchy, and a global, general self-concept (also known as self-esteem) at the apex (see Figure 6.1). These self-perceptions influence the way one acts, and these acts in turn influence one's self-perceptions.

Self-evaluations of competence in a particular domain can be made against many standards of comparison (Marsh & Seaton, 2015; Skaalvik & Skaalvik, 2002): for example, an absolute ideal (e.g., the 5-minute mile), social comparisons (e.g., results of classmates on a test), temporal comparisons (e.g., improvement over time, a personal best), or dimensional comparisons (e.g., accomplishments in one domain relative to those in others).

Widely used multidimensional self-concept instruments, stimulated at least in part by Shavelson and colleagues (1976), differ in the self-concept dimensions addressed (see review by Byrne, 1996) but typically include at least one or more factors representing academic (e.g., Math self-concept [MSC], verbal self-concept [VSC], and global academic self-concept [ASC]), social (e.g., relations with friends, relations with parents), physical (e.g., physical competence,

attractiveness) or emotional domains of self-concept, as well as a global self-esteem (general self-concept) scale, as posited in the Shavelson and colleagues model. Hence, self-concept is considered in this chapter to be a central operationalization of competence perceptions.

Self-Efficacy

As emphasized by Bong and Skaalvik (2003) and others (e.g., Marsh, 2007; Schunk & Pajares, 2005), academic self-efficacy and academic self-concept (ASC) constructs have much in common: an emphasis on perceived competence; a multidimensional and hierarchical structure; content specificity; and the prediction of future performance, emotion, and motivation. Historically, self-concept was argued to be a global measure, whereas self-efficacy was seen as being very domain-specific (Bandura, 1986). However, in modern approaches to self-concept, it is reasonable to conceptualize and measure self-concept facets that are as domain-specific as typical self-efficacy measures, while some researchers focus on global measures of self-efficacy. Nevertheless, self-efficacy researchers have not developed or tested multidimensional, hierarchical models of self-efficacy that integrate global and increasingly specific components of self-efficacy, such as those underlying self-concept theory (e.g., Figure 6.1). Indeed, on a theme that is similar to related discussion on the usefulness of global versus domain-specific measures of self-concept in this chapter, Maddux (2009) suggests that global measures of self-efficacy are less useful than more specific measures, and posits their continued use as an unresolved issue for further research. Hence, this distinction between self-efficacy and self-concept would not appear to be very useful.

For the present purposes we focus on two key characteristics that do distinguish between self-efficacy and self-concept. First, self-efficacy responses are prospective, in terms of what one is able to accomplish in the future, relative to a specific task in a particular context. Hence, Bandura (1997) and others (e.g., Schunk & Pajares, 2005) suggest that self-efficacy refers to beliefs about

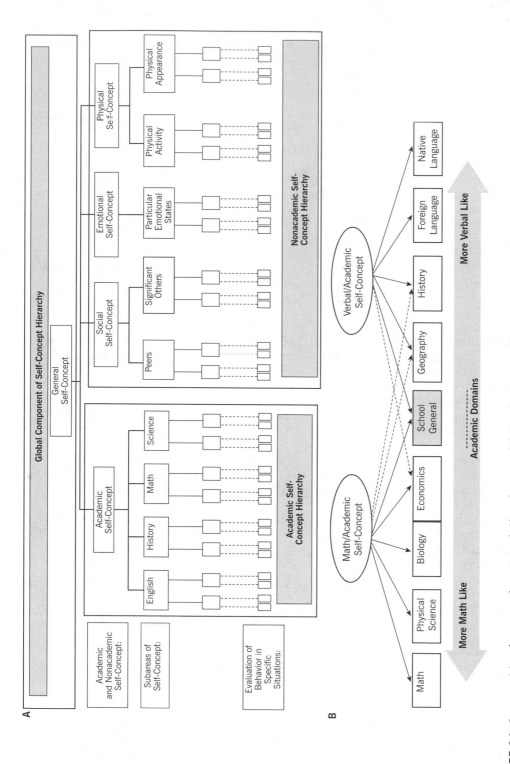

FIGURE 6.1. Juxtaposition between the original Shavelson model (A) depicting self-concept as a multidimensional, hierarchical model and the Marsh–Shavelson revision (B) of the original Shavelson model for the academic component of the self-concept hierarchy, in which there are two higher-order academic self-concepts (math self-concept and verbal self-concept) rather than just one (academic self-concept). The revision was brought about by the finding that math and verbal self-concepts are nearly uncorrelated. The revised model posits a continuum of academic domains that vary along a continuum, ranging from more math-like academic domains to more verbal-like academic domains. The model also posits that relations between all these core academic domains can be explained in terms of just two higher-order academic components.

"what I can do": cognitive, goal-referenced, relatively context-specific, future-oriented judgments in relation to success in a narrowly defined task (Bong & Skaalvik, 2003; Schunk & Pajares, 2005). In contrast, although self-concept is predictive of future behavior and outcomes, it is largely based on past accomplishments. However, logically, we note that competence self-perceptions are also a reflection of past performances, which are predictive of future choices and behaviors. At least in this regard, competence self-perceptions are more logically operationalized in relation to self-concept than to self-efficacy.

Second, as emphasized by Bong and Skaalvik (2003) and others, paradigmatic, appropriately constructed self-efficacy items "solicit goal referenced evaluations and do not directly ask students to compare their abilities to those of others" (p. 9) and "provide respondents with a specific description of the required referent against which to judge their competence" (p. 9), whereas "assessing one's capability in ASC relies heavily on social comparison information" (p. 9). Similarly, Bandura (1986) emphasized that self-esteem and self-concept—but not self-efficacy—are partly determined by "how well one's behavior matches personal standards of worthiness" (p. 410). Thus, for example, in a typical operationalization of self-efficacy, students are shown example math test items and asked the probability of correctly answering such items; their responses are based on an absolute criterion that does not require them to compare their own performances with those of other students (also see Bong & Skaalvik, 2003).

Consistent with this distinction, Marsh (Marsh & Seaton, 2015; Marsh, Walker, & Debus, 1991; also see discussion by Marsh, 2007) found that relatively pure measures of self-efficacy are much less affected by frame of reference effects and social comparisons than are self-concept responses. For example, being in an academically selective school with other academically gifted classmates should not have much effect on academic self-efficacy measures, but it does have a negative effect on ASC. However, in discussion of this distinction, Marsh (2007) argued that much of the power of self-beliefs to motivate and predict future behavior

depends on the evaluation one makes of a purely performance expectation. Whereas the self-efficacy belief that I can run 100 meters in 13 seconds in the next school track meet might be descriptive in nature, the self-evaluation of this outcome—whether this represents a great result or a terrible one—has important implications. Relatedly, Bong and Clark (1999) acknowledge that "self-concept is judged to be more inclusive . . . because it embraces a broader range of descriptive and evaluative inferences with ensuing affective reactions" (p. 142).

Nevertheless, even these distinctions between self-concept and self-efficacy depend on how the constructs are measured. Thus, when comparing the self-concept and self-efficacy measures typically used in applied research (as opposed to relatively pure self-efficacy measures, consistent with the design features originally posited by Bandura and colleagues), Marsh and colleagues (1991) also note that measures purporting to measure self-efficacy are sometimes based on stimuli likely to invoke social comparisons with other students (e.g., "I'm certain I can do an excellent job on assignments and tests," where the term "excellent" might imply a comparison with the work of others). Hence, the empirically demonstrated distinction between self-concept and self-efficacy responses is likely to depend on the nature and wording of the items rather than on the label assigned to the construct. Thus, for example, Marsh, Trautwein, Lüdtke, and Köller (2008) argue that the generalized self-efficacy items in the Program for International Student Assessment (PISA) 2000 were more like self-concept items, in that the criterion of successful performance was not an explicit part of these items. It is for this reason that they found a negative effect of school-average ability (the big-fish-little-pond effect, BFLPE) for self-efficacy responses, albeit one that was smaller than for ASC responses. Apparently for reasons such as this, in their meta-analysis of how well self-belief constructs predict future academic achievement, Valentine and colleagues (Valentine & DuBois, 2005; Valentine, DuBois, & Cooper, 2004) found that there were no differences between domain-specific ASC and self-efficacy measures, although both did systematically better than more global measures of these constructs or self-esteem.

Self-Confidence

The *Oxford Advanced Learner's Dictionary* defines *self-confidence* as a feeling of trust in one's abilities, qualities, and judgment—as in confidence in oneself and one's abilities. In a sporting context, Horn (2004) defined *self-confidence* as positive self-beliefs about abilities or expectations about being able to achieve success. She distinguishes between self-confidence in relation to winning (outcome); performance in relation to standards; self-regulation of thoughts, emotions, and resilience; and physical skills. In psychology more generally, self-confidence is often operationalized as self-esteem, self-efficacy, self-concept, positive self-beliefs, and optimism. In a recent series of studies, Stankov (see overview by Stankov & Lee, 2015) developed an alternative perspective of confidence, as a mindset of having done well on a previously completed task (e.g., "I am sure that I have done this correctly"), in contrast to perceptions of self-efficacy ("I can do this") in relation to a future activity. This notion of confidence in relation to an activity that has already been performed, such as the likelihood or subjective probability that one correctly answered each question on an achievement test, is different to notions predicting what one might be able to accomplish on a specific task.

In marked contrast to domain-specific measures of self-concept, Stankov and Lee (2015) present evidence that confidence is a global construct that generalizes over diverse activities, somewhat akin to the "big-G" factor for cognitive tasks, and that it is empirically distinguishable from other self-belief constructs such as self-efficacy, self-concept, and anxiety. Not surprisingly, perhaps, confidence in relation to each item on a test more accurately predicts test performance than do other self-belief items, but confidence remains a significant predictor of subsequent school grades 3 months later, even after researchers control for test scores and other self-belief constructs. However, although more research into confidence as defined by Stankov and Lee is clearly warranted, it seems to be conceptually and operationally distinct from other self-belief constructs that are used to represent competence self-perceptions.

Effectance

Effectance is, perhaps, the most rudimentary of competence perceptions. Indeed, much current research on competence perceptions stems from White's (1959) concept of effectance, in which a sense of competence is the most fundamental source of motivation. Thus, Elliot, McGregor, and Thrash (2002) argue that, as operationalized in Deci and Ryan's (1991) self-determination theory (SDT; see subsequent discussion), "the terms 'competence' and 'effectance' are used interchangeably in explanations of need for competence" (p. 361). Building on White, from a developmental perspective, Harter (1998, 2012) posited the need for successful mastery of challenging tasks that leads to a sense of competence and intrinsic motivation. However, it is only with age and life experience that young children become more realistic about competence self-perceptions. Particularly for Harter, competence self-perceptions are operationalized as domain-specific self-concept responses. More generally, much of the work on intrinsic motivation and interest stems from White's seminal work. In this respect White was also highly influential in the development of expectancy–value theory (EVT; Eccles & Wigfield, 2002; Wigfield & Eccles, 1992), although effectance motivation or need for competence can be thought of as a value component in EVT rather than the expectancy component that represents competence perceptions.

Competence Expectancy in EVT

The construct of competence expectancy has been important since early theoretical work by Tolman (1932), who studied cognitive representations of habit in early animal learning studies, and Lewin, Dembo, Festinger, and Sear's (1944) concept of level of aspiration, which individuals set for themselves in task performance. These notions were subsequently incorporated into Atkinson's model of achievement motivation, which emphasized that motivation is a function of expectations of success in a given situation and the value placed on the outcome (e.g., Atkinson, 1964; Feather, 1982). In particular, Atkinson (1964) posited that expectancy and value interact such that motivation is maximized when both are high.

Modern versions of EVT, based substantially on the work of Eccles and colleagues (e.g., Eccles & Wigfield, 2002), have greatly expanded on this historical theoretical framework, incorporating a wide variety of psychosocial and sociocultural variables. Of particular relevance, Eccles initially posited ASC to be distinct from expectations of success; whereas ASCs were posited as domain-specific competence beliefs, expectations of success were operationalized as more narrowly defined task-specific expectations of the likelihood of success on an upcoming task. Schunk and Pajares (2005) noted that this conceptualization of expectancy is similar to that used in self-efficacy research, but they also emphasized that expectancy–value theorists have subsequently concluded that expectations of success (which are like the self-efficacy construct) and ASC are not empirically separable (Eccles & Wigfield, 2002; Wigfield & Eccles, 1992). Furthermore, Wigfield, Eccles, Schiefele, Roeser, and Davis-Kean (2006) emphasized that competence beliefs in EVT, as in self-concept research (e.g., Harter, 1998; Marsh, 1990), are defined in relation to how good one is at a particular activity and other activities relative to other individuals, an approach that is somewhat different than that used in self-efficacy research. Indeed, many recent EVT studies use ASC responses to operationalize expectations of success (e.g., Eccles, 2009; Guo, Marsh, Morin, Parker, & Kaur, 2015; Guo, Parker, Marsh, & Morin, 2015; Fredricks & Eccles, 2002; Jacobs, Lanza, Osgood, Eccles, & Wigfield, 2002; Nagengast et al., 2011; Trautwein et al., 2012).

EVT also makes an important distinction between ASC and value that clarifies an issue of confusion in ASC research, in which these constructs are sometimes combined to form a single construct. Thus, EVT theorists (e.g., Eccles, 2009) argue for the conceptual distinction between ASC as a relatively pure measure of competence self-perceptions, and multiple components of value (attainment, intrinsic, utility, and cost). Interestingly, this conceptual distinction is in accord with recent self-concept theory and research, which has delineated the cognitive and affective components of the self-concept construct whereby cognitive self-competence perceptions (e.g., "I am good at math") may be conceptualized and operationalized as separate from affective self-perceptions (e.g., "I like math"; Arens, Yeung, Craven, & Hasselhorn, 2011; Marsh, Craven, & Debus, 1999; Pinxten, Marsh, De Fraine, Van Den Noortgate, & Van Damme, 2013).

The work of Harter (1986, 1998, 2012) in particular has focused on students' perceptions of their own competence. However, like Eccles and Wigfield (2002), and similar to the perspective taken in this chapter, Harter operationalized competence perceptions as self-concept responses. Thus, Pintrich and Schunk (1996) argue that Harter's definition of self-perceptions of competency is isomorphic with task-specific self-concept in EVT (Wigfield, Eccles, et al., 2002). In this respect, competency self-beliefs are operationalized as self-concept responses in research by Harter (1998), Marsh (1990), and in EVT (Wigfield & Eccles, 2002).

Need for Competence Satisfaction in SDT

Self-perceptions of competence, operationalized as self-concept, are closely related to the need for competence satisfaction in SDT, which postulates that this need is a major reason why people seek out optimal stimulation and challenging activities (Deci & Ryan, 1985, 2012). However, there is possibly a subtle distinction between competence self-perceptions and competence need satisfaction. It seems to be difficult to maintain high self-perceptions in a particular domain if competence need satisfaction continues to be low. In order to have competence need satisfaction, individuals need to evaluate their performance in relation to some standard, which might be as follows:

- Social comparisons with others in their context (e.g., classmates in schools).
- Externally established standards of excellence (which are probably based on a form of social comparison against a "generalized" other (Marsh et al., 2008).

- Temporal comparisons based past performances in the same domain, which may or may not involve social comparison (i.e., a personal best; Marsh & Martin, 2011; Martin & Liem, 2010).
- Relative to performances in another domain (dimensional comparison; e.g., "I am not really great at sports but I am a *lot* better at sports than schoolwork," although even this probably involves a complex form of social comparison).
- Feedback from significant others that probably involves one of the above.

Although competence need satisfaction might be posited to lead to self-concept, it is more likely that they are reciprocally related (see related discussion below of the reciprocal effects model of relations between academic achievement and self-concept, in which each is a cause and an effect of the other); need satisfaction–dissatisfaction is likely to result in increased–decreased self-concept, but increased–decreased self-concept is likely to result in higher/lower need satisfaction. Furthermore, perhaps the distinction might be like the distinction between self-concept and expectations of success in EVT; the conceptual distinction is difficult to operationalize in relation to empirical research.

Perceived Competence and Recent Advances in Achievement Goal Theory

Recent extensions of achievement goal theory represent another perspective that is relevant to perceived competence. Achievement goals represent a mastery and performance distinction (Elliot, 2005). *Mastery goals* involve striving to develop competence and attain task mastery, whereas *performance goals* involve striving to attain or demonstrate competence relative to others (Elliot, 2005). Subsequent theorizing has emphasized bifurcating mastery and performance goals into an approach–avoidance distinction, with the predominant representation in terms of 2 × 2 achievement goal models comprising mastery-approach, mastery-avoidance, performance-approach, and performance-avoidance goals (Elliot & McGregor, 2001). The need to be seen as competent and to avoid being seen as incompetent is directed through goals to achieve more specific outcomes in relation to self (e.g., previous performance), the task (task mastery), or levels of competence displayed by others (e.g., social comparison). Indeed, early work emphasized the role of perceived competence in achievement goals. For example, perceived competence has been identified as a moderator of performance goal effects by Dweck (1986) and as an antecedent of achievement goal adoption by Elliot (1999).

More recently, achievement goal theory has been expanded to include self-based goals. In a recent special issue of *British Journal of Educational Psychology* (Martin, 2015b) focusing on academic growth (including trajectories in self-concept; Parker, Marsh, Morin, Seaton, & Van Zanden, 2015), Elliot, Murayama, Kobeisy, and Lichtenfeld (2015) explored self-based (growth) goals (i.e., using one's own personal trajectory as a standard of evaluation), with a particular focus on potential-based goals. This emanated from their earlier expansion of the 2 × 2 achievement goal framework to the 3 × 2 framework, which included self-based (growth) goals alongside task-based and other-based goals (Elliot, Murayama, & Pekrun, 2011). In an article in that special issue, Martin (2015b) also explored growth goals, but with a focus on personal best (PB) goals directed at outperforming one's previous best efforts or performance.

As work into growth goals and the 3 × 2 framework expands, three questions to address are centrally connected to perceived competence. First, it has been suggested that positive perceptions of self-competence are required for a student to raise the bar on him- or herself and to set a goal that exceeds his or her best level of effort or performance (Martin, 2011). To what extent is this the case? Second, to the extent that perceived competence does play into one's self-set growth goals, what is the impact of attaining a personally set growth goal on one's perceived competence? Presumably it is positive—but reciprocal effects models (REMs) to test this are now needed (Martin & Liem, 2010). Third, Martin (2015a, 2015b) has raised questions about the impact on perceived competence if one fails to attain one's self-set growth goal. Relative to failing to attain a mastery or performance goal, might failure to attain one's own personal standards be more damaging to perceived competence? Clearly, advances and future directions in goal theory and growth goals bring into sharp focus and highlight the relevance of the role of perceived competence.

UNIDIMENSIONAL VERSUS MULTIDIMENSIONAL MODELS OF SELF-CONCEPT

As noted earlier, in this chapter, we operationalize competence perceptions as the competence component of self-concept—a multidimensional, hierarchical construct. Although James (1890/1963) originally conceived of self-concept as a multidimensional construct, there has been much debate on the value of unidimensional perspectives that emphasize a single, global domain of self-concept, often referred to as *self-esteem,* versus multidimensional perspectives based on multiple distinct components of self-concept (Marsh & Craven, 2006). Early self-concept research was generally dominated by a unidimensional perspective in which self-concept was represented by a single, general self-esteem score (Rosenberg, 1979). Indeed, the difference between self-esteem and self-concept has long been a source of confusion and controversy. Particularly since the development of the Shavelson and colleagues (1976) model, researchers (e.g., Hattie, 1992; Kernis, 2006; Marsh, 2007) have viewed general self-esteem as a global construct that appears at the apex of the hierarchy, thus reflecting the broad view that an individual has about him- or herself (see Figure 6.1). Marsh (2007) argued that self-esteem items such as those on the widely used Rosenberg's Self-Esteem Scale (1979) are specifically constructed so that they do not refer to any specific domain. Historically, some theoretical models distinguished between self-esteem as the evaluative component of self-concept, and self-concept—posited to be the descriptive component. However, following Shavelson and colleagues, it is generally accepted that self-concept is both descriptive and evaluative (e.g., Byrne, 1996; Marsh, 2007), so that this is not a useful distinction (Marsh

& Craven, 2006). Consistent with the Shavelson and colleagues model, in this chapter, we refer to self-esteem as the global component of self-concept, and discuss it further in relation to advances in self-concept theory, research, and practice emanating from unidimensional versus multidimensional conceptualizations of the self-concept construct.

Support for a Multidimensional Perspective on Self-Concept

Marsh and Craven (1997) argue that "if the role of self-concept research is to better understand the complexity of self in different contexts, to predict a wide variety of behaviors, to provide outcome measures for diverse interventions, and to relate self-concept to other constructs, then the specific domains of self-concept are more useful than a general domain" (p. 191).

Marsh and Craven (2006; Marsh, Xu, & Martin, 2012) note that in many psychological disciplines (e.g., educational, developmental, and sports psychology) the multidimensional perspective of self-concept is now widely accepted. However, support is strongest in educational psychology research, where diverse academic outcomes are systematically related to academic components of self-concept but are nearly unrelated to self-esteem and nonacademic components of self-concept. This extreme multidimensionality was highlighted by Marsh, Trautwein, Lüdtke, Köller, and Baumert (2005, 2006), who showed that nine academic outcomes (e.g., standardized test scores, school grades, and coursework selection in different school subjects) were systematically related to corresponding ASCs. For example, MSC was substantially related to math school grades ($r = .71$), math standardized achievement test scores ($r = .59$), and taking advanced math courses ($r = .51$). In contrast, the academic outcomes were nearly unrelated to global self-esteem (r's ranging from $-.03$ to $.05$), as well as nine other nonacademic specific domains of self-concept.

The need for a multidimensional perspective on self-concept, and for competence beliefs more generally, is evident in other psychological disciplines as well (see review by Marsh & Craven, 2006; Marsh et al.,

2012). For example, in developmental psychology, research has shown differentiation between multiple domains of self-concept in children as young as age 5 (Marsh, Craven, & Debus, 1998; Marsh et al., 2002). In mental health research, Marsh, Parada, and Ayotte (2004) demonstrated that relations between 11 self-concept factors and seven mental health problems varied substantially (r's +.11 to −.83; mean $r = -.35$), demonstrating an a priori multivariate pattern of relations that support a multidimensional perspective. In sports psychology, Marsh and Peart (1988) demonstrated that the results of a physical fitness intervention, and physical fitness indicators, were substantially related to physical self-concept but nearly uncorrelated with nonphysical components of self-concept. Gender differences in self-esteem are small (Wylie, 1979), but these small gender differences mask larger, counterbalancing gender-stereotypical differences in specific components of self-concept (e.g., boys have higher MSCs, girls have higher MSCs) that are reasonably consistent from early childhood to adulthood (e.g., Crain, 1996; Eccles & Wigfield, 2002; Jacobs et al., 2002; Marsh, 1989, 2007). In social psychology and sociology there is a rich theoretical literature on the agreement between self-ratings of self-concept and inferred self-concept ratings by significant others. However, support for the convergent and discriminant validity of these ratings is good when both participants and significant others make ratings on specific self-concept factors based on multi-item scales with strong psychometric properties. In summary, across many disciplines there is growing support for a multidimensional perspective of self-concept.

Support for a Global Self-Esteem Construct

It is also important to emphasize that we are not claiming that self-esteem is never a useful construct (see Kernis, 2006). Rather, to be consistent with the specificity-matching principle (Swann, Chang-Schneider, & McClarty, 2007), we conclude that when the focus of a study is on educational outcomes, for example, it is important to focus on academic components of self-concept. Swann and colleagues (2007) also reviewed other research that is consistent with the specificity-matching principle, showing that self-esteem significantly but weakly predicted specific outcomes and more strongly predicted global outcomes. For example, using a prospective, longitudinal design based on a large birth cohort study, Trzesniewski and colleagues (2006) reported that adolescents with low self-esteem subsequently (10 years later) had poorer mental and physical health, worse economic prospects (more likely to leave school early and to have money problems; less likely to attend university), and higher levels of criminal behavior during adulthood compared to adolescents with high self-esteem—even after they controlled for adolescent depression, gender, socioeconomic status (SES), IQ, and body mass index. However, recognizing that many of the effect sizes were modest, they concluded that low adolescent self-esteem was one of many potentially modifiable risk factors for a wide variety of adult adjustment problems.

THE RELATION OF COMPETENCE TO ACHIEVEMENT: CAUSAL ORDERING OF SELF-CONCEPT AND PERFORMANCE

The Reciprocal Effects Model

ASC and academic achievement are substantially correlated, but this does not answer the critical question of the temporal ordering of these two constructs. This question is important because of not only the theoretical implications for self-concept theory but also the practical implications for determining the teaching practices that are most effective in enhancing student educational outcomes and beliefs given that ASC has motivational properties that contribute to achievement (Byrne, 2002). Traditional approaches to this issue (Calsyn & Kenny, 1977) took an either–or approach—either prior achievement leads to subsequent ASC (a skills development model) or prior ASC leads to subsequent achievement (a self-enhancement model). However, integrating theoretical and statistical perspectives, Marsh (1990) argued for a dynamic REM that incorporates both the skills development and self-enhancement models, such that both ASC and achievement are causes and also effects of each other (see Figure 6.2).

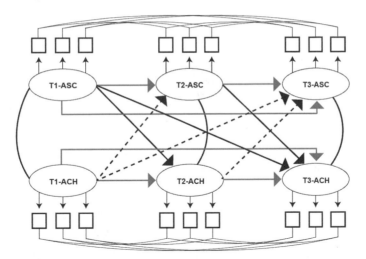

FIGURE 6.2. In this full-forward, multiwave, multivariable model, multiple indicators of academic self-concept (ASC) and achievement (ACH) are collected in three successive waves (T1, T2, and T3). Each latent construct (represented by ovals) has paths leading to all latent constructs in subsequent waves. Within each wave, ASC and ACH are assumed to be correlated; in the first wave, this correlation is a covariance between two latent constructs, and in subsequent waves, it is a covariance between residual factors. Curved lines at the top and bottom of the figure reflect correlated uniquenesses between responses to the same measured variable (represented by boxes) collected on different occasions. Paths connecting the same variable on multiple occasions reflect stability (the solid gray paths), but these coefficients typically differ from the corresponding test–retest correlations (which do not include the effects of other variables). Dashed lines reflect effects of prior achievement on subsequent self-concept, whereas solid black lines reflect the effects of prior self-concept on subsequent achievement.

Generalizability

Subsequent to Marsh (1990), there have been increasingly sophisticated developments in the statistical methodology measures used to test the REM, and substantial support has been garnered for the generalizability of the findings over age, nationality, different self-concept instruments, and different ways of measuring achievement (Marsh, 2007; Marsh & Craven, 2006; also see meta-analyses by Huang, 2011; Valentine, DuBois, & Cooper, 2004). In particular, Valentine and colleagues (Valentine & DuBois, 2005; Valentine et al., 2004) reported that the effect of prior self-beliefs on subsequent achievement, after controlling for the effects of prior achievement, was highly significant overall and positive in 90% of the studies they considered. Furthermore, and consistent with a multidimensional perspective, the effects of prior self-beliefs were significantly stronger when the measure of self-belief was based on a domain-specific measure of self-concept, and achievement measures were matched in terms of subject area (e.g., mathematics achievement and MSC). In contrast, they reported little evidence of the effects of generalized self-beliefs, such as self-esteem, on academic achievement. They concluded that the REM relating academic self-beliefs and achievement is consistent with theories of learning and human development that view the self as a causal agent (e.g., Bandura, 2008b; Carver & Scheier, 2002; Deci & Ryan, 1985, 2012). Indeed, Valentine and DuBois (2005) concluded that support for the REM is equally strong for domain-specific ratings of ASC and self-efficacy. Based on similar findings in a subsequent meta-analysis, Huang (2011) concluded that "as high self-concept is related to high academic performance and vice versa, intervention programs that combine self-enhancement and skill development should be integrated" (p. 505). Demonstrating the importance of the separation of competence and affect, Pinxten and colleagues (2013) demonstrated that although competence and intrinsic motivation, and competence and achievement, were reciprocally related over time, intrinsic motivation had no positive effects on subsequent achievement in their REM study.

Generalizing support to the physical arena, Marsh, Papaionannou, and Theodorakis (2006) demonstrated the REM in a study investigating the causal ordering of physical self-concept and exercise behavior, while Marsh, Chanal, and Sarrazin (2006) found support for an REM of self-concept and gymnastics performance. These findings are further supported by Marsh and Perry's (2005) study of self-concept and performance in a large sample of many of the top-ranked swimmers in the world, in which prior self-concept was a significant positive predictor of subsequent performance in international championships, beyond what could be explained by previous PB performances.

Challenges to the REM

The REM is consistent with positive psychology perspectives, in that positive self-beliefs are posited to be associated with enhanced life outcomes. Baumeister, Campbell, Krueger, and Vohs (2003) challenged this premise in an influential review commissioned for the journal *Psychological Science in the Public Interest,* arguing that efforts to boost people's self-esteem are of little value in fostering academic achievement or preventing undesirable behavior. In a critique of these claims, Marsh and Craven (2006) argued that these conclusions were problematic in the context of recent advances in methodological and theoretical understandings of self-concept. In particular, Baumeister and colleagues relied on a unidimensional perspective that emphasized self-esteem, largely ignoring the research based on a multidimensional perspective focusing on ASC. From a multidimensional perspective, it is reasonable that self-esteem would have little or no relation with academic achievement, even though ASC and achievement are reciprocally related (Marsh & Craven, 2006). Marsh and O'Mara

(2008) subsequently provided clear support for this theoretical claim by juxtaposing the negligible effects of self-esteem with the substantial effects of ASC, in a reanalysis of the classic Youth in Transition study used by Baumeiser and colleagues in support of their claims (in relation to self-esteem) and by Marsh and Craven (2006) in support of their REM (in relation to ASC). This conclusion is also consistent with meta-analytic research indicating consistent support for a reciprocal relation between ASC and achievement, but little to no reciprocal effect between achievement and self-esteem (Valentine & DuBois, 2005; Valentine et al., 2004; also see Huang, 2011). Importantly, the apparent controversy and the challenge to the REM are easily resolved when they are placed within the appropriate multidimensional perspective of self-concept theory (Marsh et al., 2012) supported by more appropriate statistical evidence.

In summary, the REM has been a critical development in self-concept theory. First, the REM established that positive self-concept and achievement are mutually reinforcing. Second, this finding supports the notion that positive self-concept is an integral part of success and achievement. Finally, these findings have important implications for educators. Since self-concept and achievement are mutually reinforcing and reciprocally related, interventions aimed at improving performance should not only strive to promote skills development but also seek simultaneously to enhance self-concept to encourage achievement.

COMPETENCE AND FRAME-OF-REFERENCE MODELS: INTERNAL COMPARISON PROCESSES

Theoretical Background

Shavelson and colleagues (1976) posited that different domains of ASC should be substantially correlated and form a single higher-order ASC factor, consistent with similar theoretical models of achievement and the substantial positive correlations routinely observed between achievements in different school subjects (Marsh, 2007). However, subsequent research revealed that MSC and VSC in particular, were nearly uncorrelated.

This led to the Marsh–Shavelson revision, in which Marsh and Shavelson (1985; Marsh, Byrne, & Shavelson, 1988) posited two higher-order ASC factors (math and verbal) and a continuum of core ASC factors ranging from MSC at one end to VSC at the other end (Figure 6.1). From these findings the internal/external frame-of-reference (I/E) model was developed to explain why MSC and VSC are almost uncorrelated (Marsh, 1986). However, it was subsequently expanded to incorporate a more general framework, in the form of dimensional comparison theory (DCT; Marsh, Möller, et al., 2015; Marsh, Parker, & Craven, 2015; Möller & Marsh, 2013).

The I/E model posited what initially seemed to be a paradoxical effect: that while achievement in each domain has a positive effect on self-concept in the matching domain (e.g., mathematics achievement on MSC), there is a negative (contrast) effect on self-concept in the nonmatching domain (e.g., mathematics achievement on VSC). Theoretically, the external comparison process predicts assimilation: that good math skills lead to higher MSCs and that good verbal skills lead to higher VSCs. According to the internal dimensional comparison process, however, good math skills lead to lower VSCs once the positive effects of good verbal skills are controlled: "The better I am at mathematics, the poorer I am at verbal subjects, relative to my good math skills." Similarly, better verbal skills lead to lower MSCs once the positive effects of good math skills are controlled. Summarizing the results of 13 studies, Marsh (1986) reported that in the I/E process (Figure 6.3A), the (horizontal) paths from math achievement to MSC and from verbal achievement to VSC, are substantial and positive. However, the (cross) paths from math achievement to VSC and from verbal achievement to MSC are significant and negative.

Support and Generalizability

Subsequent research provides strong support for the generalizability of I/E predictions. For example, in a large cross-cultural study, Marsh and colleagues (Marsh & Hau, 2004; Marsh, Hau, Artelt, Baumert, & Peschar, 2006) demonstrated that support for these theoretical predictions generalized over large, nationally representative samples of 15-year-olds from 26 countries based on PISA data. In a meta-analysis of 69 data sets, Möller, Pohlmann, Köller, and Marsh (2009) reported that math and verbal achievements were highly correlated ($r = .67$), but self-concepts were nearly uncorrelated ($r = .10$). The horizontal paths from achievement to ASC in the matching domains were positive (beta = .61 for math, beta = .49 for verbal), but crosspaths were negative from math achievement to VSC (beta = −.21) and verbal achievement to MSC (beta = −.27).

There is also experimental research in support of the causal hypotheses of the I/E model. For example, Möller and Köller (2001) found that manipulation of feedback on achievement in one subject area had an inverse effect on self-concept in the subject at the opposite end of the verbal–mathematics continuum. Furthermore, diary studies have also confirmed that students spontaneously undertake dimensional comparisons on a day-to-day basis. Importantly, these dimensional comparisons have been shown to predict postschool education and career pathways (Parker et al., 2012; Parker, Marsh, et al., 2014; Parker, Nagy, Trautwein, & Lüdtke, 2014). The I/E model has also been heuristic in relation to other major theoretical models, such as Pekrun's (2006) control–value theory of achievement emotions and Eccles's expectancy–value theory for the prediction of gender differences in academic and career choice (e.g., Eccles, Vida, & Barber, 2004; Parker et al., 2012). Extensions of the I/E model also show how it is integrated with some of the major theoretical models of ASC (see Marsh, Parker, et al., 2015): The Marsh–Shavelson multidimensional, hierarchical model of ASC (Figure 6.1), the longitudinal REM of the causal ordering of relations between self-concepts and accomplishments (Figure 6.2), and the BFLPE model of negative (contrast) social comparison effects associated with attending academically selective schools and classes (see discussion below).

Commenting on ongoing debates about how self-concept and self-efficacy are impacted by different frames of reference in relation to the meta-analysis of I/E studies, Möller and colleagues (2009) found that the

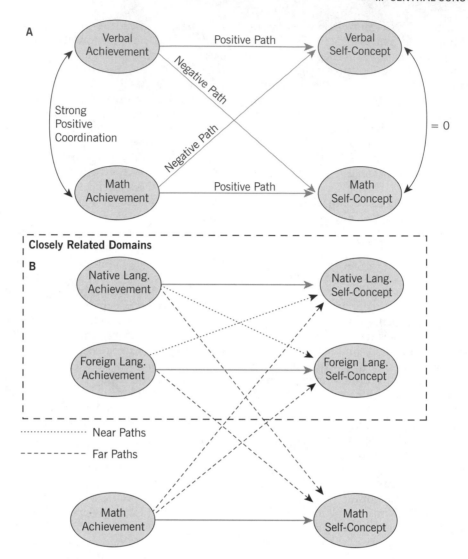

FIGURE 6.3. Juxtaposing the internal/external frame-of-reference (I/E) model (A) and the dimensional comparison theory (DCT) model (B). The "classic" I/E model relates verbal and math achievement to verbal and math self-concept. According to predictions from the I/E model, the horizontal paths from achievement to self-concept in the matching domains (content area) are predicted to be substantial and positive, whereas the crosspaths from achievement in one domain area to self-concept in a nonmatching domain are predicted to be negative (i.e., contrast). In the DCT model the I/E model is extended to include two closely related verbal domains. Far crosspaths (relating math and the two verbal domains) are again predicted to be negative. However, the near crosspaths (relating the two verbal domains) are predicted to be significantly less negative, nonsignificant, or even positive (assimilation).

correlation between math and verbal self-efficacy measures ($r = .50$) is much higher than the correlation between self-concept measures (between $r = -.09$ and $.17$), and nearly as high as the corresponding achievement correlation ($r = .70$). More generally, strong support for the generalizability of the I/E predictions led Möller and colleagues to conclude that "the results of our meta-analyses indicate that the relations described in the classical I/E model are not restricted to a particular achievement or self-concept measure or to specific age groups, gender groups, or countries" (p. 1157).

Domain Specificity

A salient and critical feature of the self-concept construct and of competence perceptions more generally is the domain specificity that underpins the I/E model and DCT more generally. Support for domain specificity is based on the low positive (or even negative) correlations among self-concepts in different domains (e.g., MSC and VSC). To what extent does this domain specificity, so evident in self-concept responses, generalize to other motivation constructs?

To address this question, Marsh, Martin, and Debus (2001) evaluated the domain specificity of 22 academic motivational constructs (e.g., self-concept, attributions, persistence, academic plans, self-regulation, motivational orientation, self-handicapping, defensive pessimism, implicit theories). For each of these 22 constructs, separate scales were constructed for the math and verbal domains. There was clear support for the domain specificity of self-concept and, to a lesser extent, self-concept-like constructs (e.g., future plans; ability attributions for success and failure), in that correlations were modest. However, many other constructs were domain general, in that correlations between the math and verbal scales were extremely large (e.g., external attributions to success and failure; entity and incremental implicit theories; self-handicapping; avoidance orientation; ego orientation).

Partly on the basis of constructs from PISA 2000 (see Marsh, Hau, et al., 2006), Xu and colleagues (2013) reached similar conclusions with Hong Kong secondary students: In a study of 17 motivational constructs in math, Chinese and English domain specificity (evidenced by low correlations) was evident for self-concept, interest, and self-efficacy constructs, while the other constructs were all more domain general. In terms of domain specificity, these results have important implications for theory, methodology, applied research, and practice. Of particular relevance to our chapter, they suggest that support for the I/E model is likely to be specific to competence constructs such as self-concept, but may not generalize to other motivational constructs.

Dimensional Comparison Theory

Möller and Marsh (2013; Marsh, Möller, et al., 2015; Marsh, Parker, et al., 2015) extended the I/E model to incorporate a more general theoretical framework that they called dimensional comparison theory (DCT). In the broader psychological literature, the two most frequently posited frames of reference for forming self-perceptions are temporal comparisons (how current accomplishments compare with past performances) and social comparisons (comparison with the accomplishments of others in one's immediate context; e.g., classmates in one's school or class). However, in DCT, Möller and Marsh (2013) proposed an additional comparison process, dimensional comparisons, based on how accomplishments in one domain compare with those in different domains—an extension of the internal comparison process in the I/E model.

Extending the traditional tests of the I/E model, DCT predicts strong contrast effects only for contrasting domains at opposite ends of the theoretical continuum of ASC (far comparisons; e.g., the negative effect of math achievement on VSC), but much weaker negative contrast or even positive assimilation effects for complementary domains that are close to each other (near domains; e.g., positive effects of math achievement on physics self-concept; positive effects of native language on foreign language self-concept). This ordering of school subjects along an a priori verbal-to-math continuum is based on theoretical and empirical research that led to the Marsh–Shavelson revision (Figure

6.1), thus integrating DCT with established self-concept theory and empirical results. Recent studies (Jansen, Schroeders, Lüdtke, & Marsh, 2015; Marsh, Kuyper, Seaton, et al., 2014; Marsh, Lüdtke, Nagengast, Trautwein, & Abduljabbar, 2015) were explicitly designed to test DCT theoretical predictions based on a comprehensive range of academic domains. All these studies provide clear support for the critical prediction that paths from achievement to ASC, based on near comparisons, were less negative than those based on far comparisons. These results have important implications for theory, research, and practice. The results extend self-concept theory in new and nuanced ways and provide a fertile foundation for further research. More broadly, DCT theory posits dimensional comparison as a critical basis for the formation of self-perceptions, in addition to temporal and social comparisons. The results imply that educators, parents, and significant others need to be aware of these effects when attempting to shore up students' ASCs (see Van Zanden et al., 2016), and to discourage comparisons in which good achievement in one results in poorer self-concepts in contrasting domains.

COMPETENCE PERCEPTIONS AND FRAME-OF-REFERENCE MODELS: THE BFLPE

Theoretical Background

As noted earlier, psychologists from the time of William James (1890/1983) have recognized that objective accomplishments are evaluated in relation to frames of reference. Here the focus is the widely studied BFLPE model, which emphasizes the frame of reference of the relative performance of classmates, and the negative effect of school- or class-average achievement on ASC (Figure 6.4). Although the initial inspiration came from psychophysical research (Marsh, 1974), Marsh (1984; see also Marsh & Parker, 1984; Marsh, Seaton, et al., 2008) proposed the BFLPE to capture frame-of-reference effects on ASCs, based on an integration of theoretical models and empirical research from diverse disciplines: relative deprivation theory, sociology, psychophysical judgment, social judgment,

and social comparison theory (Festinger, 1954). According to the BFLPE, students compare their own academic abilities with the abilities of their classmates and use this social comparison as the basis of their ASCs (Huguet et al., 2009). In the BFLPE, students who attend high-ability classes and schools tend to have lower ASCs than equally able students who attend mixed- or low-ability classes and schools. Thus, the BFLPE explains how students with equal ability can have differing ASCs as a result of their educational setting.

Support and Generalizability

Since the initial BFLPE study (Marsh & Parker, 1984) there has been a wealth of support for BFLPE predictions based on studies that used differing experimental and analytical approaches (Alicke, Zell, & Bloom, 2010; Marsh, 1987; Marsh & Craven, 1997; see reviews by Marsh & Seaton, 2015; Marsh, Seaton, et al., 2008; Marsh, Xu, et al., 2012). Indeed, based on a very large sample of U.K. schools, Tymms (2001) reported support for the BFLPE in 7-year-old students. Furthermore, Marsh (1991) demonstrated that students attending higher-ability high schools were likely not only to have depleted ASCs but also lower GPAs, lower educational aspirations, lower occupational aspirations, and lower standardized test scores. They were also more likely to select less demanding coursework than their equally able peers attending schools with lower average abilities. These findings are significant given that they have important implications for parents, teachers, and policymakers; they counter the commonly held belief that it is advantageous to send students to schools where the average ability level is high. Instead, Marsh argues, the BFLPE findings indicate that many students attending such schools are not reaching their full academic potential.

Local Dominance Effects: Class versus School Social Comparison Processes

BFLPE studies typically are based either on the class or the school, but almost none have contrasted the two in the same study. Alicke, Zell, and Bloom (2010) provided support for

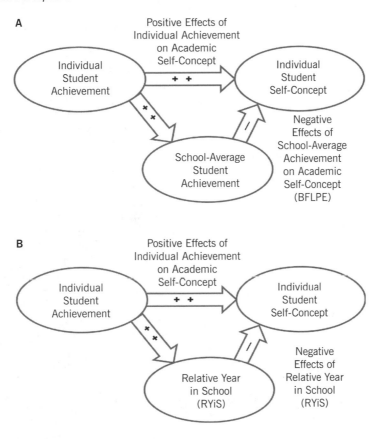

FIGURE 6.4. A. Conceptual model of the big-fish-little-pond effect. [Adapted with permission from Marsh, H. W. (2007). *Self-concept theory, measurement and research into practice: The role of self-concept in educational psychology.* Leicester, UK: British Psychological Society.] B. Conceptual model of the relative year in school effect (RYiSE).

the BFLPE by experimentally manipulating the frame of reference in relation to the feedback given to participants about their performances compared to others. When they pitted "local" against more "general" comparison standards, participants consistently used the most local comparison information available to them, even when they were told that the local comparison was not representative of the broader population, and when they were provided with more appropriate normative comparison data. Extending this theoretical research on the local dominance effect because class-average achievement is a more proximally relevant frame of reference than the school-average achievement, class-average achievement should be more locally dominant. Based on new (latent three-level) statistical models and theoretical predictions integrating BFLPEs and local dominance effects, Marsh, Kuyper, Morin, Parker, and Seaton (2014) found that significantly negative BFLPEs at the school level were largely eliminated and were absorbed into even larger BFLPEs at the class level. Students accurately perceived large achievement differences between different classes within their school and across different schools. However, consistent with the local dominance effect, ASCs and the BFLPE were largely determined by comparisons with students in their own class, not by objective or subjective comparisons with other classes or schools. Because the majority of BFLPE studies have been conducted at the school level rather than the class level, these results suggest that many studies have underestimated the size of the BFLPE.

Cross-Cultural Generalizability

Further support for the BFLPE was also found in the quasi-experimental setting that arose after the fall of the Berlin Wall (Marsh, Köller, & Baumert, 2001). Essentially, the fall provided researchers an opportunity to compare the effects of attending school systems that differed in the extent to which they segregated students by ability. While West German students had previously attended academically differentiated schools, East German students had not been exposed to an academically differentiated school system. Results of the study supported the BFLPE predictions. The BFLPE was significantly larger for West German students at the start of reunification of the schooling systems. Importantly, as time passed, the difference in the size of the BFLPE between East and West German students was reduced, and eventually disappeared after the East German students had been exposed to the West German schooling system for a year. According to Marsh, Köller, and Baumert (2001), these findings are a testament to how national educational policy differences impact the ASCs of individual students.

In research reviewed by Marsh, Seaton, and colleagues (2008; Marsh, Abduljabbar, et al., 2014), there is consistent cross-cultural support for the BFLPE, based on studies from many different countries. Three successive PISA data collections (103,558 students from 26 countries: Marsh & Hau, 2003; 265,180 students from 41 countries: Seaton, Marsh, & Craven, 2009, 2010;: 265,180 students from 41 countries; 397,500 students from 57 countries: Nagengast & Marsh, 2012) showed that the effect of school-average achievement on ASC was negative in all but one of the 123 samples, and significantly so in 114 samples.

Moderation and Generalizability: Two Sides of the Same Coin

One approach to testing the generalizability of the BFLPE is to evaluate potential moderators—particularly those of sufficient strength to eliminate the BFLPE or even to change its direction (i.e., positive effects of school-average achievement for students with certain characteristics). Of course, moderation is an important focus for research: (1) Significant moderators contribute to understanding the nature of the BFLPE and are potentially heuristic in terms of reducing the negative consequences; (2) conversely, the failure to find substantial moderators argues for the broad generalizability and robustness of the effects.

Based on PISA 2003 (41 countries, 10,221 schools, 265,180 students), Seaton and colleagues (2010; also see Marsh & Seaton, 2015) found that the BFLPE was not substantially moderated by any of 16 individual student characteristics (e.g., SES, individual ability, intrinsic and extrinsic motivation, self-efficacy, study methods, anxiety, competitive and cooperative learning orientations, sense of school belonging, teacher–student relationships). Seaton and colleagues concluded "that the BFLPE was an extremely robust effect" (p. 390). Jonkman, Becker, Marsh, Lüdtke, and Trautwein (2012) evaluated whether the BFLPE was moderated by personality factors (Big Five traits and narcissism). They found that students high in narcissism had exaggerated ASCs and smaller BFLPEs, while noting, of course, that enhancing narcissism to reduce the negative consequences of the BFLPE would be counterproductive. In contrast, students high in neuroticism experienced more negative BFLPEs. However, these moderation effects were modest, in that they did not change the direction of the BFLPE; this again supports the robustness of the BFLPE.

Achievement Goal Theory

Achievement goal theory, and related theoretical approaches, might suggest that the BFLPE would be accentuated by performance, ego, or competitive orientations, but be lower for students who have a mastery or learning approach. However, results by Seaton and colleagues (2010; also see Marsh & Seaton, 2015) failed to support these suggestions. In a particularly strong test of these predictions, Wouters, Colpin, Van Damme, and Verschueren (2015) evaluated the extent to which the BFLPE varied as a function of individual-student and class-average constructs from achievement goal theory (mastery, performance-approach, and performance-avoidance; N = 2,987 grade 6 students from 174 elementary school classes). There was clear support for the BFLPE (class-average effect size = –.34). However, there were also small moderating effects of each of the individual goal constructs, such that students who more strongly endorsed any of these goals experienced larger BFLPEs (effect sizes = –.07 to –.10). The authors suggested that students who are more academically engaged are more susceptible to BFLPEs, regardless of their reasons for being engaged. However, somewhat surprisingly, when all three academic goals were included in the same model, mastery was the only goal that significantly interacted with class-average ability (effect size = –.07) and the direction of this effect was the opposite of what one might anticipate. Cheng, McInerney, and Mok (2014) also evaluated whether the BFLPE was moderated by any of seven goal orientations (intrinsic: task, effort, social concern, affiliation; extrinsic: competition, social power, praise and token; N = 7,334 Hong Kong high school students from 201 math classes). Again they found a substantial BFLPE (effect size = –.62). Although all but one of the goal orientations (affiliation) interacted significantly with the negative effect of class-average ability, the authors concluded that the sizes of these moderating effects were very small (–.05 to –.09) and consistently negative. Similar to Wouters and colleagues (2015), Cheng and colleagues (2014) suggested that "students who were more motivated in general, irrespective of the types of goal constructs, experienced stronger BFLPE" (pp. 575–576). In summary, there is little evidence that goal theory orientations at the individual-student, class, or school level, moderate effects of the BFLPE.

Individual Student Ability

Perhaps the most extensive research on moderators of the BFLPE has focused on individual student ability, exploring whether high ability is a protective factor in relation to the BFLPE. Indeed, the theoretical debate regarding the substantive issue of whether the BFLPE is moderated by

individual student achievement (e.g., Coleman & Fults, 1985; Marsh, Kuyper, Morin, et al., 2014; Marsh, Seaton, et al., 2008) has important policy/practice implications for gifted education research. However, according to the theoretical model underpinning the BFLPE (Marsh, 1984, 2007; also see Marsh & Seaton, 2015; Marsh, Seaton, et al., 2008), the frame of reference is largely determined by class/school-average achievement, which is necessarily the same for all students within a given school or class. This theoretical rationale is similar to that in classical psychophysical models, such as Helson's (1964) adaptation-level theory. Thus, the BFLPE should be similar for the brightest and the weakest students within a given class or school. Consistent with these theoretical predictions, a growing body of empirical research (Marsh, 1984; Marsh, Kuyper, Morin, et al., 2014; Marsh & Seaton, 2015; Marsh, Seaton, et al., 2008) shows that interactions between school- or class-average achievement and individual student achievement are consistently small or nonsignificant, and not even consistent in direction—that bright, average, and less bright students experience negative BFLPEs to a similar extent.

Explicit Tracking: BFLPEs for Gifted and Academically Disadvantaged Students

Much of the support for the BFLPE is based on de facto selection processes that result in naturally occurring differences between schools and classes in terms of school- or class-average achievement. However, a number of studies have also considered explicit tracking, in which students are specifically selected to attend special schools, classes, or programs for academically gifted or disadvantaged students. Hence, a critical issue with important theoretical, substantive, and policy implications is whether these results based on de facto selection generalize to settings in which students are specifically selected to be in classes and schools with other students of similar abilities—as in the case of ability grouping, streamed classes, and academically selective schools. In addressing this issue in relation to gifted and talented primary school classes, Marsh, Chessor, Craven, and Roche (1995) used pretest data (age, sex, IQ) collected prior to an intervention to match students who subsequently moved to gifted and talented classes, with students from mixed-ability classes. In two separate studies, students in the gifted program experienced significant declines in all three domains of ASC over time and in relation to matched comparison students. In both studies, this general pattern of results was reasonably consistent across gender, age, and initial ability. Also consistent with a priori predictions, participation in gifted programs had little or no effect on non-ASC or global self-esteem.

BFLPE studies have mostly focused on the negative effects of ability grouping, tracking, and school/class-average achievement on the ASC of high-ability students who attend high-ability schools and classes. However, the BFLPE also has important theoretical and practical implications for less able students in low-ability tracks or special schools/classes for academically disadvantaged students. Marsh, Tracey, and Craven (2006; see also Tracey, Marsh, & Craven, 2003) contrasted predictions from two different theoretical perspectives: Labeling theory predicts that special class placement with other disadvantaged students undermines self-concept; the BFLPE predicts that mainstreaming disadvantaged students into regular classes with more able students will have negative effects that are specific to ASC. They found that, compared to mainstreamed students, those in the special classes not only had significantly higher ASCs (consistent with BFLPE predictions) but also higher peer self-concepts. Thus, disadvantaged students in regular mixed-ability classes did not feel as included as proponents of the inclusion movement would have hoped. In their subsequent review of research in this area from different countries, Marsh and Seaton (2015) concluded that "mainstreaming has potentially negative consequences for the academic and social self-concepts of academically disadvantaged students, suggesting that integration policies should be reconsidered. Appropriate strategies are needed to counter these negative effects of inclusion on ASC rather than accepting the largely unsupported inference from labeling theory that the effects of inclusion on ASC are positive" (p. 155).

Juxtaposition of School-Average Achievement and Year in School

The BFLPE effect is based on the assumption that the academic accomplishments of classmates form a frame of reference or standard of comparison that students use to form their own academic self-concepts. However, being in a school environment with highly able students, as operationalized by school-average achievement, is not the only way in which a student's frame of reference can be altered. For a variety of reasons, such as acceleration or starting school at an early age, students can find themselves in classes with older, more academically advanced students who form a potentially more demanding frame of reference than would same-age classmates. Similarly, due to starting school at a later age or being held back to repeat a grade, students may find themselves in classes with younger, less academically advanced students. Based on the logic of the BFLPE, Marsh (2016; see also Marsh et al., 2016) posited and found that the relative year in school had a negative effect on ASC (i.e., being 1 or more years ahead of same-age classmates had a negative effect, while being 1 or more years behind had a negative effect). The effects on ASC were negative for de facto acceleration (e.g., starting early and skipping grades) and positive for de facto retention (e.g., starting late and repeating grades). Based on PISA 2003 (276,165 fifteen-year-old students from 10,274 schools in 41 countries) the negative effects of relative year in school were

- Cross-culturally robust across the 41 PISA countries.
- Neither substantially explained nor moderated by a diverse range of control variables (e.g., gender, school starting age, repeating grades, home language, immigrant status, SES, achievement).
- Independent of the negative BFLPEs also demonstrated with these data.

The negative effects of de facto acceleration and the positive effects of de facto retention are consistent with a priori predictions based on the logic of the BFLPE and the social comparison processes upon which it is based. The results also have important policy implications, in that the findings are apparently inconsistent with some popular beliefs about policy/practice in relation to acceleration and retention.

Addressing Measurement Issues

Particularly for responses by young children, the failure to identify the intended factors may reflect problems with the particular instrument, or the inability of children to reflect their self-concepts accurately with conventional paper-and-pencil tests. Marsh and colleagues (1998) have suggested that the problem might be resolved by the development of better measurement procedures. They described a new, adaptive procedure for assessing multiple dimensions of self-concept for children ages 5–8, using an individual interview format. At each age level, CFA identified all a priori self-concept factors. In their study of even younger preschool children, ages 4 and 5 years, Marsh and colleagues (2002) reported good psychometric properties, in that the self-concept scales were reliable (ranging from .75 to .89; median = .83), first- and higher-order confirmatory factor-analytic models fitted the data well, and correlations among the scales were moderate (r's −.03 to .73; median = .29). Achievement test scores correlated modestly with academic self-concept factors (r's .15 to .40), but were nonsignificantly or significantly negatively related to nonacademic self-concept scales.

Changes in Self-Concept during Early Childhood

Shavelson and colleagues (1976) hypothesized that the domain specificity of self-concept would increase with age (i.e., correlations among multiple domains of self-concept would decrease with age). Marsh and Ayotte (2003) reviewed previous tests of this hypothesis, but suggested that the results were more complex than initially posited. In particular, they proposed and found support for a differential distinctiveness hypothesis; with increasing age and cognitive development, there are counterbalancing processes of self-concept integration and differentiation. *Integration* occurs when closely related areas of self-concept become

more strongly related; *differentiation* refers to the increasing differentiation of disparate areas of self-concept (math and verbal self-concepts). Interestingly, this distinction is similar to the distinction between "near" and "far" domains posited in DCT.

A host of theories aim to explain the changes in self-concept that occur across the lifespan. According to Marsh and Craven (1997), children's self-concepts decrease with age as the result of increased exposure to situations that challenge the high self-concepts of childhood. Other researchers argue that the tumultuous transitions during puberty lead to radical decreases in self-perceptions (see Harter, 1998). Furthermore, others have posited that improved social skills, autonomy, and maturity may lead to increased self-concept (Hart, Fegley, & Brengelman, 1993). Based on empirical evidence, Marsh (1989) described a curvilinear relation between age and self-concept, whereby self-concept declines during preadolescence and early adolescence, levels out in middle adolescence, and then increases in late adolescence through to at least early adulthood. This curvilinear relation was subsequently replicated by Cole and colleagues (2001) and by Jacobs and colleagues (2002), but the findings were more nuanced, depending in part on the specific domain and on the potential confounding between age and transition to different levels of schooling.

Support for the REM with Young Children

Guay, Marsh, and Boivin (2003) tested the developmental generalizability of the REM of the causal ordering of academic self-concept and academic achievement. Participants were young children in grades 2, 3, and 4: three age cohorts, each tested once a year over a 3-year period. Through the use of a sophisticated multicohort (cross-sectional) multioccasion (longitudinal) design, Guay and colleagues found support for the REM for three age groups.

In summary, research with young children supports the feasibility and validity of appropriately constructed self-report instruments for young children as the basis for validating claims based on theoretical models of self-concept development, and suggests that children as young as 4 and 5 years of age should be able to distinguish among multiple dimensions of self-concept. The combination of more appropriate measurement tools, better methodology, and stronger statistical procedures should facilitate a resurgence of good-quality self-concept research with young children, as has been the case for self-concept research with older children, adolescents, and adults.

SELF-CONCEPT INTERVENTIONS

According to a multidimensional perspective of self-concept, interventions should impact in ways that map onto specific, relevant dimensions of self-concept. Hence, intervention studies provide a strong test of the construct validity of a multidimensional perspective on self-concept. To the extent that an intervention has the predicted pattern of effects on multiple dimensions of self-concept, there is even stronger support for the construct validity of interpretations of the intervention. This construct validation approach is evident in academic interventions in which successful interventions impact ASCs more than nonacademic and global components (e.g., Craven, Marsh, & Debus, 1991; Marsh, Martin, & Hau, 2006), and physical interventions in which the effects are greater for physical components of self-concept (Marsh & Peart, 1988). This construct validity approach was highlighted in the juxtaposition of two Outward Bound studies, in which students experienced a residential wilderness intervention. The "standard" outdoor wilderness course focused largely on nonacademic outcomes (Marsh, Richards, & Barnes, 1986a, 1986b); effects were significantly larger for domains posited a priori to be most relevant to the intervention, were consistent across 27 different programs, and were maintained over 18 months. The Outward Bound "bridging" course (Marsh & Richards, 1988) was designed to produce significant gains in the academic domain for underachieving adolescents; ASC effects were significantly more positive than nonacademic effects, and there were corresponding effects on math and reading achievement. If these studies had taken a unidimensional perspective and only measured global self-esteem,

both interventions would have been judged much weaker, and a rich understanding of the match between specific intended goals and actual outcomes would have been lost.

Haney and Durlak (1998), in their meta-analysis of self-concept interventions, found significantly positive effect sizes, leading to the conclusion that "it is possible to significantly improve children's and adolescents' levels of SE/SC [self-esteem and self-concept] and to obtain concomitant positive changes in other areas of adjustment. There is even the suggestion that SE/SC programs do at least as well as other types of interventions in changing other domains" (p. 429).

Consistent with typical approaches to meta-analysis, Haney and Durlak (1998) considered only one effect size per intervention—the mean effect size averaged across different self-concept dimensions, where more than one had been considered—an implicitly unidimensional approach. Taking a multidimensional perspective, O'Mara, Marsh, Craven, and Debus (2006) updated and extended this meta-analysis to embrace a multidimensional perspective, coding the relevance of each self-concept domain in relation to the aims of the intervention. Similar to Haney and Durlak, they found that the interventions were significantly effective ($d = 0.51$, 460 effect sizes) overall. However, in support of a multidimensional perspective, interventions targeting a specific self-concept domain and subsequently measuring that domain, were much more effective ($d = 1.16$). O'Mara and colleagues also found that studies designed to enhance global self-esteem were much less successful compared to those that targeted specific components of self-concept. These results demonstrate that the Haney and Durlak meta-analysis substantially underestimated the effectiveness of self-concept interventions and provide further support the usefulness of a multidimensional perspective of self-concept in intervention research.

SUMMARY

In a fast-changing world, the development of learners' sense of competence may be more beneficial than developing specific and specialized skills that could be obsolete in the next decade. Thus, Marsh and Yeung (1997a, 1997b), for example, demonstrated that whereas self-concepts in specific school subjects and matching school grades were substantially correlated, the specific components of academic self-concept predicted subsequent coursework selection better than did school grades or more general components of self-concept (e.g., self-esteem). Similarly, Marsh and O'Mara (2008) showed that an ASC formed in high school contributed to the prediction of long-term educational attainment 8 years later, beyond the effects of school grades, standardized achievement tests, IQ, and SES. More generally, the behavioral implications of having higher levels of perceived competence include a reduction in test anxiety (e.g., Zeidner & Schleyer, 1999), taking advanced course work (e.g., Marsh, 1993; Marsh & Yeung, 1997a, 1997b), lower levels of school attrition (e.g., House, 1993), and higher levels of long-term educational attainment (Marsh & O'Mara, 2008). This is because a sense of competence is dynamic in facilitating a range of other psychological attributes that may benefit personal development in various ways (e.g., happiness, academic motivation, career aspiration, resilience when faced with difficulty). Hence, competence perceptions serve as an influential platform for facilitating life potential and getting the most out of life.

Competence perceptions as operationalized in the self-concept construct have had a long and distinguished history. Research over the last 35 years has demonstrated that self-concept, once conceptualized as unidimensional, is indeed a multidimensional construct. As Marsh and Hattie (1996) aptly declared, in relation to academic outcomes, "there appears to be no support at all for the unidimensional perspective of self-concept or, apparently, even a unidimensional perspective of academic self-concept" (p. 44). Indeed, self-concept research has blossomed in this period; it spans issues as varied as developmental perspectives to gender differences, the effects of differing frames of reference on self-concept, self-concept's association with personality, and the reciprocal relation that it has with achievement. These advances in self-concept are exciting and augur well for the future of the discipline.

Perhaps more importantly, they demonstrate how crucial a positive self-concept is in many areas of human functioning, and endorse Marsh and Craven's (2006) description of self-concept as a "hot variable that makes good things happen, facilitating the realization of full human potential in a range of settings" (p. 134).

We conclude with a set of questions and issues for future research:

1. Further jingle-jangle studies on the distinction/nondistinction between similar self-belief constructs that have been posited to reflect competence self-perceptions.
2. Positive competence self-perceptions and related self-beliefs are important in facilitating and, perhaps, mediating diverse positive outcomes, but more work is needed on the psychological processes underlying change. What is the role of goals, different types of value, intentions, and other sources of motivation?
3. Are there situations or research questions for which global competence self-perceptions (e.g., self-esteem) are more useful than relevant specific competence self-perceptions, or should global measures only be considered in combination with domain-specific measures (consistent with a multidimensional, hierarchical perspective)?
4. Do "collective" competence perceptions have a role in relation to organizational and societal change, as posited in self-efficacy research and positive psychology more generally (Bandura, 2008a, 2008b; Maddux, 2009), and what are the implications for organizational contextual and climate research (Marsh, Lüdtke, et al., 2012)?
5. In EVT there is a need for further development of the value components (Gaspard et al., 2015): what they are, whether they can be discriminated, their domain-specificity, and how they are related to competence self-beliefs.
6. Relative to DCT, more research is needed on the nature of dimensional comparisons in relation to assimilation and contrast effects in competence self-perceptions; the nomographic and

idiographic bases of what constitutes "near" and "far" comparisons; and the generalizability of results based largely on academic domains to nonacademic domains of competence.

7. How do the reciprocal relations among competence self-perceptions, interest, extrinsic motivation, autonomy, and reinforcement from significant others develop and vary across the lifespan from early childhood to old age?

8. Competence self-perceptions can be made through various processes: social comparisons (in relation to performances by others), temporal comparisons (in relation to one's own previous performances in the same domain), dimensional comparisons (in relation to one's own previous performances in the different domains), or absolute standards (external standards of excellence or task-specific criteria). However, more research is needed that will juxtapose these alternative processes, the extent that they vary as a function of context, and how they can be optimally used to enhance outcomes.

9. Needed is exploration of perceived competence in recent extensions of achievement goal theory and growth goals; in particular, the role of perceived competence in self-based goals, potential-based goals, and PB goals. This would investigate both the extent to which perceived competence underpins students' inclination to set more demanding growth goals for themselves and the extent to which meeting (or failing to meet) these self-set growth goals enhances (or reduces) perceived competence.

10. Recent research suggests that relative year in school (being a year ahead or behind same-age students) has negative effects on academic self-concept and related psychosocial constructs that have a similar theoretical rationale as the BFLPE, but further research is needed to tease out the effects of starting age, repeating a school year, and skipping a school year, as well as the implications for academic achievement.

11. More research is needed on the measurement and development of self-concept with young children.

12. Whereas some interventions can enhance actual competence (e.g., academic achievement), others can enhance competence perceptions (e.g., ASC). However, there is insufficient research—or even appropriate methodology—to evaluate underlying processes in interventions designed to enhance both in a way that is reciprocally beneficial to competence and competence perceptions.

REFERENCES

Alicke, M. D., Zell, E., & Bloom, D. (2010). Mere categorization and the frog pond effect. *Psychological Science, 2,* 174–177.

Arens, A. K., Yeung, A. S., Craven, R. G., & Hasselhorn, M. (2011). The twofold multidimensionality of academic self-concept: Domain specificity and separation between competence and affect components. *Journal of Educational Psychology, 103*(4), 970–981.

Atkinson, J. W. (1964). *An introduction to motivation.* Oxford, UK: Van Nostrand.

Bandura, A. (1986). *Social foundations of thought and action: A social cognitive theory.* Englewood Cliffs, NJ: Prentice Hall.

Bandura, A. (1997). *Self-efficacy: The exercise of control.* New York: Freeman/Times Books/Holt.

Bandura, A. (2008a). An agentic perspective on positive psychology. In S. J. Lopez (Ed.), *Positive psychology: Exploring the best in people: Vol. 1. Discovering human strengths* (pp. 167–196). Westport, CT: Praeger/Greenwood.

Bandura, A. (2008b). Toward an agentic theory of the self. In H. Marsh, R. G. Craven, & D. M. McInerney (Eds.), *Advances in self research: Vol. 3. Self-processes, learning, and enabling human potential* (pp. 15–49). Charlotte, NC: Information Age.

Baumeister, R. F., Campbell, J. D., Krueger, J. I., & Vohs, K. D. (2003). Does high self-esteem cause better performance, interpersonal success, happiness, or healthier lifestyles? *Psychological Science in the Public Interest, 4,* 1–44.

Bong, M., & Clark, R. E. (1999). Comparison between self-concept and self-efficacy in academic motivation research. *Educational Psychologist, 34,* 139–154.

Bong, M., & Skaalvik, E. M. (2003). Academic self-concept and self-efficacy: How different are they really? *Educational Psychology Review, 15*(1), 1–40.

Bruner, J. (1996). A narrative model of self construction. *Psyke and Logos, 17,* 154–170.

Byrne, B. M. (1996). *Measuring self-concept across the life span: Issues and instrumentation.* Washington, DC: American Psychological Association.

Byrne, B. M. (2002). Validating the measurement and structure of self-concept: Snapshots of past, present, and future research. *American Psychologist, 57,* 897–909.

Calysn, R., & Kenny, D., 1977. Self-concept of ability and perceived evaluations by others: Cause or effect of academic achievement? *Journal of Educational Psychology, 69,* 136–145.

Carver, C. S., & Scheier, M. F. (2002). Control processes and self-organization as complementary principles underlying behaviour. *Personality and Social Psychology Review, 6,* 304–315.

Chen, S., Yeh, Y., Hwang, F., & Lin, S. S. J. (2013). The relationship between academic self-concept and achievement: A multicohort–multioccasion study. *Learning and Individual Differences, 23,* 172–178.

Cheng, R. W.-Y., McInerney, D. M., & Mok, M. M. C. (2014). Does big-fish-little-pond effect always exist?: Investigation of goal orientations as moderators in the Hong Kong context. *Educational Psychology, 34*(5), 561–580.

Cole, D. A., Maxwell, S. E., Martin, J. M., Peeke, L. G., Seroczynski, A. D., Tram, J. M., et al. (2001). The development of multiple domains of child and adolescent self-concept: A cohort sequential longitudinal design. *Child Development, 72,* 1723–1746.

Coleman, J. M., & Fults, B. A. (1985). Special class placement, level of intelligence, and the self-concepts of gifted children: A social comparison perspective. *Remedial and Special Education, 6,* 7–11.

Crain, R. M. (1996). The influence of age, race, and gender on child and adolescent multidimensional self-concept. In B. A. Bracken (Ed.), *Handbook of self-concept* (pp. 395–420). Oxford, UK: Wiley.

Craven, R. G., Marsh, H. W., & Debus, R. L. (1991). Effects of internally focused feedback and attributional feedback on enhancement of academic self-concept. *Journal of Educational Psychology, 83*(1), 17–27.

Davis-Kean, P. E., & Sandler, H. M. (2001). A meta-analysis of measures of self-esteem for young children: A framework for future measures. *Child Development, 72,* 887–906.

Deci, E. L., & Ryan, R. M. (1985). *Intrinsic motivation and self-determination in human behavior.* New York: Plenum Press.

Deci, E. L., & Ryan, R. M. (1991). A motivational approach to self: Integration in personality. In R. Dienstbier (Ed.), *Nebraska Symposium on Motivation: Vol. 38. Perspectives on motivation* (pp. 237–288). Lincoln: University of Nebraska Press.

Deci, E. L., & Ryan, R. M. (2012). Motivation, personality, and development within embedded social contexts: An overview of self-determination theory. In R. M. Ryan (Ed.), *The Oxford handbook of human motivation* (pp. 85–107). New York: Oxford University Press.

Donahue, E. M., Robins, R. W., Roberts, B. W., & John, O. P. (1993). The divided self: Concurrent and longitudinal effects of psychological adjustment and social roles on self-concept differentiation. *Journal of Personality and Social Psychology, 64,* 834–846.

Dweck, C. S. (1986). Motivational processes affecting learning. *American Psychologist, 41,* 1040–1048.

Eccles, J. S. (2009). Who am I and what am I going to do with my life?: Personal and collective identities as motivators of action. *Educational Psychologist, 44,* 78–89.

Eccles, J. S., Vida, M. N., & Barber, B. (2004). The relation of early adolescents' college plans and both academic ability and task-value beliefs to subsequent college enrollment. *Journal of Early Adolescence, 24*(1), 63–77.

Eccles, J. S., & Wigfield, A. (2002). Motivational beliefs, values, and goals. *Annual Review of Psychology, 53*(1), 109–132.

Elliot, A. J. (1999). Approach and avoidance motivation and achievement goals. *Educational Psychologist, 34,* 169–189.

Elliot, A. J. (2005). A conceptual history of the achievement goal construct. In A. J. Elliot & C. S. Dweck (Eds.), *Handbook of competence and motivation* (pp. 52–72). New York: Guilford Press.

Elliot, A. J., & Dweck, C. S. (2005). Competence and motivation: Competence as the core of achievement motivation. In A. J. Elliot & C. S. Dweck (Eds.), *Handbook of competence and motivation* (pp. 3–12). New York: Guilford Press.

Elliot, A. J., & McGregor, H. A. (2001). A 2 × 2 achievement goal framework. *Journal of Personality and Social Psychology, 80,* 501–519.

Elliot, A. J., McGregor, H. A., & Thrash, T. M. (2002). The need for competence. In E. L. Deci & R. M. Ryan (Eds.), *Handbook of self-determination research* (pp. 361–387). Rochester, NY: University of Rochester Press.

Elliot, A. J., Murayama, K., Kobeisy, A., & Lichtenfeld, S. (2015). Potential-based achievement goals. *British Journal of Educational Psychology, 85,* 192–206.

Elliot, A. J., Murayama, K., & Pekrun, R. (2011).

A 3 × 2 achievement goal model. *Journal of Educational Psychology, 103*(3), 632–648.

Fantuzzo, J. W., McDermott, P. A., Manz, P. H., Hampton, V. R., & Burdick, N. A. (1996). The Pictorial Scale of Perceived Competence and Social Acceptance: Does it work with low-income urban children? *Child Development, 67,* 1071–1084.

Feather, N. T. (1982). Expectancy-value approaches: Present status and future directions. In N. T. Feather (Ed.), *Expectations and actions: Expectancy–value models in psychology* (pp. 395–420). Hillsdale, NJ: Erlbaum.

Festinger, L. (1954). A theory of social comparison processes. *Human Relations, 7,* 117–140.

Fredricks, J. A., & Eccles, J. S. (2002). Children's competence and value beliefs from childhood through adolescence: Growth trajectories in two male-sex-typed domains. *Developmental Psychology, 38*(4), 519–533.

Gaspard, H., Dicke, A.-L., Flunger, B., Schreier, B., Häfner, I., Trautwein, U., et al. (2015). More value through greater differentiation: Gender differences in value beliefs about math. *Journal of Educational Psychology, 107*(3), 663–677.

Guay, F., Marsh, H. W., & Boivin, M. (2003). Academic self-concept and academic achievement: Developmental perspectives on their causal ordering, *Journal of Educational Psychology, 95,* 124–136.

Guo, J., Marsh, H. W., Morin, A. J. S., Parker, P. D., & Kaur, G. (2015). Directionality of the associations of high school expectancy–value, aspirations, and attainment: A longitudinal study. *American Educational Research Journal, 52*(2), 371–402.

Guo, J., Parker, P. D., Marsh, H. W., & Morin, A. J. S. (2015). Achievement, motivation, and educational choices: A longitudinal study of expectancy and value using a multiplicative perspective. *Developmental Psychology, 51*(8), 1163–1176.

Haney, P., & Durlak, J. A. (1998). Changing self-esteem in children and adolescents: A meta-analytic review. *Journal of Clinical Child Psychology, 27,* 423–433.

Hart, D., Fegley, S., & Brengelman, D. (1993). Perceptions of past, present and future selves among children and adolescents. *British Journal of Developmental Psychology, 11,* 265–282.

Harter, S. (1986). Processes underlying the construction, maintenance and enhancement of self-concept in children. In J. Suls & A. Greenwald (Eds.), *Psychological perspectives on the self* (Vol. 3, pp. 136–182). Hillsdale, NJ: Erlbaum.

Harter, S. (1998). The development of self-representations. In W. Damon & N. Eisenberg (Eds.), *Handbook of child psychology: Vol. 3. Social, emotional, and personality development* (5th ed., pp. 553–618). Hoboken, NJ: Wiley.

Harter, S. (2012). New directions in self development: Resurrecting the I-self. In D. McInerney (Ed.), *Theory driving research: New wave perspectives on self-processes and human development* (pp. 1–30). Charlotte, NC: Information Age.

Hattie, J. (1992). *Self-concept.* Hillsdale, NJ: Erlbaum.

Helson, H. (1964). *Adaptation-level theory.* New York: Harper & Row.

Horn, T. S. (2004). Developmental perspectives on self-perceptions in children and adolescents. In M. R. Weiss (Ed.), *Developmental sport and exercise psychology: A lifespan perspective* (pp. 101–143). Morgantown, WV: Fitness Information Technology.

House, J. D. (1993). The relationship between academic self-concept and school withdrawal. *Journal of Social Psychology, 133,* 125–127.

Huang, C. (2011). Self-concept and academic achievement: A meta-analysis of longitudinal relations. *Journal of School Psychology, 49,* 505–528.

Huguet, P., Dumas, F., Marsh, H. W., Regner, I., Wheeler, L., Suls, J., et al. (2009). Clarifying the role of social comparison in the Big-Fish-Little-Pond Effect (BFLPE): An integrative study. *Journal of Personality and Social Psychology, 97,* 671–710.

Hunter, J. P., & Csikszentmihalyi, M. (2003). The positive psychology of interested adolescents. *Journal of Youth and Adolescence, 32,* 27–35.

Jacobs, J. E., Lanza, S., Osgood, D. W., Eccles, J. S., & Wigfield, A. (2002). Changes in children's self-competence and values: Gender and domain differences across grades one through twelve. *Child Development, 73,* 509–527.

James, W. (1963). *The principles of psychology.* New York: Holt, Rinehart & Winston. (Original work published 1890)

Jansen, M., Schroeders, U., Lüdtke, O., & Marsh, H. W. (2015). Contrast and assimilation effects of dimensional comparisons in five subjects: An extension of the I/E model. *Journal of Educational Psychology, 107*(4), 1086–1101.

Jonkmann, K., Becker, M., Marsh, H. W., Lüdtke, O., & Trautwein, U. (2012). Personality traits moderate the big-fish-little-pond effect of academic self-concept. *Learning and Individual Differences, 22,* 736–746.

Kagen, S. L., Moore, E., & Bredekamp, S. (1995). *Considering children's early development and learning: Toward common views and vocabulary* (Report N. 95-03). Washington, DC: National Education Goals Panel.

Kernis, M. H. (Ed.). (2006). *Self-esteem issues and answers.* New York: Psychological Press.

Lewin, K., Dembo, T., Festinger, L., & Sears, P. S. (1944). Level of aspiration. In J. M. Hunt (Ed.), *Personality and the behavior disorders* (pp. 333–378). Oxford, UK: Ronald Press.

Maddux, J. E. (2009). Self-efficacy: The power of believing you can. In S. J. Lopez & C. R. Snyder (Eds.), *Oxford handbook of positive psychology* (2nd ed., pp. 335–343). New York: Oxford University Press.

Marsh, H. W. (1974). *Judgmental anchoring: Stimulus and response variables.* Unpublished doctoral dissertation, University of California, Los Angeles, CA.

Marsh, H. W. (1984). Self-concept: The application of a frame of reference model to explain paradoxical results. *Australian Journal of Education, 28,* 165–181.

Marsh, H. W. (1986). Verbal and math self-concepts: An internal/external frame of reference model. *American Educational Research Journal, 23,* 129–149.

Marsh, H. W. (1987). The big-fish-little-pond effect on academic self-concept. *Journal of Educational Psychology, 79*(3), 280–295.

Marsh, H. W. (1989). Age and sex effects in multiple dimensions of self-concept: Preadolescence to early adulthood. *Journal of Educational Psychology, 81,* 417–430.

Marsh, H. W. (1990). The causal ordering of academic self-concept and academic achievement: A multiwave, longitudinal panel analysis. *Journal of Educational Psychology, 82,* 646–656.

Marsh, H. W. (1991). The failure of high ability schools to deliver academic benefits: The importance of academic self-concept and educational aspirations. *American Educational Research Journal, 28,* 445–480.

Marsh, H. W. (1993). Academic self-concept: Theory, measurement and research. In J. Suls (Ed.), *Psychological perspectives on the self* (pp. 59–98). Hillsdale, NJ: Erlbaum.

Marsh, H. W. (1994). Sport motivation orientations: Beware of the jingle-jangle fallacies. *Journal of Sport and Exercise Psychology, 16,* 365–380.

Marsh, H. W. (2007). *Self-concept theory, measurement and research into practice: The role of self-concept in educational psychology.* Leicester, UK: British Psychological Society.

Marsh, H. W. (2016). Cross-cultural generalizability of year in school effects: Negative effects of acceleration and positive effects of retention on academic self-concept. *Journal of Educational Psychology, 108*(2), 256–273.

Marsh, H. W., Abduljabbar, A. S., Parker, P. D., Morin, A. J., Abdelfattah, F., & Nagengast, B. (2014). The big-fish-little-pond effect in mathematics: A cross-cultural comparison of US and Saudi Arabian TIMSS responses. *Journal of Cross-Cultural Psychology, 45*(5), 777–804.

Marsh, H. W., & Ayotte, V. (2003). Do multiple dimensions of self-concept become more differentiated with age?: The differential distinctiveness hypothesis. *Journal of Educational Psychology, 95,* 687–706.

Marsh, H. W., Byrne, B. M., & Shavelson, R. J. (1988). A multifaceted academic self-concept: Its hierarchical structure and its relation to academic achievement. *Journal of Educational Psychology, 80,* 366–380.

Marsh, H. W., Chanal, J. P., & Sarrazin, P. G. (2006). Self-belief does make a difference: A reciprocal effects model of the causal ordering of physical self-concept and gymnastics performance. *Journal of Sports Sciences, 24,* 101–111.

Marsh, H. W., Chessor, D., Craven, R. G., & Roche, L. (1995). The effects of gifted-and-talented programs on academic self-concept: The big fish strikes again. *American Educational Research Journal, 32,* 385–319.

Marsh, H. W., & Craven, R. (1997). Academic self-concept: Beyond the dustbowl. In G. Phye (Ed.), *Handbook of classroom assessment: Learning, achievement, and adjustment* (pp. 131–198). Orlando, FL: Academic Press.

Marsh, H. W., & Craven, R. G. (2006). Reciprocal effects of self-concept and performance from a multidimensional perspective: Beyond seductive pleasure and unidimensional perspectives. *Perspectives on Psychological Science, 1,* 133–163.

Marsh, H. W., Craven, R. G., & Debus, R. L. (1998). Structure, stability, and development of young children's self-concepts: A multicohort–multioccasion study. *Child Development, 69,* 1030–1053.

Marsh, H. W., Craven, R., & Debus, R. (1999). Separation of competency and affect components of multiple dimensions of academic self-concept: A developmental perspective. *Merrill–Palmer Quarterly, 45,* 567–601.

Marsh, H. W., Craven, R. G., Hinkley, J. W., & Debus, R. L. (2003). Evaluation of the big-two-factor theory of academic motivation orientations: An evaluation of jingle-jangle fallacies. *Multivariate Behavioral Research, 38*(2), 189–224.

Marsh, H. W., Ellis, L. A., & Craven, R. G.

(2002). How do preschool children feel about themselves?: Unraveling measurement and multidimensional self-concept structure. *Developmental Psychology, 38,* 376–393.

Marsh, H. W., & Hattie, J. A. (1996). Theoretical perspectives on the structure of self-concept. In B. A. Bracken (Ed.), *Handbook of self-concept: Developmental, social and clinical considerations* (pp. 38–90). Hoboken, NJ: Wiley.

Marsh, H. W., & Hau, K. T. (2003). Big-fish-little-pond effect on academic self-concept: A cross-cultural (26 country) test of the negative effects of academically selective schools. *American Psychologist, 58,* 364–376.

Marsh, H. W., & Hau, K. T. (2004). Explaining paradoxical relations between academic self-concepts and achievements: Cross-cultural generalizability of the internal/external frame of reference predictions across 26 countries. *Journal of Educational Psychology, 96,* 56–67.

Marsh, H. W., Hau, K. T., Artelt, C., Baumert, J., & Peschar, J. L. (2006). OECD's brief self-report measure of educational psychology's most useful affective constructs: Cross-cultural, psychometric comparisons across 25 countries. *International Journal of Testing, 6,* 311–360.

Marsh, H. W., Köller, O., & Baumert, J. (2001). Reunification of East and West German school systems: Longitudinal multilevel modeling study of the big-fish-little-pond effect on academic self-concept. *American Educational Research Journal, 38*(2), 321–350.

Marsh, H. W., Kuyper, H., Morin, A. J. S., Parker, P. D., & Seaton, M. (2014). Big-fish-little-pond social comparison and local dominance effects: Integrating new statistical models, methodology, design, theory and substantive implications. *Learning and Instruction, 33,* 50–66.

Marsh, H. W., Kuyper, H., Seaton, M., Parker, P. D., Morin, A. J. S., Möller, J., et al. (2014). Dimensional comparison theory: An extension of the internal/external frame of reference effect on academic self-concept formation. *Contemporary Educational Psychology, 39,* 326–341.

Marsh, H. W., Lüdtke, O., Nagengast, B., Trautwein, U., & Abduljabbar, A. S. (2015). Dimensional Comparison Theory: Paradoxical relations between self-beliefs and achievements in multiple domains. *Learning and Instruction, 35,* 16–32.

Marsh, H. W., Lüdtke, O., Nagengast, B., Trautwein, U., Morin, A. J. S., Abduljabbar, A. S., et al. (2012). Classroom climate and contextual effects: Conceptual and methodological issues in the evaluation of group-level effects. *Educational Psychologist, 47*(2), 106–124.

Marsh, H. W., Martin, A., & Debus, R. (2001). Individual differences in verbal and math self-perceptions: One factor, two factors, or does it depend on the construct? In R. Riding & S. Rayner (Eds.), *Self-perception: International perspectives on individual differences* (pp. 149–170). Westport, CT: Able.

Marsh, H. W., & Martin, A. J. (2011). Academic self-concept and academic achievement: Relations and causal ordering. *British Journal of Educational Psychology, 81,* 59–77.

Marsh, H. W., Martin, A. J., & Hau, K. (2006). A multimethod perspective on self-concept research in educational psychology: A construct validity approach. In M. Eid & E. Diener (Eds.), *Handbook of multimethod measurement in psychology* (pp. 441–456). Washington, DC: American Psychological Association.

Marsh, H. W., Möller, J., Parker, P., Xu, M. K., Nagengast, B., & Pekrun, R. (2015). Academic internal/external frame of reference model. In J. D. Wright (Ed.), *International encyclopedia of the social and behavioral sciences* (2nd ed., pp. 425–432). Oxford, UK: Elsevier.

Marsh, H. W., & O'Mara, A. (2008). Reciprocal effects between academic self-concept, self-esteem, achievement, and attainment over seven adolescent years: Unidimensional and multidimensional perspectives of self-concept. *Personality and Social Psychology Bulletin, 34,* 542–552.

Marsh, H. W., Papaionannou, A., & Theodorakis, Y. (2006). Causal ordering of physical self-concept and exercise behavior: Reciprocal effects model and the influence of physical education teachers. *Health Psychology, 25,* 316–328.

Marsh, H. W., Parada, R. H., & Ayotte, V. (2004). A multidimensional perspective of relations between self-concept (Self Description Questionnaire II) and adolescent mental health (Youth Self Report). *Psychological Assessment, 16,* 27–41.

Marsh, H. W., Parada, R. H., Craven, R. G., & Finger, L. (2004). In the looking glass: A reciprocal effects model elucidating the complex nature of bullying, psychological determinants and the central role of self-concept. In C. S. Sanders & G. D. Phye (Eds.), *Bullying: Implications for the classroom* (pp. 63–109). Orlando, FL: Academic Press.

Marsh, H. W., & Parker, J. (1984). Determinants of student self-concept: Is it better to be a relatively large fish in a small pond even if you don't learn to swim as well? *Journal of Personality and Social Psychology, 47,* 213–231.

Marsh, H. W., Parker, P., & Craven, R. G. (2015). Dimensional comparisons theory: An extension of the internal/external frame of reference model. In F. Guay, H. W. Marsh, R. G. Craven, & D. McInerney (Eds.), *Self-concept, motivation, and identity: Underpinning success with research and practice* (International Advances in Self Research; Vol. 5, pp. 115–151). Charlotte, NC: Information Age.

Marsh, H. W., & Peart, N. (1988). Competitive and cooperative physical fitness training programs for girls: Effects on physical fitness and on multidimensional self-concepts. *Journal of Sport and Exercise Psychology, 10*, 390–407.

Marsh, H. W., Pekrun, R., Murayama, K., Guo, J., Dicke, T., & Litchenfeld, S. (2016). Long-term positive effects of repeating a year in school. Six-year longitudinal study of self-beliefs, anxiety, social relations, school grades, and test scores. *Journal of Educational Psychology*. [Epub ahead of print]

Marsh, H. W., & Perry, C. (2005). Self-concept contributes to winning gold medals: Causal ordering of self-concept and elite swimming performance. *Journal of Sport and Exercise Psychology, 27*, 71–91.

Marsh, H. W., & Richards, G. (1988). The outward bound bridging course for low achieving high-school males: Effect on academic achievement and multidimensional self-concepts. *Australian Journal of Psychology, 40*, 281–298.

Marsh, H. W., Richards, G., & Barnes, J. (1986a). Multidimensional self-concepts: A long term follow-up of the effect of participation in an Outward Bound program. *Personality and Social Psychology Bulletin, 12*, 475–492.

Marsh, H. W., Richards, G., & Barnes, J. (1986b). Multidimensional self-concepts: The effect of participation in an Outward Bound program. *Journal of Personality and Social Psychology, 45*, 173–187.

Marsh, H. W., & Seaton, M. (2015). The big-fish-little-pond effect, competence self-perceptions, and relativity: Substantive advances and methodological innovation. In A. Elliot (Ed.), *Advances in motivation science* (Vol. 2, pp. 127–184). Waltham, MA: Academic Press.

Marsh, H. W., Seaton, M., Trautwein, U., Ludtke, O., Hau, K. T., O'Mara, A. J., et al. (2008). The big-fish-little-pond-effect stands up to critical scrutiny: Implications for theory, methodology, and future research. *Educational Psychology Review, 20*, 319–350.

Marsh, H. W., & Shavelson, R. (1985). Self-concept: Its multifaceted, hierarchical structure. *Educational Psychologist, 20*, 107–125.

Marsh, H. W., Tracey, D. K., & Craven, R. G. (2006). Multidimensional self-concept structure for preadolescents with mild intellectual disabilities: A hybrid multigroup-mimic approach to factorial invariance and latent mean differences. *Educational and Psychological Measurement, 66*, 795–818.

Marsh, H. W., Trautwein, U., Lüdtke, O., & Köller, O. (2008). Social comparison and big-fish-little-pond effects on self-concept and other self-belief constructs: Role of generalized and specific others. *Journal of Educational Psychology, 100*, 510–524.

Marsh, H. W., Trautwein, U., Lüdtke, O., Köller, O., & Baumert, J. (2005). Academic self-concept, interest, grades and standardized test scores: Reciprocal effects model of causal ordering. *Child Development, 76*, 397–416.

Marsh, H. W., Trautwein, U., Lüdtke, O., Köller, O., & Baumert, J. (2006). Integration of multidimensional self-concept and core personality constructs: Construct validation and relations to well-being and achievement. *Journal of Personality, 74*(2), 403–456.

Marsh, H. W., Walker, R., & Debus, R. (1991). Subject-specific components of academic self-concept and self-efficacy. *Contemporary Educational Psychology, 16*, 331–345.

Marsh, H. W., Xu, M., & Martin, A. J. (2012). Self-concept: A synergy of theory, method, and application. In K. R. Harris, S. Graham, T. Urdan, C. B. McCormick, G. M. Sinatra, & J. Sweller (Eds.), *APA educational psychology handbook: Vol. 1. Theories, constructs, and critical issues* (pp. 427–458). Washington, DC: American Psychological Association.

Marsh, H. W., & Yeung, A. S. (1997a). Causal effects of academic self-concept on academic achievement: Structural equation models of longitudinal data. *Journal of Educational Psychology, 89*, 41–54.

Marsh, H. W., & Yeung, A. S. (1997b). Coursework selection: The effects of academic self-concept and achievement. *American Educational Research Journal, 34*, 691–720.

Martin, A. J. (2011). Personal best (PB) approaches to academic development: Implications for motivation and assessment. *Educational Practice and Theory, 33*, 93–99.

Martin, A. J. (2015a). Growth approaches to academic development: Research into academic trajectories and growth assessment, goals and mindsets. *British Journal of Educational Psychology, 85*, 133–137.

Martin, A. J. (2015b). Implicit theories about intelligence and growth (personal best) goals: Exploring reciprocal relationships. *British Journal of Educational Psychology, 85*, 207–223.

Martin, A. J., & Liem, G. A. (2010). Academic

personal bests (PBs), engagement, and achievement: A cross-lagged panel analysis. *Learning and Individual Differences, 20,* 265–270.

Möller, J., & Köller, O. (2001). Dimensional comparisons: An experimental approach to the internal/external frames of reference model. *Journal of Educational Psychology, 93,* 826–835.

Möller, J., & Marsh, H. W. (2013). Dimensional comparison theory. *Psychological Review, 120*(3), 544–560.

Möller, J., Pohlmann, B., Köller, O., & Marsh, H. W. (2009). A meta-analytic path analysis of the internal/extern frame of reference model of academic achievement and academic self-concept. *Review of Educational Research, 79,* 1129–1167.

Nagengast, B., & Marsh, H. W. (2012). Big fish in little ponds aspire more: Mediation and cross-cultural generalizability of school-average ability effects on self-concept and career aspirations in science. *Journal of Educational Psychology, 104,* 1033–1053.

Nagengast, B., Marsh, H. W., Scalas, L. F., Xu, M. K., Hau, K.-T., & Trautwein, U. (2011). Who took the "×" out of expectancy–value theory?: A psychological mystery, a substantive–methodological synergy, and a cross-national generalization. *Psychological Science, 22*(8), 1058–1066.

O'Mara, A. J., Marsh, H. W., Craven, R. G., & Debus, R. (2006). Do self-concept interventions make a difference?: A synergistic blend of construct validation and meta-analysis. *Educational Psychologist, 41,* 181–206.

Parker, P. D., Marsh, H. W., Ciarrochi, J., Marshall, S., & Abduljabbar, A. S. (2014). Juxtaposing math self-efficacy and self-concept as predictors of long-term achievement outcomes. *Educational Psychology, 34,* 29–48.

Parker, P. D., Marsh, H. W., Morin, A. J. S., Seaton, M., & Van Zanden, B. (2015). If one goes up the other must come down: Examining ipsative relationships between math and English self-concept trajectories across high school. *British Journal of Educational Psychology, 85,* 172–191.

Parker, P. D., Nagy, P. D., Trautwein, U., & Lüdtke, O. (2014). The internal/external frame of reference as predictors of career aspirations and university majors. In I. Eccles & I. Schoon (Eds.), *Gender differences in aspirations and attainment* (pp. 224–246). Cambridge, UK: Cambridge University Press.

Parker, P. D., Schoon, I., Tsai, Y., Nagy, G., Trautwein, U., & Eccles, J. (2012). Achievement, agency, gender, and socioeconomic background as predictors of postschool choices: A multi-context study. *Developmental Psychology, 48,* 1629–1642.

Pekrun, R. (2006). The control–value theory of achievement emotions: Assumptions, corollaries, and implications for educational research and practice. *Educational Psychology Review, 18,* 315–341.

Pintrich, P. R., & Schunk, D. H. (1996). *Motivation in education: Theory, research, and applications.* Englewood Cliffs, NJ: Merrill/Prentice Hall.

Pinxten, M., Marsh, H. W., De Fraine, B., Van Den Noortgate, W., & Van Damme, J. (2013). Enjoying mathematics or feeling competent in mathematics?: Reciprocal effects on mathematics achievement and perceived math effort expenditure. *British Journal of Educational Psychology, 84*(1), 152–174.

Rosenberg, M. (1979). *Conceiving the self.* New York: Basic Books.

Schunk, D. H., & Pajares, F. (2005). Competence perceptions and academic functioning. In A. J. Elliot & C. S. Dweck (Eds.), *Handbook of competence and motivation* (pp. 85–104). New York: Guilford Press.

Seaton, M., Marsh, H. W., & Craven, R. G. (2009). Earning its place as a pan-human theory: Universality of the big-fish-little-pond effect across 41 culturally and economically diverse countries. *Journal of Educational Psychology, 101,* 403–419.

Seaton, M., Marsh, H. W., & Craven, R. G. (2010). Big-fish-little-pond effect: Generalizability and moderation—two sides of the same coin. *American Educational Research Journal, 47,* 390–433.

Seligman, M. E. P., & Csikszentmihalyi, M. (2000). Positive psychology: An introduction. *American Psychologist, 55,* 5–14.

Shavelson, R. J., Hubner, J. J., & Stanton, G. C. (1976). Self-concept: Validation of construct interpretations. *Review of Educational Research, 46,* 407–441.

Skaalvik, E. M., & Skaalvik, S. (2002). Internal and external frames of reference for academic self-concept. *Educational Psychologist, 37,* 233–244.

Stankov, L., & Lee, J. (2015). Confidence: Is it different from self-efficacy? In F. Guay, H. W. Marsh, R. G. Craven, & D. McInerney (Eds.), *Self-concept, motivation, and identity: Underpinning success with research and practice* (International Advances in Self Research; Vol. 5, pp. 225–248). Charlotte, NC: Information Age.

Swann, W. B., Jr., Chang-Schneider, C., & McClarty, K. L. (2007). Do people's self-views matter?: Self-concept and self-esteem in everyday life. *American Psychologist, 62,* 84–94.

Tolman, E. C. (1932). *Purposive behavior in animals and men.* New York: Century.

Tracey, D. K., Marsh, H. W., & Craven, R. G. (2003). Self-concepts of preadolescent students with mild intellectual disabilities: Issues of measurement and educational placement. In H. W. Marsh, R. G. Craven, & D. M. McInerney (Eds.), *Self-concept, motivation, and identity: Underpinning success with research and practice* (pp. 203–230). Charlotte, NC: Information Age.

Trautwein, U., Marsh, H. W., Nagengast, B., Lüdtke, O., Nagy, G., & Jonkmann, K. (2012). Probing for the multiplicative term in modern expectancy–value theory: A latent interaction modeling study. *Journal of Educational Psychology, 104*(3), 763–777.

Trzesniewski, K., Donnellan, B., Moffitt, T., Robins, R., Poulton, R., & Caspi, A. (2006). Low self-esteem during adolescence predicts poor health, criminal behavior, and limited economic prospects during adulthood. *Developmental Psychology, 42,* 381–390.

Tymms, P. (2001). A test of the big fish in a little pond hypothesis: An investigation into the feelings of seven-year-old pupils in school. *School Effectiveness and School Improvement, 12,* 161–181.

Valentine, J. C., & DuBois, D. L. (2005). Effects of self-beliefs on academic achievement and vice-versa: Separating the chicken from the egg. In H. W. Marsh, R. G. Craven, & D. M. McInerney (Eds.), *Self-concept, motivation, and identity: Underpinning success with research and practice* (Vol. 2, pp. 53–78). Charlotte, NC: Information Age.

Valentine, J. C., DuBois, D. L., & Cooper, H. (2004). The relations between self-beliefs and academic achievement: A systematic review. *Educational Psychologist, 39,* 111–133.

Van Zanden, B. E., Marsh, H. W., Seaton, M., Parker, P. D., Guo, J., & Duineveld, J. J. (2016). How well do parents know their adolescent children?: Extending the internal/external frame of reference model of self-concept to parents. *Learning and Instruction, 47,* 25–32.

Wells, L. E., & Marwell, G. (1976). *Self-esteem: Its conceptualisation and measurement.* Beverly Hills, CA: Sage.

White, R. W. (1959). Motivation reconsidered: The concept of competence. *Psychological Bulletin, 66,* 297–333.

Wigfield, A., & Eccles, J. S. (1992). The development of achievement task values: A theoretical analysis. *Developmental Review, 12*(3), 265–310.

Wigfield, A., & Eccles, J. S. (2002). The development of competence beliefs and values from childhood through adolescence. In A. Wigfield & J. S. Eccles (Eds.), *Development of achievement motivation* (pp. 92–120). San Diego, CA: Academic Press.

Wigfield, A., Eccles, J. S., Schiefele, U., Roeser, R. W., & Davis-Kean, P. (2006). Development of achievement motivation. In N. Eisenberg, W. Damon, & R. M. Lerner (Eds.), *Handbook of child psychology: Vol. 3. Social, emotional, and personality development* (6th ed., pp. 933–1002). Hoboken, NJ: Wiley.

Wouters, S., Colpin, H., Van Damme, J., & Verschueren, K. (2015). Endorsing achievement goals exacerbates the big-fish-little-pond effect on academic self-concept. *Educational Psychology, 35*(2), 252–270.

Wylie, R. C. (1979). *The self-concept* (Vol. 2). Lincoln: University of Nebraska Press.

Xu, M. K., Marsh, H. W., Hau, K.-T., Ho, I. T., Morin, A. J. S., & Abduljabbar, A. S. (2013). The internal/external frame of reference of academic self-concept: Extension to a foreign language and the role of language of instruction. *Journal of Educational Psychology, 105*(2), 489–503.

Zeidner, M. H., & Schleyer, E. J. (1999). The big-fish-little-pond effect for academic self-concept, test anxiety, and school grades in gifted children. *Contemporary Educational Psychology, 24*(4), 305–329.

CHAPTER 7

Achievement Values
Interactions, Interventions, and Future Directions

ALLAN WIGFIELD
EMILY Q. ROSENZWEIG
JACQUELYNNE S. ECCLES

In this chapter we summarize recent research on the achievement values construct in the Eccles and colleagues expectancy–value theory (EEVT) developed over 30 years ago (Eccles-Parsons et al., 1983), and tested in a variety of studies over the intervening years. In the past decade, there has been exciting new work on individuals' achievement values, notably studies looking at how expectancies and values interact to influence outcomes, a deeper examination of the "cost" construct in EEVT, and a variety of intervention studies that are designed to enhance different-age students valuing of achievement for different subject areas. We devote much of this chapter to these three areas of research on values. We believe that the ways in which individuals value or devalue their achievement strongly influence the ways in which "people learn to use their self-regulatory tools to channel their general desire for competence towards specific outcomes and experiences" (Elliot & Dweck, 2005, p. 6). To state our argument as cogently as we can, when students do not value achievement activities, they have little competence motivation for them. We begin with a brief look at how the values construct

has been defined in the motivation field, particularly in expectancy–value theories of motivation.

A BRIEF HISTORY OF EEVT

The constructs of expectancy and value have a long history in the motivation field (Higgins, 2007; Roese & Sherman, 2007; Weiner, 1992; Wigfield & Eccles, 1992; see Wigfield, Tonks, & Klauda, 2016, for more detailed review), beginning with the work of Lewin (1938) on valence and that of Tolman (1932) on expectancies. Although in this chapter we focus primarily on values, we include expectancies in this first section because the two constructs have been linked in much of the work in the field (see Marsh, Martin, Yeung, & Craven, Chapter 6, this volume, for an in depth review of competence-related beliefs, such as expectancies). Lewin discussed how the value (or valence) of an activity influenced whether individuals would engage in the activity, and Tolman studied how expectancies for success influenced later action in both animals and humans. Atkinson (1957) developed an expectancy–value model of achievement motivation in an attempt to explain how individuals' need for achievement, expectancies, and values affected different kinds of achievement-related behaviors, such as striving for success, choice among achievement tasks, and persistence. In his model, he defined values as the inverse of expectancy; that is, tasks for which one has low expectancies for success should be the ones that are most valued. We return to this point later in our discussion of how expectancies and values interact.

MODERN EXPECTANCY–VALUE MODELS IN ACHIEVEMENT MOTIVATION

Modern expectancy value theories of achievement motivation, or motivation for activities in which there are standards for performance (e.g., Barron & Hulleman, 2015; Eccles, 2005; Eccles-Parsons et al., 1983; Pekrun, 2000, 2009; Wigfield & Eccles, 1992, 2000; see Wigfield et al., 2009, 2016), are based in Atkinson's (1957) work, in that they link achievement performance, persistence, and choice most proximally to individuals' expectancy-related and task value beliefs. However, they differ from Atkinson's model in that both the expectancy and value components are defined in richer ways, and are linked to a broader array of more distal psychological, social, and cultural determinants. We focus throughout this chapter primarily on Eccles and colleagues' EEVT model, but in this section we also discuss Pekrun's control–value approach.

Eccles and colleagues' EEVT model is presented in Figure 7.1. They initially developed the model to help understand gender differences in adolescents' achievement choices, such as why girls do not take as many advanced high school math courses or pursue math and science careers (for further discussion, see Eccles, 1984, 2005). They and other researchers have built on this work by examining how students' values predict their choices in a variety of domains, and have also looked at the developmental course of individuals' expectancies and values (e.g., Durik, Vida, & Eccles, 2006; Jacobs, Lanza, Osgood, Eccles, & Wigfield, 2002; Simpkins, Davis-Kean, & Eccles, 2006). As

can be seen by looking at the right side of the model in Figure 7.1, they postulated that expectancies and values influence performance and task choice directly. Expectancies and values themselves are influenced by individuals' task-specific beliefs, such as their self-concepts of ability, and their goals and self-schemas, along with their affective memories for different achievement-related events. These beliefs, goals, and affective memories are in turn influenced by individuals' perceptions of other peoples' attitudes and expectations for them, and by their own interpretations of their previous achievement outcomes. These perceptions and interpretations are influenced by a broad array of social and cultural factors, which include socializers' (especially parents and teachers) beliefs and behaviors, children's prior achievement experiences and aptitudes, and the cultural milieu in which they live.

The "static" nature of Figure 7.1 does not capture its full complexity. Eccles (2005) discussed four particular points about this issue. First, she discussed how students' choices based in their values have some conscious and some unconscious aspects; that is, they engage in rational decision making about their choices based on their conscious values, but there are many other socialization, cultural, and other influences of which they are not always aware that also influence their decisions. Second, individuals consider a limited array of options when making achievement choices; they may be unaware of other options available to them. Third, students make their choices in a complex social environment, and choices are often made in the context of other choices ("If I take this advanced class, I can't take this other one"; "If I do my homework, I will miss out on what is happening on Instagram"). This means that students have to weigh positive and negative aspects of their choices; Eccles states, "thus it is the hierarchy of Subjective Task Values that matter rather than the absolute values attached to the various options under consideration" (p. 107). Fourth, the processes in the model are dynamic, and the relations among the constructs in the model are developmental; that is, they change over time. We consider next how values are defined in the EEVT model.

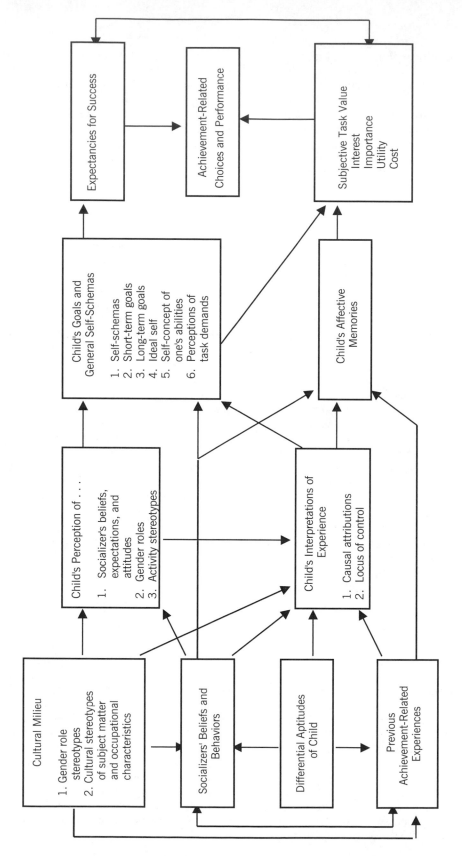

FIGURE 7.1. Eccles and colleagues' expectancy–value model of achievement choice.

Defining the Achievement Values Construct

In the motivation field, researchers have defined values in both broad and task-specific ways (for detailed discussion, see Higgins, 2007; Rohan, 2000; Wigfield & Eccles, 1992). Rokeach (1973) took a "broad" approach to human and achievement values, distinguishing between *terminal* values or desired end states (e.g., wisdom, freedom, equality, and happiness), and *instrumental* values, which are ways to attain the terminal values (e.g., honesty, responsibility, and independence). Feather (1988) found that college students' instrumental values, as defined by Rokeach (1973), predicted the value they attached to different college courses in math and English, and that the course-specific values predicted choice of college major.

Other researchers have focused more on values related to specific *tasks* than on overall values. Higgins (2007) defined *values* as the relative worth of a commodity, activity, or person, and also as the psychological experience of being attracted to (or repulsed by) an object or activity. Similarly, Eccles and her colleagues define values with respect to the qualities of different achievement tasks and how those qualities influence the individual's desire to do the tasks (Eccles, 2005; Eccles-Parsons et al., 1983; Wigfield & Eccles, 1992). Their definition, like that of Higgins (2007), stresses the motivational aspects of task value. Furthermore, values in the EEVT model are *subjective* because various individuals assign different values to the same activity; math achievement is valuable to some students but not to others.

Eccles-Parsons and colleagues (1983) proposed that one's overall subjective task value for an activity is a function of three components: attainment value or importance, intrinsic value, and utility value or usefulness of the task (for a more detailed discussion of these components, see Eccles, 2005; Eccles-Parsons et al., 1983; Wigfield & Eccles, 1992). Eccles-Parsons and colleagues defined *attainment value* as the importance of doing well on a given task. Attainment value incorporates identity issues; tasks are important when individuals view them as central to their own sense of themselves, or as allowing them to express or confirm important aspects of self. For example, if high school athletes have high attainment value in sports, this means they define themselves at least in part in terms of their success at sports, see sports as an important part of who they will be in the future, and feel that sports success is very important to them.

Intrinsic value is the enjoyment one gains from doing the task. This component is similar in certain respects to notions of intrinsic motivation and interest (see Hidi & Renninger, 2006; Ryan & Deci, 2009; Schiefele, 2009), but it is important to acknowledge that these constructs come from different theoretical traditions. Eccles (2005) discusses in some detail not only the similarities but also the distinctions between intrinsic value, intrinsic motivation, as defined by Ryan and Deci, and interest, as defined by researchers such as Hidi and Schiefele. When children intrinsically value an activity, they often become deeply engaged in it and can persist at it for a long time.

Utility value, or usefulness, refers to how a task fits into an individual's future plans, for instance, taking a math class to fulfill a requirement for a science degree. In certain respects, utility value is similar to extrinsic motivation because when doing an activity out of utility value, the activity is a means to an end rather than an end in itself (see Ryan & Deci, 2009; Ryan & Moller, Chapter 12, this volume). However, the activity also can reflect some important goals that the person holds deeply, such as attaining a certain occupation. In this sense, utility value also connects to personal goals and sense of self, and so has some ties to attainment value. These three all exert positive influences on the overall subjective value the individual has for a given achievement activity.

Eccles-Parsons and colleagues (1983) also discussed other things that influence individuals' subjective task values: sex role identity, their previous affective experiences with different activities, and perceptions of the cost of doing the activity. We focus here on cost, which Eccles-Parsons and colleagues described in terms of cost–benefit ratio for different activities. If an activity "costs" too much, the individual won't do it (see also Eccles, 2005). They described different kinds or types of costs: individuals' perceptions of how much effort they would need to exert to complete a task and whether it is worth doing, how much engaging in one activity means that other valued activities cannot be done (e.g., "Do I do my math homework or check Instagram?"), and the emotional or psychological costs of pursuing the task, particularly the cost of failure (e.g., "Will taking this advanced course make me feel emotionally drained?"). Over the last few years, researchers have done important work on the nature of cost; we discuss this work later.

Pekrun's Control–Value Model

Pekrun (1993, 2000, 2006, 2009) developed a model of achievement motivation based in the expectancy–value tradition (see also Pekrun, Chapter 14, this volume). He calls his theory a control–value theory, defining *control* as individuals' appraisals of how much control they think they have over their achievement outcomes. This sense of control is based on their expectancies for success in a given achievement situation, as well as their attributions for their performance (e.g., "Was my outcome due to my own actions or something else?"). He also distinguished different kinds of achievement values, or *value cognitions,* to use his term; one example of this is that he differentiates between the value of outcomes and the value of actions, and further separates intrinsic and extrinsic aspects of each. *Intrinsic outcome values* concern the intrinsic enjoyment of an outcome, whereas *extrinsic outcome values* reflect the instrumentality of an outcome (i.e., how useful that outcome is for the future). In the same vein, *intrinsic action values* relate to the inherent value of the action to the individual, whereas *extrinsic action values* have to do with actions that lead to an instrumental outcome (e.g., studying to get a good grade on a test in order to maximize one's chances of getting into graduate school).

One important aspect of this model is Pekrun's (1993) specification of how individuals' appraisals of different activities lead to motivation to undertake an action or not, and also to their performance. The process starts with an appraisal of the value of a given outcome; if it is valued, then the

individual forms expectancies of success for it. Ultimately, individuals' motivation to engage in the activity is determined by the complex interplay of their values, expectancies, and control beliefs (see Pekrun, Chapter 14, this volume, for further discussion of these beliefs and values and their ties to achievement emotions).

RELATIONS OF VALUES TO OUTCOMES: MAIN EFFECTS

As specified in the EEVT model, Eccles-Parsons and colleagues (1983) proposed that individuals' expectancies and values are the strongest direct predictors of different achievement outcomes, performance, and choices. Many studies in different domains show that individuals' expectancies for success are (relative to values) particularly strong predictors of their subsequent performance (e.g., Bong, Cho, Ahn, & Kim, 2012; Durik et al., 2006; Meece, Wigfield, & Eccles, 1990; Musu-Gillette, Wigfield, Harring, & Eccles, 2015).

Students' subjective task values predict both intentions and actual decisions to persist at different activities, such as taking mathematics and English courses, and engaging in sports. For instance, Meece and colleagues (1990) looked at the longitudinal relations of students' expectancies for success at math and the importance of math to their subsequent performance and intentions to continue taking math courses. Students' expectancies were the strongest direct predictor of performance, whereas their math importance ratings were the strongest predictors of their intentions to keep taking math when the option to stop became available. Importantly, because expectancies and values relate positively to one another, each also has indirect effects on both performance and intentions; we return to this point later.

The relations of values to choice extend over time. Durik and colleagues (2006) found that the importance children gave to reading in fourth grade related significantly to the number of English classes they took in high school. Also, children's interest in reading measured in fourth grade indirectly predicted (through interest measured in 10th grade) high school leisure-time reading, career aspirations, and course selections. Simpkins and colleagues (2006) found that children's participation in math and science activities in late elementary school related to their subsequent expectancies and values in these subjects, which in turn predicted the number of math and science courses they took through high school. Interestingly, in this study, children's ability-related beliefs in high school predicted choice more strongly than did their values; Simpkins and colleagues speculated that this may have occurred because most students know the importance of such courses for college entrance and are more likely to take them when they expect to do well in them. Finally, Musu-Gillette and colleagues (2015) found that students' valuing of math measured in high school predicted their college major choice.

THE INTERACTIONS OF EXPECTANCIES AND VALUES IN PREDICTING OUTCOMES

Much of the work examining how expectancies and values predict outcomes has not examined the potential interactions between the two; however, this has changed over the last few years. In an initial study, Trautwein and colleagues (2012) examined the main effects of expectancies, different aspects of values, and their interaction on the math and English performance of a large sample of German high school students, noting that the interaction of expectancies and values was an important part of Atkinson's (1957) original expectancy–value model. Both expectancies and the different aspects of values (interest, attainment, and utility) predicted performance. When students' values were entered into the model after expectancies, values were no longer a significant predictor of performance. However, the expectancies × values interaction term positively predicted performance; in other words, having higher value increased the positive effect of expectancies on performance. Nagengast and colleagues (2011) found this same interaction effect when studying engagement in science and intention to pursue science careers in a sample of nearly 400,000 high school students from 57 countries.

Since this initial work, both Guo, Parker, Marsh, and Morin (2015) and Nagengast, Trautwein, Kelava, and Lüdtke (2013) found that the interaction of students' expectancies and values predicted a variety of student outcomes in different academic domains. Nagengast and colleagues used multilevel modeling to test how high school students' expectations and values predicted their homework engagement in different subjects; rather than testing the effects of these variables between students, the researchers evaluated intraindividual differences in students' expectations and values for one of six subjects relative to others. They found that a latent within-student interaction between expectations and values predicted homework engagement. Students engaged more with their homework in a particular subject when their expectancies and values were both high in that subject. Guo, Parker, and colleagues found that high school students' choices to take advanced math courses, math achievement, and whether students entered college were predicted by a positive expectancy–value interaction as well. That is, the interaction effects build on the individual main effects of both expectancies and values on outcomes.

By contrast, other researchers have found interaction effects suggesting that the value students have for some achievement activities predicts their achievement behavior more strongly when their self-concepts of ability for that activity are low. These effects have been found for both maladaptive and positive achievement outcomes. Lee, Bong, and Kim (2014) found that Korean middle school students with high intrinsic or utility value for learning English were more likely to procrastinate and to cheat in their English as a foreign language class as their self-efficacy decreased. Hensley (2014) found a similar interaction for procrastination among undergraduate anatomy students, and Lee, Lee, and Bong (2013) also found this effect among Korean eighth- and ninth-grade students on test stress and academic self-handicapping. Guo, Marsh, Parker, Morin, and Yeung (2015) found that utility value predicted students' scores on an international standardized math exam and their intentions to pursue advanced education more strongly when their self-concepts were low.

Why do interactive effects of expectancies and values look different across these studies? Perhaps the age of students, students' overall levels of achievement on the task or activity being measured, the academic domain, or facets of school culture, such as a norm for performance versus mastery, influenced whether expectations and values interacted positively or negatively with each other. Recall that Atkinson (1957) originally proposed that expectancies and values are inversely related and sum to one, meaning that the tasks students value most are the ones at which they have low expectancies for success. Furthermore, resultant motivation is highest when expectancies and values are both .50. The interaction effect found by Lee and colleagues (2014) provides some support for the inverse relation of expectancies and values; at least on *maladaptive* achievement behaviors, middle school students who valued English were more likely to cheat if their self-efficacy was low rather than high. It is important to note, however, that researchers studying how expectancies and values interact do not assume, as Atkinson did, that the two are inversely related; indeed, all of the correlational work to date shows that students' interest, attainment, and utility values relate positively to their expectancies for success. Wigfield and Eccles (1992) discussed in detail reasons why we should expect positive relations of expectancies and values in "real-world" situations in which most individuals likely value tasks at which they have a much higher probability of succeeding than the "optimum" .50 in Atkinson's model.

Although these findings add to our understanding of how expectancies and values predict outcomes, it is important to note that the overall amount of variance explained by the interactions in most of the previously discussed studies was small and likely detected because researchers used very large samples. Trautwein and colleagues (2012) argued that a small effect size does not mean that an effect is unimportant, which is true. However, many researchers may not be able to find such interactions unless they use large samples of students in their analyses. Researchers should keep this in mind when considering how many students to use in studies of interactions between expectations and values.

Researchers also may want to consider alternative ways to explore the interplay between values and expectations, such as manipulating both of these constructs experimentally rather than simply measuring them (e.g., Durik, Schechter, Noh, Rozek, & Harackiewicz, 2014); manipulations often cause larger effects because these variables are more salient to students, so this paradigm might require fewer students to observe an expectancy–value interaction (Trautwein et al., 2012). Another idea is to employ person-centered approaches to analyze these variables (e.g., Conley, 2012; Rosenzweig & Wigfield, in press; Simpkins & Davis-Kean, 2005). Person-centered approaches can separate students into profiles based on their combinations of expectations and values; the relationship of the different profiles with achievement can provide insight into what combinations of these constructs might be adaptive for students, as well as information about what combinations are most common for certain groups.

COST: EXPANDING ITS COMPONENTS

In a number of review chapters that Wigfield, Eccles, and others have written on EEVT, they described cost as a "component" of achievement values, and stated that it has been the least studied. With respect to the first point, both Barron and Hulleman (2015) and Flake, Barron, Hulleman, McCoach, and Welsh (2015) recently have described cost as something that influences values rather than as a "component" of values. As noted earlier, this view actually corresponds more to the way in which Eccles-Parsons and colleagues (1983) defined cost in their original presentation of the model (see also Eccles, 2005). Eccles-Parsons and colleagues stated that individuals think about the cost–benefit ratio of doing an activity when determining its value to them. Thus, in their conceptualization, cost *impacts* values but is not a *component* of values (despite the fact that it often is included in the subjective task values box in figures depicting the model).

Researchers have shown that cost is empirically distinct from the interest, importance, and utility aspects of task values. Furthermore, using confirmatory factor analysis, Conley (2012), Kosovich, Hulleman, Barron, and Getty (2015), and Trautwein and colleagues (2012) all demonstrated that cost, expectancies, and values are separate factors. Additionally, there is some work suggesting that cost relates more highly to individuals' expectancies than to their values. Barron and Hulleman (2015) conducted a thoughtful and comprehensive historical review of how cost is conceptualized in the EEVT model, and proposed an expectancy–value–*cost* motivation model, in which cost is a separate construct from values. We concur that viewing cost as something that impacts values rather than being a component of values is theoretically more in line with the EEVT model as originally proposed by Eccles-Parsons and colleagues. However, we do not at this point believe that cost should be added to the name of the theory. We also encourage researchers to continue to examine the relations among these constructs.

Also as mentioned earlier, Eccles-Parsons and colleagues (1983) and Eccles (2005) discussed several different types of cost, as have Baron and Hulleman (2015), Battle and Wigfield (2003), and Perez, Cromley, and Kaplan (2014). *Opportunity cost* refers to valued alternatives that an individual has to give up to do a task (e.g., "Do I do my math homework or go on Facebook?"). *Effort cost* is the individual's sense of whether the perceived effort he or she needs to put into task completion is worth it (e.g., "Is working this hard to get an A in math worth it?"). Baron and Hulleman (2015) proposed adding another aspect of effort cost, the amount of effort needed to complete other valued activities and its impact on one's ability to complete the task at hand. They called this *effort unrelated cost*. The example they used is faculty members trying to balance the effort needed to complete both research and teaching activities. *Psychological cost* concerns the potentially negative psychological or emotional consequences of participating in an academic activity, such as performance anxiety and fear of success or failure (e.g., "Will I feel stupid if I don't do well on the math test?"). In our recent discussions of cost while preparing this chapter, Eccles noted another kind of cost, *sunk cost*, which refers

to one's evaluation of how much effort one already has put into an activity, and given that, whether it makes sense to continue or to quit. There also can be *economic costs* of completing some activities, and *social costs* as well ("Will doing this activity impact my standing with important others?"). In Figure 7.2 we present a graphic representing the way we see intrinsic, attainment, utility, and these other aspects of cost influencing individuals' overall valuing of a given activity.

A number of researchers have developed and tested some interesting expanded measures of task values and cost. Based on a review of existing literature, Gaspard, Dicke, Flunger, Schreier, and colleagues (2015) expanded the operationalization of task values, proposing that the importance, utility, and intrinsic components of values, and cost, can be differentiated further. They proposed that attainment value consists of the overall importance of achieving good grades, and personal importance, or the importance of mastering the material and how it relates to one's identity. They proposed five components of utility: utility for school, or the usefulness of one's education; utility for job, or future career opportunities; utility of math for different parts of one's daily life; social utility, or how being knowledgeable in math impacted being accepted by one's peers; and general utility for the future. They subdivided cost into opportunity cost, effort cost, and psychological cost. Their new measure assessed these proposed new dimensions, and Gaspard and colleagues gave it to 1,900 German ninth-grade students. Their confirmatory factor analysis supported the separation of cost into the separate components they defined. The measurement of cost was invariant between males and females, but females were found to perceive more psychological and effort cost than males.

Perez and colleagues (2014) adapted Battle and Wigfield's (2003) measure of cost and developed questions to assess effort cost, opportunity cost, and psychological cost in the domain of college science. These aspects of cost are similar to those defined by Gaspard, Dicke, Flunger, Schreier, and colleagues (2015), but Perez and colleagues' items are mostly about specific barriers that students are likely to encounter during college (i.e., student loans, choosing majors).

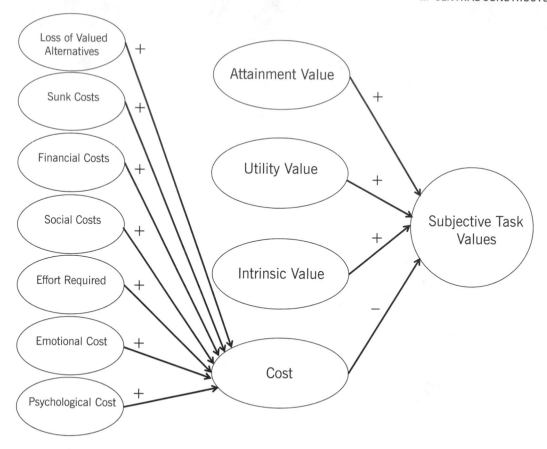

FIGURE 7.2. How value components and cost influence individuals' overall subjective valuing of achievement tasks.

They also defined *opportunity cost* as how much schoolwork interfered with students' relationships, whereas Gaspard, Dicke, Flunger, Schreier, and colleagues considered opportunity cost more broadly, as sacrificing time spent on one activity to do another. They found that these three aspects of cost were empirically distinct.

Flake and colleagues (2015) also developed a new measure of cost that was intended to apply to a broader variety of students than the Perez and colleagues (2014) scale, such as college or noncollege students, and students who were studying a particular class instead of pursuing a specific major. Opportunity and psychological cost in these models were defined similarly to Gaspard, Dicke, Flunger, Schreier, and colleagues' (2015) definitions, but as we just discussed, Flake and colleagues' measure separated effort cost into two aspects, related and unrelated effort. They found that these four components of cost formed separate factors empirically. However, they were highly correlated and a higher-order model of "overall" cost also fit the data well.

Researchers have examined how strongly cost predicts outcomes in different academic domains. Battle and Wigfield (2003), Flake and colleagues (2015), Kirkpatrick, Chang, Lee, Tas, and Anderman (2013), Perez and colleagues (2014), Safavian, Conley, and Karabenick (2013), and others have found that cost negatively predicts adolescents' and college students' achievement, plans to take Advanced Placement (AP) courses, and plans to pursue science courses or careers, or graduate school in general. Some work suggests that students' perceptions of cost may be an especially important predictor of adaptive academic achievement. Barron and Hulleman (2015) reported that students' expectations predicted their grades in biology, and their values predicted their interest in the subject, but their perceptions of cost predicted both outcomes. Conley (2012) conducted cluster analyses on variables from expectancy–value theory and goal orientation theory. Cost was a key variable differentiating groups of students with high and low combinations of goals, values, and competence beliefs, and the groups that perceived high cost showed less adaptive patterns of math test scores and positive affect than did the groups that perceived low cost. One study in the sports domain had different findings. Chiang, Byrd, and Molin (2011) found that cost did not predict students' self-reports of exercising as strongly as did the other components of task values. However, they used a measure of cost with only three items looking at perceptions of effort and opportunity cost, and the measure had relatively low reliability. Thus, taken together, this variety of recent findings suggests that cost should be consistently included in studies exploring the effects of values on students' achievement outcomes. This work also suggests, as Eccles-Parsons and colleagues (1983) stated, that cost should be considered an influence on values rather than an aspect of values. We are excited that researchers have done this important work on cost and believe it will lead to further important work. Like Barron and Hulleman (2015), we urge researchers to include appropriate measures of cost in their studies based in expectancy–value theory.

INTERVENING TO ENHANCE CHILDREN'S VALUES: FROM FOCUSED TO BROAD APPROACHES

Children's experiences in school, including classroom climate and the specific interactions students have with their teachers and peers, strongly influence their developing values (Eccles & Midgley, 1989; Wigfield, Eccles, & Rodriguez, 1998). Researchers increasingly have begun to conduct intervention studies designed to enhance students' achievement values in different academic areas. These interventions range in scope from targeting only one type of achievement value to targeting multiple types of values, to targeting values in addition to other motivational variables. Some of the interventions are quite brief, in the tradition of other recently developed social psychological interventions designed to enhance students' motivation (Yeager & Walton, 2011), while others last longer and are fully embedded in teachers' classroom practices. We review both types of work in this section.

Interventions Targeting One Aspect of Values

Researchers implementing brief interventions usually have focused on enhancing one aspect of students' achievement values. Most of this work has targeted utility value and has been conducted in science, technology, engineering, and math (STEM) fields (for reviews, see Harackiewicz, Tibbits, Canning, & Hyde, 2014; Rosenzweig & Wigfield, 2016). For instance, Hulleman and Harackiewicz (2009; Hulleman, Godes, Hendricks, & Harackiewicz, 2010) conducted experiments in which they had one group of high school or college students write a brief essay, either once in the lab or in class every 3 or 4 weeks, about the relevance of what they were learning to their lives. A control group completed an unrelated task, such as summarizing what they learned (students were learning science, psychology, or a new mental math technique). Results showed that (relative to the control group) the intervention boosted students' utility value and interest in the topics they were learning, as well as their achievement; there were also stronger effects for students who started with lower expectations for their performance.

Brown, Smith, Thoman, Allen, and Muragishi (2015), Canning and Harackiewicz (2015), Durik and colleagues (2014), and Shechter, Durik, Miyamoto, and Harackiewicz (2011) have studied the effects of interventions that directly tell students about utility value of a topic, instead of asking students to come up with utility value connections themselves. For instance, in a laboratory study, Canning and Harackiewicz found that directly communicating utility value information to low-confidence students undermined their math performance and interest, but when these students received this information *and* generated their own examples of utility value, they performed better and were more interested in the math technique than when they only generated their own examples. They also found that low-confidence students preferred to read examples of how utility value connected to their everyday lives versus to their careers or academics. Brown and colleagues proposed an additional way to frame utility value information; college students in a laboratory study were more interested in a biomedical career after reading about how biomedical research helped others than when they read only about the personal utility of the research.

Harackiewicz, Rozek, Hulleman, and Hyde (2012) targeted high school students' utility value by intervening with their parents. Parents were randomly assigned to treatment and control groups; treatment parents received brief materials a few times over 2 years regarding how to help their children make decisions about their futures; the materials emphasized the importance of math and science. Students whose parents received the materials took significantly more math and science courses than did those in the control group. Furthermore, mothers' perceived utility value of math and science partially mediated these effects. Interestingly, though, follow-up analyses of this data by Rozek, Hyde, Svoboda, Hulleman, and Harackiewicz (2015) indicated that the intervention only improved course taking for lower-achieving boys and higher-achieving girls. The authors discussed how parents of daughters who are achieving less well may succumb to the stereotype that girls generally do less well in math and science, so a utility intervention may not be effective with them.

In their utility value intervention work, Orthner, Jones-Sanpei, Akos, and Rose (2013) and Wooley, Rose, Orthner, Akos, and Jones-Sanpei (2013) evaluated at the school level CareerStart, a schoolwide intervention focused on emphasizing the relevance of instruction for students' careers. Middle school teachers in core academic domains provided students with examples of careers that were related to course content; these examples represented careers from the labor markets of the schools that were participating in the program. The authors found that students in schools randomly assigned to CareerStart reported more utility and importance of school, and earned higher state math test scores (but not reading scores), than did students in control schools.

To date, no researchers have solely targeted students' attainment or intrinsic value, or perceptions of cost, in their interventions; however, some broader interventions may have improved these aspects of task value without the authors intending to do so. Specifically, Cohen, Garcia, Apfel, and Master (2006), Cohen, Garcia, Purdie-Vaughns, Apfel, and Brzustoski (2009), Cook, Purdie-Vaughns, Garcia, and Cohen (2012), Harackiewicz, Canning, and colleagues (2014), Miyake and colleagues (2010), Sherman and colleagues (2013), and others conducted interventions that likely targeted cost using interventions focused on personally meaningful values, and Walkington (2013), Renninger and colleagues (2014), and others may have targeted intrinsic value in interventions targeting interest. For instance, Miyake and colleagues asked students to affirm personal values in order to mitigate negative psychological experiences that might occur when taking physics. Intervention students wrote brief essays about personal values that were important to them, such as family. Women, who are typically negatively stereotyped for science, showed higher achievement versus women in a control group, and the achievement gap between men and women in the physics class narrowed. This intervention was thought to buffer women against identity threat associated with participation in STEM fields by having them write about social belonging (Cohen & Sherman, 2014; Shnabel, Purdie-Vaughts, Cook, Garcia, & Cohen, 2013). Although uncertainty about social belonging experiences relates to psychological cost, reducing cost was not an explicit goal of the study. Future research might consider using these types of methods to target students' experiences of cost in a class.

Interventions Targeting Multiple Types of Values

Gaspard, Dicke, Flunger, Brisson, and colleagues (2015) designed an intervention program targeting achievement values (called Motivation for Mathematics, or MoMa) focused on enhancing ninth-grade students' math utility value. They implemented in 25 German high schools a 1-hour intervention either encouraging students to write a brief essay connecting math to their lives or asking them to read and respond to quotations from fellow students about the relevance of math. The study utilized a cluster randomized control design. Compared to a waiting-list control condition, students in both intervention conditions reported higher utility value for math, but effects were stronger in the quotation condition than in the essay condition. Also, even though the intervention focused on utility value, students in the quotation condition reported higher perceptions of intrinsic and attainment value (but not lower perceptions of cost) than students in the control group. Female students benefited from the intervention more than males on some measures.

Acee and Weinstein (2010) conducted an intervention that explicitly targeted three aspects of values defined in Eccles-Parsons and colleagues' (1983) EEVT model. These researchers asked college statistics students to complete a 100-minute computer session containing activities designed to target attainment, utility, and intrinsic value. For example, to increase attainment value, students read a passage about the importance of understanding why course content would be personally valuable; they brainstormed a list of skills that they could develop by learning statistics. Intervention group students showed higher perceptions of statistics value and instrumentality than did control group students, and they were more likely than control group students to access a supplemental website about statistics, provided a few weeks after the intervention. One class section of two that received the intervention also earned higher statistics test scores.

Interventions Targeting Values and Other Motivational Constructs

Some researchers have targeted students' values as part of interventions that also target other motivational variables, such as expectations or perceptions of autonomy. In a series of studies, Weisgram and Bigler (2006a, 2006b, 2007) targeted the variables from expectancy–value theory (women's self-efficacy, measured in place of expectations in this study, and values) by recruiting middle and high school girls to attend workshops or camps about science and engineering. They embedded into these programs activities designed to target self-efficacy (e.g., students successfully completed hands-on science activities) and values (e.g., students received information about scientific careers). These researchers targeted achievement values broadly rather than focusing on just one of the aspects of task value. They found that their programs improved students' values and self-efficacy compared to comparison groups of students who did not attend, or based on a comparison of the same students before and after the intervention programs.

In their intervention, Yang and Wu (2012) also targeted students' achievement values broadly, along with expectations, but they focused on English rather than math and science. High school students who received a digital storytelling intervention for 22 weeks, in which they created stories based on course content, had higher self-efficacy and values (measured as a composite score based on attainment, utility, and intrinsic value items), English achievement, and critical thinking than did students who heard lectures on course content. The authors argued that the storytelling intervention allowed students to experience mastery (increasing their competence beliefs) and to connect the material to their personal experiences (increasing their task value).

Falco, Summers, and Bauman (2010), Feng and Tuan (2005), Guthrie and colleagues (2004); Guthrie, Wigfield, and Klauda (2012), Marinak (2013), Martin (2005, 2008), and others (see Wigfield, Mason-Singh, Ho, & Guthrie, 2014, for a recent review) have conducted motivation interventions designed to foster a variety of aspects of students' motivation, including their achievement values. All of these researchers took an eclectic approach in their interventions, in that they utilized multiple motivation theories in selecting intervention practices, and most measured multiple aspects of motivation as outcome measures. We describe in some detail one example of this kind of work, Guthrie and colleagues' (2004; Guthrie, Klauda, & Morrison, 2012) work on concept-oriented reading instruction (CORI).

The purpose of CORI is to help children and adolescents become engaged readers; that is, to become strategic, knowledge-driven, motivated, and socially interactive in their reading activities (Guthrie et al., 2004; Guthrie, Klauda, & Morrison, 2012; Guthrie & Wigfield, 2000). CORI is based in Guthrie and Wigfield's (2000) engagement model of reading comprehension, in which they describe how teaching and classroom practices impact students' motivation, which then influences their reading comprehension. In designing CORI and developing teaching practices to promote students' motivation Guthrie, Wigfield and their colleagues (e.g., Guthrie, Wigfield, & Klauda, 2012; Guthrie, Wigfield, & Perencevich, 2004) took an eclectic approach to motivation, including major constructs from a variety of motivation theories, including EEVT, social-cognitive theory, and self-determination theory. Table 7.1 presents the motivation support strategies included in CORI at both the elementary and middle school levels (see Wigfield et al., 2014, for more detailed discussion of these practices). The motivation practices differ at the different grade levels in order to reflect children's motivational characteristics and the issues they face at that developmental phase. For our purposes in this chapter, the most important thing to note is that practices related to students' valuing of reading are more prominent at middle school; there, the relevance of reading to students and its importance receive greater emphasis. The reason for this is that in an interview study conducted by Guthrie, Klauda, and Morrison (2012), seventh-grade students expressed in no uncertain terms how the science reading in their classrooms was boring and irrelevant to them.

To describe these practices in more detail, when *emphasizing importance,* teachers help students to recognize why information text reading is useful to their future lives and careers. For example, a teacher might point out to students that of the five classroom activities they did that day, reading gave them the most information about the day's topic. *Affording relevance* means helping students connect their reading with personal experiences. For example, teachers might show brief video clips to introduce scientific phenomena and historical events to students in a dynamic and memorable way. The videos help students form their own questions and interests related to the conceptual theme of a particular unit, which they then explore further by reading books, articles, and Web resources in depth.

Much research has been conducted on CORI. Guthrie and colleagues (2007) conducted a meta-analysis of 11 quasi-experimental studies that investigated how CORI impacted third- through fifth-grade students. The results showed moderate-to-strong positive effects of CORI on motivation, reading comprehension, reading strategy use, science knowledge, word recognition speed, and oral reading fluency. Similarly, using a comparison group pretest–posttest quasi-experimental design, Guthrie, Klauda, and Ho (2013) found that a 6-week iteration of CORI improved middle school students' motivation, engagement, and information text comprehension; CORI was also associated indirectly with information text comprehension through motivation. Finally, a 4-week CORI unit that integrated history and reading/language arts instruction produced increased information text comprehension in comparison to traditional instruction, and

TABLE 7.1. Motivational and Strategy Instructional Practices for Elementary and Middle School Implementations of CORI

Elementary school	Middle school
• Knowledge content goals	• Thematic unit
• Optimizing student choice	• Relevance
• Hands-on experiences relating to text and reading activities	• Reading importance
• Collaboration	• Success
• Many interesting texts	• Choice
• Support for student collaboration	• Collaboration

accounted for positive changes in students' motivation and engagement in a study using a switching replications design (Guthrie & Klauda, 2014). Thus, CORI has been implemented successfully at both elementary and middle school levels, and has had positive effects on students' reading motivation and comprehension.

Conclusions and Future Directions for Intervention Work

Generally, the intervention work to date that has focused on enhancing different-age students' achievement values and other motivational constructs has shown strong positive effects on the motivational constructs that they target. Some interventions have demonstrated that targeting only utility value can improve performance, although there are moderating variables that influenced these results, such as students' competence-related beliefs and their achievement at the beginning of the intervention. Other interventions have targeted multiple types of values, and the work of Gaspard, Dicke, Flunger, Brisson, and colleagues (2015) suggests interventions that only target one aspect of students' achievement values actually can improve several aspects simultaneously. Finally, there is evidence that broader motivation interventions targeting a number of variables also can improve students' values in different subject areas.

There are several important directions that future researchers should consider for values-focused interventions. To date, we have found no study that solely targets students' attainment value, intrinsic value, or attempts to reduce perceptions of cost in any academic domain. Interventions specifically focused on utility value have provided many important insights as to the best practices for improving this variable and the types of students for whom these practices work best. Researchers should conduct similar work with respect to the other values-related constructs (for examples of related work, see Harackiewicz, Tibbetts, et al., 2014; Renninger et al., 2014).

A second important future direction is paying more attention to moderating variables that might limit the efficacy of values interventions. In previous studies, students'

confidence, previous ability, gender, and ethnicity moderated the effects of different interventions (for a review, see Rosenzweig & Wigfield, 2016). One critical moderating variable to which researchers have paid little attention is age; it is likely that developmental differences affect the results of interventions. Some researchers have replicated successful interventions with different ages of students (e.g., CORI, utility value essay interventions); however, few researchers have specifically evaluated whether age moderates the results of values interventions or examined how motivation intervention practices "match" the motivation-related challenges different-aged students face.

There are also moderating variables associated with the classroom context, such as teacher–student relationships, the domain of interventions, and school culture, that may affect how well values-focused interventions work. These types of variables have received less research attention than have individual-level variables, yet they are quite likely to moderate interventions' results (Rosenzweig & Wigfield, 2016). For instance, it may be difficult for a teacher to convince students that learning math is important when students do not have a positive, trusting relationship with that teacher. Researchers should assess these variables when conducting values interventions and take care to replicate successful interventions with multiple types of schools and classrooms, and across different academic domains.

Finally, measurement and design characteristics of interventions should be improved in future research. With few exceptions, intervention researchers have measured motivation using self-report questionnaires completed by participants. This can be difficult because students' self-reports of motivation do not always match their experiences. Researchers should explore new ways to assess students' motivation and use a variety of types of measures to gain a more complete picture of students' values. Two research design issues that warrant attention are intervention length (i.e., how long interventions last) and dosage (i.e., how many motivation supports, or what amount of motivation supports, are given to students during each intervention session). Few researchers have systematically explored these variables or justified their choices of particular intervention lengths or dosages to date (Rosenzweig & Wigfield, 2016). Understanding these effects can improve the effect sizes of interventions that target students' values.

CONCLUSION

As we hope is clear from the studies reviewed in this chapter, work on achievement values has been a vibrant part of the research on competence motivation. We are particularly excited about two aspects of this work. First is the burgeoning work on cost. The cost construct is no longer "understudied," although, clearly, more work on it is needed (utilizing the recently developed, more elaborate questionnaire measures) to understand its relations to the three components of achievement values and various academic outcomes. Second is the new intervention work on utility and other components of students' values for tasks in different subject areas. Much of this work is in the tradition of other brief, focused psychological interventions that have proven remarkably successful (Yeager & Walton, 2011). While we are encouraged by this, more work is needed on the long-term effectiveness of such interventions, the variables that moderate their effects, and the processes that explain why simple interventions can be effective.

We have discussed individuals' achievement values separately from the other constructs in EEVT in this chapter. As research on values moves forward, it will be critical to look at values and their relations to various outcomes in conjunction with individuals' expectancies, goals, and other achievement-related beliefs. We look forward to participating in the work on these topics.

ACKNOWLEDGMENTS

Much of the research on the development of children's competence beliefs and values was conducted by Jacquelynne S. Eccles, Allan Wigfield, and colleagues with support from Grant No. HD-17553 from the National Institute of Child Health and Human Development (NICHD). Other research discussed in this chapter was supported by Grant No. MH-31724 from the National Institute of Mental Health, Grant No. HD-17296 from NICHD, Grant No. BNS-8510504, and Graduate Research Fellowship No. DGE1322106 from the National Science Foundation, and grants from the Spencer Foundation. The research on CORI was funded by Grant No. 0089225 from the Interagency Educational Research Initiative (funding through the National Science Foundation) and Grant No. R01HD052590 from NICHD.

REFERENCES

Acee, T. W., & Weinstein, C. E. (2010). Effects of a value-reappraisal intervention on statistics students' motivation and performance. *Journal of Experimental Education, 78*(4), 487–512.

Atkinson, J. W. (1957). Motivational determinants of risk-taking behavior. *Psychological Review, 64,* 359–372.

Barron, K. E., & Hulleman, C. S. (2015). Expectancy–value–cost model of motivation. In J. S. Eccles & K. Salmelo-Aro (Eds.), *International encyclopedia of social and behavioral sciences: Motivational psychology* (2nd ed., pp. 503–509). New York: Elsevier.

Battle, A., & Wigfield, A. (2003). College women's value orientations toward family, career, and graduate school. *Journal of Vocational Behavior, 62,* 56–75.

Bong, M., Cho, C., Ahn, H. S., & Kim, H. J. (2012). Comparison of self-beliefs for predicting student motivation and achievement. *Journal of Educational Research, 105,* 336–352.

Brown, E. R., Smith, J. L., Thoman, D. B., Allen, J. M., & Muragishi, G. (2015). From bench to bedside: A communal utility value intervention to enhance students' biomedical science motivation. *Journal of Educational Psychology, 107*(4), 1116–1135.

Canning, E. A., & Harackiewicz, J. M. (2015). Teach it, don't preach it: The differential effects of directly communicated and self-generated utility–value information. *Motivation Science, 1*(1), 47–71.

Chiang, E. S., Byrd, S. P., & Molin, A. J. (2011). Children's perceived cost for exercise: Application of an expectancy–value paradigm. *Health Education and Behavior, 38*(2), 143–149.

Cohen, G. L., Garcia, J., Apfel, N., & Master, A. (2006). Reducing the racial achievement gap: A social-psychological intervention. *Science, 313,* 1307–1310.

Cohen, G. L., Garcia, J., Purdie-Vaughns, V., Apfel, N., & Brzustoski, P. (2009). Recursive processes in self-affirmation: Intervening to close the minority achievement gap. *Science, 324,* 400–403.

Cohen, G. L., & Sherman, D. K. (2014). The psychology of change: Self-affirmation and social-psychological intervention. *Annual Review of Psychology, 65,* 333–371.

Conley, A. M. (2012). Patterns of motivation beliefs: Combining achievement goal and expectancy–value perspectives. *Journal of Educational Psychology, 104*(1), 32–47.

Cook, J. E., Purdie-Vaughns, V., Garcia, J., & Cohen, G. L. (2012). Chronic threat and contingent belonging: Protective benefits of values affirmation on identity development. *Journal of Personality and Social Psychology, 102,* 479–496.

Durik, A. M., Shechter, O. G., Noh, M., Rozek, C. S., & Harackiewicz, J. M. (2014). What if I can't?: Success expectancies moderate the effects of utility value information on situational interest and performance. *Motivation and Emotion, 39*(1), 104–118.

Durik, A. M., Vida, M., & Eccles, J. S. (2006). Task values and ability beliefs as predictors of high school literacy choices: A developmental analysis. *Journal of Educational Psychology, 98,* 382–393.

Eccles, J. S. (1984). Sex differences in achievement patterns. *Nebraska Symposium on Motivation, 32,* 97–132.

Eccles, J. S. (2005). Subjective task values and the Eccles et al. model of achievement related choices. In A. J. Elliott & C. S. Dweck (Eds.), *Handbook of competence and motivation* (pp. 105–121). New York: Guilford Press.

Eccles, J. S., & Midgley, C. (1989). Stage/environment fit: Developmentally appropriate classrooms for early adolescents. In R. Ames & C. Ames (Eds.), *Research on motivation in education* (Vol. 3, pp. 139–181). New York: Academic Press.

Eccles-Parsons, J. S., Adler, T. F., Futterman, R., Goff, S. B., Kaczala, C. M., Meece, J. L., et al. (1983). Expectancies, values, and academic behaviors. In J. T. Spence (Ed.), *Achievement and achievement motivation* (pp. 75–146). San Francisco: Freeman.

Elliot, A. J., & Dweck, C. S. (Eds.). (2005). *Handbook of competence and motivation.* New York: Guilford Press.

Falco, L. D., Summers, J. J., & Bauman, S. (2010). Encouraging mathematics participation through improved self-efficacy: A school counseling outcomes study. *Educational Research and Evaluation, 16*(6), 529–549.

Feather, N. T. (1988). Values, valences, and course enrollment: Testing the role of personal values within expectancy–value framework. *Journal of Educational Psychology, 80,* 381–391.

Feng, S. L., & Tuan, H. L. (2005). Using ARCS model to promote 11th graders' motivation and achievement in learning about acids and bases. *International Journal of Science and Mathematics Education, 3*(3), 463–484.

Flake, J. K., Barron, K. E., Hulleman, C., McCoach, D. B., & Welsh, M. E. (2015). Measuring cost: The forgotten component of expectancy–value theory. *Contemporary Educational Psychology, 41,* 232–244.

Gaspard, H., Dicke, A., Flunger, B., Brisson, B., Hafner, I., Nagengast, B., et al. (2015). Fostering adolescents' value beliefs for mathematics with a relevance intervention in the classroom. *Developmental Psychology, 51*(9), 1226–1240.

Gaspard, H., Dicke, A., Flunger, B., Schreier, B., Hafner, I., Trautwein, U., et al. (2015). More value through greater differentiation: Gender differences in value beliefs about math. *Journal of Educational Psychology, 107*(3), 663–677.

Guo, J., Marsh, H. W., Parker, P. D., Morin, A. J. S., & Yeung, A. S. (2015). Expectancy–value in mathematics, gender and socioeconomic background as predictors of achievement and aspirations: A multi-cohort study. *Learning and Individual Differences, 37,* 161–168.

Guo, J., Parker, P. D., Marsh, H. W., & Morin, A. J. (2015). Achievement, motivation, and educational choices: A longitudinal study of expectancy and value using a multiplicative perspective. *Developmental Psychology, 51*(8), 1163–1176.

Guthrie, J. T., & Klauda, S. L. (2014). Effects of classroom practices on reading comprehension, engagement, and motivations for adolescents. *Reading Research Quarterly, 49,* 387–416.

Guthrie, J. T., Klauda, S. L., & Ho, A. (2013). Modeling the relationships among reading instruction, motivation, engagement, and achievement for adolescents. *Reading Research Quarterly, 48,* 9–26.

Guthrie, J. T., Klauda, S., & Morrison, D. (2012). Motivation, achievement, and classroom contexts for information book reading. In J. T. Guthrie, A. Wigfield, & S. L. Klauda (Eds.), *Adolescents' engagement in academic literacy* (pp. 1–51). College Park: University of Maryland.

Guthrie, J. T., McRae, A. C., & Klauda, S. L. (2007). Contributions of Concept-Oriented Reading Instruction to knowledge about interventions for motivations in reading. *Educational Psychologist, 42,* 237–250.

Guthrie, J. T., & Wigfield, A. (2000). Engagement and motivation in reading. In M. L. Kamil, P. B. Mosenthal, P. D. Pearson, &

R. Barr (Eds.), *Handbook of reading research* (Vol. 3, pp. 403–422). Mahwah, NJ: Erlbaum.

Guthrie, J. T., Wigfield, A., Barbosa, P., Perencevich, K. C., Taboada, A., Davis, M. H., et al. (2004). Increasing reading comprehension and engagement through concept-oriented reading instruction. *Journal of Educational Psychology, 96*(3), 403–423.

Guthrie, J. T., Wigfield, A., & Klauda, S. L. (Eds.). (2012). *Adolescents' engagement in academic literacy.* College Park: University of Maryland.

Guthrie, J. T., Wigfield, A., & Perencevich, K. (Eds.). (2004). *Motivating reading comprehension: Concept-oriented reading instruction.* Mahwah, NJ: Erlbaum.

Harackiewicz, J. M., Canning, E. A., Tibbetts, Y., Giffen, C. J., Blair, S. S., Rouse, D. I., et al. (2014). Closing the social class achievement gap for first-generation students in undergraduate biology. *Journal of Educational Psychology, 106*(2), 375–389.

Harackiewicz, J. M., Rozek, C. S., Hulleman, C. S., & Hyde, J. S. (2012). Helping parents motivate adolescents in mathematics and science: An experimental test of a utility–value intervention. *Psychological Science, 23,* 899–906.

Harackiewicz, J. M., Tibbetts, Y., Canning, E. A., & Hyde, J. S. (2014). Harnessing values to promote motivation in education. In S. Karabenick and T. Urdan (Eds.), *Advances in motivation and achievement* (Vol. 18, pp. 71–105). Bingley, UK: Emerald Group.

Hensley, L. C. (2014). Reconsidering active procrastination: Relations to motivation and achievement in college anatomy. *Learning and Individual Differences, 36,* 157–164.

Hidi, S., & Renninger, K. A., (2006). The four-phase model of interest development. *Educational Psychologist, 41,* 111–127.

Higgins, E. T. (2007). Value. In A. W. Kruglanski & E. T. Higgins (Eds.), *Handbook of social psychology* (2nd ed., pp. 454–472). New York: Guilford Press.

Hulleman, C. S., Godes, O., Hendricks, B. L., & Harackiewicz, J. M. (2010). Enhancing interest and performance with a utility value intervention. *Journal of Educational Psychology, 102,* 880–895.

Hulleman, C. S., & Harackiewicz, J. M. (2009). Promoting interest and performance in high school science classes. *Science, 326,* 1410–1412.

Jacobs, J., Lanza, S., Osgood, D. W., Eccles, J. S., & Wigfield, A. (2002). Ontogeny of children's self-beliefs: Gender and domain differences across grades one through 12. *Child Development, 73,* 509–527.

Kirkpatrick, K. M., Chang, Y., Lee, Y. J., Tas, Y., Anderman, E. M. (2013, April). *The role of perceived social cost of math and science learning in academic expectations and intentions.* Paper presented at the annual meeting of the American Educational Research Association, San Francisco, CA.

Kosovich, J. J., Hulleman, C. S., Barron, K. E., & Getty, S. (2015). A practical measure of student motivation: Establishing validity evidence for the expectancy–value-cost scale in middle school. *Journal of Early Adolescence, 35*(5–6), 790–816.

Lee, J., Bong, M., & Kim, S. (2014). Interaction between task values and self-efficacy on maladaptive achievement strategy use. *Educational Psychology, 34,* 538–560.

Lee, J., Lee, M., & Bong, M. (2013). High value with low perceived competence as an amplifier of self-worth threat. In D. M. McInerney, H. W. Marsh, R. G. Craven, & F. Guay (Eds.), *Theory driving research* (pp. 205–231). Charlotte, NC: Information Age.

Lewin, K. (1938). *The conceptual representation and the measurement of psychological forces.* Durham, NC: Duke University Press.

Marinak, B. A. (2013). Courageous reading instruction: The effects of an elementary motivation intervention. *Journal of Educational Research, 106*(1), 39–48.

Martin, A. J. (2005). Exploring the effects of a youth enrichment program on academic motivation and engagement. *Social Psychology of Education, 8*(2), 179–206.

Martin, A. J. (2008). Enhancing student motivation and engagement: The effects of a multidimensional intervention. *Contemporary Educational Psychology, 33*(2), 239–269.

Meece, J. L., Wigfield, A., & Eccles, J. S. (1990). Predictors of math anxiety and its consequences for young adolescents' course enrollment intentions and performances in mathematics. *Journal of Educational Psychology, 82,* 60–70.

Miyake, A., Kost-Smith, L. E., Finkelstein, N. D., Pollock, S. J., Cohen, G. L., & Ito, T. A. (2010). Reducing the gender achievement gap in college science: A classroom study of values affirmation. *Science, 330,* 1234–1237.

Musu-Gillette, L. E., Wigfield, A., Harring, J., & Eccles, J. S. (2015). Trajectories of change in student's self-concepts of ability and values in math and college major choice. *Educational Research and Evaluation, 21*(4), 343–370.

Nagengast, B., Marsh, H. W., Scalas, L. F., Xu, M. K., Hau, K.-T., & Trautwein, U. (2011). Who took the "×" out of expectancy–value theory?: A psychological mystery, a substantive-methodological synergy, and a cross-national generalization. *Psychological Science, 22,* 1058–1066.

Nagengast, B., Trautwein, U., Kelava, A., & Lüdtke, O. (2013). Synergistic effects of expectancy and value on homework engagement: The case for a within-person perspective. *Multivariate Behavioral Research, 48,* 428–460.

Orthner, D. K., Jones-Sanpei, H., Akos, P., & Rose, R. A. (2013). Improving middle school student engagement through career-relevant instruction in the core curriculum. *Journal of Educational Research, 106*(1), 27–38.

Pekrun, R. (1993). Facets of adolescents' academic motivation: A longitudinal expectancy-value approach. In P. Pintrich & M. L. Maehr (Eds.), *Advances in motivation and achievement* (Vol. 8, pp. 139–189). Greenwich, CT: JAI Press.

Pekrun, R. (2000). A social-cognitive, control-value theory of achievement emotions. In J. Heckhausen (Ed.), *Motivational psychology of human development* (pp. 143–163). Oxford, UK: Elsevier.

Pekrun, R. (2006). The control–value theory of achievement emotions: Assumptions, corollaries, and implications for education and practice. *Educational Psychology Review, 18,* 315–341.

Pekrun, R. (2009). Emotions at school. In K. R. Wentzel & A. Wigfield (Eds.), *Handbook of motivation at school* (pp. 575–604). New York: Routledge.

Perez, T., Cromley, J. G., & Kaplan, A. (2014). The role of identity development, values, and costs in college STEM retention. *Journal of Educational Psychology, 106,* 315–329.

Renninger, K. A., Austin, L., Bachrach, J. E., Chau, A. Emmerson, M., King, R. B., et al. (2014). Going beyond Whoa! That's cool!: Achieving science interest and learning with the ICAN intervention. In T. C. Urdan & S. A. Karabenick (Eds.), *Advances in motivation and achievement* (Vol. 18, pp. 107–138). Bingley, UK: Emerald Group.

Roese, N. J., & Sherman, J. W. (2007). Expectancy. In A. W. Kruglanski & E. T. Higgins (Eds.), *Handbook of social psychology* (2nd ed., pp. 91–115). New York: Guilford Press.

Rohan, M. J. (2000). A rose by any name?: The values construct. *Personality and Social Psychology Review, 4,* 255–277.

Rokeach, M. (1973). *The nature of human values*. New York: Free Press.

Rosenzweig, E. Q., & Wigfield, A. (2016). STEM motivation interventions for adolescents: A systematic review and future directions. *Educational Psychologist, 51*(2), 146–163.

Rosenzweig, E. Q., & Wigfield, A. (in press). What if reading is easy but unimportant?: How students' patterns of affirming and undermining motivation for reading information text predict different reading outcomes. *Contemporary Educational Psychology.*

Rozek, C. S, Hyde, J. S., Svoboda, R. C., Hulleman, C. S., & Harackiewicz, J. M. (2015). Gender differences in the effects of a utility-value intervention to help parents motivate adolescents in mathematics and science *Journal of Educational Psychology, 107*(1), 195–206.

Ryan, R. M., & Deci, E. L. (2009). Promoting self-determined school engagement: Motivation, learning, and well being in school. In K. R. Wentzel & A. Wigfield (Eds.), *Handbook of motivation at school* (pp. 171–196). New York: Routledge.

Safavian, N., Conley, A., & Karabenick, S. (2013, April). *Examining mathematics cost value among middle school youth.* Paper presented at the annual meeting of the American Educational Research Association, San Francisco, CA.

Schiefele, U. (2009). Situational and individual interest. In K. R. Wentzel & A. Wigfield (Eds.), *Handbook of motivation at school* (pp. 197–223). New York: Routledge.

Shechter, O. G., Durik, A. M., Miyamoto, Y., & Harackiewicz, J. M. (2011). The role of utility value in achievement behavior: The importance of culture. *Personality and Social Psychology Bulletin, 37*(3), 303–317.

Sherman, D. K., Hartson, K. A., Binning, K. R., Purdie-Vaughns, V., Garcia, J., Taborsky-Barba, S., et al. (2013). Deflecting the trajectory and changing the narrative: How self-affirmation affects academic performance and motivation under identity threat. *Journal of Personality and Social Psychology, 104*(4), 591–618.

Shnabel, N., Purdie-Vaughns, V., Cook, J. E., Garcia, J., & Cohen, G. L. (2013). Demystifying values-affirmation interventions writing about social belonging is a key to buffering against identity threat. *Personality and Social Psychology Bulletin, 39*(5), 663–676.

Simpkins, S. D., & Davis-Kean, P. E. (2005). The intersection between self-concepts and values: Links between beliefs and choices in high school. *New Directions for Child and Adolescent Development, 110,* 31–47.

Simpkins, S. D., Davis-Kean, P. E., & Eccles, J. S. (2006). Math and science motivation: A longitudinal examination of the links between choice and beliefs. *Developmental Psychology, 42,* 70–83.

Tolman, E. C. (1932). *Purposive behavior in animals and men.* New York: Appleton-Century-Crofts.

Trautwein, U., Nagengast, B., Nagy, G., Jonkmann, K., Marsh, H. W., & Ludtke, O. (2012).

Probing for the multiplicative term in modem expectancy–value theory: A latent interaction modeling study. *Journal of Educational Psychology, 104,* 763–777.

Walkington, C. A. (2013). Using adaptive learning technologies to personalize instruction to student interests: The impact of relevant contexts on performance and learning outcomes. *Journal of Educational Psychology, 105*(4), 932–945.

Weiner, B. (1992). *Human motivation: Metaphors, theories, and research.* Newbury Park, CA: Sage.

Weisgram, E. S., & Bigler, R. S. (2006a). Girls and science careers: The role of altruistic values and attitudes about scientific tasks. *Journal of Applied Developmental Psychology, 27*(4), 326–348.

Weisgram, E. S., & Bigler, R. S. (2006b). The role of attitudes and intervention in high school girls' interest in computer science. *Journal of Women and Minorities in Science and Engineering, 12,* 325–336.

Weisgram, E. S., & Bigler, R. S. (2007). Effects of learning about gender discrimination on adolescent girls' attitudes toward and interest in science. *Psychology of Women Quarterly, 31*(3), 262–269.

Wigfield, A., & Eccles, J. (1992). The development of achievement task values: A theoretical analysis. *Developmental Review, 12,* 265–310.

Wigfield, A., & Eccles, J. S. (2000). Expectancy–value theory of motivation. *Contemporary Educational Psychology, 25,* 68–81.

Wigfield, A., Eccles, J. S., & Rodriguez, D. (1998). The development of children's motivation in school contexts. In A. Iran-Nejad & P. D. Pearson (Eds.), *Review of research in education* (Vol. 23, pp. 73–118). Washington, DC: American Educational Research Association.

Wigfield, A., Mason-Singh, A., Ho, A., & Guthrie, J. T. (2014). Intervening to improve children's reading motivation and comprehension: Concept oriented reading instruction. In S. Karabenick & T. Urdan (Eds.), *Advances in motivation and achievement* (Vol. 18, pp. 37–70). Bingley, UK: Emerald Group.

Wigfield, A., Tonks, S. M., & Klauda, S. L. (2016). Expectancy–value theory. In K. R. Wentzel & D. B. Miele (Eds.), *Handbook of motivation at school* (2nd ed., pp. 55–74). New York: Routledge.

Woolley, M. E., Rose, R. A., Orthner, D. K., Akos, P. T., & Jones-Sanpei, H. (2013). Advancing academic achievement through career relevance in the middle grades: A longitudinal evaluation of CareerStart. *American Educational Research Journal, 50*(6), 1309–1335.

Yang, Y. C., & Wu, W. I. (2012). Digital storytelling for enhancing student academic achievement, critical thinking, and learning motivation: A year-long experimental study. *Computers and Education, 59*(2), 339–352.

Yeager, D. S., & Walton, G. M. (2011). Social-psychological interventions in education: They're not magic. *Review of Educational Research, 81,* 267–301.

CHAPTER 8

Mindsets

Their Impact on Competence Motivation and Acquisition

CAROL S. DWECK
DANIEL C. MOLDEN

Achievement motivation is about striving for competence. Thus, a major part of understanding achievement motivation is understanding people's beliefs about competence—what competence is and what it means about the self.

Why do people want competence? First, there appears to be an inborn desire to acquire and exercise competence. From the beginning, its acquisition is readily initiated, inherently sustained, and intrinsically rewarded. This is simply part of our survival. Later, this can become a more conscious valuing of learning and growth. A second reason that people want competence is that it becomes part of the self-concept, part of what people measure themselves by, and what other people esteem them for. Thus, achievement motivation is powered by the valuing of both competence acquisition (learning goals) and competence validation (performance goals).

People's *mindsets* about competence help us understand which of these two facets of competence—competence acquisition or competence validation—becomes most valued. This is important, for we will show how an overemphasis on competence validation can drive out learning. By illuminating the valuing of different competence goals,

mindsets can also give us entrée into the *meaning systems* people use to understand and act in competence-relevant situations. Often, motivational variables are considered in isolation. Rarely do researchers look at a network of beliefs and goals that work together to produce important behaviors and outcomes; that is, rarely do they look at the meaning systems that give rise to the behaviors and outcomes we care about.

In this chapter, we begin by showing how mindsets about competence create meaning systems—how they attract or highlight certain competence goals and certain attributions (explanations for difficulty), which go on to foster particular strategies (see also Molden & Dweck, 2006). These processes, in turn, can result in different levels of interest, self-esteem, and competence, especially in the face of challenge or threat. We show how these mindset-based meaning systems operate in the areas of academic achievement, sports, relationships, and organizations. We also describe how socialization practices can foster different mindsets, and how altering people's mindsets has a cascade of effects, altering their meaning systems and their academic outcomes. Finally, we close by showing how thinking in terms of mindsets and the meaning systems they engender can link competence and motivation to other important areas of psychology.

FIXED AND GROWTH MINDSETS

The mindsets we focus on in this chapter involve people's beliefs about the fixedness or malleability of their personal qualities, such as their intelligence: Do people believe that their intelligence is a fixed trait ("You have it or you don't") or a malleable quality that they can cultivate through learning? These mindsets are typically measured by asking people to agree or disagree with a series of statements, such as "Your intelligence is something basic about you that you can't really change" or "No matter who you are, you can substantially change your level of intelligence." Agreement with statements like the first reflects a *fixed mindset,* that is, the idea that intelligence is a fixed entity. In contrast, agreement with statements like the second reflects a *growth mindset,* that is, the idea that intellectual ability can be increased through learning (Dweck, 1999).

Although many people think fixed mindsets are dominant in our society, it turns out that both mindsets are equally popular. When they are assessed in children or adults, about 40% of people tend to endorse a fixed mindset, about 40% tend to endorse a growth mindset, and about 20% are undecided. Furthermore, these mindsets have, at most, a small relationship to people's actual level of intelligence (Spinath, Spinath, Riemann, & Angleitner, 2003).

Mindsets can also be induced experimentally; that is, although they can reflect relatively stable beliefs that individuals hold (see, e.g., Robins & Pals, 2002), they can also be taught or primed. In many studies, researchers have taught their participants a fixed or growth mindset, often by means of persuasive articles (e.g., Miele & Molden, 2010; Niiya, Crocker, & Bartmess, 2004; Nussbaum & Dweck, 2008). These articles depict the attribute in question, such as intelligence or personality, as a relatively inborn trait that is resistant to change or, alternatively, as a quality that can be developed throughout one's life. Researchers have also manipulated mindsets by portraying the task on which people are about to embark as one that measures (or requires)

either inherent abilities or skills that can be acquired through practice. This has been done for diverse abilities, including intellectual (e.g., Martocchio, 1994), physical (e.g., Jourden, Bandura, & Banfield, 1991), and managerial skills (e.g., Wood & Bandura, 1989). Finally, as we will see, people's mindsets can be changed in a more long-term way through targeted interventions (Aronson, Fried, & Good, 2002; Blackwell, Dweck, & Trzesniewski, 2007; Good, Aronson, & Inzlicht, 2003; Miu & Yeager, 2015; Panuesku et al., 2015; Yeager et al., 2014).

Can people hold different mindsets about different attributes? Can they believe that their intelligence is fixed but their personality is malleable? Yes, people can and often do hold different mindsets about different personal qualities (Dweck, Chiu, & Hong, 1995). They can even hold different mindsets about different intellectual skills, for example, believing that their math ability is fixed but their verbal abilities can be developed. And, as indicated by the experiments mentioned, people can be "triggered" into adopting different mindsets in different situations.

Which mindset is correct? Historically, psychologists have heatedly argued both sides of the issue, and they are still at it today. As with most issues, the answer may lie somewhere in between, but evidence suggests that important parts of many abilities can be acquired (see Brown, 1997; Diamond & Lee, 2011; Ericsson, Krampe, & Tesch-Römer, 1993; Sternberg, 1985). This trend is clear not only in the research literature but also in popular literature, where we see more and more documented cases of disadvantaged or previously low-achieving students learning calculus (Mathews, 1988) or reading and discussing Shakespeare (Collins, 1992; Levin, 1987). In Marva Collins's inner-city Chicago school, all 4-year-olds who entered in September were reading by Christmas. These were children who might often reach high school without knowing how to read.

In this context, it is interesting to note that even Alfred Binet, the inventor of the IQ test, was a strong proponent of a growth mindset of intelligence. Although his test was later used to measure fixed intelligence, that was far from his intention. His life's work was devoted not to pigeonholing failing students, but to devising educational programs that would help them become smarter:

A few modern philosophers . . . assert that an individual's intelligence is a fixed quantity which cannot be increased. We must protest and react against this brutal pessimism. . . . With practice, training, and above all method, we manage to increase our attention, our memory, our judgment, and literally to become more intelligent than we were before. (Binet, 1909/1973, pp. 105–106)

However, this is not simply an issue of intellectual interest to psychologists. In the sections that follow, we see the profound consequences of adopting one mindset or the other. We see the way in which believing in fixed attributes leads people to become highly concerned (sometimes overconcerned) with measuring those attributes, often to the detriment of their learning. It leads people to interpret setbacks as a reflection of their underlying incompetence and to show defensive or ineffective self-regulatory strategies in the face of threat. In contrast, we see how believing in malleable attributes leads people to place a priority on learning and self-development, to interpret setbacks as a reflection of their effort or learning strategies, and to mobilize effective self-regulatory strategies in the face of threat.

MINDSETS AND MEANING SYSTEMS

There is now considerable evidence that mindsets of intelligence form the core of motivationally important meaning systems. This evidence comes from multiple longitudinal studies (Blackwell et al., 2007; Robins & Pals, 2002; Romero, Master, Paunesku, Dweck, & Gross, 2014; Trzesniewski & Robins, 2003; Yeager et al., 2014) and a recent meta-analysis assessing the critical components of these meaning systems and their implications for performance or self-worth (Burnette, O'Boyle, VanEpps, Pollack, & Finkel, 2013). The results of these analyses are clear: These mindsets are associated with unique constellations of related motivations, beliefs, and attributions that arise when facing challenge and can cumulatively affect achievement, stress, and self-esteem.

Mindsets and Achievement

In one study, Blackwell and colleagues (2007) followed several hundred seventh graders across the transition to junior high school. At the beginning of seventh grade, they assessed the students' mindsets of intelligence, along with a host of other motivational variables, and monitored math grades over the next 2 years. Math is perhaps the subject that poses the greatest difficulty for many students as they find themselves in new conceptual realms during these years. In many studies, students show a sharp decline in grades as they go from elementary school to junior high, and this decline continues throughout junior high.

Effects on Goals

What did they find? First, students' mindsets of intelligence predicted other key motivational variables. Specifically, a growth versus a fixed mindset of intelligence was associated with holding strong learning goals. Students with a growth mindset more strongly endorsed statements such as "It is much more important for me to learn things in my classes than it is to get the best grades"; that is, when students believed their intelligence could be developed, they sought learning as a means to do so. When they believed their intelligence was fixed, they were diverted from learning by the need to validate their intelligence through their performance.[1]

Effects on Effort Beliefs

In this study, students' mindsets of intelligence also strongly predicted their beliefs about effort. For those with a growth mindset, effort was positive, a means to become smarter: "The harder you work at something, the better you'll be at it." However, for those with a fixed mindset, effort was negative: "To tell the truth, when I work hard at my schoolwork, it makes me feel like I'm not very smart." Within this fixed intelligence mindset, effort reflected deficient ability. Since effort is the path to achievement, it is clear how such a belief could set up roadblocks (see also Miele & Molden, 2010).

Effects on Attributions

Beyond goals and effort beliefs, students' mindset of intelligence was a significant predictor of their explanations for their difficulties as well. Students with a fixed mindset saw setbacks (just as they saw effort) as a sign of deficient ability: "I wasn't smart enough" or "I'm just not good at this subject." When you are oriented toward measuring your ability, mistakes signal failure and inadequacy.

Effects on Strategies

What would students do after a setback? What were their strategies? In line with the belief that they could develop their competence, after a failure on a test, those with a growth mindset more often said, "I would work harder in this class from now on" and "I would spend more time studying for the tests." Perfectly sensible. However, those with a fixed mindset—with their lack-of-ability attributions and their concern over exposing deficiencies—more often said, "I would spend less time on this subject from now on"; "I would try not to take this subject ever again"; or "I would try to cheat on the next test." A fixed mindset leaves students with no good recipe for success. If you lack ability and if further effort will just confirm it, there are few constructive strategies left at your disposal.

Effects on Grades

Finally, did students' mindsets of intelligence predict their math grades? Those with fixed versus growth mindsets entered junior high with equivalent math achievement, but their grades increasingly diverged over the 2-year period. Students with growth mindsets earned higher grades after only one term, and this gap grew larger over time. Moreover, despite the often-reported tendency for all students' grades to decline over this period, the grades of those with growth mindsets actually rose every semester (for related findings, see Romero et al., 2014; Yeager et al., 2014).

Meaning Systems Analysis

The most important question about these findings from a meaning systems perspective, however, is how all of the motivational variables worked in concert to produce these differences in achievement. Path analyses showed that a growth mindset, by encouraging learning goals and positive effort beliefs and attributions, gave rise to positive, *mastery-oriented* strategies. These strategies, in turn, predicted increasing math scores across the junior high years. Interestingly, students' entering achievement test scores did not predict increasing or decreasing grades. Only the mindsets and related variables did that.[2]

The question then becomes whether other studies yield evidence for the same meaning system. Trzesniewski and Robins (2003) conducted a similar study, following children from their last semester of elementary school (in this case, grade 5) through three semesters of middle school. They assessed students' mindsets of intelligence, as well as other motivational variables, then monitored their math grades during middle school. Aside from the fact that Trzesniewski and Robins did not measure effort beliefs or mastery-oriented strategies, the path analysis looked highly similar to that of Blackwell and colleagues (2007). A growth mindset, by orienting students toward learning goals rather than performance goals, led to more positive attributions for setbacks, and from there to increasing math grades. Again, despite the fact that math grades were declining for the sample as a whole, students with a growth mindset showed a rise in grades over the course of the study.

Our meaning systems analysis is further bolstered by a recent meta-analysis that specifically examined the cumulative evidence for all of the separate links among mindsets, achievement goals, helpless- versus mastery-oriented strategies, and negative emotions and expectations (Burnette et al., 2013). The meta-analysis provided robust confirmation of the role of growth mindsets in producing the overall pattern of adaptive goals, behaviors, and outcomes detailed earlier. Furthermore, this meta-analysis confirmed that such meaning systems were most important in circumstances where people were faced with challenges and setbacks (see Blackwell et al., 2007; Grant & Dweck, 2003).

Mindsets and Self-Esteem

In addition to scholastic achievement, can mindsets and their allied meaning systems predict the course of other important outcomes? Robins and Pals (2002) used a similar set of variables to predict changes in self-esteem. They followed 363 students at the University of California at Berkeley across their college years, another challenging time. Would the same meaning systems that predicted students' grade trajectories predict their self-esteem trajectories?

First, students' mindsets of intelligence were significant predictors of other important variables. Those with growth mindsets were more focused on learning goals, whereas those with fixed mindsets were more focused on performance goals. Further, those with growth mindsets made more attributions to effort and study skills, while those with fixed mindsets made more attributions to lack of ability when explaining setbacks.[3] Looking at responses to challenge, a growth mindset was highly predictive of positive, mastery-oriented responses ("When something I am studying is difficult, I try harder"), while a fixed mindset was highly predictive of more "helpless" responses to setbacks ("When I fail to understand something, I become discouraged to the point of wanting to give up"). Finally, those with fixed mindsets were on a downward self-esteem trajectory relative to those with growth mindsets, and this tendency was independent of any differences in their average level of self-esteem. This difference was also independent of their grades. Thus, mindsets were able to predict self-esteem trajectories, in addition to the grade trajectories found in the previous studies.[4]

Impact on affective outcomes has been found for other mindsets as well, such as mindsets about personality. Yeager and colleagues (2014) showed that adolescents who hold growth versus fixed mindsets concerning personality generally experience less stress during the transition to high school, and Miu and Yeager (2015) found that teaching new high school students a growth mindset of personality led to a significant reduction in the emergence of depression, an affliction that typically increases dramatically over that year.

Implications

In effect, a very similar meaning system to the one found to govern grade changes was found to predict self-esteem changes.

Motivational variables, rather than working in isolation, were repeatedly seen to work together to create favorable or unfavorable outcomes: Mindsets lead to goals, which (sometimes together with the mindsets) lead to attributions and strategies, which in turn lead to achievement and self-esteem outcomes. These findings raise several important issues. For example, attributions have long been known to be important predictors of self-related affect and coping in the face of setbacks (Abramson, Seligman, & Teasdale, 1978; Dweck & Reppucci, 1973; Weiner, 1986), and this was found in the studies reviewed as well. Thus, the importance of attributional processes was confirmed. However, the attributions in each case were predicted by the mindsets and goals; that is, the attributions appear to grow out of the meaning systems in which people are operating. When people believe intelligence is fixed and are oriented toward competence validation, negative outcomes speak to a lack of ability. When, instead, people believe intelligence can grow and are oriented toward competence acquisition, negative outcomes speak to effort and strategy. Therefore, it becomes important to understand the origins and impact of attributions in terms of the meaning systems that appear to give rise to them.

In a related vein, much research has been directed toward styles of coping, for example, coping through active problem solving versus more passive avoidance. Typically, these styles are not analyzed in the context of people's beliefs and goals, but rather as styles that have somehow emerged over time. However, the research reviewed so far suggests that some of the very coping styles that researchers have been most interested in may stem from the meaning systems we have been describing. Meaning systems built around growth mindsets appear to promote active, direct, and constructive coping, whereas those built around fixed mindsets appear to foster more avoidant, indirect, and defensive coping. As with attributions, then, a full understanding of coping styles should include an examination of the core beliefs that lead people to cope in characteristic ways.

Thus, a meaning systems analysis has the potential to illuminate key processes of interest to psychologists, such as affect, esteem, and coping, and bring them into the realm of motivation.

WHAT IS COMPETENCE?

We have shown how mindsets affect whether people are primarily focused on competence validation or competence acquisition. Yet, beyond these effects, mindsets set up different meaning systems to the point that the very idea of competence is quite different (see Molden & Dweck, 2000). Butler (2000) examined this issue of what constitutes competence with a sample of junior high school students and their math teachers. For some of the participants, Butler simply measured their existing mindsets of intelligence; for others, she induced a fixed or growth mindset of math ability. Those in the fixed condition were told, "People differ in mathematical ability. Studies show that people's mathematical ability does not change much throughout life." In contrast, those in the growth condition were told, "Studies show that people acquire math ability through learning and practice; people who learn as they work develop higher ability."

Half of the participants were then shown a student's performance that started high and declined over a series of days, whereas the other half were shown a student's performance that started lower, but rose over time, and everyone judged his ability. Those with a fixed mindset thought the student with declining performance had higher ability. He had the competence right away, without working; no matter that he slacked off later on. However, those with a growth mindset thought the student with ascending performance had higher ability. He presumably had worked hard and acquired competence.

These findings are important because educators and employers are often in the position of judging people's competence. If they have a fixed mindset, they may well make an immediate judgment based on initial performance. If they have a growth mindset, they will instead value and recognize growth and what people can learn over time (see Heslin, Latham, & VandeWalle, 2005). In fact, Rheinberg (1980) found that teachers with fixed beliefs ("According to my experience, students' achievement mostly keeps constant

in the course of a year"; "As a teacher, I have no influence on students' intellectual ability") did not produce maximal growth in students who came into their classroom with lower achievement. These students remained low achievers. In contrast, teachers with more of a growth mindset promoted growth in achievement among those who were initially behind, to the point that many of them caught up to the higher achievers.

A second study by Butler (2000) showed that people's mindsets affect not only their definitions of competence when they observe others but also their definition of competence for themselves. Students worked on a task and were given feedback indicating either a decline in performance over time or an improvement over time. Their intrinsic motivation was then assessed by asking them: How interesting did you find the problems? How interested are you in receiving more problems like the ones you worked on? How interested would you be in working on extra problems during recess? Those with growth mindsets displayed higher interest when their performance had improved rather than declined, but those with fixed mindsets showed a trend in the opposite direction.

These findings are important because they suggest that those with fixed mindsets may not enjoy something fully unless they are good at it right away, whereas those with growth mindsets can take pleasure in things they've worked hard to master over time. This is further supported by research that monitored people's affect and enjoyment as they learned a variety of difficult tasks (e.g., a perceptual–motor task: Jourden et al., 1991; computer skills: Martocchio, 1994; managerial skills: Tabernero & Wood, 1999). For example, in the study by Jourden and colleagues (1991), people learned a challenging perceptual–motor skill. For half of them, a fixed mindset was induced by telling them that their performance reflected inherent aptitude; for the other half, a growth mindset was induced by telling them that their performance reflected an acquirable skill.

On this difficult task, people in the fixed mindset condition showed no growth in confidence over learning trials, negative reactions to their performance, and low interest in the activity—even though they were improving. Since they were not good at it right away, they could not enjoy the task or any progress they were making on it. As a result, their final skill level was limited. In contrast, those in the growth mindset condition showed growth in confidence, positive reactions to their performance, and widespread interest in the activity. Since a growth mindset orients people toward learning, their progress was a source of pride and enjoyment. In line with this, they displayed a high level of skill acquisition.

In summary, mindsets change the very meaning of competence. With a fixed mindset, competence is something people simply have and display right away. If it does not emerge at once, they may lose interest or become distressed. But with a growth mindset, competence is something that develops over time through effort. That growth of competence over time is then the occasion for growing confidence, pride, and interest.

IMPLICATIONS OF MEANING SYSTEMS

Handling Threats to Competence

We have already seen how the different mindsets and the meaning systems that grow up around them affect people's self-esteem and performance as they grapple with the threat of difficult tasks and difficult transitions. Here we see how these same mindsets affect the self-esteem and performance of people who may be particularly prone to threat because their race or gender makes them the target of negative stereotypes.

Studies have now shown that a growth mindset can protect students from the debilitating effects of negative stereotypes on performance. As Steele and Aronson (1995) point out in their groundbreaking work on stereotype threat, the activation of a negative stereotype about a group's ability poses a threat because it makes group members concerned that they might confirm the negative stereotype. It makes sense that some of the sting of that stereotype would be removed when people believe that the ability in question is one that they can develop.

The first study to suggest this was a study by Aronson and colleagues (2002). In this research, African American and European

American college students were taught different mindsets of intelligence. One group was taught a growth mindset that intelligence is expandable, and that every time they learn new things, their brains form new connections. They saw a film on this, they discussed it, and, in order to stamp in the message, the students went on to mentor younger students using the growth message. Another group was taught the theory of multiple intelligences, with the message being not to worry if you lack intelligence in one area, you may still have it in another area. They, too, mentored younger children in terms of this theory. Finally, a third group was a no-treatment control group.

At the end of the semester, Aronson and colleagues (2002) looked at the students' grade-point averages, and assessed both their valuing of academics and their enjoyment of academic work. They found that those students who learned a growth mindset subsequently earned significantly higher grades than the students in the other two groups. Importantly, among African American students, the growth mindset also led to a significant increase in students' valuing of academics (with these students reporting that, in the larger scheme of things, their academic work was more important to them) and a significant increase in their enjoyment of their academic work (e.g., doing homework assignments, studying for tests, writing papers). It is noteworthy that the African American students in the growth mindset condition did not report any less exposure to negative stereotypes in their academic environment than did the African Americans in other groups. This mindset simply armed them to deal with these experiences without harm to their academic attitudes and performance. This analysis has received support from experimental studies by Aronson (1998) and Dar-Nimrod and Heine (2006).

Extending these studies, Good, Rattan, and Dweck (2012) went on to examine the impact of a fixed- versus growth-mindset-oriented classroom culture on female college students' sense of belonging in mathematics (i.e., the feeling that they were valuable and accepted members in their math environment). They asked: Which students would be most vulnerable to stereotyped messages of lower ability in females? As they followed female students through their calculus course, they found that those who (1) believed that people in their math classes held a fixed mindset of math ability and (2) perceived a high degree of stereotyping in their environment showed a decline over the course of the semester in their sense of belonging in math, their confidence in their math ability, and their enjoyment of math. The lowered sense of belonging also led to lower final grades. This was true even though their entering math SAT scores were as high as those in the other groups.

In contrast, when female students perceived a growth mindset culture in their math classes, even a high degree of negative stereotyping in their environment did not lead them to question their membership in the math community, to lose their confidence in their math abilities, or to suffer a decline in their interest in math. As in the Aronson and colleagues (2002) study, holding a growth mindset did not blind them to the fact that negative stereotypes exist, but it allowed them to function more effectively in the face of them (see also Emerson & Murphy, 2015).

Online Attentional and Self-Regulatory Strategies

Beyond establishing the basic elements of the meaning systems in terms of the goals and attributions that emerge from different mindsets, research has also examined the more fine-grained attentional, learning, and self-regulatory strategies that arise from the meaning systems. These too are important to consider, for it is through them that such meaning systems come to affect performance.

Online Deployment of Attention

The first study we examine (Mangels, Butterfield, Lamb, Good, & Dweck, 2006) used event-related potentials (ERPs) in the brain to track people's deployment of attention as they worked on a task. College students were asked a series of difficult questions, one at a time, on a computer. They were given time to type in their answer, and shortly thereafter were told whether they were right or wrong (ability-oriented feedback). Then,

a short time later, they were told the correct answer (learning-oriented feedback). By tracking students' brain activity during the different stages of the task, researchers could assess the strategies people were using to deploy their attention in anticipation of the feedback.

Regardless of whether students held a fixed or a growth mindset of intelligence, their ERPs showed that they all displayed heightened attention when anticipating the initial feedback about whether their answer was right or wrong. This information is important for those with fixed mindsets, who want to validate their ability, but it is also important to those with growth mindsets, who put a premium on learning. However, those with fixed mindsets did not show this heightened attention in preparation for the right answer. Apparently, once they learned whether they had been right or wrong, their job was over. This is clearly not a stance that fosters learning. In contrast, those with growth mindsets still showed heightened attention for information about the right answer—whether they had been right or wrong. They were apparently interested in seeing and thinking about the correct answer even when they had already gotten the right answer.

These findings were replicated and extended in another study that examined college students' online processing of errors on a perceptual task (Moser, Schroder, Heeter, Moran, & Lee, 2011). On this task, the ERP activity of those with growth mindsets revealed heightened attention to and processing of their errors, which then mediated increased performance on the next trials; that is, in a matter of milliseconds, those with growth mindsets attended more to an error and exerted greater control to correct it compared to those with fixed mindsets. Thus, the impact of mindsets can be seen at the most basic attentional level in the brain activity that prepares people to learn.

A final set of studies by Ehrlinger, Mitchum, and Dweck (2016) examined the strategic deployment of attention and its consequences. Ehrlinger and colleagues found that as people worked on a task, those with more of a fixed mindset directed their attention toward the easier problems rather than the harder ones. As a result, they ended up with a distorted, overly high view of their abilities on the task. Those with a growth mindset, by attending to hard problems as well as easy ones, had a more realistic view of their abilities, one that could direct their learning more effectively.

Online Reactions to Effort Cues

As we saw earlier, people's general interpretation of their effort—as something negative or positive—is part of their mindset-related meaning system. Is it possible to monitor the repercussion of these effort beliefs in a more online fashion? To find this out, Miele and his colleagues (Miele, Finn, & Molden, 2011; Miele & Molden, 2010) used a variety of methods to alter the effort college students experienced while performing a variety of reading comprehension and memory tasks. These methods included altering the text to make the syntax more awkward or making the text font smaller or blurrier.

In each case, students with fixed mindsets of intelligence (or for whom this mindset had been temporarily induced) tended to interpret their experience of effort as indicating poor comprehension and memory. In line with the Blackwell and colleagues (2007) research, these individuals presumably viewed these experiences of effort as signaling that they were approaching the limits of their fixed abilities. In contrast, students with growth mindsets of intelligence did not show this pattern and at times even interpreted increased effort as signaling or leading to improved performance. Intriguingly, these differences in students' perceptions of their comprehension and memory did not reflect actual differences in their ability—just differences in their mindsets.

In short, studies of students' online reactions to error cues, difficulty cues, or effort cues can give us more insight into how mindsets and their allied meaning systems work to affect performance.

Strategies of Self-Esteem Repair

Much has been written about how people repair their self-esteem after a threat or a failure but most typically it has been assumed that everyone does it in roughly the same way (Gollwitzer & Wicklund,

1985; Tesser, 2000). For example, Tesser (2000) has shown that after a failure, people want to compare themselves to or associate with people who are less competent than they are. Gollwitzer and Wicklund (1985), in their program of research on symbolic self-completion, also show the humiliating lengths to which people will go after a failure to restore their sense of self.

However, it stands to reason that people will use different strategies of self-repair when the self that has been undermined consists of fixed qualities rather than expandable ones. When the traits are perceived as fixed and, therefore, there is nothing people can do to truly improve them, then they have to turn to defensive strategies—they must expose themselves to information, even distorted information, that will make them feel good about themselves again (cf. Ehrlinger et al., 2016, described earlier). However, when the trait in question can be developed, then the most sensible strategy for repairing the failure and the blow to self-esteem is to rededicate oneself to such development. In this framework, it is basically a waste of time to artificially prop yourself up when you could be remedying the deficit.

In three studies, Nussbaum and Dweck (2008) showed that students working within fixed versus growth mindsets repair their self-esteem in very different ways. In one study, students first read articles that induced either a fixed or a growth mindset of intelligence. They then worked on a very difficult task on which they initially failed, and, before the next trial, were given the option of examining strategies used by previous students. They could examine strategies of students who either had done better than they had on the task or had done as poorly or worse. To repair their self-esteem, students primed with a fixed mindset looked at the strategies of students who had also done poorly on the task. However, students primed with a growth mindset looked at strategies of students who had done substantially better than they had, presumably in an effort to remedy their deficit and improve on the next trial. A second, follow-up study replicated this effect and confirmed that defensive, downward comparisons were more effective at making those with fixed mindsets feel better following their own failure, whereas remedial, upward comparisons were more effective at making those with growth mindsets feel better.

In a third study, engineering students were given a difficult test of engineering ability with four sections. They received feedback that they had done well on three sections and poorly on one. On which sections did they want to work further? Those primed with a fixed mindset chose the sections they were already good at—missing an opportunity to address a weakness in the area that was central to their identity (engineering). However, students primed with a growth mindset overwhelmingly chose the section they failed, presumably to try to master the skills they lacked.

Similarly Rhodewalt (1994) has shown that those with fixed mindsets act to protect their self-esteem even before failure occurs by using "self-handicapping" strategies, such as not studying until the last minute. Although these strategies make failure more likely, they allow people to see a failure as less indicative of their true abilities: "I could have done well if I had studied earlier." Specifically, Rhodewalt found that students with fixed mindsets of intelligence (and who pursued performance goals) were more likely to engage in self-handicapping than students with growth mindsets of intelligence (and who pursued learning goals). Once again, a fixed mindset fosters strategies that protect self-esteem at the expense of learning, whereas a growth mindset fosters strategies that are conducive to the growth of competence.

SOCIALIZATION OF MEANING SYSTEMS

Where do mindsets come from? How are mindsets and their associated meaning systems socialized? One way is through the praise and criticism children receive. Multiple studies have shown that "person" feedback that focuses on and judges the child's traits or abilities (whether in a positive or negative way) fosters a fixed mindset and its associated meaning systems, whereas "process" feedback that focuses on the child's work process or learning (e.g., effort or strategy) fosters a growth mindset and its associated meaning system (Kamins & Dweck, 1999;

Mueller & Dweck, 1998). Furthermore, in these studies, different types of praise had direct causal effects on children's mindsets and meaning systems (see also Cimpian, Arce, Markman, & Dweck, 2007).

Several additional studies have now extended such findings to real-world behaviors. In one, parents of children ages 8–12 took part in daily interviews in which they reported whether their child had some kind of success at school and how they had responded (Pomerantz & Kempner, 2013). These responses were coded as either person praise (telling a child he or she is smart or a "good kid") or process praise (telling a child he or she tried hard or must have really enjoyed the schoolwork). Then, 6 months later, children reported their mindset of intelligence. The more person praise parents reported giving, the stronger children's fixed mindset had become and the less the children reported enjoying challenging work at school.

Another study conducted with much younger children confirmed the broad effects of process versus person praise, not only on fixed versus growth mindsets of intelligence, but on the other components of the larger meaning systems that grow out of these mindsets as well (Gunderson et al., 2013). Parents' spontaneous interactions with their children at home were recorded for 90 minutes when the children were 14, 26, and 38 months old. These interactions were coded for performance praise ("You're good at that") or effort praise ("Good job trying to put that back in"). Then, 4–5 years later, the children reported their mindsets of intelligence, achievement goals, attributions for success, and strategies for success. The more process praise parents delivered (as a proportion of total praise) when the children were ages 1–3, the more these children reported (1) stronger growth mindsets of intelligence, and (2) motivations and attributions consistent with mastery-oriented responses to challenge (i.e., stronger learning goals, effort attributions for performance, and generation of strategies for improvement).

Rather than examining specific praise or criticism practices, Haimovitz and Dweck (2016) assessed parents' general beliefs about failure and their reactions to their children's failures. They found that parents who believed that failure was harmful (e.g., "The effects of failure are negative and should be avoided") responded to their child's setbacks with anxiety and concern about their child's ability. In contrast, parents who believed that failure was beneficial (e.g., "Experiencing failure facilitates learning and growth") responded with learning-oriented suggestions. In turn, these reactions fostered fixed and growth mindsets of intelligence, respectively, in their children. Furthermore, the parents' own mindsets of intelligence were only weakly correlated with their children's (also see Gunderson et al., 2013). This suggests that it is parents' overt practices (their praise, their reactions to the child's setbacks) that is molding their child's mindset, rather than the less visible mindsets that might be in parents' heads.

Despite the power of mindsets to affect children's motivation, and despite the work showing the practices that instill them, there has been a general lack of attention to mental representations, such as children's beliefs, in the study of social development and socialization (see Dweck & London, 2004; Olson & Dweck, 2008). Certainly, children build up mindsets about themselves and the world as they develop, and these mindsets play a critical role in their behavior and adjustment. Yet social-developmental psychologists, with the exception of attachment researchers, have paid scant attention to such mindsets. Given their broad impact, further research on mindsets and their development could be a fruitful place to correct this deficit.

BEYOND ACADEMIC COMPETENCE: MEANING SYSTEMS ACROSS MULTIPLE SKILLS DOMAINS

Most of the work reviewed thus far has dealt with motivation and competence in students facing challenging academic tasks. Although academic competence is of great interest and importance to many people, the impact of mindsets and their attendant meaning systems is not limited to this domain. In this section, therefore, we present work that shows the generality of our conceptualization and its utility for understanding for competence in other areas.

Organizational Behavior

Wood and his colleagues (Tabernero & Wood, 1999; Wood & Bandura, 1989; Wood, Phillips, & Tabernero, 2002) introduced mindsets into the realm of organizational behavior (see also Maurer, Wrenn, Pierce, Tross, & Collins, 2003) by examining their impact on the acquisition of managerial skills. The managerial skills task involved matching employee attributes to the different jobs in an organization, and, over time, learning how best to guide and motivate each employee so as to reach the production quota. To discover the best solutions, managers had to continue testing hypotheses and revising their decisions as a function of the feedback they received.

In the Wood and Bandura (1989) study, participants worked as individuals and their mindsets were induced by telling them either that their performance was a function of their underlying capacities (fixed mindset induction) or that the skills were developed through practice (growth mindset condition). Although both groups confronted the task with a relatively strong sense of managerial efficacy, the people in the fixed mindset group showed a progressive decrease in self-efficacy across trials as they continued to try to meet the challenging production quota. In addition, they set less and less challenging goals across trials, became less and less efficient in their use of analytic strategies, and showed a marked decline in performance over time. Those in the growth mindset group, in contrast, were able to maintain their sense of efficacy, became increasingly systematic in their use of strategies, and sustained a high level of organizational performance.

In the study by Wood and colleagues (2002), people's mindsets of managerial ability were assessed and work groups were formed consisting of three individuals with growth mindsets or three individuals with fixed mindsets. After working together for some weeks, the groups completed the same managerial decision-making task described earlier. Although at the start both groups were quite similar, they diverged over the course of the task. They differed in their goals (with growth mindset groups setting more challenging goals for themselves), they made different attributions for their setbacks (with fixed mindset groups blaming the task, their ability, and their luck, but growth mindset groups questioning their strategies, which they could readily alter), and they differed in their self-regulatory strategies (e.g., attention and time management)—all of which led to increasingly superior performance by the growth mindset groups over time.

In a complementary line of work, Heslin and colleagues (2005) examined the impact of managers' fixed or growth mindsets on their perceptions and treatment of their employees. Results showed that, compared to managers with a fixed mindset, who stuck more to their original perceptions of employees, managers with a growth mindset were more sensitive to actual changes in employees performance over time (Heslin et al., 2005). Moreover, teaching managers a growth mindset made them more willing to coach and mentor their employees and more effective doing so (Heslin, VandeWalle, & Latham, 2006). They no longer saw poor performance as permanent and now felt they had a role in fostering their employees' improvement.

Finally, Murphy and Dweck (2010) found that organizations as a whole can have cultures that reflect more of a fixed or growth mindset, which can affect their employees. In a series of experiments, people prepared a job application for a hypothetical organization. When applying to an organization portrayed as having a pervasive fixed mindset, people emphasized their intelligence and ability; however, when applying to an organization portrayed has having a pervasive growth mindset, people emphasized their motivations and dedication to learning. This is not surprising, but the self-presentations had sticky effects: Participants later reported that the attributes emphasized in their applications (intelligence and ability vs. motivation and dedication to learn) were central to who they were. Moreover, when judging people for a different job in a different organization, participants used these attributes to decide whom to hire. Thus the perceptions of what an environment values can shape our own values.

In summary, similar mindset-related processes appear to be at play in organizational settings as well. Given that organizations create broader cultures and social structures,

the mindsets held by organizations and their leaders can have wide-ranging effects.

Social Relationships

A number of researchers have now examined the role of mindsets in social relationships among children (Erdley, Cain, Loomis, Dumas-Hines, & Dweck, 1997; Rudolph, 2010), adolescents (Yeager, Trzesniewski, Tirri, Nokelanian, & Dweck, 2011), and adults (Beer, 2003; Knee & Petty, 2013). Importantly, many of the same patterns have been found, with goals, attributions, affective responses, and coping strategies affecting meaningful outcomes.

For example, Beer's (2003) studies of peer relationships in adults beautifully illustrate the role of mindset in influencing people's response to threat, and speak to the impact of threat on social competence. In her studies, Beer measured people's mindsets about shyness, with items such as "My shyness is something about me that I can't change very much" (fixed mindset) and "I can change aspects of my shyness if I want to" (growth mindset). She also had people report on their own level of shyness. In three studies, Beer found that holding a growth versus fixed mindset of shyness led to many of the same processes we have described in other realms and mitigated the negative effects of shyness on both the shy person's sense of well-being and the interactions in which the person participated.

Research on the role of mindsets in more intimate relationships also illustrates the impact of the larger meaning systems. First, people with a fixed mindset (who believe that intimate relationships are largely fixed and are "destined to be" or not) tend to adopt the goal of evaluating their partner. Accordingly, the length of and their satisfaction with their relationship are associated with their early positive impressions and how closely their partner matches their ideals (e.g., Burnette & Franiuk, 2010; see Knee & Petty, 2013, for a review). In contrast, people with a growth mindset (who believe that intimate relationships can be developed and are not simply destined) tend to adopt goals of cultivating these relationships and their satisfaction, and willingness to remain is not associated with first impressions or consistency with their preformed ideal.

Beyond approaching relationships with different goals, people with fixed or growth mindsets of relationships also form different attributions when conflicts inevitably arise. For those with fixed mindsets, conflict can be a major threat because it raises doubts that the relationship is actually destined to endure. As such, those with fixed mindsets initially attempt to ignore or deny the conflict (e.g., Kammrath & Dweck, 2006), but, if the conflict remains unresolved, they show reduced commitment and forgiveness. However, for those with growth mindsets, conflict is a more natural part of relationship development. Therefore, they more actively acknowledge and attempt to address conflicts in a way that sustains commitment (see Knee & Petty, 2013).

Based on these findings, it is clear that possessing a growth mindset generally benefits relationships but, interestingly, a few studies have identified one possible cost. When focused on growth and development, people tend to be optimistic that their partners can change. However, if the partner does not display sufficient effort at improvement, as time goes on, individuals with growth mindsets become upset and less satisfied with the relationship (Hui, Bond, & Molden, 2012). Individuals with fixed mindsets, who do not expect change, do not show the same reduction in satisfaction (see also Kammrath & Peetz, 2012). Future research should explore how to temper expectations, on the part of those with a growth mindset, that change should be quicker, easier, and more linear than might often be possible.

In summary, in the area of both peer and adult relationships, people's mindsets are linked to other motivational variables, such as goals (Beer, 2003; Erdley et al. 1997), attributions (Erdley et al., 1997; Rudolph, 2010; Yeager et al., 2011, 2014), and mastery-oriented versus helpless responses to threat (Beer, 2003; Kammrath & Dweck, 2006; Knee & Petty, 2013), and, in this way, have their impact on relationship outcomes.

Sports

Biddle and his colleagues (Biddle, Wang, Chatzisaray, & Spray, 2003; Sarrazin et al., 1996) studied the impact of theories of sports ability on young people's motivation for sports and physical activity. They devised a questionnaire to assess mindsets, containing questions such as "You have a certain level of ability in sports and you cannot really do much to change that level" (fixed mindset) and "How good you are at sports will always improve if you work harder at it" (growth mindset). Results showed that a growth mindset was associated with feeling successful when learning goals were achieved ("When I improve and master new things") and to greater enjoyment of sports. In contrast, a fixed mindset was linked to feeling successful when performance goals were achieved ("When I beat out others") and to "amotivation" (the belief that participating in sports is a waste of time).

Following up on this work, Ommundsen (2001, 2003) showed that a growth mindset predicted effective self-regulatory strategies in sports, such as generalizing effective strategies across activities, and both varying learning strategies and being willing to ask for help when necessary. A fixed mindset predicted not taking an analytic stance toward one's learning strategies, not asking for help, and giving up when the activities were difficult. This mindset also predicted increased levels of anxiety, reduced enjoyment of physical activity, and a tendency to use self-handicapping strategies, just as in the academic domain.

Finally, studies have further shown that following a brief manipulation of mindsets of athletic ability, individuals in the growth condition were more likely to adopt learning goals and less likely to adopt performance goals or attribute their athletic failure to a lack of ability than individuals in the fixed condition (Spray, Wang, Biddle, Chatzisarantis, & Warbuton, 2006). Thus, in the domain of sports as well, growth mindsets have been linked through cross-sectional, longitudinal, and experimental evidence to the broader meaning systems outlined earlier, including learning versus performance goals, mastery-oriented versus helpless learning strategies, and intrinsic motivation versus amotivation or anxiety (Stevenson & Lochbaum, 2008).

Weight Management

Paralleling the research on mindsets of athletic performance, Burnette (2010), in a large and diverse sample of dieters, demonstrated that a growth mindset of body weight predicted higher expectations for weight loss success, which in turn predicted more mastery-oriented responses when coping with dieting setbacks and greater weight loss success 8 weeks later. These results held even when controlling for many other factors that are typically related to weight loss success, such as self-efficacy for exercise and nutrition or previous dieting history.

Further illustrating the unique contributions of mindsets, Burnette and Finkel (2012) showed that a growth mindset intervention in which dieters learned about the malleability of body weight produced more mastery-oriented behavior and eliminated weight gain following dieting setbacks, whereas an intervention in which dieters merely learned practical advice about behaviors that facilitate weight loss (e.g., good nutrition and exercise) did not protect against weight gain in the face of such setbacks. Thus, mindsets can play an important role in behaviors involved in reaching and maintaining a healthy life style (see also Lyons, Kaufman, & Rima, 2013).

Self-Control

Finally, much recent research has begun to show that mindsets have broader implications for how and when people exert self-control. Some of this research has examined mindsets about whether the amount of willpower one has is fixed or can be developed, as has been the primary focus of this chapter, but, as detailed below, some of this research has investigated closely related but distinct mindsets about whether willpower is highly limited and easily depleted, or whether it is potentially abundant and self-energizing.

Mrazek, Molden, Mrazek, and Schooler (2016) conducted several studies in which participants' mindsets of "mental control" were manipulated by having them read research articles suggesting that mental control is something fixed and stable (the fixed mindset condition) or something that can grow and be developed (the growth mindset condition). Participants next completed tasks that required mental effort, including solving anagram problems or closely monitoring their breathing. Results showed that those with growth mindsets exerted more control and persisted longer on these tasks.

In a subsequent study, Mrazek and colleagues (2016) conducted a 6-week intervention in which people learned a growth mindset of self-control and practical suggestions for improving their control. Compared to a control condition in which people received instruction on improvement in another domain that did not include a growth mindset, individuals in the growth mindset condition were more likely to (1) spontaneously recognize the need to exert self-control, (2) attempt to exert such control, (3) report that this exertion required less effort, and (4) report successful control.

In an extended program of research, Job and colleagues have demonstrated that mindsets about the limited versus abundant, self-energizing nature of willpower have similarly important consequences for self-control. Individuals with a mindset that willpower is limited show diminished effort and attention even after exerting effort on one short attention-demanding task, whereas individuals with a mindset that willpower is not limited tend to sustain their effort or attention even after a series of attention-demanding tasks (Job, Dweck, & Walton, 2010; Miller et al., 2012). Indeed, students with limited mindsets of willpower reported engaging in less self-control in the face of academic demands (e.g., procrastinated more) and, as a result, earned poorer grades than people with nonlimited mindsets of willpower (Job, Walton, Bernecker, & Dweck, 2015). These two emerging lines of research on mindsets of willpower thus suggest another important route by which mindsets may influence competence and performance.

ALTERING MEANING SYSTEMS: INTERVENTIONS

One important implication of a meaning systems approach is that altering people's mindsets should produce effects on their meaning systems and alter their learning and achievement. It is often difficult for people to believe that simply changing these mindsets will have much impact given the many things that affect students' learning (see Yeager & Walton, 2011). However, if these mindsets are a key to students' motivation, it can have more impact than one would expect. We have already seen how the relatively short growth mindset intervention by Aronson and colleagues (2002) succeeded in changing students' valuing and enjoyment of their schoolwork and their grade-point averages. Several other studies, with junior high and high school students, have now yielded similarly encouraging findings.

In one study, Blackwell and colleagues (2007, study 2) gave seventh graders an eight-session workshop. All of the students in the workshop were given lessons on study skills, but half of them were also taught a growth mindset of intelligence and how to apply it to their schoolwork. As in the Aronson and colleagues (2002) study, students were taught that the brain grows new connections every time they learn and that, in this sense, they are in charge of how smart they become. Students' math grades were monitored over the course of the semester and, at the end, teachers' reports on the students in the workshop were solicited.

First, the growth mindset workshop, but not the control workshop, halted and even reversed the decline in math grades shown prior to the intervention. Second, the teachers, who had no idea which group the different children were in, singled out significantly more of the children in the growth mindset group as showing positive motivational change. Moreover, what the teachers reported about these students was precisely in line with our meaning systems analysis. Teachers pinpointed changes in the valuing of learning and improvement and in the belief in effort, the very factors that were found to lead to enhanced achievement in the studies described at the outset (e.g., Blackwell et al., 2007, Study 1).

In another study, Good and colleagues (2003) taught junior high school students a growth mindset of intelligence during a course in computer skills. Students were mentored by college students, who delivered the growth mindset message and helped them design a Web page that conveyed this message. The message was reinforced throughout the year through e-mail correspondence between the mentors and the students. The control group also received a constructive message (an antidrug message) and engaged in similar activities with respect to this message. At the end of the year, the groups were compared on their performance on standardized reading and math achievement tests, and the growth mindset group showed significantly better performance than the control group on both. Another interesting finding was that although the growth mindset intervention was beneficial to all, it was particularly beneficial to females. Although there was a gender gap in math achievement in the control group, this gap was reduced in the growth mindset group. Once again, this mindset seems to have helped students combat stereotypes.

In studies by Yeager and colleagues (2014), students in their first months of high school received an online growth mindset intervention, in which (1) they learned that people's behaviors and the neural circuits that control them can change, (2) read testimonials from upperclassmen about how this information had helped them, and (3) constructed their own narratives on this theme to share with other students in the future. In both studies, compared to a control group that learned about the malleability of athletic skills, students who learned a broad growth mindset not only had higher grades at the end of the year but also lower levels of global stress and better health.

Finally, a study by Paunesku and colleagues (2015) with high school students not only further replicated these types of effects but also provided initial evidence that manipulating mindsets could be practically implemented as a large-scale intervention to improve student performance. Students from 13 high schools, diverse in their size and student population, completed a 45-minute online module on growth mindsets that was condensed from the Blackwell and colleagues (2007) materials. Compared to a control condition, struggling students who learned this mindset earned significantly higher grades by the end of the semester.

Thus, in a number of studies, a relatively modest but very carefully crafted intervention yielded encouraging changes. The Blackwell and colleagues (2007) study suggests that these changes came about by boosting students' valuing of learning and improvement, and their belief in the efficacy of their efforts. And the Paunesku and colleagues (2015) study provides preliminary evidence that such interventions can be practically implemented on a large scale in school settings and, importantly, might be most beneficial to the students who most need help.

SUMMARY AND CONCLUSIONS

We have seen that mindsets form the core of meaning systems, attracting goals and beliefs (attributions, effort beliefs) that work in concert to produce outcomes across important realms: school, work, sports, relationships, and health. Fixed mindsets create a meaning system focused on the goal of measuring and validating competence, and are therefore associated with ability-oriented performance goals, ability attributions for setbacks, and the belief that effort indicates low ability. These goals and beliefs in turn lead to helpless reactions to difficulty and to diminished self-esteem, intrinsic motivation, and learning in the face of difficulty. Growth mindsets, in contrast, create a meaning system built around the acquisition of competence, and are therefore linked to learning goals, effort and strategy attributions for setbacks, and the belief that effort increases ability. These goals and beliefs then promote mastery-oriented strategies in the face of challenge and lead to enhanced self-esteem, intrinsic motivation, and learning. We have also seen that changing people's mindsets can lead to a cascade of changes in their motivation, behavior, and outcomes. Thus, the mindsets provide powerful psychological frames that influence what people try to accomplish, how they go about it, and how successful they are likely to be.

The fact that mindsets can be induced experimentally and altered through interventions suggests a dynamic view of the associated motivational systems. Although, as noted at the outset, mindsets can be relatively stable over long periods of time (e.g., Robins & Pals, 2002), they are knowledge structures and, as such, their accessibility can be changed by powerful situations and interventions; that is, people may be familiar with both fixed- and growth-oriented outlooks and can apply either to a task or domain when faced with potent cues. This dynamic view may provide a window into how personality often operates: People may have relatively stable tendencies based on chronic beliefs and goals, but they are attuned to cues from the environment that shape the beliefs and goals that they apply to a given situation (cf. Dweck & Leggett, 1988; Grant & Dweck, 2000; Mischel & Shoda, 1995).

This view, as noted earlier, can also link the study of motivation and competence to the literature on coping, since coping styles can clearly arise from mindsets. Indeed, interventions to aid coping would profit from altering the mindsets from which maladaptive coping may arise rather than simply attempting to alter the strategies directly. For example, rather than trying to discourage the avoidant or defensive coping we have seen in those with fixed mindsets and teaching more direct, problem-focused coping, one might, in conjunction with this, encourage more of a growth mindset in the relevant domains (see also Mrazek et al., 2016).

In the same vein, this approach may hold promise of insight into emotions and emotion regulation. As we saw, different emotions seem to arise more readily within particular meaning systems. For example, anxiety seems to arise more quickly and subside more slowly within fixed mindsets, whereas interest and enjoyment seem to be hardier and longer-lasting within growth mindsets. As we also saw, people appear to be using different self-regulatory strategies to deal with their negative emotions, for example, following blows to their self-esteem. Although the idea of cognitive appraisal processes leading to emotions has received much attention (e.g., Lazarus & Folkman, 1984), less attention has been paid to the meaning systems that may facilitate these emotions and that may, in addition, affect their regulation (but see Park & Folkman, 1997). Combining the study of emotion and emotion regulation with the study of mindsets—begun by Tamir, John, Srivastava, and Gross (2007; see also Romero et al., 2014)—is an important endeavor that will strengthen the link between the study of emotion and the study of motivation, and increase our understanding of both.

In conclusion, the study of mindsets has shed light on how people strive for competence and the degree to which they attain it across a variety of domains. The study of mindsets also holds promise of linking the study of motivation and competence to other key areas of psychology.

NOTES

1. Another study, examining students making the transition to college, also highlighted how mindsets of intelligence orient students toward different goals. Hong, Chiu, Dweck, Lin, and Wan (1999) surveyed students who were entering the University of Hong Kong, where all of the classes were conducted in English, but not all of the entering students were proficient in English. As the students filled out their registration materials, Hong and colleagues asked them whether they would take a remedial English course if the faculty offered it. Students who held a growth mindset of intelligence replied with a resounding "yes"— they wanted to learn—but students with a fixed mindset of intelligence were not at all enthusiastic. They perhaps preferred to live with their deficiency, even if it put their college careers in jeopardy, rather than expose it, for in that framework a deficiency can reflect a permanent inadequacy.

2. An elegant set of studies by Cury, Elliot, Da Fonseca, and Moller (2006) lends further support to this analysis. In their first study, they showed that mindsets of intelligence predicted adolescents' math grades, and that this was mediated through students' achievement goals. In their second study, they showed that manipulating adolescents' mindsets of intelligence affected their IQ scores, through their achievement goals and their mastery-oriented strategies.

3. Robins and Pals (2002) also measured affective responses to failure (which were not assessed in the previous studies), and found that even equating for grades, those with growth mindsets more often felt determined and enthusiastic, whereas those with fixed mindsets more often felt distressed or ashamed.

4. Trzesniewski and Robins (2003) also measured self-esteem. They found that the same meaning system that predicted change in math grades predicted change in self-esteem.

REFERENCES

Abramson, L. Y., Seligman, M. E., & Teasdale, J. D. (1978). Learned helplessness in humans: Critique and reformulation. *Journal of Abnormal Psychology, 87,* 49–74.

Aronson, J. (1998). *The effects of conceiving ability as fixed or improvable on responses to stereotype threat.* Unpublished manuscript.

Aronson, J., Fried, C., & Good, C. (2002). Reducing the effects of stereotype threat on African American college students by shaping theories of intelligence. *Journal of Experimental Social Psychology, 38,* 113–125.

Beer, J. S. (2003). Implicit mindsets of shyness. *Journal of Personality and Social Psychology, 83,* 1009–1024.

Biddle, S., Wang, J., Chatzisaray, N., & Spray, C. M. (2003). Motivation for physical activity in young people: Entity and incremental beliefs about athletic ability. *Journal of Sports Sciences, 21,* 973–989.

Binet, A. (1973). *Les idées modernes sur les enfants* [Modern ideas on children]. Paris: Flamarion. (Original work published 1909)

Blackwell, L. S., Dweck, C. S., & Trzesniewski, K. (2007). Implicit theories of intelligence predict achievement across an adolescent transition: A longitudinal study and an intervention. *Child Development, 78,* 246–263.

Brown, A. L. (1997). Transforming schools in to communities of thinking and learning about serious matters. *American Psychologist, 52,* 399–413.

Burnette, J. L. (2010). Implicit theories of body weight: Entity beliefs can weigh you down. *Personality and Social Psychology Bulletin, 36,* 410–422.

Burnette, J. L., & Finkel, E. J. (2012). Buffering against weight gain following dieting setbacks: An implicit theory intervention. *Journal of Experimental Social Psychology, 48*(3), 721–725.

Burnette, J. L., & Franiuk, R. (2010). Individual differences in implicit theories of relationships and partner fit: Predicting forgiveness in developing relationships. *Personality and Individual Differences, 48*(2), 144–148.

Burnette, J. L., O'Boyle, E. H., VanEpps, E. M., Pollack, J. M., & Finkel, E. J. (2013). Mindsets matter: A meta-analytic review of implicit theories and self-regulation. *Psychological Bulletin, 139*(3), 655–701.

Butler, R. (2000). Making judgments about ability: The role of implicit theories of ability in moderating inferences from temporal and social comparison information. *Journal of Personality and Social Psychology, 78,* 965–978.

Cimpian, A., Arce, H.-M. C., Markman, E. M., & Dweck, C. S. (2007). Subtle linguistic cues affect children's motivation. *Psychological Science, 18*(4), 314–316.

Collins, M. (1992). *Ordinary children, extraordinary teachers.* Charlottesville, VA: Hampton Roads.

Cury, F., Elliot, A. J., Da Fonseca, D., & Moller, A. C. (2006). The social-cognitive model of achievement motivation and the 2 × 2 achievement goal framework. *Journal of Personality and Social Psychology, 90,* 666–679.

Dar-Nimrod, I., & Heine, S. J. (2006). Exposure to scientific theories affects women's math performance. *Science, 314,* 435.

Diamond, A., & Lee, K. (2011). How can we help children succeed in the 21st century?: What the scientific evidence shows aids executive function development in children 4–12 years of age. *Science, 333,* 959–964.

Dweck, C. S. (1999). *Self-theories: Their role in motivation, personality, and development.* Philadelphia: Psychology Press.

Dweck, C. S., Chiu, C., & Hong, Y. (1995). Implicit theories and their role in judgments and reactions: A world from two perspectives. *Psychological Inquiry, 6,* 267–285.

Dweck, C. S., & Leggett, E. L. (1988). A social-cognitive approach to motivation and personality, *Psychological Review, 95,* 256–273.

Dweck, C. S., & London, B. E. (2004). The role of mental representation in social development. *Merrill–Palmer Quarterly (50th Anniversary Issue), 50,* 428–444.

Dweck, C. S., & Reppucci, N. D. (1973). Learned helplessness and reinforcement responsibility in children. *Journal of Personality and Social Psychology, 25*(1), 109–116.

Ehrlinger, J., Mitchum, A., & Dweck, C. S. (2016). Understanding overconfidence: Theories of intelligence, preferential attention, and distorted self-assessment. *Journal of Experimental Social Psychology, 63,* 94–100.

Emerson, K. T., & Murphy, M. C. (2015). A company I can trust?: Organizational lay theories moderate stereotype threat for women. *Personality and Social Psychology Bulletin, 41*(2), 295–307.

Erdley, C., Cain, K., Loomis, C., Dumas-Hines, F., & Dweck, C. S. (1997). The relations among children's social goals, implicit personality theories and response to social failure. *Developmental Psychology, 33,* 263–272.

Ericsson, K. A., Krampe, R. T., & Tesch-Römer, C. (1993). The role of deliberate practice in the acquisition of expert performance. *Psychological Review, 100*(3), 363–403.

Gollwitzer, P. M., & Wicklund, R. A. (1985). The pursuit of self-defining goals. In J. Kuhl & J. Beckmann (Eds.), *Action control: From cognition to behavior* (pp. 101–128). Heidelberg, Germany: Springer-Verlag.

Good, C., Aronson, J., & Inzlicht, M. (2003). Improving adolescents' standardized test performance: An intervention to reduce the effects of stereotype threat. *Journal of Applied Developmental Psychology, 24,* 645–662.

Good, C., Rattan, A., & Dweck, C. S. (2012). Why do women opt out?: Sense of belonging and women's representation in mathematics. *Journal of Personality and Social Psychology, 102*(4), 700–717.

Grant, H., & Dweck, C. S. (2003). Clarifying achievement goals and their impact. *Journal of Personality and Social Psychology, 85,* 541–553.

Gunderson, E. A., Gripshover, S. J., Romero, C., Dweck, C. S., Goldin-Meadow, S., & Levine, S. C. (2013). Parent praise to 1- to 3-year-olds predicts children's motivational frameworks 5 years later. *Child Development, 84*(5), 1526–1541.

Haimovitz, K., & Dweck, C. S. (2016). What predicts children's fixed and growth intelligence mind-sets?: Not their parents' views of intelligence but their parents' views of failure. *Psychological Science, 27*(6), 859–869.

Heslin, P. A., Latham, G. P., & VandeWalle, D. (2005). The effect of implicit person theory on performance appraisals. *Journal of Applied Psychology, 90*(5), 842–856.

Heslin, P. A., VandeWalle, D., & Latham, G. P. (2006). Keen to help?: Manager's implicit person theories and their subsequent employee coaching. *Personnel Psychology, 59*(4), 871–890.

Hong, Y. Y., Chiu, C., Dweck, C. S., Lin, D., & Wan, W. (1999). Implicit theories, attributions, and coping: A meaning system approach. *Journal of Personality and Social Psychology, 77,* 588–599.

Hui, C. M., Bond, M. H., & Molden, D. C. (2012). Why do(n't) your partner's efforts at self-improvement make you happy?: An implicit theories perspective. *Personality and Social Psychology Bulletin, 38*(1), 101–113.

Job, V., Dweck, C. S., & Walton, G. M. (2010). Ego depletion—Is it all in your head?: Implicit theories about willpower affect self-regulation. *Psychological Science, 21,* 1686–1693.

Job, V., Walton, G. M., Bernecker, K., & Dweck, C. S. (2015). Implicit theories about willpower predict self-regulation and grades in everyday life. *Journal of Personality and Social Psychology, 108*(4), 637–647.

Jourden, F. J., Bandura, A., & Banfield, J. T. (1991). The impact of conceptions of ability on self-regulatory factors and motor skill acquisition. *Journal of Sport and Exercise Psychology, 13,* 213–226.

Kamins, M., & Dweck, C. S. (1999). Person vs. process praise and criticism: Implications for contingent self-worth and coping. *Developmental Psychology, 35,* 835–847.

Kammrath, L. K., & Dweck, C. (2006). Voicing conflict: Preferred conflict strategies among incremental and entity. *Personality and Social Psychology Bulletin, 32*(11), 1497–1508.

Kammrath, L. K., & Peetz, J. (2012). You promised you'd change: How incremental and entity theorists react to a romantic partner's promised change attempts. *Journal of Experimental Social Psychology, 48*(2), 570–574.

Knee, C. R., & Petty, K. N. (2013). Implicit theories of relationships: Destiny and growth beliefs. In J. A. Simpson, L. Campbell, J. A. Simpson, & L. Campbell (Eds.), *The Oxford handbook of close relationships* (pp. 183–198). New York: Oxford University Press.

Lazarus, R., & Folkman, S. (1984). *Stress, appraisal, and coping.* New York: Springer-Verlag.

Levin, H. M. (1987). New schools for the disadvantaged. *Teacher Education Quarterly, 14,* 60–83.

Lyons, C., Kaufman, A. R., & Rima, B. (2013). Implicit theories of the body among college women: Implications for physical activity. *Journal of Health Psychology, 20,* 1142–1153.

Mangels, J. A., Butterfield, B., Lamb, J., Good, C., & Dweck, C. S. (2006). Why do beliefs about intelligence influence learning success?: A social cognitive neuroscience model. *Social Cognitive and Affective Neuroscience, 1*(2), 75–86.

Martocchio, J. J. (1994). Effects of conceptions of ability on anxiety, self-efficacy, and learning in training. *Journal of Applied Psychology, 79,* 819–825.

Mathews, J. (1988). *Escalante: The best teacher in America.* New York: Holt.

Maurer, T. J., Wrenn, K. A., Pierce, H. R., Tross, S. A., & Collins, W. C. (2003). Beliefs about improvability of career-relevant skills: Relevance to job/task analysis, competency modeling, and learning orientation. *Journal of Organizational Behavior, 24,* 107–131.

Miele, D. B., Finn, B., & Molden, D. C. (2011). Does easily learned mean easily remembered?: It depends on your beliefs about intelligence. *Psychological Science, 22*(3), 320–324.

Miele, D. B., & Molden, D. C. (2010). Naive theories of intelligence and the role of processing fluency in perceived comprehension. *Journal of Experimental Psychology: General, 139*(3), 535–557.

Miller, E. M., Walton, G. M., Dweck, C. S., Job, V., Trzesniewski, K. H., & McClure, S. M. (2012). Theories of willpower affect sustained learning. *PLoS ONE, 7*(6), e38680.

Mischel, W., & Shoda, Y. (1995). A cognitive-affective systems theory of personality: Reconceptualizing the invariances in personality and the role of situations. *Psychological Review, 102,* 246–268.

Miu, A. S., & Yeager, D. S. (2015). Preventing symptoms of depression by teaching adolescents that people can change: Effects of a brief incremental theory of personality intervention at 9-month follow-up. *Clinical Psychological Science, 3,* 726–743.

Molden, D. C., & Dweck, C. S. (2000). Meaning and motivation. In C. Sansone & J. M. Harackiewicz (Eds.), *Intrinsic and extrinsic motivation: The search for optimal motivation and performance* (pp. 131–153). San Diego, CA: Academic Press.

Molden, D. C., & Dweck, C. S. (2006). Finding "meaning" in psychology: A lay theories approach to self-regulation, social perception, and social development. *American Psychologist, 61,* 192–203.

Moser, J. S., Schroder, H. S., Heeter, C., Moran, T. P., & Lee, Y. H. (2011). Mind your errors: Evidence for a neural mechanism linking growth mind-set to adaptive posterior adjustments. *Psychological Science, 22,* 1484–1489.

Mrazek, A. J., Molden, D. C., Mrazek, M. D., & Schooler, J. W. (2016). *Cultivating self-control through growth mindsets.* Unpublished manuscript, Northwestern University, Evanston, IL.

Mueller, C. M., & Dweck, C. S. (1998). Intelligence praise can undermine motivation and performance. *Journal of Personality and Social Psychology, 75,* 33–52.

Murphy, M. C., & Dweck, C. S. (2010). A culture of genius: How an organization's lay theory shapes people's cognition, affect, and behavior. *Personality and Social Psychology Bulletin, 36,* 283–296.

Niiya, Y., Crocker, J., & Bartmess, E. N. (2004). From vulnerability to resilience: Learning orientations buffer contingent self-esteem from failure. *Psychological Science, 15*(12), 801–805.

Nussbaum, A. D., & Dweck, C. S. (2008). Defensiveness versus remediation: Mindsets and modes of self-esteem maintenance. *Personality and Social Psychology Bulletin, 34*(5), 599–612.

Olson, K. R., & Dweck, C. S. (2008). A blueprint for social cognitive development. *Perspectives on Psychological Science, 3,* 193–202.

Ommundsen, Y. (2001). Pupils' affective responses in physical education classes: The association of implicit theories of the nature of ability and achievement goals. *European Physical Education Review, 7,* 219–242.

Ommundsen, Y. (2003). Implicit theories of ability and self-regulation strategies in physical education classes. *Educational Psychology, 23,* 141–157.

Panuesku, D., Walton, G. M., Romero, C., Smith, E. N., Yeager, D. S., & Dweck, C. S. (2015). Mind-set interventions are a scalable treatment for academic underachievement. *Psychological Science, 26*(6), 784–793.

Park, C. L., & Folkman, S. (1997). Meaning in the context of stress and coping. *Review of General Psychology, 1,* 115–144.

Pomerantz, E. M., & Kempner, S. G. (2013). Mothers' daily person and process praise: Implications for children's theory of intelligence and motivation. *Developmental Psychology, 49*(11), 2040–2046.

Rheinberg, F. (1980). *Leistungsbewertung und Lernmotivation* [Achievement evaluation and motivation to learn]. Göttingen, Germany: Hogrefe.

Rhodewalt, F. (1994). Conceptions of ability, achievement goals, and individual differences in self-handicapping behavior: On the application of implicit theories. *Journal of Personality, 62,* 67–85.

Robins, R. W., & Pals, J. L. (2002). Implicit mindsets in the academic domain: Implications for goal orientation, attributions, affect, and self-esteem change. *Self and Identity, 1,* 313–336.

Romero, C., Master, A., Paunesku, D., Dweck, C. S., & Gross, J. J. (2014). Academic and emotional functioning in middle school: The role of implicit theories. *Emotion, 14*(2), 227–234.

Rudolph, K. D. (2010). Implicit theories of peer relationships. *Social Development, 19*(1), 113–129.

Sarrazin, P., Biddle, S., Famose, J. P., Cury, F., Fox, K., & Durand, M. (1966). Goal orientation and conceptions of the nature of sport ability in children: A social cognitive approach. *British Journal of Social Psychology, 35,* 399–414.

Spinath, B., Spinath, F. M., Riemann, R., & Angleitner, A. (2003). Implicit theories about personality and intelligence and their relationship to actual personality and intelligence. *Personality and Individual Differences, 35*(4), 939–951.

Spray, C. M., Wang, C. J., Biddle, S. J., Chatzisarantis, N. L., & Warburton, V. E. (2006). An experimental test of mindsets of ability in youth sport. *Psychology of Sport and Exercise, 7*(3), 255–267.

Steele, C. M., & Aronson, J. (1995). Stereotype threat and the intellectual test performance of African-Americans. *Journal of Personality and Social Psychology, 68,* 797–811.

Sternberg, R. J. (1985). *Beyond IQ.* New York: Cambridge University Press.

Stevenson, S. J., & Lochbaum, M. R. (2008). Understanding exercise motivation: Examining the revised social-cognitive model of achievement motivation. *Journal of Sport Behavior, 31*(4), 389–412.

Tabernero, C., & Wood, R. E. (1999). Implicit theories versus the social construal of ability in self-regulation and performance on a complex task. *Organizational Behavior and Human Decision Processes, 78*(2), 104–127.

Tamir, M., John, O. P., Srivastava, S., & Gross, J. J. (2007). Implicit theories of emotion: Affective and social outcomes across a major life transition. *Journal of Personality and Social Psychology, 92,* 731–744.

Tesser, A. (2000). On the confluence of self-esteem maintenance mechanisms. *Personality and Social Psychology Review, 4,* 290–299.

Trzesniewski, K., & Robins, R. (2003, April). *Integrating self-esteem into a process model of academic achievement.* Symposium paper presented at the binennial meeting of the Society for Research in Child Development, Tampa, FL.

Weiner, B. (1986). *An attributional theory of motivation and emotion.* New York: Springer-Verlag.

Wood, R., & Bandura, A. (1989). Impact of conceptions of ability on self-regulatory mechanisms and complex decision making. *Journal of Personality and Social Psychology, 56,* 407–415.

Wood, R. E., Phillips, K. W., & Tabernero, C. (2002). *Implicit theories of ability, processing dynamics and performance in decision-making groups.* Unpublished manuscript, University of New South Wales, Sydney, Australia.

Yeager, D. S., Johnson, R., Spitzer, B. J., Trzesniewski, K. H., Powers, J., & Dweck, C. S. (2014). The far-reaching effects of believing people can change: Implicit theories of personality shape stress, health, and achievement during adolescence. *Journal of Personality and Social Psychology, 106*(6), 867–884.

Yeager, D. S., Trzesniewski, K. H., Tirri, K., Nokelainen, P., & Dweck, C. S. (2011). Adolescents' implicit theories predict desire for vengeance after peer conflicts: Correlational and experimental evidence. *Developmental Psychology, 47*(4), 1090–1107.

Yeager, D. S., & Walton, G. M. (2011). Social-psychological interventions in education: They're not magic. *Review of Educational Research, 81*(2), 267–301.

CHAPTER 9

Understanding and Addressing Performance Anxiety

SIAN L. BEILOCK
MARJORIE W. SCHAEFFER
CHRISTOPHER S. ROZEK

Alex has been preparing all year for this moment. Her number two pencils are sharp; her breakfast was full of protein. For months, she has been drilling herself on math problems and new vocabulary words. Then the moment comes—it is time to open her test booklet to the first page. Just last night she wrote three practice essays, but as she rereads the prompt, her mind goes totally blank. Precious minutes are passing, yet she is helpless to write even a single word.

Today is an important business meeting for Josh. He has spent the last 2 hours wining and dining a very important client. He reaches for the check and begins to fill in the tip when he feels an all-too-familiar sense of anxious dread. What was the rule again? Move the decimal one place or two?

Danny's daughter started fourth grade 3 weeks ago. She has been working on her homework for nearly an hour when she finally carries a worksheet covered in fractions to Danny and asks plaintively, "Can you look at this?" Stuttering, Danny reaches for the paper, answering, "I don't know, I was never so good at fractions when I was your age. I'm just not a math person."

Throughout life, there are many situations in which we desire optimal performance.

Unfortunately, sometimes we are unable to perform up to our potential. Performing at a lower level than one is capable of in a high-stakes situation is often referred to as "choking under pressure." This poor performance is not necessarily a result of lack of motivation, effort, or even skill—poor performance can result from anxiety about the task at hand.

In this chapter, we explore why individuals are generally less likely to succeed when anxious in academic situations. We argue that performance anxiety undermines performance by leading to negative attitudes (e.g., a lack of confidence), changing behaviors (e.g., when a student avoids doing homework or studying), and decreasing cognitive resources available for the task at hand (e.g., working memory, which is our limited-capacity memory system used to store, manipulate, and manage information). A negative feedback loop occurs, wherein performance anxiety decreases performance, and poor performance increases anxiety on subsequent tasks. We focus on a discussion of math anxiety as a common example of performance anxiety and argue that findings related to this domain-specific performance anxiety can shed light on other types of performance anxieties as well. Additionally, we explain how many of the consequences of performance anxiety are reversible and may even be preventable.

A CONCEPTUAL MODEL OF PERFORMANCE ANXIETY

Performance anxiety is broadly defined as fear and apprehension connected to completion of a specific task (e.g., a test) or even engagement with a specific domain (e.g., math). It is characterized by the anticipatory reactions that individuals engage in to manage uncertainty associated with potential future threats (Grupe & Nitschke, 2013). Although related, performance anxiety is different from generalized anxiety. *Generalized anxiety* is defined as uncontrollable worry about one's welfare (and that of one's immediate family) that interferes with daily life. By definition, generalized anxiety impacts many domains (Akiskal, 1998). Performance anxiety is different from generalized anxiety because it concerns a specific domain (e.g., math) and is focused on performance.

There are two distinct components of performance anxiety: anxious apprehension and anxious arousal (Nitschke, Heller, Imig, McDonald, & Miller, 2001). *Anxious apprehension* is the cognitive aspect of anxiety (i.e., worries), whereas *anxious arousal* is characterized by somatic tension and physiological hyperarousal (Moser, Moran, & Jendrusina, 2012). Therefore, to have a full understanding of performance anxiety, we must understand anxious apprehension and anxious arousal as related, yet separate, constructs.

Our theoretical model of the relation between performance anxiety and poor performance is outlined in Figure 9.1. In this model, performance anxiety comprises the two aforementioned components: worry and physiological arousal. Although they are separate components of performance anxiety, worry and arousal often co-occur; that is, individuals tend to be both worried and aroused when they are experiencing performance anxiety. Additionally, increased worry and arousal can result in negative attitudes, avoidance behaviors, and fewer of the resources that individuals need to perform well on a task (e.g., working memory). The deleterious effect of performance anxiety on task performance creates a negative feedback loop in which performance anxiety undermines performance through negative attitudes, avoidance behaviors, and decreased resources. Poorer performance, in turn, leads to increased performance anxiety. Thus, both performance anxiety and actual performance continue to worsen over time in a negative recursive feedback loop (e.g., Cohen, Garcia, Purdie-Vaughns, Apfel, & Brzustoski, 2009).

Anxious Apprehension

Worries are commonly understood to be a major component of performance anxiety. These include concerned thoughts about performance during a task and in anticipation of a task. Importantly, worries can be distracting to individuals during a task and result in hypervigilance for problems. Some worries are situational, but worries also contribute to depression and other clinical

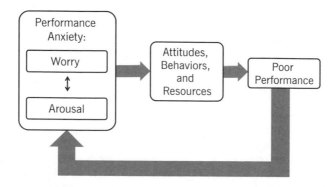

FIGURE 9.1. A conceptual model of how performance anxiety undermines task performance.

disorders (Joormann & Tran, 2009). It is therefore unsurprising that the tendency to worry in response to uncertainty may be related to maladaptive neurocognitive function and behaviors (Grupe & Nitschke, 2013).

Worries not only negatively impact performance, but they are also a distinct component of anxiety. Importantly, worries are associated with vigilance for threat in the environment. This often means that worries lead to increased attention to errors and problems. As evidence of this point, Moser and colleagues (2012) asked participants to complete the letter version of the Eriksen flanker task (Eriksen & Eriksen, 1974), in which participants are instructed to respond to the center letter (target) of a five-letter sequence and to identify whether the target letter is congruent with the rest of the letters (e.g., MMMMM) or incongruent (e.g., NNMNN). Participants are asked to work quickly, and the purpose of this task is to create a situation in which individuals make mistakes, so researchers can study what happens during incorrect responses. For example, this paradigm can be used by researchers to examine brain activity using electroencephalographic (EEG) results associated with making a mistake.

In the Moser and colleagues (2012) work, in addition to the Eriksen flanker task, participants also completed two additional measures in order to assess the two components of anxiety. Participants completed the Penn State Worry Questionnaire (PSWQ; Meyer, Miller, Metzger, & Borkovec, 1990) to measure their tendency to worry and the Anxious Arousal subscale of the Mood and Anxiety Symptoms Questionnaire (MASQ; Watson & Clark, 1991) to measure anxious arousal. Worry was highly correlated with brain activity known to be indicative of monitoring for errors. In contrast, arousal was not associated with error monitoring. These findings support the idea that anxious worries are associated with checking for problems and errors. This makes sense because worries or negative thoughts should logically result from noticing errors and might also lead to increased vigilance or even hypervigilance for errors in the future. In comparison, anxious arousal is defined by a particular physical state, which might co-occur with but is not the same as worried thoughts.

Anxious Arousal

There is evidence that not only is arousal is a component of performance anxiety, but also that anxious arousal is distinct from anxious apprehension. Everyday events such as test-taking, social interactions, or calculating a tip can cause an increase in physical arousal, such as a state of increased heart rate and blood pressure (Seery, 2013). In certain situations, physiological arousal (i.e., increased blood flow, heart rate) can be beneficial. But sometimes, physiological arousal is instead viewed as a threat, which undermines task performance. Jamieson, Mendes, and Nock (2013) use the example of a skier looking down a steep, icy slope to highlight the contrast between arousal being interpreted positively or negatively. Experienced skiers might interpret a pounding heart rate as a sign that they are excited and have the skills necessary to succeed, whereas a novice might interpret a pounding heart rate as a sign that the hill is too difficult, inciting panic. In both cases, however, the skier experiences similar increases in physiological arousal. What we know about performance anxiety would lead us to hypothesize that a skier with performance anxiety would be more likely to view arousal negatively, which can undermine performance.

There is evidence that anxious arousal is generally implicated in worse task performance. A research study showed that when participants were given a practice graduate school entrance exam in a laboratory setting, the higher their physiological arousal (as indicated by salivary alpha amylase), the worse their performance (Jamieson, Mendes, Blackstock, & Schmader, 2010). (An additional condition, in which participants were trained to reappraise their arousal, is discussed in greater detail later in the chapter.) Although this finding shows that anxious arousal might negatively impact performance for most people in high-pressure contexts, it may be that individuals high in performance anxiety respond this same way, even in low-pressure situations.

Mattarella-Micke, Mateo, Kozak, Foster, and Beilock (2011) demonstrated this by studying high- and low-math-anxious participants' performance and physiological reactivity during a math task. For participants high in math anxiety, higher levels of physiological arousal, which was assessed by measuring the stress hormone cortisol, were associated with worse task performance. For participants low in math anxiety, higher levels of physiological arousal were associated with improved task performance. Thus, the effect of physiological arousal depended on individuals' level of performance anxiety, which demonstrates that individuals' interpretation of their physiological arousal can moderate the effects of arousal on performance. This is a topic that we discuss in more detail in the intervention and treatment section of this chapter.

Is Poor Performance the Result or Cause of Performance Anxiety?

Before delving deeper into the mechanisms underlying performance anxiety, it is important to discuss whether the relationship between performance anxiety and poor performance is solely due to performance-anxious individuals lacking ability in a specific domain. Although we know performance anxiety can emerge in early childhood and is linked to decreased performance in subjects such as math (Ramirez, Gunderson, Levine, & Beilock, 2013), its developmental origins are only now beginning to be explored. One hypothesis is that performance anxiety is synonymous with low ability in a domain; that is, performance anxiety is entirely caused by (and is nothing more than) another way to measure lack of ability. A second hypothesis is that performance anxiety plays a causal role in poor performance, independent of an individual's ability level. Thus, performance anxiety is viewed as a factor that can affect individuals with high and low levels of ability. A third, competing reciprocal relationship hypothesis is that performance anxiety leads to lower performance and engagement in a domain or task, which in turn results in lower ability and higher performance anxiety over time. Given that psychological interventions (e.g., Park, Ramirez, & Beilock, 2014), which do not increase ability, can help performance-anxious individuals perform close to the level of less performance-anxious individuals, the evidence seems to favor the idea that performance anxiety is not *simply* a proxy for a lack of ability in a domain or task; that is, there is a psychological component to

performance, and performance anxiety can undermine how well individuals perform, regardless of their ability (Beilock & Maloney, 2015; Geary, 2014).

Further evidence that performance anxiety is not the same as a lack of ability comes from the work of Lyons and Beilock (2012), who focused on math anxiety (i.e., fear and apprehension about performing poorly in math) as a type of performance anxiety. Specifically, they found that some math-anxious individuals are able to perform at high levels despite their math anxiety. Participants performed a mental arithmetic task in which they identified whether an arithmetic problem had been correctly solved. They also completed a difficulty matched word-verification task in which they had to decide whether a letter string, if reversed, spelled an actual English word. All of this was done while having their brain activity recorded in a magnetic resonance imaging (MRI) scanner. Overall, high- and low-math-anxious participants scored identically on the word tasks, but the high-math-anxious participants generally scored worse than low-math-anxious individuals on the math tasks. Most interestingly, Lyons and Beilock also found that not all high-math-anxious participants showed identical neural patterns. Before each type of problem, participants were given a visual cue that indicated whether the next problem would be a math or a word trial, allowing researchers to distinguish the neural activity associated with the anticipation of doing math from that of actually doing the math. The more that high-math-anxious individuals showed activation of a frontoparietal network when anticipating math problems, including the inferior frontal junction (IFJ), the inferior parietal lobule (IPL), and the left anterior inferior frontal gyrus (IFGa), the better they performed. These regions are known to help coordinate cognitive control and motivational resources, and can indicate positive reappraisals of stress. These findings, in terms of the brain activation patterns, suggest that some performance-anxious individuals may be reappraising the situation more positively than their peers before they begin the task and that this reappraisal leads to better performance. All in all, because the different brain activation patterns of high-math-anxious participants are thought to represent something about how individuals view the task and not something about their innate ability—further evidence that suggests performance anxiety has a causal role in performance. Of course, none of the previously mentioned evidence rules out the possibility that some individuals are anxious because they start out low in ability, or the possibility that there might be a reciprocal relationship between performance anxiety and poor performance. However, it does suggest that performance anxiety is not solely due to low ability.

Summary

Performance anxiety is characterized by the anxiety experienced in the immediate context of the performance setting (e.g., a testing situation), the anticipation of having to perform a task, and even fear about future evaluation. Performance anxiety includes physiological arousal and negative cognitions or worries and may lead to negative attitudes, avoidance behaviors, decreased resources, and performance deficits (Ashcraft & Krause, 2007; Hopko, McNeil, Zvolensky, & Eifert, 2002). Moreover, experimental evidence supports performance anxiety as being a causal factor in poor performance. While there are many types of performance anxiety, we explore one specific form, math anxiety, as an exemplar of how performance anxiety works. Although math anxiety is just an example of performance anxiety within one domain, we argue that the mechanisms of math anxiety generalize to other types of performance anxiety, such as test anxiety or sports anxiety. In addition, we argue that performance anxieties are domain-specific. Thus, an individual's level of math anxiety should predict his or her math performance, but not necessarily performance in other domains, such as sports.

ONE EXAMPLE OF A DOMAIN-SPECIFIC PERFORMANCE ANXIETY: MATH ANXIETY

The fear and terror experienced by Josh in the opening anecdote while calculating a tip, is an example of the negative emotions math-anxious individuals may feel when faced with everyday math tasks. *Math anxiety* is a domain-specific performance anxiety defined by the fear and apprehension experienced by an individual when placed in a situation wherein math must be performed (Hembree, 1990). Consistent with our theoretical model of performance anxiety, these fears and negative emotions utilize cognitive resources that might otherwise be focused on math-related tasks and have deleterious effects on performance. Math anxiety also affects behavior, especially by leading individuals to avoid math whenever possible. For example, math-anxious individuals tend to avoid math classes. Furthermore, they perform worse in the math classes they do take than do less-math-anxious individuals (Ashcraft, 2002; Hembree, 1990; Ma, 1999). One study even showed that some of the same areas of the brain that are activated in response to pain become active for math-anxious individuals in anticipation of a math task (Lyons & Beilock, 2012). Thus, it is not surprising that math-anxious individuals often avoid college majors requiring math and eventually avoid math-related careers (Chipman, Krantz, & Silver, 1992).

Explaining the Relation between Math Anxiety and Poor Math Performance

Several mechanisms have been hypothesized to explain the relation between math anxiety and poor performance. Following our theoretical model, we posit that attitudes, behaviors, and reduced resources (e.g., working memory) act as key mechanisms. However, there is also evidence that a lack of basic number skills may contribute to math anxiety, resulting in a reciprocal relationship: Poor numerical skills result in math anxiety, which reduces cognitive resources, leading students to avoid situations involving math and, as a result, limiting students' opportunities to learn and master new math skills.

Research shows that high-math-anxious individuals struggle with both simple and complex math concepts and skills. In terms of the former, in one study, college-age participants were asked to identify the number of squares on a screen, ranging from one to nine. No differences between high- and low-math-anxious individuals were found when one to four squares were presented, but when presented with five or more squares, the high-math-anxious individuals were slower and less accurate at identifying the number of squares than low-math-anxious individuals (Maloney, Risko, Ansari, & Fugelsang, 2010). In another study, high-math-anxious individuals were found to exhibit a larger numerical distance effect, or were slower to judge numbers that were numerically closer together (e.g., 4 and 5 compared with 4 and 8), than were low-math-anxious individuals. This suggests that high-math-anxious individuals have less precise representations of numbers than do their low-math-anxious peers (Maloney, Ansari, & Fugelsang, 2011). Thus, one potential reason why math anxiety is related to poor math performance is that anxiety makes it more difficult to think about numbers at a basic level, which makes doing complex math problems more difficult, more anxiety-provoking, and unpleasant (Maloney & Beilock, 2012). Though experimental research rules out the possibility that math anxiety is due only to innate numerical deficits (e.g., Park et al., 2014), having poor basic number skills may lead to math anxiety, which in turn leads to worse math performance.

Another potential explanation for why math anxiety might undermine math performance is that it takes up or depletes limited cognitive resources, specifically, working memory. Similar mechanisms have been hypothesized for many types of performance anxiety (e.g., Schmader & Johns, 2003). When faced with performing math tasks, math-anxious individuals experience worries and fears, which might then compromise cognitive resources, particularly working memory. Working memory is often described as a limited-capacity system that stores, computes, and manipulates information (Baddeley, 2000; Engle, 2002; Miyake & Shah, 1999). Therefore, how we use our working memory has implications for performance. Although working memory is limited by default, it is important to recognize that there are substantial individual differences in working memory, even at different stages in development (e.g., Ramirez et al., 2013).

Performance anxieties (e.g., math anxiety, test anxiety, and other domain-specific anxieties) are hypothesized to impact working memory because anxious thoughts (e.g., "I'll never be able to do this!") may occupy the working memory resources available in that moment. Therefore, when math-anxious individuals are doing math problems, they are actually engaging in a dual task—solving the task at hand and thinking about their fears. Support for this hypothesis comes from two main types of studies: (1) studies that examine the effects of performance anxiety on tasks that are either demanding or not, in terms of working memory, and (2) studies that examine the effects of performance anxiety on individuals with higher and lower levels of working memory. The first type of study would support reduced working memory availability as a mechanism underlying performance anxiety, if performance anxiety were associated with poor performance only on highly demanding working memory tasks. The second type of study would support reduced working memory availability as a mechanism underlying performance anxiety if performance anxiety were only associated with worse performance in individuals with naturally high levels of working memory. The idea here is that individuals with low levels of working memory would not be affected by reduced working memory because they start off with such low levels that they tend not rely on working memory resources for optimal performance. On the other hand, individuals with higher levels of working memory tend to use working memory resources during performance tasks, so if their working memory is reduced due to performance anxiety, then these individuals are likely to underperform.

As an example of the first type of study, Ashcraft and Kirk (2001) asked high- and low-math-anxious participants to solve high-demand and low-demand working memory problems. On questions that were not demanding of working memory resources, both the high- and low-math-anxious groups performed similarly, but on problems that were more demanding on working memory resources, high-math-anxious participants performed significantly worse than at baseline. In fact, the drop in performance for high-math-anxious individuals was far larger than that for the low-math-anxious participants. One way to interpret these findings is that when high-math-anxious individuals are doing math, their working memory capacity is reduced because of their nervous thoughts, at least as compared to that of low-math-anxious individuals. Therefore, when considering tasks that place a high demand on working memory, individuals with high math anxiety (e.g., Alex, in the case anecdotes at the beginning of this chapter) may be disadvantaged.

These findings show that math anxiety undermines performance on high-demand working memory tasks, but another way to examine this question is to test whether individual differences in working memory play a role in the effects of math anxiety. Specifically, do individual differences in working memory capacity impact the relation between math anxiety and math performance? One study examined this in first- and second-grade children and showed that there was a clear negative relation between math anxiety and math achievement for children with high-capacity working memory (Ramirez et al., 2013). However, no such relationship existed for children with low-capacity working memory. The authors suggested that individuals with higher working memory capacities prefer to use and rely on strategies that require more working memory. Thus, when high-math-anxious children are faced with the negative thoughts associated with math anxiety, their working memory capacity is disturbed, leaving them unable to use their preferred high-capacity working memory requirement strategies. This finding—that those with the highest working memory capacity are most impacted by math anxiety—is especially troubling because these children are more likely to avoid math and math-related careers, despite their clear potential.

Math anxiety has also been found to be negatively associated with the use of more advanced problem-solving strategies, which undermines performance, because advanced strategies are associated with better math achievement. Advanced strategies might rely on working memory resources, so if math anxiety reduces available working memory, then it might block the ability of anxious individuals to utilize these useful ways of solving math problems. Following up on their previous study, Ramirez, Chang, Maloney, Levine, and Beilock (2016) investigated how math anxiety and individual differences in working memory predicted advanced strategy use in math tasks. Consistent with other studies, the negative effects

of math anxiety were limited to individuals with high-capacity working memory. Moreover, math anxiety affected strategy use in children with high-capacity working memory. High-math-anxious children with higher levels of working memory were less likely to use advanced memory-based strategies to solve math problems. In contrast, children with low-capacity working memory showed no effect of math anxiety on strategy use. The authors suggest two possibilities for why higher levels of math anxiety were associated with reduced use of advanced strategies among children with higher capacity working memory. One possibility is that these children with high-capacity working memory initially use advanced strategies, but their math anxiety interferes with these strategies, and they come to rely less on these strategies since they are no longer effective. Another possibility is that the math anxiety actually fundamentally alters children's behavior; thus, high-math-anxious children with high-capacity working memory never attempt to use the advanced memory-based strategies. In either case, there is a strong body of work to support the hypothesis that one route through which math anxiety relates to poor math performance is by occupying or depleting working memory resources.

SOCIAL FACTORS IN PERFORMANCE ANXIETY

Social Pressure and Stereotypes as Sources of Performance Anxiety

It is important to acknowledge that the source of performance anxiety is sometimes social in nature. For example, math-anxious adults often attribute their math anxiety to public embarrassment connected to math (e.g., often directly from math teachers) (Ashcraft, 2002). This is supported by a meta-analytic review of the research on social-evaluative threat, or the fear of being judged negatively by others, which has been shown to be a highly potent psychological stressor across a range of studies (Dickerson & Kemeny, 2004). Social pressure may take many forms, including pressure from higher status individuals, cultural norms that promote pressure in certain situations, and the pressure of letting down a team or group.

Although any situation can be made into a high-pressure context by, for example, adding a judgmental audience during a performance task or raising the stakes of the task by adding monetary incentives or penalties (e.g., Ramirez & Beilock, 2011), one frequently studied type of social pressure concerns stereotypes about groups of people. Stereotypes are ubiquitous in society, and some stereotypes focus on the performance of one group relative to other groups. *Stereotype threat* refers to a phenomenon whereby individuals perform below their ability when a relevant negative stereotype to the individual is made salient in a performance situation, thereby inducing performance anxiety (Steele & Aronson, 1995). For example, researchers observed a decrease in women's math performance when the stereotype "women are bad at math" was made salient (Spencer, Steel, & Quinn, 1999). Unfortunately, even minor acts, such as being asked to circle one's gender in a test booklet before a test, can activate previously established stereotypes (McQueen & Klein, 2006).

But why would stereotypes disrupt performance? The resulting poor performance is believed to be a result of the fear of confirming the negative social stereotype (e.g., a woman in a high-stakes testing situation might worry that she will confirm the stereotype that women are bad at math). Although stereotype threat is often discussed with regard to underrepresented gender and racial-minority groups, theoretically, it might affect anyone for whom a negative stereotype exists. Furthermore, research has shown that one reason why stereotype threat undermines performance is because it depletes working memory resources, similar to the mechanism by which other types of performance anxiety, such as math anxiety, affect performance (Schmader & Johns, 2003).

Person-to-Person Transmission of Performance Anxiety: Examples from Math and Test Anxiety

Not only can performance anxiety be impacted by social factors, such as social evaluation and cultural stereotypes, but an individual's performance anxiety can also influence others around him or her. For example, researchers investigated the impact of female elementary school teachers' math anxiety on their first- and second-grade students (Beilock, Gunderson, Ramirez, & Levine, 2010). Because of the stereotypes about women in math, and because female students might be more likely to identify with female teachers, one hypothesis is that young girls might be particularly likely to be influenced by their female teachers' attitudes about math. At the beginning of the school year, there was no relation between a teacher's math anxiety and her students' math achievement. However, at the end of the school year, results showed that female students in high-math-anxious teachers' classrooms learned less math over the course of the school year than female students in low-math-anxious teachers' classrooms. These students were also more likely to endorse the stereotype "boys are good at math, and girls are good at reading." In contrast, for male students, there was no relation between boys' stereotype endorsement, math achievement, and their teachers' math anxiety levels.

Given that high-math-anxious elementary school teachers can influence children's math performance and stereotype endorsement, even though they only are with children for 180 days, parents stand to make an even greater impact. Parents have varying levels of math anxiety, and this could affect their children's math performance. In one study, researchers examined parents' math anxiety in combination with how often they interacted with their first- and second-grade children about math, specifically, how frequently they helped their children with their math homework, a relatively ubiquitous part of the elementary school experience. When parents who were high in math anxiety helped their children with math homework, their children learned less over the course of the school year than did children of high-math-anxious parents who did not receive help from parents with their math homework (Maloney, Ramirez, Gunderson, Levine, & Beilock, 2015). Simply put, children of high-math-anxious parents actually performed worse when their parents helped them with math homework than did children with low-math-anxious parents, which suggests that the interactions of these math-anxious parents with their children were negative. Furthermore, children's poor performance was associated with higher levels of math anxiety. Thus, one route through which parents' math anxiety might increase their children's math anxiety is by undermining their math performance.

A similar pattern of results has also been found in other countries; therefore, the relation between parents' math anxiety and their children's math achievement is not unique to the North American context. One study in India examined the role of parents' math anxiety and attitudes in shaping their 10- to 15-year-old children's math anxiety and achievement (Soni & Kumari, 2015). Parents' math anxiety was found to be a significant positive predictor of children's math anxiety and children's math attitudes, such that parents with higher levels of math anxiety tended to have children with higher levels of math anxiety. In fact, there was a remarkably high association between parents' math anxiety and children's math anxiety, suggesting that parents might have an important and strong influence on their children's performance anxiety. In addition, children's math anxiety and math attitudes were negatively associated with their math achievement.

Taken together, these studies on the relations between teachers' and parents' math attitudes and children's math attitudes help shed light on a social-developmental model in which adults' math anxiety acts as precursor to children's math anxiety, math attitudes, and math performance. A better understanding of the connections between adults' and children's math anxiety, attitudes, and achievement will allow researchers specifically to target interventions that disrupt this relationship. We can look to research on another type of performance anxiety, test anxiety (i.e., fear and apprehension about performing well on tests), to add to our knowledge of how specific types of performance anxiety (i.e., math or test anxiety) might develop.

Sarason (1960) proposed that children develop test anxiety when they fail to meet their parents' overly high expectations and when parents react critically in an evaluative setting, which makes children sensitive to adult reactions. Adams and Sarason (1963) tested part of this hypothesis using the Test Anxiety Scale, the Need for Achievement Scale, the Lack of Protection Scale of the Autobiographical Survey, and Bendig's (1956) brief version of Taylor's Manifest Anxiety Scale. The authors found a positive correlation for female students and their mothers on all four scales. Additionally, anxiety scores of both boys and girls were more related to their mothers' anxiety levels than to their fathers' anxiety levels.

Similar effects have been shown when examining how much children fear failure, which concerns performance anxiety in general. Elliot and Thrash (2004) found that parents with higher levels of fear of failure had children with higher levels of fear of failure, which suggests that parents might be transmitting these attitudes to their children. The association between mothers' fear of failure and their children's fear of failure was mediated by love withdrawal, which was measured by asking children about how each of their parents would respond to the children's mistakes or perceived failures (e.g., "He or she would avoid looking at me when I disappointed him or her"). Children with higher levels of fear of failure were also more likely to adopt avoidance goals in the academic domain (i.e., goals to avoid performing poorly relative to others in school), which are associated with worse task performance.

Finally, once a child's performance anxiety is high, parents might be crucial factors in maintaining those high levels of anxiety. For example, in one study, the parents of high- and low-test-anxious students worked on a problem-solving task with their children. Parents of high-anxious children provided less support, rejected children's attempts for attention, and were less likely to provide reinforcement following success than did parents of low-anxious students (Hermans, ter Laak, & Maes, 1972). Thus, not only might adults be one cause of performance anxiety, but they also may play a role in the persistence and growth of these attitudes over time.

INTERVENTIONS AND TREATMENTS FOR PERFORMANCE ANXIETY

Given evidence showing that a psychological factor (i.e., performance anxiety) has a significant impact on task performance, psychologists can play a pivotal role in creating theory-driven interventions to address the problems caused by performance anxiety. Many of the techniques developed by psychologists focus on the anxiety instead of the task; that is, an intervention may work by helping to reduce an individual's worries and arousal, not by training him or her to be more skillful at the task. Because these types of interventions target underlying social and cognitive processes of anxiety, these interventions are relevant for a wide range of performance anxiety, rather than being specific only to math anxiety, for example. However, we do not want to suggest that skills and ability do not matter. It is clear that both anxiety and ability play important roles in task performance (Beilock & Maloney, 2015).

To put performance anxiety interventions in the context of our conceptual model (see Figure 9.2), the interventions we discuss target at least one of the two components of performance anxiety: worry and arousal. Interventions may work by reducing these aspects of anxiety, thereby buffering individuals from negative effects. Interventions may also work by changing how worries and arousal are connected to performance, thereby disrupting the negative link between performance anxiety and the resources needed to do well on tasks. For example, if an intervention reduces worries, then performance anxiety should have a smaller negative effect on working memory, which means that more working memory is available for the task, and performance should be improved. Importantly, this can then disrupt the negative recursive cycle that develops when poor performance leads to increased performance anxiety and subsequent even poorer performance. Table 9.1 provides an overview of a set of interventions that have been found to be successful in combating the negative effects of performance anxiety. As mentioned previously, the majority of these interventions are likely applicable for treatment of performance anxiety in a wide variety of domains. Different types of performance anxiety may manifest themselves in widely different ways, but the underlying processes are similar.

As an overview, we discuss three types of performance anxiety interventions in this chapter: exposure; mindset: anxiety-focused; and mindset: self-focused. Exposure interventions involve positive experiences in the anxiety-provoking domain. The two types of mindset interventions involve changing individuals' ways of thinking, or mindsets, about either the anxiety they are feeling (anxiety-focused) or the way they are thinking about themselves in the situation (self-focused). All three types of interventions have been shown to be promising for

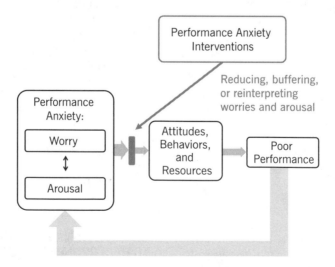

FIGURE 9.2. Interventions can disrupt the negative cycle between performance anxiety and performance.

TABLE 9.1. Performance Anxiety Interventions

Focus	Intervention	Representative study	Brief description
Exposure	Encouraging positive experiences in the threatening domain	Berkowitz et al. (2015)	This intervention works by providing scripted, positive interactions within the anxiety-provoking domain.
Exposure	Practice under pressure	Oudejans and Pijpers (2009)	Practicing under pressure can help to prevent underperformance in future high-stakes events.
Mindset: Anxiety-focused	Anxiety reappraisal	Johns, Inzlicht, and Schmader (2008)	This intervention focuses on reinterpreting anxious thoughts as helpful for task performance (e.g., worries can help you pay attention during a test).
Mindset: Anxiety-focused	Arousal reappraisal	Jamieson et al. (2010)	This intervention asks individuals to reinterpret the arousal that comes with anxious situations as helpful for task performance (e.g., a faster heart rate means increased energy).
Mindset: Anxiety-focused	Expressive writing	Ramirez and Beilock (2011)	This brief writing intervention consists of writing about and off-loading worries before a stressful situation.
Mindset: Anxiety-focused	Labeling the worries	Johns, Schmader, and Martens (2005)	This intervention involves explicitly focusing attention on the existence of a threatening stereotype and acknowledging that it is only a stereotype.
Mindset: Anxiety-focused	Mindfulness	Mrazek et al. (2013)	This intervention involves regularly practicing mindfulness mediation and learning to focus on different aspects of thoughts and sensations.
Mindset: Anxiety-focused	Reattribution of uncertainty	Wilson and Linville (1982)	This intervention focuses on teaching individuals to view ambiguous cues, such as a low grade on a test, as common to everyone and as temporary in nature.
Mindset: Self-focused	Perspective broadening	Critcher and Dunning (2015)	This intervention asks individuals to think about multiple aspects of their identities in order to decrease their focus on the threatening domain or task.
Mindset: Self-focused	Self-affirmation	Cohen et al. (2009)	This brief writing exercise increases individuals' self-integrity by asking them to write about important interests and activities.

reducing the negative effects of performance anxiety (though more research is needed) and are described in more detail below.

Exposure Interventions

One of the most intuitive methods for reducing the impact of performance anxiety on performance is exposure interventions. One example of exposure interventions involves having individuals practice in the anxiety-provoking domain. However, practice alone is not enough to overcome performance anxiety. Individuals need to practice under pressure to see a reduced impact of performance anxiety. As evidence for this, in one study, expert basketball players and dart throwers practiced with or without induced performance pressure for 5 weeks. Only those participants who practiced under pressure showed an improvement in performance during a high-pressure posttest (Oudejans & Pijpers, 2009).

Performance anxiety can affect others beyond the individual with performance anxiety. For example, children of parents who are anxious about math perform worse in math than children with less-math-anxious parents (Maloney et al., 2015; Soni & Kumari, 2015). One way to lessen the impact of parents' math anxiety on their children's math performance is to provide parents with scripted ways to talk about math with their children in order to create more positive math interactions in the home. One recent study involved providing parents of elementary school-age children with access to either an iPad math app (intervention condition) or a reading app (control condition). The math app provided a nightly word problem; that is, a written script with problems and solutions for parents' use to engage in math discussions and increase positive math talk in the home. Being assigned to the intervention condition improved the academic performance of children of high-math-anxious parents. In fact, the achievement gap between children of high- and low-math-anxious parents was greatly diminished. Therefore, providing a scripted way for families to have positive math interactions offered a way to block the negative effects of parents' math anxiety on their children's math performance. The app may give parents, especially high-math-anxious parents, more (and better) ways to talk to their children about math not only during app usage but also in other everyday interactions (Berkowitz et al., 2015).

Mindset

Anxiety-Focused Interventions

Exposure interventions are an intuitive and straightforward strategy for managing performance anxiety; however, other, less intuitive strategies involve helping individuals to think about the performance anxiety or themselves in different ways in order to allow them to perform well even when anxious. These psychological-based mindset interventions often involve giving individuals new information and teaching them to change how they think about a task or themselves, which can occur in an intervention as brief as reading a paragraph before taking a test or completing a short writing exercise at the beginning of a school year (Wilson, 2011). Mindset interventions can focus directly on how to think about the anxiety (anxiety-focused) or they can focus on how individuals view themselves in situations in which anxiety might occur (self-focused).

One type of mindset intervention focuses on reappraisal. Reappraisal interventions can work by reframing anxiety in general or by targeting one specific component of anxiety, such as arousal or worries. To demonstrate the effectiveness of reappraisal, one study examined how reappraisal might help participants when they were experiencing performance anxiety because of stereotype threat, which is the fear of being judged because of negative stereotypes about one's group, such as the stereotype about women being worse at math than men (Johns, Inzlicht, & Schmader, 2008). The authors hypothesized that the performance deficit associated with stereotype threat could be reduced (or eliminated) when individuals' performance anxiety was reframed more positively. Specifically, when participants were told that anxiety could help, rather than harm, performance on a math task (e.g., by increasing their attention during the task), subsequent performance improved compared to that of the control group. Importantly, the reappraisal manipulation did not reduce self-reported anxiety; instead, it helped participants turn the anxiety into a positive for task performance.

Some other treatments try to curtail the negative impacts of performance anxiety by reappraising or reframing just the arousal component of anxiety. In one study, students completed a practice version of an upcoming high-stakes test (Jamieson et al., 2010). Before the test, half of the participants (the reappraisal condition) were informed that the physical arousal that they would feel (e.g., sweaty palms and a fast heartrate) is actually helpful for test performance (e.g., because it indicates that their bodies are energizing them for the task). Participants in the control condition were given no additional information. The participants in the reappraisal group who were told that arousal was positive outperformed participants in the control group on the practice test. This change in mindset, or the way in which students thought about physiological arousal before a test, seemed to persist, as the students in the reappraisal group also had better performance on the actual test, outside of the lab, several months later, which suggests that teaching individuals about this reappraisal mindset once could have long-lasting effects. These effects were later confirmed and replicated in a study showing the positive effects of the arousal reappraisal intervention on test performance for remedial math students in community college (Jamieson, Peters, Greenwood, & Altose, 2016). A related study indicated that arousal reappraisal interventions can also have positive effects on physiological stress responses, such as improved immune functioning (John-Henderson, Rheinschmidt, & Mendoza-Denton, 2015).

A different way of reframing an anxiety-provoking task is to educate individuals explicitly about and label the source of the worries. Johns, Schmader, and Martens (2005) did this by teaching women about the concept of stereotype threat in the math domain. Specifically, researchers told participants in a stereotype threat awareness condition the definition of stereotype threat (i.e., that *stereotype threat* is defined as worrying that if you are a woman and perform poorly in math, then you will confirm the negative stereotype that women are worse at math than men, and that stereotype threat has been shown to undermine performance). The hypothesis was that the stereotype threat awareness condition could reduce the amount of performance anxiety experienced by participants by giving them a known external source for the pressure (i.e., stereotype threat). Put another way, making participants aware of stereotype threat could give them a ready-made excuse for underperformance, which might alleviate the performance anxiety that they would experience (Brown & Josephs, 1999). Both men and women were asked to complete math problems, described either as a "problem-solving task" (control group) or as a "math test" (so-called to induce the pressure associated

with stereotype threat, the stereotype threat group). One additional group was informed that the task was a math test (stereotype induction), but participants in this group were also given information defining stereotype threat, and they were informed that stereotype threat might make women feel more anxious (stereotype-threat-aware group). Women in the stereotype-threat-aware group performed identically to men; in the unaware-stereotype-threat condition, women performed significantly worse than men. In other words, simply labeling and explaining the effects of stereotype threat to women enabled them to perform better. As mentioned previously, this is hypothesized to be because they could attribute the worries and arousal associated with performance anxiety to stereotype threat rather than attributing it to a high degree of pressure to succeed, consequently inoculating them against stereotype threat. A more recent study found comparable results with high school students using a similar intervention (Moè, 2012).

A third way of reframing anxiety focuses on the attributions individuals make about ambiguous situations. *Attributions* are the reasons or causes individuals give to events, and much research has been conducted on how attributions can affect performance. Importantly, attributions can either be stable or unstable. For example, if individuals believe that their performance is due to an immutable ability they were either born with or without (stable), then when they perform poorly at that task, they are likely to interpret that poor performance as a signal that they should quit the task because they have low ability levels that cannot be changed. Conversely, if individuals believe that their performance is due to effort or another malleable factor (unstable), then even when they perform poorly, they should persist on a task because low task performance only indicates a lack of effort, which can be increased (Dweck, 1986).

Intervention work has shown that teaching students that perceived failure in school is due to unstable causes can help them react better when they feel anxious about their performance. For example, Wilson and Linville (1982) recruited a sample of first-year college students who were anxious about their performance in college. Students in an intervention condition were taught that poor performance during their first year of college was common and generally became less of a problem over time for students, which was done to teach students in the intervention condition to make unstable attributions about performance. As compared to a control group, students in the intervention group had a higher grade-point average (GPA) and were less likely to drop out of college. More recent studies have replicated these findings with groups of students who suffer from performance anxiety due to their race (Walton & Cohen, 2011), socioeconomic status (Yeager et al., 2016), and the transition to middle school (Rozek, Pyne, Hanselman, Feldman, & Borman, 2016). Thus, reframing individuals' attributions about perceived failure is another way to help mitigate the effects of performance anxiety.

Instead of reframing the meaning of performance anxiety, other types of mindset interventions focus on reducing worries during the task. One method for reducing worries involves mindfulness meditation techniques. In one study, participants were given a 2-week mindfulness training course designed to lessen anxiety and the associated mind wandering or distraction (e.g., thinking about worries), especially during assessments (Mrazek, Franklin, Philips, Baird, & Schooler, 2013). At the end of the training, participants showed improved performance on the Graduate Record Exam (GRE) Reading Comprehension subtest, as well as increased working memory capacity, which is consistent with the idea that this intervention might work to reduce the negative effects of performance anxiety by targeting the worry component of anxiety. Additionally, participants who completed the training reported the reduced occurrence of distracting thoughts during assessments. This work suggests that training underlying cognitive processes (e.g., mindfulness) can prevent the cycle of negative ruminations that leads to a drain on cognitive resources, which are necessary for performance. Relatedly, a randomized trial of mindfulness Kindness Curriculum in preschool classrooms showed further support for the positive effects of mindfulness interventions in educational settings in a much younger age group (Flook, Goldberg, Pinger, & Davidson, 2015).

Instead of training for 2 weeks, another option for targeting the cognitive worry component of anxiety is to do a specific activity directly before the task to regulate anxious thoughts. Across several studies, Ramirez and Beilock (2011) demonstrated that expressive writing (i.e., writing about one's thoughts and feelings about an upcoming task or event) can alleviate the negative impact of test anxiety on exam performance. This intervention is theorized to work by off-loading worries, which should then reduce the number of intrusive thoughts that are experienced while one is anxious. In one of the studies, on the day of the final exam in ninth-grade science courses, the researchers asked half of the students either to think about a topic not on the exam (control condition) or to write about their thoughts and feelings regarding the upcoming exam (expressive writing condition) for 10 minutes. Students given the opportunity to write about their worries had higher overall scores than those students who were in the control condition. However, the most striking finding was that students with the highest reported levels of test anxiety benefited the most from expressive writing. In fact, the expressive writing exercise was able to close the achievement gap between students high and low in test anxiety.

This same idea—that expressive writing dampens the impact of performance anxiety—has been shown to lessen the impact of math anxiety as well (Park et al., 2014). For high-math-anxious participants, engaging in an expressive writing exercise before completing math problems resulted in improved performance on those math problems. This positive effect of expressive writing narrowed the performance gap between high- and low-math-anxious individuals. A third study showed similar positive effects of expressive writing on Medical College Admission Test (MCAT) and Law School Admission Test (LSAT) scores, and also on participants' depressive symptoms before the exams (Frattaroli, Thomas, & Lyubomirsky, 2011).

Self-Focused Interventions

Although changing how individuals think about anxiety can be helpful for reducing the negative effects of performance anxiety, another type of mindset intervention focuses on how individuals think about themselves in situations that create high performance anxiety. The hypothesis is that when in a high-performance-anxiety situation, such as a math test for a high-math-anxious individual, attention becomes narrowed and focused on the anxiety-provoking task or stimuli to the exclusion of everything else. That is, threats, like performance anxiety, constrict the working self-concept, or what is salient in individuals' minds, to focus on threatened self-aspects (Critcher & Dunning, 2015). For example, when individuals are worried about their academic performance, they put more of their attention on that particular domain (i.e., academics), even though remembering that they care about other domains or that they are good in other areas of life might reduce their anxiety levels.

Critcher and Dunning (2015) found that helping individuals to broaden their perspective in high-performance-anxiety situations could help reduce the negative effects of performance anxiety. First, performance pressure was manipulated for participants. Then, all participants completed a task in which they were asked to think and write about various aspects of their identity. Before beginning that task, participants in the perspective-broadening condition were asked to think about the actions, talents, characteristics, and tasks that define who they are as a person because this was hypothesized to remind them about nonthreatened aspects of their identities. Supporting this hypothesis, participants in the perspective-broadening condition were more able to identify multiple aspects of their self-concepts than participants in the control condition. They also responded in a less anxious manner (e.g., less defensively) on the task at hand. Alternatively, participants who were not given the opportunity to engage in a perspective-broadening writing activity displayed a constricted self-concept, which is indicative of anxiety, and responded more defensively during the task. Performance anxiety alone (without the opportunity for perspective-broadening writing) left participants unable to recognize their own full potential and instead left them distracted and focused mainly on feeling threatened. These results demonstrate the potential

for low-cost interventions to combat performance anxiety through engagement in perspective-broadening writing activities before high-performance-anxiety tasks.

With a related self-focused intervention, Cohen, Garcia, Purdie-Vaughns, Apfel, and Brzustoski (2009) have done groundbreaking work to reduce racial achievement gaps by using an intervention called self-affirmation to buffer minority students from the negative effects of performance anxiety (for a review of self-affirmation studies, see Hanselman, Rozek, Grigg, & Borman, 2016). In a study with middle school students, those students assigned to the intervention group completed brief, structured writing assignments designed to allow them to affirm important values (e.g., liking sports or caring about their families). Control group students wrote about values that were important to other people. Students only completed a few of these writing exercises over the course of the school year, but results showed that intervention group students potentially susceptible to stereotype threat had higher grades for up to 2 years after the intervention took place. The authors suggest that an initial boost in performance disrupted the negative recursive cycle between performance anxiety and poor performance, placing students on a new and positive performance trajectory. As further support of these findings, another study showed positive effects of self-affirmation on physiological stress responses directly by randomly assigning some participants to a self-affirmation condition and others to a control writing condition before having them engage in a high-pressure publicly evaluated speech (Creswell et al., 2005). Participants in the self-affirmation condition showed smaller physiological stress responses (i.e., cortisol responses) than participants in the control condition, suggesting that self-focused interventions such as self-affirmation may improve performance by dampening the physiological stress response.

CONCLUSION

Performance anxiety has myriad and long-reaching effects. It can impact academic performance, social interactions, and even life decisions, such as college major and career choices. The roots and mechanisms of performance anxiety are complex and multifaceted, but research across different domains of performance anxiety (e.g., math anxiety and test anxiety) can be used to provide a clearer picture of how performance anxiety develops and works in general. Research points to multiple mechanisms, including negative attitudes (e.g., negative affect), specific behaviors (e.g., avoidance), and decreased resources (e.g., working memory impairment). Although more research is needed to understand better how performance anxiety develops, current findings suggest an important role for both social evaluation and relevant adults (e.g., parents, teachers) during childhood.

Current research is also developing both treatments and preventive measures, including interventions that focus on exposure, on anxiety itself, and on changing the way people think about themselves in situations that evoke performance anxiety. Performance anxiety treatment studies point to the benefit of decreasing working memory load through tasks such as expressive writing and mindfulness mediation. Preventive measures have also proven helpful. For instance, providing positive scripts for anxious adults to use when working with children can help reduce the transmission of performance anxiety to young children, which could stop performance anxiety before it develops. In summary, performance anxiety is an important factor to take into account in promoting optimal task performance and developing competence in a domain over time.

REFERENCES

Adams, E. B., & Sarason, I. G. (1963). Relation between anxiety in children and their parents. *Child Development, 34,* 237–246.

Akiskal, H. S. (1998). Toward a definition of generalized anxiety disorder as an anxious temperament type. *Acta Psychiatrica Scandinavica Supplementum, 393*(98), 66–73.

Ashcraft, M. H. (2002). Math anxiety: Personal, educational, and cognitive consequences. *Current Directions in Psychological Science, 11*(5), 181–185.

Ashcraft, M. H., & Kirk, E. P. (2001). The relationships among working memory, math anxiety, and performance. *Journal of Experimental Psychology: General, 130*(2), 224–237.

Ashcraft, M. H., & Krause, J. (2007). Working memory, math performance, and math anxiety. *Psychonomic Bulletin and Review, 14,* 243–248.

Baddeley, A. (2000). The episodic buffer: A new component of working memory? *Trends in Cognitive Sciences, 4*(11), 417–423.

Beilock, S. L., Gunderson, E. A., Ramirez, G., & Levine, S. C. (2010). Female teachers' math anxiety affects girls' math achievement. *Proceedings of the National Academy of Sciences USA, 107*(5), 1860–1863.

Beilock, S. L., & Maloney, E. A. (2015). Math anxiety: A factor in math achievement not to be ignored. *Policy Insights from the Behavioral and Brain Sciences, 2*(1), 4–12.

Bendig, A. W. (1956). The development of a short form of the Manifest Anxiety Scale. *Journal of Consulting Psychology, 20*(5), 384.

Berkowitz, T., Schaeffer, M. W., Maloney, E. A., Peterson, L., Gregor, C., Levine, S. C., et al. (2015). Math at home adds up to achievement in school. *Science, 350,* 196–198.

Brown, R. P., & Josephs, R. A. (1999). A burden of proof: Stereotype relevance and gender differences in math performance. *Journal of Personality and Social Psychology, 76*(2), 246–257.

Chipman, S. F., Krantz, D. H., & Silver, R. (1992). Mathematics anxiety and science careers among able college women. *Psychological Science, 3*(5), 292–295.

Cohen, G. L., Garcia, J., Purdie-Vaughns, V., Apfel, N., & Brzustoski, P. (2009). Recursive processes in self-affirmation: Intervening to close the minority achievement gap. *Science, 324,* 400–403.

Creswell, J. D., Welch, W. T., Taylor, S. E., Sherman, D. K., Gruenewald, T. L., & Mann, T. (2005). Affirmation of personal values buffers neuroendocrine and psychological stress responses. *Psychological Science, 16*(11), 846–851.

Critcher, C. R., & Dunning, D. (2015). Self-affirmations provide a broader perspective on self-threat. *Personality and Social Psychology Bulletin, 41*(1), 3–18.

Dickerson, S. S., & Kemeny, M. E. (2004). Acute stressors and cortisol responses: A theoretical integration and synthesis of laboratory research. *Psychological Bulletin, 130*(3), 355–391.

Dweck, C. S. (1986). Motivational processes affecting learning. *American Psychologist, 41*(10), 1040–1048.

Elliot, A. J., & Thrash, T. M. (2004). The intergenerational transmission of fear of failure. *Personality and Social Psychology Bulletin, 30*(8), 957–971.

Engle, R. W. (2002). Working memory capacity as executive attention. *Current Directions in Psychological Science, 11*(1), 19–23.

Eriksen, B. A., & Eriksen, C. W. (1974). Effects of noise letters upon the identification of a target letter in a nonsearch task. *Perception and Psychophysics, 16*(1), 143–149.

Flook, L., Goldberg, S. B., Pinger, L., & Davidson, R. J. (2015). Promoting prosocial behavior and self-regulatory skills in preschool children through a mindfulness-based kindness curriculum. *Developmental Psychology, 51*(1), 44–51.

Frattaroli, J., Thomas, M., & Lyubomirsky, S. (2011). Opening up in the classroom: Effects of expressive writing on graduate school entrance exam performance. *Emotion, 11*(3), 691–696.

Geary, D. C. (2014). *Learning mathematics: Findings from the National (U.S.) Mathematics Panel.* Presentation at the 3rd National Conference Dyscalculia and Maths LD, Columbia, MO.

Grupe, D. W., & Nitschke, J. B. (2013). Uncertainty and anticipation in anxiety: An integrated neurobiological and psychological perspective. *Nature Reviews Neuroscience, 14*(7), 488–501.

Hanselman, P., Rozek, C. S., Grigg, J., & Borman, G. D. (2016). New evidence on self-affirmation effects and theorized sources of heterogeneity from large-scale replications. *Journal of Educational Psychology.* [Epub ahead of print]

Hembree, R. (1990). The nature, effects, and relief of mathematics anxiety. *Journal for Research in Mathematics Education, 21*(1), 33–46.

Hermans, H. J., ter Laak, J. J., & Maes, P. C. (1972). Achievement motivation and fear of failure in family and school. *Developmental Psychology, 6*(3), 520–528.

Hopko, D. R., McNeil, D. W., Zvolensky, M. J., & Eifert, G. H. (2002). The relation between anxiety and skill in performance-based anxiety disorders: A behavioral formulation of social phobia. *Behavior Therapy, 32*(1), 185–207.

Jamieson, J. P., Mendes, W. B., Blackstock, E., & Schmader, T. (2010). Turning the knots in your stomach into bows: Reappraising arousal improves performance on the GRE. *Journal of Experimental Social Psychology, 46*(1), 208–212.

Jamieson, J. P., Mendes, W. B., & Nock, M. K. (2013). Improving acute stress responses: The power of reappraisal. *Current Directions in Psychological Science, 22*(1), 51–56.

Jamieson, J. P., Peters, B. J., Greenwood, E. J., & Altose, A. J. (2016). Reappraising stress arousal improves performance and reduces evaluation anxiety in classroom exam situations. *Social Psychological and Personality Science, 7*(6), 579–587.

John-Henderson, N. A., Rheinschmidt, M. L., & Mendoza-Denton, R. (2015). Cytokine responses and math performance: The role of stereotype threat and anxiety reappraisals. *Journal of Experimental Social Psychology, 56*, 203–206.

Johns, M., Inzlicht, M., & Schmader, T. (2008). Stereotype threat and executive resource depletion: Examining the influence of emotion regulation. *Journal of Experimental Psychology: General, 137*(4), 691.

Johns, M., Schmader, T., & Martens, A. (2005). Knowing is half the battle: Teaching stereotype threat as a means of improving women's math performance. *Psychological Science, 16*(3), 175–179.

Joormann, J., & Tran, T. B. (2009). Rumination and intentional forgetting of emotional material. *Cognition and Emotion, 23*(6), 1233–1246.

Lyons, I. M., & Beilock, S. L. (2012). When math hurts: Math anxiety predicts pain network activation in anticipation of doing math. *PLoS ONE, 7*(10), e48076.

Ma, X. (1999). A meta-analysis of the relationship between anxiety toward mathematics and achievement in mathematics. *Journal for Research in Mathematics Education, 30*(5), 520–540.

Maloney, E. A., Ansari, D., & Fugelsang, J. A. (2011). The effect of mathematics anxiety on the processing of numerical magnitude. *Quarterly Journal of Experimental Psychology, 64*(1), 10–16.

Maloney, E. A., & Beilock, S. L. (2012). Math anxiety: Who has it, why it develops, and how to guard against it. *Trends in Cognitive Sciences, 16*(8), 404–406.

Maloney, E. A., Ramirez, G., Gunderson, E. A., Levine, S. C., & Beilock, S. L. (2015). Intergenerational effects of parents' math anxiety on children's math achievement and anxiety. *Psychological Science, 26*(9), 1–9.

Maloney, E. A., Risko, E. F., Ansari, D., & Fugelsang, J. (2010). Mathematics anxiety affects counting but not subitizing during visual enumeration. *Cognition, 114*(2), 293–297.

Mattarella-Micke, A., Mateo, J., Kozak, M. N., Foster, K., & Beilock, S. L. (2011). Choke or thrive?: The relation between salivary cortisol and math performance depends on individual differences in working memory and math-anxiety. *Emotion, 11*(4), 1000–1005.

McQueen, A., & Klein, W. M. (2006).

Experimental manipulations of self-affirmation: A systematic review. *Self and Identity, 5*(4), 289–354.

Meyer, T. J., Miller, M. L., Metzger, R. L., & Borkovec, T. D. (1990). Development and validation of the Penn State Worry Questionnaire. *Behaviour Research and Therapy, 28*(6), 487–495.

Miyake, A., & Shah, P. (1999). *Models of working memory: Mechanisms of active maintenance and executive control.* New York: Cambridge University Press.

Moè, A. (2012). Gender difference does not mean genetic difference: Externalizing improves performance in mental rotation. *Learning and Individual Differences, 22*(1), 20–24.

Moser, J. S., Moran, T. P., & Jendrusina, A. A. (2012). Parsing relationships between dimensions of anxiety and action monitoring brain potentials in female undergraduates. *Psychophysiology, 49*(1), 3–10.

Mrazek, M. D., Franklin, M. S., Phillips, D. T., Baird, B., & Schooler, J. W. (2013). Mindfulness training improves working memory capacity and GRE performance while reducing mind wandering. *Psychological Science, 24*(5), 776–781.

Nitschke, J. B., Heller, W., Imig, J. C., McDonald, R. P., & Miller, G. A. (2001). Distinguishing dimensions of anxiety and depression. *Cognitive Therapy and Research, 25*(1), 1–22.

Oudejans, R. R., & Pijpers, J. R. (2009). Training with anxiety has a positive effect on expert perceptual–motor performance under pressure. *Quarterly Journal of Experimental Psychology, 62*(8), 1631–1647.

Park, D., Ramirez, G., & Beilock, S. L. (2014). The role of expressive writing in math anxiety. *Journal of Experimental Psychology: Applied, 20*(2), 103–111.

Ramirez, G., & Beilock, S. L. (2011). Writing about testing worries boosts exam performance in the classroom. *Science, 331,* 211–213.

Ramirez, G., Chang, H., Maloney, E. A., Levine, S. C., & Beilock, S. L. (2016). On the relationship between math anxiety and math achievement in early elementary school: The role of problem solving strategies. *Journal of Experimental Child Psychology, 141,* 83–100.

Ramirez, G., Gunderson, E. A., Levine, S. C., & Beilock, S. L. (2013). Math anxiety, working memory, and math achievement in early elementary school. *Journal of Cognition and Development, 14*(2), 187–202.

Rozek, C. S., Pyne, J. R., Hanselman, P., Feldman, R. C., & Borman, G. D. (2016, January). *Reappraising adversity improves students' academic achievement, behavior, and well-being.* Poster presented at the annual meeting of the Society for Personality and Social Psychology, San Diego, CA.

Sarason, I. G. (1960). Empirical findings and theoretical problems in the use of anxiety scales. *Psychological Bulletin, 57*(5), 403–415.

Schmader, T., & Johns, M. (2003). Converging evidence that stereotype threat reduces working memory capacity. *Journal of Personality and Social Psychology, 85*(3), 440–452.

Seery, M. D. (2013). The biopsychosocial model of challenge and threat: Using the heart to measure the mind. *Social and Personality Psychology Compass, 7*(9), 637–653.

Soni, A., & Kumari, S. (2015). The role of parental math anxiety and math attitude in their children's math achievement. *International Journal of Science and Mathematics Education, 5*(4), 159–163.

Spencer, S. J., Steele, C. M., & Quinn, D. M. (1999). Stereotype threat and women's math performance. *Journal of Experimental Social Psychology, 35*(1), 4–28.

Steele, C. M., & Aronson, J. (1995). Stereotype threat and the intellectual test performance of African Americans. *Journal of Personality and Social Psychology, 69*(5), 797–811.

Walton, G. M., & Cohen, G. L. (2011). A brief social-belonging intervention improves academic and health outcomes of minority students. *Science, 331,* 1447–1451.

Watson, D., & Clark, L. A. (1991). *The Mood and Anxiety Symptoms Questionnaire (MASQ).* Unpublished manuscript, University of Iowa, Iowa City, IA.

Wilson, T. D. (2011). *Redirect: The surprising new science of psychological change.* London: Penguin.

Wilson, T. D., & Linville, P. W. (1982). Improving the academic performance of college freshmen: Attribution therapy revisited. *Journal of Personality and Social Psychology, 42*(2), 367–376.

Yeager, D. S., Walton, G. M., Brady, S. T., Akcinar, E. N., Paunesku, D., Keane, L., et al. (2016). Teaching a lay theory before college narrows achievement gaps at scale. *Proceedings of the National Academy of Sciences, 113*(24), E3341–E3348.

PART III

RELEVANT PROCESSES

CHAPTER 10

Challenge and Threat Appraisals

JEREMY P. JAMIESON

Extending back to the formative years of psychology as a science, William James and Wilhelm Wundt believed mental processes were rooted in bodily processes. Thus, scientists have long theorized that the mind and body are not ontologically distinct, but changes in one directly affect the other. Many major advances in psychological theory and treatment research over the past 50+ years are predicated on a belief in mind–body monism. For instance, the idea that the mind and body operate in concert to produce psychological states is evident in modern models of emotion. Specifically, conceptual act theory argues that appraisal processes transform internal states into emotional experiences by integrating bodily changes with external sensory information and knowledge of the situation (see Barrett, 2014, for a review). Along similar lines, empirically based cognitive-behavioral therapies are predicated on the belief that changing cognitive appraisals are often sufficient to improve downstream mental (and physical) health outcomes (see Hofmann, Asnaani, Vonk, Sawyer, & Fang, 2012, for a review).

The research presented in this chapter builds on ideas of monism and mind–body processes to understand how cognitive appraisal processes interact with situational factors to determine motivational, physiological, and behavioral responses, with the goal of informing future avenues of exploration. More specifically, the work presented here relies on the *biopsychosocial model of challenge and threat* (e.g., Blascovich & Mendes, 2010) as an organizing framework though which to understand how cognitive appraisal processes can produce affective, physiological, and behavioral responses in motivated performance situations, and how altering appraisals can be used to optimize responses to acute social stressors.

THE APPRAISAL THEORY OF STRESS AND COPING

Schachter and Singer (1962) pioneered the idea that appraisals are contextually grounded. Specifically, their seminal research suggests that perceptions of bodily states can shape emotional experiences. To illustrate, participants who were injected with epinephrine (adrenaline), but were led to believe the injection would have no impact on their stress arousal, labeled their affective states consistent with situational cues. Subsequent appraisal models of emotional experience were based on the idea that situational and cognitive processes interact to determine emotions.

In classic work on the *appraisal theory of emotion,* Lazarus and colleagues introduced notions of *challenge* and *threat* states experienced in stressful situations (see Lazarus, 1991, for a review). The notion was that no single process—psychological, biological, or situational—undergirded stress responses. Instead, the appraisal theory of emotion argued for multiple processes derived from bodily sensations, past experience, and situational factors, to name a few, that contributed to stress appraisals and subsequent emotional experiences (e.g., Lazarus, DeLongis, Folkman, & Gruen, 1985). Considering stress responses as a *system* required categorizing responses into general rubrics rather than using single processes to define stress. Central to the model is the malleability of stress responses rooted in cognitive appraisal processes; that is, stress responses can be altered by changing how individuals perceive stressors.

Lazarus's model specified two levels or stages of cognitive appraisal processes: primary and secondary. Primary appraisals address whether a situation is relevant to well-being and emotion. For instance, primary appraisal processes assess whether situations are irrelevant, benign, or stressful. Irrelevant situations are those that do not require instrumental responding and have no impact on well-being or health outcomes. Benign-positive situations *only* signal positive outcomes with relatively involvement (i.e., no instrumental action is needed to obtain good outcomes). The stressful type of primary appraisal, however, is further subdivided into *threat* and *challenge*. Threatening situations are those that involve potential for harm/loss, whereas challenging situations refer to opportunities for growth, mastery, or gain (Lazarus, 1991). Primary appraisal processes alone, however, are not sufficient to determine affective responses. Secondary appraisals inform affective responses by evaluating available coping resources and response options available. Essentially, secondary appraisals seek to establish how to address or cope with stressors (e.g., Folkman & Lazarus, 1985).

Primary appraisals are not "primary" because these necessarily come first in the temporal sequence (though they usually do). Primary appraisals are primary because these appraisals confer personal relevance and have the potential to elicit emotional responses (Lazarus & Smith, 1988). Similarly, primary and secondary appraisals can be interdependent (e.g., Folkman & Lazarus, 1980). For example, primary appraisals might suggest a threatening situation with the potential for harm, such as the sudden escalation of an interpersonal conflict in which one is in danger of being physically assaulted. However, if secondary appraisals indicate one can cope with the threat, such as martial arts training in the earlier example, the experience of threat is diminished. Alternatively, challenging situations can become threatening if coping resources are not sufficient to meet perceived situational demands. To illustrate, a high-achieving student is about to take an important exam. Because of her high level of prior performance, this situation is initially appraised as challenging. However, she has not studied at all for this particular exam. So, during the test, her secondary appraisal processes indicate that she does not have the requisite knowledge to perform well on this particular test, causing her to experience threat.

In summary, the appraisal theory of stress and coping established challenge and threat profiles across two levels of appraisals—primary and secondary. Building on this model, researchers sought to refine the appraisal processes and ground *challenge* and *threat* predictions in physiological systems. This led to the development of the biopsychosocial (BPS) model of challenge and threat (e.g., Blascovich, 1992; Blascovich & Tomaka, 1996; Tomaka, Blascovich, Kelsey, & Leitten, 1993).

THE BPS MODEL OF CHALLENGE AND THREAT

A fundamental principle of the BPS model of challenge and threat is the idea that appraisals of situational demands and coping resources interact to elicit challenge- and threat-type responses in motivated performance contexts—those that present acute demands that require instrumental responding (see Mendes & Park, 2014, for a review). In Lazarus's appraisal model, challenge and threat referred to types of primary appraisals rooted in perceptions of gain (challenge) and loss (threat) potential. Then, secondary appraisal processes acted on this information by assessing one's capacity to cope and delineating response options. The BPS model of challenge and threat integrates primary and second appraisal levels such that an individual appraises situational demands and available coping resources in concert. Appraisals of resources and demands then produce challenge or threat responses. Note that challenge–threat responses represent anchors along a continuum in the context of the BPS model of challenge and threat (e.g., Jamieson, Koslov, Nock, & Mendes, 2013).

In the BPS model (as well as Lazarus's appraisal theory), *challenge* and *threat* are experienced during motivated performance situations but differ in antecedent appraisals and downstream motivational and physiological processes. Individuals experience challenge when appraisals of personal coping resources exceed situational demands. Alternatively, threat manifests when perceived demands exceed resources. To demonstrate, consider a skier staring down a steep, narrow, icy slope lined with imposing trees. There is no other way off the mountain other than navigating this treacherous trail. Regardless of one's affinity for skiing, this situation is acutely stressful. There is an immediate demand (the difficult trail) that requires instrumental responding (navigating down it). Expert skiers might appraise the situation as challenging, believing that their skill, training, and experience (i.e., resources) allow them to handle the demands of the difficult trail, whereas novices are more likely to experience threat because the difficulty of the trail is appraised as outweighing their (low) skill level. Thus, the general increase in stress arousal experienced by skiers standing at the top of the slope is semantically and psychologically fuzzy (Blascovich, 1992)—arousal is simply the consequence of engagement within a motivated-performance situation. The form the arousal takes—threat or challenge—depends on appraisals of situational demands in relation to coping resources.

An important advance the BPS model of challenge and threat has made beyond existing appraisal theories is the grounding of challenge and threat predictions and psychological states in physiology. Theoretical physiological underpinnings were based on models of *physiological toughness* (Dienstbier, 1989), which targeted primary stress systems active in motivated performance (i.e., stressful) situations: the sympathetic–adrenal–medullary (SAM) and hypothalamic–pituitary–adrenal–cortical (HPA; also known as pituitary–adrenocortical [PAC]) axes. Broadly, the SAM system can be conceived as reflecting general sympathetic nervous system activation (e.g., "fight-or-flight" response). The HPA system, on the other hand, is more conservative, coming online after longer exposures to (usually more negative) stressors.

Activation of the SAM system stimulates release of epinephrine (also known as adrenaline) from the adrenal medulla, which produces important changes relevant for challenge–threat responding. For example, epinephrine increases heart rate, dilates blood vessels, and stimulates release of glucose from the liver. HPA activation results in the release of cortisol from the *zona fasciculata* of the adrenal gland. Given the chemical signaling sequence of the HPA axis—the hypothalamus releases corticotropin, which triggers the pituitary gland to release adrenocorticotropin, which then travels through bloodstream to the adrenal glands to stimulate cortisol release; levels of cortisol typically peak 15–20 minutes after the onset of stress (e.g., Dickerson & Kemeny, 2004). Challenge *and* threat appraisals are each hypothesized to activate the SAM, but only threat is also accompanied by HPA activation, thus inhibiting vasodilation (see Blascovich, 2008, for a review).

More downstream, the physiological consequences of challenge and threat appraisals can be clearly observed in differential patterns of cardiovascular (CV) responding. The BPS model of challenge and threat originally focused on stress axes (SAM and HPA), but it has evolved and been refined to include CV as means to assess task engagement and differentiate challenge and threat states (e.g., Blascovich, Mendes, Hunter, & Salomon, 1999; Jamieson, Valdesolo, & Peters, 2014; Seery, Weisbuch, & Blascovich, 2009). The most common CV measures used to index task engagement are heart rate (HR) and pre-ejection period (PEP). HR is simply the rate of left ventricle contraction. Increases in task engagement produce increases in HR primarily through increased sympathetic tone, but vagal withdrawal (decrease parasympathetic tone) can also contribute to increases in HR observed under situations involving cognitive effort (e.g., Appelhans, & Luecken, 2006). PEP assesses time from left ventricle contraction to the opening of the aortic valve, and is therefore an index of ventricular contractility (VC) or the contractile force of the left ventricle. More forceful contractions yield shorter PEP intervals.

To differentiate challenge and threat responses following from appraisals of situational demands and coping resources, research has most frequently focused on cardiac output (CO) and total peripheral resistance (TPR) (see Seery, 2011, for a review). CO is a measure of cardiac efficiency that reflects the amount of blood pumped per minute (usually in liters) and is calculated by first estimating stroke volume (SV), which is the amount of blood ejected during each beat, and multiplying SV by HR. Challenge states are marked by an increase in CO resulting from increases in cardiac activity combined with vasodilation, whereas CO either declines or exhibits little change in threat states because cardiac activity increases but is not accompanied by dilation of the vasculature. To directly assess net resistance in peripheral vasculature, researchers use TPR, which is often calculated using the following validated formula: TPR = (mean arterial pressure/CO) *80 (see Sherwood, Turner, Light, & Blumenthal, 1990). When threatened, vascular resistance increases, limiting blood flow to the periphery and producing high TPR scores. On the other hand, vasodilation (i.e., reduced TPR) accompanies challenge states so as to facilitate delivery of oxygenated blood to the brain and periphery.

The BPS model of challenge and threat is an appraisal-based model that has clear physiological underpinnings, but it should be noted that challenge–threat are *psychological* states encompassing appraisals, physiology, motivation, and behavior. Although challenge–threat response patterns are often indexed using physiological responses, it is important to remember that the physiological response is a manifestation of the psychological state.

The breadth of challenge and threat states can be seen in research examining the motivational and behavioral consequences of these processes. For instance, and importantly for research on competence and motivation, challenge and threat states direct motivational orientation (e.g., Jamieson, Nock, & Mendes, 2013). When challenged, resource appraisals are sufficient to meet demands (i.e., "I can handle this") and the body enacts changes (e.g., vasodilation increases delivery of blood and oxygen to the brain) to enable people to actively address stressors. Thus, challenge predicts approach motivation. Threat, on the other hand, is rooted in demand appraisals exceeding resources (i.e., "I can't handle this") and prepares the body for damage or social defeat. This signals an avoidance orientation (Mendes, Blascovich, Hunter, Lickel, & Jost, 2007). Whereas challenge typically is associated with positive behavioral and performance outcomes (e.g., Blascovich et al., 1999; Dienstbier, 1989; Jamieson, Mendes, Blackstock, & Schmader, 2010), threat impairs decision making in the short term and in the long term is associated with accelerated "brain aging," cognitive decline, and cardiovascular disease (Jefferson et al., 2010; Matthews, Gump, Block, & Allen, 1997).

APPRAISAL DYNAMICS

Challenge and threat appraisals and responses are not constrained to a single point in time or to within-individual processes only. Appraisals operate dynamically to shape responses to future situations (e.g., Jamieson et al., 2010) and to influence cognitions and responses in those with whom we interact (e.g., Mendes, Blascovich, et al., 2007). Along these lines, the *extended process model of emotion regulation* emphasizes the temporal dynamics of appraisal processes for determining affective or emotional responses (Gross, 2015; Ochsner & Gross, 2014; Sheppes, Suri, & Gross, 2015). Central to this update to Gross's (1998) process model of emotion regulation is the notion that a valuation system—which includes appraisal processes—can be activated for extended periods of time (Oschner & Gross, 2014). To demonstrate, as shown in Figure

10.1, attributes of the external environment ("the world" in the extended process model) necessitate engagement of perception processes (or selective attention mechanisms). Perceptions then trigger the valuation system, which produce action outputs (behaviors, decisions, physiological responses, etc.). Targets of actions are attributes of "the world," and the resulting change in situational or external factors directly leads to a second cycle that is perceived, valued, and acted upon (e.g., Sheppes et al., 2015). This cyclical process then repeats itself in a dynamical nature over time and across situations. For instance, a valuation process at Cycle 1 can feed forward and "snowball" to influence situations, attentional processes, valuations, and actions in future cycles. Such a regulatory system helps explain how appraisal-based cognitive-behavioral therapies can have long-lasting benefits (e.g., Barrett, Duffy, Dadds, & Rapee, 2001).

Valuations in the extended process model of emotion regulation may be consider similar to, albeit more general than, appraisal processes in the BPS model of challenge and threat because valuations are appraisals that involve integrating perceptions of internal and situational processes to determine the functional utility of situations; that is, values, like challenge–threat appraisals, are based on weighting perceived costs and benefits derived from prior experience and perceptions of demands versus resources to inform approach or avoidance actions. Slightly different from challenge–threat appraisal processes in BPS models, however, the feed-forward effect of valuations is emphasized by the extended process model. As shown in Figure 10.1, the physiological, behavioral, and experiential output of the valuation system at Cycle 1 can activate a second cycle. This requires valuation processes at Cycle 2 to act on the outputs of the first cycle. Thus, targets of valuations can be previous valuations. In current conceptualizations of the BPS model of challenge and threat, challenge–threat appraisals are situation-specific. Although BPS researchers would certainly agree that appraisals produce outcomes that influence subsequent appraisal processes and behaviors (e.g., Jamieson et al., 2010), the appraisal processes themselves are tied to specific situations, as resources to cope are considered in the context of situational demands.

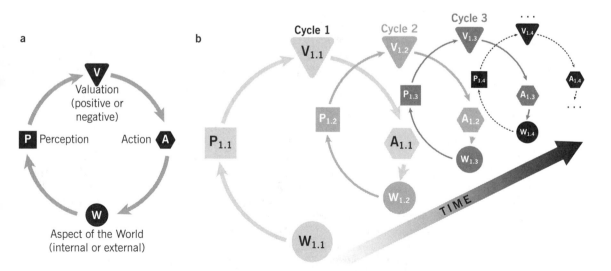

FIGURE 10.1. (a) The world (W) (notably, motivated performance situations) give rise to perception (P) processes. Valuations (V) based on perceptions give rise to actions (A) that alter situational factors (i.e., "the World"). (b) Valuation processes, which include appraisals, take place over time (see cycles 1, 2, 3, etc.), as shown in this spiral depiction. Data from Gross (2015), Oschner and Gross (2014), and Sheppes, Suri, and Gross (2015).

To consider fully the role of appraisals in producing challenge and threat states in a dynamical nature, one must also integrate interpersonal processes. Valuations and challenge–threat appraisals are often conceptualized as intrapsychic processes that interact with external factors. However, appraisal processes have direct interpersonal consequences. Not only do appraisals of demands and resources affect one's own physiological responses and behaviors, but appraisals and physiology can feed forward to impact those with whom one interacts. The dyadic effects of challenge–threat appraisals and responses are highlighted in recent research that measured interpersonal effects of expressive suppression online during interactions (Peters, Overall, & Jamieson, 2014). More specifically, an emotion regulation paradigm that required unacquainted dyads to watch a film and discuss their emotional responses (for a full description, see Butler et al., 2003) was utilized to study the transmission of challenge–threat processes between individuals. Prior to the emotional conversation, one member of the dyad was given additional instructions either to express affective displays normally or to suppress affective displays, whereas the other member of the dyad was given no instructions and was unaware of the instructions his or her partner received. Physiological, affective, and behavioral responses were measured to assess partner effects of suppressing affective displays; that is, the research sought to demonstrate how regulatory processes enacted in one person can impact naive interaction partners. Suppression is an effortful regulatory process, thus creating task demands (and threat) for the regulator (e.g., Gross, 1998; Gross & Levenson, 1997; Peters et al., 2014; for reviews, see English, John, & Gross, 2013; Gross, 2002). Physiological responses associated with the experience of threat also "spilled over" to impact interaction partners of expressive regulators (Peters et al., 2014). These data demonstrate that dynamical appraisal–valuation processes can operate at the interpersonal level.

Thus, the "cycles" captured in the extended process model of emotion may operate not only within a person across time but also *between* people *and* across time.

For example, as suggested in Figure 10.2, in Cycle 1, Person 1's appraisal processes (or attentional allocation) produce physiological and behavioral responses (e.g., suppression of affective displays elicits threat responses). The downstream responses of these appraisals (e.g., challenge–threat responses) can then "spill over" to directly impact Person 2's appraisals–valuations and subsequent responses in what could be considered his or her Cycle 1. Then, the outcomes–behavior of Person 2 might feed back to influence Person 1 in Cycle 2, and so on.

CHALLENGE AND THREAT REAPPRAISAL

Recent advances in emotion regulation dynamics (see Koole & Veenstra, 2015) indicate that appraisal processes can exert long-lasting effects on individuals and those with whom they interact. A pertinent question then becomes can appraisal processes be manipulated to optimize outcomes? This is a particularly important question in the context of acutely stressful motivated performance situations. Building on research from emotion (e.g., Barrett, 2006), emotion regulation (e.g., Gross, 2015), and the BPS model of challenge and threat (e.g., Mendes & Park, 2014), this section presents a method for improving appraisal processes during acute stress: reappraising arousal.

Upstream, the BPS model of challenge and threat argues that appraisals of demands and resources determine physiological and behavioral responses in motivated performance situations. Recall, however, that BPS theory is consistent with beliefs in mind–body monism (Blascovich & Mendes, 2010). Thus, signals from the body can feed back and influence appraisal processes (Gross, 2015); that is, physiological responses to motivated performance situations can influence challenge–threat appraisal processes that determine subsequent response patterns.

Using the BPS model of challenge and threat as a framework, recent researchers have sought to optimize responses in motivated performance situations by altering appraisals of bodily states (e.g., Beltzer, Nock, Peters, & Jamieson, 2014; Jamieson et al., 2010; Jamieson, Mendes, & Nock,

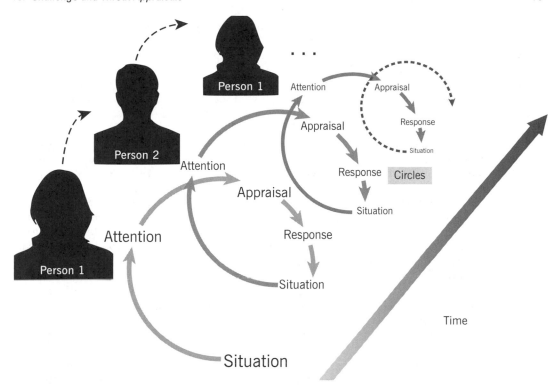

FIGURE 10.2. Dyadic process model of emotion regulation. Cycles operate between people and across time such that attention and appraisal processes enacted by Person 1 at Cycle 1 can feed forward to impact Person 2 at Cycle 1, which can then produce effects in Person 1 at Cycle 2, and so on.

2013; Jamieson, Nock, & Mendes, 2012, 2013; John-Henderson, Rheinschmidt, & Mendoza-Denton, 2015). In this line of research, the arousal experienced during stressful situations is presented as a functional *coping resource* that aids performance; that is, signs of stress arousal are reinterpreted as coping tools, which facilitate challenge appraisals that have effects on subsequent physiological, affective, and motivational processes.

Research on reappraising stress arousal extended seminal work on emotion regulation (Gross, 1998, 2002, 2015) and cognitive-behavioral therapy (CBT) (Hofmann & Smits, 2008). Underpinning these theories is that changing cognitive appraisal processes can alter downstream affective responding, and improve mental and physical health outcomes. To provide context, reappraisal, as specified by emotion regulation models, typically involves the reinterpretation of the affective meaning of contextual cues, which

can include physical stimuli, attributes of situations, and actions–words of other people, to name a few. In other words, emotionally charged stimuli are presented, and participants are instructed to reinterpret those stimuli (e.g., "The disturbing movie I'm watching is fake") or distance themselves from the stimuli (e.g., by adopting a third-person perspective; Kross & Ayduk, 2011; Ochsner & Gross, 2008). Clinical researchers developed CBT to help improve patient outcomes by modifying faulty affective responses and cognitions (Barlow, 2004). For instance, patients with depression are taught to identify errors in thinking (e.g., "Everyone hates me and always will") and replace them with more rational thoughts.

In the "classic" emotion regulation literature, reappraisal has often (but not always) centered on decreasing sympathetic arousal in passive situations (e.g., Gross, 2002). For example, an individual might reinterpret the meaning of affective videos. No instrumental responding is needed when watching a movie. It is a "passive receiving" situation, not a motivated performance one, and therefore falls outside the bounds of the BPS model of challenge and threat. Similarly, reappraisal processes in clinical psychological science typically either seek to decrease arousal (e.g., mindfulness meditation; Cincotta, Gehrman, Gooneratne, & Baime, 2011) or encourage individuals to accept heightened arousal in acute stress situations (e.g., interoceptive exposure; Levitt, Brown, Orsillo, & Barlow, 2004). Across these approaches, decreased arousal should be construed as adaptive when no instrumental cognitive or physical responses are required. However, motivated performance situations necessitate instrumental responding, and *increased* sympathetic arousal can be functional. As touched on before, a hallmark of challenge- and threat-type responses is activation of the SAM axis and increased cardiac activity. Harkening back to Dienstbier's (1989) physiological toughness model, SAM axis activation can facilitate mobilization of oxygenated blood to the brain and periphery via dilation of the vasculature, thereby improving performance under challenge states. Thus, contrary to popular beliefs, stress arousal itself is not harmful for performance, nor does it signal a negative affective state during motivated performance situations.

Arousal reappraisal narrows in on situations of acute stress that require active responding and identifies bodily responses, specifically, signs of sympathetic arousal (e.g., racing heart or "butterflies in my stomach") as coping tools; that is, stress reappraisal seeks to alter cognitive construal of bodily signals to promote adaptive, challenge type responses during acute social stress (Dienstbier, 1989; Mendes & Jamieson, 2011). Stress reappraisal is not aimed at eliminating or dampening stress arousal but instead focuses on changing the *type* of acute stress response (Brooks, 2014; Crum, Salovey, & Achor, 2013). As can be seen in Figure 10.3, arousal reappraisal operates after the instantiation of stress (i.e., engagement), but severs the (almost automatic) tie between acute stress and negative appraisal processes. People taught to reinterpret the meaning of stress and their body's response to stressors no longer experience stressful situations as negative. Stress becomes a coping resource, not a demand to be eliminated.

Laboratory studies of reappraisal of stress arousal provide mechanistic evidence for how appraisals shape downstream performance outcomes. To demonstrate, one study examined how reappraising arousal might alter responses to a well-controlled, laboratory evaluation task (Jamieson et al., 2012). After a resting baseline, participants were informed that they were going to complete a public speaking task (the Trier Social Stress Test; Kirschbaum, Pirke, & Hellhammer, 1993). Just prior to the task, one-third of the participants were randomly assigned to a stress reappraisal condition; another one-third received the "placebo" materials ("ignore stress"); and the remaining one-third were given no instructions. During the stressful social evaluative task, reappraisal participants exhibited a more challenge-type CV profile, indexed by less vascular resistance and greater cardiac output, compared with participants assigned to the other conditions. Moreover, immediately after the public speaking task, attentional bias for negative information was assessed using an emotional Stroop task (e.g., Williams, Mathews, & MacLeod, 1996). Reappraisal participants exhibited less vigilance for potentially threatening cues than did participants assigned to the other two groups. This has important implications for how changing appraisals processes in response to one situation can feed forward to positively impact affective, physiological, and behavioral responses in future situations (i.e., a positive "snowball" effect in the extended process model of emotion regulation; Gross, 2015).

Importantly for research on competence and achievement motivation, benefits of reappraising arousal have been observed in academic contexts. For instance, a double-blind randomized field study conducted in community college classrooms demonstrated that teaching students to appraise their stress arousal as a coping tool reduced test anxiety and improved exam performance. Mediation analyses indicated that reappraisal improved academic performance by increasing students' perceptions of their ability to cope with the stressful testing situation (Jamieson, Peters, Greenwood, & Altose,

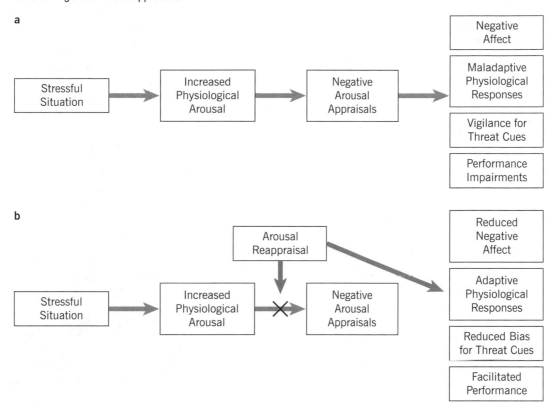

FIGURE 10.3. In panel (a), stressful situations elicit physiological arousal, which is typically construed negatively. These negative appraisals feed forward to produce negative outcomes. In panel (b), arousal reappraisal manipulations break the association between stress-based arousal and negative appraisals. By severing this link, arousal reappraisal techniques help shift negative acute stress states (threat) to more positive ones (challenge), leading to a reduction in negative affect, more adaptive patterns of physiological reactivity, reduced attentional bias for threat cues, and improved performance. From Jamieson, Mendes, and Nock (2013). Copyright © 2013 Association for Psychological Science. Adapted by permission.

2016). In other words, the stress reappraisal materials increased challenge appraisals by specifically targeting the resource, not the demand, side of the appraisal process.

Benefits of arousal reappraisal have also been shown to improve long(er)-term academic achievement outcomes. To demonstrate, the first empirical test of arousal reappraisal examined potential benefits of the approach for students preparing to take the Graduate Record Examination (GRE)—a standardized test used to assess applicants to graduate school (Jamieson et al., 2010). The research included laboratory and "field" components. First, students preparing to take the GRE reported to the lab for a practice GRE study, where they were randomly assigned to read arousal reappraisal materials or to receive no instructions prior to taking a practice test. Reappraisal students outperformed no-instruction controls on the quantitative section of the practice GRE. Participants then completed the GRE within 3 months of the lab session and reported back to the lab after completing their "real" tests. Similar to the pattern observed in the lab, participants who reappraised stress as a coping resource scored higher on the quantitative section of the actual GRE. This performance effect was achieved without the delivery of any intervention "boosters" after the lab session.

How, then, did a laboratory reappraisal manipulation operate to improve GRE scores up to 3 months later? Although daily diaries (or similar event-sampling methods) were not used to track psychological processes leading up to the "real" exams, self-reported psychological experiences of the GRE testing experience indicated that the reappraisal participants were less concerned with being anxious, believed arousal aided performance, and were more sure of themselves compared to no-instruction controls. Building on the recent work on appraisal dynamics, these findings might suggest that the reappraisal materials delivered in the lab fed forward to impact test-takers' future appraisal and attention processes (perceptions and valuations) in a future academic performance situation. However, it should be emphasized that no direct evidence has demonstrated *how* arousal reappraisal feeds forward to operate within the context of the extended process model of emotion regulation. In fact, this endeavor would be an interesting area of future research on this topic.

INTEGRATION AND FUTURE DIRECTIONS

The previous sections have delineated how appraisal processes operate in the context of the BPS model of challenge and threat, have explicated the dynamical nature of appraisal processes, and have highlighted a method for optimizing appraisals and subsequent responses in acutely stressful situations. This section explores avenues for integrating BPS-derived work on challenge–threat appraisals with other prominent theories from the social-psychological literature on competence and motivation.

In the context of the BPS model of challenge and threat, an individual appraises situational demands and personal coping resources in motivated performance situations. Because challenge and threat responses are thought to follow from a ratio of perceive demands and resources, these appraisals should operate in parallel or at nearly the same cognitive stage. Appraisal processes then predict patterns of challenge–threat response patterns with important implication for motivation (challenge = approach,

threat = avoidance), physiological responses, and behavioral outcomes.

Broadly, appraisals in the context of the BPS model can be conceived of as situation-specific. Situational demands versus personal resources are appraised in a motivated performance context and are unique to that context because demands necessarily vary situation-to-situation and assessments of coping resources vary across domains. For instance, one may consider oneself an adept skier. Presented with a demanding trail (e.g., steep, icy, and narrow), the expert skier may perceive one's coping resources (ability, training, experience, etc.) to exceed task demands. However, when the same expert skier is placed in a mathematics achievement context, such as when taking an important standardized test, he or she may perceive the demands as exceeding his or her abilities to cope successfully in this domain (math knowledge, experience, etc.). So, whereas the demanding skiing situation produced challenge appraisals, the demanding math situation produced threat appraisals, and the two are independent of each other. Multiple other cognitive processes, however, can operate on appraisal processes to influence or moderate patterns of responding.

Little research, though, has sought to explicate how more meta-level cognitive processes interact with, shape, and are shaped by proximal challenge–threat appraisals. Even less research (actually, none as of this writing) has integrated work on appraisal dynamics with proximal and distal influences on situation-specific challenge–threat appraisal processes. Two promising lines of research that are ripe for integration with BPS-derived challenge–threat appraisal processes in motivated performance situations are achievement goals (Elliot, 1999; Elliot & Thrash, 2001; Pekrun, Elliot, & Maier, 2009) and implicit theories (Dweck, 1996; Dweck, Chiu, & Hong, 1995; Yeager et al., 2014).

Similar to the BPS model of challenge and threat, achievement goal theory is rooted in concepts of approach and avoidance (see Elliot, 1999, for a review). This may not be surprising given that a fundamental, evolved process observed across all organisms is the ability to assess the adaptive significance of environmental stimuli (via myriad sensory mechanisms) and to respond accordingly (e.g., Orians & Heerwagen, 1992). Even amoebas will avoid harmful stimuli (Schneirla, 1959). In humans, and in the context of BPS models, appraisal processes function to assess demands–resources and direct behavioral outputs. Assessment and direction of behavior can also be achieved via other cognitive processes. Prominently, achievement goal models place an emphasis on goals for assessment of the situation and one's ability to cope (i.e., competence; for a review, see Elliot & Hulleman, Chapter 4, this volume).

Achievement goals vary along two dimensions: valance and definition (or evaluative standard). Goals may focus on either approaching positive outcomes or avoiding negative outcomes, and are evaluated using mastery or normative–performance standards (Elliot & McGregor, 2001). For instance, a performance-avoidance goal might manifest as a student trying to avoid performing poorly on an exam relative to the rest of the class. Or a mastery-approach goal could result from a student learning course material purely to increase knowledge in the domain. Whereas performance goals require evaluative standards—performance either meets the goal or falls short—mastery goals do not necessarily involve evaluation. In the previous example, the student striving to learn could do so without setting a standard to assess his or her learning progress. Given the greater evaluative demands that accompany performance-based goals relative to mastery-based goals, performance-based goals are more easily integrated with appraisal processes derived from the BPS model of challenge and threat.

Similar to challenge–threat appraisals, performance-approach and performance-avoidance goals are determined by situational and cognitive factors, and produce downstream responses and behaviors (Elliot & McGregor, 2001). The antecedent factors that give rise to challenge–threat appraisals and performance-approach–performance-avoidance goals may also likely overlap in many cases. For instance, higher assessments of competence can predict performance-approach goals (e.g., Elliot & Church, 1997; Urdan & Schoenfelder, 2006), and competence can also be construed as a coping resource, which elicits challenge. However,

do goals give rise to appraisals, do appraisals give rise to goals, or do the two processes operate independently (or dependently) in parallel? For instance, high perceptions of competence could prompt performance-approach goal adoption, which is predictive of proximal resource–demand appraisals (Elliot & Reis, 2003). Or competence could be appraised as a coping resource, predicting a challenge response that includes the pursuit of performance-based goals.

Given the structure and function of achievement goal and BPS models, it may be more likely that appraisals function more upstream from task-specific goals. Appraisals in the context of the BPS model are situation-specific but general. Challenge and threat responses stem from broad-based resource–demand assessments. For example, "resources" include myriad factors such as individual resources (e.g., competence, ability/knowledge, or experience), social resources (i.e., others to help, network of people to tap), or even institutional resources (e.g., equipment/tools). Similarly, task demands can encompass multiple domains, from perceptions of difficulty to time/evaluative pressure to concurrent tasks, to name a few. Performance-based goals, too, are context bound. Goals based on performance standards require an evaluative situation in which to apply the goal. Slightly different from BPS conceptualizations of challenge–threat appraisals, though, performance-based goals are more specific in their focus and application. For example, a performance-approach goal in an academic achievement context might take the form of trying to surpass a specific score or trying to outperform one's classmates on an exam. To summarize, antecedent factors, such perceived competence, might *cause* goal adoption, whereas these antecedent factors are *part of* (not separate from) challenge–threat appraisal processes. Alternatively, BPS researchers have specifically stated that achievement motivation "may capture motivational underpinnings of the demand-to-resource ratio" (Blascovich, Mendes, Tomaka, Salomon, & Seery, 2003, p. 239). So, instead of appraisals predicting goals, goals may operate as factors (like competence assessments) that give rise to challenge–threat appraisals.

As highlighted earlier, interesting avenues for future research could seek to explicate how appraisal processes shape and are shaped by goal adoption, or whether these processes might unfold independently in parallel. To date, however, few studies have sought to examine temporal relationships between achievement goals and BPS-derived challenge–threat appraisals. The little research on this topic that exists has focused on athletics. For example, theories of athlete performance have sought to link achievement goals to physiological response patterns associated with challenge and threat states (Jones, Meijen, McCarthy, & Sheffield, 2009). Along similar lines, an imagery intervention for athletes sought to promote approach goals and challenge responses (Williams, Cumming, & Balanos, 2010) but did not provide direct insight into temporal associations between the goals and appraisals in athletes. Future studies on achievement goals and challenge–threat appraisals are relevant for advancing theories of competition, emotion regulation, and close relationships.

Whereas goals may, at least at times, be more specific than BPS-derived challenge–threat appraisals, other processes likely consistently operate at a more general level than situation-specific appraisals. Implicit theories, specifically, warrant consideration for integration with concepts of challenge and threat (see Dweck & Leggett, 1988, for a review). Dweck's model broadly organizes implicit theories into one of two types: *entity* and *incremental* theories. An individual holding an entity theory endorses the belief that traits, intelligence, and so forth, are fixed and immutable. For instance, an *entity* theorist believes that people are innately intelligent or not. He or she would not endorse the belief that one's intellectual ability can grow across the lifespan with study and hard work. Rather, an individual who believes in the potential for growth and change in traits, intelligence, and so forth, would hold an *incremental* theory.

A large corpus of research indicates that individuals who endorse an incremental theory of intelligence and ability are more resilient, have better social interactions, and demonstrate improved academic performance relative to individuals holding an entity theory (for reviews, see Burnette, O'Boyle, VanEpps, Pollack, & Finkel, 2013; Yeager & Walton, 2011). Importantly for integrating implicit theories with work on challenge–threat appraisals, entity or incremental beliefs may be conceptualized as operating at the "global belief" level, which is more broad and general than situation-specific appraisal processes. Whereas challenge–threat appraisals vary substantially from situation to situation within domains (e.g., social processes), implicit theories are more likely to be stable across situations. If one believes in an entity theory of intelligence, for example, one is also likely to endorse an entity theory of personality (e.g., morality) (see Dweck et al., 1995, for a review).

Implicit theories may be conceptualized as a "lens" that focuses situation-specific challenge–threat appraisal processes. To illustrate, if one perceives ability (i.e., resources) as fixed in a given domain, then challenge–threat appraisals will be particularly sensitive to perceptions of demands; that is, the "action" in challenge–threat response patterns will be rooted in the demand side of the resource-to-demand ratio. Similarly, appraisal-based interventions that target resource appraisals, such as the arousal reappraisal method highlighted earlier, will be less effective for those holding an entity theory.

Fortunately, global belief systems are not "set for life." Methods have been developed to modify implicit theories so as to maximize the instantiation of an incremental theory. For example, a brief (20-minute) intervention teaches individuals to endorse incremental theory through educational material and written "endorsements." Experimental research demonstrates that incremental theory interventions can exert long-lasting and powerful benefits for individuals randomly assigned to complete those materials (e.g., Yeager et al., 2014). Building on these previous implicit theories intervention studies, recent research has begun to explore the interplay between belief-level implicit theories and situation-level challenge–threat appraisals (Yeager, Lee, & Jamieson, 2016). More specifically, high school students were taught an incremental theory or control message prior to completing a stressful evaluative laboratory task—an age-modified Trier

Social Stress Test (TSST; Kirschbaum et al., 1993). Prior to beginning the TSST, but after intervention materials, adolescents completed challenge–threat appraisal measures. Then, physiological responses were tracked online during task performance. Adolescents assigned to complete incremental theory materials reported greater challenge appraisals relative to those who completed control materials. Moreover, the incremental theory intervention also produced improvements in physiological indices of challenge and threat—cortisol, CO, and TPR—compared to controls. These data demonstrate that instantiating a global belief in the capacity for growth and change can directly impact situation-specific appraisal processes relevant to challenge–threat response patterns. Additional research, however, is needed to elucidate *how* changing global beliefs functions to alter situation-specific appraisals, and the generalizability of effects across different types of situations. For instance, altering global beliefs could possibly impact performance situations more strongly than social situations.

SUMMARY AND CONCLUSION

The BPS model of challenge and threat is based on classic work on appraisal processes (Lazarus & Folkman, 1991) and delineates two *types* of organized responses to motivated performance situations: challenge and threat, which have clear physiological underpinnings (e.g., Dienstbier, 1989). Physiological responses associated with approach-oriented challenge states are considered benign compared to avoidance-oriented threat states because of higher levels of anabolic (dehydroepiandosterone [DHEA]) relative to catabolic (cortisol) hormones (e.g., Mendes, Gray, Mendoza-Denton, Major, & Epel, 2007), dilation in the peripheral vasculature (e.g., Dienstbier, 1989), and rapid recovery to homeostasis after stress (e.g., Jamieson et al., 2014). Challenge–threat response patterns flow directly from cognitive appraisal processes that assess situational demands and perceived coping resources (Blascovich, 1992; Blascovich & Tomaka, 1996). Challenge manifests when an individual appraises that he or she has

the resources to meet demands successfully, whereas threat is marked by the opposite pattern: when demands exceed resources. The goal of this review is to provide an overview of theoretical and empirical work on appraisal processes in the context of the BPS model of challenge and threat, and to suggest avenues for future research on challenge–threat appraisals, with an emphasis on dynamics and integration with other theories of motivation.

At its core, the BPS model of challenge and threat is a model of motivation. Challenge and threat appraisals and responses facilitate an approach (challenge) or avoidance (threat) orientation to stressors or task demands, respectively. Although research frequently conceptualizes challenge and threat states as positive and negative, respectively, it is important to note that the BPS model is not necessarily a valanced model. A clear example of this can be observed in research on responses associated with the experience of anger. Anger is clearly negatively valanced but approach motivated. When one examines the appraisal processes and physiological responses of individuals experiencing anger, these appear similar to responses in individuals who are "excited" or more classically challenged because of the concordance in motivation–orientation between anger and positive challenge (e.g., Jamieson, Koslov, et al., 2013; for a review, see Blascovich & Mendes, 2010).

The motivational emphasis of the BPS model of challenge and threat makes it ideal for integration with emotion regulatory processes in the context of the *extended process model of emotion regulation* (Gross, 2015) or the *modal model of emotion* (Gross & Barrett, 2011). Such integrations can help inform future work on the BPS model that more fully captures the dynamical nature of challenge–threat appraisals across situations and across people. As highlighted in this review, challenge–threat appraisals fit well with the conceptualization of the "valuation" process in the extended process model. Explicitly incorporating challenge–threat concepts into the valuation process has the potential to better explicate how appraisals of resources and demands can feed forward to exert potent, long-lasting effects. Research along these lines may also help inform future development of the extended process model by emphasizing physiological (and motivational) underpinnings of effects of valuations on emotions, behaviors, and behavioral responses in situations of high affective intensity.

Research on reappraising arousal has started to scratch the surface on utilizing challenge–threat appraisals to regulate affective responses (see Jamieson, Mendes, & Nock, 2013, for a review). In fact, a number of distinct lines of research are emerging that suggest altering appraisal processes to capitalize on the plurality of stress responses is effective at improving health and performance outcomes (e.g., Brooks, 2014; Crum et al., 2013; Jamieson et al., 2010, John-Henderson et al., 2015). This review highlights the BPS-grounded arousal reappraisal method (see Jamieson, Mendes, et al., 2013, for a review), but similar lines of research demonstrate the effectiveness of reappraising anxiety as excitement (Brooks, 2014) and changing more general stress mindsets (Crum et al., 2013), for example. These and other similar psychosituational intervention approaches are examples of research using an established, well-validated model, such as the BPS model of challenge and threat, to develop interventions targeting mechanisms (e.g., resource appraisals). Process-focused interventions are much preferred to outcome-focused approaches that are less well grounded in psychophysiological theory (e.g., Lilienfeld, 2007). This perspective is shared by the recent Research Domain Criteria (RDoC) initiative undertaken at National Institute of Mental Health (NIMH), which advocates first identifying mechanisms of mental health problems, then developing diagnostic methods and treatments to target those mechanisms (e.g., Franklin, Jamieson, Glenn, & Nock, 2015; Insel et al., 2010).

More broadly, challenge–threat appraisal processes are relevant for myriad other models and theories of motivation, including achievement goal and implicit theory models. The iterative processes through which appraisals shape and are shaped by achievement goals is an unexplored area ripe for study. Research on this topic has the potential to refine our understanding of how achievement goals and appraisals operate to impact outcomes, particularly performance outcomes in achievement contexts. Although challenge–threat appraisals are best conceptualized as situation-specific processes, this does not mean that they are not subject to effects of more general belief systems. For example, altering implicit theories of personality can directly affect challenge–threat appraisal processes during motivated performance situations (Yeager et al., 2016).

In the approximately 25 years since the introduction of the BPS model of challenge and threat (e.g., Blascovich, 1992), it has been applied to diverse and important domains, ranging from stereotyping, prejudice, and discrimination to academic and athletic performance, to behavioral economics, to name a few. The relationship between resource and demand appraisals is believed to mediate the link between motivated performance situations and physiological, motivational, and behavioral responses. This review has emphasized the importance of challenge–threat appraisal processes for predicting downstream outcomes and potential integrations with other theories and models of motivation. Researchers have just started exploring the dynamics of challenge–threat appraisals and developing process-focused interventions to optimize responses under acute stress. As always, further inquiries into these and other topics relevant to challenge and threat appraisals are needed to advance and extend theory.

REFERENCES

Appelhans, B. M., & Luecken, L. J. (2006). Heart rate variability as an index of regulated emotional responding. *Review of General Psychology, 10*(3), 229–240.

Barlow, D. H. (2004). *Anxiety and its disorders: The nature and treatment of anxiety and panic.* New York: Guilford Press.

Barrett, L. F. (2006). Solving the emotion paradox: Categorization and the experience of emotion. *Personality and Social Psychology Review, 10*(1), 20–46.

Barrett, L. F. (2014). The conceptual act theory: A précis. *Emotion Review, 6*(4), 292–297.

Barrett, P. M., Duffy, A. L., Dadds, M. R., & Rapee, R. M. (2001). Cognitive-behavioral treatment of anxiety disorders in children: Long-term (6-year) follow-up. *Journal of Consulting and Clinical Psychology, 69*(1), 135–141.

Beltzer, M. L., Nock, M. K., Peters, B. J., & Jamieson, J. P. (2014). Rethinking butterflies: The affective, physiological, and performance effects of reappraising arousal during social evaluation. *Emotion, 14,* 761–768.

Blascovich, J. (1992). A biopsychosocial approach to arousal regulation. *Journal of Social and Clinical Psychology, 11,* 213–237.

Blascovich, J. (2008). Challenge and threat. In A. J. Elliot (Ed.), *Handbook of approach and avoidance motivation* (pp. 431–445). New York: Psychology Press.

Blascovich, J., & Mendes, W. B. (2010). Social psychophysiology and embodiment. In S. T. Fiske & D. T. Gilbert (Eds.), *Handbook of social psychology* (5th ed., pp. 194–227). New York: Wiley.

Blascovich, J., Mendes, W. B., Hunter, S. B., & Salomon, K. (1999). Social "facilitation" as challenge and threat. *Journal of Personality and Social Psychology, 77*(1), 68–77.

Blascovich, J., Mendes, W. B., Tomaka, J., Salomon, K., & Seery, M. (2003). The robust nature of the biopsychosocial model challenge and threat: A reply to Wright and Kirby. *Personality and Social Psychology Review, 7*(3), 234–243.

Blascovich, J., & Tomaka, J. (1996). The biopsychosocial model of arousal regulation. *Advances in Experimental Social Psychology, 28,* 1–52.

Brooks, A. W. (2014). Get excited: Reappraising pre-performance anxiety as excitement. *Journal of Experimental Psychology: General, 143*(3), 1144–1158.

Burnette, J. L., O'Boyle, E. H., VanEpps, E. M., Pollack, J. M., & Finkel, E. J. (2013). Mindsets matter: A meta-analytic review of implicit theories and self-regulation. *Psychological Bulletin, 139*(3), 655–701.

Butler, E. A., Egloff, B., Wlhelm, F. H., Smith, N. C., Erickson, E. A., & Gross, J. J. (2003). The social consequences of expressive suppression. *Emotion, 3*(1), 48–67.

Cincotta, A. L., Gehrman, P., Gooneratne, N. S., & Baime, M. J. (2011). The effects of a mindfulness-based stress reduction programme on pre-sleep cognitive arousal and insomnia symptoms: A pilot study. *Stress and Health, 27*(3), e299–e305.

Crum, A. J., Salovey, P., & Achor, S. (2013). Rethinking stress: The role of mindsets in determining the stress response. *Journal of Personality and Social Psychology, 104*(4), 716–733.

Dickerson, S. S., & Kemeny, M. E. (2004). Acute stressors and cortisol responses: A theoretical integration and synthesis of laboratory research. *Psychological Bulletin, 130*(3), 355–391.

Dienstbier, R. A. (1989). Arousal and physiological toughness: Implications for mental and physical health. *Psychological Review, 96*(1), 84–100.

Dweck, C. S. (1996). Implicit theories as organizers of goals and behavior. In P. M. Gollwitzer & J. A. Bargh (Eds.), *The psychology of action: Linking cognition and motivation to behavior* (pp. 69–90). New York: Guilford Press.

Dweck, C. S., Chiu, C. Y., & Hong, Y. Y. (1995). Implicit theories and their role in judgments and reactions: A word from two perspectives. *Psychological Inquiry, 6*(4), 267–285.

Dweck, C. S., & Leggett, E. L. (1988). A social-cognitive approach to motivation and personality. *Psychological Review, 95*(2), 256–273.

Elliot, A. J. (1999). Approach and avoidance motivation and achievement goals. *Educational Psychologist, 34*(3), 169–189.

Elliot, A. J., & Church, M. A. (1997). A hierarchical model of approach and avoidance achievement motivation. *Journal of personality and social psychology, 72*(1), 218–232.

Elliot, A. J., & McGregor, H. A. (2001). A 2 × 2 achievement goal framework. *Journal of Personality and Social Psychology, 80*(3), 501–519.

Elliot, A. J., & Reis, H. T. (2003). Attachment and exploration in adulthood. *Journal of Personality and Social Psychology, 85*(2), 317–331.

Elliot, A. J., & Thrash, T. M. (2001). Achievement goals and the hierarchical model of achievement motivation. *Educational Psychology Review, 13*(2), 139–156.

English, T., John, O. P., & Gross, J. J. (2013). Emotion regulation in close relationships. In J. A. Simpson & L. Campbell (Eds.), *The Oxford handbook of close relationships* (pp. 500–513). New York: Oxford University Press.

Folkman, S., & Lazarus, R. S. (1980). An analysis of coping in a middle-aged community sample. *Journal of Health and Social Behavior, 21*(3), 219–239.

Folkman, S., & Lazarus, R. S. (1985). If it changes it must be a process: Study of emotion and coping during three stages of a college examination. *Journal of Personality and Social Psychology, 48*(1), 150–170.

Franklin, J. C., Jamieson, J. P., Glenn, C. R., & Nock, M. K. (2015). How developmental psychopathology theory and research can inform the research domain criteria (RDoC) project. *Journal of Clinical Child and Adolescent Psychology, 44*(2), 280–290.

Gross, J. J. (1998). The emerging field of emotion regulation: An integrative review. *Review of General Psychology, 2*(3), 271–299.

Gross, J. J. (2002). Emotion regulation: Affective,

cognitive, and social consequences. *Psychophysiology, 39*(3), 281–291.

Gross, J. J. (2015). The extended process model of emotion regulation: Elaborations, applications, and future directions. *Psychological Inquiry, 26*(1), 130–137.

Gross, J. J., & Barrett, L. F. (2011). Emotion generation and emotion regulation: One or two depends on your point of view. *Emotion Review, 3*(1), 8–16.

Gross, J. J., & Levenson, R. W. (1997). Hiding feelings: The acute effects of inhibiting negative and positive emotion. *Journal of abnormal psychology, 106*(1), 95–103.

Hofmann, S. G., Asnaani, A., Vonk, I. J., Sawyer, A. T., & Fang, A. (2012). The efficacy of cognitive behavioral therapy: A review of meta-analyses. *Cognitive Therapy and Research, 36*(5), 427–440.

Hofmann, S. G., & Smits, J. A. (2008). Cognitive-behavioral therapy for adult anxiety disorders: a meta-analysis of randomized placebo-controlled trials. *Journal of Clinical Psychiatry, 69*(4), 621–632.

Insel, T., Cuthbert, B., Garvey, M., Heinssen, R., Pine, D. S., Quinn, K., et al. (2010). Research domain criteria (RDoC): Toward a new classification framework for research on mental disorders. *American Journal of Psychiatry, 167*(7), 748–751.

Jamieson, J. P., Koslov, K., Nock, M. K., & Mendes, W. B. (2013). Experiencing discrimination increases risk taking. *Psychological Science, 24,* 131–139.

Jamieson, J. P., Mendes, W. B., Blackstock, E., & Schmader, T. (2010). Turning the knots in your stomach into bows: Reappraising arousal improves performance on the GRE. *Journal of Experimental Social Psychology, 46*(1), 208–212.

Jamieson, J. P., Mendes, W. B., & Nock, M. K. (2013). Improving acute stress responses: The power of reappraisal. *Current Directions in Psychological Science, 22*(1), 51–56.

Jamieson, J. P., Nock, M. K., & Mendes, W. B. (2012). Mind over matter: Reappraising arousal improves cardiovascular and cognitive responses to stress. *Journal of Experimental Psychology: General, 141*(3), 417–422.

Jamieson, J. P., Nock, M. K., & Mendes, W. B. (2013). Changing the conceptualization of stress in social anxiety disorder affective and physiological consequences. *Clinical Psychological Science, 1,* 363–374.

Jamieson, J. P., Peters, B. J., Greenwood, E. J., & Altose, A. J. (2016). Reappraising stress arousal improves performance and reduces evaluation anxiety in classroom exam situations. *Social Psychological and Personality Science, 7,* 579–587.

Jamieson, J. P., Valdesolo, P., & Peters, B. J. (2014). Sympathy for the devil?: The physiological and psychological effects of being an agent (and target) of dissent during intragroup conflict. *Journal of Experimental Social Psychology, 55,* 221–227.

Jefferson, A. L., Himali, J. J., Beiser, A. S., Au, R., Massaro, J. M., Seshadri, S., et al. (2010). Cardiac index is associated with brain aging: The Framingham Heart Study. *Circulation, 122,* 690–697.

John-Henderson, N. A., Rheinschmidt, M. L., & Mendoza-Denton, R. (2015). Cytokine responses and math performance: The role of stereotype threat and anxiety reappraisals. *Journal of Experimental Social Psychology, 56,* 203–206.

Jones, M., Meijen, C., McCarthy, P. J., & Sheffield, D. (2009). A theory of challenge and threat states in athletes. *International Review of Sport and Exercise Psychology, 2*(2), 161–180.

Kirschbaum, C., Pirke, K. M., & Hellhammer, D. H. (1993). The "Trier Social Stress Test"—a tool for investigating psychobiological stress responses in a laboratory setting. *Neuropsychobiology, 28*(1–2), 76–81.

Koole, S. L., & Veenstra, L. (2015). Does emotion regulation occur only inside people's heads?: Toward a situated cognition analysis of emotion-regulatory dynamics. *Psychological Inquiry, 26*(1), 61–68.

Kross, E., & Ayduk, O. (2011). Making meaning out of negative experiences by self-distancing. *Current Directions in Psychological Science, 20*(3), 187–191.

Lazarus, R. S. (1991). Progress on a cognitive-motivational-relational theory of emotion. *American Psychologist, 46*(8), 819–834.

Lazarus, R. S., DeLongis, A., Folkman, S., & Gruen, R. (1985). Stress and adaptational outcomes: The problem of confounded measures. *American Psychologist, 40*(7), 770–779.

Lazarus, R. S., & Folkman, S. (1991). The concept of coping. In A. Monat & R. S. Lazarus (Eds.), *Stress and coping: An anthology* (3rd ed., pp. 189–206). New York: Columbia University Press.

Lazarus, R. S., & Smith, C. A. (1988). Knowledge and appraisal in the cognition—emotion relationship. *Cognition and Emotion, 2*(4), 281–300.

Levitt, J. T., Brown, T. A., Orsillo, S. M., & Barlow, D. H. (2004). The effects of acceptance versus suppression of emotion on subjective and psychophysiological response to carbon dioxide challenge in patients with panic disorder. *Behavior Therapy, 35*(4), 747–766.

Lilienfeld, S. O. (2007). Psychological treatments that cause harm. *Perspectives on Psychological Science, 2*(1), 53–70.

Matthews, K. A., Gump, B. B., Block, D. R., & Allen, M. T. (1997). Does background stress heighten or dampen children's cardiovascular responses to acute stress? *Psychosomatic Medicine, 59*(5), 488–496.

Mendes, W. B., Blascovich, J., Hunter, S. B., Lickel, B., & Jost, J. T. (2007). Threatened by the unexpected: Physiological responses during social interactions with expectancy-violating partners. *Journal of Personality and Social Psychology, 92*(4), 698–716.

Mendes, W. B., Gray, H. M., Mendoza-Denton, R., Major, B., & Epel, E. S. (2007). Why egalitarianism might be good for your health physiological thriving during stressful intergroup encounters. *Psychological Science, 18*(11), 991–998.

Mendes, W. B., & Jamieson, J. (2011). Embodied stereotype threat: Exploring brain and body mechanisms underlying performance impairments. In M. Inzlicht & T. Schmader (Eds.), *Stereotype threat: Theory, process, and application* (pp. 51–68). New York: Oxford University Press.

Mendes, W. B., & Park, J. (2014). Neurobiological concomitants of motivational states. *Advances in Motivation Science, 1*, 233–270.

Ochsner, K. N., & Gross, J. J. (2008). Cognitive emotion regulation insights from social cognitive and affective neuroscience. *Current Directions in Psychological Science, 17*(2), 153–158.

Ochsner, K. N., & Gross, J. J. (2014). The neural bases of emotion and emotion regulation: A valuation perspective. In J. J. Gross (Ed.), *Handbook of emotion regulation* (2nd ed., pp. 23–41). New York: Guilford Press.

Orians, G. H., & Heerwagen, J. H. (1992). Evolved responses to landscapes. In J. H. Barkow, L. Cosmides, & J. Tooby (Eds.), *The adapted mind: Evolutionary psychology and the generation of culture* (pp. 555–597). New York: Oxford University Press.

Pekrun, R., Elliot, A. J., & Maier, M. A. (2009). Achievement goals and achievement emotions: Testing a model of their joint relations with academic performance. *Journal of Educational Psychology, 101*(1), 115–135.

Peters, B. J., Overall, N. C., & Jamieson, J. P. (2014). Physiological and cognitive consequences of suppressing and expressing emotion in dyadic interactions. *International Journal of Psychophysiology, 94*(1), 100–107.

Schachter, S., & Singer, J. (1962). Cognitive, social, and physiological determinants of emotional state. *Psychological Review, 69*(5), 379–399.

Schneirla, T. C. (1959). An evolutionary and developmental theory of biphasic processes underlying approach and withdrawal. In M. Jones (Ed), *Nebraska Symposium on Motivation* (Vol. 4, pp. 1–44). Lincoln: University of Nebraska Press.

Seery, M. D. (2011). Challenge or threat?: Cardiovascular indexes of resilience and vulnerability to potential stress in humans. *Neuroscience and Biobehavioral Reviews, 35*(7), 1603–1610.

Seery, M. D., Weisbuch, M., & Blascovich, J. (2009). Something to gain, something to lose: The cardiovascular consequences of outcome framing. *International Journal of Psychophysiology, 73*(3), 308–312.

Sheppes, G., Suri, G., & Gross, J. J. (2015). Emotion regulation and psychopathology. *Annual Review of Clinical Psychology, 11*, 379–405.

Sherwood, A., Turner, J. R., Light, K. C., & Blumenthal, J. A. (1990). Temporal stability of the hemodynamics of cardiovascular reactivity. *International Journal of Psychophysiology, 10*(1), 95–98.

Tomaka, J., Blascovich, J., Kelsey, R. M., & Leitten, C. L. (1993). Subjective, physiological, and behavioral effects of threat and challenge appraisal. *Journal of Personality and Social Psychology, 65*(2), 248–260.

Urdan, T., & Schoenfelder, E. (2006). Classroom effects on student motivation: Goal structures, social relationships, and competence beliefs. *Journal of School Psychology, 44*(5), 331–349.

Williams, J. M. G., Mathews, A., & MacLeod, C. (1996). The emotional Stroop task and psychopathology. *Psychological Bulletin, 120*(1), 3–24.

Williams, S. E., Cumming, J., & Balanos, G. M. (2010). The use of imagery to manipulate challenge and threat appraisal states in athletes. *Journal of Sport and Exercise Psychology, 32*, 339–358.

Yeager, D. S., Johnson, R., Spitzer, B. J., Trzesniewski, K. H., Powers, J., & Dweck, C. S. (2014). The far-reaching effects of believing people can change: Implicit theories of personality shape stress, health, and achievement during adolescence. *Journal of Personality and Social Psychology, 106*(6), 867–884.

Yeager, D. S., Lee, H. Y., & Jamieson, J. P. (2016). How to improve adolescent stress responses: Insights from integrating implicit theories of personality and biopsychosocial models. *Psychological Science, 27*(8), 1078–1091.

Yeager, D. S., & Walton, G. M. (2011). Social-psychological interventions in education They're not magic. *Review of Educational Research, 81*(2), 267–301.

CHAPTER 11

Competence Assessment, Social Comparison, and Conflict Regulation

FABRIZIO BUTERA
CÉLINE DARNON

Life is punctuated by important decisions that involve estimating whether one is able to do something. They can be important in the short term, like deciding to cook a *chevreuil grand veneur* for one's guests or helping one's children with their math homework, or they can have long-term consequences, like deciding to enroll in a graduate course or apply for a demanding professional position. How do people decide whether they can do it or not? How do people estimate to what extent they are competent?

In this chapter, we overview what it takes to reach self-knowledge about one's competence, and the consequences of such knowledge in terms of social interactions and performance. We first describe how research on social comparison (Festinger, 1954) has noted that objective standards for assessing one's competence are scarce; therefore, individuals need to compare themselves with other individuals. Second, we discuss the consequences of such comparisons, in particular whether they are functional in satisfying people's need to achieve positive competence, or are threatening for self-evaluation. Third, we turn to action. Individuals do more than passively compare themselves with other individuals; they also

interact with them. Competence, that is, "an organism's capacity to interact effectively with its environment" (White, 1959, p. 297), requires interacting with both the task at hand and relevant others. If a student wants to know whether he or she has competently addressed the topic of an essay, that student has to not only reflect on his or her work but also compare that work with what others have done. In this process, it may very well happen that the student disagrees with his or her fellow students because a single topic is likely to be viewed in multiple ways. Thus, we discuss how disagreements with others about a task, called *sociocognitive conflicts* (Doise & Mugny, 1984), are linked to individuals' assessment of their own and others' competence, and how these factors determine how effectively individuals interact with their environment in terms of performance and learning. Fourth, we review a line of work that uncovers the motivational precursors, in particular achievement goals, of such sociocognitive conflicts and their relative conflict regulation processes. Finally, we discuss some potential applications of this research, in particular for group work, training, and education.

COMPETENCE ASSESSMENT AND SOCIAL COMPARISON

The basic tenet of the theory of social comparison, and Festinger's first hypothesis in his seminal 1954 article, is that individuals are motivated to evaluate their opinions and abilities. Because this chapter is concerned with competence, we focus on abilities in the remainder of our argument. The origin of this motivation has been largely debated, and research has pointed to two nonexclusive factors. On the one hand, competence has been described as a basic psychological need (White, 1959; see also Deci & Ryan, 2000), a "persistent motivator that, if satisfied, promotes health and, if thwarted, results in ill-being" (Deci & Moller, 2005, p. 582). On the other hand, competence is reinforced and rewarded for cultural reasons, especially in Western countries, because it is linked to production in society; thus, individuals are motivated to comply with such societal expectations (Tesser, 1988).

However, assessing one's own competence is a rather tricky endeavor. Although people may hold positive illusions about the level of their abilities (Taylor & Brown, 1988), accurate assessment of what one can do is needed to avoid "punishing or even fatal" consequences (Festinger, 1954, p. 117), such as embarrassment or physical injury. Moreover, objective measures of competence may be difficult to obtain. How does one measure one's competence in swimming in open water? This is why Festinger's second and third founding hypotheses of social comparison theory state that, in the absence of objective measures, individuals evaluate their abilities in comparison with others, preferably, similar others. Indeed, comparing oneself with others can be a useful substitute for the absence of an objective standard. As explained by Wheeler, Martin, and Suls (1997), the question "Can I do X?", say, swim in the sea during a windy day, may be answered by comparing with a person—termed a *proxy*—who has similar attributes (e.g., years of experience) and has already attempted X. The reasoning behind this comparison is that if the proxy has succeeded at doing X, then it is likely that one can also do X (Wheeler & Suls, 2005; see also Bandura, 1977). In summary, social

comparison theory recognized from its inception that the evaluation of competence (ability) is a fundamental human motivation that cannot be limited to the instances in which either the task itself or a precise measurement instrument provide accurate feedback. Instead, social comparison targets are readily available in most social settings in which an assessment of competence is needed (e.g., at school, at work, in sports), and these targets are used as standards.

INSPIRING AND THREATENING SOCIAL COMPARISONS

Self-assessment is a rather descriptive and operational motive. It aims at obtaining accurate information about one's competence, and we have seen that this may be of capital importance. However, competence is also a valued commodity, especially in Western societies (Plaut & Markus, 2005), because the higher the competence the better the overall evaluation. Education, professional training, athletic training—all are institutionalized practices that convey the notion that competence should gradually increase. And indeed, the theory of social comparison, in Festinger's (1954) original formulation, also claims that individuals are motivated to increase their abilities gradually (a "unidirectional drive upward"). This is a motive that is qualitatively different from self-assessment and later was studied under the term "self-improvement" (Taylor, Neter, & Wayment, 1995). Again, relevant others are needed to serve as standards, not so much to assess the extent of one's improvement compared with the past, but because they may constitute an example or provide useful information for future improvement. In particular, it was proposed that if individuals want to improve themselves, comparison should target others who are slightly better off. This particular point of the reasoning is important because it implies that if an individual compares him- or herself with another individual who is better off ("upward comparison"), the comparison—however useful and informative it may be—also highlights the inferiority of the first individual. Thus, would this individual feel that his or her motive for self-improvement is fulfilled because the comparison target was inspiring, or would he or she feel threatened by the target's superiority? This question has occupied an entire stream of research, and whereas earlier research on social comparison focused on its function, a great deal of later research has been devoted to the study of its consequences (for a historical account of this evolution, see Suls & Wheeler, 2000).

Positive Consequences of Social Comparison

It has been noted that people do seek out social comparison with better-off targets (Collins, 1996), especially when they are motivated by self-improvement (Smith & Sachs, 1997), and that upward social comparison may afford positive consequences in terms of self-esteem and actual self-improvement. Taylor and Lobel (1989), for instance, in a classic study, have shown that contact with upward comparison targets may increase self-evaluation and optimism. Buunk, Peiro, and Griffioen (2007) showed that "a positive role model may stimulate career-oriented behaviors," as they summarize in the title of their article. And both Blanton, Buunk, Gibbons, and Kuyper (1999), and Huguet, Dumas, Monteil, and Genestoux (2001) have shown that students who compared upwards with other students improve their academic performance in the course of the school year. More generally, it has been shown that upward social comparison results in positive effects when an individual cognitively construes the relation with the target in terms of similarity (Collins, 1996), when the information about the target is included in the self (Schwarz & Bless, 2007), for example, when the relation with the target is one of cooperation (Colpaert, Muller, Fayant, & Butera, 2015), or even when the individual's mindset is just oriented toward similarity for other reasons (e.g., priming; Mussweiler, 2003).

It has also been noted that there are situations in which people seek out downward social comparison, choosing targets who are worse off (Wills, 1981). The seminal work by Hakmiller (1966) showed that this is the case when people's self-esteem is threatened, an effect later confirmed by several additional studies (e.g., Friend & Gilbert, 1973). Wood, Taylor, and Lichtman (1985)

discussed how downward social comparison may help in coping with threat, and serve a self-enhancement motive; indeed, it has been argued that emotions such as pride, contempt, or *schadenfreude* may emerge when individuals compare away from worse-off targets (Smith, 2000). For the moment, we retain from this brief overview that both upward and downward comparisons may yield positive effects for self-esteem, and that upward comparison also yields positive effects for performance.

Negative Consequences of Social Comparison

The literature on social comparison has also produced a wealth of results showing that upward social comparison may be threatening for self-esteem (for a review, see Muller & Fayant, 2010). Pictures of attractive, relative to unattractive, women led female college students to lower their evaluations of their own looks (Cash, Cash, & Butters, 1983). Comparison with a socially desirable, relative to socially undesirable, target produced a reduction in self-esteem in a set of job applicants (Morse & Gergen, 1970). Participants outperformed by a similar other felt more jealous of their comparison target and more depressed, especially when the outperformance occurred on a self-definitional dimension (Salovey & Rodin, 1984). However, it should be noted that upward social comparison results in negative self-evaluations when the individual cognitively construes the relation with the target in terms of dissimilarity (Collins, 1996). This conclusion is also supported by Mussweiler's (2003) selective accessibility process model: Dissimilarity between the individual and the comparison target is assumed to lead to a contrast effect, which in the case of an upward comparison target would result in a decrease in self-evaluation.

Along the same lines, it is possible that downward comparison may result in depletion rather than a boost of self-esteem; according to Mussweiler's (2003) model, this is possible when contextual reasons lead the individual to perceive some similarity with the downward comparison target, thereby prompting an assimilation effect. Indeed, Wood and colleagues (1985) found that although the majority of the participants in their breast cancer study used downward social comparison to cope with threat, some felt threatened by such comparison, to the extent that they felt some level of similarity with the target ("Is this going to be me, this kind of future?"; p. 1174). In summary, as expressed by Buunk, Collins, Taylor, Van Yperen, and Dakof (1990) in the title of their article on the consequences of both upward and downward social comparison, "either direction has its ups and downs."

The Question of Threat

Now that we have clarified that social comparison is not threatening as a function of its direction (upward or downward), we are left to clarify the nature of the threat involved in social comparison and why it matters. In the 1980s, two theoretical models concomitantly proposed the idea that individuals are motivated to achieve positive self-competence, namely, Steele's (1988) self-affirmation theory and Tesser's (1988) self-evaluation maintenance model. For our purpose of defining the nature of the threat in social comparison, we highlight three elements that are common to both models. First, individuals are motivated to hold a positive view of themselves. Second, threat occurs when an individual fails to reach the expected or hoped-for self-evaluation. In an article in which he discusses the similarities between the self-evaluation maintenance model and self-affirmation theory, Tesser (2000) noted that both theories stress that individuals' ability to match their behavior to a standard (be it another individual's level of performance or an important value) is a fundamental source of positive self-evaluation, which explains why not reaching those standards (e.g., by being outperformed by a relevant other) is threatening for self-evaluation. Third, when self-evaluation is threatened, individuals are motivated to put into place self-regulatory strategies to maintain or restore a positive self-evaluation.

The third element is particularly important to explain why clearly defining the nature of the threat matters. Stating that an individual tries to restore his or her self-evaluation if, say, a threatening social comparison has occurred, implies that this individual's cognitive system will be loaded with this goal.

Consistent with this inference, Martin and Tesser (1996) demonstrated that a mismatch between one's current self-evaluation and a relevant standard predicts the emergence of ruminative thoughts, which may interfere with cognitive processes otherwise devoted to an individual's activity (e.g., performance). This is why Muller and Butera (2007) defined self-evaluation threat as the "situations in which performance level is not high enough to reach relevant standards used to evaluate performance" (p. 196), and set out to investigate the consequences of such a threat relative to cognitive processes.

The guiding hypothesis of this work is that comparison with a standard may lead to an enhancement of attentional focusing as long as there is a threat, or a potential threat, to self-evaluation. Attentional focusing is an important part of this hypothesis. Threat is a theoretical construct that poses a number of measurement challenges. This long-standing problem dates back to dissonance theory (Festinger, 1957) and has been discussed by many theorists who have used threat as one of their central concepts; in particular, Tesser, Millar, and Moore (1988) pointed out that threats to self-evaluation should be detected as a result of the outcomes that they produce. One such outcome is the impairment of attention. Muller and Butera (2007) reasoned that because self-evaluation threat produces ruminative thoughts, these thoughts should create an attentional disturbance (Muller & Fayant, 2010), that is, reduce the attention in a task that could be devoted to peripheral cues, thereby creating an attentional focusing on central cues. Thus, self-evaluation threat should induce attentional focusing. To test this hypothesis, Muller and Butera (2007; see also Muller, Atzeni, & Butera, 2004) chose a perceptual task known to reveal attentional focusing, namely, illusory conjunctions (Treisman, 1998).

In their first experiment, Muller and Butera (2007) showed that comparison with a co-actor, whether present or absent, resulted in more attentional focusing when the co-actor allegedly outperformed rather than underperformed the participant. These results are consistent with the work reviewed earlier that showed upward comparison may be threatening. Interestingly, this experiment also featured a condition without social comparison (no information about the participant's and the co-actor's respective scores), again with a co-actor either being present or absent; the results showed that when the co-actor was present, but not when he or she was absent, the level of attentional focusing was similar to that in the condition where the co-actor outperformed the participant. In other words, the mere possibility that the co-actor could outperform the participant, like upward comparison, appeared to be threatening.

The authors' hypothesis was that self-evaluation threat is induced by any situation in which comparison with a standard does not satisfy the need for positive self-evaluation, and not by upward comparison per se. In their second experiment, Muller and Butera (2007) showed that self-evaluation is indeed a matter of standards: Without any social comparison information, they manipulated the performance feedback given to participants, either above or below the midpoint of an evaluative scale. The results showed that, without a co-actor, the focusing effect was stronger when participants allegedly scored below than when they scored above the symbolic midpoint of the scale. Then, the third and fourth experiments demonstrated that the observed effects were indeed a matter of threat, by respectively showing that (1) attentional focus could be increased in a downward social comparison condition when low performance feedback was given to the participant, and (2) attentional focus could be reduced in an upward social comparison condition when the participant was told that his or her score was good in comparison with the results of the general population. In summary, a threatening social comparison, or a threatening comparison to a standard, or even a potentially threatening comparison, can induce attentional focusing (i.e., a distraction that reduces the amount of attention that the cognitive system can devote to the task at hand).

In line with these hypotheses, a complementary stream of research has studied the effect of performance-approach goals on working memory (Crouzevialle & Butera, 2013). Performance-approach goals are interesting for the present contention because they have been characterized as the goal to outperform relevant others, to get better grades, or to do better than meaningful comparison targets (Elliot & Church, 1997). In other words, and to provide a link with the previous line of research, performance-approach goals express a desired state in which an individual seeks a comparatively positive self-evaluation, whose outcome is uncertain, such as the comparison with a co-actor whose relative standard is not known by the participant (Muller & Butera, 2007). Working memory is also interesting because, like attention, it comes in finite quantities (Baddeley, 1986) and it is likely to be disrupted by ruminations induced by threat (Beilock, Rydell, & McConnell, 2007; Schmader & Johns, 2003). Indeed, Crouzevialle and Butera (2013) showed in their first experiment that inducing performance-approach goals reduced performance, compared with a control condition, on a task that was sensitive to the available amount of working memory (the modular arithmetic problems; Beilock & Carr, 2005). Moreover, their third experiment confirmed that ruminations about the attainment of the goal were indeed responsible for these effects. These results reinforce the notion that comparison-induced evaluative threat has the potential to reduce the cognitive resources that should otherwise be devoted to the task.

Summary

Taken as a whole, the results presented in this section show that social comparison is indeed an important mechanism in the assessment of self-competence. However, it is also important to recognize that the direction of social comparison in itself is not sufficient to predict whether the need to hold a positive view of one's competence is fulfilled. It was demonstrated that self-evaluation threat may emerge, and may be reduced, with either direction of social comparison. These results also indicate a supplementary conclusion: that self-evaluation threat has consequences, in particular, for the extent to which the cognitive system can attend to all aspects of the task. This argument is important in the next section, in which we discuss how threatening social comparisons can affect the outcomes of social interaction during task engagement.

SOCIAL COMPARISON AND SOCIOCOGNITIVE CONFLICT

In everyday life outside the laboratory, social comparison targets are not passive reference points: They are coworkers, friends, and family members with whom people interact. For example, students compare with each other, particularly when they study together and share ideas, solutions to problems, and other relevant information. Coworkers spend a great deal of time comparing their relative performance, but they often do so in the context of working together on common tasks and joint decisions. In this section, we describe what happens when people compare their answers, and present a model that allows prediction of the outcomes of comparisons that take place in such social interaction contexts.

The notion of sociocognitive conflict was first studied to understand the effects of disagreement on children's cognitive progress (Doise & Mugny, 1984) and was later extended to disagreement among adults (Mugny, Butera, & Falomir, 2001; Quiamzade, Mugny, & Butera, 2013). *Sociocognitive conflict* refers to the social and cognitive disequilibrium that follows disagreement between two (or more) individuals; the conflict is both social, as it involves the confrontation between individuals, and cognitive, as it involves questioning the validity of each answer (Darnon, Buchs, & Butera, 2002; Darnon, Butera, & Mugny, 2008). This notion is particularly useful to study social interactions in situations where aptitudes and competence are concerned, for two reasons. First, it is very likely that disagreement emerges in people's everyday activities when jointly working on a task, given people's diversity in training, knowledge, and points of view (Butera, Darnon, & Mugny, 2011). Second, as mentioned earlier, the study of sociocognitive conflict extends the study of social comparison by including, in addition to the appraisal of the relative competence of partners, the appraisal of the relative validity of their answers.

Conflict and Conflict Regulation

The study of sociocognitive conflict began in the 1970s, following Piaget's (1975/1985) theory of equilibration, with the intention to show that social interaction, and the sociocognitive conflict inherent to that interaction, is a source of progress over and beyond cognitive development (Doise & Mugny, 1984). For instance, Doise and Mugny (1979) confronted two children with a developmental task aimed at assessing the acquisition of spatial transformation skills. In this experiment, dyads of children had to look at a target village laid out on a table and copy it on another table, but after a rotation. The authors composed dyads by putting together children who manifested the same difficulties during a pretest and did not solve the problem. However, they also created the conditions for the two children to be in conflict by positioning them on each side of the table, thereby creating opposing points of view. In a control condition, the participants worked alone and experienced the two points of view by moving from one side of the table to the other. Results showed that significantly more children in the interindividual conflict condition progressed in the acquisition of spatial transformation skills, compared to the children in the intraindividual conflict condition.

However, they also found some anomalies. Indeed, in another study, they confronted children with a similar task, but this time the dyads comprised children who displayed different levels of competence during the pretest (Mugny & Doise, 1978). Children in each dyad were on the same side of the table. Results showed that low-competence children who were paired with children of equal competence (no conflict) did not progress, consistent with the theory (no conflict, no progress). Moreover, low-competence children paired with children who were slightly superior (thereby introducing a conflicting point of view) did progress, again consistent with the theory, and consistent with social comparison theory. Interestingly, low-competence children paired with high-competence children did not progress at all. The high-competence children knew the correct answer, and presented it with great self-assurance to the low-competence children, who accepted it out of compliance but also without any real information processing. Owing to these results, the theory of sociocognitive conflict integrated a supplementary concept, namely, conflict regulation. Sociocognitive conflict is a crucial condition for progress to occur, but it is not sufficient: Conflict needs to be regulated (i.e., socially construed), and this regulation can be either epistemic or relational. *Epistemic conflict regulation* refers to a focus on knowledge, on the reasons that may explain why two different answers have emerged from the same task. In other words, epistemic regulation leans toward the cognitive side of sociocognitive conflict, leading partners to ask themselves and each other questions about the validity of their answers. *Relational conflict regulation* refers to a focus on relative status, on who is right and who is wrong. In other words, relational regulation leans toward the social side of the sociocognitive conflict, leading partners to ask themselves and each other questions about their relative competence. It is worth noting that relational conflict regulation is assumed to be the most threatening because, in line with the work on self-evaluation threat (Muller & Butera, 2007), such regulation focuses the individual on the possibility, or even the certainty, of being outperformed by his or her partner.

The distinction between two forms of conflict regulation is important because it allows us to predict when sociocognitive conflict may lead to progress and learning, namely, when it is regulated in an epistemic way, and when it may not, namely, when it is regulated in a relational way. Research in this area has, by and large, been supportive of this prediction (for reviews, see Butera et al., 2011; Butera & Mugny, 2001). For example, with adults as participants, Darnon, Doll, and Butera (2007) directly manipulated the regulation of conflict during a learning task through the presence of a bogus partner who regulated conflict in either an epistemic or a relational way. Results showed that not only did relational conflict regulation appear to be perceived as more threatening, but it also elicited lower levels of learning than did epistemic conflict regulation.

Conflict and Social Comparison of Competences

An assumption of the early work on sociocognitive conflict was that relational regulation would occur with a high-competence partner, and epistemic regulation with a more similar or slightly superior partner. The assumption was based on results like the ones presented by Mugny and Doise (1978), as well as the classic idea that in social influence, high-status sources induce compliance. However, as noted earlier, social comparison research had already shown that it is not the competence of the comparison target per se that matters, but the target's competence relative to that of the individual.

Based on these considerations, a 2×2 model was devised to predict the outcomes of conflict as a function of the high versus low competence of the influence source and the high versus low competence of the influence target (Butera, Gardair, Maggi, & Mugny, 1998). Two important elements are worth noting. First, in this model, the two individuals in interaction are termed *source* and *target* of influence, due to the fact that this model was a spinoff, so to speak, of a more general theory of social influence, called conflict elaboration theory (Pérez & Mugny, 1996). This theory was intended to predict the outcomes of the various kinds of social influence that occur in various domains of human knowledge and behavior; the Butera and colleagues (1998) model was limited to social influence occurring in "aptitude tasks," those tasks that are concerned with performance, problem solving, decision making, and all the activities that involve competence. This is relevant for this chapter, as it focuses on not only competence assessment but also the argument that we laid out at the beginning of this section: When people interact with each other, not only do they compare their relative competence but they also compare their answers to the task at hand. This may in turn produce changes in knowledge, decisions, and representations (i.e., produce social influence). Second, research has long pointed out that social influence can have an effect at not only an immediate and manifest level but also, or only, at a delayed and latent level (e.g., on a related task; Moscovici, 1980).

In this respect, conflict elaboration theory was devised to make predictions on the level of influence that would result from specific social influence dynamics.

The 2 × 2 model included four different influence dynamics.

1. When the source's competence is high and the target's competence is low, *informational constraint* is expected to occur: At the manifest level the target imitates the answer or solution given by the target, as the target assumes that the difference in competence implies that the source is right. This reasoning based on status, and not on the task, is not likely to produce a great deal of processing, and it is not expected that influence results in any long-lasting effects or generalization to related tasks. This is actually what Mugny and Doise (1978) had observed.

2. However, when the source's competence is high and the target's competence is also high, compliance is not an option, and a *conflict of competences* is expected to occur. In this case, which had not been studied in previous research, the competition for high status implies that the target will disregard the source's point of view and even try to invalidate it. Such a focus on competition is not expected to be conducive to any deep processing of the task or any influence.

3. The case in which the source's competence is low and the target's competence is high, called *absence of conflict,* is also not expected to be conducive to any influence, but for a different reason. Because the target is superior in competence, self-evaluation is not threatened (Muller & Butera, 2007), and disagreement with the point of view of a source that is believed to be wrong is likely to produce sociocognitive apathy and no change.

4. Even more interesting, when the source's competence is low and the target's competence is also low, a *conflict of incompetences* is expected to occur. Comparison of relative status is not particularly informative here: The low-competence source's answer is probably wrong and cannot be imitated, but the low-competence target's answer is also probably wrong, and the source's answer cannot be completely rejected. Because status does not help, the target is expected to engage in deep processing, reconsider the problem, and articulate the two answers, which should result in delayed, latent change. This is indeed what Doise and Mugny (1979) had observed when they positioned two low-competence children, one on each side of the table, in a spatial orientation task: The two children were forced to articulate the two opposing incorrect views, which resulted in reconsidering their knowledge on spatial orientation, and eventually in progress (see also Ames & Murray, 1982).

This model has received extensive empirical support, and here we report only a study that tested some of the model's prediction (Maggi, Butera, & Mugny, 1996). Participants had to estimate the length of a series of vertical bars; upon completion of this task, they received bogus feedback indicating that their competence in the task was either high (78/100) or low (24/100). Then again they had to estimate the length of a series of vertical bars, this time accompanied by the answer given by another participant whose competence level was either 78 or 24. Importantly, the estimates given by this influence source were systematically much lower than the real length of the bars, conflicting with the participants' estimates. A control condition was also added, with no feedback and no influence source. Then followed a posttest in which participants again had to estimate the length of a series of vertical bars, then draw an 8-cm line with paper and pencil. Manifest influence was measured by the reduction in estimated length of the bars between the pre- and the posttest. The measure of latent influence was the length of the 8-cm line: The longer the line, the higher the influence. Indeed, because the source was systematically underestimating the length of the bars, one could infer that his or her representation of the centimeter was longer than normal. If the participants are influenced by the source, and therefore develop a longer representation of what a centimeter is, then they will draw a longer line when asked to draw 8 cm. The results showed that in the *informational constraint* condition (high-competence source–low-competence target) influence occurred at the manifest but not at the latent level, whereas in the *conflict of competences* condition (high-competence source–high-competence target) influence was blocked at both levels. Moreover, in the *conflict of incompetences* condition (low-competence source–low-competence target), although no manifest influence appeared, the participants did draw a longer line, a latent influence that did not appear for participants in the *absence of conflict* condition (low-competence source–high-competence target). These results show an important cross-fertilization between social comparison and social influence research, and point to the relevance of taking into account the relative competence of partners when sociocognitive conflict arises.

Conflict, Competence Threat, and Social Comparison of Competences

Relative standing in terms of competence is an important feature when trying to predict the outcomes of a given interaction. At school, for example, pupils are aware of the competence of each of their classmates, in each subject, at least in broad terms (e.g., strong–weak), because teachers generally hand out the graded tests in class, and pupils talk with each other and have reputations. Thus, relative standing in terms of competence is likely a salient feature and is likely to influence the outcome of an interaction. However, one of the conclusions of the work conducted on self-evaluation threat is that social comparison information does not determine per se whether a partner or a co-actor is threatening. The crucial factor is whether the desired standards of competence are reached (Muller & Butera, 2007).

In the study reported earlier (Maggi et al., 1996), and in the relative model, it is assumed that high-competence sources of influence are threatening because they challenge the target's competence, and that low-competence sources are not. This is likely the case in the majority of interactions because in Western cultures competence is associated with status and with all the material and symbolic benefits that derive from it (Kasser, Cohn, Kanner, & Ryan, 2007), and people are used to competing for status (as in conflict of competence), or submitting

(as in informational constraint). However, an analysis of real-life situations, and of the literature, reveals that this picture is limited. For a high-competence target, it is likely that disagreement with a high-competence source is perceived as threatening and leads to a sterile conflict of competencies. However, many buildings and machines that we use every day have been designed by engineers who have worked constructively by pooling their high and complementary competences. And indeed, a long-standing tradition in cooperative learning has shown that working with complementary experts may be beneficial to everybody's learning (e.g., Aronson & Patnoe, 1997). For a low-competence target, it is also likely that disagreement with a high-competence source is perceived as threatening and leads to informational constraint and to compliance without further elaboration; however, we know that many teachers manage to have a profound influence on the knowledge and values of their pupils and students (e.g., Guimond, 2001). Also, a low-competence target would probably be puzzled and not threatened by disagreement with a low-competence source, and likely engage in a conflict of incompetence and in deep processing of the task. However, this is possible to the extent that the environment is competition-free. If not, partners distrustfully withhold their information and stick to their own points of view, thereby jeopardizing the task (e.g., Toma & Butera, 2009).

These considerations point to the conclusion that in order to predict the nature of conflict in social interactions, it is important to study not only the specific social comparison dynamics that take place but also the extent to which such social comparison is threatening. Thus, in 2001, Mugny and colleagues adapted the 2×2 model to include threat. The resulting $2 \times 2 \times 2$ model presented the hypothesized conflicts, and their effects, that should arise from the confrontation of high- and low-competence targets with high- and low-competence sources in social comparisons that are either threatening or not. The full model can be found in the aforementioned publication, and here we only discuss the changes in conflict generated by the presence versus absence of threat.

Let us start with conflict of competences. Two high-competence partners may feel threatened when they disagree because they assume that if one is right, the other is wrong and, therefore, incompetent. However, as mentioned earlier, high-competence individuals may work without threatening each other's self-evaluation if they assume that their competences and answers may be complementary. This type of conflict has been called *informational interdependence*. Quiamzade and Mugny (2009) have provided a compelling illustration of the mechanisms that allow switching from conflict of competences to informational interdependence. In their first study, participants answered a few questions on economy and received bogus feedback that declared them excellent. Then, they were presented, or not, with a decentering task designed to suggest that different, even seemingly incompatible answers, may in fact be complementary and refer to a more complex reality (Butera & Buchs, 2005). They continued the experiment with a new task in which they were asked to make a specific economic prediction, and were provided with the answer of a bogus source, allegedly also excellent, who contradicted their answer. The authors also included a control condition without influence. Results revealed that the conflict of competencies condition (both target and source were declared excellent) did not yield any influence because the change in answer in this condition was the same as that in the control condition. However, in the informational interdependence condition (both target and source were declared excellent + the decentering task meant to promote complementarity of points of view)—when the threat inherent to the social comparison between two high-competence individuals was removed by the suggestion that different answers may be complementary—influence was significantly higher than in the two other conditions. In summary, the conflict of competencies appears to be threatening because one's own competence is construed as the negation of the other's competence, and vice versa; the decentering procedure allowed removal of this threat and moving from an exclusively relational conflict regulation (who is right and who is wrong) to an epistemic conflict regulation that allowed information to be processed and influence to emerge.

If we now turn to informational constraint, we may ask whether it is also possible to remove the threat experienced by a low-competence target when in disagreement with a high-competence source, which should allow deeper processing and integration of information to emerge. This type of conflict has been called *informational dependence*. Mugny, Tafani, Butera, and Pigière (1998) presented their participants, psychology students, with a task designed to capture the participants' beliefs regarding group dynamics. A bogus study was then presented that contradicted the participant's beliefs; either a researcher or a student like themselves had allegedly conducted the study (but let us focus on the researcher because we are now concerned with comparison with higher-competence sources). In this experiment, the threat involved in social comparison was directly manipulated: Participants were asked to rate their competence and that of the source in one of two ways. In the negative interdependence condition, participants had 100 points to distribute between them and the source; this implied that what was given to the source was subtracted from the target, and vice versa, thereby mimicking the functioning of a competitive social comparison. In the independence condition, participants had up to 100 points to allocate to themselves and up to 100 points to allocate to the target; in this case, the competence of one had no impact on the competence of the other. Finally, their beliefs about group dynamics were assessed again, to measure the extent to which the position of the source was integrated into their answers. Results concerning the high-competence source, the researcher, showed that an independent assessment of the source's and the target's competencies resulted in a higher integration of information in the posttest than when competencies were seen as excluding each other. Again, threat and its inhibiting effects seem to be associated not so much with a specific direction of social comparison but rather with the inability of social comparison to grant a positive view of one's own competence.

Let us conclude with conflict of incompetencies (and let us skip the case of the absence of conflict, which has not received much empirical attention). This conflict is described as conducive to epistemic conflict regulation and deep processing because targets focus on the task rather than on the uninformative social comparison information. We might, however, ask a question that is complementary to the one asked in the previous paragraph: Is it also possible to induce threat in a low-competence target who is in disagreement with a low-competence source, which should impair deeper processing and integration of information? Butera and Mugny (1995) asked their participants to solve a set of inductive reasoning problems and measured the extent to which they used disconfirmation in hypothesis testing, an infrequent behavior that requires integrating alternative mental models (Johnson-Laird, 1983). Participants were also presented the conflicting answer proposed by a novice (participants were also low in competence) and had to distribute competence points in a negatively interdependent versus independent fashion. Results revealed that participants who disagreed with the novice and were asked to rate their competence in an independent fashion appeared to use disconfirmation to a greater extent than did participants who compared themselves competitively. Participants in the latter condition clearly felt threatened in their self-evaluation because they displayed a focusing effect, in the form of the well-known confirmation bias in hypothesis testing (Wason, 1960).

Summary

People often disagree with their partners in tasks that require the use of a certain degree of competence. The outcomes of such conflicts depend on the way conflict is regulated: Relational regulation focuses individuals on issues of status and rank and turns attention away from the task, whereas epistemic regulation focuses individuals on the validity of their answer and on the quest for the most accurate answer or solution. The research presented in this section argues that the specific type of regulation that will be adopted is determined by not only the high versus low competence of both the target and the source participating in a social influence interaction, but also the threatening versus nonthreatening nature of the social comparison involved. The various

types of conflict that result from such a $2 \times 2 \times 2$ model are a sign of the complexity of the mechanisms at work in achievement settings if one wants to account for the dynamics that influence both the assessment of competence and the outcomes of the interaction in terms of actual processing of the task and performance. This stated, such theoretical complexity can be useful to fine-tune interventions aiming at fostering deep processing and facilitate performance, as we see in the final section of this chapter.

ACHIEVEMENT GOALS, CONFLICT REGULATION, AND SOCIAL COMPARISON

Conflict regulation is a regulatory process that helps individuals cope with the disequilibrium created by sociocognitive conflict. We have already discussed one important source of disequilibrium: An individual holding a piece of knowledge needs to make sense of the disagreement introduced by another individual who holds a different piece of knowledge. We have also argued that such a disequilibrium is likely to become threatening and then regulated in a relational way. This is notably what happens when conflict involves a threatening social comparison (e.g., in competitive settings). Another source that potentially renders social comparison threatening during sociocognitive conflict can also be found in the reasons one has to engage in and achieve the task. Indeed, in achievement settings—at school, at work—an individual may very well be motivated to achieve, to succeed (Atkinson, 1957). If the individual's achievement goal is to acquire competence, conflict signals that more work is needed to reach the desired competence level, and it is therefore not threatening. If the individual's achievement goal is to demonstrate competence, conflict signals that another individual may be demonstrating more competence and, as such, becomes an important source of threat to the self. In this section, we discuss the relationship between achievement goals and conflict regulation.

Achievement Goals and Conflict Regulation

The achievement goals to which we just alluded have been characterized as the purpose of task engagement (Maehr, 1989), and divided by early researchers into mastery goals—aimed at mastering the task and developing competence—and performance goals—aimed at demonstrating competence compared with relevant others (Ames & Archer, 1988; Dweck, 1986; Nicholls, 1984). The very definitions we used earlier suggest that these goals refer to appetitive forms of motivation, aimed at reaching, approaching the desired state; later research has shown that some additional specifications are necessary, but we introduce them in the following pages. Because mastery goals are concerned with reaching an accurate knowledge about the task, when conflict arises, it is likely that the individual's doubts will concern the nature of the task, the validity of each conflicting answer, and the development of new knowledge. If this is the case, then it is reasonable to think that epistemic regulation would be a relevant coping strategy when conflict has thwarted mastery goals. Symmetrically, as performance goals are concerned with positioning one's competence in comparison with others, when conflict arises it is likely that the individual's doubts will concern his or her rank, reputation, and the pursuit of status. If this is the case, then it is reasonable to think that relational regulation would be a relevant coping strategy when conflict has thwarted performance goals.

The first test of the hypothesis that some relation should be found between achievement goals and conflict regulation was provided by Darnon, Muller, Schrager, Pannuzzo, and Butera (2006). In their first study, these authors measured the mastery and performance goals (in their approach form; Elliot & McGregor, 2001) of their psychology students, then confronted them with a vignette in which another student contradicted the usual interpretation of a well-known social psychology experiment. The participants had to imagine the discussion, write down the arguments that they would put forward, then answer a conflict regulation scale in which they were to indicate to what extent they would regulate conflict in an epistemic and relational way, in the imagined discussion. The items of these scales were developed to pattern the theoretical characteristics of these two forms of conflict regulation. In the epistemic conflict regulation scale, students were asked to what extent they would "try to think about the text again in order to understand better," "try to examine the conditions under which each point of view could help you understand," and "try to think of a solution that could integrate both points of view." In the relational conflict regulation scale, students were asked to what extent they would "try to show you were right," "try to resist by maintaining your initial position," and "try to show your partner was wrong." The results showed that, indeed, mastery goals were associated with epistemic regulation but not relational regulation, and that performance goals were associated with relational regulation but not epistemic regulation. In other words, the more students strove to master the task and improve their competence, the more they said they would try to make sense of a sign that their knowledge may not be as accurate as they thought by going back to the task. Symmetrically, the more students strove to assert their competence over others, the more they said they would try to make sense of a sign that their knowledge might not be as accurate as they thought by stressing that their answer was the good one.

This study measured the general orientation of students toward mastery and performance goals, but a wealth of research has shown that achievement goals can be the results of specific environments or "climates," with, for instance, diversity-oriented contexts promoting mastery goals (e.g., Ames, 1992), and competition-oriented contexts promoting performance goals (e.g., Murayama & Elliot, 2012). Thus, in another study, the association between achievement goals and conflict regulation was investigated by manipulating goals (Darnon & Butera, 2007). Participants were given mastery-enhancing or performance-enhancing instructions or were placed in a control condition without goal instructions, then grouped in dyads. In order to create sociocognitive conflict, each dyad was asked to discuss a particular topic in psychology, but the two members were given two different texts that presented conflicting results (e.g., primacy vs. recency effects). After the discussion, participants were asked to rate the level of disagreement that occurred during the discussion, as well as the conflict regulation scales. The results showed that perceived disagreement predicted epistemic conflict regulation in the mastery goal condition but not in the performance goal and control conditions. Moreover, perceived disagreement also predicted relational conflict regulation in the performance goal condition, but not in the mastery goal and control conditions. Thus, sociocognitive conflict was regulated—so the participants reported—in a fashion that matched the motivational climate that had been experimentally induced.

Achievement Goals, Conflict, and Performance

Why does all this matter? Research on achievement goals, since its inception, has pointed out that these goals predict a host of cognitive, emotional, and behavioral outcomes, including performance in several achievement domains (work, sports and education; Van Yperen, Blaga, & Postmes, 2014). This research has shown that mastery goals typically predict effort, task interest, and deep studying (e.g., Dweck, 1986; Pintrich & Schunk, 2002), although they only moderately and inconsistently predict performance (e.g., Dompnier, Darnon, & Butera, 2009; Hulleman, Schrager, Bodmann, & Harackiewicz, 2010). Performance-approach goals have been shown to predict surface learning, low persistence after failure, negative affects and, more consistently, performance and academic achievement (Elliot & Church, 1997; Senko, Hulleman, & Harackiewicz, 2011). Many of these predominantly prospective studies, however, do not account for the group dynamics that occur during progress toward achievement, such as encountering other students or other coworkers who disagree with one's understanding. What happens to performance when sociocognitive conflict occurs during the pursuit of mastery and performance goals?

Darnon, Butera, and Harackiewicz (2007) asked their participants to work on an alleged computer-mediated cooperative learning session. Achievement goals were manipulated through instructions emphasizing either mastery or performance goals (or no instructions). Participants then read

a text, answered a series of questions related to the text and, after each answer, received a (bogus) answer given by the partner, who either agreed or disagreed. At the end of the session, each participant answered a multiple-choice questionnaire on the text, which constituted the measure of learning. When the partner agreed, no differences across goal conditions were observed. When the partner disagreed, however, the mastery goal condition displayed a higher learning score than the performance goal and control conditions. Moreover, consistent with work that has showed the constructive effects of sociocognitive conflict on cognitive progress (Doise & Mugny, 1984), these results showed that a partner's disagreement tended to lead to better learning than agreement; however, the authors specify that this was the case only when participants were instructed to pursue mastery goals. Under performance goal and no instructions, partner's disagreement tended to lead to worse learning than agreement.

A "Trichotomous" View on Achievement Goals and Conflict Regulation

In a caveat presented at the beginning of this section, we noted that we were presenting research concerned with achievement goals that refer to appetitive forms of motivation, aimed at reaching or approaching the desired state. Elliot and Harackiewicz (1996) remarked that this interpretation had been dominant from the beginning of achievement goal theory, until their article was published, in which they proposed a "trichotomous" model that divides performance goals into their approach and avoidance components. Their work and that of Elliot and Church (1997) showed that mastery goals, performance-approach goals, and performance-avoidance goals are indeed three separate constructs that predict separate outcomes. In particular, whereas performance-approach goals positively predict performance, performance-avoidance goals predict performance negatively.[1]

Sommet and colleagues (2014) reconsidered the relationship between achievement goals and conflict regulation from the point of view of the trichotomous model and devised a series of studies aiming at dividing relational conflict regulation into its "competitive" and "protective" components. The reasoning was based on two elements: the existing evidence on relational conflict regulation on the one hand, and the parallel with achievement goals on the other. First, the literature has documented various forms of regulation that have traditionally been termed *relational conflict regulation*. Some studies have reported that conflict was regulated by trying to impose one's own point of view (Psaltis & Duveen, 2006), whereas other studies reported attempts to regulate conflict based on the imitation of the partner's answer, without any further elaboration (Mugny & Doise, 1978). Both types of regulation focus on the relative status of the partners, but they are qualitatively different: In the former case, individuals assume that they are right (or want to appear so), whereas in the latter, they assume that the partner is right. This remark leads to the second element, the parallel with the partition of performance goals in their approach and avoidance components. Asserting that one is right (and the other is wrong) may very well be motivated by the performance-approach goal of outperforming others—this is precisely what Darnon and colleagues (2006) had shown, as the performance goals they used were in fact performance-approach goals. Complying with the partner and imitating his or her answer, on the contrary, may proceed from performance-avoidance goals, as imitation of the partner allows one to avoid failure, or at least to avoid being inferior to one's partner.

In their first experiment, Sommet and colleagues (2014) measured participants' performance-approach and performance-avoidance goals (extracted from Elliot and McGregor's [2001] Achievement Goal Questionnaire), then assigned them to dyads to work on the relationship between the position of a word in a list and the probability that it would be recalled. One partner received a text on the primacy effect and the other, a text on the recency effect, which created sociocognitive conflict. Finally, participants filled in a behavioral measure of conflict regulation: They were to rate, on a scale from 1 to 7, the extent to which four models referring to four possible relationships between the position of a word

and the probability of recall were "correct, defendable, and convincing." The four models depicted: "(1) A decreasing curve (corresponding to the primacy effect); (2) An increasing curve (corresponding to the recency effect); (3) A U-shaped curve (corresponding to the serial position effect); and (4) An inverse U-shaped curve (corresponding to an incorrect alternative answer)" (p. 138). From these four mean scores, two proportional indices were computed: (1) participants' preference for their own answer, which refers to competitive conflict regulation, and (2) preference for the partner's answer, which refers to protective conflict regulation. The analyses revealed that performance-approach goals positively predicted the preference for a model depicting one's own answer (competitive conflict regulation), and that performance-avoidance goals positively predicted the preference for a model depicting the partner's answer (protective conflict regulation).

In their third experiment, Sommet and colleagues (2014) manipulated performance-approach and performance-avoidance goals through the experimental instructions. Then participants were assigned to dyads, experienced conflict induced by two texts reporting contradictory results, and rated their perceived disagreement, as well as the extent to which they used competitive and protective conflict regulation. The competitive conflict regulation scale included items similar to those used by Darnon and colleagues (2006). The protective conflict regulation scale was built on the basis of the aforementioned theoretical elements, and included three items: to what extent did you (1) "think your partner was certainly more correct than you," (2) "comply with his(her) proposition," and (3) "agree with his(her) own way of viewing things." It appeared that disagreement more positively predicted competitive conflict regulation under performance-approach than performance-avoidance goal instructions, whereas it more positively predicted protective conflict regulation under performance-avoidance than performance-approach goal instructions. In summary, the distinction between performance-approach and performance-avoidance goals also helped generate novel hypotheses on the structure of relational conflict regulation, and led to the identification of two separate constructs, namely competitive and protective conflict regulations.

Again, it is important to ask what happens to performance when sociocognitive conflict occurs during the pursuit of, this time, performance-approach and performance-avoidance goals. Darnon, Harackiewicz, Butera, Mugny, and Quiamzade (2007) manipulated the two kinds of performance goals through experimental instructions, and once again the alleged computer-mediated cooperative learning session was used to create, or not, a sociocognitive conflict. Participants read a text, answered a series of questions, and received the answer given by their partner, who either agreed or disagreed. The learning measure consisted of a multiple-choice questionnaire on the text. The significant interaction between goals and conflict revealed that when the partner agreed, performance-approach goals induced a higher learning score than performance-avoidance goals, but when the partner disagreed, both goals induced the same low level of learning. This result stimulates an important consideration. A wealth of research has shown that performance-approach goals are positive predictors of performance, whereas performance-avoidance goals are negative predictors (e.g., Hulleman et al., 2010; Murayama & Elliot, 2012). However, most of these studies investigated the performance goals—performance link either prospectively, or in experiments where participants were required to work alone. Consistent with these findings, when in this study the partner did not pose any particular challenge (agreement), performance-approach goals did induce better performance than performance-avoidance goals. This was not the case when the partner introduced a sociocognitive conflict (disagreement). Thus, it appears that sociocognitive conflict disrupts task processing when it intervenes during the pursuit of either performance goals. This is in line with the results showing that both conflict regulations associated with performance goals (i.e., competitive and protective conflict regulation) orient attention toward relational concerns rather than toward a deep processing of the task (Sommet et al., 2014).

Social Comparison, Performance Goals, and Conflict Regulation

When one reads the articles on the relation between performance goals and relational conflict regulation, it appears that the hypotheses are based on an important assumption: The disagreeing partner is, or might be, superior in competence. This assumption is evident in the characterization of protective conflict regulation, which is described as a form of deferential compliance, but it also applies to competitive conflict regulation, as one needs to struggle to show that one is right and the other is wrong when it is possible that the hierarchy goes in the other direction. This assumption is coherent with the self-evaluation threat hypothesis, to the extent that a more competent other may be perceived as a source of threat, which is potentially distracting and impairs performance in complex tasks. But it had remained an assumption until very recently.

Sommet, Darnon, and Butera (2015) tested the hypothesis that performance-approach goals lead to competitive conflict regulation and performance-avoidance goals lead to protective conflict regulation when conflict arises with a more competent rather than an equally competent other. Four studies supported this hypothesis with various types of conflict elaboration measures, including self-report scales, preference for models, and even conflict regulation behaviors coded during interaction. In other words, social comparison seems to affect the extent to which performance goals give way to relational conflict regulation: It is the comparison with a more threatening other that leads performance-approach-oriented individuals to regulate conflict in a competitive way and performance-avoidance-oriented individuals to regulate conflict in a protective way.

Summary

In this section, we have presented a line of research that points to the role of achievement goals in the emergence of specific forms of conflict regulation. This work has led to a refined classification of conflict regulation and a rather precise picture of how achievement goals are associated with conflict regulation: Mastery goals predict epistemic regulation, performance-approach goals predict competitive relational regulation, and performance-avoidance goals predict protective relational regulation. The very last part of the section also indicated that achievement goals may interact with social comparison in the prediction of conflict regulation and, more precisely, that both performance goals predict relational conflict regulation, especially when social comparison is threatening. As noted already in the previous section, this level of complexity is a sign of the maturity of the research program presented here, and a promise of precision in recommendations for applied research and interventions.

CONCLUSIONS AND PRACTICAL APPLICATIONS

In this chapter we have highlighted the complexity of assessing one's competence. We have argued that people do not assess their competence by statically looking to their self-concept, but rather by dynamically evaluating their competence against relevant social standards, and against the reality check of disagreement with relevant others. In the first two sections, we dove into the research area of social comparison and noted that one's competence needs to be evaluated in relation to relevant others or to relevant normative standards (which are also socially defined targets of comparison). We also noted that in comparing oneself with others, the extent to which a given comparison is threatening seems to organize the consequences for not only self-evaluation but also the cognitive processes devoted to the task at hand. Social comparisons are threatening whenever they prevent individuals from reaching a valued or desired standard, and when this happens, attention and other cognitive functions are diverted from at least part of the task. In the third section we extended these views to take into account the fact that people compare themselves with each other while also interacting with each other. We reviewed a research program that studied the emergence of conflict from social influence interactions, and the various forms that

conflict takes as a function of the source's competence, the target's competence, and the threat involved in social comparison. The resulting model allows a high degree of precision in predicting the specific conflicts and the specific conflict regulations that are likely to emerge from a given situation, as well as the likely consequences in terms of task processing and performance. Finally, in the fourth section, we reviewed a research program that studied the motivational antecedents of conflict regulation. Interestingly, the motivational antecedents under study were achievement goals, the cognitive-dynamic manifestations of competence-relevant motives (Elliot & Church, 1997). This program, too, provides a great deal of detail as to which achievement goal predicts which conflict regulation, and under which conditions. We argue that this level of complexity and precision is a valuable asset for tailoring applied research and training programs.

Let us start with the benefits of precision in the use of sociocognitive conflict. Research on sociocognitive conflict assumes that intellectual confrontation is good. A host of publications in this area have presented countless examples of areas in which the use of sociocognitive conflict can be constructive (see, e.g., Buchs, Butera, Mugny, & Darnon, 2004, for practical advice on how to use sociocognitive conflict in educational settings). The same conclusion comes from the cognate area of constructive controversy, which also refers to intellectual conflict. In his latest book, Johnson (2015) reviews several domains of intervention in which constructive controversy can solve social and societal problems, including industrial and organizational decision making, education, political discourse, and building and maintaining peace. We fully agree with this perspective, and we view the $2 \times 2 \times 2$ model of conflict elaboration in achievement settings as an important practical contribution to the careful use of conflict in social interactions. Indeed, the model proposes that conflict may sometimes result in epistemic conflict regulation, which has been shown to yield positive outcomes, and at other times in relational regulation, which has been shown to yield negative outcomes.

An important area of application for this model is group composition, which is used daily in educational (Cohen & Lotan, 1995) and organizational settings (e.g., Argote, 2012) to pool together individuals who possess specific competences. Group composition is often used by educators and managers to maximize diversity—which increases the likelihood for conflict to emerge—in order to avoid closed-mindedness and self-confirmation (Janis, 1982). Importantly, the model proposes three variables that determine whether sociocognitive conflict will be constructive, and that are easy to monitor during group composition, namely, two personal characteristics (the source's and the target's competence) and a contextual characteristic (threatening social comparison). With these three variables, and the results presented in the third section of this chapter, it is then possible to fine-tune group composition. For example, one might want to have two seasoned lawyers (or two graduate students) work on the same case (the same research project), hoping that informational interdependence might emerge because they have complementary competencies and one might see details the other does not see. However, if they perceive that they are up for promotion to the same position, one might expect that conflict of competencies might emerge instead, which would result in more rigidity instead of divergent thinking when discussing the case (research). Another example involves parents. Parents might want to decide who should help their son with his math homework, and choose a parent or a private teacher who has followed the most advanced curriculum in mathematics, hoping that informational dependence might emerge and facilitate learning. However, if the child is threatened by the unattainable level of the high-competence parent–teacher, it is more likely that informational constraint would lead him to nod throughout the explanation of the foundations of trigonometry, without remembering a single word the day after. In this sense, a peer, or a less advanced referent, would certainly be of better help. In summary, we believe that this theoretical model may be used for crafting practical, tailor-made recommendations on how to implement sociocognitive conflict in group composition effectively.

The research program presented in the fourth section of this chapter is also quite precise in predicting which achievement goal predicts which conflict regulation and when. We believe that this may be particularly useful when devising practices whose aim is to create a particular climate, either in the classroom or at work—for example, in training courses for teachers and managers. At school, in particular, this endeavor has generated an impressive amount of research aimed at identifying the factors that shape classroom goal structure, and influence student motivation and academic achievement (Meece, Anderman, & Anderman, 2006). As classroom and school environments influence students' academic motivation and achievement, the factors that influence the structure of these environments are particularly interesting for teacher training and professional training courses for administrators (e.g., Ames, 1992; Midgley & Maehr, 1999). The work presented in the fourth section contributes to this endeavor by drawing attention to the fact that students interact with each other and very often disagree, and that a given goal structure may have different effects as a function of the specific conflict regulation that emerges. For instance, a teacher may be tempted to set up a dynamic and competitive environment to promote performance goals in order to boost students' performance. However, considering that classes are social environments in which students interact, argue, and potentially disagree with each other (Darnon, Dompnier, & Poortvliet, 2012), such a goal structure in a classroom may very well annihilate the positive effects conflict could have on performance (as shown by Darnon, Harackiewicz, et al., 2007). Importantly, this research suggests that a mastery goal structure would represent a more appropriate environment for the emergence of epistemic conflict regulation and learning (Darnon, Butera, & Harackiewicz, 2007).

It is worth noting on this front that creating a mastery goal climate in the classroom requires more than just telling students that they *should* endorse mastery goals. Indeed, such recommendations are likely to increase the already high social desirability of mastery goals, without leading students to genuinely and personally endorse such goals. This could even be counterproductive for students, as recent research has shown that mastery goals endorsed to garner the teacher's appreciation do not predict actual achievement (Dompnier et al., 2009, 2015). Instead, creating a mastery goal climate implies organizing and structuring the class in such a way that what is really expected from students (what is "socially useful") is learning and self-improvement (Ames, 1992). This should in turn focus students on the content of what they are studying and thereby increase the likelihood that conflicts are regulated in an epistemic manner.

We have one last suggestion for application. In this research program, it is assumed that achievement goals influence conflict regulation, which is a sensible assumption— because conflict regulation takes place among students who come with preexisting dispositions and are inserted into classrooms with preoriented goal structures. Moreover, this assumption has been supported by the results of the studies presented earlier. However, it is also possible that practicing certain types of conflict regulation may in the long run create corresponding achievement goals. Let us take for example the study by Darnon, Doll, and Butera (2007) presented earlier. It showed that the use of a rhetoric typical of epistemic conflict regulation resulted in increased learning during collaborative work. The appendix to that article provides examples of what such a rhetoric may be (e.g., "I thought that . . ." instead of "No, you didn't get it . . ."; "It seemed weird to me . . ." instead of "Excuse me, but . . ."; p. 238). Actually, the development of an extended version of these examples may serve to devise a protocol that could be offered as training for peer tutoring (Damon & Phelps, 1989). It could also serve as a basis for devising a training module that could be integrated into teacher training or offered as a continuing education course. Such a protocol could have two categories of benefits. On the one hand, it might suggest how to help give students personalized feedback in a nonthreatening way, especially low-achieving students who may be particularly sensitive to disagreement and interpret conflict as failure. In this respect, it would be quite a different method than the very popular conflict resolution training

(e.g., Segal & Smith, 2015), in that the goal would not be to reduce or eliminate conflict, but rather to create it and make sure it is regulated in an epistemic way. On the other hand, if, indeed, a similar protocol made it into teacher training and was used in class, it might—as mentioned earlier—habituate teachers and pupils to argue about the task, and eventually contribute to a mastery-goal-oriented classroom structure. We hope that these suggestions inspire new research and useful interventions.

ACKNOWLEDGMENT

The preparation of this chapter was supported by the Swiss National Science Foundation.

NOTE

1. Since publication of the trichotomous model, two more sophisticated models of achievement goals have been developed: (1) a 2 × 2 model separating mastery-approach from mastery-avoidance goals (Elliot & McGregor, 2001), and (2) a 3 × 2 model that organizes achievement goals as a function of their definition (absolute, intrapersonal, interpersonal) and valence (approach and avoidance; Elliot, Murayama, & Pekrun, 2011). The goals stemming from these models have not (yet) been related to conflict regulation, and we therefore do not discuss them in this chapter.

REFERENCES

Ames, C. (1992). Classrooms: Goals, structures, and students' motivation. *Journal of Educational Psychology, 84,* 261–271.

Ames, C., & Archer, J. (1988). Achievement goals in the classroom: Students' learning strategies and motivation processes. *Journal of Educational Psychology, 80,* 260–267.

Ames, G. J., & Murray, F. B. (1982). When two wrongs make a right: Promoting cognitive change by social conflict. *Developmental Psychology, 18,* 894–897.

Argote, L. (2012). *Organizational learning.* New York: Springer.

Aronson, E., & Patnoe, S. (1997). *The jigsaw classroom: Building cooperation in the classroom.* Upper Saddle River, NJ: Scott, Foresman.

Atkinson, J. W. (1957). Motivational determinants of risk-taking behavior. *Psychological Review, 64,* 359–372.

Baddeley, A. D. (1986). *Working memory.* Oxford, UK: Oxford University Press.

Bandura, A. (1977). Self-efficacy: Toward a unifying theory of behavioral change. *Psychological Review, 84,* 191–215.

Beilock, S. L., & Carr, T. H. (2001). On the fragility of skilled performance: What governs choking under pressure? *Journal of Experimental Psychology: General, 130,* 701–725.

Beilock, S. L., Rydell, R. J., & McConnell, A. R. (2007). Stereotype threat and working memory: Mechanisms, alleviation, and spillover. *Journal of Experimental Psychology: General, 136,* 256–276.

Blanton, H., Buunk, B. P., Gibbons, F. X., & Kuyper, H. (1999). When better-than-others compare upward: Choice of comparison and comparative evaluation as independent predictors of academic performance. *Journal of Personality and Social Psychology, 76,* 420–430.

Buchs, C., Butera, F., Mugny, G., & Darnon, C. (2004). Conflict resolution and cognitive outcomes. *Theory Into Practice, 43,* 23–30.

Butera, F., & Buchs, C. (2005). Reasoning together: From focussing to decentring. In V. Girotto & P. N. Johnson-Laird (Eds.), *The shape of reason* (pp. 193–203). Hove, UK: Psychology Press.

Butera, F., Darnon, C., & Mugny, G. (2011). Learning from conflict. In J. Jetten & M. Hornsey (Eds.), *Rebels in groups: Dissent, deviance, difference and defiance* (pp. 36–53). Oxford, UK: Wiley-Blackwell.

Butera, F., Gardair, E., Maggi, J., & Mugny, G. (1998). Les paradoxes de l'expertise: Influence sociale et (in)compétence de soi et d'autrui [Paradoxes of expertise: Social influence and self- and other-(in)competence]. In J. Py, A. Somat, & J. Baillé (Eds.), *Psychologie sociale et formation professionnelle: propositions et regards critiques* (pp. 109–123). Rennes, France: Presses Universitaires de Rennes.

Butera, F., & Mugny, G. (1995). Conflict between incompetences and influence of a low competence source in hypothesis testing. *European Journal of Social Psychology, 25,* 457–462.

Butera, F., & Mugny, G. (2001). Conflicts and social influences in hypothesis testing. In C. De Dreu & N. De Vries (Eds.), *Group consensus and minority influence: Implications for innovation* (pp. 160–182). Oxford, UK: Blackwell.

Buunk, A. P., Peiró, J. M., & Griffioen, C. (2007). A positive role model may stimulate career-oriented behavior. *Journal of Applied Social Psychology, 37,* 1489–1500.

Buunk, B. P., Collins, R. L., Taylor, S. E., Van Yperen, N. W., & Dakof, G. A. (1990). The affective consequences of social comparison: Either direction has its ups and downs. *Journal of Personality and Social Psychology, 59,* 1238–1249.

Cash, T. F., Cash, D. W., & Butters, J. W. (1983). "Mirror, mirror, on the wall . . . ?": Contrast effects and self-evaluations of physical attractiveness. *Personality and Social Psychology Bulletin, 9,* 351–358.

Cohen, E. G., & Lotan, R. A. (1995). Producing equal-status interaction in the heterogeneous classroom. *American Educational Research Journal, 32,* 99–120.

Collins, R. L. (1996). For better or worse: The impact of upward social comparison on self-evaluations. *Psychological Bulletin, 119,* 51–69.

Colpaert, L., Muller, D., Fayant, M. P., & Butera, F. (2015). A mindset of competition versus cooperation moderates the impact of social comparison on self-evaluation. *Frontiers in Psychology, 6,* 1337.

Crouzevialle, M., & Butera, F. (2013). Performance-approach goals deplete working memory and impair cognitive performance. *Journal of Experimental Psychology: General, 142,* 666–678.

Damon, W., & Phelps, E. (1989). Critical distinctions among three approaches to peer education. *International Journal of Educational Research, 13,* 9–19.

Darnon, C., Buchs, C., & Butera, F. (2002). Epistemic and relational conflict in sharing information during cooperative learning. *Swiss Journal of Psychology, 61,* 139–151.

Darnon, C., & Butera, F. (2007). Learning or succeeding?: Conflict regulation with mastery or performance goals. *Swiss Journal of Psychology, 66,* 145–152.

Darnon, C., Butera, F., & Harackiewicz, J. (2007). Achievement goals in social interactions: Learning within a mastery vs. performance goal. *Motivation and Emotion, 31,* 61–70.

Darnon, C., Butera, F., & Mugny, G. (2008). *Des conflits pour apprendre* [Conflicts for learning]. Grenoble, France: Presses Universitaires de Grenoble.

Darnon, C., Doll, S., & Butera, F. (2007). Dealing with a disagreeing partner: Relational and epistemic conflict elaboration. *European Journal of Psychology of Education, 22,* 227–242.

Darnon, C., Dompnier, B., & Poortvliet, M. (2012). Achievement goals in educational contexts: A social psychology perspective. *Social and Personality Psychology Compass, 6,* 760–771.

Darnon, C., Harackiewicz, J., Butera, F., Mugny, G., & Quiamzade, A. (2007). Performance-approach and performance-avoidance goals:

When uncertainty makes a difference. *Personality and Social Psychology Bulletin, 33,* 813–827.

Darnon, C., Muller, D., Schrager, S., Pannuzzo, N., & Butera, F. (2006). Mastery and performance goals predict epistemic and relational conflict regulation. *Journal of Educational Psychology, 98,* 766–776.

Deci, E. L., & Moller, A. C. (2005). The concept of competence: A starting place for understanding intrinsic motivation and self-determined extrinsic motivation. In A. J. Elliot & C. S. Dweck (Eds.), *Handbook of competence and motivation* (pp. 579–597). New York: Guilford Press.

Deci, E. L., & Ryan, R. M. (2000). The "what" and "why" of goal pursuits: Human needs and the self-determination of behavior. *Psychological Inquiry, 11,* 227–268.

Doise, W., & Mugny, G. (1979). Individual and collective conflicts of centrations in cognitive development. *European Journal of Social Psychology, 9,* 105–108.

Doise, W., & Mugny, G. (1984). *The social development of the intellect.* Oxford, UK: Pergamon Press.

Dompnier, B., Darnon, C., & Butera, F. (2009). Faking the desire to learn: A clarification of the link between mastery goals and academic achievement. *Psychological Science, 20,* 939–943.

Dompnier, B., Darnon, C., Meier, E., Brandner, C., Smeding, A., & Butera, F. (2015). Improving low achievers' academic performance at university by changing the social value of mastery goals. *American Education Research Journal, 52,* 720–749.

Dweck, C. S. (1986). Motivational processes affecting learning. *American Psychologist, 41,* 1040–1048.

Elliot, A. J., & Church, M. A. (1997). A hierarchical model of approach and avoidance achievement motivation. *Journal of Personality and Social Psychology, 72,* 218–232.

Elliot, A. J., & Harackiewicz, J. M. (1996). Approach and avoidance achievement goals and intrinsic motivation: A mediational analysis. *Journal of Personality and Social Psychology, 70,* 461–475.

Elliot, A. J., & McGregor, H. A. (2001). A 2 × 2 achievement goal framework. *Journal of Personality and Social Psychology, 80,* 501–519.

Elliot, A. J., Murayama, K., & Pekrun, R. (2011). A 3 × 2 achievement goal model. *Journal of Educational Psychology, 103,* 632–648.

Festinger, L. (1954). A theory of social comparison processes. *Human Relations, 7,* 117–140.

Festinger, L. (1957). *A theory of cognitive dissonance.* Evanston, IL: Row & Peterson.

Friend, R. M., & Gilbert, J. (1973). Threat and fear of negative evaluation as determinants of locus of social comparison. *Journal of Personality, 41,* 328–340.

Guimond, S. (2001). Epistemic authorities in higher education: The relative influence of peers, faculty and courses on attitude formation and change. In F. Butera & G. Mugny (Eds.), *Social influence in social reality* (pp. 211–223). Göttingen, Germany: Hogrefe & Huber.

Hakmiller, K. L. (1966). Threat as a determinant of downward comparison. *Journal of Experimental Social Psychology, 1*(1), 32–39.

Huguet, P., Dumas, F., Monteil, J.-M., & Genestoux, N. (2001). Social comparison choices in the classroom: Further evidence for students' upward comparison tendency and its beneficial impact on performance. *European Journal of Social Psychology, 31,* 557–578.

Hulleman, C. S., Schrager, S. M., Bodmann, S. M., & Harackiewicz, J. M. (2010). A meta-analytic review of achievement goal measures: Different labels for the same constructs or different constructs with similar labels? *Psychological Bulletin, 136,* 422–449.

Janis, I. L. (1982). *Groupthink: Psychological studies of policy decisions and fiascoes* (2nd ed.). Boston: Houghton Mifflin.

Johnson, D. W. (2015). *Constructive controversy: Theory, research, practice.* Cambridge, UK: Cambridge University Press.

Johnson-Laird, P. N. (1983). *Mental models: Towards a cognitive science of language, inference, and consciousness.* Cambridge, MA: Harvard University Press.

Kasser, T., Cohn, S., Kanner, A. D., & Ryan, R. M. (2007). Some costs of American corporate capitalism: A psychological exploration of value and goal conflicts. *Psychological Inquiry, 18,* 1–22.

Maehr, M. L. (1989). Thoughts about motivation. In C. Ames & R. Ames (Eds.), *Research on motivation in education: Goals and cognitions* (Vol. 3, pp. 299–315). San Diego, CA: Academic Press.

Maggi, J., Butera, F., & Mugny, G. (1996). Conflict of incompetences: Direct and indirect influences on representation of the centimetre. *International Review of Social Psychology, 9,* 91–105.

Martin, L. L., & Tesser, A. (1996). Some ruminative thoughts. In R. S. Wyer, Jr. (Ed.), *Ruminative thoughts: Advances in social cognition* (Vol. 9, pp. 1–47). Mahwah, NJ: Erlbaum.

Meece, J. L., Anderman, E. M., & Anderman, L. H. (2006). Classroom goal structure, student motivation and academic achievement. *Annual Review of Psychology, 57,* 487–503.

Midgley, C., & Maehr, M. (1999). Using motivation theory to guide school reform. In A. J. Reynolds, H. J. Walberg, & R. P. Weissberg (Eds.), *Promoting positive outcomes: Issues in children's and families' lives* (pp. 129–159). Washington, DC: Child Welfare League.

Morse, S., & Gergen, K. J. (1970). Social comparison, self-consistency, and the concept of self. *Journal of Personality and Social Psychology, 16,* 148–156.

Moscovici, S. (1980). Toward a theory of conversion behavior. In L. Berkowitz (Ed.), *Advances in experimental social psychology* (Vol. 13, pp. 209–239). New York: Academic Press.

Mugny, G., Butera, F., & Falomir, J. M. (2001). Social influence and threat in social comparison between self and source's competence: Relational factors affecting the transmission of knowledge. In F. Butera & G. Mugny (Eds.), *Social influence in social reality* (pp. 225–237). Bern, Germany: Hogrefe & Huber.

Mugny, G., & Doise, W. (1978). Socio-cognitive conflict and structure of individual and collective performances. *European Journal of Social Psychology, 8,* 181–192.

Mugny, G., Tafani, E., Butera, F., & Pigière, D. (1998). Contrainte et dépendance informationnelles: Influence sociale sur la représentation du groupe d'amis idéal [Informational constraint and dependence: Social influence on the representation of the ideal group of friends]. *Connexions, 72,* 55–72.

Muller, D., Atzeni, T. & Butera, F. (2004). Coaction and upward social comparison reduce the illusory conjunction effect: Some support for distraction-conflict theory. *Journal of Experimental Social Psychology, 40,* 659–665.

Muller, D., & Butera, F. (2007). The distracting effect of self-evaluation threat in coaction and social comparison. *Journal of Personality and Social Psychology, 93,* 194–211.

Muller, D., & Fayant, M. P. (2010). On being exposed to superior others: Consequences of self-threatening upward social comparisons. *Social and Personality Psychology Compass, 4,* 621–634.

Murayama, K., & Elliot, A. J. (2012). The competition–performance relation: A meta-analytic review and test of the opposing processes model of competition and performance. *Psychological Bulletin, 138,* 1035–1070.

Mussweiler, T. (2003). Comparison processes in social judgment: Mechanisms and consequences. *Psychological Review, 110,* 472–489.

Nicholls, J. G. (1984). Achievement motivation: Conceptions of ability, subjective experience, task choice, and performance. *Psychological Review, 91,* 328–346.

Pérez, J. A., & Mugny, G. (1996). The conflict elaboration theory of social influence. In E. H. Witte & J. H. Davis (Eds.), *Understanding group behavior: Vol. 2. Small group processes and interpersonal relations* (pp. 191–210). Hillsdale, NJ: Erlbaum.

Piaget, J. (1985). *The equilibration of cognitive structures: The central problem of intellectual development.* Chicago: University of Chicago Press. (Original work published 1975)

Pintrich, P., & Schunk, D. (2002). *Motivation in education: Theory, research, and applications.* Upper Saddle River, NJ: Merrill/Prentice Hall.

Plaut, V. C., & Markus, H. R. (2005). The "inside story": A cultural–historical analysis of being smart and motivated, American style. In A. J. Elliot & C. S. Dweck (Eds.), *Handbook of competence and motivation* (pp. 457–488). New York: Guilford Press.

Psaltis, C., & Duveen, G. (2006). Social relations and cognitive development: The influence of conversation type and representations of gender. *European Journal of Social Psychology, 36,* 407–430.

Quiamzade, A., & Mugny, G. (2009). Social influence and threat in confrontations between competent peers. *Journal of Personality and Social Psychology, 97,* 652–666.

Quiamzade, A., Mugny, G., & Butera, F. (2013). *Psychologie sociale de la connaissance: Fondements théoriques* [Social psychology of knowledge: Theoretical foundations]. Grenoble, France: Presses Universitaires de Grenoble.

Salovey, P., & Rodin, J. (1984). Some antecedents and consequences of social-comparison jealousy. *Journal of Personality and Social Psychology, 47,* 780–792.

Schmader, T., & Johns, M. (2003). Converging evidence that stereotype threat reduces working memory capacity. *Journal of Personality and Social Psychology, 85,* 440–452.

Schwarz, N., & Bless, H. (2007). Mental construal processes: The inclusion/exclusion model. In D. A. Stapel & J. M. Suls (Eds.), *Assimilation and contrast in social psychology* (pp. 119–141). New York: Psychology Press.

Segal, J., & Smith, M. (2015). Conflict resolution skills. Retrieved from *www.helpguide. org/articles/relationships/conflict-resolution-skills.htm#resources.*

Senko, C., Hulleman, C. S., & Harackiewicz, J. M. (2011). Achievement goal theory at the crossroads: Old controversies, current challenges, and new directions. *Educational Psychologist, 46,* 26–47.

Smith, R. H. (2000). Assimilative and contrastive emotional reactions to upward and downward social comparison. In J. Suls & L. Wheeler (Eds.), *Handbook of social comparison* (pp. 173–200). New York: Kluwer Academic.

Smith, W. P., & Sachs, P. R. (1997). Social comparison and task prediction: Ability similarity and the use of a proxy. *British Journal of Social Psychology, 36,* 587–602.

Sommet, N., Darnon, C., & Butera, F. (2015). To confirm or to conform?: Performance goals as a regulator of conflict with more competent others. *Journal of Educational Psychology, 107,* 580–598.

Sommet, N., Darnon, C., Mugny, G., Quiamzade, A., Pulfrey, C., Dompnier, B., et al. (2014). Performance goals in conflictual social interactions: Toward the distinction between two modes of relational conflict regulation. *British Journal of Social Psychology, 53,* 134–153.

Steele, C. M. (1988). The psychology of self-affirmation: Sustaining the integrity of the self. In L. Berkowitz (Ed.), *Advances in experimental social psychology* (Vol. 21, pp. 261–302). San Diego, CA: Academic Press.

Suls, J., & Wheeler, L. (2000). A selective history of classic and neo-social comparison theory. In J. Suls & L. Wheeler (Eds.), *Handbook of social comparison* (pp. 3–19). New York: Kluwer Academic.

Taylor, S. E., & Brown, J. D. (1988). Illusion and well-being: A social psychological perspective on mental health. *Psychological Bulletin, 103,* 193–210.

Taylor, S. E., & Lobel, M. (1989). Social comparison activity under threat: Downward evaluation and upward contacts. *Psychological Review, 96,* 569–575.

Taylor, S. E., Neter, E., & Wayment, H. A. (1995). Self-evaluation processes. *Personality and Social Psychology Bulletin, 21,* 1278–1287.

Tesser, A. (1988). Toward a self-evaluation maintenance model of social behavior. In L. Berkowitz (Ed.), *Advances in experimental social psychology* (Vol. 21, pp. 181–227). San Diego, CA: Academic Press.

Tesser, A. (2000). On the confluence of self-esteem maintenance mechanisms. *Personality and Social Psychology Review, 4,* 290–299.

Tesser, A., Millar, M., & Moore, J. (1988). Some affective consequences of social comparison and reflection processes: The pain and pleasure of being close. *Journal of Personality and Social Psychology, 54,* 49–61.

Toma, C., & Butera, F. (2009). Hidden profiles and concealed information: Strategic information sharing and use in group decision making. *Personality and Social Psychology Bulletin, 35,* 793–806.

Treisman, A. (1998). Feature binding, attention and object perception. *Philosophical Transactions of the Royal Society of London B: Biological Sciences, 353,* 1295–1306.

Van Yperen, N. W., Blaga, M., & Postmes, T. (2014). A meta-analysis of self-reported achievement goals and nonself-report performance across three achievement domains (work, sports, and education). *PLoS ONE, 9,* e93594.

Wason, P. C. (1960). On the failure to eliminate hypotheses in a conceptual task. *Quarterly Journal of Experimental Psychology, 12,* 129–140.

Wheeler, L., Martin, R., & Suls, J. (1997). The proxy model of social comparison for self-assessment of ability. *Personality and Social Psychology Review, 1,* 54–61.

Wheeler, L., & Suls, J. (2005). Social comparison and self-evaluations of competence. In A. J. Elliot & C. S. Dweck (Eds.), *Handbook of competence and motivation* (pp. 566–578). New York: Guilford Press.

White, R. W. (1959). Motivation reconsidered: The concept of competence. *Psychological Review, 66,* 297–333.

Wills, T. A. (1981). Downward comparison principles in social psychology. *Psychological Bulletin, 90,* 245–271.

Wood, J. V., Taylor, S. E., & Lichtman, R. (1985). Social comparison in adjustement to breast cancer. *Journal of Personality and Social Psychology, 49,* 1169–1183.

CHAPTER 12

Competence as Central, but Not Sufficient, for High-Quality Motivation
A Self-Determination Theory Perspective

RICHARD M. RYAN
ARLEN C. MOLLER

Every motivational theory in psychology emphasizes perceived competence as playing a central role in intentional behaviors. The feeling or expectation that one *can* successfully perform an action or achieve is rightly seen as an important, even necessary, element in goal-directed activities (e.g., Bandura, 1989). Furthermore, the satisfaction of being competent or effective can itself be a motivation for learning and achievement (Deci & Ryan, 1985; Koestner & McClelland, 1990; White, 1959). In the case of intrinsically motivated actions, for example, feelings of competence can play a strong proximate role in energizing behaviors, and can even be an explicit reason for acting (Deci, 1975; Elliot & McGregor, 2001).

Clearly, this is not the case for most activities. The motivation for most behaviors requires more than merely competence expectations—there must be other rewards or satisfactions for behaviors to be energized and maintained. Thus, although competence-focused theorists are no doubt correct in emphasizing that people often gravitate toward activities and domains in which they can experience competence, and

avoid areas in which competence is lacking, this still leaves the explanation of behavioral motivations quite incomplete. There are many behaviors one might perform highly competently that nevertheless hold no interest or value for the individual. One may have the competence to play high-level chess, but find it boring. One might have excellent reading skills and comprehension, yet find novels tedious. Alternatively, many an unskilled photographer can be found prolifically taking photos. In short, any comprehensive theory of motivation needs to consider more than competence to understand why people select and persist at some acts over others. The element of *volition* in behavior—why people choose to do what they do—cannot be explained by focusing on competence alone.

One perspective linking competence and motivation to other satisfactions and incentives is offered by *self-determination theory* (SDT; Ryan & Deci, 2000), which is a macrotheory of human motivation and personality development. SDT distinguishes several basic psychological needs, the satisfaction of which are essential to optimal functioning and well-being. These include a basic *need for competence* (Deci & Ryan, 1985; Elliot & McGregor, 2001), which is a core focus of this volume, as well as needs for *autonomy* and *relatedness* (Deci & Ryan, 2000). Although SDT sees competence as playing a central role in intentional motivation, it provides substantial evidence of the importance of considering all three of these needs in distinguishing the sources and consequences of varied types of human motivation, and explaining why people do what they do.

In this chapter, we (1) outline different types of intrinsically and extrinsically motivated behaviors and their varied consequences; (2) consider how basic psychological needs, including the need for competence, are differentially satisfied in different types of motivated actions; (3) present theoretical predictions and empirical evidence relating basic need satisfaction and thwarting to different forms of human motivation; and (4) investigate several important and common contexts involving competence-related goals and aspirations as they affect persistence, performance, and wellness.

DIFFERING TYPES MOTIVATION AND THEIR CONSEQUENCES

Motivation simply means to be moved to act, but what moves people to act varies greatly from person to person and from situation to situation. People can be moved to act by external rewards and punishments, by internalized pressures and standards, or even by values and interests. Among theories of motivation, SDT is relatively unique in distinguishing different types and subtypes of motivation and self-regulation. The value of making these distinctions is supported by decades of careful SDT research indicating that different types of motivation differentially predict success, perseverance, and emotions in a wide range of achievement and competence-related contexts (Deci & Ryan, 1985, 2011; Ryan & Deci, 2000). To understand how types of motivation produce these varied outcomes, and the role of competence within each, we begin with a taxonomy of motivation as understood within SDT.

Distinguishing Intrinsic and Extrinsic Motivation

An early distinction drawn by SDT contrasts the categories of intrinsic motivation and extrinsic motivation (Deci & Ryan, 1980, 1985). *Intrinsic motivation* is represented by activities in which the individual finds inherent satisfactions; he or she finds the activity interesting and enjoyable in its own right. In this sense, the "rewards" are intrinsic to the activity, which is supported by the fact that intrinsically motivated activities activate reward areas of the brain (e.g., Lee, Reeve, Xue, & Xiong, 2012; Murayama, Matsumoto, Izuma, & Matsumoto, 2010; Ryan & Di Domenico, in press). Functionally, SDT research has shown that what makes intrinsically motivated activities enjoyable are the satisfactions specifically associated with competence and autonomy. Opportunities to exercise and test skills and to self-organize and endorse ones actions—to feel both able and volitional—are the main satisfactions inherent in intrinsically motivated actions. Factors in contexts that disrupt experiences of competence and autonomy therefore undermine intrinsic motivation.

The concept of *extrinsic motivation,* in contrast, concerns all instrumental motivation—motivations whose rewards and incentives for participation are "extrinsic to the activity," though not necessarily external to the person (as in a tangible reward). Within SDT, in fact, extrinsic motivation is recognized as a heterogeneous category of motivation, and includes a range of motivations or forms of self-regulation.

Forms of Extrinsic Motivation

A relatively early extension of SDT involved the subclassification of multiple (four) types of extrinsic motivation that are conceptualized as differing along an *internalization continuum*, ranging from maximally controlled (least autonomous) at one extreme to maximally autonomous and well integrated at the other (Ryan & Connell, 1989; Ryan & Deci, 2000). These subclassifications include external, introjected, identified, and integrated self-regulation.

The most controlled form of extrinsic motivation, *external regulation*, is motivation propelled by external contingencies, such as acts to obtain tangible external rewards (e.g., monetary payments) or to avoid threatened punishments. Here, the activity has an external *perceived locus of causality* (DeCharms, 1968), as the individual experiences his or her behavior as being controlled by the external agent. *Introjected regulation* when an individual controls him- or herself with internal rewards and punishments. Articulations of introjected regulation often involve words such as "should" (as in "I don't really want to, but I really should do _____"). As with external regulation, introjection is characterized by a sense of pressure to act. With introjection, this pressure is experienced internally and is often associated with internal conflict and defenses.

Moving along the internalization continuum, two relatively more autonomous forms of extrinsic motivation are *identified regulation* and *integrated regulation*. Each of these subtypes of self-regulation involve a person being motivated because he or she values the activity, or sees it as contributing to some personally meaningful goal. Thus, identified motivation has an internal perceived locus of causality; it is relatively autonomous. Even more autonomous is integrated regulation; here, the personally meaningful goal is also consistent with other goals and life pursuits the person finds meaningful. The relatively nuanced distinctions between these four forms of extrinsic motivation are illustrated in Figure 12.1a, along with concrete examples of each type of self-regulation in a competence-related context (completing a math problem assigned for homework in Figure 12.1b).

Also included in this SDT taxonomy is a category called *amotivation*, in which the

Amotivation	Controlled Motivation		Autonomous Motivation		
Amotivation	Extrinsic Motivation				Intrinsic Motivation
Amotivation	External Regulation	Introjected Regulation	Identified Regulation	Integrated Regulation	Intrinsic Regulation

←————————— **Internalization Continuum** —————————→

Most Controlled   Most Autonomous

FIGURE 12.1a. Superordinate and subordinate categories of motivation and self-regulation as defined by self-determination theory (SDT).

Amotivation	External Regulation	Introjected Regulation	Identified Regulation	Integrated Regulation	Intrinsic Regulation
Student is not motivated to complete the math problem.	Student's parents will pay $50 for an A in math class. Student wishes to avoid loss of privileges for bad grades.	Student will be ashamed of herself if she doesn't get an A in math class. Student likes to show off skills to feel good about himself.	Student values developing her math skills so she can pursue a career in engineering.	Student values developing his math skills so he can pursue a career in environmental engineering. This career aspiration fits with his wider interest in hiking and promoting environmental sustainability.	The math problem is optimally challenging and novel, and the student finds solving it interesting and enjoyable.

FIGURE 12.1b. Examples of self-regulation of students completing a math problem assigned for homework.

person is unwilling or unable to engage in an action and is therefore neither intrinsically nor extrinsically motivated. Most theories of lack of motivation focus exclusively on helplessness and external locus of control, suggesting that amotivation is mainly a result of a lack competence or positive efficacy expectations. Yet SDT, which is concerned with volition, also sees amotivation as sometimes resulting from another source—lack of interest or value. This is equally important as an explanation because an absence of autonomy to act can be just as amotivating as a lack of competence. Effectively intervening in situations where people lack motivation, in fact, requires distinguishing these two sources of unmotivated (amotivated) behavior.

Although for many research purposes one can focus on these specific types of motivation, a more broad-stroke distinction within SDT is to sort these subtypes into three larger categories of motivation: *autonomous, controlled,* and *amotivated.* Autonomous motivation includes identified, integrated, and intrinsic regulation; controlled motivation includes external and introjected regulation; and amotivated is yet a third category (see Figure 12.1a).

Rationale for Distinguishing Different Types and Subtypes of Motivation and Regulation

Researchers working within the SDT framework have developed a variety of measures and methods to assess these types and subtypes of motivation and self-regulation in a wide range of contexts, including academic and professional work settings, and in relation to prosocial behavior, health care, learning, exercise, sports, religion, politics, work, and friendship. Collectively, the findings from this research literature show first that individuals can be strongly motivated by either autonomous or controlled forms of motivation. Yet there are distinct consequences. More autonomous forms of motivation are associated with more positive emotions accompanying the activity in question, more creative output, deeper processing of information, and more sustainable persistence. In contrast, more controlled forms of motivation tend to predict more negative emotions (i.e., anxiety and tension)

accompanying an activity, shallower processing of information, and higher rates of burnout (Deci & Ryan, 2014; Ryan & Deci, 2000).

BASIC PSYCHOLOGICAL NEEDS

SDT has further postulated the existence of various basic psychological needs, including competence, as satisfactions that are both differentially associated with the varied forms of motivation we outlined earlier, and predictive of the qualities of action and experience associated with them (Chen et al., 2015; Deci & Ryan, 1985, 2011; Ryan & Deci, 2000, 2008). The experience of psychological need satisfaction can be assessed at multiple levels of analysis, including at the state-level in a particular moment (e.g., a single tennis match), averaged across experiences while performing a particular activity (e.g., playing tennis in general), with a particular person, in particular contexts (e.g., playing sports), or even aggregated across one's entire life (e.g., "in my life"). Need satisfaction is even implicated in the structure of people's episodic memories for events (Philippe, Koestner, Beaulieu-Pelletier, Lecours, & Lekes., 2012). Furthermore, psychological need satisfaction plays both a proximate role in the motivation of behavior (producing state-level positive affect, interest, and enjoyment) and a more pervasive role in long-term health and development (producing greater satisfaction with life, personality integration, and growth); that is, the satisfaction of basic psychological needs robustly predicts mental and physical health (Ratelle & Duchesne, 2014; Ryan, Deci, & Vansteenkiste, 2016).

The term *basic* refers to the assertion that these needs are functionally critical elements in organismic thriving and wellness. As such, a sometimes controversial feature of SDT involves the assertion that all people share these basic psychological needs. This assertion that basic needs are universal, however, includes a recognition that the satisfaction of basic needs (internal experiences) can be accomplished in varied ways through different cultural forms (Chen et al., 2015). Nonetheless, the theory suggests that lacking autonomy, competence, or relatedness in any activity or domain of activity has detectable costs for both quality of motivation and well-being.

Defining a Basic Need for Competence

SDT's definition of a basic need for competence can be traced back to White's (1959) seminal work introducing the concept of *effectance motivation*. White used the term *competence* to connote people's capacity to interact effectively with their environment—to understand the effects they have on the environment and the effects the environment has on them. According to White, to attain greater competence defines human development. Importantly, White also emphasized that effectance motivation is not drive-derivative; rather he speculated that competence-promoting behavior "satisfies *an intrinsic need* to deal with the environment" (p. 318, emphasis added), behavior that is persistent and "occupies the spare waking time between episodes of homeostatic crisis" (p. 321).

Consistent with White's conceptualization of effectance motivation, SDT posits that the need for competence is evident in people's seeking out and mastering challenges, and finding experiences of mastery and effectiveness to be intrinsically rewarding (Deci & Ryan, 1985; Moller & Elliot, 2009). The concept helps to explain a variety of activities that fall under categories including play, exploration, and manipulation of novel stimuli or environments, as people simply enjoy the experience of challenging themselves and exercising new capacities.

It may also be helpful to distinguish the concept of competence need satisfaction as employed in SDT from the concept of *self-efficacy*, a centerpiece of social-cognitive theory (SCT; Bandura, 1977, 1997). In SCT, self-efficacy "refers to beliefs in one's capabilities to organize and execute the courses of action required to produce given attainments" (Bandura, 1997, p. 3). Thus, whereas competence need satisfaction concerns the intrinsic satisfaction a person feels when effectively meeting a challenge, self-efficacy is a cognition that concerns the degree to which a person believes (accurately or not)

that he or she has the power to be effective in the future. As such, someone might report very high self-efficacy for an easy task; yet in such a circumstance, SDT would not expect positive feedback to enhance feelings of competence. In general, people do not enjoy masterfully completing very easy tasks (e.g., an adult completing a puzzle designed for a small child); correspondingly, these experiences would not satisfy their needs for competence. Studies by Rodgers, Markland, Selzer, Murray, and Wilson (2014) have shown that measures of self-efficacy and competence satisfaction have both unique and overlapping variance in motivation, with self-efficacy measures generally moderately associated with perceived competence, but unrelated to either autonomy or relatedness need satisfactions.

Defining a Basic Need for Autonomy

A second basic psychological need identified within SDT is the need for autonomy. At its core, the experience of autonomy need satisfaction is defined by wholeheartedly or congruently endorsing one's action(s). This psychological experience has alternatively been referred to as feeling choiceful and "ownership" of one's actions, and by the absence of feeling controlled or coerced by internal or external forces (e.g., by guilt and shame, or by externally controlled rewards and punishments, respectively).

It is especially noteworthy that in earlier theoretical formulations by White (1959), Angyal (1941), de Charms (1968), and Deci (1971, 1975), the two needs for competence and autonomy were essentially treated as a single need, and it was not until 1980 that Deci and Ryan argued for the utility of distinguishing these competence and autonomy needs to better account for emerging experimental evidence. In the decades since, evidence for the utility of articulating this distinction has accumulated, and this literature is a central focus of this chapter. Clearly, people can experience some behaviors as within their competence, yet have no willingness or volition to perform them. Conversely, one might have a willingness to act in some contexts, yet lack the ability or confidence to do so.

Defining a Basic Need for Relatedness

A third basic psychological need included in SDT is the need for relatedness. The satisfaction of this need involves feeling a sense of connection with other human beings, and of mutual trust and concern for others' well-being; this need includes a desire to form and maintain strong, stable social bonds over time (Baumeister & Leary, 1995; Deci & Ryan, 2011; Maslow, 1954/1987). SDT first argues that relatedness, like competence and autonomy, is an intrinsic satisfaction, explaining, for example, the enhancements in wellness associated with merely connecting with others, even without benefits (e.g., Ryan & Hawley, 2016). SDT further argues that people gravitate toward and more readily internalize practices and values embraced by those with whom they experience (or wish to experience) more relatedness.

THE ROLE OF BASIC NEEDS, INCLUDING COMPETENCE, IN DIFFERENT TYPES OF MOTIVATION

Different types of motivations satisfy each of these basic needs to different degrees. Indeed, the qualities and persistence of motivation associated with each type of regulation detailed by SDT reveal the differential role of basic needs in each.

First consider *intrinsic motivation,* which is a type of motivation characterized by high satisfaction of both autonomy and competence needs. In fact, both are necessary for intrinsic motivation to occur when intrinsically motivated people enjoy the exercise of their abilities and capacities. Yet, they are only intrinsically motivated when they also feel autonomous. SDT uniquely shows, using both experimental and field data, how factors that undermine autonomy functionally undermine intrinsic motivation (Deci & Moller, 2005; Moller & Deci, 2014; Ryan & Deci, 2013).

We now turn to the various forms of extrinsic motivation. First, consider the most classic form of extrinsic motivation, *external regulation,* in which one is motivated by externally controlled rewards and punishments. For example, a child who does

homework to avoid parental wrath, or to get a tangible contingent reward, is externally regulated. Here, the perceived locus of causality is likely to be external, and the child's sense of autonomy is low. The child experiences the behavior as driven or controlled by others, rather than as something he or she wants to do. With external regulation, motivation is therefore dependent on the proximal salience of the external contingencies (e.g., so long as the parent is standing over the child, motivation for doing homework may be very high). Furthermore, because the work is done for the rewards, it will likely be done in a minimally sufficient manner; in external regulation one takes the shortest route to the outcome. Here, one is unlikely to stretch or push the limits of one's competence, as there is no motivation to do so. Indeed, when behavior is externally regulated, effort and engagement, and quality of output tend to be minimal, and felt competence need satisfactions are therefore low (e.g., in elementary school children: Katz, Eilot, & Nevo, 2014; in medical students: Kusurkar, Ten Cate, Vos, Westers, & Croiset, 2013; in high school and college students: Taylor et al., 2014). Finally, because the person feels controlled by the other, relatedness satisfactions are also often absent or diminished. Feeling controlled tends to disrupt rather than support feelings of relatedness (Deci, La Guardia, Moller, Scheiner, & Ryan, 2006; Soenens, Sierens, Vansteenkiste, Dochy, & Goossens, 2012).

Introjected regulation is more complex in relation to basic need satisfactions. People introject regulations because, ultimately, they seek to please or receive approval from important others. They attempt to live up to the standards they perceive the others to have. Thus, introjection relies on a desire to be connected with the other. It is the child who is desperate for parental approval who feels guilty or bad when performing poorly. It is the athlete who wants coaches' approval, and is most internally driven by those expectations. In introjection, then, developing and exhibiting competence is not intrinsically satisfying, but it is instrumental to getting the self- or other approval one seeks (Assor, Roth, & Deci, 2004). Introjected regulation is therefore a controlled form of motivation, absent of or even thwarting autonomy need satisfaction.

Identified and integrated forms of regulation, in contrast, entail a strong sense of autonomy. In these forms of motivation, there is a personal value for the action, and one therefore feels autonomy in engagement. In addition, personal value supports the desire to do the behaviors well and to be competent in enacting them. Effort and interest therefore characterize identified regulations. Finally, identifications are based in values that often are highly social in nature; therefore, there is no antithesis between autonomy and relatedness in these forms of regulation. Often, the things people identify with and value most are indeed values of caring and connecting with others. A person who identifies with and values contributing to community, for example, will feel autonomy, competence, and relatedness in such actions.

Finally, we mentioned several forms of amotivation. One is based in lack of efficacy or even helplessness. Here, no basic psychological needs are satisfied. One lacks a sense of competence, one lacks relatedness, and there is no autonomy. However, lack of motivation can also stem from lack of value. Here, one might actually have self-efficacy but simply not want to engage in action. Here, too, no competence need satisfactions are derived, although one can sometimes feel autonomous in electing not to act (Vansteenkiste, Lens, De Witte, De Witte, & Deci, 2004), for example, when workers decide to go on strike and not work. People may also feel controlled when electing not to act, for example, in cases of oppositional defiance (Van Petegem, Soenens, Vansteenkiste, & Beyers, 2015). In summary, types of amotivation are distinguished by different mixes of competence, relatedness, and autonomy need satisfactions.

SDT's differentiated taxonomy of motivations is thus systematically connected with patterns of basic need satisfactions. In amotivation, little or no need satisfactions need be entailed. In external regulation one is motivated to get rewards or avoid aversive contingencies. Doing so may engender feelings of competence (though often impoverished ones), but not autonomy or relatedness.

In introjection, one needs both some sense of competence and (at least desire for) relatedness, but autonomy is low. Finally, in identified and integrated motivations, all three needs can be satisfied—which helps explain why these autonomous forms of motivation are associated with the highest quality of behaviors (sustainability, depth of processing, creativity) and positive experience.

The Satisfaction of Basic Psychological Needs Is Mutually Supportive

Looking with hindsight, one of the factors that likely contributed to early theorists' conflating the needs for competence and autonomy concerns the empirically supported observation that satisfaction of basic psychological needs often seems to be synergistic or mutually supportive. For example, de Charms (1968) wrote that "man's primary motivational propensity is to be effective in producing changes in his environment. Man strives to be a causal agent, . . . to experience personal causation" (p. 269). In conflating the needs for competence and autonomy, he was correctly pointing out that competence need satisfaction supports autonomy need satisfaction.

We would argue that the reverse is equally true; that is, autonomy need satisfaction supports competence need satisfaction. Indeed, patterns of reciprocal or mutually supportive relations between different psychological needs have been observed across a wide range of contexts. As a result, at increasingly global units of analysis (i.e., aggregating across time or contexts), researchers tend to finding increasingly stronger correlations between basic needs; thus, it is more common for investigators to use basic psychological need satisfaction as a single construct (Milyavskaya, Philippe, & Koestner, 2013). By contrast, at smaller and more elemental units of analysis—as in a specific situation or moment (Ryan, Bernstein, & Brown, 2010), or when one is with a specific partner (e.g., La Guardia, Ryan, Couchman, & Deci., 2000; Lynch, La Guardia, & Ryan, 2009)—factor analyses support a three-factor solution (Brown & Ryan, 2006; Deci & Ryan, 2011; Johnston & Finney, 2010).

Competing Needs

Another contribution of SDT has been to point out that not only does the relative satisfaction of different needs vary from situation-to-situation, but many situations pit the satisfaction of different basic psychological needs against each other. Under such circumstances, SDT predicts that even the need that is prioritized will be satisfied in a degraded, less than optimal way. A poignant example of this from the research literature concerns the case of children who are subjected to "parental conditional regard" (PCR; see Roth, Assor, Niemiec, Ryan, & Deci, 2009), a socializing strategy that is used, and sometimes even strongly endorsed by parents, to promote achievement. It involves providing affection especially when a child meets the parents' standards of behavior (e.g., getting A's in school; a common competence-related goal), and withholding affection when the child does not. Under these conditions, children must essentially choose between satisfying their need for relatedness (e.g., love from their parent) and competence (e.g., by performing well in school) or experience autonomy (e.g., by resisting the manipulative pressures). Research indicates that children exposed to PCR pay significant costs in terms of the quality of satisfaction experienced with respect to all three needs. For example, Assor and colleagues (2004) found that college students' perceptions of their mothers' and fathers' having used conditional regard in four domains (including academic achievement) was positively associated with behavioral enactment, yet with costs to children's self-esteem, a greater sense of parental disapproval, and a continuing resentment of parents.

In short, numerous programs of research have demonstrated the individual contributions of the three basic needs identified by SDT (autonomy, competence, and relatedness) toward predicting well-being and quality of motivation (Reis, Sheldon, Gable, Roscoe, & Ryan, 2000; Sheldon & Filak, 2008; Sheldon, Ryan, & Reis, 1996). These studies all suggest that for people to experience energy and well-being as they engage in motivated behaviors, a sense of efficacy or competence is not enough.

CONTEXTUAL FACTORS THAT PROMOTE OPTIMAL COMPETENCE NEED SATISFACTION

As described earlier, the optimal conditions for satisfying a person's basic need for competence typically involve finding activities that are both volitional and well suited to stretching one's ability (i.e., optimal challenges). Activities vary not only in terms of not only how challenging they are, but also in their flexibility with regard to affording variable levels of challenge and sources of feedback as individuals' gain experience and skills over time. Activities that afford variability in levels of challenge generally have greater potential for sustaining long-term engagement and deeper, more intrinsically rewarding need satisfactions.

SDT argues that the feedback and structures in most achievement contexts have both informational and controlling elements (Deci & Ryan, 1980, 2011). *Informational elements* are those that provide effectance-relevant feedback and therefore speak directly to the satisfaction of a person's need for competence. Informational feedback can vary in terms of source (task-oriented, self-oriented, or normative), level of refinement, and timing or responsiveness. Yet, in general, more refined and responsive feedback is most effective for enhancing feelings of competence (Rigby & Ryan, 2011). Yet feedback within many contexts can also communicate pressure toward specified outcomes, and have controlling salience. SDT predicts that even successfully meeting challenges in controlling contexts will feel less satisfying, engender less work and life satisfaction, and less sustained high-quality engagement over time.

Standards and Yardsticks

The standards, metrics, or "yardsticks" used to assess and provide feedback about competence can take a variety of forms. A *task-oriented standard of competence* involves focusing on elements of the activity itself. Some activities have task-oriented standards of success; for example, a Rubik's cube or crossword puzzle can be completed to varying degrees that are visually apparent;

similarly, a particular mountain can be scaled to varying degrees. Task-oriented standards are naturally employed in development, as illustrated by young children at play (a prototypical example of intrinsic motivation). Here, the activities of play themselves provide immediate and self-evident success and failure feedback. *Self-oriented standards of competence* involve comparing one's past performance at a given activity with one's current performance. Informational feedback based on self-oriented standards has the advantage of being potentially more refined (e.g., one might summit the same mountain in more or less time on consecutive attempts), and does not carry some of the controlling features of social comparisons. Yet self-related comparisons can be used either informationally (as competence feedback) or controllingly (as a basis for self-disparagement or self-inflation), as is common in perfectionism (Soenens et al., 2008).

A third type of competence yardstick offers even more vulnerability to having controlling significance, namely, *normative standards,* in which feedback is focused on one's performance relative to that of other people. Examples of normative feedback include percentile rankings on the Graduate Record Exam (GRE), posted finishing times, and ranks after a marathon.

As understood within SDT, the issue with normative feedback is its motivational significance to the recipient. In some circumstances, normatively focused feedback can be *informational,* helping the learner gage improvement. This is especially easy when the comparative information is impersonal and not ego-threatening (e.g., pinball board scores). Many video games have been engineered to provide responsive, refined feedback about competence using multiple standards, including normative data, thereby promoting high levels of competence need satisfaction and intrinsic motivation (Przybylski, Rigby, & Ryan, 2010; Rigby & Ryan, 2011). However normative comparisons can also have *controlling* significance and readily engender both ego-involvement and self-esteem concerns (Ryan, 1982). In extreme cases they can be a focus of obsessive self-control and rigid self-regulation (Ryan et al., 2016; Soenens, Vansteenkiste, Duriez, & Goossens, 2006). Here, again,

SDT highlights the importance of distinguishing between the controlled pursuit of competence ("I have to outperform others") and the informational use of normative comparisons in gauging volitional progress (see also Vallerand, 2015). In general, emphasis on normatively oriented standards of competence, relative to task- and self-oriented standards, runs a higher risk of being experienced as evaluative and controlling.

Achievement Goals

A widely researched issue related to source of feedback is the distinction between performance- and mastery-focused goals. *Mastery goals* are those on which the focus is on enhancing one's own competence (i.e., using task- or self-oriented standards); *performance goals* focus on performing well relative to others (i.e., normatively oriented standards) (Elliot, Murayama, & Pekrun, 2011). Both mastery and performance goals can be further differentiated into approach and avoidance types (Elliot & McGregor, 2001; Murayama, Elliot, & Friedman, 2012). A good deal of evidence suggests that whereas mastery goals have many adaptive aspects, performance goals can be problematic. For example, whereas performance-approach goals have been associated with improved performance, performance-avoidance goals are linked with greater susceptibility to helplessness and poorer well-being (Elliot, 2005; Elliot & Moller, 2003).

Applying SDT's concepts of autonomous and controlled motives to these achievement goals allows a fuller understanding of such effects. SDT specifically suggests that performance goals have a higher probability of stemming from, and/or engendering, controlled motivations. In contrast, mastery goals are much more likely to be associated with autonomous pursuits. In line with this, Vansteenkiste and colleagues (2010) showed that although performance-approach goals sometimes predict positive educational outcomes, this is largely mediated by the autonomous versus controlled motives people have for pursuing these goals. In other words, the effects of performance-approach goals were largely accounted for by the autonomous or controlled motives underlying them. Research by Vansteenkiste, Lens,

Elliot, Soenens, and Mouratidis (2014) has similarly supported this idea. Assessing both the strength of performance-approach goals and the motives for pursuing them across several studies using SDT's distinctions, they found that distinguishing autonomous and controlled motives for goal pursuits helped substantially in accounting for goal-related outcomes.

Extending this idea, Benita, Roth, and Deci (2014) examined autonomous versus controlled motivations in relation to mastery(-approach) goals. Their results showed that when students adopted mastery goals in autonomy-supportive contexts, they were associated with more interest and engagement than when these goals were adopted in controlling contexts. Thus, research is increasingly suggesting that people's motives for pursuing achievement goals are more critical to understanding the goals' effects than are the goals themselves (see also Gillet, Lafrenière, Huyghebaert, & Fouquereau, 2015).

The practical importance of these theoretical ideas is manifold. For example, consider that the grading schemes so widely used in education are typically activating (indeed, intended to activate) performance-based goals and, more importantly, often feel like forms of external regulation. When applied in classrooms, these performance-based goals can affect students strongly, and unlike most laboratory experiments, many students do poorly at the goal and receive negative feedback. In SDT terms, when normative goals are experienced as controlling, they negatively affect *both* autonomy and competence, and can diminish both motivation and performance (Grolnick & Ryan, 1987). For example, Pulfrey, Buchs, and Butera (2011) examined what happened to students when they expected to be graded, and found that it resulted in lower autonomy and a greater tendency to adopt performance-avoidance goals.

Interpersonal Context

Often, information about competence is conveyed by a person (e.g., parent, teacher, coach, or boss), and how he or she conveys it influences the quality of need satisfaction. Specifically, when the interpersonal source

of competence-related information has a history of having been controlling, individuals tend to have more controlled motivation in their pursuit of competence, and are at greater risk for burnout. This pattern has been observed in many contexts, including with parents in relation to children's self-regulation and competence in school (Grolnick & Ryan, 1989), with teachers in relation to elementary-, high school-, undergraduate-, and graduate-level student education (Hagger & Chatzisarantis, 2016; Roth, 2014; Taylor et al., 2014), with coaches in relation to athletes' performance in competitive sports or students in physical education (Adie, Duda, & Ntoumanis, 2012; Jõesaar, Hein, & Hagger, 2012; Standage & Ryan, 2012; Van den Berghe, Vansteenkiste, Cardon, Kirk, & Haerens, 2014), and with managers in relation to people's achievement in the workplace (Deci & Ryan, 2014).

Tangible Rewards

In some contexts, leaders attempt to convey competence-related information through the provision of tangible rewards. Often, tangible rewards involve money, as in raises at work, bonuses, grants, and so on, but tangible rewards also include things like trophies and prizes (food or merchandise). Intuitively, many people assume that receiving a tangible reward in recognition of competence would be uniformly positive in terms of its affective and motivational consequences—and to the extent that rewards provide informational feedback, indeed, such rewards can support competence need satisfaction and promote intrinsic motivation. Yet tangible rewards often set off a parallel psychological process that involves diminishing autonomy (Moller, McFadden, Hedeker, & Spring, 2012), which has the potential to "undermine" intrinsic motivation. As such, SDT holds that the net effect of tangible rewards will be determined by which of these two opposing psychological processes (the informational competence feedback vs. the controlling element inherent in the contingency) is more salient.

Summarizing research from over 100 lab and field experiments in a meta-analysis, Deci, Koestner, and Ryan (1999) found that, on average, offering tangible rewards that are expected and salient results in less intrinsic motivation (i.e., "undermining"); that is, on average, the degree to which expected and salient tangible rewards thwart autonomy often supersedes the degree to which rewards support competence satisfactions. Yet Deci and colleagues' analysis further revealed that reward contingencies that convey more informational feedback regarding competence are relatively less likely to undermine intrinsic motivation. For example, the strongest undermining effects were observed in studies that used either *engagement-contingent* or *completion-contingent* rewards. These reward contingencies tend to convey little by way of effectance-relevant information, yet clearly they are often used to control behavior. *Performance-contingent rewards,* in contrast, were more complex in their effects. When well administered, performance-contingent rewards can be used to recognize mastery or competence, and therefore do not undermine. Yet they can be very controlling, for example, when they imply that one must live up to the reward-giver's standards, in which case they have a strong undermining effect. Findings also show no undermining effects from *unexpected rewards,* as SDT predicts, because unexpected rewards are not salient as controls and can be a strong acknowledgment of good performance.

Based on such findings, one would expect that the best-case scenario when it comes to tangible rewards, psychological need satisfaction, and autonomous motivation would involve an unexpected reward that conveys a great deal of informational feedback about one's competence. An illustrative example of one such reward involves the prestigious MacArthur Fellows Program (or "Genius Grant"), a prize awarded to individuals who "show exceptional merit and promise for continued and enhanced creative work." According to the Foundation's website, "the fellowship is not a reward for past accomplishment, but rather an investment in a person's originality, insight, and potential." The award allows no applications (thus, no undermining of "losers"), yet because of this, its receipt is necessarily unexpected; furthermore, the award does not *require* future productivity. As such, the award has been called "one of the most significant awards that is truly '*no strings attached*'" (Harris, 2007, emphasis added, p. 85). For these reasons,

although no systematic investigation has yet been undertaken, we would expect that such a reward would not undermine the recipient's subsequent intrinsic motivation.

In contrast, consider the situation of elite athletes in a highly performance-contingent world. Analyzing records from the National Basketball Association and Major League Baseball, White and Sheldon (2014) examined players' careers over a baseline year, a contract year, and a postcontract year. Their focus was on whether the salience of the players' monetary rewards highlighted during the contract year would impact their motivation. White and Sheldon found that, after the contract award (Year 3) performance was poorer than that during the first 2 years, indicating that the emphasis on rewards in the contract year led to a decrease in intrinsic motivation, as manifested in statistics such as points scored, batting averages, and defensive performance. Rewards do motivate, but when controlling, not always in ways that sustain competence or interest.

Verbal Rewards/Praise

Verbal rewards, more commonly referred to as *praise,* represent another common method of conveying competence-related information. Praise is conveyed by parents, teachers, work supervisors, and peers, and has the potential to strongly support competence need satisfaction and downstream intrinsic motivation. Consistently, Deci and colleagues' (1999) meta-analysis found a net positive relation between praise and intrinsic motivation. Nevertheless, SDT maintains that different kinds of praise can convey more or less information about competence; furthermore, some forms of praise can be readily interpreted as controlling, thus disrupting competence need satisfaction and downstream intrinsic motivation (Deci & Ryan, 1985; Henderlong & Lepper, 2002). For example, Koestner, Zuckerman, and Koestner (1987) experimentally varied the type of praise offered in relation to different types of tasks. They found that ability praise increased intrinsic motivation more than effort praise (or no praise), presumably because it generally convened more information about competence. Furthermore, higher intrinsic motivation following praise predicted the choice of a higher level of challenge and better performance at a related but more complex task. Kanouse, Gumpert, and Canavan-Gumpert (1981) reported that in order for praise to support competence need satisfaction and intrinsic motivation, it must be interpreted as sincere; again, this is consistent with the premise that effective praise conveys information. Similarly, others have demonstrated that when praise is offered for exceptionally easy tasks, it can negatively influence perceived competence and future motivation (Graham, 1990; Meyer et al., 1979).

Praise can be interpreted as relatively controlling for a variety of reasons, including the interpersonal context, individual features of the communicator and recipient, and linguistic features of the praise itself. For example, a linguistically controlling form of praise might involving telling someone, "You did very well, just as I expected of you." Research shows that this type of praise tends to be perceived as controlling, and undermines competence need satisfaction and intrinsic motivation (Ratelle, Baldwin, & Vallerand, 2005; Ryan, 1982).

Competition

Like tangible rewards and praise, competition represents another common method of seeking and conveying competence-related information. Competition can take a variety of forms (e.g., between individuals or teams; zero-sum, positive-sum, or negative-sum), and individuals vary considerably in terms of seeking (or avoiding) opportunities to engage competitively (Houston, Harris, McIntire, & Francis, 2002; Newby & Klein, 2014). As with other sources of competence-related information, SDT maintains that the affect of competition will be moderated by not only the quality of the information but also the context's tendency to support or thwart the satisfaction of other psychological needs, namely, autonomy and (in this case, more than others) relatedness. At its best, competition can provide a naturalistic opportunity for rapidly delivered, rich information about one's competence; well-matched opponents can push each other to achieve higher levels of mastery. Furthermore, many activities

that people choose to pursue, by their very design, virtually require competition (e.g., competitive sports). Nevertheless, competitive situations can thwart other psychological needs. For example, competing against an opponent who is either much more skilled or much less skilled at an activity is unlikely to provide on optimal challenge or satisfy one's need for competence. Competition can also thwart autonomy need satisfaction when individuals feel pressured to engage or become preoccupied with the outcome (winning or losing) rather than satisfaction of play (Reeve & Deci, 1996). Furthermore, interpersonal competition has the potential to thwart relatedness need satisfaction. For example, insults or "trash talking" with opponents is a common features of competitive sports (Conmy, Tenenbaum, Eklund, Roehrig, & Filho, 2013; Dixon, 2007; Kassing, Sanderson, Avtigs, & Rancer, 2010). On the other hand, team-oriented competition creates opportunities for cooperation and may even facilitate relatedness need satisfaction within teams. Tauer and Harackiewicz (2004) demonstrated that the combination of competition and cooperation (intergroup competition) could promote higher levels of intrinsic motivation and even enhanced performance. Thus, similar to our discussion of rewards, praise, and achievement goals, understanding the effects of competition requires going beyond merely its implications for competence, to its impacts on autonomy and relatedness as well.

NOT ALL ATTAINABLE GOALS ARE CREATED EQUAL

The heavy focus on perceived competence and efficacy across theories of motivation might suggest that competence is uniformly laudable: Greater competence is always good thing. Clearly, SDT suggests that this general truth requires considerable qualifications. Whether competence enhances one's life and wellness requires looking beyond competence per se to consider what other need satisfactions and outcomes might result from one's competence. There are many high-achieving persons who do more damage than good to themselves and those around them. SDT, in fact, argues that high competence without autonomy and related-ness will not enhance well-being.

Recently, researchers embracing a "eudai-monic" perspective have suggested that well-being will most reliably result from the pursuit of what is intrinsically worthwhile to humans, such as the expression of virtues and the actualization of human values (see, e.g., Ryan, Curren, & Deci, 2013). Eudai-monic hypotheses have been particularly tested in SDT research on aspirations and life goals. Kasser and Ryan (1996) distinguished between *extrinsic aspirations* focused on external attainments (e.g., gaining wealth, popularity, or image) and *intrinsic aspi-rations* (e.g., goals relationships, commu-nity and personal growth), with the latter assumed to be more eudaimonic and more likely to satisfy basic psychological needs. They found that the more people emphasized extrinsic relative to intrinsic aspirations, the lower their well-being, a result that has been widely researched and replicated (Kasser, 2002). This observation takes on special rel-evance in cultures that strongly emphasize the accumulation of material wealth as a (or even "the") yardstick for assessing one's competence (e.g., "He who dies with the most toys wins," a popular sentiment attrib-uted to billionaire Malcolm Forbes).

Relevant to the current thesis, evidence suggests that even when people highly value extrinsic attainments and are competent and successful at realizing them, positive well-ness outcomes do not reliably obtain. For example, Niemiec, Ryan, and Deci (2009) followed college postgraduates over a 2-year period. Among these young adults, those who were focused on extrinsic aspirations "got what they wished for"—they made progress on their extrinsic goals. This was also true of those with intrinsic aspirations. Yet, whereas competence and progress at intrinsic goals was associated with enhanced well-being, competence at and attainment of extrinsic goals was not. These findings were mediated by basic need satisfactions, with extrinsic goal pursuits being associated with lower autonomy and relatedness satisfac-tions.

In a more recent demonstration, Sheldon and Krieger (2014) identified more than 1,000 lawyers with high-paying jobs within a money-focused firm (e.g., corporate law, securities work), and a similar number of lawyers doing public service or serving the public good (e.g., doing sustainability-related work for nonprofit organizations). Lawyers in the money-focused jobs, who presumably embraced extrinsic goals, had significantly larger incomes than those in the service-focused jobs. They were apparently successful! Nonetheless, those with more money-focused practices reported more negative affect, lower well-being, and more alcohol consumption. They also reported less autonomy in their work.

Here, again, we see that competence alone, even toward a valued goal, and even when attained, is not enough. When a per-son's achievement and attainments do not satisfy autonomy or relatedness, they do not produce the expected positive effects on well-being. Understanding what make human successes beneficial necessitates looking beyond mere competence and effi-cacy to what is being achieved, and the other needs and life goals one's actions satisfy or frustrate.

CONCLUSION

Competence-related strivings are ubiqui-tous: Humans find themselves striving to behave competently in nearly all phases and waking hours of life. Whether in edu-cational settings (at every level), at work, or in play or leisure, people are frequently concerned about, and sometimes directly pursue, competence. Yet despite this ubiq-uity, our overarching goal in this chapter has been to highlight some ways in which com-petence and its satisfactions are not enough, even in these settings, to explain either moti-vation or wellness. First, we suggested that as the sources of an individual's motivation differ, competence and competence feedback matters differently as well. For example, in externally regulated behaviors, competence is often just a means to an end, whereas in intrinsically motivated actions, competence is an inherent satisfaction and energizer of action. In fact, we have argued that dif-ferent forms of motivation (e.g., external, introjected, integrated, identified, or intrin-sic) are differentially associated with basic psychological need (competence, autonomy, and relatedness) satisfactions, with more volitional forms of motivation being more fulfilling of all needs. This fact helps to explain the higher quality and greater persistence of autonomous motivations. Furthermore, we have discussed how a range of different contextual features, including tangible rewards, praise, competition, and interpersonal dynamics, might support different needs, and as a result, more autonomous and therefore competence-seeking forms of motivation.

As the varied contributions in this handbook attest, many theoretical frameworks rightly emphasize the centrality of competence-related strivings to human progress and achievements. SDT's organismic view shares with these perspectives an appreciation of the deep adaptive roots of people's striving for competence; furthermore, it suggests that competence satisfactions represent an evolved internal support for ongoing learning and development. At the same time, as a dynamic theory of human needs in motivation and wellness, SDT argues that different types and styles of feedback, praise, and reward differentially affect motivation, as a function of both their informational and controlling properties. Furthermore, it is clear that competence satisfactions alone cannot meaningfully account for high-quality motivation, or the positive effects of accomplishment on wellness. What a person is striving for matters; thus, it is when activities are autonomously engaged, and invested with interest or value, that a person's competencies most effectively develop, and energy for applying them most easily is mobilized by the individual. It is then that a person's accomplishments contribute most to personal and social wellness.

REFERENCES

Adie, J. W., Duda, J. L., & Ntoumanis, N. (2012). Perceived coach-autonomy support, basic need satisfaction and the well- and ill-being of elite youth soccer players: A longitudinal investigation. *Psychology of Sport and Exercise, 13*(1), 51–59.

Angyal, A. (1941). *Foundations for a science of personality*. New York: Commonwealth Fund.

Assor, A., Roth, G., & Deci, E. L. (2004). The emotional costs of parents' conditional regard: A self-determination theory analysis. *Journal of Personality, 72*(1), 47–88.

Bandura, A. (1977). Self-efficacy: Toward a unifying theory of behavioral change. *Psychological Review, 84*(2), 191–215.

Bandura, A. (1989). Human agency in social cognitive theory. *American Psychologist, 44*(9), 1175–1184.

Bandura, A. (1997). *Self-efficacy: The exercise of control*. New York: Freeman.

Baumeister, R. F., & Leary, M. R. (1995). The need to belong: Desire for interpersonal attachments as a fundamental human motivation. *Psychological Bulletin, 117*(3), 497–529

Benita, M., Roth, G., & Deci, E. L. (2014). When are mastery goals more adaptive?: It depends on experiences of autonomy support and autonomy. *Journal of Educational Psychology, 106*(1), 258–267.

Brown, K. W., & Ryan, R. M. (2006). Multilevel modeling of motivation: A Self-determination Theory analysis of basic psychological needs. In A. D. Ong & M. van Dulmen (Eds.), *Oxford handbook of methods in positive psychology* (pp. 1158–1183). New York: Oxford University Press.

Chen, B., Vansteenkiste, M., Beyers, W., Boone, L., Deci, E. L., Van der Kaap-Deeder, J., et al. (2015). Basic psychological need satisfaction, need frustration, and need strength across four cultures. *Motivation and Emotion, 39*(2), 216–236.

Conmy, B., Tenenbaum, G., Eklund, R., Roehrig, A., & Filho, E. (2013). Trash talk in a competitive setting: Impact on self-efficacy and affect. *Journal of Applied Social Psychology, 43*(5), 1002–1014.

de Charms, R. (1968). *Personal causation*. New York: Plenum Press.

Deci, E. L. (1971). Effects of externally mediated rewards on intrinsic motivation. *Journal of Personality and Social Psychology, 18*(1), 105–115.

Deci, E. L. (1975). *Intrinsic motivation*. New York: Plenum Press.

Deci, E. L., Koestner, R., & Ryan, R. M. (1999). A meta-analytic review of experiments examining the effects of extrinsic rewards on intrinsic motivation. *Psychological Bulletin, 125*(6), 627–668.

Deci, E. L., La Guardia, J. G., Moller, A. C., Scheiner, M. J., & Ryan, R. M. (2006). On the benefits of giving as well as receiving autonomy support: Mutuality in close friendships. *Personality and Social Psychology Bulletin, 32*(3), 313–327.

Deci, E. L., & Moller, A. C. (2005). The concept of competence: A starting place for understanding intrinsic motivation and self-determined extrinsic motivation. In A. J. Elliot & C. S. Dweck (Eds.), *Handbook of competence and motivation* (pp. 579–597). New York: Guilford Press.

Deci, E. L., & Ryan, R. M. (1980). The empirical exploration of intrinsic motivational processes. In L. Berkowitz (Ed.), *Advances in experimental social psychology* (Vol. 13, pp. 39–80). New York: Academic Press.

Deci, E. L., & Ryan, R. M. (1985). *Intrinsic motivation and self-determination in human behavior*. New York: Plenum Press.

Deci, E. L., & Ryan, R. M. (2000). The "what" and "why" of goal pursuits: Human needs and the self-determination of behavior. *Psychological Inquiry, 11*(4), 227–268.

Deci, E. L., & Ryan, R. M. (2011). Levels of analysis, regnant causes of behavior and well-being: The role of psychological needs. *Psychological Inquiry, 22*(1), 17–22.

Deci, E. L., & Ryan, R. M. (2014). The importance of universal psychological needs for understanding motivation in the workplace. In M. Gagné (Ed.), *Oxford handbook of work engagement, motivation, and self-determination theory* (pp. 13–32). New York: Oxford University Press.

Dixon, N. (2007). Trash talking, respect for opponents and good competition. *Sport, Ethics and Philosophy, 1*(1), 96–106.

Elliot, A. J. (2005). A conceptual history of the achievement goal construct. In A. J. Elliot & C. S. Dweck (Eds.), *Handbook of competence and motivation* (pp. 52–72). New York: Guilford Press.

Elliot, A. J., & McGregor, H. A. (2001). A 2 × 2 achievement goal framework. *Journal of Personality and Social Psychology, 80*(3), 501–519.

Elliot, A. J., & Moller, A. C. (2003). Performance-approach goals: Good or bad forms of regulation? *International Journal of Educational Research, 39*(4–5), 339–356.

Elliot, A. J., Murayama, K., & Pekrun, R. (2011). A 3 × 2 achievement goal model. *Journal of Educational Psychology, 103*(3), 632–648.

Gillet, N., Lafrenière, M.-A. K., Huyghebaert, T., & Fouquereau, E. (2015). Autonomous and controlled reasons underlying achievement goals: Implications for the 3 × 2 achievement goal model in educational and work settings. *Motivation and Emotion, 39*(6), 858–875.

Graham, S. (1990). On communicating low ability in the classroom: Bad things good teachers sometimes do. In S. Graham & V. Folkes (Eds.), *Attribution theory: Applications to achievement, mental health, and interpersonal conflict* (pp. 17–36). Hillsdale, NJ: Erlbaum.

Grolnick, W. S., & Ryan, R. M. (1987). Autonomy in children's learning: An experimental and individual difference investigation. *Journal of Personality and Social Psychology, 52*(5), 890–898.

Grolnick, W. S., & Ryan, R. M. (1989). Parent styles associated with children's self-regulation and competence in school. *Journal of Educational Psychology, 81*(2), 143–154.

Hagger, M. S., & Chatzisarantis, N. L. D. (2016). The trans-contextual model of autonomous motivation in education: Conceptual and empirical issues and meta-analysis. *Review of Educational Research, 86*(2), 360–407.

Harris, D. (2007). *The complete guide to writing effective and award winning grants: Step-by-step instructions*. Ocala, FL: Atlantic.

Henderlong, J., & Lepper, M. R. (2002). The effects of praise on children's intrinsic motivation: A review and synthesis. *Psychological Bulletin, 128*(5), 774–795.

Houston, J., Harris, P., McIntire, S., & Francis, D. (2002). Revising the competitiveness index using factor analysis. *Psychological Reports, 90*(1), 31–34.

Jõesaar, H., Hein, V., & Hagger, M. S. (2012). Youth athletes' perception of autonomy support from the coach, peer motivational climate and intrinsic motivation in sport setting: One-year effects. *Psychology of Sport and Exercise, 13*(3), 257–262.

Johnston, M. M., & Finney, S. J. (2010). Measuring basic needs satisfaction: Evaluating previous research and conducting new psychometric evaluations of the Basic Needs Satisfaction in General Scale. *Contemporary Educational Psychology, 35*, 280–296.

Kanouse, D. E., Gumpert, P., & Canavan-Gumpert, D. (1981). The semantics of praise. In J. H. Harvey, W. Ickes, & R. F. Kidd (Eds.), *New directions in attribution research* (pp. 97–115). Hillsdale, NJ: Erlbaum.

Kasser, T. (2002). *The high price of materialism*. Cambridge, MA: MIT Press.

Kasser, T., & Ryan, R. M. (1996). Further examining the American dream: Differential correlates of intrinsic and extrinsic goals. *Personality and Social Psychology Bulletin, 22*(3), 280–287.

Kassing, J. W., Sanderson, J., Avtigs, T. A., & Rancer, A. S. (2010). Trash talk and beyond: Aggressive communication in the context of sports. In T. A. Avtgis & A. S. Rancer (Eds.), *Arguments, aggression, and conflict: New directions in theory and research* (pp. 253–266). London: Routledge.

Katz, I., Eilot, K., & Nevo, N. (2014). "I'll do it later": Type of motivation, self-efficacy and homework procrastination. *Motivation and Emotion, 38*(1), 111–119.

Koestner, R., & McClelland, D. C. (1990). Perspectives on competence motivation. In L. Pervin (Ed.), *Handbook of personality: Theory and research* (pp. 527–548). New York: Guilford Press.

Koestner, R., Zuckerman, M., & Koestner, J. (1987). Praise, involvement, and intrinsic motivation. *Journal of Personality and Social Psychology, 53*(2), 383–390.

Kusurkar, R. A., Ten Cate, T. J., Vos, C. M. P., Westers, P., & Croiset, G. (2013). How motivation affects academic performance: A structural equation modelling analysis. *Advances in Health Sciences Education, 18*(1), 57–69.

La Guardia, J. G., Ryan, R. M., Couchman, C., & Deci, E. L. (2000). Within-person variations in attachment style and their relations to psychological need satisfaction. *Journal of Personality and Social Psychology, 79*(3), 367–384.

Lee, W., Reeve, J., Xue, Y., & Xiong, J. (2012). Neural differences between intrinsic reasons for doing versus extrinsic reasons for doing: An fMRI study. *Neuroscience Research, 73*, 68–72.

Lynch, M. F., La Guardia, J. G., & Ryan, R. M. (2009). On being yourself in different cultures: Ideal and actual self-concept, autonomy support, and well-being in China, Russia, and the United States. *Journal of Positive Psychology, 4*(4), 290–304.

Maslow, A. H. (1987). *Motivation and personality* (3rd ed.). New York: Harper & Row. (Original work published 1954)

Meyer, W. U., Bachmann, M., Biermann, U., Hempelmann, M., Ploger, F. O., & Spiller, H. (1979). The informational value of evaluative behavior: Influences of praise and blame on perceptions of ability. *Journal of Educational Psychology, 71*, 259–268.

Milyavskaya, M., Philippe, F. L., & Koestner, R. (2013). Psychological need satisfaction across levels of experience: Their organization and contribution to general well-being. *Journal of Research in Personality, 47*(1), 41–51.

Moller, A. C., & Deci, E. L. (2014). The psychology of getting paid: An integrated perspective. In E. H. Bijleveld & H. Aarts (Eds.), *The psychological science of money* (pp. 189–211). New York: Springer.

Moller, A. C., & Elliot, A. J. (2009). Competence. In D. Matsumoto (Ed.), *Cambridge dictionary of psychology* (pp. 121–122). Cambridge, UK: Cambridge University Press.

Moller, A. C., McFadden, H. G., Hedeker, D., & Spring, B. (2012). Financial motivation undermines maintenance in an intensive diet and activity intervention. *Journal of Obesity.* [Epub ahead of print]

Murayama, K., Elliot, A. J., & Friedman, R. (2012). Achievement goals and approach-avoidance motivation. In R. M. Ryan (Ed.), *The Oxford handbook of human motivation* (pp. 191–207). Oxford, UK: Oxford University Press.

Murayama, K., Matsumoto, M., Izuma, K., Matsumoto, K. (2010). Neural basis of the undermining effect of monetary reward on intrinsic motivation. *Proceedings of the National Academy of Sciences USA, 107*(49), 20911–20916.

Niemiec, C. P., Ryan, R. M., & Deci, E. L. (2009). The path taken: Consequences of attaining intrinsic and extrinsic aspirations in post-college life. *Journal of Research in Personality, 73*(3), 291–306.

Newby, J. L., & Klein, R. G. (2014). Competitiveness reconceptualized: Psychometric development of the competitiveness orientation measure as a unified measure of trait competitiveness. *Psychological Record, 64*, 1–17.

Philippe, F. L., Koestner, R., Beaulieu-Pelletier, G., Lecours, S., & Lekes, N. (2012). The role of episodic memories in current and future well-being. *Personality and Social Psychology Bulletin, 38*(4), 505–519.

Przybylski, A. K., Rigby, C. S., & Ryan, R. M. (2010). A motivational model of video game engagement. *Review of General Psychology, 14*(2), 154–166.

Pulfrey, C., Buchs, C., & Butera, F. (2011). Why grades engender performance-avoidance goals: The mediating role of autonomous motivation. *Journal of Educational Psychology, 103*(3), 683–700.

Ratelle, C. F., Baldwin, M. W., & Vallerand, R. J. (2005). On the cued activation of situational motivation. *Journal of Experimental Social Psychology, 41*(5), 482–487.

Ratelle, C. F., & Duchesne, S. (2014). Trajectories of psychological need satisfaction from early to late adolescence as a predictor of adjustment in school. *Contemporary Educational Psychology, 39*, 388–400.

Reeve, J., & Deci, E. L. (1996). Elements of the competitive situation that affect intrinsic motivation. *Personality and Social Psychology Bulletin, 22*(1), 24–33.

Reis, H. T., Sheldon, K. M., Gable, S. L., Roscoe, J., & Ryan, R. M. (2000). Daily well-being: The role of autonomy, competence, and relatedness. *Personality and Social Psychology Bulletin, 26*(4), 419–435.

Rigby, S., & Ryan, R. M. (2011). *Glued to games: How video games draw us in and hold us spellbound.* Santa Barbara, CA: Praeger.

Rodgers, W. M., Markland, D., Selzer, A.-M., Murray, T. C., & Wilson, P. M. (2014). Distinguishing perceived competence and self-efficacy: An example from physical exercise. *Research Quarterly for Exercise and Sport, 85,* 527–539.

Roth, G. (2014). Antecedents and outcomes of teachers' autonomous motivation: A self-determination theory analysis. In P. W. Richardson, H. M. G. Watt, & S. A. Karabenick (Eds.), *Teacher motivation: Theory and practice* (pp. 36–51). New York: Routledge.

Roth, G., Assor, A., Niemiec, C. P., Ryan, R. M., & Deci, E. L. (2009). The emotional and academic consequences of parental conditional regard: Comparing conditional positive regard, conditional negative regard, and autonomy support as parenting practices. *Developmental Psychology, 45*(4), 1119–1142.

Ryan, R. M. (1982). Control and information in the intrapersonal sphere: An extension of cognitive evaluation theory. *Journal of Personality and Social Psychology, 43*(3), 450–461.

Ryan, R. M., Bernstein, J. H., & Brown, K. W. (2010). Weekends, work, and well-being: Psychological need satisfactions and day of the week effects on mood, vitality, and physical symptoms. *Journal of Social and Clinical Psychology, 29*(1), 95–122.

Ryan, R. M., & Connell, J. P. (1989). Perceived locus of causality and internalization: Examining reasons for acting in two domains. *Journal of Personality and Social Psychology, 57*(5), 749–761.

Ryan, R. M., Curren, R. R., & Deci, E. L. (2013). What humans need: Flourishing in Aristotelian philosophy and self-determination theory. In A. S. Waterman (Eds.), *The best within us: Positive psychology perspectives on eudaimonia* (pp. 57–75). Washington, DC: American Psychological Association.

Ryan, R. M., & Deci, E. L. (2000). Self-determination theory and the facilitation of intrinsic motivation, social development, and well-being. *American Psychologist, 55*(1), 68–78.

Ryan, R. M., & Deci, E. L. (2008). Self-determination theory and the role of basic psychological needs in personality and the organization of behavior. In O. P. John, R. W. Robins, & L. A. Pervin (Eds.), *Handbook of personality: Theory and research* (3rd ed., pp. 654–678). New York: Guilford Press.

Ryan, R. M., & Deci, E. L. (2013). Toward a social psychology of assimilation: Self-determination theory in cognitive development and education. In B. W. Sokol, F. M. E. Grouzet, & U. Muller (Eds.), *Self-regulation and autonomy: Social and developmental dimensions of human conduct* (pp. 191–207). New York: Cambridge University Press.

Ryan, R. M., Deci, E. L., & Vansteenkiste, M. (2016). Autonomy and autonomy disturbance in self-development and psychopathology: Research on motivation, attachment, and clinical process. In D. Cicchetti (Ed.), *Developmental psychopathology: Vol. 1. Theory and method* (3rd ed., pp. 385–438). Hoboken, NJ: Wiley.

Ryan, R. M. & Di Domenico, S. I. (in press). Distinct motivations and their differentiated mechanisms: Reflections on the emerging neuroscience of human motivation. In S. Kim, J. Reeve, & M. Bong (Eds.), *Advances in motivation and achievement: Vol. 19. Recent developments in neuroscience research on human motivation.* Bingley, UK: Emerald Group.

Ryan, R. M., & Hawley, P. (2016). Naturally good?: Basic psychological needs and the proximal and evolutionary bases of human benevolence. In K. W. Brown & M. Leary (Eds.), *The Oxford handbook of hypo-egoic phenomena* (pp. 205–222). New York: Oxford University Press.

Sheldon, K. M., & Filak, V. (2008). Manipulating autonomy, competence, and relatedness support in a game-learning context: New evidence that all three needs matter. *British Journal of Social Psychology/British Psychological Society, 47,* 267–283.

Sheldon, K. M., & Krieger, L. S. (2014). Service job lawyers are happier than money job lawyers, despite their lower income. *Journal of Positive Psychology, 90*(3), 219–226.

Sheldon, K. M., Ryan, R., & Reis, H. T. (1996). What makes for a good day?: Competence and autonomy in the day and in the person. *Personality and Social Psychology Bulletin, 22*(12), 1270–1279.

Soenens, B., Sierens, E., Vansteenkiste, M., Dochy, F., & Goossens, L. (2012). Psychologically controlling teaching: Examining outcomes, antecedents, and mediators. *Journal of Educational Psychology, 104*(1), 108–120.

Soenens, B., Vansteenkiste, M., Duriez, B., & Goossens, L. (2006). In search of the sources of psychologically controlling parenting: The role of parental separation anxiety and parental maladaptive perfectionism. *Journal of Research on Adolescence, 16*(4), 539–559.

Soenens, B., Vansteenkiste, M., Luyckx, K., Luyten, P., Duriez, B., & Goossens, L. (2008). Maladaptive perfectionism as an intervening variable between psychological control and adolescent depressive symptoms: A three-wave longitudinal study. *Journal of Family Psychology, 22,* 465–474.

Standage, M., & Ryan, R. M. (2012). Self-determination theory and exercise motivation:

Facilitating self-regulatory processes to support and maintain health and well-being. In C. Roberts & D. C. Treasure (Eds.), *Advances in motivation in sport and exercise* (pp. 233–270). Champaign, IL: Human Kinetics.

Tauer, J. M., & Harackiewicz, J. M. (2004). The effects of cooperation and competition on intrinsic motivation and performance. *Journal of Personality and Social Psychology, 86*(6), 849–861.

Taylor, G., Jungert, T., Mageau, G. A., Schattke, K., Dedic, H., Rosenfield, S., et al. (2014). A self-determination theory approach to predicting school achievement over time: The unique role of intrinsic motivation. *Contemporary Educational Psychology, 39*(4), 342–358.

Vallerand, R. J. (2015). *The psychology of passion: A dualistic model.* Oxford, UK: Oxford University Press.

Van den Berghe, L., Vansteenkiste, M., Cardon, G., Kirk, D., & Haerens, L. (2014). Research on self-determination in physical education: Key findings and proposals for future research. *Physical Education and Sport Pedagogy, 19*(1), 97–121.

Van Petegem, S., Soenens, B., Vansteenkiste, M., & Beyers, W. (2015). Rebels with a cause?: Adolescent defiance from the perspective of reactance theory and self-determination theory. *Child Development, 86*(3), 903–918.

Vansteenkiste, M., Lens, W., De Witte, S., De Witte, H., & Deci, E. L. (2004). The "why" and "why not" of job search behaviour: Their relation to searching, unemployment experience, and well-being. *European Journal of Social Psychology, 34*(3), 345–363.

Vansteenkiste, M., Lens, W., Elliot, A. J., Soenens, B., & Mouratidis, A. (2014). Moving the achievement goal approach one step forward: Toward a systematic examination of the autonomous and controlled reasons underlying achievement goals. *Educational Psychologist, 49*(3), 153–174.

Vansteenkiste, M., Smeets, S., Soenens, B., Lens, W., Matos, L., & Deci, E. L. (2010). Autonomous and controlled regulation of performance-approach goals: Their relations to perfectionism and educational outcomes. *Motivation and Emotion, 34*(4), 333–353.

White, M., & Sheldon, K. M. (2014). The contract year syndrome in the NBA and MLB: A classic undermining pattern. *Motivation and Emotion, 38*(2), 196–205.

White, R. W. (1959). Motivation reconsidered: The concept of competence. *Psychological Review, 66*(5), 297–333.

CHAPTER 13

Competence and Pay for Performance

BARRY GERHART
MEIYU FANG

In the first edition of the *Handbook of Competence and Motivation*, Elliot and Dweck (2005) defined *competence* as behaviors characterized by effectiveness, ability, sufficiency, or success, and they defined *competence motivation* as the energization and direction of such behaviors. Goals, ability, motivation (mostly intrinsic), and personality were key areas of focus.[1] Kanfer and Ackerman (2005) contributed the chapter that was most geared toward competence in the workplace. They, too, focused primarily on goals, motivation, and person-oriented determinants (abilities and motivational traits). The work motivation literature has had a similar focus (Gerhart & Fang, 2015; Rynes, Gerhart, & Parks, 2005). For example, a recent review of the broad topic of work motivation (Schmidt, Beck, & Gillespie, 2013) was organized around the following major topics: overview of goals and goal processes; expectancies, self-efficacy, and related concepts; affect; individual differences related to the self and personality; temporal dynamics; and multiple goals and decision making.

What is largely absent from these scholarly treatments of competence and motivation is the role played by *compensation*, which is how much and how people are paid in work organizations (e.g., Gerhart &

Rynes, 2003; Newman, Gerhart, & Milkovich, 2016). Our focus in this chapter is primarily on the effects of how people are paid, primarily the effects of pay for performance (PFP). We also provide a shorter discussion of the effects of how much organizations pay (pay level). PFP can take many forms (e.g., merit pay, merit bonuses, piece rates, commissions, gainsharing, profit sharing, stock options) and is sometimes referred to in generic terms such as *incentives, extrinsic incentives,* or *performance-contingent pay.* But the common principle is that employee pay is higher or lower depending on some combination of individual and/or group/organization measures of performance.

In work organizations, employee performance is arguably an especially important type of competence and it (as well as organization performance) is the primary focus of our chapter.

OVERVIEW OF THIS CHAPTER AND DEFINITION OF COMPENSATION

We begin by placing compensation and PFP in the broader context of human resource (HR) or people management decisions and strategies. We then discuss the effects of pay level, followed by a description and evaluation of PFP that includes its use, importance, effects, and potential pitfalls. We give special attention to the well-known concern that PFP undermines intrinsic motivation. In addressing these issues, we draw on our previous related work (e.g., Fang & Gerhart, 2012; Gerhart & Fang, 2014, 2015; Gerhart & Milkovich, 1992; Gerhart & Rynes, 2003; Gerhart, Rynes, & Fulmer, 2009; Rynes et al., 2005).

PFP is one of several aspects of a pay strategy, which also includes decisions about how much to pay (pay level), and the form of pay (direct pay such as wages/salaries, bonuses, incentives vs. indirect pay/benefits such as retirement, medical care, paid vacation) and the mix of monetary (e.g., extrinsic) and nonmonetary (e.g., intrinsic) rewards. We briefly discuss pay level, but not the question of form of pay/benefits, except to address extrinsic and intrinsic motivation issues.

Our perspective on the topic of PFP may be different than what readers of this handbook may encounter elsewhere in at least two respects. First, our focus is very applied, with a primary focus on policy and practice in work organizations. Second, we have observed elsewhere (Rynes et al., 2005) that in the rare case when compensation and/or PFP is discussed in the psychology literature, it often seems to be in a negative light, as though it is something more likely to cause problems than to play a positive role in achieving competence. Our perspective, based on our reading and evaluation of theory and evidence as it applies to the workplace, is different. We suggest that PFP is a valuable tool for building competence and probably a necessary tool for organizations to execute their business strategies successfully. This does not mean there are not risks in using PFP. There are. But, those risks must be balanced against the significant, average positive effects of PFP.

COMPENSATION AND PFP IN THE BROADER MANAGEMENT CONTEXT

It is useful to ground compensation/PFP in the broader context of managing people/HR in work organizations because the effects of PFP may depend on or be constrained by decisions regarding design and execution of other aspects of an employment/HR system. In the management literature, a standard approach to studying individual, unit, and organization performance is to specify its determinants as employee ability (A), employee motivation (M), and employee opportunity (O) to contribute to performance. This has come to be known as the "AMO" model (Appelbaum, Bailey, Berg, & Kalleberg, 2000; Bailey, 1993; Boxall & Purcell, 2003; Gerhart, 2007; Huselid, 1995; Jiang, Lepak, Hu, & Baer, 2012; Katz, Kochan, & Weber, 1985; Macduffie, 1995).

Ability has, of course, long been studied in psychology, and Chapter 2 by Sternberg and Chapter 19 by Kanfer and Ackerman, for example, in the previous edition of this handbook addressed this aspect of competence. In the HR and work psychology literatures, there is extensive evidence of the (positive) relationship between cognitive abilities (as well as some personality traits) and job performance (e.g., Barrick & Mount, 1991; Judge, Rodell, Klinger, Simon, & Crawford, 2013; Ployhart & Moliterno, 2011; Schmidt & Hunter, 1998). In the AMO literature, the focus is on how HR policies such as high selectivity in employee selection and significant investment in employee training and development can build the ability component.

There is also a vast literature on work motivation in psychology (Adams, 1963; Bandura, 1977; Kanfer, 1990; Latham, 2007; Latham & Pinder, 2005; Lawler, 1971; Locke & Latham, 1990; Vroom, 1964), as well as specific attention in psychology to achievement motivation and competence (Dweck & Leggett, 1988; Elliot & Church, 1997; McClelland, Atkinson, Clark, & Lowell, 1953; Nicholls, 1984; Ryan & Deci, 2000; White, 1959). Again, what will be less familiar to readers may be the focus in the HR literature on how workplace policies/practices such as compensation (e.g., PFP) can be used to influence motivation (and ability, performance, and competence).

The opportunity component (Blumberg & Pringle, 1982), although dealt with to some degree in applied psychology in terms of its role as a constraint on performance (e.g., Campbell, 1990; Peters & O'Connor, 1980) or as an important source of internal, intrinsic, and/or self-determined/autonomous work motivation (Deci & Ryan, 1985; Gagné & Deci, 2005; Hackman & Oldham, 1976; Ryan & Deci, 2000), has been more systematically addressed elsewhere (see earlier cites that refer to AMO logic) as a determinant of performance in work organizations. A key finding is that policies/practices that design workplace structures to allow greater decision input on the part of employees and give them more responsibility for and autonomy in decisions, can result in better plant- and organization-level performance (and possibly more positive employee attitudes).

The AMO model is useful because when competence is defined as success or performance in the workplace, it helps us to keep in mind that there are at least three main "levers" (i.e., policy/practice areas) that can be used to influence performance and that the impact of any one of these policy choices may depend on choices in the other two areas. As one example, an organization that wishes to improve average ability of its workforce may wish to do so by being more selective in its hiring. But, greater selectivity requires a larger and/or better applicant pool, which may depend on compensation. It may be necessary to increase pay level and/ or more strongly emphasize PFP to improve the applicant pool.

PAY LEVEL

Pay level can be defined as the average total compensation (including direct and indirect pay) per employee. Pay level can describe organizations, units within organizations, or jobs within organizations. Thus, Google may have a higher pay level than other organizations, but perhaps how much higher also varies according to product line and/ or whether we are talking about programmers or accountants. Total labor cost for an organization is a function of pay level and its staffing level (i.e., number of employees). We also note that organizations do not always use their own employees to get work done. They can, for example, contract out work (e.g., as Apple does to Foxconn to assemble iPhones and iPads overseas). Pay level matters for competence because pay level is a major determinant of attraction and selection of employees. Higher pay levels allow organizations to be more selective in hiring/ retention. Thus, all else being equal, higher paying organizations can achieve a labor force with higher levels of competence and performance, and possibly higher levels of motivation by choosing higher pay levels (see, e.g., the summary and review of efficiency wage and related theories in Gerhart & Rynes, 2003, Chapters 2 and 3). Whether the benefits of attracting and selecting a more competent and possibly more motivated workforce more than make up for the higher costs can be addressed using utility analysis (e.g., Brogden, 1949; Cascio & Boudreau, 2011) and is thought to depend on the nature of the organization's strategy and how that translates into the design of work roles and the opportunity to contribute (see AMO) of a workforce high in ability and motivation.

We also know that the main way that employees maximize their career earnings is by moving to higher-level, more impactful, higher-paying jobs. That can occur either through promotion in one's current organization or by moving to another organization (i.e., turnover) that offers higher paying job opportunities (e.g., Gerhart & Fang, 2014). There is solid evidence that opportunities for higher pay at other organizations do contribute significantly to employee turnover/retention. For example, Newman and colleagues (2016, Chapter 7) summarize five studies showing that employee turnover is 8.5–35.0% lower when pay level is 10% higher. Gerhart and Rynes (2003, Chapter 3) reviewed studies on what happens to employees' pay level when they do quit. One study showed that pay level for MBA graduates was 20% higher if they had quit and changed employers at least once (Dreher & Cox, 2000), and another reported that pay level was 25% higher among college and university faculty for each employer change they had made (Gomez-Mejia & Balkin, 1992). A third study, using a national sample of adults, found that pay was 8–11% higher among those who had changed employers at least once, and 14–18% higher among those who searched for another job prior to quitting and changing employers (Keith & McWilliams, 1999). These results point to the central importance of pay in achieving workforce competence and competence motivation. We return to this topic shortly.

Although we discuss pay level and PFP in separate sections, it is important to realize that they are (or should be) closely related decisions. We have seen in a variety of industries (e.g., airlines, automobiles) that a high pay level without a commensurate high level of organization performance is a recipe for failure, including bankruptcy. In a competitive market, high organization pay levels are sustainable only if employee and organization performance are also high. Successful use of PFP can help achieve that joint goal.

PAY FOR PERFORMANCE

We organize the following discussion of PFP around definition, use and importance, effects, and risks (what can go wrong) in using PFP.

Definition

PFP may be said to exist when pay level changes for an individual are positively related to changes in performance at the individual and/or aggregate level. PFP may take many forms and is referred to using a variety of terms, including *merit pay, merit bonuses, incentives, piece rates, stock options, stock grants,* and *gainsharing* (Newman et al., 2016). PFP plans can be classified on the basis of at least three dimensions. Traditionally, two dimensions are: degree of emphasis on objective and subjective performance measures and degree of emphasis on individual- versus aggregate-level (team, unit, organization) performance measures. For example, merit pay uses a subjective and individual level of performance, whereas profit sharing uses an objective, organization-level measure of performance. Additionally, the increased emphasis on variable pay suggests a third dimension: Does the pay become part of base pay/salary/wages (as with merit pay) or is it paid as variable pay (e.g., a merit bonus), which must be reearned in the future? A fourth dimension, *incentive intensity,* refers to how much pay level for individual employees varies in response to changes in performance. As a rule, incentive intensity is a classic case of a "double-edged sword." On the positive side, higher incentive intensity can generate

significantly (even dramatically) higher levels of (extrinsic) motivation; on the negative side, the higher the extrinsic motivation, the greater the risk that the PFP plan will have negative, unintended consequences.

The considerations in choosing a PFP strategy (which is often a combination of PFP plans) are many and we do not attempt to cover them here. Rather, let us highlight a few interesting observations from theory and research (Gerhart & Rynes, 2003). First, PFP plans using individual-level performance measures are thought to be more likely to generate high levels of motivation because the "line of sight" between individual effort and performance (and pay) is generally stronger. High performers are more likely to gravitate to organizations using such plans. Also, there are not social loafing (e.g., Shepperd, 1993) or what is also called "free rider problems" with such plans. On the other hand, an exclusive focus on individual performance may not elicit the level of cooperation and teamwork necessary in organizations. So some mix of individual and collective performance measures are often used. Second, incentive intensity is usually stronger when objective (vs. subjective) performance measures are used. This may be because of their higher reliability and credibility. Higher incentive intensity is positively associated with intensity of motivation. However, higher intensity also increases the risk of unintended consequences (e.g., achieving performance objectives and incentive payouts through gaming or another unacceptable means). Behavioral measures of performance can be used in conjunction with objective measures to help ensure that not only are objective performance goals achieved, but also achieved using acceptable means/behaviors. Third, according to agency theory, the larger the share of employees' pay that is at risk (i.e., based on PFP rather than guaranteed base pay and benefits), the higher their pay level will need to be to compensate them (compensating risk differential) for taking on that increased risk. Fourth, variable pay is not only relevant to motivation, but it is also a key part of how organizations align labor costs with the economic ups and downs of their business. *Profit sharing,* for example, is a variable pay plan that allows labor costs to increase when profits increase, but it ensures that labor costs will decrease when profits decrease.

Use and Importance

PFP is used widely, both in the United States and elsewhere (Gerhart & Fang, 2014; Gerhart et al., 2009; Newman et al., 2016). In a survey of 1,080 mostly U.S. organizations (WorldatWork, 2012), 92% reported that base pay increases depended on employee performance, with 92% of those organizations giving pay increases to top performers that are 1.25–2 times larger than those given to average performers. In the same survey, 84% of employers reported that they used variable pay (other than sales commissions) for employees (e.g., programs such as individual incentives, goal sharing, merit bonuses, gainsharing, and profit sharing). Thus, the typical organization uses multiple types of PFP programs. It is noteworthy that not all of the surveyed organizations were from the private, for-profit sector. Indeed, not-for-profit and/or public-sector organizations accounted for roughly one-third of the responses. Although responses were not reported separately by sector, it was reported that private sector organizations were more likely to use PFP and to use it with greater intensity (e.g., more strongly differentiating size of pay increase based on differences in employee performance). Thus, it may be that nearly 100% of private sector organizations use PFP. The strength of PFP also varies according to other factors, but perhaps most important is job level, with PFP representing a much larger share of total compensation as one moves to higher job levels (e.g., Gerhart & Fang, 2014).

Pay is very important to employees (Rynes, Gerhart, & Minette, 2004). Evidence of this takes two main forms: how important people say it is, and its effects on organization objectives (e.g., performance). We saw earlier that pay level has important effects on retention, and therefore on workforce competence. We review the effects of PFP later. We focus here on how important employees state that pay is. Rynes and colleagues (2004) reviewed evidence to indicate that when asked directly, people sometimes underreport the importance of pay, perhaps because of social desirability (e.g., meaningful work may be considered a loftier goal than making more money). But even when asked directly, employees often indicate that pay is most important. As an example, the Society for Human Resource Management (2014) has surveyed employees for many years regarding which of 21 job attributes (including "opportunities to use skills/abilities," "relationship with immediate supervisor," "communication between employees and senior management") are most important to them (in deciding whether to stay with the organization). Over the course of 10 years (2004–2013) of these surveys, the three job attributes most often rated as "very important" were, in order: job security, benefits, and compensation/pay—all of which relate to compensation.

To evaluate their compensation, employees compare themselves to others. Thus, in the workplace, employee attitudes and behaviors are driven to an important degree by perceptions of fairness and equity, which in turn rely on social comparisons. Equity theory (Adams, 1963), for example, specifies that people compare the ratio of their outcomes (e.g., pay) to inputs (e.g., effort, performance) to the ratios of others (or themselves in previous jobs). To the degree they perceive they are being treated inequitably (especially in the case of underreward equity), they take actions (behavioral or cognitive) to restore equity. Many of these actions (e.g., lower effort, turnover) are undesirable from an organization's point of view. Equity theory also raises the question of what fair or equitable pay looks like to people. The answer is that, on average, people believe that pay should be based on performance (e.g., Dyer, Schwab, & Theriault, 1976; see Gerhart & Fang, 2015, for a review). Thus, not using PFP is likely to violate an important and widely held workplace norm and result in perceived inequity, which we know can lead to a number of undesirable outcomes (Adams, 1963; Gerhart & Rynes, 2003). To the degree that high performers expect their pay to be commensurate with their performance, and that expectation is not met, an organization will face the potential negative consequences of perceived inequity among this key employee group. We return to this issue in our discussion below (e.g., on sorting effects).

Effects on Performance: Incentive and Sorting Effects

Does Use Imply Effectiveness?

As we have seen, PFP is used widely in the in the United States, especially in the private sector. It is also used in much of the rest of the world, including in the largest economies (e.g., Newman et al., 2016, Chapter 16). Although it is true that widespread use of a practice does not necessarily mean it is effective, it is also true that over time, market forces are expected to select out less competitive organizations, which, by definition, are less likely to use competence-enhancing practices. If surviving organizations, which have met the market test, widely use a PFP strategy, then this suggests a positive role of PFP in survival. Of course, it remains possible that more or less PFP, or a different form of PFP, could result in greater survival and success and/or a lower risk of something unintended/negative happening as a result of PFP. That is the focus of much of the literature on PFP (e.g., Gerhart & Rynes, 2003).

As we have seen, there are some sectors (e.g., the public sector) in which PFP is used less. Of course, competition and market forces also play less of a role in the public sector. It may be that private-sector organizations, which are less likely to be insulated from market forces, are less likely to be able to compete successfully and survive without practices such as PFP that play a key role in competing for and motivating top talent. Another sector in which PFP is rare is among workers who are union members.[2] We also know that in the United States, the percentage of the private-sector workforce that is union members has declined dramatically over time. Although there are likely multiple reasons for the decline in unionized firms and unionized workers, one reason often given is that productivity of union workers has not been high enough to offset the higher wages and benefits that union workers receive on average, and as heavily unionized sectors have either been deregulated (e.g., trucking, airlines) or faced growing competition from other sources (e.g., entry of international competitors, as in automobiles and electronics), business and union jobs have been lost because union worker productivity has not

been high enough to offset the higher labor costs of union workers.

Direct Evidence on PFP Effects: Incentive and Sorting

We now turn to a review, necessarily limited in its scope, of more direct evidence on the effects of PFP, primarily on performance (for more complete reviews, see Gerhart & Rynes, 2003; Gerhart et al., 2009). There are two general pathways by which PFP influences performance: incentive effects and sorting effects (Gerhart & Milkovich, 1992; Gerhart & Rynes, 2003; Lazear, 1986). First, the incentive effect describes how PFP changes the attitudes and behaviors (including competence/performance and sometimes competence motivation) of the current workforce. For example, if an organization implements a new PFP policy (e.g., merit pay or stronger merit pay), does it find that employees present both before and after implementation of the new PFP policy now have higher motivation and performance?

In terms of internal validity, the strongest evidence on this point comes from a meta-analysis of 47 effect sizes from 39 studies that included 3,124 employees (Jenkins, Mitra, Gupta, & Shaw, 1998). Importantly, among the criteria for inclusion were that a study use objective performance measures, focus on financial incentives tied to individual performance, and "have a control group or a premeasure with an explicit manipulation of the performance contingency of the incentive" (p. 779). Based on 41 effect sizes covering 2,773 employees, the mean correlation between use of financial incentives and performance quantity was $r = .32$, which converts to $d = 0.68$. In other words, employees receiving higher pay for achieving higher objective performance were 0.68 standard deviations higher on that performance measure than employees not receiving financial incentives based on their performance. Jenkins and colleagues (1998) also reported that the mean effect size based on field/workplace settings ($r = .46$, $d = 1.04$) was roughly twice as large as the mean effect size from laboratory studies ($r = .23$, $d = 0.47$). They also used type of task as a moderator. The effect size for tasks with more intrinsic interest ($r = .33$, $d = 0.72$) was nearly identical to the effect size for less interesting tasks ($r = .34$, $d = 0.72$), which appears to conflict with a key hypothesis from cognitive evaluation theory (e.g., Deci, Koestner, & Ryan, 1999; see our later discussion) that extrinsic performance-contingent rewards are best used for boring tasks.[3] Finally, based on a small number ($k = 6$) of effect sizes, no statistically significant correlation was found between incentive use and quality of performance. Thus, financial incentives were associated with higher performance quantity, without any detrimental impact on performance quality.

An important limitation of the preceding findings is that the types of jobs studied may not be very representative (Gerhart & Fang, 2014). Of the 47 effect sizes covering 3,124 employees examined by Jenkins and colleagues (1998), only eight studies were conducted in a field setting, covering 470 employees. The performance measures in the eight studies were number of trees planted (2), number of animals trapped (2), task completion time (1), number of items tested in a manufacturing setting (1), and observer assessments of behaviors (2). There is a much larger body of evidence (again, for reviews, see Gerhart & Rynes, 2003; Gerhart et al., 2009) that finds support for a positive relationship between PFP and performance in a wide range of jobs (including managerial and executive; e.g., Gerhart & Milkovich, 1990). But, the Jenkins and colleagues study is the most straightforward. It also makes for a useful comparison with other meta-analytic results on cognitive evaluation theory that we review later in this chapter.

Second, PFP can influence performance/competence via what Lazear (1986) described as a "sorting" effect (Gerhart & Milkovich, 1992; Gerhart & Rynes, 2003; Lazear, 1986, 2000; Rynes, 1987). This refers to a change in PFP strategy that influences employee performance not by changing the motivation and behavior of the current workforce, but instead refers to changing the composition of the current workforce: who the employees are and their attributes. Lazear (2000), in his study of worker productivity at an automobile glass installation company, provides what is probably the best illustration of how incentive and sorting effects can operate, and how overlooking

sorting effects can greatly underestimate the total impact of a change in PFP strategy. He took the opportunity to measure productivity (number of windshields installed per installer) both before and after the change from a fixed pay system, in which installers were paid a flat rate regardless of productivity. to a system in which installers who installed more windshields per hour were paid more. Lazear observed a 44% increase in productivity when the company implemented PFP. When he compared the productivity of individual workers present both before and after the pay system change, he found that the average increase in productivity was 22% (or about one-half of the total increase). This represents the incentive effect. What accounted for the other one-half (the other 22%) of the increase in productivity? Lazear found that this other one-half of the effect could be explained by the fact that less productive workers became more likely to quit under the new PFP system (because they now earned less money than their peers), and these less productive workers were replaced by newly hired workers who had higher productivity.

This sorting effect is consistent with attraction–selection–attrition (ASA) theory (Schneider, 1987) and related theories that emphasize that individuals and organizations match in a nonrandom fashion based on fit, including a fit between employee PFP preferences and organization PFP policy. Indeed, abundant empirical evidence now exists to document how pay systems that vary in their emphasis on PFP contribute to variations in the characteristics (including personality and performance) of those they attract (Cable & Judge, 1994; Trank, Rynes, & Bretz, 2002). Laboratory evidence, where subjects are permitted to choose the pay system under which they work, indicates that high performers are much more likely to choose PFP over fixed pay (Cadsby, Song, & Tapon, 2007; Dohmen & Falk, 2011). In addition, field work shows that high-performing employees are more likely than low-performing employees to quit when the pay–performance link is weak (Harrison, Virick, & William, 1996; Lazear, 2000; Nyberg, 2010; Salamin & Hom, 2005; Shaw, Dineen, Fang, & Vellella, 2009; Trevor, Gerhart, & Boudreau, 1997). Thus, an organization with weak PFP would be expected to disproportionately lose its high performers, keep its lower performers, and replace departing high performers with more low performers.

To get a sense of just how nonrandom the person–organization matching process is, consider the study in which Schneider, Smith, Taylor, and Fleenor (1998) estimated the magnitude of organization differences in personality traits. They found that 24% of the variance in employee personality (using the four Myers–Briggs-type indicator personality variables) occurred between organizations. The degree to which organization differences in PFP explained this pattern was not addressed. Fang and Gerhart (2012), however, also found significant organization differences (19% of the variance was between organizations) in motivation-related traits (extrinsic motivation orientation, intrinsic motivation, and internal work locus of control) and additionally demonstrated that PFP played a key role, such that extrinsic motivation orientation and internal work locus of control were higher in organizations that more strongly emphasized PFP (there was no relationship between PFP strength and intrinsic motivation orientation).

Pitfalls and Risks of PFP: What Can Go Wrong?

Even if PFP "works" on average (via positive incentive and sorting effects), we know that few situations are average, and that PFP potentially has both upsides and downsides (Gerhart & Fang, 2015). Indeed, it has been observed of PFP that "when 'it works,' it seems capable of producing spectacularly good results and when it does not work, it can likewise produce spectacularly bad results" (Gerhart et al., 2009, p. 253). The use of PFP having a strong incentive intensity (i.e., the degree to which the payoff to high and low performance is different) can be thought of as a high-risk, high-return strategy (Gerhart & Fang, 2015; Gerhart, Trevor, & Graham, 1996). This refers to the fact that using strong incentives (i.e., high incentive intensity) increases the probability of not only strong motivation and performance (the "return") but also unintended

negative consequences (the "risk"). Many scholars (e.g., Kerr, 1975; Kohn, 1993; Lawler, 1971; Milgrom & Roberts, 1992; Pfeffer, 1998; Roy, 1952; Sanders & Hambrick, 2007) have documented the risks (what can go wrong) when PFP is used, including excessive risk taking, excessive competition within the firm, focusing too little on performance measures (e.g., quality, customer service, long-term performance) not explicitly included in the PFP plan, and focusing too much on performance measures that are explicitly included in the PFP plan, including how people sometimes seek to "game" the plan to achieve incentivized performance objectives in an unacceptable manner.[4] Let us look at a few specific examples.

One way to understand the risk is to recall that motivation is not only about intensity/level of effort but also how that effort is directed. A choice is made regarding which goals to pursue and the amount of effort to be devoted to each of them (Vroom, 1964). We know that goals play a major role in motivating and directing behavior (Elliot, 2006; Locke & Latham, 2002) and in self-regulation (Bandura, 1997; Lord, Diefendorff, Schmidt, & Hall, 2010). The fact that cognitive resources are limited means that employees must choose and assign priorities to goals (Kanfer & Ackerman, 1989). In understanding what motivates employee choice, it is useful to keep in mind what Milgrom and Roberts (1992) define as the *equal compensation principle*:

> If an employee's allocation of time or attention between two different activities cannot be monitored by the employer, then either the marginal rate of return to the employee from time or attention spent in each of the two activities must be equal, or the activity with the lower marginal rate of return receives no time or attention. (p. 228)

There is a related economics literature on "multitasking" (Prendergast, 1999) and this issue has also been addressed in psychology (e.g., Lawler, 1971, p. 171; Schmidt & DeShon, 2007; Wright, George, Farnsworth, & McMahan, 1993; for a review, see Gerhart & Rynes, 2003). In plain English, the implication is that when faced with multiple performance objectives, employees choose those that bring the most rewards, which are often in the form of pay. Of course, we know that employees are not motivated only by money. Nevertheless, the equal compensation principle is ignored at one's peril.

Consider an example. Perhaps in an effort to grow the business, a well-known company implemented a new PFP plan in its automobile repair centers that paid managers more if revenue grew. There are a few basic ways to grow revenue in the automobile repair business. One way is to attract a greater share of customers needing auto repairs or maintenance. Another way is to increase the cost of the average repair per customer. Both avenues face the challenge that cars have become more reliable, less repair-prone over time. There is often information asymmetry in the repair shop–customer relationship, such that the repair shop knows what needs to be repaired, but the customer does not know. In the case of this particular company, this information asymmetry, together with a strong incentive to grow revenue, was alleged to have resulted in some auto repair centers telling customers they needed repairs that they did not actually need. This helped grow revenue. But it also brought customer complaints, and subsequently in both New York and California, the attorneys general took legal action against the company. According to California's Bureau of Automotive Repair, in its 18-month undercover investigation and in 38 visits to 27 auto repair shops, "unnecessary service and repairs were recommended 34 times" (Fisher, 1992, p. D1). The Bureau found that the company set daily sales targets (e.g., a specific number of alignments, brake jobs) for each repair shop, and if these targets were not met, there were negative consequences. The company's CEO at the time denied the fraud allegation but acknowledged "isolated incidents" and that they "could have been the result of rigid attention to goals, or . . . aggressive selling" (p. D1). He stated that the company would no longer set sales goals for specific repairs and that the incentive system would be replaced with a system that would reward employees based on customer satisfaction.

Another concern with PFP is that it can encourage/cause excessive risk-taking behavior (Devers, McNamara, Wiseman, & Arrfelt, 2008; Sanders & Hambrick, 2007). For example, Wall Street incentivized employees to develop "innovative" new financial investment vehicles and to take the kinds of risks (e.g., selling mortgages to high-risk borrowers) that could earn the biggest investment returns (as long as the risk, higher mortgage default rates, did not come to pass). For a while, everything went well. The firms and their employees made a lot of money and investors did well, too. Then, things suddenly went wrong, and a chain of events (e.g., the economy contracted, people lost their jobs, and one of many things that happened is that high-risk borrowers defaulted on their mortgages at higher rates) led to the Global Financial Crisis of 2007–2008. Blue Chip firms such as Lehman Brothers went bankrupt, and other firms (e.g., Bear Stearns and Merrill Lynch) survived because other firms (J. P. Morgan and Bank of America, respectively) bought them. The former director of corporate finance policy at the U.S. Treasury wrote that "misaligned incentive programs are at the core of what brought our financial system to its knees" (Jacobs, 2009). The former vice-chairman of the U.S. Federal Reserve has made similar comments (Blinder, 2009). The President and the Congress of the United States apparently agreed that incentives, especially how they influenced risk-taking behavior, played a key role in the Global Financial Crisis. They put into place legislation, the Troubled Asset Relief Program (TARP), which included restrictions on executive pay that were designed to discourage executives from taking "unnecessary and excessive risks." Why wasn't there more and/or earlier concern among Wall Street firms and their employees about taking such risks? One reason could be the belief that Wall Street firms were "too big to fail." If things really went badly, perhaps they believed that the government would bail them out (which turned out to be true to some extent). This is another example of an unintended (perverse) incentive effect, in that there was no expected penalty for failure, only an expected reward for success. To the degree that this was true, there was no downside risk to worry about. Similarly, perhaps there was a belief among employees (e.g., brokers) that they would not personally suffer the negative consequences of such investment risks (investors or the firm would—but later, after the firm's employees had already made their money). Many years after the Global Financial Crisis, incentives and how they influence risk-taking behavior continue to be a concern. Recently, for example, U.S. Federal Reserve officials advised firms to be aware of "warning signs of excessive risk taking and other cultural breakdowns" (Glazer & Rexrode, 2015).

PFP has also been identified as a culprit in test-cheating scandals in education. The *Washington Post* (Strauss, 2015) reported that "an Atlanta jury convicted 11 teachers of racketeering and other crimes in a standardized test-cheating scandal believed to be the worst of a wave of test cheating in nearly 40 states and Washington, D.C.—not by students but by teachers and principals who were under pressure to meet certain score goals at the risk of sanction if they failed." According to the grand jury indictment, the then-Superintendent of Atlanta Public Schools (APS), Beverley Hall, set teacher and administrator performance targets that were "largely based on students' performance on the Criterion Referenced Competency Test, a standardized test given annually to elementary and middle school students in Georgia." These targets are reported to have "often" been more difficult than those required under the No Child Left Behind Act of 2001. The indictment further states that "APS principals and teachers were frequently told by Beverly Hall and her subordinates that excuses for not meeting targets would not be tolerated. When principals and teachers could not reach their targets, their performance was criticized, their jobs were threatened and some were terminated." The indictment went on to say:

> To satisfy annual targets and AYP [adequate yearly progress], test answer sheets were altered, fabricated, and falsely certified. Test scores that were inflated as a result of cheating were purported to be the actual achievement of targets through legitimately obtained improvements in students' performance when, in fact, the conspirators knew those results had been obtained through cheating and did not reflect students' actual academic performance. . . . As part of the conspiracy, employees of APS who failed to satisfy targets were

terminated or threatened with termination, while others who achieved targets through cheating were publicly praised and financially rewarded. For example, teachers who reported other teachers who cheated were terminated, while teachers who were caught cheating were only suspended. The message from Beverly Hall was clear: there were to be no exceptions and no excuses for failure to meet targets.

We have gone into some detail regarding what can go wrong with PFPs. We think that this is necessary in the interest of painting an accurate picture that includes not only the generally positive effects of PFP but also how things may not just go wrong, but go very wrong. It is also worth noting that if ineffective organizational practices are less likely to survive the test of time, then there may be a multitude of failed PFP plans that have been tried in organizations (Gerhart et al., 1996). However, we rarely hear about these, so they tend to be excluded from consideration when we look at evidence on the effectiveness of PFP. We hope these examples help make the point that any decision regarding whether to use PFP plans, and what type, should depend not only on the mean expected effect but also on the variance (i.e., risk) associated with such a decision, and the recognition that selection bias may preclude us from accurately estimating both the mean and the variance of the PFP effect (Gerhart et al., 1996).

Avoiding the Pitfalls

Clearly, ignoring the means used to achieve ends is one way that PFP plans go wrong. As such, many organizations instead monitor not just outcomes (e.g., student achievement test results), but also how those results are achieved (e.g., the means and the behaviors used). Leaving out important objectives of the PFP plan runs afoul of the equal compensation principle. Unreasonably high performance objectives, especially when employees are not given what they need (training/development, restructuring of work responsibilities, adequate resources) is likely to lead to problems. Structuring PFP plans so that risks are taken with other people's money, and such that the employee can only gain from success but not lose when there is failure, is another clear path to problems. All of these risks are magnified to the extent that PFP/incentive intensity is high.[5] In this situation, it is essential that behaviors (not just results) be monitored to ensure to the degree possible that objective/results-based performance goals are being achieved using acceptable means and behaviors.

Intrinsic Motivation

Perhaps the risk of PFP that has received the most attention in the psychology and management literatures is that it may harm/undermine intrinsic motivation. We accordingly address this issue in greater depth, drawing in particular on our recent review on this topic (Gerhart & Fang, 2015). Those writing for management audiences have regularly argued that a key reason not to use PFP is that it will harm intrinsic motivation and/or creativity (e.g., Kohn, 1993; Pfeffer, 1998; Pink, 2009). The seminal work (and the work that is most often cited by those writing for management audiences about this concern) in this area has been conducted by Deci, Ryan, and colleagues, beginning with the development of cognitive evaluation theory (CET; Deci, 1975; Deci & Ryan, 1985; Ryan, Mims, & Koestner, 1983) and the following program of empirical research that was summarized in a meta-analysis (Deci et al., 1999). CET, and later self-determination theory (SDT), distinguishes between "intrinsic motivation, which refers to doing something because it is inherently interesting or enjoyable, and extrinsic motivation, which refers to doing something because it leads to a separable outcome" (Ryan & Deci, 2000, p. 55) such as a monetary reward. Earlier, Deci and Ryan (1985) stated that intrinsic motivation is derived from "innate . . . needs for competence and self-determination" (p. 33) and occurs when a person is motivated to conduct "an activity in the absence of a reward contingency or control" (p. 35).

Although it is generally acknowledged (including by CET scholars) that PFP has a positive effect on extrinsic motivation, the concern is that PFP may negatively influence (or "undermine") intrinsic motivation. Although PFP can have either positive or negative effects on intrinsic motivation under CET, depending on how it influences

two intervening mechanisms, perceived self-competence and perceived autonomy (e.g., Ryan et al., 1983), PFP is typically seen as having a net negative effect on intrinsic motivation. Although either a positive or negative effect on self-competence is possible, it is generally argued that a negative effect on perceived autonomy (i.e., PFP is often thought to be experienced as controlling) is likely, and this negative effect will dominate even if PFP has a positive effect on self-competence.[6] In this most commonly assumed case under CET, using PFP will not be very effective if, while increasing extrinsic motivation, it at the same time decreases intrinsic motivation.

Furthermore, and this is of great importance, intrinsic motivation is seen as being a higher-quality form of motivation than extrinsic motivation (Gerhart & Fang, 2015). So, a unit decrease in intrinsic motivation is not likely to be offset by a unit increase in extrinsic motivation. For example, Ryan and Deci (2000, p. 69) argue that the more autonomous the motivation, the higher its quality and the more authentic it is, which means that people "have more interest, excitement, and confidence, which in turn is manifest . . . as enhanced performance, persistence, and creativity" (see also Gagné & Deci, 2005; Sheldon & Elliot, 1999; Sheldon, Ryan, Deci, & Kasser, 2004; Vansteenkiste, Sierens, Soenens, Luyckx, & Lens, 2009). In their Proposition 1, Gagné and Deci (2005, p. 348) argue that "autonomous extrinsic motivation will be more effective in predicting persistence on uninteresting but effort-driven tasks, whereas intrinsic motivation will be more effective in predicting persistence on interesting tasks." Typically, the latter are more important, higher-impact types of tasks that are more central to work in a knowledge-based economy. In her earlier work, Amabile (1998, p. 78) likewise argued that "not all motivation is created equal. An inner passion to solve the problem at hand leads to solutions far more creative than do external rewards such as money." Thus, to summarize, under SDT, an increase of one unit in extrinsic motivation and a decrease of one unit in intrinsic motivation do not offset each other. Rather, this scenario represents a change for the worse because higher-quality motivation is replaced by lower-quality motivation.

The evidence on CET's hypothesized undermining effect of PFP on intrinsic motivation from the Deci and colleagues (1999) meta-analysis relied entirely on experimental evidence that used either children or college students as subjects. There do not appear to have been any studies included from ongoing work settings. Based on 128 effect sizes, contingent rewards did have a negative relationship with intrinsic motivation. In the specific case of performance-contingent rewards, $d = -0.28$ (95% confidence interval of -0.38 to -0.18) for the free-choice measure of intrinsic motivation and $d = -0.01$ (95% confidence interval of -0.10 to 0.08) for the self-reported interest measure of intrinsic motivation.

Deci and colleagues (1999) do not report the effect of contingent rewards on either extrinsic motivation or on performance (Gerhart & Fang, 2015). Therefore, the meta-analysis does not tell us the net effect of contingent rewards on overall motivation or performance. What it tells us is that there is essentially no effect of contingent rewards on self-reported intrinsic motivation, and that use of contingent rewards was associated with subjects spending 0.28 standard deviations less time working on the experimental task during their free time (not during "work" time). Recall that the Jenkins and colleagues (1998) meta-analysis did use performance as a dependent variable, and found a much larger and positive effect size of $d = 0.68$ for the association between PFP/incentive use and performance.

By not including extrinsic motivation or performance (and/or especially relevant aspects of performance under CET/SDT expected to be most influenced by intrinsic motivation such as creativity) as dependent variables, the Deci and colleagues (1999) meta-analysis also cannot shed any light on whether intrinsic motivation is of higher quality than intrinsic motivation. For example, is intrinsic motivation more strongly related to creativity than is extrinsic motivation (for a review, see Gerhart & Fang, 2015)? A meta-analysis (Byron & Khazanchi, 2012) finds that the use of PFP incentives (which presumably mainly increases extrinsic motivation) does *not* diminish creativity.[7] In fact, it found that incentive use and creativity were actually positively related.

But perhaps intrinsic motivation has an even stronger positive relationship with creativity. It should also be noted that PFP (or, for that matter, any monetary payment) is *not* the norm in settings such as schools, the source of many of the studies summarized by Deci and colleagues (or in volunteer/charity situations, the situation addressed in the related "motivational crowding" literature, e.g., Frey & Jegen, 2001). In contrast, monetary payment is the norm in the workplace. Moreover, as noted earlier, surveys indicate that most people believe that employees' pay should be based on their performance. Thus, not using PFP would mean paying everyone in a job the same, regardless of their performance (Gerhart & Fang, 2015). In most cases, this would violate widely held workplace norms and cause perceptions of inequity, especially among the top performers, which is likely to result in more job dissatisfaction (Williams, McDaniel, & Nguyen, 2006) and a higher probability of turnover among top performers (perhaps to organizations that use PFP), or what might be called *negative sorting effects* (see our earlier discussion).

Gerhart and Fang (2015) also observe that in organizations, there does not necessarily seem to be a trade-off between extrinsic and intrinsic motivators. Google, for example, is regularly ranked the best company to work for on the Fortune list of the "100 Best Companies to Work For." One reason is that the nature of the work at Google is described as very interesting, challenging, and cutting edge. Yet Google is also known as a company that has very high pay levels and believes strongly in PFP. For example, Google was recently ranked Number 1 on Glassdoor's list of Top Companies for Compensation and Benefits (Newman et al., 2016, Chapter 2). Glassdoor shows that the average salary for a senior software engineer at Google is $162,637, compared to a national average of $106,675. Regarding, PFP, Laszlo Bock (2015), Google's Head of People Operations, says that Google follows the following principle: "Pay unfairly (it's more fair!)." That phrasing is used to get people's attention. In fact, Bock states that a small percentage of employees create a large percentage of the value, and that Google makes sure that their pay is very high in relative terms to recognize their disproportionate contributions to company success. In other words, employees are paid fairly (i.e., according to their performance contributions/inputs), consistent with equity theory, and consistent with research evidence from field settings, employees do not view being paid well and being paid for their performance at odds with also doing work that is intrinsically motivating and autonomy-enhancing (Gerhart & Fang, 2015).

The fact that sorting effects operate in the labor market is another factor that may significantly limit the degree to which PFP will have negative effects on intrinsic motivation. The standard CET paradigm randomly assigns subjects to performance-contingent pay condition (yes or no), which is intended to ensure that groups are equivalent (i.e., there are no omitted variables). However, it also ensures that there will be a significant degree of mismatch, significantly more than would be found in an actual workplace, between subjects' PFP preferences and how they are paid because in the labor market, people do not match to organizations in a random manner. In fact, the matching process is decidedly nonrandom, such that people and organizations seek to match (or achieve fit) on a variety of dimensions, including between PFP preferences of individuals and actual PFP practice of the organization. By implication, any negative effects of PFP found in a laboratory study where subjects are randomly assigned to PFP conditions (i.e., their PFP preferences are ignored) are likely to be more pronounced than in actual organizations (Fang & Gerhart, 2012; Gerhart & Fang, 2015).

A recent meta-analysis (Cerasoli, Nicklin, & Ford, 2014) examined the relationship between intrinsic motivation and performance, with and without incentives in place. In contrast to the Deci and colleagues (1999) meta-analysis, all included studies used a "correlational" rather than experimental design and included not only nonwork settings (e.g., schools) but also a significant number of effect sizes that were coded as taken from a "work" setting (no description was provided for what qualified as a work setting). As noted, although an experimental design has key advantages, random assignment in this case may be an important limitation in that it eliminates sorting/matching of PFP practice and individual preferences. So results from correlational designs, where random assignment does not take place (and matching/sorting have taken place), are of significant interest. Another key difference is that the Cerasoli and colleagues (2014) meta-analysis used performance (not intrinsic motivation) as its dependent variable. Based on 183 effect sizes, intrinsic motivation (used as an independent variable) and performance (used as a dependent variable) were positively correlated ($r = .21$). In a subset of 74 studies in which the use of extrinsic incentives (compensation) could be clearly determined,[8] the correlation of intrinsic motivation with performance was $r = .21$ when there was no compensation, and $r = .27$ when there was compensation. Thus, a possible interpretation is that there was either no undermining effect of extrinsic incentives (PFP) on intrinsic motivation or, if there was, it was more than offset by the larger positive effect on performance via extrinsic motivation. In their Table 4, Cerasoli and colleagues also reported meta-analytic regression results showing that both intrinsic motivation and extrinsic incentives had positive standardized regression weights in predicting performance quantity ($b = .24$ for intrinsic motivation, $b = .33$ for extrinsic incentives) and performance quality ($b = .35$ for intrinsic motivation performance, $b = .06$ for extrinsic incentives), but that the coefficient for intrinsic motivation in predicting quality, as we see, was considerably larger.[9] This may be taken as evidence that intrinsic motivation is a higher quality of motivation, consistent with SDT (see below). But when it came to predicting a combination of performance quality and quantity ("both"), the regression weights were identical ($b = .29$) for intrinsic motivation and extrinsic incentives.

Cerasoli and colleagues (2014) included a moderator called *salience* (of extrinsic incentives) in an effort to assess the CET-based expectation that more salient incentives are likely to be experienced as more controlling and are therefore more likely to have negative effects. Cerasoli and colleagues concluded that this is the case, stating that "as incentives become larger and more directly salient, teamwork and creativity will be disincentivized, intrinsic motivation and its importance to performance will be crowded out, and unethical or counterproductive behaviors may become more likely" (p. 1000). We note, however, that Cerasoli and colleagues actually presented no empirical evidence on incentive intensity, teamwork, or creativity. With respect to their conclusion that more directly salient rewards lead to reduced intrinsic motivation, none of their main results speak directly to that question either. What their results do show is that the relationship between intrinsic motivation and performance was r = .21 under directly salient incentives, and r = .34 under indirectly salient incentives. Thus, it does not appear that the use of directly salient incentives reduced the influence intrinsic motivation compared to not using directly salient incentives. However, it does appear that the use of directly salient incentives, compared to the use of indirectly salient incentives, was associated with a smaller positive relationship between intrinsic motivation and performance.

Thus, the Cerasoli and colleagues (2014) meta-analysis, the first to incorporate workplace studies, did not find that PFP undermines intrinsic motivation. Likewise, in our review of the literature (Gerhart & Fang, 2015), we found no evidence of an undermining effect in workplace settings and additionally, found little conceptual reason given key attributes of workplace settings that differ from other settings (the norm to be paid for one's work, the norm that higher performers get paid more, the tendency for employees to view intrinsic and extrinsic outcomes as intertwined, not separable career success goals, the operation of sorting/matching/fit processes), to expect an undermining effect. Indeed, one can argue, as just one example, that violating the workplace norm of paying for performance would cause far larger problems than the potential for lowered intrinsic motivation.

Before wrapping up this discussion, we note that SDT, at least in some forms, especially the work by Gagné and Deci (2005), takes a less negative view on the role of PFP in the workplace and indeed recognizes that PFP can enhance intrinsic motivation under some circumstances. One reason is that some forms of extrinsic motivation are now conceptualized under SDT as positively contributing to feelings of autonomy and self-determination (Ryan & Deci, 2000). However, as noted, intrinsic motivation continues to be seen as a higher quality of motivation than extrinsic motivation, which continues to be seen, even in its relatively autonomous forms, as contributing less than intrinsic motivation to the experience of autonomy and self-determination. This important proposition, in our opinion, remains in need of further empirical testing (Gerhart & Fang, 2015).

SUMMARY

In this chapter, we have addressed the role of compensation and how it influences competence in the workplace. Our primary focus has been on the PFP aspect of compensation and on competence defined in terms of performance. We have seen that PFP is widely used in organizations, especially in the private sector, where market forces are strongest, arguably requiring, at least to some significant degree, the use of practices that contribute to efficiency and effectiveness, or what we might call *organization competence*.

In addition, our reading of the evidence (some of which we reviewed here) is that PFP generally has positive effects, contrary to the impression one may develop based on reading some strands of the psychological literature. Nevertheless, no discussion of PFP would be complete without recognizing that the use of PFP can have negative effects, sometimes very negative effects. We suggested that the stronger the intensity of PFP and/or the more of that intensity that is aimed at a specific performance (often objective) goal, the greater the risk of negative, unintended consequences of PFP. We sought to identify some of the factors that make PFP more at risk of causing serious problems and we hope these can be used in improving the design of PFP plans.

We dealt in some depth with one often-discussed unintended negative effect of PFP, which is the concern that PFP, while increasing extrinsic motivation, will often undermine intrinsic motivation, which is seen as being especially problematic because intrinsic motivation under SDT is seen as being a higher-quality form of motivation than extrinsic motivation. Our reading of the evidence is that such undermining effects are small in nonwork settings (based on Deci et al.'s [1999] meta-analytic findings) and that there is no evidence in workplace settings that such an undermining effect takes place. This is not to say that such undermining effects cannot occur in the workplace. But, for reasons (e.g., the norm that work is compensated and that compensation is based on individual performance) that we have described here and elsewhere (Gerhart & Fang, 2015), this seems less likely in workplace settings. Finally, we suggest that future research focus on examining SDT in workplace settings, both to determine whether and under what conditions undermining effects occur, as well as to better establish whether intrinsic motivation is indeed a higher-quality form of motivation than extrinsic motivation.

NOTES

1. Using the "look inside" search function in Google Books of the *Handbook* (*https://books. google.com/books?id=B14TMHRtYBcC*), the term "goal" (or "goals") and "trait" (or "traits") appeared over 100 times; "motivation" appeared 100 times ("intrinsic motivation," 78 times); "ability" appeared 90 times, and "personality," 81 times. The term "employer" appeared one time and the term "employee" appeared two times. The term "compensation" and terms pertaining to its key aspects (e.g., "pay for performance," "merit pay") each appeared zero times. (Actually, there were two instances of the word "compensation" appearing. However, both were in reference lists, and the term was not used to apply to how people are paid.)

2. There are important exceptions. For example, professional sports players' unions in the United States strongly support individual players being paid as much as possible, which is most likely when they are the best performers.

3. On the other hand, a more recent meta-analysis by Weibel, Rost, and Osterloh (2010, Table 2) reports that financial incentives did have a negative effect, $d = -0.13$, in "difficult and/or interesting" tasks. That Weibel

and colleagues obtained a result different from that of Jenkins and colleagues (1998) may stem from the fact that the two meta-analyses include somewhat different primary studies. In any case, using the 15 studies in Table 1 of Weibel and colleagues, which used a "difficult and/or interesting" task, we computed the mean effect size to be +0.21 and the sample-weighted mean effect size to be +0.28. Thus, we were unable to reproduce the negative effect size of incentives on performance in tasks coded as "difficult and/or uninteresting" reported in Weibel and colleagues' Table 2. (One final note is that Webeil et al. did not explain why effect sizes for difficult and interesting tasks were combined.)

4. PFP has also been claimed not to fit with teamwork, and with certain national cultures. Gerhart and Fang (2014) critically evaluate these concerns.

5. A key aspect of the Milgrom and Roberts (1992) incentive intensity principle (p. 221) states: "Incentives should be most intense when agents are able most able to respond to them. Generally, this happens when they have discretion about more aspects of their work, including the pace of work, the tools and methods they use, and so on."

6. One can also challenge the assumption that PFP will typically have a negative effect on perceived autonomy. Fang and Gerhart (2012) did not find this, but instead found a positive effect. Others have also recognized that PFP can have a positive effect on feelings of autonomy (see, e.g., Eisenberger, Rhoades, & Cameron, 1999; Gagné & Deci, 2005).

7. Gerhart and Fang (2015) have noted some limitations when one attempts to draw inferences from the Byron and Khazanchi (2012) meta-analysis for workplace settings given the way creativity was typically defined and measured (e.g., asking children to imagine they are a kernel of popcorn and the heat is being turned on) in most of the studies in the meta-analysis.

8. For example, "when there was any prize, credit, or financial compensation surrounding task performance" (Cerasoli et al., 2014, p. 986).

9. Cerasoli and colleagues (2014, p. 986) coded performance as quality "when output was compared with some evaluative performance standard other than quantity (e.g., creativity, assembly quality, research proposal)" and coded as quantity "when performance was evaluated by counting discrete units of output (e.g., number of points, number of errors

detected, number of problems solved." Performance was coded as "both" for "any criteria that were considered to have elements of *both* (e.g., academic performance). Productivity was included in this category" (p. 986).

REFERENCES

Adams, J. S. (1963). Towards an understanding of inequity. *Journal of Abnormal and Social Psychology, 67,* 422–436.

Amabile, T. M. (1998). How to kill creativity. *Harvard Business Review, 76*(5), 76–87.

Appelbaum, E., Bailey, T., Berg, P., & Kalleberg, A. (2000). *Manufacturing advantage: Why high performance work systems pay off.* Ithaca, NY: Cornell University Press.

Bailcy, T. (1993). *Discretionary effort and the organization of work: Employee participation and work reform since Hawthorne.* Unpublished manuscript, Teachers College, Columbia University, New York.

Bandura, A. (1977). Self-efficacy: Toward a unifying theory of behavioral change. *Psychological Review, 84,* 191–215.

Barrick, M. R., & Mount, M. K. (1991). The Big Five personality dimensions and job performance: A meta-analysis. *Personnel Psychology, 44,* 1–26.

Blinder, A. S. (2009, May 28). Crazy compensation and the crisis. *Wall Street Journal,* p. A15.

Blumberg, M., & Pringle, C. D. (1982). The missing opportunity in organizational research: Some implications for a theory of work performance. *Academy of Management Review, 7*(4), 560–569.

Bock, L. (2015, March). Google's 10 things to transform your team and your workplace. *Fortune,* pp. 136–137.

Boxall, P., & Purcell, J. (2003). *Strategy and human resource management.* Hampshire, UK: Palgrave/Macmillan.

Brogden, H. E. (1949). When testing pays off. *Personnel Psychology, 2,* 171–185.

Byron, K., & Khazanchi, S. (2012). Rewards and creative performance: A meta-analytic test of theoretically derived hypotheses. *Psychological Bulletin, 138,* 809–830.

Cable, D. M., & Judge, T. A. (1994). Pay preferences and job search decisions: A person–organization fit perspective. *Personnel Psychology, 47,* 317–348.

Cadsby, C. B., Song, F., & Tapon, F. (2007). Sorting and incentive effects of pay-for-performance: An experimental investigation. *Academy of Management Journal, 50,* 387–405.

Campbell, J. P. (1990). Modeling the performance prediction problem in industrial and organizational psychology. In M. D. Dunnette & L. M. Hough (Eds.), *Handbook of industrial and organizational psychology* (2nd ed., Vol. 1, pp. 687–732). Palo Alto, CA: Consulting Psychologists Press.

Cascio, W. F., & Boudreau, J. W. (2011). *Investing in people: Financial impact of human resource initiatives* (2nd ed.). Upper Saddle River, NJ: Pearson.

Cerasoli, C. P., Nicklin, J. M., & Ford, M. T. (2014). Intrinsic motivation and extrinsic incentives jointly predict performance: A 40-year meta-analysis. *Psychological Bulletin, 140,* 980–1008.

Deci, E. L. (1975). *Intrinsic motivation.* New York: Plenum Press.

Deci, E. L., Koestner, R., & Ryan, R. M. (1999). A meta-analytic review of experiments examining the effects of extrinsic rewards on intrinsic motivation. *Psychological Bulletin, 25,* 627–668.

Deci, E. L., & Ryan, R. M. (1985). *Intrinsic motivation and self-determination in human behavior.* New York: Plenum Press.

Devers, C. E., McNamara, G., Wiseman, R. M., & Arrfelt, M. (2008). Moving closer to the action: Examining compensation design effects on firm risk. *Organization Science, 19,* 548–566.

Dohmen, T., & Falk, A. (2011). Performance pay and multidimensional sorting: Productivity, preferences, and gender. *American Economic Review, 101,* 556–590.

Dreher, G. F., & Cox, T. H. (2000). Labor market mobility and cash compensation: The moderating effects of race and gender. *Academy of Management Journal, 43*(5), 890–900.

Dweck, C. S., & Leggett, E. L. (1988). A social-cognitive approach to motivation and personality. *Psychological Review, 95,* 256–273.

Dyer, L., Schwab, D. P., & Theriault, R. D. (1976). Managerial perceptions regarding salary increase criteria. *Personnel Psychology, 29,* 233–242.

Eisenberger, R., Rhoades, L., & Cameron, J. (1999). Does pay for performance increase or decrease perceived self-determination and intrinsic motivation? *Journal of Personality and Social Psychology, 77,* 1026–1040.

Elliot, A. J. (2006). The hierarchical model of approach–avoidance motivation. *Motivation and Emotion, 30,* 111–116.

Elliot, A. J., & Church, M. A. (1997). A hierarchical model of approach and avoidance achievement motivation. *Journal of Personality and Social Psychology, 72,* 218–232.

Elliot, A. J., & Dweck, C. S. (2005). Competence as the core of achievement motivation. In A.

J. Elliot & C. S. Dweck (Eds.), *Handbook of competence and motivation* (pp. 3–12). New York: Guilford Press.

Fang, M., & Gerhart, B. (2012). Does pay for performance diminish intrinsic interest? *International Journal of Human Resource Management, 23,* 1176–1196.

Fisher, L. M. (1992, June 23). Sears Auto Centers halt commissions after flap. *New York Times,* pp. D1–D2.

Frey, B. S., & Jegen, R. (2001). Motivation crowding theory. *Journal of Economic Surveys, 15,* 589–611.

Gagné, M., & Deci, E. L. (2005). Self-determination theory and work motivation. *Journal of Organizational Behavior, 26,* 331–362.

Gerhart, B. (2007). Horizontal and vertical fit in human resource systems. In C. Ostroff & T. A. Judge (Eds.), *Perspectives on organizational fit* (pp. 317–348). Mahwah, NJ: Erlbaum.

Gerhart, B., & Fang, M. (2014). Pay for (individual) performance: Issues, claims, evidence and the role of sorting effects. *Human Resource Management Review, 24,* 41–52.

Gerhart, B., & Fang, M. (2015). Pay, intrinsic motivation, extrinsic motivation, performance, and creativity in the workplace: Revisiting long-held beliefs. *Annual Review of Organizational Psychology and Organizational Behavior, 2,* 489–521.

Gerhart, B., & Milkovich, G. T. (1990). Organizational differences in managerial compensation and financial performance. *Academy of Management Journal, 33,* 663–691.

Gerhart, B., & Milkovich, G. T. (1992). Employee compensation: Research and practice. In M. D. Dunnette & L. M. Hough (Eds.), *Handbook of industrial and organizational psychology* (2nd ed., pp. 481–569). Palo Alto, CA: Consulting Psychologists Press.

Gerhart, B., & Rynes, S. (2003). *Compensation: Theory, evidence, and strategic implications.* Thousand Oaks, CA: Sage.

Gerhart, B., Rynes, S. L., & Fulmer, I. S. (2009). Pay and performance: Individuals, groups, and executives. *Academy of Management Annals, 3,* 251–315.

Gerhart, B., Trevor, C., & Graham, M. (1996). New directions in employee compensation research. In G. R. Ferris (Ed.), *Research in personnel and human resources management* (Vol. 14, pp. 143–203). Greenwich, CT: JAI Press.

Glazer, E., & Rexrode, C. (2015, February 2). As regulators focus on culture, Wall Street struggles to define it. *Wall Street Journal,* p. A1.

Gomez-Mejia, L. R., & Balkin, D. B. (1992). Determinants of faculty pay: An agency theory perspective. *Academy of Management Journal, 35*(5), 921–955.

Hackman, J. R., & Oldham, G. R. (1976). Motivation through the design of work: Test of a theory. *Organizational Behavior and Human Performance, 16,* 250–279.

Harrison, D. A., Virick, M., & William, S. (1996). Working without a net: Time, performance, and turnover under maximally contingent rewards. *Journal of Applied Psychology, 81,* 331–345.

Huselid, M. A. (1995). The impact of human resource management practices on turnover, productivity, and corporate financial performance. *Academy of Management Journal, 38,* 635–672.

Jacobs, M. (2009, April 24). Opinion: How business schools have failed business. *Wall Street Journal,* p. A13.

Jenkins, D. G., Jr., Mitra, A., Gupta, N., & Shaw, J. D. (1998). Are financial incentives related to performance?: A meta-analytic review of empirical research. *Journal of Applied Psychology, 83,* 777–787.

Jiang, K., Lepak, D. P., Hu, J., & Baer, J. C. (2012). How does human resource management influence organizational outcomes?: A meta-analytic investigation of mediating mechanisms. *Academy of Management Journal, 55,* 1264–1294.

Judge, T. A., Rodell, J. B., Klinger, R. L., Simon, L. S., & Crawford, E. R. (2013). Hierarchical representations of the five-factor model of personality in predicting job performance: Integrating three organizing frameworks with two theoretical perspectives. *Journal of Applied Psychology, 98,* 875–925.

Kanfer, R. (1990). Motivation theory and industrial/organizational psychology. In M. D. Dunnette & L. M. Hough (Eds.), *Handbook of industrial and organizational psychology* (2nd ed., Vol. 1, pp. 75–170). Palo Alto, CA: Consulting Psychologists Press.

Kanfer, R., & Ackerman, P. L. (1989). Motivation and cognitive abilities: An integrative/aptitude-treatment interaction approach to skill acquisition. *Journal of Applied Psychology, 74,* 657–690.

Kanfer, R., & Ackerman, P. L. (2005). Work competence. In A. J. Elliot & C. S. Dweck (Eds.), *Handbook of competence and motivation* (pp. 336–353). New York: Guilford Press.

Katz, H. C., Kochan, T. A., & Weber, M. R. (1985). Assessing the effects of industrial relations systems and efforts to improve the quality of working life on organizational effectiveness. *Academy of Management Journal, 28,* 509–526.

Keith, K., & McWilliams, A. (1999). The returns

to mobility and job search by gender. *Industrial and Labor Relations Review, 52*(3), 460–477.

Kerr, S. (1975). On the folly of rewarding A, while hoping for B. *Academy of Management Journal, 18*, 769–783.

Kohn, A. (1993, September). Why incentive plans cannot work. *Harvard Business Review*, pp. 54–63.

Latham, G. P. (2007). *Work motivation: History, theory, research, and practice.* Thousand Oaks, CA: Sage.

Latham, G. P., & Pinder, C. C. (2005). Work motivation theory and research at the dawn of the twenty-first century. *Annual Review of Psychology, 56*, 485–516.

Lawler, E. E., III. (1971). *Pay and organizational effectiveness: A psychological view.* New York: McGraw-Hill.

Lazear, E. P. (2000). Performance pay and productivity. *American Economic Review, 90*, 1346–1361.

Lazear, E. P. (1986). Salaries and piece rates. *Journal of Business, 59*, 405–431.

Locke, E. A., & Latham, G. P. (1990). *A theory of goal setting and task performance.* New York: Prentice Hall.

Locke, E. A., & Latham, G. P. (2002). Building a practically useful theory of goal setting and task motivation. *American Psychology, 57*, 705–717.

Lord, R. G., Diefendorff, J. M., Schmidt A. M., & Hall, R. J. (2010). Self-regulation at work. *Annual Review of Psychology, 61*, 543–568.

Macduffie, J. P. (1995). Human resource bundles and manufacturing performance: Organizational logic and flexible production systems in the world auto industry. *Industrial and Labor Relations Review, 48*(2), 197–221.

McClelland, D. C., Atkinson, J. W., Clark, R. A., & Lowell, E. L. (1953). *The achievement motive.* Oxford, UK: Irvington.

Milgrom, P., & Roberts, J. (1992). *Economics, organization, and management.* Englewood Cliffs, NJ: Prentice Hall.

Newman, J., Gerhart, B., & Milkovich, G. T. (2016). *Compensation* (12th ed.). New York: McGraw-Hill/Irwin.

Nicholls, J. G. (1984). Achievement motivation: Conceptions of ability, subjective experience, task choice, and performance. *Psychological Review, 91*, 328–346.

Nyberg, A. J. (2010). Retaining your high performers: Moderators of the performance–job satisfaction–voluntary turnover relationships. *Journal of Applied Psychology, 95*, 440–53.

The origins of the financial crisis: Crash course. (2013, September 7). *The Economist*, p. 74.

Peters, L. H., & O'Connor, E. J. (1980). Situational constraints and work outcomes: The influences of a frequently overlooked construct. *Academy of Management Review, 5*, 391–397.

Pfeffer, J. (1998). *The human equation: Building profits by putting people first.* Boston: Harvard Business School Press.

Pink, D. (2009). *Drive: The surprising truth about what motivates us.* New York: Penguin.

Ployhart, R. E., & Moliterno, T. P. (2011). Emergence of the human capital resource: A multilevel model. *Academy of Management Review, 36*, 127–150.

Prendergast, C. (1999). The provision of incentives in firms. *Journal of Economic Literature, 37*, 7–63.

Roy, D. (1952). Quota restriction and gold bricking in a machine shop. *American Journal of Sociology, 57*, 427–442.

Ryan, R. M., & Deci, E. L. (2000). Intrinsic and extrinsic motivations: Classic definitions and new directions. *Contemporary Educational Psychology, 25*, 54–67.

Ryan, R. M., Mims, V., & Koestner, R. (1983). Relation of reward contingency and interpersonal context to intrinsic motivation: A review and test using cognitive evaluation theory. *Journal of Personality and Social Psychology, 45*, 736–750.

Rynes, S. L. (1987). Compensation strategies for recruiting. *Topics in Total Compensation, 2*, 185–196.

Rynes, S. L., Gerhart, B., & Minette, K. A. (2004). The importance of pay in employee motivation: Discrepancies between what people say and what they do. *Human Resource Management, 43*, 381–394.

Rynes, S. L., Gerhart, B., & Parks, L. (2005). Personnel psychology: Performance evaluation and pay for performance. *Annual Review of Psychology, 56*, 571–600.

Salamin, A., & Hom, P. W. (2005). In search of the elusive U-shaped performance turnover relationship: Are high performing Swiss bankers more liable to quit? *Journal of Applied Psychology, 90*, 1204–1216.

Sanders, W. G., & Hambrick, D. C. (2007). Swinging for the fences: The effects of CEO stock options on company risk taking and performance. *Academy of Management Journal, 50*, 1055–1078.

Schmidt, A. M., Beck, J. W., & Gillespie, J. Z. (2013). Motivation. In N. W. Schmitt, S. Highhouse, & I. Weiner (Eds.), *Handbook of psychology: Industrial and organizational psychology* (Vol. 12, pp. 311–340). Hoboken, NJ: Wiley.

Schmidt, A. M., & DeShon, R. P. (2007). What to do?: The effects of discrepancies, incentives, and time on dynamic goal prioritization. *Journal of Applied Psychology, 92,* 928–41.

Schmidt, F. L., & Hunter, J. E. (1998). The validity of selection methods in personnel psychology: Practical and theoretical implications of 85 years of research findings. *Psychological Bulletin, 124,* 262–274.

Schneider, B. (1987). The people make the place. *Personnel Psychology, 40,* 437–453.

Schneider, B., Smith, D. B., Taylor, S., & Fleenor, J. (1998). Personality and organizations: A test of the homogeneity of personality hypothesis. *Journal of Applied Psychology, 83,* 462–470.

Shaw, J. D., Dineen, B. R., Fang, R., & Vellella, R. F. (2009). Employee–organization exchange relationships, HRM practices, and quit rates of good and poor performers. *Academy of Management Journal, 52,* 1016–1033.

Sheldon, K. M., & Elliot, A. J. (1999). Goal striving, need-satisfaction, and longitudinal well-being: The self-concordance model. *Journal of Personality and Social Psychology, 76,* 482–497.

Sheldon, K. M., Ryan, R. M., Deci, E. L., & Kasser, T. (2004). The independent effects of goal contents and motives on well-being: It's both what you pursue and why you pursue it. *Personal and Social Psychology Bulletin, 30,* 475–486.

Shepperd, J. A. (1993). Productivity loss in performance groups: A motivation analysis. *Psychological Bulletin, 113,* 67–81.

Society for Human Resource Management. (2014). Job satisfaction and engagement survey. Retrieved from *www.shrm.org/research/surveyfindings/documents/14–0028%20job-satengage_report_full_fnl.pdf.*

Strauss, V. (2015, April 1). How and why convicted Atlanta teachers cheated on standardized tests. *Washington Post.* Retrieved from *www. washingtonpost.com/news/answer-sheet/wp/2015/04/01/how-and-why-convicted-atlanta-teachers-cheated-on-standardized-tests.*

Trank, C. Q., Rynes, S. L., & Bretz, R. D., Jr. (2002). Attracting applicants in the war for talent: Differences in work preferences among high achievers. *Journal of Business and Psychology, 16,* 331–345.

Trevor, C. O., Gerhart, B., & Boudreau, J. W. (1997). Voluntary turnover and job performance: Curvilinearity and the moderating influences of salary growth and promotions. *Journal of Applied Psychology, 82,* 44–61.

Vansteenkiste, M., Sierens, E., Soenens, B., Luyckx, K., & Lens, W. (2009). Motivational profiles from a self-determination theory perspective: The quality of motivation matters. *Journal of Educational Psychology, 101,* 671–688.

Vroom, V. H. (1964). *Work and motivation.* New York: Wiley.

Weibel, A., Rost, K., & Osterloh, M. (2010). Pay for performance in the public sector—Benefits and (hidden) costs. *Journal of Public Administration Research and Theory, 20,* 387–412.

White, R. W. (1959). Motivation reconsidered: The concept of competence. *Psychological Review, 66,* 297–333.

Williams, M. L., McDaniel, M. A., & Nguyen, N. T. (2006). A meta-analysis of the antecedents and consequences of pay level satisfaction. *Journal of Applied Psychology, 91,* 392–413.

WorldatWork. (2012). *Compensation programs and practices 2012.* Scottsdale, AZ: Author.

Wright, P. M., George, J. M., Farnsworth, R., & McMahan, G. C. (1993). Productivity and extra-role behavior: The effects of goals and incentives on spontaneous helping. *Journal of Applied Psychology, 78,* 374–381.

CHAPTER 14

Achievement Emotions

REINHARD PEKRUN

Emotions are ubiquitous in achievement settings. Remember the last time you took an important exam? You may have hoped for success, feared failure, or felt desperate because you were unprepared, but you likely did not feel indifferent. Furthermore, these emotions affected your motivation, concentration, and strategies used for studying—even if you were unaware of these effects. Similarly, think of the last time you worked on a project. Depending on the goals, tasks, and social interactions involved, you may have enjoyed working on it or felt bored, experienced a sense of flow or frustration about never-ending obstacles, and felt proud of the outcome or ashamed of lack of accomplishment. Again, these emotions likely had profound effects on your interest in the project, motivation to persist, and strategies for approaching the tasks involved.

Until recently, these emotions did not receive much of researchers' attention, except for studies on test anxiety (Zeidner, 2014). Early work on achievement emotions remained largely unattended (e.g., Hersey, 1932). During the past 20 years, however, there has been growing recognition that emotions are central to human achievement strivings. Emotions are no longer regarded as epiphenomena that may occur in achievement settings but lack any instrumental relevance. Across disciplines, there is growing recognition that emotions are critically important for performance and the productivity of individuals, organizations, and cultures (Ashkanasy & Humphrey, 2011; Pekrun & Linnenbrink-Garcia, 2014b). In fact, authors in educational research and management science alike have recently claimed that there is an affective turn in their fields (Barsade, Brief, & Spataro, 2003; Pekrun & Linnenbrink-Garcia, 2014a).

In this chapter, I provide an overview of theories, findings, and applications related to achievement emotions. To begin, I discuss concepts of emotion and achievement emotions. In the next sections I address the functions and origins of achievement emotions, as well as reciprocal causation, regulation, and relative universality of these emotions. Finally, I discuss implications for practice, including implications for understanding achievement emotions, the design of tasks and achievement settings, the assessment of achievement, and treatment interventions aiming to enhance adaptive and reduce maladaptive achievement emotions.

CONCEPTS OF EMOTION AND ACHIEVEMENT EMOTION

In current emotion research, *emotions* are defined as multifaceted phenomena

251

involving sets of coordinated psychological processes, including affective, cognitive, physiological, motivational, and expressive components (Scherer, 2009). For example, a student's anxiety before an exam may comprise nervous, uneasy feelings (affective); worries about failing the exam (cognitive); increased physiological activation (physiological); impulses to escape the situation (motivation); and anxious facial expression (expressive). As compared to intense emotions, *moods* are of lower intensity and lack a specific referent. Some authors define emotion and mood as categorically distinct (see Rosenberg, 1998). Alternatively, since moods show a similar profile of components and similar qualitative differences as emotions (as in cheerful, angry, or anxious mood), they can be regarded as low-intensity emotions (Pekrun, 2006).

Achievement emotions are defined as emotions that relate to achievement activities (e.g., participating in a competition) or achievement outcomes (success and failure; see Table 14.1). As such, achievement emotions are defined by their object focus and differ from other types of emotions in terms of object focus. Most emotions pertaining to studying, working, or participating in sports are seen as achievement emotions, since they relate to activities and outcomes that are typically judged according to competence-based standards of quality. However, not all of the emotions experienced in achievement settings are achievement emotions. Specifically, *social emotions* are frequently experienced in these same settings, such as empathy for a coworker. Achievement and social emotions

may overlap, as in emotions directed toward the achievement of others (e.g., contempt, envy, empathy, or admiration instigated by the success or failure of others). Similarly, *epistemic emotions,* such as surprise, curiosity, or confusion that relate to the generation of knowledge, also frequently occur in achievement situations like preparing for a test (Muis et al., 2015; Pekrun, Vogl, Muis, & Sinatra, 2016).

Past research focused on emotions induced by achievement outcomes, such as hope and pride related to success, or anxiety and shame related to failure. Two important traditions of research on outcome emotions are test anxiety studies (Zeidner, 1998, 2014) and studies on emotions following success and failure (e.g., Weiner, 1985). Certainly outcome emotions are of critical importance for achievement strivings. However, herein I argue that emotions directly pertaining to the performance of achievement activities are also to be considered achievement emotions and are of equal relevance for achievement strivings. The excitement arising from the commencement of a challenging project, boredom experienced when performing monotonous routine tasks, or anger felt when task demands seem unreasonable are examples of activity-related achievement emotions. These emotions have traditionally been neglected but have received more attention recently (see, e.g., Tze, Daniels, & Klassen, 2016).

In Pekrun, Goetz, Titz, and Perry's (2002; Pekrun & Perry, 2014) three-dimensional taxonomy of achievement emotions, the differentiation of activity versus outcome

TABLE 14.1. A Three-Dimensional Taxonomy of Achievement Emotions

Object focus	Positive[a]		Negative[b]	
	Activating	Deactivating	Activating	Deactivating
Activity	Enjoyment	Relaxation	Anger	Boredom Frustration
Outcome: prospective	Hope Joy[c]	Relief[c]	Anxiety	Hopelessness
Outcome: retrospective	Joy Pride Gratitude	Contentment Relief	Shame Anger	Sadness Disappointment

[a]Positive, pleasant emotion; [b]negative, unpleasant emotion; [c]anticipatory joy/relief.

emotions pertains to the *object focus* of these emotions. In addition, as emotions more generally, achievement emotions can be grouped according to their *valence* and to the degree of *activation* implied (Table 14.1). In terms of valence, positive emotions can be distinguished from negative emotions, such as pleasant enjoyment versus unpleasant anxiety. In terms of activation, physiologically activating emotions can be distinguished from deactivating emotions, such as activating excitement versus deactivating contentment. By using the dimensions valence and activation, the taxonomy is consistent with circumplex models that arrange affective states in a two-dimensional (valence × activation) space (Barrett & Russell, 1998).

Exploratory research has documented that the emotions organized in this taxonomy are experienced frequently in achievement settings. For example, in a series of interview and questionnaire studies with high school and university students, we found that anxiety was the emotion reported most often, constituting 15–27% of all emotional episodes reported across various academic situations (e.g., attending class, studying, taking tests and exams; Pekrun et al., 2002). This prevalence of anxiety corroborates the importance of test anxiety research. However, the vast majority of emotions reported in these studies pertained to emotion categories other than anxiety, with episodes of enjoyment, satisfaction, hope, pride, relief, anger, boredom, and shame reported frequently as well.

FUNCTIONS FOR MOTIVATION AND PERFORMANCE

Are emotions functionally important for human performance? Experimental mood research suggests the answer is "yes." In this research, mood and emotions have been found to influence a wide range of cognitive processes, including attention, memory storage and retrieval, social judgment, decision making, and cognitive problem solving (Clore & Huntsinger, 2007, 2009; Lewis, Haviland-Jones, & Barrett, 2008). Specifically, it has been shown that both positive and negative emotional states consume *cognitive resources* by focusing attention on the object of emotion (Ellis & Ashbrook, 1988). Consumption of cognitive resources for task-irrelevant purposes implies that fewer resources are available for task completion, thereby negatively impacting performance (Meinhardt & Pekrun, 2003). Second, mood can influence *memory processes*, such as mood-congruent memory recall and retrieval-induced facilitation and forgetting. Mood-congruent recall implies that positive mood supports retrieval of positive self-related and task-related information, and negative mood supports the retrieval of negative information (e.g., Olafson & Ferraro, 2001). Retrieval-induced facilitation and forgetting imply that practicing learned materials promotes or inhibits recall of nonpracticed materials. Positive mood can support retrieval-induced facilitation, and negative mood can reduce retrieval-induced forgetting (see Kuhbandner & Pekrun, 2013), thus influencing success at learning.

Finally, mood has been shown to influence *cognitive problem solving*, with positive mood promoting flexible and creative ways of solving problems, and negative mood promoting more focused, detail-oriented, and analytical ways of thinking (Clore & Huntsinger, 2007, 2009; Fredrickson, 2001). In mood-as-information approaches (Clore & Huntsinger, 2007), this finding is explained by assuming that positive affective states signal that "all is well," implying safety and the discretion to engage in creative exploration, whereas negative states indicate that something is going wrong, making it necessary to focus on problems in analytical, cognitively cautious ways.

Experimental mood research has generally been conducted in laboratory settings and has tended to disregard ecological validity for real-life achievement. It is open to question whether laboratory findings are generalizable to the more intense emotions experienced in school, work, and sports settings; different mechanisms may be operating under natural conditions, and these mechanisms may interact in different ways. By contrast, field research in education, business, and sports has directly analyzed links between emotions and real-life performance. Though most of this research has focused on achievement-related anxiety (see Beilock, Schaeffer, & Rozek, Chapter 9, this volume), a few studies have analyzed other emotions as well. The valence and activation dimensions of emotions may be most important for explaining the findings of these studies, implying that four emotion categories should be distinguished for doing so (positive-activating, positive-deactivating, negative-activating, negative-deactivating; Table 14.1). Emotions from these four categories can influence the various mechanisms underlying effects on performance, such as the availability of cognitive resources enabling individuals to focus attention on achievement tasks; interest and motivation to perform these tasks; memory processes; and use of cognitive and metacognitive strategies for solving task problems, including the self-regulation of achievement behavior.

Positive Emotions: Enjoyment, Hope, Pride, and Relief

In experimental mood research, it was traditionally assumed that positive emotions can be maladaptive as a result of inducing unrealistic appraisals, fostering superficial information processing, and reducing motivation to pursue challenging goals. This perspective implied that "our primary goal is to feel good, and feeling good makes us lazy thinkers who are oblivious to potentially useful negative information and unresponsive to meaningful variations in information and situation" (Aspinwall, 1998, p. 7). However, positive mood has typically been regarded as a unitary construct in this research. Such a view fails to distinguish between activating versus deactivating moods and emotions (also see Ashkanasy, Härtel, & Daus, 2002).

As detailed in Pekrun's (2006) cognitive–motivational model of emotion effects, *deactivating* positive emotions may well have negative effects on the investment of effort, whereas *activating* positive emotions, such as task enjoyment or pride, may have positive effects. Specifically, task enjoyment can preserve cognitive resources and focus attention on the task; promote the development of interest and intrinsic motivation; support retrieval-induced facilitation; and enhance the use of flexible cognitive strategies (e.g., elaboration and organization of task material) and self-regulation, thus exerting positive effects on overall performance under

many task conditions (Fredrickson, 2001; Kuhbandner & Pekrun, 2013). By contrast, deactivating positive emotions, such as relief and relaxation, can reduce task attention, can have variable motivational effects by undermining current motivation while at the same time reinforcing motivation to reengage with the task (Sweeny & Vohs, 2012), and can lead to superficial information processing, thus likely making effects on overall performance more variable.

Empirical evidence on the effects of positive achievement emotions is scarce, but supports the view that activating positive emotions can enhance performance. Specifically, enjoyment of learning was found to correlate positively with K–12 and college students' interest, use of flexible learning strategies, self-regulation of learning, and academic performance (e.g., Pekrun et al., 2002). Consistent with evidence on discrete emotions, general positive affect has also been found to correlate positively with students' cognitive engagement, as well as with workers' success on the job (Fisher, 2010; Linnenbrink, 2007). However, some studies have found null relations between activating positive emotions (or affect) and individual engagement and performance (Linnenbrink, 2007; Pekrun, Elliot, & Maier, 2009). Also, caution should be exercised in interpreting the reported correlations. Links between emotions and performance are likely due not only to performance effects of emotions but also to effects of performance attainment on emotions, implying reciprocal rather than unidirectional causation (Pekrun, Lichtenfeld, Marsh, Murayama, & Goetz, in press).

Negative Activating Emotions: Anxiety, Shame, and Anger

Emotions such as anger, anxiety, and shame produce task-irrelevant thinking, thus reducing cognitive resources available for task purposes, and they undermine intrinsic motivation. On the other hand, these emotions can induce motivation to avoid failure, reduce retrieval-induced forgetting, and facilitate the use of more rigid learning strategies. By implication, the effects on resulting performance depend on task conditions and may well be variable, similar to the proposed effects of positive deactivating emotions. The available evidence supports this position. Specifically, it has been shown that *test anxiety* impairs performance on complex or difficult tasks that demand cognitive resources, such as difficult intelligence test items, whereas performance on easy, less complex, and repetitive tasks may not suffer or is even enhanced (Hembree, 1988; Zeidner, 1998, 2014). Theories explaining this finding have focused on the effects of anxiety on task-irrelevant thinking that interferes with performance on tasks requiring cognitive resources (interference and attentional deficit models; see Chang & Beilock, 2016; Eysenck, 1997).

In line with experimental findings, field studies have shown that test anxiety correlates moderately negatively with students' academic performance. Typically, 5–10% of the variance in students' achievement scores is explained by self-reported anxiety (Hembree, 1988; Zeidner, 2014). Similarly, a few studies in occupational and sports psychology have found that anxiety relates negatively to overall performance in the workplace (Warr, 2007) and in sports involving complex sensorimotor skills (e.g., Wilson, Smith, & Holmes, 2007).

Again, in explaining the correlational evidence, reciprocal causation of emotion and performance has to be considered. Links between test anxiety and achievement may be caused by effects of success and failure on the development of test anxiety, in addition to effects of anxiety on performance, as shown in longitudinal studies of causal ordering (Meece, Wigfield, & Eccles, 1990; Pekrun, 1992; Pekrun et al., in press). Furthermore, correlations with performance variables have not been uniformly negative across studies; zero and positive correlations have sometimes been found. Anxiety likely has deleterious effects in many individuals, but it may induce motivation to invest more effort, thus facilitating overall performance in those who are more resilient to the devastating aspects of anxiety (e.g., Perkins & Corr, 2005).

Few studies have addressed the effects of negative activating emotions other than anxiety. Similar to anxiety, *shame* related to failure shows negative overall correlations with students' effort and academic achievement (Pekrun, Goetz, Frenzel, Barchfeld,

& Perry, 2011) and negatively predicts exam performance (Pekrun et al., 2009). However, as with anxiety, shame likely exerts variable motivational effects. Turner and Schallert (2001) showed that students who experienced shame following negative exam feedback increased their motivation when they continued to be committed to future academic goals and believed these goals were attainable. Baggozi, Verbeke, and Gavino (2003) found that shame either decreased or increased salespeople's performance, depending on culture-linked ways of regulating the emotion.

Similarly, while achievement-related *anger* correlated positively with task-irrelevant thinking and negatively with self-efficacy, interest, self regulation of learning, and performance in a few studies (Boekaerts, 1993; Pekrun, Goetz, et al., 2011), the underlying mechanisms can be complex. In a study by Lane, Whyte, Terry, and Nevill (2005), anger was related to improved performance in students who reported no depressive mood symptoms—presumably because they were able to maintain motivation and invest necessary effort. It has also been found that anger can support performance in the management of projects (Lindebaum & Fielden, 2010; Thiel, Connelly, & Griffith, 2012). In summary, the findings for anxiety, shame, and anger support the notion that performance effects of negative activating emotions are complex, although relationships with overall performance are negative for many task conditions and individuals.

Negative Deactivating Emotions: Boredom and Hopelessness

In contrast to negative activating emotions, negative deactivating emotions, such as boredom and hopelessness, may uniformly impair performance by reducing cognitive resources, undermining both intrinsic and extrinsic motivation, and promoting superficial information processing (Pekrun, 2006). The scant evidence available today corroborates that boredom and hopelessness relate uniformly negatively to students' and employees' motivation and achievement (e.g., Ahmed, van der Werf, Kuyper, & Minnaert, 2013), and longitudinal research has confirmed that boredom negatively predicts performance (Pekrun, Goetz, Daniels, Stupnisky, & Perry, 2010; Pekrun, Hall, Goetz, & Perry, 2014).

In summary, theoretical expectations, the evidence produced by experimental studies, and findings from field studies imply that achievement emotions have profound effects on engagement and performance. As such, educators, supervisors, and coaches should pay attention to the emotions experienced by their students, employees, and athletes. Most likely, the effects of enjoyment of achievement activities are beneficial, whereas hopelessness and boredom are detrimental for engagement. The effects of emotions such as anger, anxiety, or shame are more complex, but for the average individual, these emotions typically also have negative overall effects.

INDIVIDUAL AND SOCIAL ORIGINS

Appraisal Antecedents

Emotions can be influenced by numerous individual factors, including genetic dispositions, temperament, situational perceptions, cognitive appraisals, neurohormonal processes, and sensory feedback from nonverbal expression (Lewis et al., 2008). Among these factors, cognitive appraisals of situational demands, personal competencies, and the value of success and failure outcomes likely play a major role in the arousal of achievement emotions. In contrast to emotions induced in phylogenetically older and more constrained situations (e.g., enjoyment of physiological need fulfilment; anxiety of falling when perceiving heights; Campos, Bertenthal, & Kermoian, 1992), achievement emotions pertain to culturally defined demands in settings that are a recent product of civilization. In these settings, the individual has to learn how to adapt to situational demands while preserving individual autonomy—inevitably a process guided by appraisals. Thus, research on the determinants of achievement emotions from early on has focused on appraisals.

Test Anxiety

In research on test anxiety, appraisals concerning threat of failure have been addressed as causing anxiety. Using R. S. Lazarus's transactional stress model (Lazarus & Folkman, 1984) for explaining test anxiety, threat in a given achievement setting is evaluated in a *primary appraisal* related to the likelihood and subjective importance of failure. If failure is appraised as possible and subjectively important, ways to cope with the situation are evaluated in a *secondary appraisal*. A student may experience anxiety when his or her primary appraisal indicates that failure on an important test is likely, and when his or her secondary appraisal indicates that this threat is not sufficiently controllable. Empirical research confirms that test anxiety is closely related to perceived lack of control over performance. Specifically, numerous studies have shown that students' academic self-concept, self-efficacy expectations, and control beliefs correlate negatively with their test anxiety (Zeidner, 1998, 2014).

Attributional Theory

Extending the perspective beyond test anxiety, Weiner (1985) proposed an attributional approach to the appraisal antecedents of emotions related to success and failure (see Perry & Hamm, Chapter 5, this volume). In Weiner's theory, causal achievement attributions—explanations about the causes of success and failure (e.g., ability, effort, task difficulty, luck)—are considered primary determinants of these emotions. More specifically, it is assumed that achievement outcomes are first subjectively evaluated as success or failure. This outcome appraisal immediately leads to cognitively less elaborated, "attribution-independent" emotions, namely, happiness following success, and frustration and sadness following failure. Following the outcome appraisal and immediate emotional reaction, causal ascriptions are sought that lead to differentiated, attribution-dependent emotions.

Three dimensions of causal attributions are assumed to play key roles in determining attribution-dependent emotions: the perceived locus of causality differentiating internal versus external causes of achievement (e.g., ability and effort vs. environmental circumstances or chance); the perceived controllability of causes (e.g., subjectively controllable effort vs. uncontrollable ability);

and the perceived stability of causes (e.g., stable ability vs. unstable chance). Weiner posits that pride should be experienced when success is attributed to internal causes (e.g., effort or ability); that shame should be experienced when failure is attributed to uncontrollable, internal causes (e.g., lack of ability); and that gratitude and anger should be experienced when success or failure, respectively, are attributed to external, other-controlled causes. Consistent with the retrospective nature of causal attributions for success and failure, Weiner's theory focuses primarily on retrospective emotions following success and failure. However, some predictions for prospective, future-related emotions are also put forward. Specifically, hopefulness and hopelessness are expected to be experienced when past success and failure are attributed to stable causes (e.g., stable ability). Empirical research has generally supported the propositions of Weiner's theory (Perry & Hamm, Chapter 5, this volume).

Control–Value Theory

While test anxiety theories and attributional theories have addressed emotions pertaining to success and failure outcomes, they have neglected activity-related achievement emotions. In Pekrun's (2006; Pekrun & Perry, 2014) control–value theory of achievement emotions, propositions of the transactional stress model (Lazarus & Folkman, 1984), expectancy–value approaches to emotion (Pekrun, 1992; Turner & Schallert, 2001), and attributional theories are expanded to explain a broader variety of achievement emotions, including both outcome emotions and activity emotions. The theory posits that achievement emotions are induced when an individual feels in control of, or out of control of, activities and outcomes that are subjectively important—implying that appraisals of control (i.e., perceived controllability) and value (i.e., perceived importance; see Wigfield, Rosenzweig, & Eccles, Chapter 7, this volume) are the proximal determinants of these emotions (Figure 14.1).

Different kinds of control and value appraisals are posited to instigate different kinds of achievement emotions (Table 14.1). *Prospective, anticipatory joy* and *hopelessness* are expected to be triggered when there

is high perceived control (joy) or a complete lack of perceived control (hopelessness). For example, a scientist who believes he has the necessary resources to publish an article on an important discovery may feel joyous about the prospect of seeing his work in print. Conversely, a CEO who believes she is incapable of preventing her company from going bankrupt may experience hopelessness. *Prospective hope and anxiety* are instigated when there is uncertainty about control, with the attentional focus on anticipated success in the case of hope and on anticipated failure in the case of anxiety. For example, a student who is unsure about being able to succeed may hope for success, fear failure, or both. *Retrospective joy and sadness* are considered control-independent emotions that immediately follow success and failure (in line with Weiner's [1985] propositions). *Disappointment and relief* are thought to depend on the perceived match between expectations and the actual outcome, with disappointment arising when anticipated success does not occur, and relief when anticipated failure does not occur. Finally, *pride, shame, gratitude,* and *anger* are assumed to be instigated by causal attributions of success and failure to oneself or others, respectively.

Furthermore, the control–value theory proposes that these outcome-related emotions also depend on the subjective importance of achievement outcomes, implying that they are a joint function of perceived control and value. For instance, an advertising executive should feel worried if she judges herself incapable of coordinating a campaign (low controllability) for an important client (high value). In contrast, if she feels that she is able to coordinate the campaign (high controllability) or is indifferent about the client (low value), her anxiety should be low.

Regarding activity emotions, *enjoyment of achievement activities* is proposed to depend on a combination of positive competence appraisals and positive appraisals of the intrinsic value of the action (e.g., studying) and its reference object (e.g., learning material). For example, a student is expected to enjoy learning if he feels competent to meet the demands of the learning task and values the learning material. If he feels

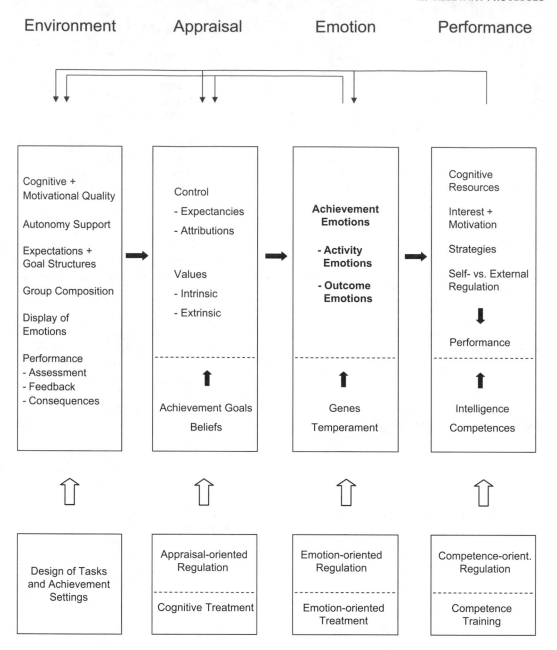

FIGURE 14.1. Basic propositions of the control–value theory of achievement emotions.

incompetent, or is disinterested in the material, studying is not enjoyable. *Anger* and *frustration* are aroused when the intrinsic value of the activity is negative (e.g., when working on a difficult project is perceived as taking too much effort that is experienced as aversive). Finally, *boredom* is experienced when the activity lacks any intrinsic incentive value (Pekrun et al., 2010).

Empirical studies have confirmed that perceived control over achievement relates positively to achievement-related enjoyment, hope, and pride, and negatively to anger, anxiety, shame, hopelessness, and boredom (for a summary, see Pekrun & Perry, 2014). Furthermore, several of these studies have shown that the perceived value of achievement related positively to both positive and negative achievement emotions except boredom, indicating that the importance of success and failure amplifies these emotions. For boredom, negative links with perceived value have been found, suggesting that boredom is reduced when individuals value achievement (Pekrun et al., 2010). Finally, recent research has confirmed that control and value interact in the arousal of achievement emotions, with positive emotions being especially pronounced when both control and value are high, and negative emotions being pronounced when value is high but control is lacking (e.g., Goetz, Frenzel, Stoeger, & Hall, 2010).

Nonreflective Induction of Emotions

Importantly, emotions need not always be mediated by conscious appraisals. Rather, recurring appraisal-based induction of emotions can become automatic and nonreflective over time. When achievement activities are repeated over and over again, appraisals and the induction of emotions can become routinized to the extent that there is no longer any conscious mediation of emotions—or no longer any cognitive mediation at all (Reisenzein, 2001). In the procedural emotion schemas established by routinization, situation perception and emotion are directly linked, such that perceptions can automatically induce the emotion (e.g., the mere smell of a chemistry lab inducing joy). However, when the situation changes or attempts are made to change the emotion (as in psychotherapy), appraisals come into play again.

The Role of Achievement Goals

To the extent that cognitive appraisals are proximal determinants of achievement emotions, more distal individual antecedents, such as gender or achievement-related beliefs, should affect these emotions by first influencing appraisals (Figure 14.1; Pekrun, 2006). This can also be assumed for the influence of achievement goals, which are thought to direct attentional focus in the course of control and value appraisals. Achievement goals are viewed as the competence-relevant aims that individuals strive for in achievement settings (Elliot & Hulleman, Chapter 4, this volume) and can

relate to different definitions of achievement. Specifically, achievement can be defined by task-based, absolute criteria or self-based individual standards (jointly called *mastery* in achievement goal research) or by other-based standards comparing performance across individuals (called *performance*), thus leading to a differentiation of mastery goals versus performance goals. In addition, both types of achievement goals can either focus on approaching success or on avoiding failure, thus rendering four types of goals within a 2 × 2 taxonomy as proposed by Elliot and McGregor (2001; mastery-approach, mastery-avoidance, performance-approach, performance-avoidance). The taxonomy has been further refined by considering the distinction between task-based and self-based goals (3 × 2 taxonomy; Elliot, Murayama, & Pekrun, 2011).

Because achievement goals are central to achievement motivation, understanding the relationship between these goals and achievement emotions is of specific importance for explaining achievement strivings. In a theoretical model linking achievement goals to emotions, Pekrun, Elliot, and Maier (2006, 2009) argued that mastery-approach goals focus attention on the ongoing mastery of the activity and the positive value of the activity itself, thus fostering positive activity emotions such as enjoyment of learning, and reducing negative activity emotions such as boredom. By contrast, performance-approach goals were posited to focus attention on the perceived controllability and positive value of outcomes, implying they should facilitate positive outcome emotions such as hope and pride. Performance-avoidance goals were posited to focus attention on the perceived uncontrollability and negative value of negative outcomes, suggesting they should evoke negative outcome emotions such as anxiety, shame, and hopelessness.

The available evidence is largely in line with these propositions. Whereas relations between achievement goals and omnibus variables of general positive and negative affect have been inconsistent (Linnenbrink & Pintrich, 2002; Pekrun et al., 2006, 2009), achievement goals show clear linkages with discrete achievement emotions. The relation between performance-avoidance goals and test anxiety is best documented, but recent research also shows clear relations for mastery-approach goals and activity emotions (positive for enjoyment, negative for boredom), and for performance goals and outcome emotions other than anxiety, such as pride, shame, and hopelessness (Huang, 2011; Pekrun et al., 2006, 2009). The close relation between achievement-related goals and subsequent emotions also implies that emotions can function as mediators of the performance effects of achievement goals. For example, in studies by Elliot and McGregor (1999) and Pekrun and colleagues (2009), performance-avoidance goals predicted anxiety, which in turn was a negative predictor of achievement, implying that anxiety mediated the effects of performance-avoidance goals on achievement.

The Influence of Tasks and Environments

The impact of task design and environments on achievement emotions has primarily been explored in research on the antecedents of test anxiety (for reviews, see Wigfield & Eccles, 1990; Zeidner, 1998, 2014). Factors influencing control and value appraisals have been found to impact test anxiety arousal, such as lack of structure and clarity in exams, excessively high task demands, time pressure, negative feedback on performance, or a lack of second chances. For emotions other than anxiety, factors that have been addressed include the cognitive and motivational quality of tasks and achievement settings, social expectations and goal structures in these settings, autonomy support, the composition of groups, and the transmission of emotions in social interaction. As all of these factors can be changed and used to influence achievement emotions, they are discussed in more detail in the sections on implications for practice.

RECIPROCAL CAUSATION AND EMOTION REGULATION

Achievement emotions influence engagement and achievement, but achievement outcomes are expected to reciprocally influence emotions, underlying appraisals, and the environment (Pekrun, 2006; see Figure 14.1). As such, achievement emotions, their antecedents, and their effects

are thought to be linked by reciprocal causation over time. Reciprocal causation may involve different kinds of feedback loops, including the following three that may be especially important. First, achievement environments shape individual appraisals and emotions, but these emotions reciprocally affect environments and the behavior of teachers, supervisors, and coaches. For example, teachers' and students' enjoyment of classroom instruction are likely linked in reciprocal ways, emotional contagion being one of the mechanisms producing these links (Frenzel, Goetz, Lüdtke, Pekrun, & Sutton, 2009). Second, emotions impact achievement behavior, and this behavior in turn influences the arousal of emotions. For example, enjoyment can facilitate use of creative problem-solving strategies, as outlined earlier. Creative involvement with tasks may in turn promote enjoyment, suggesting that enjoyment and strategy use are reciprocally linked. Similarly, emotions influence individual engagement in terms of adopting achievement goals, but these goals reciprocally influence emotion (Linnenbrink & Pintrich, 2002). Third, by impacting behavior, emotions have an influence on achievement. Achievement outcomes, however, are primary forces shaping the development of achievement emotions, again suggesting reciprocal causation (for empirical evidence, see Pekrun, Hall, et al., 2014; Pekrun et al., in press).

In line with perspectives of dynamical systems theory (Turner & Waugh, 2007), it is assumed that such reciprocal causation can take different forms and extend over fractions of seconds (e.g., in linkages between appraisals and emotions), days, weeks, months, or years. Positive feedback loops likely are commonplace (e.g., with supervisors' and employees' anger reciprocally reinforcing each other), but negative feedback loops can also be important (e.g., when a lost tournament induces anxiety in basketball team, motivating the team to avoid being defeated again in the next tournament).

Reciprocal causation has implications for the regulation of achievement emotions. Since emotions, their antecedents, and their effects can be reciprocally linked over time, emotions can be regulated by addressing any of the elements involved in these cyclic feedback processes. Regulation can target (1) the emotion itself (*emotion-oriented* regulation and treatment, e.g., using drugs and relaxation techniques to cope with anxiety or employing interest-enhancing strategies to reduce boredom; Sansone, Weir, Harpster, & Morgan, 1992); (2) the control and value appraisals underlying emotions (*appraisal-oriented* regulation); (3) the competencies determining individual agency (*competence-oriented* regulation and treatment; e.g., training of learning skills); and (4) tasks and achievement settings (*design of tasks and environments*). Empirical evidence on ways to regulate achievement emotions is still largely lacking, with few exceptions (see Diefendorff, Richard, & Yang, 2008; Nett, Goetz, & Hall, 2011; Zeidner, 1998, 2014).

UNIVERSALITY VERSUS SPECIFICITY OF ACHIEVEMENT EMOTIONS

As for emotions more generally, it can be assumed that general functional mechanisms of achievement emotions are bound to universal, species-specific characteristics of our mind (functional universality). By contrast, specific reference objects of these emotions, as well as specific process parameters (e.g., intensity of emotions), may be specific to different individuals, genders, achievement settings, and cultures. The basic structures and causal mechanisms of achievement emotions are expected to follow nomothetic principles, whereas reference objects, intensity, and duration of emotions may differ, implying that their description may require the use of idiographic principles. For example, it was found that the relationships between girls' and boys' appraisals and their achievement emotions in mathematics are structurally equivalent across the two genders (Frenzel, Pekrun, & Goetz, 2007). However, perceived control in this domain was substantially lower for girls. As a consequence, girls reported less enjoyment in mathematics, as well as more anxiety and shame (also see Goetz, Bieg, Lüdtke, Pekrun, & Hall, 2013). Similarly, in a cross-cultural comparison of Chinese and German students' achievement emotions, we found that mean levels of emotions differed between cultures, with Chinese students reporting more achievement-related enjoyment, pride, anxiety, and shame, and less anger. Nevertheless, the

functional linkages of these emotions with perceived control, important others' expectations, and academic achievement were equivalent across cultures (Frenzel, Thrash, Pekrun, & Goetz, 2007).

Concerning situational specificity, the control and value appraisals underlying achievement emotions may be specific to different achievement domains (e.g., mathematics) or subdomains within these domains (e.g., geometry vs. algebra). There is robust evidence of the situational specificity of variables related to control and value, such as competence appraisals, achievement goals, and interests (Bong, 2001). For example, students' self-concepts in math and languages often show zero correlations, as predicted by H. Marsh's (1987) internal/external frame of reference model (I/E model; see Marsh, Martin, Yeung, & Craven, Chapter 6, this volume). In line with such situational specificity, the resulting achievement emotions have also been found to be organized in domain-specific ways. Students' emotions, such as their enjoyment and anxiety, show zero to small correlations across math versus languages, and the emotional differences between these subjects were found to be mediated by students' self-concepts (see e.g., Goetz, Frenzel, Hall, & Pekrun, 2008; Goetz, Frenzel, Pekrun, Hall, & Lüdtke, 2007). However, despite situational specificity, the internal structures and linkages of emotions with academic achievement were equivalent across domains in these studies, in line with principles of functional universality.

IMPLICATIONS FOR PRACTICE

Understanding Achievement Emotions

Emotions impact motivation and performance, and they are core components of personal identity and psychological well-being. Accordingly, practitioners such as teachers, supervisors, coaches, and administrators are well advised to attend to the emotions experienced in achievement settings. To this end, it may be helpful for practitioners to develop an understanding of the variation, functions, and origins of achievement emotions. This may be especially important given that some of the scientific evidence on these emotions, as summarized in the preceding sections, is counter to widely held everyday beliefs about emotions.

Diversity of Achievement Emotions

Traditionally, research has focused on only a few achievement emotions, with test anxiety receiving the most attention. In classical achievement motivation research, four emotions were considered: hope, pride, fear, and shame related to success and failure (Heckhausen, 1991). However, current research documents that a broad range of emotions may occur in achievement settings. It is helpful for practitioners to know that there is next to no human emotion that may not be triggered by success and failure (e.g., Pekrun et al., 2002), including individual emotions as well as social and moral emotions.

Individual Specificity

Emotional responses show substantial variation between persons in achievement settings, even within the same setting and group of individuals. For example, the difference between boys' and girls' emotions in mathematics has been found to be much smaller than the differences within genders, and the differences across cultures are much smaller than the differences within cultures (e.g., Frenzel, Pekrun, et al., 2007; Goetz et al., 2013). Generally, only a minor part of individual differences in achievement emotions can be explained in terms of culture, ethnicity, gender, institution, or group membership. Because emotional reactions may differ widely, even among individuals sharing gender and group membership, it is best to avoid stereotype phrases that relate to group membership, such as "girls are afraid of math." It is more useful to pay attention to the uniqueness of each individual's emotions.

Situational Specificity

Traditionally, achievement emotions such as test anxiety have been considered as trait-like characteristics that are stable over time and generalize across different achievement settings (see Zeidner, 1998). However, the within-person variation of achievement-related emotions can be even larger than the between-person variation. Furthermore, as outlined earlier, achievement emotions are typically organized in domain-specific ways. Accordingly, it is important to attend to the situational specificity of these emotions. For example, teachers should know that it is not possible to infer from a student's enjoyment or anxiety in math to what extent the student enjoys, or has trepidations about, other subjects, such as language classes. It can be quite misleading to label a student as "anxious," "bored," or "enthusiastic" based on his or her emotional reactions to one specific school subject. Therefore, stereotypes that suggest an individual always reacts with the same emotion over time and across different achievement settings should be avoided.

Functions of Positive versus Negative Emotions

As noted by Hu and Kaplan (2015, p. 39), "Feeling good is good. This belief is so intuitive to be almost axiomatic." Similarly, there are widely held beliefs that negative emotions are simply bad. These beliefs are mirrored in traditional experimental mood research that only considered differences between broadly defined positive versus negative affect, without attending to the functional differences between discrete emotions within these categories. However, the effects of positive and negative emotions are more variable than suggested by these beliefs. As outlined earlier, task-related positive emotions focus attention on the task, promote motivation to achieve, and facilitate use of flexible behavioral strategies. In contrast, positive emotions that do not relate to the task can draw attention away and lower performance, and deactivating positive emotions, such as relief and relaxation, do not necessarily have positive effects either. For negative emotions, the evidence implies that these emotions can strongly obstruct task performance. As noted, test anxiety, hopelessness, or boredom can lead individuals to withdraw attention, avoid effort, procrastinate in doing assignments, fail exams, and drop out of school or quit their jobs. Negative emotions are a major factor explaining why many individuals do not live up to their potential and fail to pursue careers that correspond to their abilities and interests. Moreover, these emotions also jeopardize personality development and health. However, in some instances, negative emotions may be helpful to restore motivation to invest effort, and sometimes negative emotions may even be required to achieve satisfactory solutions, such as productive confusion aroused by an unresolved scientific problem that fuels researchers' motivation to persist (also see D'Mello, Lehman, Pekrun, & Graesser, 2014).

Accordingly, practitioners can help students, employees, and athletes to achieve by promoting their task-related positive emotions. However, it is better not to rely on triggering positive emotions that do not relate to the task. It may not be sufficient just to experience good feelings; rather, positive emotional experience needs to be linked to task performance. Furthermore, practitioners should help to prevent negative achievement emotions, and to reduce these emotions if they occur, especially if these emotions occur with high intensity and frequency. However, it is also important to consider that negative emotions cannot always be avoided in achievement settings, and that they can be used productively if suitable precautions are taken. As noted, less intense versions of anxiety, self-related anger, or shame can even promote task performance provided that there is sufficient confidence in success, and some amount of confusion about cognitive problems can facilitate change and the development of more advanced competencies.

Origins of Emotions: The Importance of Appraisals

The research on the antecedents of achievement emotions cited earlier implies that appraisals can be considered as main proximal determinants of these emotions, with two factors being especially important: self-confidence in one's abilities, as implied by perceived control over achievement, and the perceived value of achievement. Given that self-confidence generally promotes positive achievement emotions and reduces negative emotions, strengthening students', employees', and athletes' self-confidence is an important way to promote their adaptive emotions. However, pushing self-confidence to extremes should be avoided because overconfidence can have negative side effects,

such as increased boredom (Pekrun et al., 2010).

Whereas self-confidence differentially influences positive versus negative emotions, the perceived value of achievement activities and their outcomes (Wigfield et al., Chapter 7, this volume) amplifies both positive and negative emotions (except for boredom). Accordingly, increasing the importance of achievement is a double-edged sword. Specifically, emphasizing the negative consequences of failure can exarcebate emotions such as anxiety. It is more advisable to increase the intrinsic value of achievement activities per se, which can help to foster positive activity-related emotions, engagement, and resulting performance.

Design of Tasks and Achievement Settings

Similar to the role of distal individual antecedents such as achievement goals, the impact of task demands and environments on achievement emotions is thought to be mediated by individual control and value appraisals. Features of tasks and achievement settings that affect these appraisals should influence the resulting emotions as well. The following groups of factors may be relevant for a broad variety of achievement emotions (Figure 14.1) and may be used by practitioners to influence achievement emotions.

Cognitive Quality

The cognitive quality of tasks, as defined by their structure, clarity, and potential for cognitive stimulation, likely has a positive influence on actual and perceived competence as well as the perceived value of tasks (e.g., Cordova & Lepper, 1996), thus positively influencing achievement emotions. In addition, the relative difficulty of tasks can influence perceived control, and the match between task demands and competencies can influence subjective task value, thus also influencing emotions. If demands are too high or too low, the intrinsic value of tasks may be reduced to the extent that boredom is experienced (Csikszentmihalyi, 1975; Pekrun et al., 2010). Accordingly, achievement emotions can likely be positively influenced by providing instruction and tasks that are well structured, clear, and cognitively stimulating. For example, this can involve use of structured examples (Atkinson, Derry, Renkl, & Wortham, 2000), as well as material involving cognitive incongruity to stimulate interest and support intrinsic motivation (also see Harackiewicz & Knogler, Chapter 18, this volume; Muis et al., 2015).

Motivational Quality

Teachers, parents, supervisors, and coaches deliver both direct and indirect messages conveying information about achievement-related control and values. Direct messages inform about abilities, opportunities to succeed, and the importance of achievement. An example is fear appeals that remind students about the importance of exams and their consequences. Research has shown that fear appeals are often employed by educators and may not only trigger motivation to invest effort to avoid failure but also exacerbate anxiety about failure (see Putwain & Symes, 2011). As such, fear appeals are a double-edged sword that should be used with caution.

Indirect ways of inducing emotionally relevant appraisals including the following. First, control appraisals can be influenced by suggesting causal explanations for success and failure, with ability attributions for failure undermining perceived control and effort attributions preserving control (Perry & Hamm, Chapter 5, this volume). Second, if tasks and environments are shaped such that they meet individual needs, positive activity-related emotions and the value of achievement activities should be fostered. For example, work environments that support cooperation should help employees fulfill their needs for social relatedness, thus making work more enjoyable. Third, the value of achievement activities, such as studying for one's classes, can likely be increased by using tasks that relate to individual interests or have utility value for the individual's everyday life and future goals (Wigfield et al., Chapter 7, this volume).

Autonomy Support

Tasks and environments supporting autonomy can increase perceived control and,

by meeting needs for autonomy, the intrinsic value of related activities (Tsai, Kunter, Lüdtke, Trautwein, & Ryan, 2008). However, these beneficial effects likely depend on the match between individual competencies and needs for autonomy on the one hand, and task demands on the other. In case of a mismatch in terms of high demands on self-regulation and low competencies to meet these demands, loss of control and negative emotions might result. For example, if an employee who has difficulties in adequately planning and monitoring her work activities is left alone to deal with difficult assignment, she may experience a loss of control, along with anxiety and hopelessness, in not reaching her work goals.

Expectations and Goal Structures

Different standards for defining achievement can imply task- and self-related (mastery), competitive (normative performance), or cooperative expectations and goal structures (Johnson & Johnson, 1974). The expectations and goal structures provided in achievement settings conceivably influence emotions in two ways. First, to the extent that these structures are adopted, they influence individual achievement goals and any emotions mediated by these goals (e.g., Kaplan & Maehr, 1999). Second, goal structures determine relative opportunities for experiencing success and perceiving control, thus influencing control-dependent emotions. Specifically, competitive goal structures imply, by definition, that some individuals have to experience failure, thus inducing negative outcome emotions such as anxiety and hopelessness in these individuals. Similarly, the demands implied by an important other's unrealistic expectancies for achievement can lead to negative emotions resulting from reduced subjective control.

Ability Composition of Groups

It seems reasonable to assume that membership in a high-ability group, such as a Champions League-winning soccer team, may promote self-confidence and pride (*reflected glory effect*; Marsh, Kong, & Hau, 2000), and that membership in a low-ability group may undermine confidence and triggers shame. However, the ability level of groups determines the likelihood of performing well relative to one's peers. All things being equal, chances for performing well in one's group are higher in a low-ability group, which should result in perceived competence being higher in low-ability groups (*big-fish-little-pond effect* [BFLPE]; Marsh, 1987). Research has found that the BFLPE on self-concept is typically stronger than the reflected glory effect, implying a negative relation between group-level ability and the individual's self-perceived competence (Marsh et al., Chapter 6, this volume). Because perceived competence influences achievement emotions, the BFLPE of group ability on self-concept could prompt similar effects on these emotions. In fact, students' test anxiety has been found to be higher in high-ability classrooms than in low-ability classrooms, controlling for individual ability (e.g., Preckel, Zeidner, Goetz, & Schleyer, 2008), whereas their positive emotions are higher in low-ability classrooms (Pekrun, Murayama, et al., 2011). This is counter to widely held beliefs that being a member of high-status groups generally promotes happiness, and being a member of low-status groups undermines happiness. These beliefs need to be revised accordingly, and in making decisions about the composition of groups and the placement of individuals in groups, the psychosocial costs of these decisions need to be taken into account.

Transmission of Emotions in Social Interaction

Emotions can be transmitted in social interaction. For example, math anxiety in parents who help their children doing math homework can exacerbate their children's anxiety in this domain (Maloney, Ramirez, Gunderson, Levine, & Beilock, 2015; see Beilock, Schaeffer, & Rozek, Chapter 9, this volume), and teachers' displayed enthusiasm facilitates students' enjoyment in the classroom (Frenzel et al., 2009). Observational learning and emotional contagion may be prime mechanisms mediating these effects (Hatfield, Cacioppo, & Rapson, 1994). Accordingly, teachers, supervisors, and coaches can influence students', employees', and athletes' emotions through displaying their own emotions (Ashkanasy & Humphrey, 2011). Specifically, displaying positive emotions can promote enjoyment of achievement activities, thus likely facilitating engagement and performance. However, enacting displays that are not congruent to felt emotion involves emotional labor that can contribute to burnout (Kennworthy, Fay, Frame, & Petree, 2014).

Assessment of Achievement

Tests, exams, and other types of achievement assessments can have a profound impact on the development and occurrence of achievement emotions. Again, it seems likely that these effects are mediated by individual appraisals related to achievement, such as perceived control and value. In turn, emotions occurring before or during the assessment can impact individual performance and the psychometric quality of the assessment.

Design of Assessments

Lack of structure and transparency (e.g., lack of information regarding demands, materials, and grading practices), as well as excessive task demands, are associated with students' elevated test anxiety (Zeidner, 1998, 2014). These links are likely mediated by students' expectancies of low control and failure (Pekrun, 1992). Furthermore, the format of test items has been found to be relevant. Specifically, open-ended formats, such as essay questions, induce more anxiety than multiple-choice formats (Zeidner, 1998), possibly because open-ended formats require more attentional resources (i.e., working memory capacity). In addition, there is evidence that practices such as permitting students to choose between test items, relaxing time constraints, and giving second chances (e.g., opportunities to retake a test) may reduce test anxiety (Zeidner, 1998), presumably because perceived control and achievement expectancies are enhanced under these conditions.

Standards to Evaluate Achievement

As outlined earlier, achievement may be defined and evaluated by different standards.

Important standards include the following: (1) *task-based*, absolute criteria related to the attainment of task mastery (e.g., as defined in criterion-oriented testing); (2) *self-based* criteria involving intraindividual comparisons of present versus past performance (progress made), present performance versus current and future potential to perform, or performance across different domains (internal frame of reference in Marsh's I/E model; see Marsh et al., Chapter 6, this volume); (3) *other-based* standards involving interindividual comparison with others' performance (e.g., in normative grading on the curve); and (4) *group-based* standards involving an evaluation of the performance of groups. Use of task-based and self-based standards is likely to promote mastery goal adoption and positive emotions, whereas use of other-based, competitive standards can exacerbate achievement-related anxiety, shame, and hopelessness (Elliot et al., 2011; Pekrun, Cusack, Murayama, Elliot, & Thomas, 2014). Accordingly, practitioners are well advised to employ task- and self-based standards rather than other-based standards.

Feedback and Consequences of Achievement

Feedback on success and failure can trigger positive and negative achievement emotions, respectively (see, e.g., Peterson, Brown, & Jun, 2015). Furthermore, cumulative success is likely to strengthen perceived control, and cumulative failure may undermine control, implying that repeated feedback on achievement can be a prime driver of the long-term development of achievement emotions. A few longitudinal studies have confirmed the importance of success and failure feedback (e.g., in terms of grades in the classroom) for the development of achievement emotions (Meece et al., 1990; Pekrun, 1992; Pekrun et al., in press). In addition, the actual and perceived consequences of success and failure are likely to be important because these consequences affect the value of achievement outcomes. Positive outcome emotions (e.g., hope for success) can be increased if success produces beneficial long-term outcomes (e.g., acceptance to an esteemed university), provided that there is sufficient contingency between one's own efforts, success,

and these outcomes. Negative consequences of failure, such as unemployment, however, may increase achievement-related anxiety and hopelessness (Pekrun, 1992).

Because evaluative feedback can have negative emotional effects, it is more recommendable to provide informational feedback, which may be better suited to help the individual to develop mastery and maintain adaptive achievement emotions. Furthermore, it may be helpful to implement a culture of considering errors as opportunities to learn rather than as evaluative feedback on lack of capability. Finally, it is important to decouple assessments from serious consequences, such as career decisions, whenever possible. High-stakes testing can increase positive achievement emotions in successful individuals, but for those who fail, it likely increases frustration and shame about failure, as well as anxiety and hopelessness related to the future.

Impact of Achievement Emotions on Assessments

Emotions can impact the validity of assessments. Specifically, the validity of an assessment may be reduced if examinees with equal levels of ability but different emotional experiences have different probabilities of correctly answering test items. For example, as noted earlier, the worry cognitions implied by test anxiety can reduce performance on complex and difficult cognitive tests, and the reduction of motivation involved by hopelessness can similarly reduce test performance. Accordingly, it seems important to prevent excessive negative emotions during assessments. More research is needed to better understand these effects, such as experimental studies inducing emotional states to investigate their influence on processes and outcomes of assessment (Bornstein, 2011).

Treatment Interventions

Excessive negative achievement emotions may be modified using psychotherapy. The development of suitable treatments has focused on interventions to reduce test anxiety. Research on these interventions shows that test anxiety is treatable; in fact, some of the treatments for test anxiety are among the most successful psychological therapies available, with effect sizes above $d = 1.0$ (Hembree, 1988). Similar to individual regulation of achievement emotions, different test anxiety treatments focus on different manifestations and antecedents of this emotion (Figure 14.1), including affective–physiological symptoms of anxiety (emotion-oriented therapy), cognitive appraisals (cognitive therapy), and competence deficits (skills training; Zeidner, 1998, 2014).

Emotion-oriented therapy includes anxiety induction (e.g., flooding), biofeedback procedures, relaxation techniques (e.g., progressive muscle relaxation; Jacobson, 1938), and systematic desensitization. *Cognitive therapies* aim to modify anxiety-inducing control beliefs, values, and styles of self-related thinking. Examples are cognitive–attentional training, cognitive restructuring therapy, and stress-inoculation training. *Competence training* teaches individuals to understand and use problem-solving strategies that promote success and therefore decrease anxiety. Finally, *multimodal therapies* integrate different procedures to address different symptoms and antecedents of anxiety within one treatment.

Cognitive and multimodal therapies have proven especially effective at both reducing test anxiety and enhancing performance (Zeidner, 1998). Study skills training has been shown to successfully reduce test anxiety in students with deficits in their learning strategies. Therapy focusing exclusively on emotion-oriented procedures has been shown to successfully reduce anxiety, but it has proven less effective at improving academic achievement. These kinds of therapy address the affective and physiological components of anxiety, but not the underlying cognitive components of anxiety that are primarily responsible for the performance-debilitating effects of this emotion.

Research on treatment interventions targeting a broader range of achievement emotions is largely lacking to date. Development of such interventions might be based on methods currently explored to enhance achievement motivation (Harackiewicz, Tibbetts, Canning, & Hyde, 2014). Some of these methods aim to enhance control and value appraisals, which should affect

not only motivation but also emotions. Two examples are attributional retraining that serves to modify maladaptive causal attributions for success and failure, and value interventions that enhance the intrinsic value and utility value of achievement activities (Harackiwiecz & Knogler, Chapter 18, this volume). There is evidence from a few studies that attributional retraining can enhance positive achievement emotions and reduce negative emotions (Perry, Chipperfield, Hladkyj, Pekrun, & Hamm, 2014), suggesting that attributional retraining may be used to address a broader range of emotions in achievement settings.

CONCLUSION

Across research disciplines and throughout the 20th century, achievement emotions have been neglected, with the single exception of achievement anxiety, which has attracted researchers' attention since the 1950s (Beilock et al., Chapter 9, this volume; Zeidner, 2014). However, in current emotion research, as well as applied studies in management science, education, and sports, achievement-related emotions have received increasing attention. As outlined in this chapter, the findings of the nascent science of achievement emotions suggest that these emotions profoundly impact motivational engagement and achievement behavior, as well as important outcomes such as performance attainment at school, on the job, and in sports. The available evidence also indicates that it is possible to disentangle the multiple individual and social origins of these emotions; subjective appraisals of achievement activities and their outcomes, as well as features of achievement settings influencing these appraisals, are especially promising candidates. However, for most achievement emotions, only a handful of studies are available to derive validated conclusions on functions, origins, and related treatment interventions; test anxiety is the only major exception. Accordingly, except for achievement-related anxiety, it is still difficult to derive recommendations for practice that are firmly based on evidence.

As such, more research on achievement emotions, both achievement anxiety and emotions beyond anxiety, is clearly needed, including replication of existing findings. Research is needed to better understand the structures of achievement emotions; the variation of these emotions within and between individuals and across different types of achievement settings, institutions, and cultures; the functions of different emotions for motivation and performance, beyond global positive and negative affect; their functions for the development of personality, psychological health, and physical health; their origins and development across the lifespan; and ways to enhance adaptive and reduce maladaptive emotions (Pekrun & Linnenbrink-Garcia, 2014b). Furthermore, at present, research efforts of different disciplines to examine achievement emotions are fragmented. Better integration of research traditions from different disciplines is needed, including basic research on achievement emotions in psychology and the neurosciences, as well as research in applied fields. In the years to come, such research and conceptual integration should make it possible to derive better scientific understanding, as well as recommendations for practice that are based on multiple sources of evidence and cumulative findings. In this way, robust knowledge of achievement emotions, as well as recommendations for evidence-based practice, could be extended beyond the well-researched emotion of achievement-related anxiety.

REFERENCES

Ahmed, W., van der Werf, G., Kuyper, H., & Minnaert, A. (2013). Emotions, self-regulated learning, and achievement in mathematics: A growth curve analysis. *Journal of Educational Psychology, 105,* 150–161.

Ashkanasy, N. M., Härtel, C. E. J., & Daus, C. S. (2002). Diversity and emotion: The new frontiers in organizational behavior research. *Journal of Management, 28,* 307–338.

Ashkanasy, N. M., & Humphrey, R. H. (2011). Current emotion research in organizational behavior. *Emotion Review, 3,* 214–224.

Aspinwall, L. (1998). Rethinking the role of positive affect in self-regulation. *Motivation and Emotion, 22,* 1–32.

Atkinson, R. K., Derry, S. J., Renkl, A., & Wortham, D. (2000). Learning from examples: Instructional principles from the worked

examples research. *Review of Educational Research, 70,* 181–214.

Bagozzi, R. P., Verbeke, W., & Gavino, J. C. (2003). Culture moderates the self-regulation of shame and its effects on performance: the case of salespersons in The Netherlands and the Philippines. *Journal of Applied Psychology, 88,* 219–233.

Barrett, L. F., & Russell, J. A. (1998). Independence and bipolarity in the structure of current affect. *Journal of Personality and Social Psychology, 74,* 967–984.

Barsade, S. G., Brief, A. P., & Spataro, S. E. (2003). The affective revolution of organizational behaviour: The emergence of a paradigm. In J. Greenberg (Ed.), *Organizational behaviour: The state of the science* (pp. 3–52). Mahwah, NJ: Erlbaum.

Boekaerts, M. (1993). Anger in relation to school learning. *Learning and Instruction, 3,* 269–280.

Bong, M. (2001). Between- and within-domain relations of motivation among middle and high school students: Self-efficacy, task value and achievement goals. *Journal of Educational Psychology, 93,* 23–34.

Bornstein, R. F. (2011). Toward a process-focused model of test score validity: Improving psychological assessment in science and practice. *Psychological Assessment, 23,* 532–544.

Campos, J. J., Bertenthal, B. I., & Kermoian, R. (1992). Early experience and emotional development: The emergence of wariness of heights. *Psychological Science, 3,* 61–64.

Chang, H., & Beilock, S. L. (2016). The math anxiety–math performance link and its relation to individual and environmental factors: A review of current behavioral and psychophysiological research. *Current Opinion in Behavioral Sciences, 10,* 33–38.

Clore, G. L., & Huntsinger, J. R. (2007). How emotions inform judgment and regulate thought. *Trends in Cognitive Sciences, 11,* 393–399.

Clore, G. L., & Huntsinger, J. R. (2009). How the object of affect guides its impact. *Emotion Review, 1,* 39–54.

Cordova, D. I., & Lepper, M. R. (1996). Intrinsic motivation and the process of learning: Beneficial effects of contextualization, personalization, and choice. *Journal of Educational Psychology, 88,* 715–730.

Csikszentmihalyi, M. (1975). *Beyond boredom and anxiety.* San Francisco: Jossey-Bass.

Diefendorff, J. M., Richard, E. M., & Yang, J. (2008). Linking emotion regulation strategies to affective events and negative emotions at work. *Journal of Vocational Behavior, 73,* 498–508.

D'Mello, S., Lehman, B., Pekrun, R., & Graesser, A. (2014). Confusion can be beneficial for learning. *Learning and Instruction*, *29*, 153–170.

Elliot, A. J., & McGregor, H. (1999). Test anxiety and the hierarchical model of approach and avoidance achievement motivation. *Journal of Personality and Social Psychology*, *76*, 628–644.

Elliot, A. J., & McGregor, H. A. (2001). A 2 × 2 achievement goal framework. *Journal of Personality and Social Psychology*, *80*, 501–519.

Elliot, A. J., Murayama, K., & Pekrun, R. (2011). A 3 × 2 achievement goal model. *Journal of Educational Psychology*, *103*, 632–648.

Ellis, H. C., & Ashbrook, P. W. (1988). Resource allocation model of the effect of depressed mood states on memory. In K. Fiedler & J. Forgas (Eds.), *Affect, cognition, and social behavior* (pp. 25–43). Toronto, Ontario, Canada: Hogrefe.

Eysenck, M. W. (1997). *Anxiety and cognition*. Hove, UK: Psychology Press.

Fisher, C. D. (2010). Happiness at work. *British Academy of Management*, *12*, 384–412.

Fredrickson, B. L. (2001). The role of positive emotions in positive psychology: The broaden-and-build theory of positive emotions. *American Psychologist*, *56*, 218–226.

Frenzel, A. C., Goetz, T., Lüdtke, O., Pekrun, R., & Sutton, R. (2009). Emotional transmission in the classroom: Exploring the relationship between teacher and student enjoyment. *Journal of Educational Psychology*, *101*, 705–716.

Frenzel, A. C., Pekrun, R., & Goetz, T. (2007). Girls and mathematics – a "hopeless" issue?: A control-value approach to gender differences in emotions towards mathematics. *European Journal of Psychology of Education*, *22*, 497–514.

Frenzel, A. C., Thrash, T. M., Pekrun, R., & Goetz, T. (2007). Achievement emotions in Germany and China: A cross-cultural validation of the Academic Emotions Questionnaire–Mathematics (AEQ-M). *Journal of Cross-Cultural Psychology*, *38*, 302–309.

Goetz, T., Bieg, M., Lüdtke, O., Pekrun, R., & Hall, N. C. (2013). Do girls really experience more anxiety in mathematics? *Psychological Science*, *24*, 2079–2087.

Goetz, T., Frenzel, A. C., Hall, N. C., & Pekrun, R. (2008). Antecedents of academic emotions: Testing the internal/external frame of reference model for academic enjoyment. *Contemporary Educational Psychology*, *33*, 9–33.

Goetz, T., Frenzel, A. C., Pekrun, R., Hall, N. C., & Lüdtke, O. (2007). Between- and within-domain relations of students' academic emotions. *Journal of Educational Psychology*, *99*, 715–733.

Goetz, T., Frenzel, A. C., Stoeger, H., & Hall, N. C. (2010). Antecedents of everyday positive emotions: An experience sampling analysis. *Motivation and Emotion*, *34*, 49–62.

Goetz, T., Preckel, F., Zeidner, M., & Schleyer, E. (2008). Big fish in big ponds: A multilevel analysis of test anxiety and achievement in special gifted classes. *Anxiety, Stress and Coping*, *21*, 185–198.

Harackiewicz, J. M., Tibbetts, Y., Canning, E., & Hyde, J. S. (2014). Harnessing values to promote motivation in education. In S. Karabenick & T. C. Urdan (Eds.), *Advances in motivation and achievement* (Vol. 18, pp. 71–105). Bingley, UK: Emerald Group.

Hatfield, E., Cacioppo, J. T. & Rapson, R. L. (1994). *Emotional contagion*. New York: Cambridge University Press.

Heckhausen, H. (1991). *Motivation and action*. New York: Springer.

Hembree, R. (1988). Correlates, causes, effects, and treatment of test anxiety. *Review of Educational Research*, *58*, 47–77.

Hersey, R. B. (1932). *Workers' emotions in shop and home*. Philadelphia: University of Pennsylvania Press.

Hu, X., & Kaplan, S. (2015). Is "feeling good" good enough?: Differentiating discrete positive emotions at work. *Journal of Organizational Behavior*, *36*, 39–58.

Huang, C. (2011). Achievement goals and achievement emotions: A meta-analysis. *Educational Psychology Review*, *23*, 359–388.

Jacobson, E. (1938). *Progressive relaxation*. Chicago: University of Chicago Press

Johnson, D. W., & Johnson, R. T. (1974). Instructional goal structure: Cooperative, competitive or individualistic. *Review of Educational Research*, *4*, 213–240.

Kaplan, A., & Maehr, M. L. (1999). Achievement goals and student well-being. *Contemporary Educational Psychology*, *24*, 330–358.

Kennworthy, J., Fay, C., Frame, M., & Petree, R. (2014). A meta-analytic review of the relationship between emotional dissonance and emotional exhaustion. *Journal of Applied Social Psychology*, *44*, 94–105.

Kuhbandner, C., & Pekrun, R. (2013). Affective state influences retrieval-induced forgetting for integrated knowledge. *PLoS ONE*, *8*(2), e56617.

Lane, A. M., Whyte, G. P., Terry, P. C., & Nevill, A. M. (2005). Mood, self-set goals and examination performance: The moderating effect of depressed mood. *Personality and Individual Differences*, *39*, 143–153.

Lazarus, R. S., & Folkman, S. (1984). *Stress, appraisal, and coping*. New York: Springer.

Lewis, M., Haviland-Jones, J. M., & Barrett, L. F. (Eds.). (2008). *Handbook of emotions* (3rd ed.). New York: Guilford Press.

Lindebaum, D., & Fielden, S. (2010). "It's good

to be angry": Enacting anger in construction project management to achieve perceived leader effectiveness. *Human Relations, 64,* 437–458.

Linnenbrink, E. A. (2007). The role of affect in student learning: A multi-dimensional approach to considering the interaction of affect, motivation, and engagement. In P. A. Schutz & R. Pekrun (Eds.), *Emotion in education* (pp. 107–124). San Diego, CA: Academic Press.

Linnenbrink, E. A., & Pintrich, P. R. (2002). Achievement goal theory and affect: An asymmetrical bidirectional model. *Educational Psychologist, 37,* 69–78.

Maloney, E. A., Ramirez, G., Gunderson, E. A., Levine, S. C., & Beilock, S. L. (2015). Intergenerational effects of low math achievement and high math anxiety. *Psychological Science, 26,* 1480–1488.

Marsh, H. W. (1987). The big-fish-little-pond effect on academic self-concept. *Journal of Educational Psychology, 79,* 280–295.

Marsh, H. W., Kong, C.-K., & Hau, K.-T. (2000). Longitudinal multilevel models of the big-fish-little-pond effect on academic self-concept: Counterbalancing contrast and reflected-glory effects on Hong Kong schools. *Journal of Personality and Social Psychology, 78,* 337–349.

Meece, J. L., Wigfield, A., & Eccles, J. S. (1990). Predictors of math anxiety and its influence on young adolescents course enrollment intentions and performance in mathematics. *Journal of Educational Psychology, 82,* 60–70.

Meinhardt, J., & Pekrun, R. (2003). Attentional resource allocation to emotional events: An ERP study. *Cognition and Emotion, 17,* 477–500.

Muis, K. R., Pekrun, R., Sinatra, G. M., Azevedo, R., Trevors, G., Meier, E., et al. (2015). The curious case of climate change: Testing a theoretical model of epistemic beliefs, epistemic emotions, and complex learning. *Learning and Instruction, 39,* 168–183.

Nett, U. E., Goetz, T., & Hall, N. C. (2011). Coping with boredom in school: An experience sampling perspective. *Contemporary Educational Psychology, 36,* 49–59.

Olafson, K. M., & Ferraro, F. R. (2001). Effects of emotional state on lexical decision performance. *Brain and Cognition, 45,* 15–20.

Pekrun, R. (1992). Expectancy–value theory of anxiety: Overview and implications. In D. G. Forgays, T. Sosnowski, & K. Wrzesniewski (Eds.), *Anxiety: Recent developments in self-appraisal, psychophysiological and health research* (pp. 23–41). Washington, DC: Hemisphere.

Pekrun, R. (2006). The control–value theory of achievement emotions: Assumptions, corollaries, and implications for educational research and practice. *Educational Psychology Review, 18,* 315–341.

Pekrun, R., Cusack, A., Murayama, K., Elliot, A. J., & Thomas, K. (2014). The power of anticipated feedback: Effects on students' achievement goals and achievement emotions. *Learning and Instruction, 29,* 115–124.

Pekrun, R., Elliot, A. J., & Maier, M. A. (2006). Achievement goals and discrete achievement emotions: A theoretical model and prospective test. *Journal of Educational Psychology, 98,* 583–597.

Pekrun, R., Elliot, A. J., & Maier, M. A. (2009). Achievement goals and achievement emotions: Testing a model of their joint relations with academic performance. *Journal of Educational Psychology, 101,* 115–135.

Pekrun, R., Goetz, T., Daniels, L. M., Stupnisky, R. H., & Perry, R. P. (2010). Boredom in achievement settings: Control-value antecedents and performance outcomes of a neglected emotion. *Journal of Educational Psychology, 102,* 531–549.

Pekrun, R., Goetz, T., Frenzel, A. C., Barchfeld, P., & Perry, R. P. (2011). Measuring emotions in students' learning and performance: The Achievement Emotions Questionnaire (AEQ). *Contemporary Educational Psychology, 36,* 36–48.

Pekrun, R., Goetz, T., Titz, W., & Perry, R. P. (2002). Academic emotions in students' self-regulated learning and achievement: A program of quantitative and qualitative research. *Educational Psychologist, 37,* 91–106.

Pekrun, R., Hall, N. C., Goetz, T., & Perry, R. P. (2014). Boredom and academic achievement: Testing a model of reciprocal causation. *Journal of Educational Psychology, 106,* 696–710.

Pekrun, R., Lichtenfeld, S., Marsh, H. W., Murayama, K., & Goetz, T. (in press). Achievement emotions and academic performance: Longitudinal models of reciprocal effects. *Child Development.*

Pekrun, R., & Linnenbrink-Garcia, L. (2014a). Conclusions and future directions. In R. Pekrun & L. Linnenbrink-Garcia (Eds.), *International handbook of emotions in education* (pp. 659–675). New York: Taylor & Francis.

Pekrun, R., & Linnenbrink-Garcia, L. (Eds.). (2014b). *International handbook of emotions in education.* New York: Taylor & Francis.

Pekrun, R., Murayama, K., Frenzel, A. C., Goetz, T., & Marsh, H. W. (2011, September). *Origins of achievement emotions: The impact of individual and class-level ability.* Paper presented at the 14th biannual conference of the European Association for Research on Learning and Instruction, Exeter, UK.

Pekrun, R., & Perry, R. P. (2014). Control–value theory of achievement emotions. In R. Pekrun & L. Linnenbrink-Garcia (Eds.), *International handbook of emotions in education* (pp. 120–141). New York: Taylor & Francis.

Pekrun, R., Vogl, E., Muis, K. R., & Sinatra, G. M. (2016). Measuring emotions during epistemic activities: The Epistemically-Related Emotion Scales. *Cognition and Emotion.* [Epub ahead of print]

Perkins, A. M., & Corr, P. J. (2005). Can worriers be winners?: The association between worrying and job performance. *Personality and Individual Differences, 38,* 25–31.

Perry, R. P., Chipperfield, J. G., Hladkyj, S., Pekrun, R., & Hamm, J. M. (2014). Attribution-based treatment interventions in some achievement settings. In S. Karabenick & T. C. Urdan (Eds.), *Advances in motivation and achievement* (Vol. 18, pp. 1–35). Bingley, UK: Emerald Group.

Peterson, E. R., Brown, G. T., & Jun, M. C. (2015). Achievement emotions in higher education: A diary study exploring emotions across an assessment event. *Contemporary Educational Psychology, 42,* 82–96.

Preckel, F., Zeidner, M., Goetz, T., & Schleyer, E. (2008). Female "big fish" swimming against the tide: The "big-fish-little-pond effect" and gender ratio in special gifted classes. *Contemporary Educational Psychology, 33,* 78–96.

Putwain, D. W., & Symes, W. (2011). Teachers' use of fear appeals in the mathematics classroom: Worrying or motivating students? *British Journal of Educational Psychology, 81,* 456–474.

Reisenzein, R. (2001). Appraisal processes conceptualized from a schema-theoretic perspective. In In K. R. Scherer, A. Schorr, & T. Johnstone, T. (Eds.), *Appraisal processes in emotion* (pp. 187–201). Oxford, UK: Oxford University Press.

Rosenberg, E. L. (1998). Levels of analysis and the organization of affect. *Review of General Psychology, 2,* 247–270.

Sansone, C., Weir, C., Harpster, L., & Morgan, C. (1992). Once a boring task always a boring task?: Interest as a self-regulatory mechanism. *Journal of Personality and Social Psychology, 63,* 379–390.

Scherer, K. R. (2009). The dynamic architecture of emotions: Evidence for the component process model. *Cognition and Emotion 23,* 1307–1351.

Sweeny, K., & Vohs, K. D. (2012). On near misses and completed tasks: The nature of relief. *Psychological Science, 23,* 464–468.

Thiel, C. E., Connelly, S., & Griffith, J. A. (2012). Leadership and emotion management for complex tasks: Different emotions, different strategies. *Leadership Quarterly, 23,* 517–533.

Tsai, Y.-M., Kunter, M., Lüdtke, O., Trautwein, U., & Ryan, R. M. (2008). What makes lessons interesting?: The role of situational and individual factors in three school subjects. *Journal of Educational Psychology, 100,* 460–472.

Turner, J. E., & Schallert, D. L. (2001). Expectancy–value relationships of shame reactions and shame resiliency. *Journal of Educational Psychology, 93,* 320–329.

Turner, J. E., & Waugh, R. M. (2007). A dynamical systems perspective regarding students' learning processes: Shame reactions and emergent self-organizations. In P. A. Schutz & R. Pekrun (Eds.), *Emotions in education* (pp. 125–145). San Diego, CA: Academic Press.

Tze, V. M. C., Daniels, L. M., & Klassen, R. M. (2016). Evaluating the relationship between boredom and academic outcomes: A meta-analysis. *Educational Psychology Review, 28,* 119–144.

Warr, P. (2007). *Work, happiness, and unhappiness.* Mahwah, NJ: Erlbaum.

Weiner, B. (1985). An attributional theory of achievement motivation and emotion. *Psychological Review, 92,* 548–573.

Wigfield, A., & Eccles, J. S. (1990). Test anxiety in the school setting. In M. Lewis & S. M. Miller (Eds.), *Handbook of developmental psychopathology: Perspectives in developmental psychology* (pp. 237–250). New York: Plenum Press.

Wilson, M., Smith, N. C., & Holmes, P. S. (2007). The role of effort in influencing the effect of anxiety on performance: Testing the conflicting predictions of processing efficiency theory and the conscious processing hypothesis. *British Journal of Psychology, 98,* 411–428.

Zeidner, M. (1998). *Test anxiety: the state of the art.* New York: Plenum Press.

Zeidner, M. (2014). Anxiety in education. In R. Pekrun & L. Linnenbrink-Garcia (Eds.), *International handbook of emotions in education* (pp. 265–288). New York: Taylor & Francis.

CHAPTER 15

The Many Questions of Belonging

GREGORY M. WALTON
SHANNON T. BRADY

One of the most important questions people ask themselves when they enter a new setting is "Do I belong here?" This is not a simple question. It involves two parties, "I" and "here," and, at least implicitly, an evaluation of who I am (or can become) and what the setting allows (or can allow). Belonging is therefore not a simple summation of the number of friends one has in a space. It is a more general inference, drawn from cues, events, experiences, and relationships, about the quality of fit or potential fit between oneself and a setting. It is experienced as a feeling of being accepted, included, respected in, and contributing to a setting, or anticipating the likelihood of developing this feeling.

How do people make this inference? People assess their fit with the social world with an array of implicit worries and questions in mind, such as "Do I have anything in common with people here?"; "Are people like me valued here, or devalued?"; and "Can I be me here?" These questions tune people to specific kinds of cues that seem to address the questions they are asking. An important consequence is that a person may be highly responsive to cues that seem minor, even invisible, to a third party who does not have the same implicit question in mind.

From this theoretical perspective, fostering a sense of belonging is not about promoting positive relationship in a setting per se. Certainly, positive relationships in and of themselves are valuable and may be a source of belonging (e.g., Shook & Clay, 2012); however, people may experience a sense of belonging even in settings in which they do not yet have strong relationships. They can also experience a lack of belonging even when they do have friends in a setting, for instance, if they feel that an important social identity of theirs is marginalized there. It is essential to go beyond personal relationships to understand the implicit worries and questions people have, and how these inform the inferences they draw from cues in an environment. Thus, interventions to bolster a feeling of belonging contend primarily with the symbolic meanings people draw from experiences.

ORGANIZATION OF THE CHAPTER

In making sense of their belonging, people seek to make sense of both the social context—including how others regard and treat oneself—and of themselves—including who they can be in that context. We organize this chapter by discussing each kind of question in turn. Importantly, the distinction between these types of questions is one of emphasis, not kind. In both cases, at stake is people's perception of fit between themselves and a setting. This "setting" we define broadly, as either a specific school or work context or a broader civic or social community.

Throughout, we emphasize distinct implicit questions people ask about their belonging, how a particular question attunes people to specific cues and gives those cues meaning, and how an understanding of this process can give rise to novel strategies that help people feel included in important settings and ultimately flourish. We discuss both laboratory and field experiments, and emphasize how interventions to address belonging can alter people's outcomes along diverse dimensions over time. Because research on belonging, especially field-experimental research, is rapidly accelerating, we include both published research and relevant unpublished work.

THEORETICAL BACKGROUND

Two properties of the social world make the processes by which people draw inferences about their social standing critical: ambiguity and recursion.

First, the world is often severely ambiguous. To make sense of even nonsocial events, people must extract meaning from partial and incomplete stimuli, a process described by Gestalt psychologists and illustrated in visual illusions (Koffka, 1935). In social contexts, this tendency to draw inferences is evident in how people transform simple movies of "interacting" shapes into complex dramas (Heider, 1958). In some cases, when making sense of their relations with others and fit in a social world, people experience relatively unambiguous cues, such as explicit prejudice. Ironically, these can be less cognitively disruptive than subtle ones that might or might not reflect bias (Salvatore & Shelton, 2007). As this example illustrates, an especially important ambiguity concerns the causes of events, termed *attributional ambiguity* (e.g., Crocker, Voelkl, Testa, & Major, 1991; Weiner, 1985), and thus what they mean for one's prospects of inclusion and success. A student may wonder why she was not invited to participate in a study group. A tech worker may wonder why a supervisor

criticized her work. A Latino student may notice that the hallways in the math department are covered with pictures of mathematicians, all of whom are white or Asian, and wonder whether this means his aspirations of becoming a math professor are unrealistic. In each case, a person may wonder if the event means that he or she does not or cannot belong in the setting, rather than attribute it to a more banal cause.

The ambiguity of everyday social life means that different people can make sense of and experience the very same event differently (Ross & Nisbett, 1991). What determines this? As people make sense of a social scene, they do so from a perspective informed by personal factors and group identities. This perspective shapes the contingencies (e.g., risks, opportunities) the person faces in daily life. One kind of contingency, for instance, is whether the person is at risk of experiencing bias or being seen through the lens of a negative stereotype in a setting (Steele, 1997; Steele, Spencer, & Aronson, 2002). An important implication of this risk is that, in addition to structural barriers faced by members of marginalized groups, such as access to fewer resources and discriminatory treatment, the awareness that one could be excluded or disrespected on the basis of group identity leaves an important mark in psychology. It sensitizes people to cues that could signal the status and treatment of their group, an experience called *social-identity threat* (Garcia & Cohen, 2013; Murphy & Taylor, 2012; Steele et al., 2002). For instance, all students may find a difficult, evaluative test aversive. But black students can experience an additional form of threat in taking an evaluative test because they—and not white students—face the prospect that a poor performance could be seen as evidence confirming the stereotype that their group is less intelligent than others (Steele & Aronson, 1995). Women (but not men) may become less interested in working for a tech company whose offices include *Star Trek* posters and empty coke cans because these objects evoke a masculine representation of the social climate that excludes them (Cheryan, Plaut, Davies, & Steele, 2009). One of the hidden advantages of being a member of a privileged group—of being white or male in these examples—is that questions about the standing of one's group, or oneself as a member of a marginalized group, rarely come to mind.

As these examples illustrate, social-identity threat can create a persistent worry about whether "people like me" belong in a valued setting (Walton & Cohen, 2007; see also Walton & Carr, 2012). This worry, called *belonging uncertainty,* is distinguished from a more simple assessment of one's level of belonging (see Walton, Cohen, Cwir, & Spencer, 2012). People can feel they do not belong in a setting simply because they do not connect to it or value it. But they can also value a setting and generally feel that they belong in it but nonetheless feel uncertain about this belonging. When a person's belonging feels insecure, they can be attentive to even subtle cues that imply they (or their group) might not belong there (Walton & Cohen, 2007).

A second reason the inferences people draw about their belonging are critical involves the inherent recursion of the social world. People often behave in ways that make their expectations and beliefs come true; thus, inferences can have lasting consequences (Rosenthal & Jacobson, 1968). In close relationships, a person who doubts his or her partner's love can, as a consequence, perceive a lack of love in routine interactions and ultimately behave in ways that drive their partner away (Murray, Rose, Bellavia, Holmes, & Kusche, 2002).

Belonging is a kind of relationship with a setting, and it has similar properties. As basic research shows, when people feel they belong, they tend to be more motivated in that setting. In one study, simply sharing a birthday with a former math major increased undergraduates' motivation in math (Walton, Cohen, et al., 2012). Moreover, a sense of belonging leads people to engage with others in ways that drive lasting change—for instance, to reach out to develop friendships and mentor relationships (Walton & Cohen, 2007). Correspondingly, a student who worries that people like her may not belong in a school context (i.e., experiences belonging uncertainty) may see adverse everyday experiences such as the receipt of critical feedback or feelings of loneliness as confirmation that she does not belong. As a result, the student may not take advantage

of opportunities for learning, such as attending office hours or meeting in study groups, and not build relationships with peers and teachers necessary for belonging and success (Mendoza-Denton, Downey, Purdie, Davis, & Pietrzak, 2002; Walton & Cohen, 2007). Such students may find their original fear confirmed, while the role of their behavior in contributing to this outcome remains obscure to them. In this way, a psychological process (beliefs about belonging) can affect interpersonal processes (e.g., the quality of relationships) that further reinforce that psychological process to affect outcomes over time. If so, altering this psychological process may cause lasting change (Walton & Cohen, 2011; Yeager et al., 2016; for reviews, see Cohen & Sherman, 2014; Kenthirarajah & Walton, 2015; Walton, 2014; Yeager & Walton, 2011).

Our theoretical analysis implies four important considerations as we review different questions people ask about belonging and corresponding strategies to help people experience a sense of belonging in important settings.

First, if belonging is fundamentally a perception of the fit between the self and a context, then, in theory, the questions people ask themselves can involve, and corresponding interventions can address, perceptions primarily of either the self or the context, or both.

Second, insofar as people are responding to perceived symbolic meanings, interventions to facilitate a sense of belonging traffic in these meanings (see Ross & Nisbett, 1991; Walton & Wilson, 2016). Thus, interventions need not go so far as to establish a positive relationship in a setting or assign people to a "team," though some do (Wing & Jeffery, 1999). Instead, many effective approaches adjust seemingly subtle cues but ones that directly shape the inferences a person draws about his or her relationships with others and a setting (e.g., Carr & Walton, 2014; Walton, Cohen, et al., 2012).

Third, given the power of recursion, inferences about belonging need not—and often do not—stay in a person's head. They tend to become self-fulfilling, and, when positive, help people build substantive relationships and accrue other assets in a setting. A further consequence of recursion is that interventions to address belonging can be most effective when delivered early in a setting and, when this is done, can cause lasting benefits (Cohen & Sherman, 2014; Walton, 2014; Yeager & Walton, 2011). As will be seen, some interventions aimed at bolstering students' sense of belonging in the critical transition to college have improved life outcomes into adulthood (see Brady, Walton, Jarvis, & Cohen, 2016).

Fourth, belonging is one of the most important human needs (Baumeister & Leary, 1995). It therefore functions as a psychological hub and facilitates diverse important outcomes—from motivation and achievement to health and well-being—and, as noted, and can do so over time. Thus, understanding belonging—including how people make sense of their belonging and how to foster it—is essential for both theory and application in diverse areas.

INTERVENTIONS THAT ADDRESS QUESTIONS ABOUT THE SOCIAL CONTEXT (AND THE SELF)

When people first enter a new setting, a primary question they ask is "What is this place like, and can I fit into it?" This question can come in many forms. For a summary, see Table 15.1.

Question 1: "Does Anyone Here Even Notice Me?"

In Disney's adaptations of *Winnie the Pooh,* the pessimistic donkey Eeyore complains, "Don't pay any attention to me. Nobody ever does" (Reinert, 1983). At a most basic level, people want to be recognized, to be seen, by others. Indeed, recognition is a precondition for forming social relationships and, therefore experiencing a sense of belonging in a setting.

When people feel invisible, they suffer (Williams, 2009). It is no accident that Eeyore is depicted as depressed. *Loneliness*—which can be defined as the subjective feeling of being alone, of being disconnected from others, of having "one's intimate and social needs . . . not adequately met" (Hughes, Waite, Hawkley, & Cacioppo, 2004, p. 656)—is one of the strongest

predictors of poor health and well-being (Cacioppo & Patrick, 2008). When people feel invisible, even small acts of social recognition can carry a powerful meaning. When Eeyore is noticed, he says, "Thanks for noticin' me" (Reitherman & Disney, 1968).

Such small acts can have powerful benefits for vulnerable populations. In one study, people released from hospitals after having been admitted for depression or suicidal ideation were randomized to receive periodic postcards from a staff member they had met at the hospital over the next 5 years. These notes simply acknowledged the person and expressed support (e.g., "Dear [former patient's name]: It has been some time since you were here at the hospital, and we hope things are going well for you. If you wish to drop us a note, we would be glad to hear from you."). Compared to a business-as-usual control group (i.e., same hospital treatment, no follow-up postcards), the postcard treatment reduced subsequent suicide rates over the next 2 years (from 3.52 to 1.80%), with effects tapering off subsequently (Motto & Bostrom, 2001). Moreover, about one in four treatment participants spontaneously expressed thanks for the postcards in written responses, which suggest the meaning the notes had for them—for example, "Thank you for your continued interest"; "I really appreciate your persistence and concern"; "Your note gave me a warm, pleasant feeling. Just knowing someone cares means a lot"; "I was surprised to get your letter. I thought that when a patient left the hospital your concern ended here"; "You will never know what your little notes mean to me. I always think someone cares about what happens to me, even if my family did kick me out. I am really grateful." In a second study, such postcards reduced readmissions for self-poisoning by 50% over the next 5 years (Carter, Clover, Whyte, Dawson, & D'Este, 2013).

Socially excluded adolescents may also feel they lack social recognition. Another area of research found that simply addressing socially excluded adolescents by first name, both in person by an experimenter and in a letter from the school principal (rather than "Dear Student"), reduced feelings of loneliness (Brummelman et al., 2016). Invisibility can also take a group form (Ellison, 1952), and gestures of inclusion

TABLE 15.1. "What Is This Place—And How Do I Fit into It?": Changing Representations of the Social Context to Promote Belonging

Belonging question/worry	Remedy	Example(s)
People feel invisible: *"Does anyone here even notice me?"*	Recognize and acknowledge people	• People released following hospitalization for suicidal or depressive thoughts were less likely to commit suicide if they received periodic supportive letters from a hospital staff member over several years after having been discharged (Motto & Bostrom, 2001).
People feel disconnected: *"Are there people here whom I connect to?"*	Facilitate a sense of personal connection to other people in a setting	• Students who found they shared a birthday with a former math major showed greater interest and motivation in math (Walton et al., 2012). • Showing teachers personal preferences they shared with individual black and Latino ninth-grade students raised course grades among those students (Gehlbach et al., 2016).
	Facilitate a sense of working toward common goals with other people in a setting	• People treated by peers as partners working together on a task showed greater intrinsic motivation, enjoying the task more, persisting longer and performing better on it, and, in some cases, choosing to do more, similar tasks 1–2 weeks later (Carr & Walton, 2014).
People worry that they are devalued: *"Do people here value (people like) me?"*	Provide a narrative with which to understand common challenges in the setting so they do not seem to impugn one's belonging	• First-year black students who learned that feelings of nonbelonging are normal in the transition to college and improve with time earned higher grades through senior year, reducing the racial achievement gap by 50%, and reported more confidence in their belonging and greater happiness at the end of college (Walton & Cohen, 2007, 2011; see also Walton et al., 2015; Yeager et al., 2016). • First-year, first-generation college students who learned about the shared and unique challenges faced by first-generation students in college and how these improve over time exhibited reduced stress, increased feelings of social acceptance, and earned higher grades over the first year of college (Stephens et al., 2014).
	Broaden representations of who belongs in the setting	• Increasing the representation of women in a math and science conference increased women's anticipated belonging in the conference, and reduced threat and vigilance (Murphy et al., 2007). • Replacing objects that evoke masculine stereotypes of computer science with neutral objects increased women's interest and anticipated belonging in the field (Cheryan et al., 2009).
	Represent specific institutional actions that could seem to threaten belonging so they do not	• Reducing the stigmatization implied in a letter placing students on academic probation reduced the likelihood that students received a more severe academic status (e.g., suspension) or dropped out a year later (Brady, Fotuhi, et al., 2016). • Encouraging teachers to adapt an empathic rather than punitive mindset toward misbehaving students increased students' respect for teachers and reduced suspension rates over an academic year (Okonofua et al., 2016).
People devalue the setting: *"Is this a setting in which I want to belong?"*	Represent the setting as offering opportunities to pursue valued goals	• People and especially women expressed greater interest in math and science when the opportunities those fields offer to fulfill communal goals—to help others and work collaboratively—were highlighted (Diekman et al., 2011).

across group lines can remedy this. In one study, being asked for directions by a white confederate, instead of observing a white or Asian person be asked, led to black and Latino (but not white or Asian) commuters to express greater interest in taking part in local political activities, which may reflect a greater sense of membership in the civic community (Howe, Bryan, & Walton, 2016). There was no such effect for white or Asian commuters.

Question 2: "Are There People Here Whom I Connect To?"

People can also feel disconnected from others in a specific setting. Yet small cues of similarity or connectedness can open the door to a potential relationship. In *The Four Loves*, C. S. Lewis (1960) writes:

> Friendship arises . . . when two or more . . . companions discover that they have in common some insight or interest or even taste which the others do not share and which, till that moment, each believed to be his own unique treasure (or burden). The typical expression of opening Friendship would be something like, "What? You too? I thought I was the only one." (p. 65)

Walton, Cohen, and colleagues (2012) use the term *mere belonging* to describe how even minor cues can create a sense of social connection to new interaction partners. Moreover, when this person represents a setting, this personal tie can singal an opportunity to connect to the setting more broadly and, in so doing, enhance motivation. In a series of studies, undergraduates expressed greater interest in math and worked longer on a math puzzle when they believed they shared a birthday with a math major (compared to simply being exposed to this person), and when they believed themselves to be part of a minimal "numbers group" (compared to being labeled "the numbers person"). These gains in motivation were mediated by a greater sense of social connection to the math department as a whole. Thus, cues of social connection themselves gave rise to socially shared motivations (see also Brannon & Walton, 2013; Cwir, Carr, Walton, & Spencer, 2011; Shteynberg & Apfelbaum, 2013; Shteynberg & Galinksy,

2011). They did so by helping people answer "yes" to the implied question, "Are there people here to whom I can connect?"

Such effects arise at an early age. Preschoolers exhibit greater motivation when assigned to a minimal "puzzles group" than when identified as the "puzzles child" (Master & Walton, 2013; see also Master, Cheryan, & Meltzoff, in press). Even 1- and 2-year-olds are sensitive to reciprocal social exchanges. Barragan and Dweck (2014) found that children showed greater altruism when a partner had first rolled a ball back and forth with them than when they had played separately. Like adults, infants and toddlers are sensitive to cues that imply to whom they are connected, and behave accordingly.

Extending this laboratory work, field research shows that facilitating opportunities for social connection in school settings can have powerful benefits, especially for students from groups that are marginalized. For instance, taking advantage of a natural experiment, Shook and Clay (2012) found that ethnic-minority first-year students in a predominantly white university assigned a white roommate rather than an ethnic-minority roommate reported a greater sense of belonging on campus at the end of the first year, and this mediated higher grades. Gehlbach and colleagues (2016) gave ninth-grade teachers information about personal preferences they shared with individual black and Latino students in their classes on the premise that doing so might facilitate better teacher–student relationships (Walton, Cohen, et al., 2012). Ethnic-minority students' course grades rose, reducing the racial achievement gap by 60% (see also Bowen, Wegmann, & Webber, 2012).

These studies examined opportunities to build relationships and personal similarities. Cues that signal an opportunity to work with others on a task or toward a common goal are also psychologically powerful. Indeed, given the benefits of working together for both individuals and society, people may generally be motivated by opportunities to work together (Tomasello, Carpenter, Call, Behne, & Moll, 2005). For instance, creating teams to support personal goal pursuits can facilitate better outcomes (e.g., weight loss; Prestwich et al., 2012; Wing & Jeffery,

1999); imagining that an otherwise boring task will be done with others rather than alone increases interest (described in Master, Butler, & Walton, in press); and knowing that people similar to oneself share a goal promotes pursuit of that goal (Shteynberg & Galinksy, 2011). Even small social acts that suggest that other people think of one as a partner working on a task can facilitate motivation (Carr & Walton, 2014). In one series of studies, participants were told they would work "together" on a challenging puzzle and received a "tip" from a peer working on the same puzzle. Being treated by a peer as working together on the puzzle increased participants' intrinsic motivation for it, leading them to persist longer on it, to report enjoying it more, to perform better on it, and, in some conditions, to choose to do more similar puzzles 1–2 weeks later. These gains were found relative to a condition in which people worked on the same puzzle, knowing that others were also working on it. However, they were not told they were working "together," and the tip they received was attributed to the experimenter, not to another participant. This latter condition represented participants' work as done in parallel to others but separately from them (for related research with young children, see Butler & Walton, 2013). The results suggest that experiences are more meaningful and motivational when they are experienced as done together, and this sense of togetherness can be created through simple symbolic social acts.

Question 3: "Do People Here Value (People Like) Me?"

An especially painful experience of nonbelonging arises when people want to belong in a valued school or work setting yet harbor persistent doubts about whether they or people like them can belong. Earlier we described this as belonging uncertainty (Walton & Cohen, 2007).

Consider the transition to college. Although this transition is difficult for all students, those from groups that are socially and economically disadvantaged in higher education, such as first-generation college students and students who face stereotypes that impugn their group's intellectual

abilities, may experience the most significant and complicated challenges to belonging. Indeed, stories from many students from disadvantaged backgrounds highlight belonging concerns. In her senior thesis, after having spent nearly 4 years in college, Michelle Obama wrote, "I sometimes feel like a visitor on campus; as if I really don't belong. . . . It often seems as if . . . I will always be Black first and a student second" (Robinson, 1985, p. 2). Justice Sonia Sotomayor has said that she felt like "a visitor landing in an alien country" in college (Ludden & Weeks, 2009). One low-income student from rural South Dakota said of her transition to a small New England college, "I kind of feel like I've been dropped on Mars. . . . I mean, it's so different" (Aries & Berman, 2013, p. 1).

Students from groups that are disadvantaged in college may experience unique kinds of challenges, such as experiences of discrimination and a cultural mismatch (e.g., Stephens, Fryberg, Markus, Johnson, & Covarrubias, 2012). Moreover, when college appears to be a foreign cultural and social place, even adversities that are experienced by many students can take on especially threatening meanings. When a student who is already worried about whether she belongs fails a first-semester midterm, has a conflict with a roommate, or feels lonely or homesick, she may wonder whether this means people like her simply do not belong in college. These worries can lead students to withdraw from the academic environment and become self-fulfilling (Mendoza-Denton et al., 2002; Walton & Cohen, 2007). In one study of graduates of a high-performing urban charter network, worries about belonging in college were more predictive of lower rates of full-time college enrollment the next year than every other "noncognitive" measure assessed (e.g., Big Five personality traits, test anxiety, grit, self-control, growth-mindset of intelligence; Yeager et al., 2016). When the burden of this recursive process falls disproportionately on students from socially disadvantaged backgrounds, it further contributes to social inequality.

When people enter settings they value but where their group is disadvantaged, how can we help them feel more secure in their belonging? Research suggests three complementary approaches.

Approach 1: Provide a Narrative with Which to Understand Common Challenges So They Do Not Impugn One's Belonging

In navigating a difficult transition like going to college, people experience a great variety of challenges that can lead them to question their prospects of belonging. Thus, it can be helpful to equip people with ways of making sense of these challenges, so that they do not seem to impugn their global belonging or potential. Just knowing that many challenges are normal can go a long way because people often experience a kind of pluralistic ignorance about struggles (Prentice & Miller, 1993). When students think that challenges are personal or specific to their group, not shared widely, they may feel like "imposters" who do not belong or cannot succeed.

One important intervention strategy is therefore to provide information that helps students see that difficulties are common early in an academic transition, that these difficulties reflect the challenges of the transition, and that they improve with time. Classic interventions conveyed stories from upper-year students to struggling first-year college students about how poor grades are common at first in college and reflect the challenges of adjusting to college (e.g., getting used to new living conditions, learning to study for college classes). This improved recipients' grades and retention over a period of years (Wilson, Damiani, & Shelton, 2002).

Extending this approach, Walton and Cohen (2007, 2011) developed a *social-belonging intervention*, which uses information and stories from older students to convey that worries about belonging and social challenges—like feeling intimidated by professors, struggling to make friends, or receiving critical academic feedback— are common at first in the transition to college (e.g., experienced by students of all racial backgrounds) and improve with time. These materials were designed to prevent students from racial-minority backgrounds from inferring that such challenges mean that "people like me" do not belong here. First-year students reflected on these materials and, then, in an effort to help them connect this process of adjustment with their own experience, wrote essays and recorded a video describing how this process of change was true for them. These materials, students were told, could be shared with future students to improve their transition to college. As predicted, this exercise, which students completed in a 1-hour session in the spring of their first year of college, improved diverse outcomes for black students, who face negative stereotypes in college. It increased black students' engagement in the academic environment over the next week: for instance, they were more likely to e-mail professors, attend office hours, and meet with study groups (Walton & Cohen, 2007). Moreover, compared to several active control conditions, the exercise raised black students' grades through the end of college, cutting the racial achievement gap by half (Walton & Cohen, 2011). At the end of college, treated black students also reported being happier, healthier, and more confident in their belonging in college. Notably, at this point, students did not remember the intervention well or credit their success in college to it. Instead, the intervention seemed to improve outcomes by instigating the predicted change in social inference. Daily diaries completed in the week after the intervention (i.e., in students' first year of college) showed that the intervention prevented black students from experiencing a lack of belonging on days when they encountered greater adversities. This change in meaning mediated the long-term effects on achievement.

Understanding everyday adversities as normal challenges that can be overcome may help a student remain engaged in the academic environment, and build relationships that support lasting success (Walton & Cohen, 2007). Consistent with this reasoning, a follow-up in young adulthood found that the intervention delivered in students' first year of college improved graduates' life and job satisfaction 5.5 years after college (8.5 years after initial study participation; Brady, Walton, et al., 2016). These gains were not mediated by better college grades. Instead, graduates reported having developed more significant and lasting mentor relationships in college, and this mediated a better postcollege life. The results underscore the power of a recursive cycle in which students make sense of adversities in more adaptive ways beginning at a critical period, sustain engagement and build better relationships, which in turn further support a sense of belonging and better life outcomes.

The social-belonging intervention has been adapted for and shown to be effective in diverse populations. Among women in male-dominated engineering majors, it raised first-year grades, eliminating gender disparities, and promoted women's friendships with male peers (Walton, Logel, Peach, Spencer, & Zanna, 2015). Among African American boys entering middle school, it reduced discipline citations over 7 years through the completion of high school apparently by improving cycles of interactions and relationships with teachers (Goyer et al., 2016). Additionally, it can be effective when delivered online to full incoming classes prior to the first year of college (Yeager et al., 2016). In three large-scale trials, prematriculation versions of the social-belonging and related interventions improved academic outcomes for full cohorts of socially and economically disadvantaged students (i.e., racial- and ethnic-minority students, first-generation college students; total $N > 9,500$), increasing full-time enrollment and grade point average over the first year. These effects correspond to reductions of 31–40% in the raw achievement gaps observed at these institutions. In several cases, these effects were mediated by gains in social capital, including greater friendship development, participation in student groups, and development of mentor relationships.

Whereas the social-belonging intervention focuses on normal challenges students encounter in a transition, it can also be helpful to help students make sense of unique challenges that arise from their group identities. For instance, Stephens, Hamedani, and Destin (2014) developed a *difference-education* intervention, which exposed first-generation college students to a panel discussion in which, among other themes, peers described how their first-generation status had affected their experience in college, and how they responded to these challenges successfully. Compared to a panel discussion without this theme, the difference-education panel led first-generation students to report feeling less stressed about college, more socially accepted, and more connected to and at home at their college at the end of

the first year. It also led to higher first-year grades and greater use of resources such as office hours and mentorship (see also Stephens, Townsend, Hamedani, Destin, & Manzo, 2015).

Approach 2: Broaden Representations of Who Belongs in a Setting

When people worry about whether people like them can belong in a valued setting, they attend to cues that communicate—sometimes subtly, sometimes overtly—who fits there (Murphy & Taylor, 2012; Steele et al., 2002). Such cues often matter most when people are first trying to make sense of a setting. With insight into people's worries and the corresponding cues to which they attend, early negative impressions can be prevented.

A basic cue is group representation. As tennis great Arthur Ashe wrote, "Like many other blacks, when I find myself in a new public situation, I will count. I always count. I count the number of black and brown faces present" (Ashe & Rampersad, 1993, p. 144). In one study, women watched a video depicting a math and science conference in which men outnumbered women, as is typical (Murphy, Steele, & Gross, 2007). Compared to women who saw a video with an equal gender balance, those who saw the gender-unbalanced video were more cognitively and physiologically vigilant, remembering more details of the video and showing a physiological stress response. They also anticipated feeling they would belong less at the conference and expressed less desire to attend it. Men were unaffected by the gender-ratio manipulation. Other studies find that when women actually work in math, science, and engineering settings dominated by men, they tend to experience a lower sense of belonging and perform worse (e.g., Dasgupta, Scircle, & Hunsinger, 2015; Inzlicht & Ben-Zeev, 2000; Walton et al., 2015). One reason a lack of ingroup representation is harmful is because it can increase pressure to "represent" one's group well. Supreme Court Justice Sandra Day O'Connor described her experience when Justice Ruth Bader Ginsburg joined the Court: "The minute Justice Ginsburg came to the court, we were nine justices. It wasn't seven and then 'the women.' We became seven and then 'the women.' We became nine. It was a great relief to me" (Woodruff, 2003).

Thus, it is beneficial to include a critical mass of people from important identity groups in school and work settings. One study found that creating female-majority or gender-equal work groups among engineering students increased women's participation, confidence, and aspirations in the field (Dasgupta et al., 2015). It is also important to depict this diversity, such as by highlighting ingroup role models who show that success and inclusion are possible for people from diverse backgrounds (e.g., McIntyre, Paulson, & Lord, 2003). In one study, simply including images of female scientists in a chemistry textbook increased learning among high school girls (Good, Woodzicka, & Wingfield, 2010; see also Rios, Stewart, & Winter, 2010). In another, exposure to an academically successful Native American increased a sense of belonging in Native American middle school students compared to an ethnically ambiguous or white role model (Covarrubias & Fryberg, 2015; see also Lockwood, 2006).

There are important outstanding questions about critical mass to pursue in future research. For instance, at what point is critical mass achieved so as to allay worries about belonging? How does this vary in different contexts, or for different people? For instance, do upper-class blacks benefit from knowing that working-class blacks are numerous in a setting? In general, the answers to questions like these will depend on the meaning numeric representation carries in a given context: Does the presence of ingroup members give a person confidence that "people like me" can belong and succeed in the setting? There is unlikely to be a magic point at which critical mass is achieved for all people from all groups or in all settings.

Beyond numeric representation, people attend to cues that imply what *type* of person belongs in a setting. One study found that a 2-minute conversation with a computer science major who embodied classic stereotypes about computer science undermined women's interest in the field up to 2 weeks later. These effects were mediated by a reduced sense of belonging, and they arose regardless of the major's gender (Cheryan,

Drury, & Vichayapai, 2013). Such cues can project a narrow stereotype of who belongs in a context, decreasing interest for people who do not fit that representation. But representations can be broadened in a number of ways. In one study we have already noted, when women completed a survey in a computer science room filled with objects that challenged geeky masculine stereotypes about computer scientists (e.g., nature posters instead of *Star Trek* poster), women saw the field as less masculine, anticipated belonging more, and expressed greater interest in it (Cheryan et al., 2009). Information that computer scientists no longer fit prevalent stereotypes can also increase women's interest in the field (Cheryan, Plaut, Handron, & Hudson, 2013; see also Cheryan, Siy, Vichayapai, Drury, & Kim, 2011). Representations of who belongs can also be shaped by curricula. Using a regression discontinuity design, one study found evidence that an ethnic studies course raised attendance, credits earned, and full-year grades among Asian and Hispanic students in ninth grade (Dee & Penner, in press).

How an organization presents itself also matters. A company that states explicitly that it values diversity, as compared to endorsing a color-blindness philosophy that denies the importance of race, can increase trust among black professionals, and do so even when they company is not (yet) diverse (Purdie-Vaughns, Steele, Davies, Ditlmann, & Crosby, 2008). Job advertisements are another important signal of who belongs at a company. Gaucher, Friesen, and Kay (2011) found that job ads for male-dominated fields tended to use more words associated with male stereotypes (e.g., *leader, competitive, dominant*). The use of these words led both men and women to perceive that there would be more men in the occupation, and it led women to find these jobs less appealing, an effect mediated by a lower anticipated belonging (see also Stout & Dasgupta, 2011; Vervecken, Hannover, & Wolter, 2013). A further way that companies signal, even inadvertently, an exclusive work environment is by promulgating a culture that prizes "talent" and "genius" over growth and development (Murphy & Dweck, 2010). The notion that some people "have it"—and others don't—can convey exclusion to people who are not stereotypically associated

& Murphy, 2015; Good, Rattan, & Dweck, 2012).

Interpersonal interactions can also make people feel personally excluded or disrespected. One series of studies found that talking about engineering with a male peer who acted in a dominant and flirty manner undermined female engineering students and their engineering performance (Logel et al., 2009). Similarly, in a field study of professional female engineers, negative conversations with male colleagues predicted feelings of threat and burnout on a day-to-day basis (Hall, Schmader, & Croft, 2015). In contrast, interactions that signal inclusion and respect as a work partner can improve outcomes for women in quantitative fields (Aguilar, Carr, & Walton, 2016). An especially important interpersonal context involves the provision of critical feedback, which provides an invaluable opportunity for learning and growth but can also appear to recipients to reflect bias or disrespect (Cohen et al., 1999). One field experiment found that a single instance of disambiguating the meaning of critical feedback by prefacing it with an explicit message that the feedback reflected the teacher's belief in the student's potential to reach a higher standard improved motivation and trust among black adolescents over months (Yeager, Purdie-Vaughns, et al., 2014).

These lines of research underscore the value of making sense of the social world from the perspective of members of groups that are marginalized in a setting. From this perspective, even subtle cues that raise the prospect of group-based devaluation, disrespect, or exclusion can undermine a sense of belonging. With an understanding of these cues and this meaning-making process, organizations can address specific aspects of the environment to include people from diverse backgrounds.

Approach 3: Represent Specific Institutional Actions That Could Seem to Threaten Belonging So They Do Not

Sometimes it is not so much subtle cues as specific actions taken by institutions or institutional actors that lead people to feel they do not belong. Disciplinary action, for instance, directly indicates to a person that he or she has not met community standards.

It may also seem to convey that the person is not valued or respected, or is seen as less worthy or capable than others, even when these meanings are not intended. However, such inferences and negative downstream consequences can be prevented.

In primary and secondary school, teachers have available to them two very different models for responding to student misbehavior. A dominant approach to discipline in many schools is punitive. Derived in part from a behaviorist psychology of rewards and punishments, this approach encourages severe punishment for even minor misbehaviors (e.g., zero-tolerance policies). This is thought to motivate students to behave well, to help teachers maintain control of the class, and therefore to promote learning. However, a punitive approach can also lead misbehaving students to believe they are not wanted in class. An alternative approach, termed *empathic discipline*, emphasizes understanding the perspectives of misbehaving students, sustaining positive relationships, and helping students improve from within the context of supportive relationships. This approach is deeply rooted in the core professional values of teachers; yet it stands in tension with a more punitive approach. Consistent with the view that teachers have access to both models, Okonofua, Paunesku, and Walton (2016) found that simply priming teachers with one model of discipline or the other radically shaped their responses to hypothetical instances of student misbehavior: When primed with a punishment model, teachers treated misbehaving students in far more punitive ways, for instance, threatening to send a child to the principal's office for a minor infraction rather than talking with him about his behavior. Moreover, when students imagined receiving paradigmatic treatment from teachers exposed to the punitive prime, they expressed far less respect for the teacher and were less motivated to behave well in the future. Finally, in an intervention field experiment, math teachers at five middle schools in three districts reviewed articles and stories from students and teachers describing the empathic mindset about discipline. Then, to promote internalization, teachers described how they use this approach with their own students. Compared to students whose math teachers completed randomized control materials, the intervention halved yearlong suspension rates, from 9.6 to 4.8%. It also bolstered the respect the most at-risk students, those who had previously been suspended, perceived from their teachers.

In a second example, a selective university approached us concerned about its academic probation process (Brady, Fotuhi, Gomez, Cohen, & Walton, 2016). This process was designed to alert students not making satisfactory academic progress to this fact and to help them improve. Yet in a survey, previous probationary students expressed considerable shame and stigma regarding probation and, specifically, the probation notification letter. Students said: "I felt incredibly alone . . . I felt like I couldn't tell anyone" and "Being on probation sucked. . . . For some time after getting the [notification] letter, I felt that I didn't belong." Therefore, we revised the notification letter to mitigate these stigmatizing inferences. The revision described probation as a process not a label; conveyed that many students experience probation and do so for a variety of valid reasons (e.g., physical health, mental health, family circumstances, adjustment difficulties, etc.); highlighted the university's positive, improvement-oriented goals for probation; and offered hope for returning to good standing. In a field experiment, students who received the revised letter were marginally more likely than those who received the prior letter to reach out to an advisor soon after notification. A year later, they were less likely to have received a more serious academic status (e.g., suspension) and more likely to still be enrolled at the university.

School discipline and academic probation are actions an institution takes toward a particular student, and may reasonably raise doubt in that student's mind about the quality of their relationship with the institution going forward. In other cases, the institutional action may be impersonal, yet bring to the fore differential group-based perspectives. Take bureaucratic red tape, a prototypical impersonal experience. Reeves, Murphy, D'Mello, and Yeager (2015) found in laboratory experiments that frustrating academic forms and confusing course selection processes were negative for all students but elicited belonging concerns specifically among first-generation college students. Students without a history of family success

in higher education may wonder whether bureaucratic difficulties mean they lack "inside knowledge" to succeed. Could cutting red tape reduce hassles for everyone and help mitigate social class inequalities?

Question 4: "Is This a Setting in Which I Want to Belong?"

Although people often see the school and work settings in which they live as desirable and therefore aspire to belong in them, in some contexts the question is not "Do I belong?" but "Do I want to belong?" It can thus be important to identify what prevents people from seeing a setting as desirable.

One obstacle to interest in math, science, and engineering fields is the perception that these fields do not allow for communal goals—opportunities to work with and/or to help others. This perception is most detrimental for women, who are more likely to hold communal goals. Correcting this misperception—by highlighting the collaborative nature of science and opportunities to contribute to the social good—can increase interest in pursuing science, especially among women (Diekman, Clark, Johnston, Brown, & Steinberg, 2011; Diekman, Weisgram, & Belanger, 2015; see also Grant, 2008; Grant & Hofmann, 2011; Yeager, Henderson, et al., 2014).

Sometimes the setting itself is stigmatized. "Developmental" (i.e., remedial) math programs in community college are an essential educational context for lower-income adults aiming to improve their life circumstances. Almost two-thirds of community college students are assigned to take at least one developmental math or reading course, yet completion rates are abysmal; some estimate that just 20% of students complete the math sequence to which they are referred (e.g., Bailey, Jeong, & Cho, 2010). Revealingly, Reeves, Yeager, and Walton (2016) found that 4-year college students distance themselves academically and socially from developmental math students, and do so as much, if not more so, than from traditionally stigmatized groups (e.g., people who are obese, people who are transgender). These findings raise important questions. Do students in developmental math also see their peers in a stigmatized light? Does this discourage students from developing friendships and study groups with classmates? If so, is it possible to mitigate this stigma, such as by acquainting students with the higher-order purposes they share with their classmates for pursuing developmental math (e.g., to gain skills, to improve their family circumstances, to contribute to their communities; cf. Schroeder & Prentice, 1998; Yeager, Henderson, et al., 2014)?

INTERVENTIONS THAT ADDRESS QUESTIONS ABOUT THE SELF (IN A SOCIAL CONTEXT)

So far, we have discussed questions about belonging that primarily address the context the person is in. But, as we noted in the introduction, belonging is a matter of the fit between a setting and the self, who one can be in that setting. Another way to promote belonging and better outcomes is thus to help people feel positively about who they are or could become in a setting. For a summary of belonging questions that focus on the self, see Table 15.2.

Question 5: "Can I Be More Than a Stereotype Here?"

When people face negative stereotypes about important social groups to which they belong, a key concern involves the possibility that they could be seen through the lens of the stereotype or reduced to token status, and not be seen as or able to be a full person in that context (Steele, 1997). Michelle Obama illustrates this concern in her thesis quoted earlier, in which she worried that she was seen as "Black first and a student second."

A strikingly powerful way to help people feel they are more than a stereotype in a setting is the *self-affirmation* intervention (Cohen & Sherman, 2014; see Cohen, Garcia, & Goyer, Chapter 35, this volume). In its most common form, *values affirmation*, people take a psychological time-out to reflect on personal values that matter to them. They review a list of values (e.g., "sense of humor," "relationships with friends and family"), select those that are most important to them, then write for 10–15 minutes about why these values

TABLE 15.2. "Who Am I/We Here?": Changing Representations of the Self to Promote Belonging

Belonging question/ worry	Remedy	Example
People feel they cannot be a full person in a setting: *"Can I be more than a stereotype here?"*	Offer opportunities for people to reflect on personally important values within a setting	• Values-affirmation exercises, in which students wrote about their most important values in an in-class exercise at the beginning of seventh grade, improved the grades of black students and reduced the likelihood that they would be recommended to remedial courses (Cohen et al., 2009). • Encouraging women enrolled in male-dominated engineering majors to incorporate values into their daily lives to maintain balance and manage stress, helped women function more effectively in the face of daily adversities and improved first-year grades, eliminating gender differences (Walton et al., 2015).
People feel that who they are is incompatible with a setting or behavior: *"Are people like me incompatible with this setting or behavior?"*	Change representations of the ingroup to facilitate a perceived fit with the setting/ behavior	• Midwestern housewives were more likely to serve organ meats to their families after participating in a small-group discussion, which highlighted a collective decision to do so, than after a persuasive lecture appeal (Lewin, 1958). • Learning that peers are less comfortable with drinking than they appear reduced drinking most among students who felt uncomfortable with drinking but feared the negative judgment of peers (Schroeder & Prentice, 1998). • Exposure to an academically successful Native American enhanced the academic belonging of Native American students (Covarrubias & Fryberg, 2015).

matter to them. Values affirmation can improve health and achievement in diverse populations. The benefits are often greatest for people who are experiencing identity threat or other kinds of acute threats. In studies with adolescents, for instance, completing several such exercises as in-class writing assignments beginning at the outset of seventh grade raised achievement among black students, with gains for the most at-risk students, those performing poorly prior to treatment, persisting through the end of eighth grade (Cohen, Garcia, Purdie-Vaughns, Apfel, & Brzustoski, 2009). The benefits of value-affirmation among students who face identity threat has been replicated many times (e.g., Bowen, Wegmann, & Webber, 2013; Cook, Purdie-Vaughns, Garcia, & Cohen, 2012; Harackiewicz et al., 2014; Miyake et al., 2010; Sherman et al., 2013; Walton et al., 2015). Hanselman, Bruch, Gamoran, and Borman (2014) tested values-affirmation exercises in a randomized trial in all middle schools in a medium-size school district; the benefits were greatest for racial- and ethnic-minority students and in schools in which they were underrepresented and achievement gaps were largest—where identity threat that arises from the awareness of negative stereotypes may be largest.

How does affirmation relate to belonging? Self-affirmation theory argues that people aim to maintain a general sense of themselves as capable and good (Steele, 1988). Psychological threats imperil this general sense of goodness and capability. Moreover, threats are focal and induce a kind of tunnel vision. They narrow people's working self-concept to the threat and cause people to respond defensively (Cohen & Sherman, 2014). When chronic, identity threat contributes to a recursive cycle in which threat breeds distraction, anxiety, and poor performance, which exacerbate threat in an ongoing cycle (Cohen et al., 2009).

Affirmation exercises signal to people that they can be more than that threatened aspect of self in the setting (Cohen & Sherman, 2014; Sherman & Hartson, 2011; Walton, Paunesku, & Dweck, 2012). In so doing, they can reduce defensiveness and open people up, facilitating positive relationships and belonging that improve outcomes over time. Consistent with this hypothesis, laboratory research finds that value-affirmation exercises expand the working self-concept and discourage people from seeing threats as self-defining (Critcher & Dunning, 2015), a finding echoed in field experiments (Sherman et al., 2013). Furthermore, affirmations evoke prosocial feelings such as love and connectedness, which can mediate benefits (Crocker, Niiya, & Mischkowski, 2008). Such feelings readily follow from the fact that people's most cherished values often represent their relationships, communities, and social identities.

Furthermore, personal values offer important opportunities to connect with others. Insofar as affirmations encourage people to express more of who they are in a setting, this may facilitate the development of positive relationships (see Aron, Melinat, Aron, Vallone, & Bator, 1997; Gehlbach et al., 2016; Walton, Cohen, et al., 2012). Indeed, affirmations are of most benefit when students write about ways that values connect them to others (Shnabel, Purdie-Vaughns, Cook, Garcia, & Cohen, 2013; see also Fotuhi, Spencer, Fong, & Zanna, 2014; cf. Tibbetts et al., 2016). This may be one reason why affirmation helps promote positive relationships and a sense of belonging. In one study, value affirmations increased students' prosocial feelings and behaviors over 3 months (Thomaes, Bushman, de Castro, & Reijntjes, 2012; see also Stinson, Logel, Shepherd, & Zanna, 2011); another found that an affirmation delivered early in the school year helped black middle school students maintain a high sense of belonging over time, and did so even when they struggled academically (Cook, Purdie-Vaughns, Garcia, & Cohen, 2012; for related effects, see Harackiewicz et al., 2014; Sherman et al., 2013). A final study examined affirmation among white first-year teachers teaching predominantly minority students, who, like their students, may experience a form of identity threat in school (Carr, Dweck, & Pauker, 2012; Goff, Steele, & Davies, 2008). Teachers who completed an affirmation exercise in the first 4 months of the school year reported better relationships with their students and a greater sense of belonging at school at the end of the year than teachers who completed control materials (Brady & Cohen, 2016).

The hypothesis that affirmation works, in part, by opening people up and encouraging them to be more of who they are in a setting, which helps them connect with others, is consistent with past research but has never been tested directly. A critical question for future research is to understand further how affirmation changes the way people interact with others in settings, how this may facilitate positive relationships, and the psychological mechanisms that contribute to these processes.

Question 6: "Are People Like Me Incompatible with This Setting or Behavior?"

In other contexts, the worry is less about stereotypes and more about whether a given behavior or activity is appropriate for "a person like me." In classic research, Lewin (1958) used a small-group discussion to encourage white, middle-class Midwestern housewives to serve underused organ meats, perceived as "ethnic foods," during the meat shortages of World War II. The facilitator led the group in discussing how serving organ meats contributed to the war effort and encouraged a collective decision to do so. At the end of the discussion, the facilitator asked for a show of hands of who would try organ meats with their families over the next few weeks, thus providing each participant a visible emblem of the changing standards of the ingroup. As compared to a persuasive lecture appeal, which advocated for the serving of such meats and provided recipes and nutrition information, the small-group discussion increased the percentage of housewives who reported serving organ meats over the next week from 3 to 32%. One reason the group discussion may have been effective is that instead of trying to persuade people to engage in behavior in violation of their perceived group identity ("People like me don't serve 'ethnic foods' "), the discussion changed the perceived standards of the ingroup (see also Miller, Brickman, & Bolen, 1975).

In other cases, interventions expand the perceived boundaries of what kinds of behavior are acceptable for the ingroup, thus allowing people to resist deleterious social influences. In classic research, Prentice and Miller (1993) showed that college students tend to misperceive norms about drinking, seeing other students as more comfortable with drinking than they really are. This led students either to drink more or to feel they did not belong on campus. Learning that other students are less comfortable with drinking than they appear can reduce this pressure (Schroeder & Prentice, 1998). By lessening students' fear of violating the perceived norm, the intervention reduced drinking, especially among students who felt less comfortable with drinking than others and feared the negative judgments of others.

Finally, although role models are often thought of as changing representations of a setting and what kinds of people can succeed there, as described earlier (e.g., Covarrubias & Fryberg, 2015; Good et al., 2010; Lockwood, 2006; McIntyre et al., 2003), role models also convey information about the self and what kind of person one could become. They may thus be most effective when the role model's success appears relevant and attainable to the recipient (Lockwood & Kunda, 1997). Jen Welter (2015), the first woman to coach in the National Football League, recalled, "There wasn't any thought about a career path with the NFL. We'd joke that it was the No Female League. So . . . it was always strange to me when people would say, 'You're in the NFL now, you're living your dream.' Well, no, this wasn't a dream I was ever even permitted to have. I think that part of what I'm most proud of is that now other little girls can have that dream" (p. 105).

CONCLUSION: LESSONS FROM FAILURES

This chapter has focused on success stories, on interventions that successfully fostered people's belonging in diverse contexts, often with positive effects on an array of important outcomes. The range of these interventions illustrates some of the different questions people ask about their belonging. At their heart, these questions involve the perceived fit between the self and a context. They therefore take as their primary form a perception of either the context (and its fit with the self) or the self (and its fit with context). As we noted at the outset, psychological interventions to address belonging primarily traffic in symbolic meanings. Most do not create a friendship per se, or simply place people on a team. Instead, they vary cues in the environment, or how people make sense of these cues or themselves, to help people build strong relationships and a secure sense of belonging in a setting. These perceived meanings are not ephemeral. The inferences people draw about their belonging can become lasting and embedded in the structure of people's lives through the power of recursion. Indeed, in several cases we have seen relatively brief exercises designed to bolster belonging cause improvements in relationships, performance, health, and well-being that extend years into the future.

There are failures, as well as successes, in efforts to promote belonging, and understanding these provides important opportunities for further theory development and more effective application. There are several principled reasons that belonging interventions can fail. First, an intervention may not target the right, precise psychological process; that is, it may not directly address the implicit question people in a given setting have in mind, which shapes how they make sense of events and inferences they draw about their belonging. For instance, whites in college in general, men in engineering, and women in gender-diverse engineering majors may not worry pervasively about whether "people like me" belong. Absent this belonging uncertainty, they may not benefit from Walton and Cohen's (2011) social-belonging intervention; indeed, they were not predicted to do so. Additionally, when students face the possibility of group-based disrespect or devaluation (identity threat), their concern may center on this prospect, and they may be highly responsive to cues that others view them as people with potential (e.g., Yeager, Purdie-Vaughns, et al., 2014). However, they may be less responsive to simple affiliative information that does not directly address this concern. Thus, in Gehlbach and colleagues' (2016) study described earlier, providing teachers information about preferences they shared with their students raised minority students' grades. Presumably, this helped teachers see a connection with their minority students that they did not see before. But providing minority students information about similarities they shared with their teachers had no effect. Minority students may not worry primarily about being similar to their teachers. They may worry instead about whether they are respected. Perhaps for similar reasons, in another study, sending new college students school-related "swag" and assuring them that they are a valued member of the college community increased a sense of belonging among white students but had no effect on black students (Hausmann, Ye, Schofield, & Woods, 2009). When there is a risk of group-based devaluation, generic efforts to promote affiliation may be less effective (see also Covarrubias & Fryberg, 2015).

A focus on the specific psychological processes that contribute to people's sense of belonging also suggests that many everyday practices intended to promote belonging may backfire or be ineffective. For one of us (Walton), the first day of high school began with a literal hug of the school—the student body circled the school, held hands and hugged the school, as though to signify our community. Yet this exercise does not address the ambiguity students may feel in making sense of critical feedback they receive or how they should make sense of initial feelings of loneliness or disrespect they may encounter in entering high school (Yeager et al., 2014). For a person consumed with a specific belonging worry, it might seem like an empty charade. Rituals may be more likely to have substantive psychological effects and foster group cohesion and belongingness when they address specific processes relevant to belonging. Understanding the role of such rituals is an important direction for research (see Pia-Maria & Risto, 2016). Additionally, many of the offhand strategies people use to promote belonging may be ineffective. We have heard department administrators assure new graduate students, "I want you to belong" and teachers ask adolescents to repeat, mantra-style, the refrain "I belong, I can do it, and it matters"; such exercises may unintentionally underscore the isolation felt by students who doubt their belonging. We *want* you to belong implies that most people feel they belong, highlights that you don't right now, and doesn't necessarily offer hope that you ever will. Additionally, when university administrators brag to incoming college students about how many of them have already started a business, written a book, or performed in the Olympics, they intend to instill a sense of school pride. But for the other 99% of students, this may only heighten imposter syndrome.

Second, even when an intervention targets the precise psychological process at hand, it must do so effectively and at the right time. For instance, if people do not engage with intervention materials actively; if the exercise seems inauthentic, stigmatizing, or coercive; or if people simply fail to connect the presented ideas to their personal experience, they may not benefit. They may also not benefit if the intervention comes too late. Early in a setting, people are often most open to new ways of making sense of their belonging. Moreover, recursive processes have not yet taken hold. Thus, in general, it may be best to bolster a sense of belonging early in transitions, helping students build relationships that can promote lasting success (Cook et al., 2012; Stephens et al., 2014; Walton & Cohen, 2011; Yeager et al., 2016).

Finally, the long-term effects of interventions to promote a sense of belonging depend on the affordances of the local context (Gibson, 1977; Walton & Wilson, 2016). Does the context allow people with a more growth-oriented mindset about belonging real opportunities to develop social relationships that facilitate this sense of belonging and improve outcomes over time? In school settings, does the context offer students learning opportunities and other resources, which a more secure sense of belonging can help them pursue? If the context lacks essential affordances, no psychological intervention will be effective.

We have outlined some of the different questions of belonging that people ask, and how these questions may be addressed. These questions and the corresponding interventions are not now fully understood, including when, for whom, and in what contexts different questions of belonging arise and may be best remedied. There are also certainly additional questions beyond those discussed here, which future research may explore. Furthermore, there are cases of failure that are not now fully understood. For instance, Dee (2015) found a positive effect of a value-affirmation intervention for black

and Latino middle school students who attended classrooms that seemed to offer students greater opportunities for academic growth. Yet in these same classrooms, there was a negative effect for girls. Additionally, in a study of college physics, Miyake and colleagues (2010) found positive effects of value affirmation on multiple indices of learning for women but, on course exam scores, a negative effect for men. Do these results have to do with how affirmations intersect with belonging? Psychological interventions are typically delivered in complex social contexts (Cohen & Sherman, 2014; Walton, 2014; Yeager & Walton, 2011). Fully understanding interventions that aim to bolster a sense of belonging requires further developing theory about both the interventions and how they change key psychological processes and social meanings and the social contexts in which the interventions are implemented and how changes in meaning play out in these contexts over time.

REFERENCES

Aguilar, L. J., Carr, P. B., & Walton, G. M. (2016). *Cues of working together reduce stereotype threat among women.* Manuscript under review.

Aries, E., & Berman, R. (2013). *Speaking of race and class: The student experience at an elite college.* Philadelphia: Temple University Press.

Aron, A., Melinat, E., Aron, E. N., Vallone, R., & Bator, R. (1997). The experimental generation of interpersonal closeness: A procedure and some preliminary findings. *Personality and Social Psychology Bulletin, 23,* 363–377.

Ashe, A., & Rampersad, A. (1993). *Days of grace.* New York: Knopf.

Bailey, T., Jeong, D. W., & Cho, S. W. (2010). Referral, enrollment, and completion in developmental education sequences in community colleges. *Economics of Education Review, 29*(2), 255–270.

Barragan, R. C., & Dweck, C. S. (2014). Rethinking natural altruism: Simple reciprocal interactions trigger children's benevolence. *Proceedings of the National Academy of Sciences USA, 111*(48), 17071–17074.

Baumeister, R., & Leary, M. (1995). The need to belong: Desire for interpersonal attachments as a fundamental human motivation. *Psychological Bulletin, 117,* 497–529.

Bowen, N. K., Wegmann, K. M., & Webber, K. C. (2012). Enhancing a brief writing intervention to combat stereotype threat among middle-school students. *Journal of Educational Psychology, 105*(2), 427–435.

Brady, S. T., & Cohen, G. L. (2016). *Self-affirmation in the transition to teaching enhances relationships, boosts rigor, and increases teacher retention.* Manuscript in preparation.

Brady, S. T., Fotuhi, O., Gomez, E., Cohen, G. L., & Walton, G. M. (2016). *Reducing stigma and facilitating student success by reframing institutional messages.* Manuscript in preparation.

Brady, S. T., Walton, G. M., Jarvis, S. N., & Cohen, G. L. (2016). *Bending the river: Downstream consequences of a social-belonging intervention in the transition to college.* Manuscript in preparation.

Brannon, T. N., & Walton, G. M. (2013). Enacting cultural interests: How intergroup contact reduces prejudice by sparking interest in an outgroup's culture. *Psychological Science, 24*(10), 1947–1957.

Brummelman, E., Thomaes, S., Walton, G. M., Reijntjes, A., Orobio de Castro, B., & Sedikides, C. (2016). *Addressing people by name reduces their loneliness, even months later: Evidence from inside and outside the laboratory.* Manuscript under review.

Butler, L. P., & Walton, G. M. (2013). Opportunities to collaborate increase preschoolers' motivation for challenging tasks. *Journal of Experimental Child Psychology, 116*(4), 953–961.

Cacioppo, J. T., & Patrick, B. (2008). *Loneliness: Human nature and the need for social connection.* New York: Norton.

Carr, P. B., Dweck, C. S., & Pauker, K. (2012). "Prejudiced" behavior without prejudice?: Beliefs about the malleability of prejudice affect interracial interactions. *Journal of Personality and Social Psychology, 103*(3), 452–471.

Carr, P. B., & Walton, G. M. (2014). Cues of working together fuel intrinsic motivation. *Journal of Experimental Social Psychology, 53*, 169–184.

Carter, G. L., Clover, K., Whyte, I. M., Dawson, A. H., & D'Este, C. (2013). Postcards from the EDge: 5-year outcomes of a randomised controlled trial for hospital-treated self-poisoning. *British Journal of Psychiatry, 202*, 372–380.

Cheryan, S., Drury, B. J., & Vichayapai, M. (2013). Enduring influence of stereotypical computer science role models on women's academic aspirations. *Psychology of Women Quarterly, 37*(1), 72–79.

Cheryan, S., Plaut, V. C., Davies, P., & Steele, C. M. (2009). Ambient belonging: How stereotypical environments impact gender participation in computer science. *Journal of Personality and Social Psychology, 97*, 1045–1060.

Cheryan, S., Plaut, V. C., Handron, C., & Hudson, L. (2013). The stereotypical computer scientist: Gendered media representations as a barrier to inclusion for women. *Sex Roles, 69*(1–2), 58–71.

Cheryan, S., Siy, J. O., Vichayapai, M., Drury, B. J., & Kim, S. (2011). Do female and male role models who embody STEM stereotypes hinder women's anticipated success in STEM? *Social Psychological and Personality Science, 2*(6), 656–664.

Cohen, G. L., Garcia, J., Purdie-Vaughns, V., Apfel, N., & Brzustoski, P. (2009). Recursive processes in self-affirmation: Intervening to close the minority achievement gap. *Science, 324*, 400–403.

Cohen, G. L., & Sherman, D. K. (2014). The psychology of change: Self-affirmation and social psychological intervention. *Annual Review of Psychology, 65*(1), 333–371.

Cohen, G. L., Steele, C. M., & Ross, L. D. (1999). The mentor's dilemma: Providing critical feedback across the racial divide. *Personality and Social Psychology Bulletin, 25*(10), 1302–1318.

Cook, J. E., Purdie-Vaughns, V., Garcia, J., & Cohen, G. L. (2012). Chronic threat and contingent belonging: Protective benefits of values affirmation on identity development. *Journal of Personality and Social Psychology, 102*(3), 479–496.

Covarrubias, R., & Fryberg, S. A. (2015). The impact of self-relevant representations on school belonging for Native American students. *Cultural Diversity and Ethnic Minority Psychology, 21*(1), 10–18.

Critcher, C. R., & Dunning, D. (2015). Self-affirmations provide a broader perspective on self-threat. *Personality and Social Psychology Bulletin, 41*, 3–18.

Crocker, J., Niiya, Y., & Mischkowski, D. (2008). Why does writing about important values reduce defensiveness?: Self-affirmation and the role of positive other-directed feelings. *Psychological Science, 19*(7), 740–747.

Crocker, J., Voelkl, K., Testa, M., & Major, B. (1991). Social stigma: The affective consequences of attributional ambiguity. *Journal of Personality and Social Psychology, 60*(2), 218–228.

Cwir, D., Carr, P. B., Walton, G. M., & Spencer, S. J. (2011). Your heart makes my heart move: Cues of social connectedness cause shared emotions and physiological states among strangers. *Journal of Experimental Social Psychology, 47*(3), 661–664.

Dasgupta, N., Scircle, M. M., & Hunsinger, M. (2015). Female peers in small work groups enhance women's motivation, verbal participation, and career aspirations in engineering. *Proceedings of the National Academy of Sciences USA, 112*(16), 4988–4993.

Dee, T. (2015). Social identity and achievement gaps: Evidence from an affirmation intervention. *Journal of Research on Educational Effectiveness, 8*(2), 149–168.

Dee, T. S., & Penner, E. K. (in press). The causal effects of cultural relevance: Evidence from an ethnic studies curriculum. *American Educational Research Journal*

Diekman, A. B., Clark, E. K., Johnston, A. M., Brown, E. R., & Steinberg, M. (2011). Malleability in communal goals and beliefs influences attraction to STEM careers: Evidence for a goal congruity perspective. *Journal of Personality and Social Psychology, 101*(5), 902–918.

Diekman, A. B., Weisgram, E., & Belanger, A. L. (2015). New routes to recruiting and retaining women in STEM: Policy implications of a communal goal congruity perspective. *Social Issues and Policy Review, 9*(1), 52–88.

Ellison, R. (1952). *Invisible man.* New York: Signet Books.

Emerson, K. T. U., & Murphy, M. C. (2015). A company I can trust?: Organizational lay theories moderate stereotype threat for women. *Personality and Social Psychology Bulletin, 41,* 295–307.

Fotuhi, O., Spencer, S., Fong, G. T., & Zanna, M. P. (2016). *Contingent affirmation intervention among smokers: Directly linking affirming values to health-specific goals.* Manuscript in preparation.

Garcia, J., & Cohen, G. L. (2013). A social psychological perspective on educational intervention. In E. Shafir (Ed.), *Behavioral foundations of policy* (pp. 329–350). New York: Russell Sage Foundation.

Gaucher, D., Friesen, J., & Kay, A. C. (2011). Evidence that gendered wording in job advertisements exists and sustains gender inequality. *Journal of Personality and Social Psychology, 101,* 109–128.

Gehlbach, H., Brinkworth, M. E., Hsu, L., King, A., McIntyre, J., & Rogers, T. (2016). Creating birds of similar feathers: Leveraging similarity to improve teacher–student relationships and academic achievement. *Journal of Educational Psychology, 108*(3), 342–352.

Gibson, J. J. (1977). The theory of affordances. In R. Shaw & J. Bransford (Eds.), *Perceiving, acting, and knowing: Toward an ecological psychology* (pp. 67–82). Hillsdale, NJ: Erlbaum.

Goff, P. A., Steele, C. M., & Davies, P. G. (2008). The space between us: Stereotype threat and distance in interracial contexts. *Journal of Personality and Social Psychology, 94*(1), 91–107.

Good, C., Rattan, A., & Dweck, C. S. (2012). Why do women opt out?: Sense of belonging and women's representation in mathematics. *Journal of Personality and Social Psychology, 102*(4), 700–717.

Good, J. J., Woodzicka, J. A., & Wingfield, L. C. (2010). The effects of gender stereotypic and counter-stereotypic textbook images on science performance. *Journal of Social Psychology, 150*(2), 132–147.

Goyer, J. P., Cohen, G. L., Cook, J. E., Master, A., Okonofua, J. A., Apfel, N., et al. (2016). *A social-belonging intervention reduces discipline citations among minority boys over seven years.* Manuscript under review.

Grant, A. M. (2008). The significance of task significance: Job performance effects, relational mechanisms, and boundary conditions. *Journal of Applied Psychology, 93,* 108–124.

Grant, A. M., & Hofmann, D. A. (2011). It's not all about me: Motivating hospital hand hygiene by focusing on patients. *Psychological Science, 22,* 1494–1499.

Hall, W. M., Schmader, T., & Croft, E. (2015). Engineering exchanges: Daily social identity threat predicts burnout among female engineers. *Social Psychological and Personality Science, 6*(5), 528–534.

Hanselman, P., Bruch, S. K., Gamoran, A., & Borman, G. D. (2014). Threat in context: School moderation of the impact of social identity threat on racial/ethnic achievement gaps. *Sociology of Education, 87,* 106–124

Harackiewicz, J. M., Canning, E. A., Tibbetts, Y., Giffen, C. J., Blair, S. S., Rouse, D. I., et al. (2014). Closing the social class achievement gap for first-generation students in undergraduate biology. *Journal of Educational Psychology, 106*(2), 375–389.

Hausmann, L. R. M., Ye, F., Schofield, J. W., & Woods, R. L. (2009). Sense of belonging and persistence in White and African American first-year students. *Research in Higher Education, 50*(7), 649–669.

Heider, F. (1958). *The psychology of interpersonal relations.* Hillsdale, NJ: Erlbaum.

Howe, L. C., Bryan, C. B., & Walton, G. M. (2016). *Mere acknowledgment: The impact of everyday interactions across racial boundaries.* Manuscript in preparation.

Hughes, M. E., Waite, L. J., Hawkley, L. C., & Cacioppo, J. T. (2004). A short scale for measuring loneliness in large surveys: Results from two population-based studies. *Research on Aging, 26,* 655–672.

Inzlicht, M., & Ben-Zeev, T. (2000). A threatening intellectual environment: Why females are susceptible to experiencing problem-solving deficits in the presence of males. *Psychological Science, 11*(5), 365–371.

Kenthirarajah, D., & Walton, G. M. (2015). How brief social-psychological interventions can cause enduring effects. In R. Scott & S. Kosslyn (Eds.), *Emerging trends in the social and behavioral sciences*. Hoboken, NJ: Wiley.

Koffka, K. (1935). *Principles of Gestalt psychology*. New York: Harcourt, Brace & World.

Lewin, K. (1958). Group decision and social change. In E. Maccoby, T. M. Newcomb, & E. L. Hartley (Eds.), *Readings in social psychology* (pp. 192–211). New York: Holt, Rinehart & Winston.

Lewis, C. S. (1960). *The four loves*. New York: Harcourt Brace.

Lockwood, P. (2006). Someone like me can be successful: Do college students need same-gender role models? *Psychology of Women Quarterly, 30*(1), 36–46.

Lockwood, P., & Kunda, Z. (1997). Superstars and me: Predicting the impact of role models on the self. *Journal of Personality and Social Psychology, 73*, 91–103.

Logel, C., Walton, G. M., Spencer, S. J., Iserman, E. C., von Hippel, W., & Bell, A. (2009). Interacting with sexist men triggers social identity threat among female engineers. *Journal of Personality and Social Psychology, 96*(6), 1089–1103.

Ludden, J., & Weeks L. (2009, May 26). Sotomayor: "Always looking over my shoulder." Retrieved from *www.npr.org/templates/story/story.php?storyId=104538436*.

Master, A., Butler, L. P., & Walton, G. M. (in press). How the subjective relationship between the self, others, and a task drives interest. In P. A. O'Keefe & J. M. Harackiewicz (Eds.), *The psychological science of interest*. New York: Springer.

Master, A., Cheryan, S., & Meltzoff, A. N. (in press). Social group membership increases STEM engagement among preschoolers. *Developmental Psychology*.

Master, A., & Walton, G. M. (2013). Membership in a minimal group increases motivation and learning in young children. *Child Development, 84*, 737–751.

McIntyre, R. B., Paulson, R. M., & Lord, C. G. (2003). Alleviating women's mathematics stereotype threat through salience of group achievements. *Journal of Experimental Social Psychology, 39*, 83–90.

Mendoza-Denton, R., Downey, G., Purdie, V. J., Davis, A., & Pietrzak, J. (2002). Sensitivity to status-based rejection: Implications for African American students' college experience. *Journal of Personality and Social Psychology, 83*(4), 896–918.

Miller, R. L., Brickman, P., & Bolen, D. (1975). Attribution versus persuasion as a means for modifying behavior. *Journal of Personality and Social Psychology, 31*(3), 430–441.

Miyake, A., Kost-Smith, L. E., Finkelstein, N. D., Pollock, S. J., Cohen, G. L., & Ito, T. A. (2010). Reducing the gender achievement gap in college science: A classroom study of values affirmation. *Science, 330*, 1234–1237.

Motto, J. A., & Bostrom, A. G. (2001). A randomized controlled trial of postcrisis suicide prevention. *Psychiatric Services, 52*(6), 828–833.

Murphy, M. C., & Dweck, C. S. (2010). A culture of genius: How an organization's lay theory shapes people's cognition, affect, and behavior. *Personality and Social Psychology Bulletin, 36*(3), 283–296.

Murphy, M. C., Steele, C. M., & Gross, J. J. (2007). Signaling threat: How situational cues affect women in math, science, and engineering settings. *Psychological Science, 18*(10), 879–885.

Murphy, M. C., & Taylor, V. J. (2012). The role of situational cues in signaling and maintaining stereotype threat. In M. Inzlicht & T. Schmader (Eds.), *Stereotype threat: Theory, process, and applications* (pp. 17–33). New York: Oxford University Press.

Murray, S. L., Rose, P., Bellavia, G. M., Holmes, J. G., & Kusche, A. G. (2002). When rejection stings: How self-esteem constrains relationship-enhancement processes. *Journal of Personality and Social Psychology, 83*(3), 556–573.

Okonofua, J. A., Paunesku, D., & Walton, G. M. (2016). Brief intervention to encourage empathic discipline cuts suspension rates in half among adolescents. *Proceedings of the National Academy of Sciences USA, 113*(19), 5221–5226.

Pia-Maria, N., & Risto, H. (2016). Enhancing students' sense of belonging through school celebrations: A study in Finnish lower-secondary schools. *International Journal of Research Studies in Education, 5*(2), 43–58.

Prentice, D. A., & Miller, D. T. (1993). Pluralistic ignorance and alcohol use on campus: Some consequences of misperceiving the social norm. *Journal of Personality and Social Psychology, 64*(2), 243–256.

Prestwich, A., Conner, M. T., Lawton, R. J., Ward, J. K., Ayres, K., & McEachan, R. R. C. (2012). Randomized controlled trial of collaborative implementation intentions targeting working adults' physical activity. *Health Psychology, 31*, 486–495.

Purdie-Vaughns, V., Steele, C. M., Davies, P. G., Ditlmann, R., & Crosby, J. R. (2008). Social identity contingencies: How diversity cues signal threat or safety for African Americans in mainstream institutions. *Journal of Personality and Social Psychology, 94*(4), 615–630.

Reeves, S. L., Murphy, M. C., D'Mello, S. K., & Yeager, D. S. (2015). *Caught up in red tape: Bureaucratic hassles undermine sense of belonging in college among first-generation students.* Manuscript in preparation.

Reeves, S. L., Yeager, D. S., & Walton, G. M. (2016). *The stigma of remediation.* Manuscript in preparation.

Reinert, R. (Producer & Director). (1983). *Winnie the Pooh and a day for Eeyore* [Motion picture]. United States: Rick Reinert Productions.

Reitherman, W. (Director), & Disney, W. (Producer). (1968). *Winnie the Pooh and the blustery day* [Motion picture]. United States: Walt Disney Productions.

Rios, D., Stewart, A. J., & Winter, D. G. (2010). "Thinking she could be the next president": Why identifying with the curriculum matters. *Psychology of Women Quarterly, 34*(3), 328–338.

Robinson, M. L. (1985). *Princeton-education blacks and the black community.* Undergraduate thesis, Princeton University, Princeton, NJ. Retrieved from *www.politico.com/pdf/080222_moprincetonthesis_1–251.pdf.*

Rosenthal, R., & Jacobson, L. (1968). Pygmalion in the classroom. *Urban Review, 3*(1), 16–20.

Ross, L., & Nisbett, R. E. (1991). *The person and the situation: Perspectives of social psychology.* New York: McGraw-Hill.

Salvatore, J., & Shelton, J. N. (2007). Cognitive costs of exposure to racial prejudice. *Psychological Science, 18,* 810–815.

Schroeder, C. M., & Prentice, D. A. (1998). Exposing pluralistic ignorance to reduce alcohol use among college students. *Journal of Applied Social Psychology, 28*(23), 2150–2180.

Sherman, D. K., & Hartson, K. A. (2011). Reconciling self-defense with self-criticism: Self-affirmation theory. In M. D. Alicke & C. Sedikides (Eds.), *Handbook of self-enhancement and self-protection* (pp. 128–151). New York: Guilford Press.

Sherman, D. K., Hartson, K. A., Binning, K. R., Purdie-Vaughns, V., Garcia, J., Taborsky-Barba, S., et al. (2013). Deflecting the trajectory and changing the narrative: How self-affirmation affects academic performance and motivation under identity threat. *Journal of Personality and Social Psychology, 104*(4), 591–618.

Shnabel, N., Purdie-Vaughns, V., Cook, J. E., Garcia, J., & Cohen, G. L. (2013). Demystifying values-affirmation interventions: Writing about social belonging is a key to buffering against identity threat. *Personality and Social Psychology Bulletin, 39*(5), 663–676.

Shook, N., & Clay, R. (2012). Interracial roommate relationships: A mechanism for promoting a sense of belonging at university and academic performance. *Journal of Experimental Social Psychology, 48*(5), 1168–1172.

Shteynberg, G., & Apfelbaum, E. (2013). The power of shared experience: Simultaneous observation with similar others facilitates social learning. *Social Psychological and Personality Science, 4*(6), 738–744.

Shteynberg, G., & Galinsky, A. D. (2011). Implicit coordination: Sharing goals with similar others intensifies goal pursuit. *Journal of Experimental Social Psychology, 47*(6), 1291–1294.

Steele, C. M. (1988). The psychology of self-affirmation: Sustaining the integrity of the self. In L. Berkowitz (Ed.), *Advances in experimental social psychology* (Vol. 21, pp. 261–302). San Diego, CA: Academic Press.

Steele, C. M. (1997). A threat in the air: How stereotypes shape intellectual identity and performance. *American Psychologist, 52,* 613–629.

Steele, C. M., & Aronson, J. (1995). Stereotype threat and the intellectual test performance of African Americans. *Journal of Personality and Social Psychology, 69*(5), 797–811.

Steele, C. M., Spencer, S. J., & Aronson, J. (2002). Contending with group image: The psychology of stereotype and social identity threat. In M. P. Zanna (Ed.), *Advances in experimental social psychology* (Vol. 34, pp. 379–440). San Diego, CA: Academic Press.

Stephens, N. M., Fryberg, S. A., Markus, H. R., Johnson, C. S., & Covarrubias, R. (2012). Unseen disadvantage: How American universities' focus on independence undermines the academic performance of first-generation college students. *Journal of Personality and Social Psychology, 102*(6), 1178–1197.

Stephens, N. M., Hamedani, M. G., & Destin, M. (2014). Closing the social class achievement gap: A difference-education intervention improves first-generation students' academic performance and all students' college transition. *Psychological Science, 25*(4), 943–953.

Stephens, N. M., Townsend, S. S. M., Hamedani, M. G., Destin, M., & Manzo, V. (2015). A difference-education intervention equips first-generation college students to thrive in the face of stressful college situations. *Psychological Science, 26*(10), 1556–1566.

Stinson, D. A., Logel, C., Shepherd, S., & Zanna, M. P. (2011). Rewriting the self-fulfilling prophecy of social rejection: Self-affirmation improves relational security and social behavior up to 2 months later. *Psychological Science, 22*(9), 1145–1149.

Stout, J. G., & Dasgupta, N. (2011). When he doesn't mean you: Gender-exclusive language as ostracism. *Personality and Social Psychology Bulletin, 37*(6), 757–769.

Thomaes, S., Bushman, B. J., de Castro, B. O., & Reijntjes, A. (2012). Arousing "gentle passions" in young adolescents: Sustained experimental effects of value affirmations on prosocial feelings and behaviors. *Developmental Psychology, 48*(1), 103–110.

Tibbetts, Y., Harackiewicz, J. M., Canning, E. A., Boston, J. S., Priniski, S. J., & Hyde, J. S. (2016). Affirming independence: Exploring mechanisms underlying a values affirmation intervention for first-generation students. *Journal of Personality and Social Psychology, 110*, 635–659.

Tomasello, M., Carpenter, M., Call, J., Behne, T., & Moll, H. (2005). Understanding and sharing intentions: The origins of cultural cognition. *Behavioral and Brain Sciences, 28*(5), 675–735.

Vervecken, D., Hannover, B., & Wolter, I. (2013). Changing (S)expectations: How gender fair job descriptions impact children's perceptions and interest regarding traditionally male occupations. *Journal of Vocational Behavior, 82*(3), 208–220.

Walton, G. M. (2014). The new science of wise psychological interventions. *Current Directions in Psychological Science, 23*(1), 73–82.

Walton, G. M., & Carr, P. B. (2012). Social belonging and the motivation and intellectual achievement of negatively stereotyped students. In M. Inzlicht & T. Schmader (Eds.), *Stereotype threat: Theory, processes, and application* (pp. 89–106). New York: Oxford University Press.

Walton, G. M., & Cohen, G. L. (2007). A question of belonging: Race, social fit, and achievement. *Journal of Personality and Social Psychology, 92*(1), 82–96.

Walton, G. M., & Cohen, G. L. (2011). A brief social-belonging intervention improves academic and health outcomes of minority students. *Science, 331*, 1447–1451.

Walton, G. M., Cohen, G. L., Cwir, D., & Spencer, S. J. (2012). Mere belonging: The power of social connections. *Journal of Personality and Social Psychology, 102*(3), 513–532.

Walton, G. M., Logel, C., Peach, J., Spencer, S., & Zanna, M. P. (2015). Two brief interventions to mitigate a "chilly climate" transform women's experience, relationships, and achievement in engineering. *Journal of Educational Psychology, 107*(2), 468–485.

Walton, G. M., Paunesku, D., & Dweck, C. S. (2012). Expandable selves. In M. R. Leary & J. P. Tangney (Eds.), *Handbook of self and identity* (pp. 141–154). New York: Guilford Press.

Walton, G. M., & Wilson, T. D. (2016). *Wise interventions: Psychological remedies for social and personal problems.* Manuscript under review.

Weiner, B. (1985). An attributional theory of achievement motivation and emotion. *Psychological Review, 92*(2), 548–573.

Welter, J. (2015). Jen Welter. *Wired, 23*(11), 105.

Williams, K. D. (2009). Ostracism: A temporal need–threat model. In M. Zanna (Ed.), *Advances in experimental social psychology* (Vol. 41, pp. 279–314). Burlington, MA: Academic Press.

Wilson, T. D., Damiani, M., & Shelton, N. (2002). Improving the academic performance of college students with brief attributional interventions. In J. Aronson (Ed.), *Improving academic achievement: Impact of psychological factors on education* (pp. 89–108). Oxford, UK: Academic Press.

Wing, R. R., & Jeffery, R. W. (1999). Benefits of recruiting participants with friends and increasing social support for weight loss and maintenance. *Journal of Consulting and Clinical Psychology, 67*(1), 132–138.

Woodruff, J. (2003). Sandra Day O'Connor: "The majesty of the law." Retrieved from *www.cnn.com/2003/allpolitics/05/20/judy.page.oconnor*.

Yeager, D. S., Henderson, M., D'Mello, S., Paunesku, D. Walton, G. M., Spitzer, B. J., et al. (2014). Boring but important: A self-transcendent purpose for learning fosters academic self-regulation. *Journal of Personality and Social Psychology, 107*(4), 559–580.

Yeager, D. S., Johnson, R., Spitzer, B., Trzesniewski, K., Powers, J., & Dweck, C. S. (2014). The far-reaching effects of believing people can change: Implicit theories of personality shape stress, health, and achievement during adolescence. *Journal of Personality and Social Psychology, 106*(6), 867–884.

Yeager, D. S., Purdie-Vaughns, V., Garcia, J., Apfel, N., Brzustoski, P., Master, A., et al. (2014). Breaking the cycle of mistrust: Wise interventions to provide critical feedback across the racial divide. *Journal of Experimental Psychology: General, 143*(2), 804–824.

Yeager, D. S., & Walton, G. M. (2011). Social-psychological interventions in education: They're not magic. *Review of Educational Research, 81*(2), 267–301.

Yeager, D. S., Walton, G. M., Brady, S. T., Akcinar, E. N., Paunesku, D., Keane, L., et al. (2016). Improving the college transition in advance: Teaching a lay theory before college narrows achievement gaps at scale. *Proceedings of the National Academy of Sciences USA, 113*, E3341–E3348.

CHAPTER 16

Stereotype Threat
New Insights into Process and Intervention

ROBERT J. RYDELL
KATIE J. VAN LOO
KATHRYN L. BOUCHER

Most people like to feel smart, capable, and confident in their abilities, and they want others to see them in this positive light. Now imagine yourself in a situation where the people around you believe you are *not* smart or capable, and they came to this judgment without consideration of your past performance, your motivation to work, or your actual skills and knowledge, but instead based their evaluation on little more than your gender, your age, or even the color of your skin. Would you feel worried and anxious? Motivated to prove them wrong? Irritated that they saw and judged you as an interchangeable member of a group, rather than an individual? This is similar to what individuals experiencing stereotype threat feel. *Stereotype threat* is a situational phenomenon that members of negatively stereotyped groups experience when they worry about confirming that stereotype with their performance (see Steele, Spencer, & Aronson, 2002).

Upon recognizing intransigent achievement gaps between blacks and whites, and that blacks' prior performance underpredicted their later performance, Claude Steele hypothesized that negative performance

stereotypes could play a role in black people's depressed academic performance through stereotype threat. From this observation, Steele (1997) suggested the proposition that these types of ability stereotypes create a "threat in the air" that exists in any situation in which an individual might be seen through the lens of a negative stereotype about his or her ingroup. Knowing that some people may think, for example, that blacks are not as smart as whites, or that women are not as good at math as men, can lead members of these stereotyped groups to be especially concerned with not appearing incompetent in these domains and motivated to prove these stereotypes wrong. Ironically, the desire to disprove, or at the very least, fail to confirm these negative stereotypes stemming from stereotype threat, ultimately leads to reduced performance in the stereotyped domain (e.g., Spencer, Steele, & Quinn, 1999; Steele & Aronson, 1995).

These stereotypes come in many forms, but of particular interest for this chapter are those pertaining to academic performance. Furthermore, stereotype threat can and does occur for any negatively stereotyped group in a variety of performance domains and can even be perceived as coming from different sources (the outgroup, the ingroup, or the self) and with different targets on which one's performance reflects (the self or the group; Shapiro & Neuberg, 2007). While stereotype threat can and does occur for any negatively stereotyped group in a variety of performance domains, the bulk of the research on stereotype threat has focused on racial and ethnic minorities in academics (e.g., blacks, Latinos) and women in math and science domains (see Inzlicht & Schmader, 2012).

To demonstrate these effects, stereotype threat researchers manipulate the extent to which the negatively stereotyped identity is salient and measures performance in the stereotyped domain. For example, Spencer and colleagues (1999) framed a math test in such a way that the negative stereotype about women and math would be brought to mind: They told men and women that there were gender differences in performance on the math test they were going to complete (*stereotype threat condition*). For other men and women, the test was framed as not showing gender differences in performance (*control condition*). All participants then completed the same math test. Women who were in the stereotype threat condition performed significantly worse on the math test than not only men but, importantly, also other women who were not made aware of their stereotyped identity via the threatening test instructions.

Since Steele and Aronson's (1995) seminal article documenting stereotype threat, a great deal of accumulted research has supporting the proposition that stereotype threat can lead to reduced performance in the stereotyped domain (see Inzlicht & Schmader, 2012) and even contributes to various residual academic achievement gaps (Walton & Spencer, 2009). Research on stereotype threat has made many great strides. Researchers have examined and found what types of cues—both explicit (e.g., Beilock, Rydell, & McConnell, 2007) and subtle (Inzlicht & Ben-Zeev, 2000; Van Loo & Rydell, 2014)—can trigger stereotype threat. In addition, various groups have been found to be susceptible to stereotype threat, based on race and ethnicity, gender, age, weight, disability, and social class (e.g., Brochu &

Dovidio, 2014; Gonzales, Blanton, & Williams, 2002; Silverman & Cohen, 2014; Spencer et al., 1999) and different types of stereotype content and performance domains (e.g., verbal, mathematical, scientific, spatial, athletic ability domains; e.g., Beilock et al., 2007; McGlone & Aronson, 2007; Stone, Lynch, Sjomeling, & Darley, 1999). Importantly, recent work on stereotype threat has also focused on ways to help mitigate the deleterious consequences of stereotype threat (e.g., Cohen, Garcia, Apfel, & Master, 2006; Good, Aronson, & Inzlicht, 2003).

The last two decades have provided us with a much greater understanding of what stereotype threat is, whom it affects, how it plays out in the real world, and what we can do to mitigate its negative impact on stereotyped group members. Despite this wealth of research examining the stereotype threat phenomenon, important questions and criticisms remain. Our aim in this chapter is to provide a background on the mechanisms of stereotype threat, research demonstrating its impact in real-world settings, and the state of interventions thus far. We also address gaps and controversies within this body of research when we see an opportunity to continue to provide insights into stereotype threat. The first half of this chapter focuses on the underlying mechanisms of stereotype threat's effect on performance; the second half examines how stereotype threat occurs in real-world situations and intervention strategies.

MECHANISMS OF STEREOTYPE THREAT

After learning when and for whom stereotype threat has an effect, researchers became interested in understanding just what is happening during the stereotype threat experience. What about stereotype threat leads to ironic performance effects? Are stereotype-threatened individuals more or less motivated to perform well? Do they believe the stereotype or develop negative performance expectations for themselves? Or are they just overwhelmed with the anxiety and self-doubt that results from worrying about the stereotype? These and other similar questions led to a shift in stereotype threat research, with significant efforts made to uncover stereotype threat's underlying mechanisms. In this section, we review the progress that has been made in understanding the mechanisms of stereotype threat, with a significant focus on the integrated process model of stereotype threat (Schmader, Johns, & Forbes, 2008) and the role of working memory in explaining stereotype threat effects on performance. We also address the point at which the stereotype threat process diverges for relatively automatic tasks compared to the more commonly studied controlled performance tasks. Finally, we end with a discussion of future directions for research on stereotype threat process.

The Integrated Process Model: Accounting for the Effect of Stereotype Threat Performance

Since effects of stereotype threat were first discovered, researchers have often included measures of various factors that they think might be related to the stereotype threat process. Some of the potential mediators targeted by threat researchers have primarily included decreased performance expectations and effort (e.g., Spencer et al., 1999); increased anxiety and evaluative concern (Gonzales et al., 2002), physiological arousal (e.g., Mendes, Blascovich, Lickel, & Hunter, 2002), and cognitive load (e.g., Beilock et al., 2007; Schmader & Johns, 2003); and the possibility of (and later differentiation from) priming or ideomotor effects on performance due to stereotype activation (e.g., Jamieson & Harkins, 2012). However, the inclusion of these measures typically targets only one potential mediator, unintentionally implying that there might be a single mediator that can explain stereotype threat, and often produces mixed results from study to study. Moreover, testing actual mediation of stereotype threat has proved difficult. In a typical mediation study, the mediator needs to be assessed after the stereotype threat manipulation, but before the measure of performance. Thinking back to the Spencer and colleagues (1999) example, a proposed mediator would need to be given to participants after they read the math test instructions and before they complete the math test. Because of the nature of this experimental

setup, a measure of performance often could not be included in a mediation study because the proposed mediator could activate stereotype threat for all participants, not just those in the stereotype threat conditions. Furthermore, there are known limitations to testing mediation in this way, as it treats the mediator as an intervening task, which can make it difficult to determine whether differences in performance are due to the effect of stereotype threat on the mediator or some other reason, such as withdrawal of effort for the (presumed) irrelevant mediating task (e.g., Jamieson & Harkins, 2011). Despite these difficulties, there have been attempts to map out what has become a somewhat complex mediational landscape (see Schmader et al., 2008).

One of the more prominent and comprehensive process models of stereotype threat that has emerged from these efforts is Schmader and colleagues' (2008) integrated process model (see Figure 16.1), which synthesizes early work on stereotype threat mediators. Their model also incorporates a balance theory perspective of self-integrity threat to explain how stereotype threat is triggered and subsequently initiates the chain of psychological reactions that result in reduced performance. This model contends that explicit and situational cues can automatically activate the relevant ability stereotype, and that this can simultaneously activate a stereotyped individual's self-concept, concept of the relevant group identity, concept of the relevant ability domain, and the propositional relationships between them. The negative stereotype about the ability of one's group creates a conflict between a person's positive views of the relationship between the self and one's ability and the relationship between the self and one's group, resulting in a cognitive imbalance that individuals are motivated to resolve. This imbalance initiates a number of processes that contribute to the reduction in cognitive resources responsible for threat effects.

If, based on the negative stereotype, a situation ultimately poses little or no risk of being evaluated, then the targets of negative stereotypes are not threatened. For example, when a woman takes a math exam with other women, she performs significantly better that when she is the only woman taking the

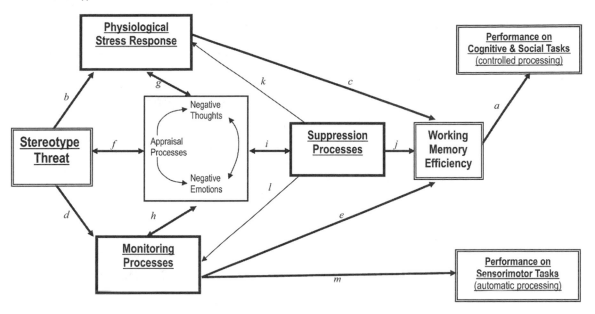

FIGURE 16.1. An integrated process model of stereotype threat effects on performance. From Schmader, Johns, and Forbes (2008). Copyright © 2008 by the American Psychological Association. Reprinted by permission.

exam (Inzlicht & Ben-Zeev, 2000). Being the only female test-taker makes salient one's gender and may indicate that the environment might be one in which women might be evaluated in light of negative stereotypes. Thus, individuals experiencing stereotype threat vigilantly monitor their environment and are especially sensitive to these types of environmental cues that indicate a situation that may be detrimental to how their performance is perceived and evaluated (e.g., Johns, Inzlicht, & Schmader, 2008; Murphy, Steele, & Gross, 2007).

When such threatening cues are perceived and the negative stereotype is activated, then the aforementioned cognitive imbalance may occur. Stereotype-threatened individuals are motivated to try to alleviate the cognitive imbalance they experience as a result of stereotype threat. One way to accomplish this is to reconcile the inconsistent relationships brought on by the activation of the negative stereotype. In their original article on stereotype threat, Steele and Aronson (1995) discovered that black students attempted to distance themselves from the negatively stereotyped group by rating stereotypical traits as less descriptive of them as individuals. Stereotype-threatened people may also activate a more negative sense of self to be in line with the negative view of the group created by the stereotype to relieve the cognitive inconsistency (Cadinu, Maass, Rosabianca, & Kiesner, 2005; Johns & Schmader, 2010).

Additionally, Rydell, McConnell, and Beilock (2009) examined what happens when stereotype-threatened individuals associate with a group membership that is not negatively stereotyped in the domain. Some female participants were made aware of the availability of not only the negative stereotype that "women are bad at math" but also the positive self-relevant stereotype that "college students are good at math." When this occurred, women's college identity was activated and their gender identity was inhibited, thus resolving the cognitive inconsistency and effectively eliminating negative stereotype threat effects on math performance. These strategies alleviate the cognitive inconsistency created by stereotype threat by changing the self, group, and domain relations to be balanced.

Stress, Vigilance, and Cognitive Monitoring

The cognitive inconsistency triggered in the stereotype threat experience initially induces a state of physiological stress, uncertainty, and vigilance. Individuals experiencing stereotype threat are worried about whether they will confirm the stereotype and how others will evaluate them in light of the stereotype. These concerns are thought to increase anxiety (e.g., Spencer et al., 1999), though research has not found consistent effects of stereotype threat on self-reported anxiety (e.g., Aronson et al., 1999; Gonzales et al., 2002; Schmader & Johns, 2003; Steele & Aronson, 1995; see also Cadinu et al., 2005). Greater success, however, using measures of physiological indicators of stress and arousal, indicates that participants under stereotype threat show a physiological threat profile (Mendes et al., 2002) and greater sympathetic nervous system activity (Murphy et al., 2007). The more consistent physiological findings suggest that people under threat feel more anxiety even though they are not always aware of and able to report it.

In addition to physiological stress responses, stereotype threat triggers a variety of negative emotions and thoughts. Individuals experiencing threat may experience feelings of self-doubt (e.g., Steele & Aronson 1995) and begin to question their ability to perform well, and develop negative expectations for their performance (e.g., Stangor, Carr, & Kiang, 1998). Stereotype threat also leads to an increase in intrusive thoughts and ruminations, including reported worries about the task, the stereotype, and one's ability and performance (e.g., Cadinu et al., 2005), which can make it difficult for women to focus on the task at hand (see Schmader et al., 2008). Furthermore, stereotype threat increases individuals' vigilance for these negative thoughts and emotions. For instance, individuals experiencing stereotype threat generally show increased attention to anxiety-related words (Johns et al., 2008). They also monitor their internal states to identify any arousal they might be experiencing and are particularly concerned with whether their arousal is related to being stereotyped (Ben-Zeev, Fein, & Inzlicht, 2005).

When experiencing stereotype threat, individuals are also sensitive to signs that they are not coping well or are confirming the negative stereotype with their behavior. Beilock and colleagues (2007) found that women experiencing stereotype threat reported monitoring their performance more than women who were not experiencing stereotype threat. Stereotype-threatened individuals are especially vigilant toward any signs of errors or mistakes in their performance (Forbes, Schmader, & Allen, 2008) and actual failure (e.g., Seibt & Forster, 2004).

Thought Suppression and Behavior Regulation

While this increased monitoring is occurring, individuals are also attempting to suppress their worries and concerns about the stereotype, and to regulate their performance and behavior. In a study by Carr and Steele (2009), women experiencing stereotype threat were given a lexical decision task in which some words were related to the gender–math stereotype. These women were significantly *slower* to respond to the stereotypical words than women who were in a no-threat control condition, which suggests that threat may lead to suppression of thoughts related to the negative stereotype. Furthermore, Logel, Iserman, Davies, Quinn, and Spencer (2009) were able to measure both stereotype suppression during a math task and postsuppression rebound after the math task was completes. They found that women experiencing stereotype threat were slower than men to respond to stereotype-related words on a lexical decision task as they were beginning the math task. However, after the task was completed, these same women showed significantly *faster* responses to stereotype-related words, indicating a post-suppression rebound for the previously suppressed stereotype.

Because of their desire not to confirm the stereotype, negatively stereotyped group members are motivated to perform well, and this increased motivation can be seen in their performance on easy and less complex tasks. For example, reduced performance on math tasks due to stereotype threat are only found on difficult math problems; women under threat perform just as well as, or better than, women not under threat on easy math problems (Beilock et al., 2007; O'Brien & Crandall, 2003). Moreover, when the correct answer is dependent on a prepotent or dominant response, as is usually the case with simpler, less complex problems, then the increased motivation individuals experience from being under stereotype threat leads to successful performance (Jamieson & Harkins, 2009). This increased motivation that stereotype-threatened individuals experience also makes them sensitive to mistakes they make (Forbes et al., 2008) and quick to correct any errors that they catch (e.g., Jamieson & Harkins, 2007).

Unfortunately, the motivation to perform well can also result in individuals under threat utilizing inefficient problem-solving strategies, such as using previously successful strategies on new problems for which they are not relevant (e.g., Carr & Steele, 2009). This is thought to be due to initiating more controlled responses during problem solving that ultimately can be detrimental to performance (see also Seibt & Forster, 2004). In other work that examined learning, Rydell, Shiffrin, Boucher, Van Loo, and Rydell (2010) found that women primed with stereotype threat failed to improve over time on a visual search task that usually leads to automatic attention attraction (a form of learning) because they persisted in using controlled visual search processes to avoid mistakes.

"Mental Overload": The Role of Working Memory

The host of physiological, psychological, and behavioral consequences of stereotype threat ultimately can overwhelm individuals' cognitive resources. It is this reduction in cognitive resources that is thought to be the proximal cause of reduced performance due to stereotype threat (Beilock et al., 2007; Schmader et al., 2008). More specifically, it is the impact that stereotype threat has on *working memory capacity* that is responsible for the effects of threat on performance. *Working memory capacity* in the stereotype threat literature is primarily conceptualized as a general and limited resource of controlled attention and executive processes (e.g., Engle, 2002; see Schmader et al., 2008). When working memory is at full

capacity, it can ensure that attention, cognition, and behavior regulation processes are coordinated and efficient. However, when working memory capacity is reduced, the efficient coordination of these processes is impaired and performance suffers. In stereotype threat, it is thought that the physiological stress, cognitive monitoring, and suppression and regulation processes that are triggered by stereotype threat usurp the working memory capacity that would otherwise be used for successful task performance.

Working memory capacity is measured in a variety of ways, but typically involves pitting relatively automatic processes against relatively more controlled processes (Engle, 2002). These tasks can assess relatively basic control processes, such as inhibiting and overriding an automatic response, to more complex and integrated control processes, such as required by dual-process tasks and complex span tasks (Engle, 2002; Miyake et al., 2000). A mixture of these methods has been used to examine the role of working memory in explaining stereotype threat effects, and the researchers supporting this role have taken two primary approaches. First, a significant amount of work has shown that stereotype threat negatively impacts working memory, and reductions in working memory account for reduced performance in response to threat in statistical mediation models (e.g., Beilock et al., 2007; Carr & Steele, 2010; Rydell, Van Loo, & Boucher, 2014; Schmader & Johns, 2003; Van Loo & Rydell, 2013).

The integrated process model (Schmader et al., 2008) allows us to conceptualize the process of stereotype threat as working through both the more distal mediators (e.g., stress, vigilance, suppression) and the more proximal mediator of working memory. Thus, the other primary approach to examining the mediational role of working memory in stereotype threat effects has focused on testing this link between proposed distal mediators and working memory. Many of these distal mediators are known to tax working memory: Stress and physiological arousal (O'Brien & Crandall, 2003), monitoring emotional information and thoughts (e.g., Beilock, Jellison, Rydell, McConnell, & Carr, 2006), suppression (e.g., Logel et al., 2009), and emotion and behavior regulation (e.g., Johns et al., 2008) have all been found to reduce working memory capacity. Together, these two approaches provide strong support for the mediational role of working memory capacity in stereotype threat effects.

WORKING MEMORY: A UNITARY CONSTRUCT?

More recently, attempts have been made to specify the subprocesses of working memory to understand better the role of working memory in stereotype threat effects. While the stereotype threat literature has tended to adopt a unitary, process-general, controlled attention definition of working memory, other more complex cognitive models exist. One of these models fractionates working memory into three specific cognitive subprocesses called *executive functions* (Miyake et al., 2000): *inhibition* (i.e., the ability intentionally to override an automatic response), *updating* (i.e., the ability to maintain relevant and delete irrelevant information in the face of interference), and *switching* (i.e., the ability to effectively switch between multiple tasks). Rydell and colleagues (2014) found that stereotype threat affects some, but not all, executive functions, and that only specific executive functions mediate threat effects on different outcomes: Only updating mediated threat-based math performance decrements, whereas only inhibition accounted for threat effects on increased risk taking. By recognizing the diversity of executive functions that make up working memory, more specific predictions can be made regarding stereotype threat effects, and a more nuanced understanding of stereotype threat process can be explored.

Automatic Tasks

Most research on stereotype threat has focused on performance tasks that require more controlled, conscious processes (e.g., academic performance, memory). However, stereotype threat effects have also been found on relatively more automatic, procedural tasks, such as the mechanics of golf-putting for expert golfers, and the process that underlies effects on these types of tasks diverges from that on more controlled

attention tasks. For these types of well-learned tasks, stereotype threat impairs performance by the initiation of more conscious, controlled attention (e.g., Beilock et al., 2006; Rydell et al., 2010). Successful performance of procedural tasks relies on these practiced, automatized processes being able to proceed uninterrupted, that is, to "flow" smoothly. When individuals are worried about performing poorly in a way that might confirm the negative stereotype, they begin to concentrate and consciously focus too much on these procedural aspects of the well-learned task. This concentration and increased monitoring actually disrupts strongly routinized performance.

Conclusions and Recommendations for Future Process Research

We have discussed several advances that have been made in our understanding of the mechanisms of stereotype threat, including a review of one of the more comprehensive stereotype threat process models and evidence in support of its proposed processes. Despite this progress, however, it is clear that some aspects of the stereotype threat process and the integrated process model are not as strongly supported by empirical evidence. We believe that addressing these areas is important to understand fully just what stereotype threat is doing, psychologically, to impair performance.

First, it is not clear whether all three concepts (i.e., self, domain, and group) proposed by the integrated process model are and must be activated in order to result in stereotype threat performance effects. Research has indicated that the stereotype is usually activated (e.g., Steele et al., 2002), implying the group and domain are accessible. Evidence for the activation of the self and domain typically comes in the form of the dependence of performance effects on the belief that one is capable or has a positive view of the domain (e.g., Schmader & Johns, 2003; Stone et al., 1999); however, this belief sometimes has no effect (e.g., Van Loo & Rydell, 2013). The concept of self and group can be made accessible (e.g., Wout, Danso, Jackson, & Spencer, 2009), but it may be an artifact of the manipulation type used in these studies (e.g., solo status;

Inzlicht & Ben-Zeev, 2000). There is less direct evidence that stereotype activation results in simultaneous domain, self, and group activation. The model would benefit from future research that directly tests the simultaneous activation of all three concepts in order to determine whether all three *must* be activated to elicit stereotype threat or, if not, when and for what types of stereotype threat experiences and manipulation is activation of different concepts necessary.

We also see room for future research in further exploring the effect of stereotype threat on the proposed distal mediators. As mentioned earlier, the evidence for the role of anxiety and stress is mixed, and few studies have found a mediational role for anxiety and stress on threat-based performance effects (see Schmader et al., 2008). Another proposed distal mediator with mixed support is decreased performance expectations; researchers have found some evidence that they do decrease (Stangor et al., 1998), but not always (Spencer et al., 1999; Stone et al., 1999). In addition to improving our understanding of stereotype threat's impact on these distal mediators, it is also important specifically to provide more *mediational* evidence for these distal mediators, in order to better support the role of these variables in the stereotype threat process.

Some of the strongest mediational evidence for stereotype threat processes has come from the examination of working memory. Though there is a good deal of evidence supporting this role of working memory in the stereotype threat process, we believe that more can be done with this aspect of the model. As alluded to earlier, utilizing more complex cognitive models can provide additional insights into how stereotype threat comes to affect different performance outcomes and increase predictive power with regard to how and when stereotype threat will affect performance. We believe it is worth continuing to pursue research that examines these and other more specific subprocesses or executive functions, how they are affected by stereotype threat, and how they can account for different threat outcomes.

While the need and desire to better understand the processes underlying stereotype threat is great, its study also creates unique

challenges. Stereotype threat research has made strides in proposing and testing a model of stereotype threat process, attempting to integrate multiple physiological, cognitive, and psychological processes. We have highlighted some of the places where there are gaps or mixed support for process and provide opportunities for future progress in stereotype threat research. But stereotype threat is interesting because it has far-reaching implications for the real world. Therefore, we shift our focus to how researchers have built on what we have learned in the laboratory to examine stereotype threat in the classroom and the effectiveness of intervention strategies to improve opportunities for stereotyped group members.

APPLYING STEREOTYPE THREAT: FROM THE LABORATORY TO THE FIELD

As discussed earlier, stereotype threat researchers have tested and provided support for multiple cognitive, physiological, and motivational pathways through which stereotype threat can impair learning, performance, and other important academic and personal outcomes. As explanations of how stereotype threat has its impact have proliferated the literature and have been synthesized into broad, overarching models, critics have questioned whether these delineated mechanisms are as influential in the real world as they are in the laboratory, and whether the models adequately characterize the process of stereotype threat in relation to other factors that can contribute to achievement gaps and reduced well-being for stigmatized groups.

In this section, we discuss how stereotype threat researchers have addressed these criticisms. We provide evidence of the generalizability of stereotype threat as a phenomenon that crosses many different contexts and impacts many different social identities, and we review efforts to demonstrate stereotype threat's relative impact in real-world settings with the (re)analysis of existing data. Moreover, we highlight work in which researchers have utilized field designs to capture stereotype threat outside of the laboratory. Last, we introduce the strongest evidence of stereotype threat's impact on students' outcomes from ambitious and promising interventions aimed at reducing performance and interest gaps outside of the laboratory. This latter work showcases how eliminating the stereotype threat that students feel by changing aspects of the situation and the attributions students make for their performance and classroom experiences has self-sustaining, long-term benefits.

Generalizability of Stereotype Threat

Stereotype threat has been shown to impact several important and basic psychological processes: It not only shapes how we view and behave in situations in which negative stereotypes can be applied to us but also influences our self-efficacy and interest in future stereotyped contexts in (e.g., Murphy & Taylor, 2012; Steele et al., 2002) and outside of academic settings (e.g., negotiations, interpersonal interactions; Kray, Thompson, & Galinsky, 2001). Stereotype threat's breadth is evidenced by the fact that it can impact anyone who is a negatively stereotyped group member—as long as people know the cultural stereotypes of their group, they are vulnerable (e.g., Kiefer & Sekaquaptewa, 2007)—and can be experienced by people at almost all points of the development trajectory, beginning as early as age 6 (McKown & Weinstein, 2003).

The reliability and magnitude of stereotype threat effects have been demonstrated in several meta-analyses examining overall stereotype threat effects and, specifically, threat effects for women and racial minorities (Nguyen & Ryan, 2008). Walton and Spencer (2009) also found that standardized tests underestimate the true ability of negatively stereotyped students, likely because of their tendency to inspire stereotype threat. In large meta-analyses of both lab experiments on stereotype threat and field interventions aimed at reducing stereotype threat, Walton and Spencer found that negatively stereotyped students consistently scored higher than nonstereotyped students when conditions that are known to reduce or eliminate stereotype threat concerns were present when performance was assessed.

Despite the results of meta-analyses such as these, critics of stereotype threat continue to assert that stereotype threat effects may not be as reliable or substantial as laboratory-based evidence suggests. One particular criticism levied against stereotype threat research is that it may not generalize to high-stakes testing situations outside of the laboratory (e.g., Sackett & Ryan, 2012). In an experimental test of stereotype threat in high stakes testing, Stricker and Ward (2004) manipulated the timing of demographic questions (i.e., either before or after the test) on Advanced Placement (AP) and college placement exams, and with a conservative threshold for statistical significance, they reported no differences in performance based on question timing.

Stereotype threat researchers have countered this criticism in several ways. First, in a reanalysis of Stricker and Ward (2004), Danaher and Crandall (2008) found statistically and practically significant findings for women's performance on the AP calculus exam: Moving the demographics survey to the end of the test would increase the number of women who score well enough to receive college credit by more than 4,700 each year. This reanalysis also highlights the importance of control conditions that sufficiently allay threat or do not activate stereotypes at all: Without such, a lack of a condition difference is not definitive evidence that threat is not impactful in high stakes settings. Second, researchers have conducted direct, experimental tests of the notion that high-stakes testing inspires stereotype threat. Aronson and Salinas (2015) found that nonelite Latino students do show stereotype-threat-based performance decrements when they are primed with a negative performance stereotype under high-stakes conditions.

Although the performance task in Aronson and Salinas (2015) was not an actual standardized test that is included in considerations such as college admissions, this work highlights the importance of experimentation when investigating stereotype threat's impact. Moreover, as described below, stereotype threat researchers have emphasized that standardized tests such as the American College Tests (ACT) and the Standard Achievement Test (SAT) are not the only critical real-world outcomes on which to assess stereotype threat. Threat has a substantial and accruing impact on course grades and other formative and influential evaluative contexts, and these effects extend beyond one test or one class to dramatically change the course of students' academic and career goals through recursive processes (e.g., Cohen, Garcia, Purdie-Vaughns, Apfel, & Brzustoski, 2009; Yeager & Walton, 2011).

A second, related criticism of stereotype threat is that researchers working within this literature underemphasize the roles of other established factors such as socialization, discrimination, and poverty (e.g., Ceci & Williams, 2010). Despite others' summaries and characterizations of stereotype threat as being the main driver of achievement gaps (see Jussim, Crawford, Anglin, Stevens, & Duarte, in press; Sackett, Hardison, & Cullen, 2004), stereotype threat researchers have long been careful to describe the effects of stereotype threat in the context of other situational factors that create and maintain achievement gaps (see Steele, 1997). Specifically, stereotype threat researchers interpret performance differences in terms of residual gaps, not raw ones by adjusting for past performance in statistical analyses. Recent research has also focused directly on how structural barriers and the biases of others can prompt perceived threats related to one's stigmatized group identity (e.g., Stephens, Hamedani, & Destin, 2014).

Stereotype Threat as a Real-World Phenomenon

In response to these early criticisms of stereotype threat as being a laboratory-based phenomenon, researchers have been motivated to demonstrate the existence and influence of stereotype threat in real-world settings and over time in longitudinal designs. In short, growing evidence clearly demonstrates that stereotype threat is a phenomenon that is pervasive in classrooms and other potentially stereotype-threatening situations. Members of racial minorities in college and female students in math and science report concerns about whether they will confirm negative stereotypes of their groups or will be viewed negatively in light

of stereotypes of their group memberships. These concerns shape and shift their identification with school and particular subjects and their future career aspirations, and negatively influence their engagement and motivation in academic work. It is unsurprising, then, that academic performance is found to be impaired for these students.

Stereotype Vulnerability or Identity Concerns in the Real World

Concerns about being viewed or evaluated in a negative light due to negative stereotypes of one's groups (i.e., stereotype vulnerability or identity concerns) have been captured in real-world settings for those of different races/ethnicities and gender. Critically, these concerns hold predictive power for students' outcomes in their actual classes and other educational settings. For example, Massey and Fischer (2005) followed several thousand college freshmen from different ethnic backgrounds and a range of colleges, and found that individual differences in stereotype vulnerability predicted almost 10% of the variation in students' grade-point averages (GPAs); this is a particularly important finding because other race-based concerns were not predictive of college achievement.

In a smaller-scale diary study conducted over 8 days, black undergraduate students who reported high stereotype vulnerability at the outset of the study showed greater fluctuations in their academic efficacy throughout the day and were less accurate in assessing their own performance on a test completed in the laboratory (Aronson & Inzlicht, 2004). Furthermore, research by Bonita London and her colleagues (London, Downey, Romer-Canyas, Rattan, & Tyson, 2012) on women's sensitivity to being evaluated negatively in terms of gender (i.e., *gender rejection sensitivity*) shows a similar pattern in terms of these concerns' impact outside of the laboratory. In a daily diary study, female first-year law students who were high in gender rejection sensitivity had greater self-doubt, felt more alienated and less motivated, and were more likely to cope in less effective ways (i.e., self-silencing themselves instead of confronting bias, not volunteering to answer questions).

Shaping and Shifting Identification, Belonging, and Motivation

Negative stereotypes can shape stigmatized group members' early identification and sense of belonging with stereotyped domains, and experiences of stereotype threat can further shift students away from these domains. For students of color who are targeted by more global stereotypes of their intelligence, their perceived belonging in academic settings may be more tenuous and more predictive of their academic outcomes. Indeed, Murphy and Zirkel (in press) showed that for black, but not white, middle schools students, belonging in school predicted academic self-efficacy and ambition. When identity concerns such as belonging are chronic, students who are identified with negatively stereotyped domains may question whether these efforts are worth pursuing. In a national longitudinal sample of racial-minority college students studying science, chronic threat was associated with disidentification with science, which then predicted lower intentions to pursue scientific careers (Woodcock, Hernandez, Estrada, & Schultz, 2012).

This disidentification process can stem from feeling that several important social identities are in conflict. Specifically, in science, technology, engineering, and mathematics (STEM) fields, where women are often underrepresented and are negatively stereotyped, women may perceive their gender and career identity to be less compatible. For instance, middle school girls who were presented with very feminine STEM role models reported lower expectations for their math performance and less interest in the subject (Betz & Sekaquaptewa, 2012).

It is important to note two caveats to this work. First, those who do have greater perceived identity compatibility may be more likely to persevere in the face of stereotype threat. Rosenthal, London, Levy, and Lobel (2011) found that female STEM majors with greater perceived identity compatibility report greater belonging and motivation, and less self-doubt in STEM classes. Greater perceived identity compatibility also reduces the likelihood of women dropping out of their STEM major. Second, female role models can have a positive impact for female students' outcomes in their actual classes. If care is taken to ensure that female students can identify and connect with present role models, having female role models in their college STEM classes can prompt female students to have more positive views of themselves in STEM, greater positivity toward STEM fields, and greater interest and motivation to pursue STEM careers (Stout, Dasgupta, Hunsinger, & McManus, 2011).

Stereotype Threat's Real-World Impact on Performance

The outcome from laboratory-based research that has drawn the most attention is stereotype threat's ironic impact on performance: Being motivated to disconfirm, or at least not confirm, group stereotypes can reduce performance, thus confirming the stereotype. This ironic effect on performance has also been examined outside of the laboratory. For instance, Mendoza-Denton and colleagues (2002) found that students who were more concerned about being rejected on the basis of their race or ethnicity earned significantly lower grades over a multiyear period. Relatedly, in a longitudinal study of women in their college math course, female students showed increases in negative implicit stereotyping of women in STEM, and this increase in stereotyping over time predicted lower course grades for them in relation to their male classmates (Ramsey & Sekaquaptewa, 2011).

As has been theorized (e.g., Steele, 1997), those who are the most identified with the negatively stereotyped domain and have had previous success within it may be the most vulnerable to stereotype threat's impact. For instance, in a longitudinal study by Osborne and Walker (2006), students of color who began high school with high levels of caring about their academics were actually more likely to drop out of high school than their peers who cared less about school. Relatedly, Good, Aronson, and Harder (2008) demonstrated that even those with high ability and past success to draw on are worried about stereotype threat in their advanced classes: Stereotype threat was eliminated on an exam for female college students in a difficult math course when they were assured that this diagnostic exam was not gender biased.

A commonality of the applied work on stereotype threat is its emphasis on chronicling the process over time. Recent research has focused on assessing stereotype threat and its effects across the years in longitudinal designs and by utilizing existing data sets. In this way, stereotype threat's long-term influence can be evidenced. Other methodologies focus on capturing the process of stereotype threat as it unfolds in the classroom or during a student's day. Experience sampling and daily diary studies have already provided rich evidence of what aspects of educational settings cue stereotype threat and what concerns, beliefs, and behaviors are invoked when stereotype threat is experienced (e.g., Zirkel, Garcia, & Murphy, 2015). As stereotype threat researchers have broadened the scope of their questions and added to their "toolkits" with these methodologies, the evidence has converged on stereotype threat's real-world impact and has furthered our knowledge of the key points to leverage for effective interventions.

Interventions to Reduce Stereotype Threat and Its Effects

Perhaps the most persuasive evidence of stereotype threat's impact on real-world outcomes and the most encouraging results from the application of the basic findings from this literature are those from recent interventions that mitigate the effects of threat. These interventions target specific maladaptive beliefs that can constrain success for negatively stereotyped groups, and work to change the way threatening contexts are construed. Specifically, these interventions challenge stereotypes of groups, stereotypes of fields, and beliefs about who belongs or fits best in certain domains or positions. By reshaping people's perceptions of stereotype-threatening situations, these interventions operate as a "workaround" to help individuals achieve success while researchers concurrently delineate ways to eliminate more structural barriers to disadvantaged groups' full participation in stereotyped domains.

Role Models and the Feedback They Give

One group of stereotype threat interventions provides role models who, through their presence and success, signal to women, racial minorities, and other stigmatized groups that they can belong and succeed. In one role model intervention, Ramsey, Betz, and Sekaquaptewa (2013) exposed female college students in STEM fields to positive messages about well-known and lesser-known women in STEM, flyers for campus events showcasing women in math, and "Women in STEM" pencils that emphasized the link between participants and other women in STEM even after the intervention. These efforts led to decreased stereotype threat concerns and increased identification with STEM fields. Relatedly, other research focusing on STEM fields showed that active collaboration with faculty mentors and participation in research laboratories helps high-achieving black and Latino undergraduate students succeed and persist in STEM (Thoman, Brown, Mason, Harmsen, & Smith, 2015). This work suggests that greater in-person interactions not only provide skills and training but also shape motivation and interest due to the exposure to positive STEM role models.

Moreover, role models, such as instructors or mentors, who communicate to students that the negative stereotypes of their group will not play a part in their evaluations, reduce the impact of stereotype threat for students. Providing black college students with critical performance feedback from an evaluator who believes the student can reach these high standards neutralizes concerns about the evaluator viewing the student in light of negative group stereotypes and increases task motivation (*wise feedback*; Cohen, Steele, & Ross, 1999). Recent interventions by Yeager, Purdie-Vaughns, and colleagues (2014) replicate these findings with middle school students and showcase the impact of teachers' wise feedback on important educational outcomes. Seventh graders who received wise feedback from their teachers were more likely to submit a revision of a class essay and turned in better final drafts of this assignment. These effects were stronger for black students, particularly those who had the greatest mistrust for their teachers and school in general (i.e., the students most vulnerable to thinking they would be viewed in line with negative stereotypes). Students can even be trained to view all feedback from their teachers as wise feedback, with the effect of raising black students' grades.

Reframing the Experience of Stereotype Threat

A similar class of interventions aimed at mitigating stereotype threat focuses on another way of reframing stereotype-threatening situations: to view threat as a challenge that can be overcome and to prompt students to reflect on their threat experiences with writing. We know that individuals experiencing stereotype threat exhibit physiological threat profiles that can hurt performance through their negative impact on working memory. Thus, intervention researchers have attempted to change the way people interpret their physiological responses, getting people to reframe their experience of stereotype threat, by testing methods for turning threat into a challenge. Interpreting physiological arousal (e.g., sweating, heart racing) as a challenge response when completing high-stakes tests such as the Graduate Record Exam (GRE) leads to better performance in the laboratory and on the actual test (Jamieson, Mendes, Blackstock, & Schmader, 2010). Interventions that inspire students to view tests in domains in which they are negatively stereotyped as challenges have a positive impact on these students' achievement. For instance, black schoolchildren for whom race was particularly salient before taking a math test performed better when it was framed as a challenge (Alter, Aronson, Darley, Rodriguez, & Ruble, 2010). Interventions that encourage this type of reframing likely reduce stereotype threat by increasing students' perceptions of their ability to deal with the stressors, and by casting doubts on the negative stereotype's relevance or veracity in the performance setting.

In addition to being able to reframe one's physiological experience of threat, writing about these concerns can be beneficial. Drawing from past research on expressive writing's ability to make sense or draw meaning from negative experiences, psychologists have asked students to write about their worries and concerns about high-stakes tests before they take them (Ramirez & Beilock, 2011). Doing so led to higher exam scores than those of students who were not asked to write and likely perseverated on their worries before the test. These effects were greater for students who had higher general test anxiety. As will become evident, the benefits of expressive writing have been extended to writing specifically about identity-threatening concerns in interventions we discuss later (e.g., belonging and affirmation interventions).

Transforming the Way Students and Teachers Think of Intelligence

The content of many negative group stereotypes includes beliefs about how intelligent members of the stereotyped group are in relation to other groups (e.g., women are bad at math). Due to our general tendency to view intelligence as an unchanging entity—one that has its predetermined limits for individuals—being reminded of negative stereotypes of the intelligence of one's group can be demotivating and impair achievement (Dweck, 2006). Whenever students experience difficulty or receive critical feedback in negatively stereotyped domains, these negative stereotypes about intelligence are especially likely to come to mind and lead to stereotype-threat-related learning and performance decrements. Similar processes are evoked when teachers or authority figures within organizations communicate these beliefs in the fixedness of intelligence (e.g., Emerson & Murphy, 2014).

A powerful way to lessen the impact of negative group stereotypes about intelligence is to reframe the experience of difficulty and receiving critical feedback by promoting a "growth mindset" (e.g., Good et al., 2003). Research in psychology and neuroscience clearly demonstrates that intelligence is more malleable than previously thought (Nisbett et al., 2012), and by challenging students' and teachers' assumptions about the fixed nature of intelligence, the effects of stereotype threat can be reduced. Growth mindset interventions convey the science of how our intelligence can be expanded and inspire participants to see obstacles in the classroom as signals that they need to put forth greater effort and seek feedback and helpful strategies.

In one of the first growth mindset interventions, Good and colleagues (2003) paired seventh graders with college students, who acted as mentors throughout the academic year. Mentors discussed similar content such as study skills with their mentees with one important exception: Mentors were randomly assigned to emphasize one particular message to their mentees. One group of mentors discussed their early difficulties with transitioning to new academic environments and how their experience and grades got better over time; in doing so, these mentors provided a less threatening external attribution for experienced difficulties. Another group of mentors specifically emphasized aspects of the growth mindset by discussing how intelligence can be expanded. These two messages powerfully impacted students' subsequent performance on standardized tests of math and reading. A gender difference in math performance for students with mentors who emphasized a control message (i.e., that male students performed better than female students in this group) was not found for students who had mentors emphasizing a growth mindset and external attributions for difficulties. Students in the two intervention conditions also had higher subsequent reading scores than controls. This intervention demonstrates that students can be taught the growth mindset and how to practice it.

Reminding Students of Positive Aspects of Their Selves

Negative stereotypes of one's group, especially those tied to intelligence, are threatening to the self because they question individuals' views of themselves as competent and good people. Self-affirmation interventions provide a way to deal with a psychological threat to one's self-worth. By considering other important aspects of the self, ones that are irrelevant to the negatively stereotyped domain, people are reminded of other aspects of their lives that are valued, and that bring meaning and afford positive views of the self. By reaffirming one's global self-integrity, adversities that could spark stereotype threat concerns are adaptively reconstrued or countered, buffering academic motivation and performance from stereotype threat's pernicious effects (Sherman et al., 2013).

In one such intervention, middle school students completed brief writing exercises in their classes; for one group of students, the writing prompt involved self-affirmation, in which students were given instructions to discuss their most important values (Cohen et al., 2006). After the intervention, black students in the self-affirmation condition had significantly improved grades, and the existing racial achievement gap was reduced by 40%. Over the next 2 years of school, self-affirmation continued to have an impact. Although there was no additional intervention, the benefits after the intervention were maintained, possibly because a positive recursive cycle of success was invoked (Cohen et al., 2009). Specifically, the GPAs of black students, especially initially low-achieving ones, improved over the 2 years.

Self-affirmation interventions can also reduce stereotype threat's effects on performance for women in STEM classes. Having women early in the college semester in an introductory physics class briefly write twice about personally important values led to a reduction in the learning and performance gap between males and females (Miyake et al., 2010). Given that introductory STEM courses are often viewed as "weeder" or "gatekeeper" courses for higher level STEM courses and admissions into professional schools, raising grades from C's to B's, like in this intervention, could have long-term impact on the women's success and persistence in STEM.

Conclusion and Recommendations for Future Applied and Intervention Research

As is evidenced from the previous review, the ways we can intervene to usurp stereotype threat's power in educational settings have grown substantially since the original laboratory studies on threat. Importantly, these interventions are often brief, they do not harm (and may benefit) students from majority and nonstigmatized groups, and they include solid control conditions for the strongest causal claims. Stereotype threat interventions are a critical and rich area for future research. A greater understanding of mechanisms may not only reveal additional intervention strategies but also help them to be more focused, more efficient, and more creative. In addition, a continued effort to create and test interventions in everyday settings can illuminate gaps and opportunities to refine and advance theory.

The future directions of this research are exciting and theoretically generative. As interest in stereotype-threat-reducing interventions has increased, researchers have focused on pinpointing the exact components of the interventions that are the most potent contributors to benefits for students and how these benefits are sustained over time (e.g., Yeager & Walton, 2011). Future research should focus specifically on providing empirical support for these proposed critical components through manipulating their presence, absence, and exact implementation within the larger intervention. Additionally, our confidence in the reach of these interventions would grow by if we captured all aspects of the proposed recursive processes as they unfold from one intervention to major milestones for participants (e.g., graduation, employment).

Stereotype threat researchers have recently placed a greater focus on examining the feasibility of scaling these interventions to different student populations in various educational contexts with initial success (e.g., Paunesku et al., 2015). This work is an important step toward understanding who can benefit from which type of intervention under which circumstances. More research should consider the boundary conditions for individual interventions and their potential interactive influence when disseminated together.

The current work in this area is leading to theoretical advances as researchers begin to examine how stereotype threat concerns relate to other social identity concerns (e.g., belonging, being authentic to oneself). Particularly, part of the impact of this research focus on how other interventions that have shown great promise to reduce achievement gaps (i.e., belonging mindset, culturally grounded interventions, and utility value interventions) is its capacity to buffer students from threat's negative consequences (e.g., Hulleman & Harackiewicz, 2009;

Walton & Cohen, 2011; Yeager, Henderson, et al., 2014). It will be important for future researchers to examine how these different social identity concerns differentially and interactively predict negative outcomes for individuals; by doing so, we can theoretically ascertain the interconnected structure of relationships between these related concerns and have the greatest opportunity to intervene to reduce or eliminate them.

Last, on a more practical level, ongoing stereotype threat research has suggested that its effects particularly on performance are not fully appreciated (Boucher, Rydell, & Murphy, 2015), so concurrent efforts have focused on translating this literature's vast knowledge to educators, parents, and policymakers (e.g., Aguilar, Walton, & Wieman, 2014; Erman & Walton, 2015). We appreciate that many stereotype threat researchers have entered into discussions and collaborations for this type of translational work. As we research best practices for teaching others to incorporate our empirically backed techniques to assuage stereotype threat's impact, future research holds great promise of sharing our science with those who can help mitigate the experience of stereotype threat for all.

REFERENCES

Aguilar, L., Walton, G., & Wieman, C. (2014). Psychological insights for improved physics teaching. *Physics Today, 67,* 43–49.

Alter, A. L., Aronson, J., Darley, J. M., Rodriguez, C., & Ruble, D. N. (2010). Rising to the threat: Reducing stereotype threat by reframing the threat as a challenge. *Journal of Experimental Social Psychology, 46,* 166–171.

Aronson, J., & Inzlicht, M. (2004). The ups and downs of attributional ambiguity: Stereotype vulnerability and the academic self-knowledge of African-American students. *Psychological Science, 15,* 829–836.

Aronson, J., Lustina, M. J., Good, C., Keough, K., Steele, C. M., & Brown, J. (1999). White men can't do math: Necessary and sufficient factors in stereotype threat. *Journal of Experimental Social Psychology, 35,* 29–46.

Aronson, J., & Salinas, M. (2015). *On the role of stereotype threat in the real world of high stakes exams.* Unpublished manuscript, New York University, New York.

Beilock, S. L., Jellison, W. A., Rydell, R. J.,

McConnell, A. R., & Carr, T. H. (2006). On the causal mechanisms of stereotype threat: Can skills that don't rely heavily on working memory still be threatened? *Personality and Social Psychology Bulletin, 32,* 1059–1071.

Beilock, S. L., Rydell, R. J., & McConnell, A. R. (2007). Stereotype threat and working memory: Mechanisms, alleviation, and spill-over. *Journal of Experimental Psychology: General, 136,* 256–276.

Ben-Zeev, T., Fein, S., & Inzlicht, M. (2005). Arousal and stereotype threat. *Journal of Experimental Social Psychology, 41,* 174–181.

Betz, D. E., & Sekaquaptewa, D. (2012). My fair physicist?: Feminine math and science role models demotivate young girls. *Social Psychological and Personality Science, 3,* 738–746.

Boucher, K. L., Rydell, R. J., & Murphy, M. C. (2015). Forecasting the experience of stereotype threat for others. *Journal of Experimental Social Psychology, 58,* 56–62.

Brochu, P. M., & Dovidio, J. F. (2014). Would you like fries (380 calories) with that?: Menu labeling mitigates the impact of weight-based stereotype threat on food choice. *Social Psychological and Personality Science, 5,* 414–421.

Cadinu, M., Maass, A., Rosabianca, A., & Kiesner, J. (2005). Why do women underperform under stereotype threat?: Evidence for the role of negative thinking. *Psychological Science, 16,* 572–578.

Carr, P., & Steele, C. (2009). Stereotype threat and inflexible perseverance in problem solving. *Journal of Experimental Social Psychology, 45,* 853–859.

Ceci, S. J., & Williams, W. M. (2010). Sex differences in math-intensive fields. *Current Directions in Psychological Science, 19,* 275–279.

Cohen, G. L., Garcia, J., Apfel, N., & Master, A. (2006). Reducing the racial achievement gap: A social-psychological intervention. *Science, 313,* 1307–1310.

Cohen, G. L., Garcia, J., Purdie-Vaughns, V., Apfel, N., & Brzustoski, P. (2009). Recursive processes in self-affirmation: Intervening to close the minority achievement gap. *Science, 324,* 400–403.

Cohen, G. L., Steele, C. M., & Ross, L. D. (1999). The mentor's dilemma: Providing critical feedback across the racial divide. *Personality and Social Psychology Bulletin, 25,* 1302–1318.

Danaher, K., & Crandall, C. S. (2008). Stereotype threat in applied settings re-examined. *Journal of Applied Social Psychology, 38,* 1639–1655.

Dweck, C. S. (2006). *Mindset.* New York: Random House.

Emerson, K. T., & Murphy, M. C. (2014). Identity threat at work: How social identity threat and situational cues contribute to racial and ethnic disparities in the workplace. *Cultural Diversity and Ethnic Minority Psychology, 20*(4), 508–520.

Engle, R. W. (2002). Working memory capacity as executive attention. *Current Directions in Psychological Science, 11,* 19–23.

Erman, W., & Walton, G. M. (2015). Stereotype threat and anti-discrimination law: Affirmative steps to promote meritocracy and racial equality. *Southern California Law Review, 88,* 307–378.

Forbes, C., Schmader, T., & Allen, J. J. B. (2008). The role of devaluing and discounting in performance monitoring: A neurophysiological study of minorities under threat. *Social Cognitive and Affective Neuroscience, 3,* 253–261.

Gonzales, P. M., Blanton, H., & Williams, K. J. (2002). The effects of stereotype threat and double-minority status on the test performance of Latino women. *Personality and Social Psychology Bulletin, 28,* 659–670.

Good, C., Aronson, J., & Harder, J. A. (2008). Problems in the pipeline: Stereotype threat and women's achievement in high-level math courses. *Journal of Applied Developmental Psychology, 29,* 17–28.

Good, C., Aronson, J., & Inzlicht, M. (2003). Improving adolescents' standardized test performance: An intervention to reduce the effects f stereotype threat. *Journal of Applied Developmental Psychology, 24,* 645–662.

Hulleman, C. S., & Harackiewicz, J. M. (2009). Promoting interest and performance in high school science classes. *Science, 326,* 1410–1412.

Inzlicht, M., & Ben-Zeev, T. (2000). A threatening intellectual environment: Why females are susceptible to experiencing problem-solving deficits in the presence of males. *Psychological Science, 11,* 365–371.

Inzlicht, M., & Schmader, T. (Eds.). (2012). *Stereotype threat: Theory, process, and application.* New York: Oxford University Press.

Jamieson, J. P., & Harkins, S. G. (2007). Mere effort and stereotype threat performance effects. *Journal of Personality and Social Psychology, 93,* 544–564.

Jamieson, J., & Harkins, S. (2009). The effect of stereotype threat on the solving of quantitative GRE problems: A mere effort interpretation. *Personality and Social Psychology Bulletin, 35,* 1301–1314.

Jamieson, J., & Harkins, S. (2011). The intervening task method: Implications for measuring mediation. *Personality and Social Psychology Bulletin, 37,* 562–661.

Jamieson, J. P., & Harkins, S. G. (2012).

Distinguishing between the effects of stereotype priming and stereotype threat on math performance. *Group Processes and Intergroup Relations, 15,* 291–304.

Jamieson, J., Mendes, W. B., Blackstock, E., & Schmader, T. (2010). Turning knots in your stomach into bows: Reppraising arousal improves performance on the GRE. *Journal of Experimental Social Psychology, 46,* 208–212.

Johns, M., & Schmader, T. (2010). Metacognitive regulation as a reaction to the uncertainty of stereotype threat. In R. M. Arkin, K. C. Oleson, & P. J. Carroll (Eds.), *The uncertain self: A handbook of perspectives from social and personality psychology* (pp. 176–192). New York: Psychology Press.

Johns, M. J., Inzlicht, M., & Schmader, T. (2008). Stereotype threat and executive resource depletion: Examining the influence of emotion regulation. *Journal of Experimental Psychology: General, 137,* 691–705.

Jussim, L., Crawford, J. T., Anglin, S. M., Stevens, S. T., & Duarte, J. L. (in press). Interpretations and methods: Towards a more effectively self-correcting social psychology. *Journal of Experimental Social Psychology.*

Kiefer, A. K., & Sekaquaptewa, D. (2007). Implicit stereotypes and women's math performance: How implicit gender-math stereotypes influence women's susceptibility to stereotype threat. *Journal of Experimental Social Psychology, 43,* 825–832.

Kray, L. J., Thompson, L., & Galinsky, A. (2001). Battle of the sexes: Gender stereotype confirmation and reactance in negotiations. *Journal of Personality and Social Psychology, 80,* 942–958.

Logel, C., Iserman, E. C., Davies, P. G., Quinn, D. M., & Spencer, S. J. (2009). The perils of double consciousness: The role of thought suppression in stereotype threat. *Journal of Experimental Social Psychology, 45,* 299–312.

London, B., Downey, G., Romero-Canyas, R., Rattan, A., & Tyson, D. (2012). Gender-based rejection sensitivity and academic self-silencing in women. *Journal of Personal and Social Psychology, 102*(5), 961–979.

Massey, D. S., & Fischer, M. J. (2005). Stereotype threat and academic performance: New findings from a racially diverse sample of college freshmen. *Du Bois Review, 2,* 45–67.

McGlone, M. S., & Aronson, J. (2007). Forewarning and forearming stereotype-threatened students. *Communication Education, 56,* 119–133.

McKown, C., & Weinstein, R. S. (2003). The development and consequences of stereotype consciousness in middle childhood. *Child Development, 74,* 498–515.

Mendes, W. B., Blascovich, J., Lickel, B., & Hunter, S. (2002). Challenge and threat during interactions with white and black men. *Personality and Social Psychology Bulletin, 28,* 939–952.

Mendoza-Denton, R., Downey, G., Purdie, V. J., Davis, A., & Pietrzak, J. (2002). Sensitivity to status-based rejection: Implications for African American students' college experience. *Journal of Personality and Social Psychology, 83,* 896–918.

Miyake, A., Friedman, N. P., Emerson, M. J., Witzki, A. H., Howerter, A., & Wager, T. (2000). The unity and diversity of executive functions and their contributions to complex "frontal lobe" tasks: A latent variable analysis. *Cognitive Psychology, 41,* 49–100.

Miyake, A., Kost-Smith, L. E., Finkelstein, N. D., Pollock, S. J., Cohen, G. L., & Ito, T. A. (2010). Reducing the gender achievement gap in college science: A classroom study of values affirmation. *Science, 330,* 1234–1237.

Murphy, M. C., Steele, C. M., & Gross, J. J. (2007). Signaling threat: How situational cues affect women in math, science, and engineering settings. *Psychological Science, 18,* 879–885.

Murphy, M. C., & Taylor, V. J. (2012). The role of situational cues in signaling and maintaining stereotype threat. In M. Inzlicht & T. Schmader (Eds.), *Stereotype threat: Theory, process, and application* (pp. 17–33). New York: Oxford University Press.

Murphy, M. C., & Zirkel, S. (in press). Race and belonging in school: How anticipated and experienced belonging affect choice, persistence, and performance. *Teachers College Record.*

Nisbett, R. E., Aronson, J., Blair, C., Dickens, W., Flynn, J., Halpern, D. F., et al. (2012). Intelligence: New findings and theoretical developments. *American Psychologist, 67,* 130–159.

Nguyen, H. H., & Ryan, A. M. (2008). Does stereotype threat affect test performance of minorities and women?: A meta-analysis of experimental evidence. *Journal of Applied Psychology, 93*(6), 131–134.

O'Brien, L. T., & Crandall, C. S. (2003). Stereotype threat and arousal: Effects on women's math performance. *Personality and Social Psychology Bulletin, 29,* 782–789.

Osborne, J. W., & Walker, C. (2006). Stereotype threat, identification with academics, and withdrawal from school: Why the most successful students of colour might be most likely to withdraw. *Educational Psychology, 26,* 563–577.

Paunesku, D., Walton, G. M., Romero, C. L., Smith, E. N., Yeager, D. S., & Dweck, C. S. (2015). Mindset interventions are a scalable treatment for academic underperformance. *Psychological Science, 26,* 784–793.

Ramirez, G., & Beilock, S. L. (2011). Writing about testing worries boosts exam performance in the classroom. *Science, 331,* 211–213.

Ramsey, L. R., Betz, D. E., & Sekaquaptewa, D. (2013). The effects of an academic environment intervention on science identification among women in STEM. *Social Psychology of Education, 16,* 377–397.

Ramsey, L. R., & Sekaquaptewa, D. (2011). Changing stereotypes, changing grades: A longitudinal study of stereotyping during a college math course. *Social Psychology of Education, 14,* 377–387.

Rosenthal, L., London, B., Levy, S. R., & Lobel, M. (2011). The roles of perceived identity compatibility and social support for women in a single-sex STEM program at a co-educational university. *Sex Roles, 65,* 725–736.

Rydell, R. J., McConnell, A. R., & Beilock, S. L. (2009). Multiple social identities and stereotype threat: Imbalance, accessibility, and working memory. *Journal of Personality and Social Psychology, 96,* 949–966.

Rydell, R. J., Shiffrin, R., Boucher, K. L., Van Loo, K., & Rydell, M. T. (2010). Stereotype threat prevents perceptual learning. *Proceedings of the National Academy of Sciences USA, 107,* 14042–14047.

Rydell, R. J., Van Loo, K. J., & Boucher, K. L. (2014). Which executive functions are impaired by stereotype threat and account for different threat-related outcomes? *Personality and Social Psychology Bulletin, 40,* 377–390.

Sackett, P. R., Hardison, C. M., & Cullen, M. J. (2004). On interpreting research on stereotype threat and test performance. *American Psychologist, 60,* 271–272.

Sackett, P. R., & Ryan, A. M. (2012). Concerns about generalizing stereotype threat research findings to operational high-stakes testing. In M. Inzlicht & T. Schmader (Eds.), *Stereotype threat: Theory, process, and application* (pp. 249–263). New York: Oxford University Press.

Schmader, T., & Johns, M. (2003). Converging evidence that stereotype threat reduces working memory capacity. *Journal of Personality and Social Psychology, 85,* 440–452.

Schmader, T., Johns, M., & Forbes, C. (2008). An integrated process model of stereotype threat on performance. *Psychological Review, 115,* 336–356.

Seibt, B., & Forster, J. (2004). Stereotype threat and performance: How self-stereotypes influence processing by inducing regulatory foci. *Journal of Personality and Social Psychology, 87,* 38–56.

Shapiro, J. R., & Neuberg, S. L. (2007). From stereotype threat to stereotype threats: Implications of a multi-threat framework for causes, moderators, mediators, consequences, and interventions. *Personality and Social Psychology Review, 11,* 107–130.

Sherman, D. K., Hartson, K. A., Binning, K. R., Purdie-Vaughns, V., Garcia, J., Taborsky-Barba, S., et al. (2013). Deflecting the trajectory and changing the narrative: How self-affirmation affects academic performance and motivation under identity threat. *Journal of Personality and Social Psychology, 104,* 591–618.

Silverman, A. M., & Cohen, G. L. (2014). Stereotypes as stumbling-blocks: How coping with stereotype threat affects life outcomes for people with physical disabilities. *Personality and Social Psychology Bulletin, 40,* 1330–1340.

Spencer, S. J., Steele, C. M., & Quinn, D. M. (1999). Stereotype threat and women's math performance. *Journal of Experimental Social Psychology, 35,* 4–28.

Stangor, C., Carr, C., & Kiang, L. (1998). Activating stereotypes undermines task performance expectations. *Journal of Personality and Social Psychology, 75,* 1191–1197.

Steele, C. M. (1997). A threat in the air: How stereotypes shape the intellectual identities and performance. *American Psychologist, 52,* 613–629.

Steele, C. M., & Aronson, J. (1995). Stereotype threat and the intellectual test performance of African Americans. *Journal of Personality and Social Psychology, 69,* 797–811.

Steele, C. M., Spencer, S. J., & Aronson, J. (2002). Contending with group image: The psychology of stereotype and social identity threat. In M. Zanna (Ed.), *Advances in experimental social psychology* (Vol. 34, pp. 379–440). New York: Academic Press.

Stephens, N., Hamedani, M. G., & Destin, M. (2014). Closing the social-class achievement gap: A difference-education intervention improves first-generation students' academic performance and all students' college transition. *Psychological Science, 25,* 943–953.

Stone, J., Lynch, C. I., Sjomeling, M., & Darley, J. M. (1999). Stereotype threat effects on Black and White athletic performance. *Journal of Personality and Social Psychology, 77,* 1213–1227.

Stout, J. G., Dasgupta, N., Hunsinger, M., & McManus, M. A. (2011). STEMing the tide:

Using ingroup experts to inoculate women's self-concept in science, technology, engineering, and mathematics (STEM). *Journal of Personality and Social Psychology, 100,* 255–270.

Stricker, L. J., & Ward, W. C. (2004). Stereotype threat, inquiring about test takers' ethnicity and gender, and standardized test performance. *Journal of Applied Social Psychology, 34,* 665–693.

Thoman, D. B., Brown, E. R., Mason, A. Z., Harmsen, A. G., & Smith, J. L. (2015). Seeing how science can help: Enhancing the participation of underrepresented minority students as biomedical researchers. *Bioscience, 65,* 183–188.

Van Loo, K. J., & Rydell, R. J. (2013). On the experience of feeling powerful: Perceived power moderates the effect of stereotype threat on women's math performance. *Personality and Social Psychology Bulletin, 39,* 287–400.

Van Loo, K. J., & Rydell, R. J. (2014). Negative exposure: Watching another woman subjected to dominant male behavior during a math interaction can induce stereotype threat. *Social Psychological and Personality Science, 5,* 601–607.

Walton, G., & Cohen, G. L. (2011). A brief social-belonging intervention improves academic and health outcomes of minority students. *Science, 331,* 1147–1151.

Walton, G. M., & Spencer, S. J. (2009). Latent ability: Grades and test scores systematically underestimate the intellectual ability of negatively stereotyped students. *Psychological Science, 20,* 1132–1139.

Woodcock, A., Hernandez, P. R., Estrada, M., & Schultz, P. W. (2012). The consequences of chronic stereotype threat: Domain disidentification and abandonment. *Journal of Personality and Social Psychology, 103,* 635–646.

Wout, D., Danso, H., Jackson, J., & Spencer, S. (2008). The many faces of stereotype threat: Group- and self-threat. *Journal of Experimental Social Psychology, 44,* 792–799.

Yeager, D. S., Henderson, M., D'Mello, S., Paunesku, D., Walton, G. M., Spitzer, B. J., et al. (2014). Boring but important: A self-transcendent purpose for learning fosters academic self-regulation. *Journal of Personality and Social Psychology, 107,* 559–580.

Yeager, D. S., Purdie-Vaughns, V., Garcia, J., Apfel, N., Pebley, P., Master, A., et al. (2014). Breaking the cycle of mistrust: Wise interventions to provide critical feedback across the racial divide. *Journal of Experimental Psychology: General, 143,* 804–824.

Yeager, D. S., & Walton, G. M. (2011). Social-psychological interventions in education: They're not magic. *Review of Educational Research, 81,* 267–301.

Zirkel, S., Garcia, J. A., & Murphy, M. C. (2015). Experience-sampling research methods and their potential for education research. *Educational Researcher, 44,* 7–16.

CHAPTER 17

The Role of Self-Efficacy and Related Beliefs in Self-Regulation of Learning and Performance

BARRY J. ZIMMERMAN
DALE H. SCHUNK
MARIA K. DiBENEDETTO

One of the most important qualities of successful students is their "sense of agency"—having the means or power to learn in a self-regulated fashion, such as when studying or practicing on their own (Bandura, 2008). As used in this chapter, *self-regulation* is the process whereby students activate and sustain behaviors, cognitions, and affects that are systematically oriented toward the attainment of their goals (Zimmerman, 2000). Social-cognitive researchers have found that students' capabilities to self-regulate depend significantly on their self-efficacy beliefs. *Self-efficacy* refers to personal judgments of one's capabilities to organize and execute courses of action to attain designated goals (Bandura, 1977, 1986), such as completing a science experiment or writing a term paper. The efficacy belief system is not a global trait but a differentiated set of self-beliefs linked to distinct realms of functioning (Bandura, 2006). We contend that self-efficacy beliefs influence and reciprocally are influenced by students' self-regulatory processes, such as goal setting, strategy use, self-monitoring, and self-judgments.

In this chapter, we describe a cyclical phase model of self-regulatory processes and beliefs, the distinctive properties of self-efficacy beliefs, assessment of these beliefs, sources and effects of self-efficacy beliefs, and cyclical relations between self-efficacy and related beliefs and self-regulatory processes. In addition, we discuss the issue of the accuracy or calibration of self-efficacy beliefs and instructional interventions to enhance their accuracy and impact on students' self-regulation of learning.

A CYCLICAL MODEL OF SELF-REGULATION

To enhance their academic performance, many students acquire and apply self-regulatory processes, especially when dealing with challenging tasks, competing attractions, and stressors (Zimmerman & Martinez-Pons, 1986, 1990). Many researchers have sought to explain self-regulation in terms of personal feedback loops that convey information about one's performance or outcomes (Hattie & Timperly, 2007). These loops produce cyclical feedback regarding students' social/environmental outcomes, such as positive or negative comments from teachers or classmates. The loops also can convey feedback

313

regarding a student's behavior, such as time spent in study. Finally, loops can convey feedback concerning covert events, such as changes in self-efficacy beliefs about one's preparation for a test due to studying. A social-cognitive model of self-regulation is used to integrate research on self-efficacy beliefs with research on self-regulatory processes because it encompasses cyclical feedback from covert personal sources, as well as from behavioral and social/environmental sources (Schunk, 2012; Zimmerman, 2000, 2008).

According to this model, feedback loops can be analyzed sequentially. As shown in Figure 17.1, feedback loops involve a cycle of three phases (Zimmerman, 2000). The first phase, *forethought,* occurs before efforts to learn and includes learning processes and motivational beliefs that influence a person's willingness and preparation to learn or perform. The second phase, *performance,* occurs during efforts to learn and includes learning and motivational processes that influence one's concentration and action. The third phase, *self-reflection,* occurs after the performance phase and involves personal reactions to performance phase outcomes. These self-reflections then affect forethought processes and beliefs about subsequent efforts to learn. This completes the self-regulatory cycle.

There are two major categories of forethought phase processes. The category of *task analysis* involves relating a task and its context to goal-setting and strategic planning processes (Winne & Hadwin, 1998). *Goal setting* involves specifying outcomes that one intends to obtain, such as writing an essay in social studies in 3 hours (Locke & Latham, 1990). Goals that are specific, proximal, or challenging are more effective

---

Performance Phase

Self-Control
Task strategies
Self-instruction
Imagery
Time management
Environmental structuring
Help seeking
Interest enhancement
Self-consequences

Self-Observation
Metacognitive monitoring
Self-recording

Forethought Phase

Task Analysis
Goal setting
Strategic planning

Self-Motivation Beliefs/Values
Self-efficacy
Outcome expectancies
Task interest/value/affect
Goal orientation

Self-Reflection Phase

Self-Judgment
Self-evaluation
Causal attribution

Self-Reaction
Self-satisfaction/affect
Adaptive/defensive

FIGURE 17.1. Relation of self-efficacy beliefs to self-regulatory beliefs and processes.

than goals that are diffused, delayed, or easy (Bandura & Schunk, 1981). There is evidence that goal systems of successful learners are structured hierarchically, with proximal process goals linked to distal outcome goals (Bandura, 1991; Carver & Scheier, 2000).

Strategic planning entails choosing or constructing advantageous learning methods that are appropriate for the task and the environmental setting (Weinstein & Mayer, 1986). Students can study or practice better when their strategic plans are tied to clear goals. For example, imagistic or self-instructional strategies improve recall (Bandura & Jeffery, 1973; Pressley, 1976). However, the effectiveness of self-regulatory strategies can vary during the course of learning. When strategies are applied without planning or adaptation, they can be ineffective, due to unfavorable shifts in personal, behavioral, or environmental conditions (Zimmerman & Kitsantas, 1999). Goal setting and strategic planning often require personal initiative and persistence; as a result, they require high levels of self-motivation (Zimmerman, 1995). A key source of self-motivation is *self-efficacy* beliefs, which are related to performance phase processes such as one's choice of activities, effort, and persistence (Schunk, 1984; Zimmerman & Kitsantas, 1996). A student's self-efficacy perceptions can affect his or her use of learning strategies in diverse areas, such as writing (Schunk & Swartz, 1993) and time management (Britton & Tesser, 1991). We discuss the defining features, theoretical properties, and assessment of self-efficacy beliefs later in this chapter.

Outcome expectancies constitute a second important source of self-motivation. *Outcome expectations* are beliefs about the ultimate consequences of one's performance, such as receiving social recognition or obtaining a desirable position. Students' outcome expectations depend on their knowledge or awareness of potential outcomes, such as salaries, quality of life, and health and retirement benefits. The motivational effect of attractive outcomes has been widely demonstrated, but these expectations also depend on one's sense of efficacy (Schunk & Zimmerman, 2008). For example, a student may want to become a

pharmacist. However, if this student lacks a sense of efficacy about passing a course in chemistry, he or she may not be motivated to pursue this career. Thus, both outcome expectations and self-efficacy beliefs play a role in the student's decision.

Task interest, valuing, and affect constitute a third source of forethought phase motivation. These motives refer to a student's liking or disliking a task and its context because of the inherent properties rather than for the instrumental qualities in gaining other outcomes. This class of motives includes measures of intrinsic motivation (Deci & Ryan, 1985), interest value (Wigfield & Eccles, 2002), and interest (Hidi & Renninger, 2006). Research by Ainley, Corrigan, and Richardson (2005) revealed that task interest can influence students' choice of learning strategies, and well as their achievement goals.

Students' *goal orientations*, or reasons for learning, is another source of motivation to self-regulate that pertains to beliefs or feelings about the purpose of learning. Although prominent theorists differ in terms of the names and number of goal orientations that they propose, there is agreement about the purpose of a learning goal orientation and a performance goal orientation. Students who hold a learning goal orientation try to improve their competence via learning, whereas students who adopt a performance goal orientation try to preserve their competence perceptions through favorable comparisons with the performance of others (Dweck & Leggett, 1988). Students' learning goal orientations are formed from the belief that their mental ability can be increased, whereas their performance goal orientations are formed from the belief that mental ability is a fixed entity. Students with a learning goal orientation tend to display higher levels of cognitive strategies than do students with a performance goal orientation (Pintrich & DeGroot, 1990).

The *performance phase* comprises two categories of self-regulatory processes: self-control and self-observation methods (Zimmerman, 2000). Self-control methods include a wide variety of strategies, such as task strategies, self-instruction, imagery, time management, environmental structuring, help-seeking methods, interest enhancements,

316 III. RELEVANT PROCESSES

and setting self-consequences. *Task strategies* are systematic processes for addressing specific components of a task, such as creating steps for editing a term paper in English or for shooting free throws in basketball. *Self-instruction* involves overt or covert self-descriptions of how to undertake a task, such as steps in solving a crossword puzzle, such as "Do the easy words first." However, the effectiveness of one's verbalizations depends on their quality and execution (Zimmerman & Bell, 1982). When these conditions are obtained, verbalizations are likely to enhance students' learning. *Imagery* is a strategy that involves forming mental pictures to facilitate learning and retention, such as converting textual material into diagrams or flow charts. There is extensive evidence that students can recover stored information from nonverbal images (Pressley, 1976). The self-control strategy of *time management* involves setting specific task goals, estimating time requirements, and monitoring progress in attaining those goals. From elementary school (Stoeger & Ziegler, 2011) to college (Schmitz & Wiese, 2006), students have benefited from instruction on time management.

Environmental structuring strategies are used to improve the supportiveness of one's immediate settings. For example, many professional writers carry a notepad with them to capture and develop ideas when they occur spontaneously (Barzun, 1964). The self-control strategy *help seeking* refers to soliciting assistance during learning or performance, such as finding a voice coach to show an aspiring actress how to project her voice. Researchers have shown that, compared with lower achievers, higher-achieving students are less likely to need help but more likely to seek help when it is needed (Karabenick, 2011). Although help seeking may be seen as a form of dependence, it can be viewed as a social form of information seeking if it leads ultimately to greater independence in learning.

Several self-control strategies are designed to improve students' motivation, such as interest enhancement and self-consequences. *Interest enhancement* involves improving the attractiveness of a task, such as by introducing competition into a dull activity (e.g.,

working out on an exercise bicycle; Wolters, Benzon, & Arroyo-Giner, 2011). The self-control strategy of setting self-consequences is another way for students to motivate themselves. Students can set rewarding or punishing contingencies for themselves, such as delaying phone calls to their friends until their homework is completed. Learners who set consequences for themselves achieve better in school (Zimmerman & Martinez-Pons, 1986).

To be effective, adaptation of self-control strategies needs to be based on learners' task outcomes. Given the importance of this strategic feedback, the accuracy of one's self-observation plays a central role in students' efforts to self-control their performance (Bandura, 1986). Self-regulated learners are distinguished by their reliance on systematic forms of self-observation to guide their efforts to self-control, whereas poorly regulated learners have trouble tracking a particular process, such as discerning a computational error when solving math problems (Zimmerman, Moylan, Hudesman, White, & Flugman, 2011).

One form of self-observation that has been studied is *metacognitive monitoring* (or *self-monitoring*), which refers to informal mental tracking of one's performance processes and outcomes. A second form of self-observation, *self-recording,* refers to creating formal records of learning processes or outcomes, such as a graph of a student's grammatical errors in his or her book reports. Records of one's efforts to learn are advantageous because they increase the reliability, specificity, and time span of self-observations. In addition, self-recording can include information about the setting, such as records of where and with whom one is studying. Experimental evidence shows that self-recording of personal outcomes enhances learning (Zimmerman & Kitsantas, 1997, 1999).

Tracking one's performance can be difficult when the amount of information exceeds one's capacity to process it. When this occurs, a student's tracking becomes disorganized or shallow. However, these limitations can be overcome by selective tracking of key processes, such as one's wrist position when hitting topspin forehand shots in tennis. Self-observation was the first of Bandura's (1986) self-regulatory subfunctions.

Self-reflection, the third phase of self-regulation, involves two self-regulatory subfunctions identified by Bandura (1986): self-judgments and self-reactions. One type of self-judgments, *self-evaluation,* refers to a student's comparisons of his or her performance against a standard. Three evaluative standards have been identified: self-comparisons with prior levels of performance, mastery comparisons with a recognized criterion of performance, and social comparisons with the performance of others (e.g., other students). Learners who are guided by specific forethought phase goals tend to self-evaluate based on attainment of those goals (Zimmerman & Kitsantas, 1997). The type of standard that is operative is determined by the setting, such as teachers' use of a mastery standard of 0–100% when grading students' tests. This standard of comparison is advantageous because it conveys self-improvement rather than social advantage or disadvantage in comparison to other students.

A second type of self-judgment is *causal attributions,* beliefs that focus on the perceived causes of personal outcomes, such as one's ability, effort, and use of strategies (Schunk, 2008; Weiner, 1992). Unfortunately, certain types of attributions for performance outcomes can undermine self-motivation. For example, attributing errors to uncontrollable factors such as insufficient talent or ability can be counterproductive. On the other hand, students who attribute errors to controllable factors, such as choice of a strategy, can maintain motivation during periods of poor performance (Zimmerman & Kitsantas, 1997, 1999).

There are two forms of self-reactions during the self-reflection phase. *Self-satisfaction* refers to cognitive and affective reactions to self-judgments, and it has been studied because students prefer learning activities that previously led to satisfaction and positive affect and tend to avoid those that produce dissatisfaction and negative affect, such as anxiety (Bandura, 1991). By contrast, *adaptive decisions* students' motivation to undertake further cycles of learning, for example, by continuing their use

of a strategy or by modifying it. *Defensive decisions* preclude further efforts to learn because they shield a student from experiencing further dissatisfaction and negative affect. Among the forms of defensiveness that have been studied are helplessness, procrastination, task avoidance, cognitive disengagement, and apathy. Both self-satisfaction and adaptive/defensive self-reactions are dependent on self-judgments during the self-reflection phase (Kitsantas & Zimmerman, 2002), for example, when students' favorable self-evaluations of their performance and attributions to controllable causes can produce increased self-satisfaction and sustained efforts to learn adaptively.

Thus, according to a social-cognitive model of self-regulation, the impact of forethought phase processes, such as self-efficacy beliefs, can extend to the performance and self-reflection phase processes and through cyclical feedback to subsequent efforts to learn. We now discuss self-efficacy beliefs.

DISTINCTIVE PROPERTIES OF SELF-EFFICACY BELIEFS

Self-efficacy measures can be distinguished from other self-belief measures on the basis of five criteria (Table 17.1). The first criterion involves the type of self-belief being assessed. Self-efficacy beliefs involve cognitive judgments of personal capability to perform specific tasks or activities, such as "I am confident that I can write essays in English." Self-efficacy measures contrast with other self-belief measures that include affective feelings of self-worth and generalized judgments of personal adequacy and competence (Pajares, 1996). A second criterion is type of self-evaluative standard. Self-efficacy measures are based on a goal-mastery standard, such as "How sure are you that you can convert a temperature reading from Centigrade to Fahrenheit in science?" Other self-belief measures are frequently interpreted on the basis of social/normative standards, such as comparisons of one's competencies to those of others (Pelham, 1995).

The third criterion concerns the temporal focus of self-judgments. Self-efficacy measures involve predicting future generative

TABLE 17.1. Comparison of Self-Efficacy Beliefs and Other Self-Beliefs

	Types of self-belief	
Comparison criteria	Self-efficacy beliefs	Other self-beliefs
Type of self-judgment	Cognitive judgments of capability	Feelings of competence, adequacy, and affect
Type of self-evaluative standard	Confidence in goal mastery	Social/normative comparisons
Temporal focus of self-judgments	Predicted generative capability	Attained competence
Relation to task outcomes	Context-dependent	Domain-dependent
Reactions to experience	Adaptively malleable	Trait-like resistance

performances, such as "I rate my confidence to learn English grammar at 80%" (Bandura, 2006, p. 326). To achieve this predictive function, Bandura (1977) cautioned researchers that self-efficacy measures should be administered prior to the performances of interest. Other self-belief measures focus instead on prior attainment of competence, such as "I am good in mathematics."

The fourth criterion deals with the relation of a self-measure to task performance outcomes. Self-efficacy measures are designed to be adaptive to specific task features and environmental contexts. Because of their emphasis on goal setting, self-efficacy measures can be assessed at varying levels of specificity depending on researchers' predictive or explanatory goals (Bandura, 2006). For example, students' academic goals in mathematics may range in specificity from a problem level to a course level. Although other self-belief measures have been designed to predict one's performance in specific domains such as academic subjects, they have not been designed to be sensitive to contextual issues.

The fifth criterion involves a student's reactions to experience, for example, to instructional training or challenging task conditions. Given that self-efficacy beliefs are designed to be malleable to experience, they contrast with self-measures that attempt to capture trait-like individual differences resistant to change from experience (Bong, 2006). Because of their sensitivity, self-efficacy beliefs can be assessed over time and provide evidence of growth. For

example, changes in self-efficacy ratings in a course can be compared with students' subsequent performance in the course. "This modifiability of self-efficacy judgments vividly contrasts with the frustration educators often experience when they strive to augment students' generalized self-perceptions" (Bong, 2006, p. 301). We next consider the issue of how to assess self-efficacy beliefs.

ASSESSING SELF-EFFICACY BELIEFS

Bandura (2006) cautioned that there is not an all-purpose measure of perceived efficacy Instead, self-efficacy scales should be tailored to the particular realm of interest. Like other self-belief measures, self-efficacy typically is assessed using rating scales. Bandura emphasized that self-efficacy is assessed optimally when a percentage response format is employed to reveal the strength of the belief. Self-efficacy beliefs can be measured most accurately when their level, strength, and generality are considered.

The early self-efficacy studies were conducted in clinical settings using self-report instruments to assess self-efficacy. For example, Bandura, Adams, and Beyer (1977) gave adults with snake phobias self-efficacy and behavioral tests whose items consisted of progressively more threatening encounters with a snake (e.g., touch it, allow it to sit in one's lap). For the self-efficacy assessment, participants initially rated the magnitude or level of self-efficacy by designating which tasks they believed they could perform.

They then rated the strength of self-efficacy by judging how sure they were that they could perform the tasks they had judged they could perform. To measure generality of self-efficacy, participants made magnitude/level and strength ratings for the same tasks but with a type of snake different from the type used on the pretest.

This methodology has been labeled "microanalytic": Self-efficacy and skill are assessed at the level of specific tasks (DiBenedetto & Zimmerman, 2013). The microanalysis involves asking participants fine-grained questions within a specific context. In the Bandura and colleagues (1977) study, participants judged whether they could perform specific tasks involving a snake, then were asked to perform those tasks. Although researchers often sum and average ratings and performance outcomes across tasks, participants were not asked for a general rating of how well they felt they could deal with snakes.

A similar methodology was used in the early educational research studies. The first application of self-efficacy theory to an educational learning setting was conducted by Schunk (1981). Children with low long-division skills judged self-efficacy, then completed an achievement test. For the self-efficacy assessment, children were shown pairs of problems; for each pair, the two problems were comparable in form and difficulty. Children judged how certain they were that they could solve problems of that type. Achievement test problems corresponded to those on the self-efficacy test in form and difficulty.

The microanalytic methodology has been used to assess self-efficacy in clinical settings (Schunk & DiBenedetto, 2014) and with athletic tasks such as basketball shooting and dart throwing (Cleary & Zimmerman, 2001; Kitsantas & Zimmerman, 2002). The first study to use microanalysis to comprehensively assess the processes of the phases of self-regulated learning (discussed later) using an academic task was conducted with high school students studying science and involved comparing low, moderate, and high achievers (DiBenedetto & Zimmerman, 2010). Students were given a passage on tornados to read, study, and be tested on

while being asked microanalytic questions. For example, students were asked questions about their self-efficacy for learning (e.g., "How self-confident do you feel in your capability to completely learn and remember all of the material in this passage?") and self-efficacy for performance (e.g., "How self-confident do you feel in your capability to earn 100% on the tornado knowledge test?").

The microanalytic methodology captured the cognitive, affective, and behavioral processes in which students engaged during a real-time learning task. Trend analyses revealed positive linear relations between students' levels of achievement and self-regulation, amount of time spent studying, and science performance. The size of each of these linear effects was large, suggesting that high-achieving students in science use more self-regulated learning processes in each self-regulated learning phase than did students who are average or at-risk. This microanalytic methodology has been shown to have construct and predictive validity when compared to previously established measures (DiBenedetto & Zimmerman, 2013).

Because self-efficacy beliefs are cast in context-specific performance terms, their relation to performance outcomes can be established empirically. For example, a *correlation* between a self-efficacy item regarding solving a mathematical problem and subsequent performance on a conceptually identical problem is an index of validity. Conversely, a *difference* between a self-efficacy rating and subsequent performance is a measure of one's accuracy in self-monitoring. Over- or underpredictions of self-efficacy can be expected to affect learning adversely. This hypothesis has led to the emergence of a body of research called *calibration* (Bol & Hacker, 2001; Hacker & Bol, 2004; Ramdass & Zimmerman, 2008; Zimmerman et al., 2011). Calibration studies are described later in this chapter, along with their pedagogical impact. When self-rating items are cast in goal-related performance terms, such as self-efficacy and self-evaluation items, it is easier to study their linkage to self-regulatory processes such as self-monitoring.

SOURCES AND EFFECTS
OF SELF-EFFICACY BELIEFS

Self-efficacy beliefs do not simply originate from nowhere. There are various sources of influence that individuals use to assess their self-efficacy in any particular situation. As originally hypothesized by Bandura (1977), self-efficacy can have diverse effects in achievement contexts. We discuss in this section discusses the sources and effects of self-efficacy beliefs.

Sources of Self-Efficacy Beliefs

Bandura (1997) postulated that learners acquire information to judge self-efficacy from four sources: actual performances, vicarious (e.g., modeled) experiences, forms of social persuasion, and physiological indices. Researchers have substantiated the importance of these four sources (Joët, Usher, & Bressoux, 2011; Usher, 2009).

The most reliable influence on self-efficacy comes from how students interpret their performances because these performances are tangible indicators of their capabilities. Performances interpreted as successful should raise self-efficacy, and those deemed as failures should lower it, although an occasional failure (success) after many successes (failures) may not have much impact on self-efficacy. Successful performances can influence achievement by enhancing motivation and continued learning (Schunk & DiBenedetto, 2014).

Students acquire information about their capabilities vicariously through knowledge of how others perform (Bandura, 1997). Similarity to others is a cue for gauging self-efficacy (Schunk, 2012). Observing similar others succeed can raise observers' self-efficacy and motivate them to try the task when they believe that if others can perform the task, then they can as well. A vicarious increase in self-efficacy, however, can be negated by subsequent performance failure because performances give the clearest information about capabilities.

Students also can develop self-efficacy beliefs as a result of social persuasions they receive from others (Bandura, 1997), for example, when a teacher tells a student, "I know you can do it." Social persuasions must be believable, and persuaders must be credible for persuasions to develop students' beliefs that success is attainable. Positive feedback can raise learners' self-efficacy, but the increase will not persist if they subsequently perform poorly (Schunk, 2012).

Students gain some self-efficacy information from physiological and emotional indicators such as anxiety and stress (Bandura, 1997). Strong emotional reactions to a task provide cues about an anticipated success or failure. When learners experience negative thoughts and fears about their capabilities (e.g., feeling nervous about speaking in front of a large group), those reactions can lower self-efficacy and trigger additional stress and agitation that can produce inadequate performances.

Information gained from these sources does not automatically affect self-efficacy because students interpret the results of events. Attribution theory predicts that people form *attributions* (perceived causes) for outcomes (Graham & Williams, 2009); for example, "They did well on a test because they studied hard." These interpretations are used to make self-efficacy judgments (Pajares, 1996). Thus, students who attribute a low test score to their feeling sick on the day of the test may hold higher self-efficacy for performing well in the course than students who attribute a low test score to their low ability to learn the content.

Effects of Self-Efficacy Beliefs

Self-efficacy can have multiple effects in educational contexts (Bandura, 1986, 1997). Self-efficacy can influence the choices students make (Patall, 2012) and the goals they set (Zimmerman, Schunk, & DiBenedetto, 2015). Self-efficacious learners are likely to set high goals and strategically plan ways to attain them. They also are likely to select tasks and activities in which they feel self-efficacious and to avoid those in which they do not. Unless they believe that their actions will produce the desired consequences, they have little incentive to engage in those actions. Self-efficacy also helps determine how much effort learners expend on an activity, how long they persevere when confronting obstacles, and how resilient they are in the face of difficulties (Joët et al., 2011;

Moos & Azevedo, 2009). In turn, higher self-efficacy affects students' motivation and predicts achievement outcomes (Fast et al., 2010; Zimmerman et al., 2015).

Self-efficacy beliefs can influence students' capability to manage their *emotions* by decreasing their stress, anxiety, and depression (Bandura, 1997). Pajares and Kranzler (1995) found a complex relation between self-efficacy and students' anxiety reactions regarding mathematics. Although the two measures were negatively correlated, only self-efficacy predicted mathematics performance using path analysis. There is also evidence that students' performance in academically threatening situations depends more on self-efficacy beliefs than on anxiety arousal. Siegel, Galassi, and Ware (1985) found that self-efficacy beliefs are more predictive of mathematics performance than is anxiety. The predictive power of self-efficacy beliefs was substantial, accounting for more than 13% of the variance in final mathematics grades. By contrast, anxiety proved to be a weak predictor of achievement. Together these results provide strong evidence of the discriminant and predictive validity of self-efficacy and imply that fostering a positive sense of personal efficacy is desirable.

Despite its importance, self-efficacy is not the only influence on behavior (Bandura, 1997). High self-efficacy will not yield a competent performance when students lack the needed skills to succeed (Schunk, 2012). Students' *values* (perceptions of importance and utility of learning) also can affect behavior (Wigfield, Cambria, & Eccles, 2012). Students who feel self-efficacious for learning mathematics are unlikely to take mathematics courses that they do not value because they believe these courses are not germane to their goal of becoming a writer. *Outcome expectations,* or beliefs about the anticipated outcomes of actions (Bandura, 1997), also are important. Students typically engage in activities that they believe will result in positive outcomes and avoid actions that they believe may lead to negative outcomes. Students who feel highly efficacious about learning the content in a course may not work diligently if they believe that no matter how well they do, they will not receive a high grade. In summary, assuming requisite skills and positive values and

outcome expectations, self-efficacy is a key influence on students' motivation, learning, self-regulation, and achievement (Schunk, 2012).

TRAINING SELF-REGULATORY PROCESSES AND SELF-EFFICACY BELIEFS

According to this cyclical perspective on self-regulation, students' self-efficacy beliefs can influence and be influenced by their use of self-regulatory processes during self-directed learning and performance. To verify the role of these processes empirically, Schunk and his colleagues conducted a series of intervention studies that involved prompting or training students to employ self-regulatory processes to enhance their academic learning and performance, and engender positive self-efficacy beliefs regarding future learning.

In an investigation of the effects of *goal setting* during the forethought phase on the acquisition of mathematical division skills, Schunk (1983b) asked students to set either a difficult goal of completing a challenging number of problems or an easier goal of completing fewer problems. To motivate the students to attempt to attain their goals, half of the students in the two goal-difficulty conditions were directly informed that they could work the designated number of problems. The other half of the students were told that similar students had been able to work the designated number of problems. Students who set difficult goals and received direct attainment information showed the highest self-efficacy and achievement. Schunk also found that direct attainment information led to higher perceptions of self-efficacy than socially comparative attainment information. Students who set more ambitious forethought phase goals and were given direct information showed higher levels of self-efficacy and division skill.

In a forethought phase intervention designed to enhance students' *valuing of a reading comprehension strategy,* Schunk and Rice (1987, Experiment 1) taught fourth- and fifth-grade remedial readers a multistep strategy for identifying main ideas in a textual passage. Some of these students were told specifically that this strategy helps children like them answer questions about main ideas. Students in a second group were told that the strategy could be used generally to answer questions about passages they read. Students in a third group were not given strategy-value information. Both the specific- and the general-value information enhanced students' self-efficacy beliefs and reading comprehension better than no-strategy value information. These results suggest that, in addition to strategy training, remedial readers need information that emphasizes the self-regulatory value of a strategy for locating main ideas.

In a second experiment, Schunk and Rice (1987) presented feedback about the effectiveness of the students' strategic performance after learners' attempted to employ the main ideas strategy. This performance phase intervention of strategic value differs from the forethought phase intervention in the first study. In the former methodology, strategy information was given before attempts to learn, whereas in the latter methodology, strategy information was given while performing. However, both self-regulatory interventions proved effective in enhancing students' self-efficacy beliefs, as well as reading comprehension.

In another performance-phase intervention study, Schunk and Rice (1993) taught students to identify main ideas during reading comprehension through *self-instruction*. These researchers investigated self-instruction training and fading with fifth-grade students with low reading skills. The instructor trained them to use a multistep comprehension strategy, teaching some students to fade their overt verbalizations to inner speech as they practiced. In addition to variations in fading, some students received feedback that linked strategy use with improved performance. The results revealed that students who faded their verbalizations and received feedback regarding their strategic success displayed higher levels of self-efficacy. Fading of verbalizations plus feedback led to higher reported strategy use and reading comprehension skill. Self-instruction during one's performance can enhance students' self-efficacy beliefs and comprehension skill.

Another self-regulatory process that has been studied in conjunction with self-efficacy is *self-evaluation*. Unlike self-efficacy, self-evaluations are collected after performance during the self-reflection phase. Reactive students do not self-evaluate their competencies spontaneously, but they can be taught to evaluate their performance more effectively.

For example, in research conducted by Schunk (1996), fourth graders were given instruction and practiced solving mathematical fraction problems. Students were asked to set either a learning goal (e.g., learn to use a strategy to solve problems) or a performance goal (e.g., solve problems). In each goal condition, half of the students evaluated their problem-solving capabilities at the end of each of six daily sessions. Students who set a learning goal, with or without self-evaluating, or who set a performance goal with self-evaluating surpassed classmates who set a performance goal without self-evaluating in skill, self-efficacy, and motivation.

Because self-evaluation was so effective, it obscured the goal-setting results. To surmount this problem, Schunk (1996) conducted a second study, in which self-evaluations were more subtle and less frequent. The students in each goal condition evaluated their progress in skill acquisition. Students who set a learning goal displayed higher motivation and achievement than did students who set a performance goal. These studies show that systematic efforts to self-evaluate can enhance perceptions of self-efficacy and the attainment of mathematical skill.

The effects of goal-setting and self-evaluating were investigated also with college students as they learned computer skills during three study sessions (Schunk & Ertmer, 1999). Students were instructed to set a learning goal and evaluate their learning progress. After the second session, students who set learning goals reported higher self-efficacy, self-judged learning progress, self-regulatory competence, and strategy use than students who set performance goals. Students' self-evaluations enhanced their self-efficacy beliefs. In a second study, self-evaluation was extended to all three sessions. Frequent self-evaluations produced comparable results for both learning and performance goals. Self-evaluating is a powerful self-regulatory process that works in conjunction with goal setting to enhance skill attainment and self-efficacy.

The impact of a self-reflection phase intervention involving ability and effort *attributional feedback* on students' self-efficacy beliefs and achievement was studied by Schunk (1983a). Third-grade children with low subtraction skills were taught subtraction operations and solved problems, after which they were informed either that they were working hard (effort attribution) or that they were good at subtraction (ability attribution). Children receiving ability attributional feedback displayed higher self-efficacy and subtraction skill than children given effort feedback. The latter children showed greater self-efficacy and subtraction attainment than students in a no-feedback control group. It should be noted that the teachers' gave feedback statements contingent on children's successful problem solving. For attributional feedback to be effective it must be credible. Attributing children's erroneous answers to high ability or effort will not enhance students' self-efficacy or achievement.

In research bearing on the self-reflection phase, Schunk (1982) provided effort attributional feedback to elementary school students who lacked subtraction skills. While these students worked on a booklet of subtraction problems, a proctor periodically asked each student what page he or she was working on and provided attributional feedback by commenting that the student had been working hard. Effort attributional feedback for achievement led to faster mastery of subtraction operations, greater subtraction skill, and higher perceptions of self-efficacy. Regression analyses also revealed that students' self-efficacy beliefs and training progress each produced a significant increase in variance in posttest subtraction skill. These results imply that students' self-efficacy was affected by self-reflection phase attributions to effort.

In addition to these limited-phase intervention studies, a growing number of multiphase intervention studies have been conducted on the role of self-efficacy and related beliefs during cyclical efforts to learn. These studies constitute a more complete test of the cyclical model of self-regulation. For example, Zimmerman and Kitsantas (1999) studied writing revision with high school girls. The task required the writer to revise highly redundant passages, and these revisions could be objectively scored for missing information and redundancies. Initially, all participants were taught a three-step revision strategy for identifying key information, eliminating redundant words, and combining the remaining words into sentences. After training was completed, a practice session was held. Participants in the learning-process goal group focused on the strategic steps for revising each writing task, whereas those in the performance-outcome group concentrated on minimizing the number of words in their revised passages. Participants in a shifting goal group initially pursued learning-process goals, then were shifted to performance-outcome goals after automaticity occurred. Half of the members in each goal group self-recorded their learning processes or performance outcomes. Girls in the process group self-recorded missing elements of the writing revision strategy; members of the outcome group self-recorded the number of words in the revision.

The results showed that girls who shifted goals from learning processes to performance outcomes after reaching automaticity surpassed the writing revision skill of girls who adhered to learning process goals. Girls who focused on outcomes displayed lower writing revision skill than girls in the shifting or process goal groups, and self-recording enhanced writing revision skill for all goal-setting groups. In addition to their acquisition of superior writing revision skill, girls who shifted goals displayed advantageous forms of self-motivation, such as greater attributions to strategy use (i.e., controllable causes), enhanced self-satisfaction, more optimistic self-efficacy beliefs, and greater task interest. Forethought phase goal setting and performance phase self-recording significantly enhanced not only writing skill but also self-reflection phase strategy attributions and self-satisfaction reactions. Goal setting influenced two forethought motivational beliefs regarding subsequent cycles of learning: self-efficacy and intrinsic interest. These findings show that self-efficacy plays an important role in predicting participants' cyclical use of important self-regulated learning processes.

In another intervention study of the role of self-efficacy and related beliefs during cyclical efforts to learn, similar self-regulation results were found with an athletic task (Zimmerman & Kitsantas, 1997). In a study of dart throwing, high school girls were taught a multistep strategy involving gripping the dart, taking the proper stance, sighting, throwing, and following through. The target involved seven concentric circles, which were assigned increasing numbers depending on their proximity to the bull's-eye. As in the prior study, the intervention involved goal setting and self-recording. Goal setting involved process goals, outcome goals, or shifting goals. The latter goal-setting group shifted from learning process goals to performance outcome goals after attaining automaticity. Self-recording for the process group involved tracking missing elements of the strategy, whereas self-recording for the outcome group involved tracking the dart-throwing points that were earned.

Participants who shifted goals from learning processes to performance outcomes surpassed the dart-throwing skill of participants who adhered to learning process goals. Participants who focused on outcomes displayed lower dart-throwing skill than the shifting or process goal groups, and self-recording enhanced acquisition for all goal groups. In addition to their acquisition of superior dart-throwing skill, girls who shifted goals displayed greater attributions to controllable causes (i.e., strategy use), enhanced self-satisfaction, more optimistic self-efficacy beliefs, and greater task interest. In short, forethought phase goal-setting and performance phase self-recording significantly affected not only dart-throwing skill but also self-reflection phase attributions and self-satisfaction reactions. Goal setting also influenced two forethought motivational beliefs regarding subsequent cycles of learning: self-efficacy and intrinsic interest. These athletic skill findings replicate those involving an academic skill, and they suggest that self-efficacy plays an important role in predicting participants' cyclical use of important self-regulated learning processes.

This experimental evidence of the differential effectiveness of learning processes and performance outcomes with both academic tasks (Zimmerman & Kitsantas, 1999) and athletic tasks (Zimmerman & Kitsantas, 1997) has led to the question of whether this differential effectiveness is evident with other self-regulation scales as well. More specifically, first, do scales that focus on learning processes form a separate composite from scales that focus on performance issues? Second, does the learning composite predict the students' academic achievement better than a performance composite factor?

In research designed to address these questions (Zimmerman & Kitsantas, 2014), performance scales focused on avoiding coping problems, such as hyperactivity, delay of gratification, and anxiety, whereas learning scales focused on developing sources of agency, such as self-efficacy, strategy use, and goal orientations. The reliability of the learning composite ($r = .91$) and performance composite ($r = .87$) were both very high, and the correlation between the composites was moderate in size ($r = .54$). These results indicate that formation of the two composites was supported empirically and that the composites were distinctive but moderately related. Hierarchical regression analyses revealed that the composite of learning scales was more predictive of the students' grade point average and performance on a statewide achievement test than the composite of performance scales. Thus, the scope of the learning and performance effects in self-regulation research appears to be wide.

IMPROVING SELF-EFFICACY CALIBRATION

Although self-efficacy is widely viewed as a motivator of learning, we have discussed its close linkage to self-regulatory processes such as goal setting, strategic feedback, and attributions. An additional issue to consider is the relation between self-efficacy and metacognitive monitoring. A compelling anecdotal example of this relation is described by Artur Rubinstein, a pianist of renown during the 20th century. He attributed his artistry and self-confidence to his close daily monitoring of his practice. "When I don't practice for a day, I know. When I don't practice for two days, the orchestra knows. When I don't practice for three days, the world knows" (Rubinstein, 2008, para. 1). The consequences of an inaccurate appraisal of his preparation for a concert were a constant concern to Rubinstein.

Metacognitive (i.e., self-) monitoring is a subtle phenomenon. A recently developed measure of this self-regulatory process shows promise. *Calibration* is a measure of the accuracy of metacognitive monitoring in terms of the congruence between one's perceptions of competence about performing a particular task and one's actual performance. Social-cognitive researchers have studied students' calibration by using measures of self-efficacy. These researchers generally have reported positive correlations between the strength of students' self-efficacy beliefs and their motivation and performance (Schunk & Pajares, 2004).

The calibration of self-efficacy perceptions can be measured when task-specific measures of self-efficacy and performance are employed, such as a student's confidence about an answer to a statistics problem. Students often overestimate their efficacy judgments (Klassen, 2002; Pajares & Miller, 1994), but underestimates also occur. The danger of overestimates is that they can lead to insufficient efforts to learn (Ghatala, Levin, Foorman, & Pressley, 1989). When people monitor more accurately, their high-quality covert feedback enables them to learn more effectively (Schunk & Pajares, 2004). DiBenedetto and Bembenutty (2013) found that among college students in biology self-efficacy at the beginning of the semester was higher than at the end, but course grades were better calibrated with end-of-semester self-efficacy, suggesting that students initially may have held unrealistic efficacy beliefs.

It is not unusual to find students who make inaccurate self-evaluations, although students who self-evaluate frequently attain higher academic outcomes than those who self-evaluate infrequently (Chen, 2003; Kitsantas, Reiser, & Doster, 2004; Schunk, 1996). It is notable, however, that low-achieving students are less accurate and more overconfident than high-achieving students who are slightly underconfident (Bol & Hacker, 2001; Kruger & Dunning, 1999). Unfortunately, interventions designed to improve students' self-evaluative accuracy

have not always been successful (Bol & Hacker, 2001; Hacker & Bol, 2004). The inability of overconfident students to improve the accuracy of their self-evaluations may be a self-regulation issue. Overconfident students are more prone to select difficult problems to solve and are more likely to fail. This error in forethought can undermine their subsequent self-efficacy to continue learning (Bandura, 1986; Schunk & Pajares, 2004).

Recent research indicates that students ranging from elementary to college levels can learn to monitor their performances more accurately and acquire greater academic skills. In a social-cognitive intervention designed to enhance elementary school students' calibration of their self-efficacy perceptions, Ramdass and Zimmerman (2008) taught a metacognitive self-monitoring strategy to fifth- and sixth-grade students learning mathematical division problems. An instructor showed all students a step-by-step problem solution. Students in the experimental group were given a strategy for self-checking their answers by multiplying the quotient by the divisor, whereas students in the control group were not. Students then practiced using a checklist to guide self-correction.

After correcting for pretest differences in division skill, the self-correction group displayed significantly higher division skill, self-efficacy, and self-evaluation than the control group. In terms of calibration, self-correction students displayed significantly greater accuracy in their self-efficacy and self-evaluation judgments, and significantly less bias (i.e., overestimation) than the control group. As expected, self-efficacy and self-evaluation beliefs correlated positively with students' mathematical performances. Self-efficacy accuracy and self-evaluation accuracy also correlated positively with performance, whereas self-efficacy bias and self-evaluation bias correlated negatively with performance. The negative direction of the bias measures indicates that quality of students' performances decreased as they became more overconfident (Chen, 2003).

These results indicate that teaching strategic planning enhanced not only forethought phase self-efficacy beliefs but also calibration of self-monitoring processes and mathematical performances. An educational

SRL Math Revision Sheet, Quiz #____ Item # ____ Student: _____ Date: _____
Instructor: _____

Now that you have received your corrected quiz, you have the opportunity to improve your score. Complete all sections thoroughly and thoughtfully. Use a separate revision sheet for each new problem.

PLAN IT								[ ] 8pts
1 a. How much time did you spend studying for this topic area? _____
    b. How many practice problems did you do in this topic area _____in preparation for this quiz?
    (circle one) 0 – 5 / 5 – 10 / 10+
    c. What did you do to prepare for this quiz? (use study strategy list to answer this question)

2. After you solved this problem, was your confidence rating too high (i.e. 4 or 5)?   yes   no

3. Explain what strategies or processes went wrong on the quiz problem.

PRACTICE IT								[ ] 8pts
4. Now re-do the original quiz problem and write the strategy you are using on the right.

	Definitely not confident	Not confident	Undecided	Confident	Very confident

5. How confident are you now that you can correctly solve this similar item?   1   2   3   4   5

6. Now use the strategy to solve the alternative problem.				[ ] 4pts

7. How confident are you now that you can correctly solve a similar problem on a quiz or test in the future?   1   2   3   4   5

FIGURE 17.2. SRL math revision sheets (i.e., self-reflection form). From Zimmerman, Moylan, Hudesman, White, and Flugman (2011, p. 127). Reprinted with permission from Pabst Publishers.

implication of these findings is that there is a need to monitor the calibration of middle school students because overestimates of personal skill can impair their learning. Fortunately, this study revealed that a self-correction strategy can be learned.

Calibration problems also have emerged with self-efficacy and self-evaluation judgments of older students. DiBenedetto and Zimmerman (2010) examined calibration among high school juniors' judgments of self-efficacy for learning and for performance. For both measures, low achievers overestimated their competence in science. High achievers showed a slight overestimation and average achievers, a moderate amount. Overestimation can occur when learners do not fully understand the task (Schunk & DiBenedetto, 2015), which may explain why the low achievers showed the poorest calibration. There is other evidence that overestimates of competence are less likely to occur when people have more relevant knowledge and expertise (Kruger & Dunning, 1999).

In a study of the effects of self-reflection training (Zimmerman et al., 2011), at-risk technical college students were taught to interpret their academic grades as self-reflective feedback rather than as signs of personal limitation. This is a challenging population of students because a majority of community college students are unprepared to engage in college-level coursework, and the dropout rate is high (Stinebrickner & Stinebrickner, 2012).

These students are often given developmental education courses to remediate their deficient skills, but there is extensive evidence that these courses do not prepare them to succeed in college-level courses (Bailey, 2009). Clearly, the problem is widespread, and alternative forms of instruction are needed. Students in developmental (remedial) mathematics or introductory college-level mathematics courses were randomly assigned to an intervention or a control classroom of their respective courses. In intervention classrooms, teachers used modeling techniques and assessment practices to enhance self-reflection processes. Frequent opportunities were given to students in intervention classrooms to improve their achievement through use of a self-reflective feedback form designed to self-regulate their learning and problem solving.

Self-reflective feedback was given during every second or third class session. A quiz composed of four or five problems provided frequent feedback to students and teachers. The quiz forms required students to make task-specific self-efficacy judgments before solving individual problems and self-evaluative judgments after attempting to solve each problem. After the quizzes were graded by the instructor, students in the intervention group were encouraged to correct their errors by completing the self-reflection forms and receiving quiz grade incentives.

The self-reflection form required students to compare their self-efficacy and self-evaluative judgments with their answers to the quiz item, explain ineffective strategies, create a more effective strategy, and rate their confidence for solving a new problem (see Figure 17.2). When the students' answers to the problem were incorrect and they were unaware of the reason, they were encouraged to seek help from other students or the instructor. At the outset of the course, the instructors demonstrated how the self-reflection forms should be completed, then allowed students to practice. Students were shown the formula for calculating bias in their self-efficacy and self-evaluation ratings of their solutions on the self-reflection forms.

The results revealed that students in self-regulation classes outperformed those in control classes on three periodic tests and a final course examination. Although there was substantial evidence of overconfidence by these at-risk students, students in self-regulation classes were better calibrated in their self-efficacy beliefs and their self-evaluative judgments than students in control classes. Significant relations among self-regulated learning processes were found. Students' self-efficacy and self-evaluation judgments regarding their performance on periodic tests were positively correlated with their achievement on the tests. Students' self-efficacy for the third and final exams, their standards for self-satisfaction, and their self-reported learning strategy use were positively correlated with final exam scores.

Teachers in self-regulated learning classes observed that students varied considerably in their use of the self-reflection form. For students in the developmental (i.e., remedial) course, high self-reflection form users (i.e., high self-reflectors) displayed significantly greater achievement on the second and third periodic tests, as well as on the final exam. High self-reflectors did not surpass low self-reflectors significantly on the first periodic test. For students in the introductory course, the high self-reflectors significantly surpassed low self-reflectors on all three periodic tests and on the final exam. It appears that students with greater background in mathematics were better able to profit from self-regulatory training on the first exam.

Because students in these classes were not admitted to this technical college as regular-status students, they were classified as at risk (or as developmental according to Bailey's [2009] criteria). To gain entrance into credit-bearing courses and make progress toward obtaining a degree, developmental students must pass a collegewide entrance test. It was discovered that 25% more of these students in the self-regulation classes passed the entrance test than students in control classes, a difference that was statistically significant. Thus, as a result of their self-regulatory training, a significantly greater percentage of these students were no longer academically at risk. These findings of success on the entrance test represent successful passage through a major gateway in the academic lives of these at-risk students. New opportunities had become available for them to take advanced courses and pursue majors that involved mathematical competence (Zimmerman et al., 2011). These life-changing results were obtained with a brief self-reflection form that could be introduced readily into the curriculum of regular classes.

FUTURE DIRECTIONS FOR RESEARCH ON SELF-REGULATED LEARNING

The purpose of a cyclical model of self-regulation is to describe the underlying processes and beliefs in order to measure sequential changes before, during, and after repeated efforts to learn. The model seeks not only to explain existing research findings but also to guide the development of new measures. These measures, termed *microanalytic,* are intended to provide a dynamic account of a student's self-regulatory strengths and limitations, and there is evidence that microanalytic measures predict academic outcomes better than a well-validated teacher rating scale of their students' self-regulation in class (DiBenedetto & Zimmerman, 2013). Furthermore, the feedback produced by microanalysis was preferred by teachers more than feedback produced by traditional measures regarding students' appraisals (Cleary & Zimmerman, 2006). The cyclical model

was also designed to provide a platform for individualized interventions that can target specific self-regulatory dysfunctions, such as overly optimistic self-efficacy beliefs, weak planning or forethought skills, and ineffective use of strategies. The Self-Regulation Empowerment Program (SREP) is an example of such an intervention grounded in the cyclical model. Broadly speaking, the SREP is an applied, academic intervention program designed to induce change in students' motivation, strategic skills, and metacognitive skills (Cleary & Zimmerman, 2004). It adheres to a semistructured instructional protocol format whereby SREP coaches use various modules and instructional guides but are afforded flexibility to adapt instruction to meet individual student needs.

The SREP has been studied with ethnically diverse and academically at-risk groups of adolescents attending urban middle school or high schools (Cleary & Platten, 2013; Cleary, Platten, & Nelson, 2008; Cleary, Velardi, & Schnaidman, 2016). These initial mixed-method case studies focused on small groups of high school students in the area of biology (Cleary & Platten, 2013; Cleary et al., 2008). Recommended by their teachers for failing or nearly failing biological science test grades and because of motivational or self-regulatory difficulties, students in these two projects received approximately 20 SREP sessions to help them learn to self-regulate their thoughts and actions as they prepared for biology tests. In addition to being exposed to foundational knowledge in self-regulated learning (SRL) processes, students received extensive instruction in SRL strategies, as well as frequent opportunities to practice using these strategies to learn course content or to manage their behaviors. The SREP coaches also guided students through self-reflection activities that enabled them to evaluate and refine use of these strategies to strive for their test grade goal. For example, following each test performance, the SREP coach asked each student, "What is the primary reason you got this score on this test?" and "What do you need to do to improve your next test score?" Asking microanalytic questions cyclically during the intervention provided self-regulation tutors or coaches with information that they could use to guide and modify the intervention. To measure changes in student motivation and self-regulation, pretest–posttest case studies were conducted involving multiple measures, such as self-report scales, teacher rating scales, microanalytic protocols, and field notes observations.

This methodology provided converging evidence regarding appropriateness of inferences regarding cyclical processes and beliefs. In these initial studies, all participants showed gains in their exam scores above the average z-score gains for their biology class during the study. One month after the SREP training was completed, seven out of nine participants exceeded the class mean score on the exam, and two of the students earned exam scores of 93 and 95%. In terms of evaluating changes in self-regulatory behaviors and cognitions using reliability change index scores, there was also some evidence for significant growth from pretest to posttest.

More recently, Cleary and colleagues (2016) conducted a field-based experiment to examine the effectiveness of SREP for improving the strategic thinking, motivation, and mathematics achievement of seventh-grade students in a middle school. There were two groups in this study, each with 22 students: SREP and an existing mathematics remediation program provided by the middle school. Although the authors used the SREP modules and procedures emphasized in the prior studies, they placed particular emphasis on engaging students in two types of feedback loops: (1) a weekly feedback loop that centered on students' learning and refining their use of strategies, and (2) a unit test feedback loop that focused more broadly on students' performance on the unit mathematics exams. Using a pretest–posttest control group design, the authors found statistically significant and medium-to-large effects of SREP in terms of the quality of students' attributions, adaptive inferences, and test preparation strategies at posttest. These effects were maintained at 2-month follow-up, except for the test preparation strategies. In terms of z-score mathematics achievement, the SREP condition, but not the alternative intervention condition, displayed a significant linear trend from pretest to 8-month follow-up, with z-scores improving from a value of -0.53 at pretest to 1.70 at 8-month follow-up. Finally, consistent with both Cleary and Platten (2013) and Cleary and colleagues (2008), the authors found strong evidence supporting the social validity of SREP; that is, both students and SREP coaches reported that the program was highly acceptable and useful in impacting important aspects of students' performance and behavior in school.

These initial efforts to validate the SREP in terms of students' academic achievement are encouraging. The greater challenge, however, is to establish the effectiveness of the intervention in teaching students to think and act in a cyclical self-regulated way as they learn biological science. By examining changes in individual students using single-subject and case study designs, SREP tutors can provide their students with a dynamic understanding of the how and why their self-regulatory processes can enhance their achievement.

REFERENCES

Ainley, M., Corrigan, M., & Richardson, N. (2005). Students, tasks and emotions: Identifying the contribution of emotions to students reading of popular culture and popular science texts. *Learning and Instruction, 15,* 433–447.

Bailey, T. (2009). Challenge and opportunity: Rethinking the role and function of developmental education in community college. *New Directions for Community Colleges, 145,* 11–30.

Bandura, A. (1977). *Social learning theory.* Englewood Cliffs, NJ: Prentice Hall.

Bandura, A. (1986). *Social foundations of thought and action: A social cognitive theory.* Englewood Cliffs, NJ: Prentice Hall.

Bandura, A. (1991). Self-regulation of motivation through anticipatory and self-reactive mechanisms. In R. A. Dienstbier (Ed.), *Perspectives on motivation: Nebraska Symposium on Motivation* (Vol. 38, pp. 69–164). Lincoln: University of Nebraska Press.

Bandura, A. (1997). *Self-efficacy: The exercise of control.* New York: Freeman.

Bandura, A. (2006). Guide for constructing self-efficacy scales. In F. Pajaras & T. Urdan (Eds.), *Self-efficacy beliefs of adolescents* (pp. 307–337). Greenwich CT: Information Age.

Bandura, A. (2008). Toward an agentic theory of the self. In H. W. Marsh, R. G. Craven, & D. McInerney (Eds.), *Self-processes, leaning, and enabling human potential: Dynamic new processes* (pp. 15–49). Charlotte NC: Information Age.

Bandura, A., Adams, N. E., & Beyer, J. (1977). Cognitive processes mediating behavioral change. *Journal of Personality and Social Psychology, 35,* 125–139.

Bandura, A., & Jeffery, R. W. (1973). Roles of symbolic and rehearsal processes in observational learning. *Journal of Personality and Social Psychology, 26,* 122–130.

Bandura, A., & Schunk, D. H. (1981). Cultivating competence, self-efficacy, and intrinsic interest through proximal self-motivation. *Journal of Personality and Social Psychology, 41,* 586–598.

Barzun, J. (1964). Calamaphobia, or hints toward a writer's discipline. In H. Hull (Ed.), *The writer's book* (pp. 84–96). New York: Barnes & Noble.

Bol, L., & Hacker, D. (2001). The effect of practice tests on students' calibration and performance. *Journal of Experimental Education, 69,* 133–151.

Bong, M. (2006). Asking the right question: How confident are you that you could successfully perform these tasks? In F. Pajaras & T. Urdan (Eds.), *Self-efficacy beliefs of adolescents* (pp. 287–305). Greenwich CT: Information Age.

Britton, B. K., & Tessor, A. (1991). Effects of time management practices on college grades. *Journal of Educational Psychology, 83,* 405–410.

Carver, C., & Scheier, M. F. (2000). On the structure of behavioral self-regulation. In M. Boekaerts, P. R. Pintrich, & M. Zeidner (Eds.), *Handbook of self-regulation* (pp. 41–84). San Diego, CA: Academic Press.

Chen, P. P. (2003). Exploring the accuracy and predictability of the self-efficacy beliefs of seventh-grade mathematics students. *Learning and Individual Differences, 14,* 79–92.

Cleary, T. J., & Platten, P. (2013). Examining the correspondence between self-regulated learning and academic achievement: A case study analysis. *Education Research International, 2013,* Article ID 272560.

Cleary, T. J., Platten, P., & Nelson, A. (2008). Effectiveness of the self-regulation empowerment program (SREP) with urban high school youth: An initial investigation. *Journal of Advanced Academics, 20,* 70–107.

Cleary, T. J., Velardi, B., & Schnaidman, B. (2016, April). *Effects of a Self-Regulated Empowerment Program (SREP) on middle school students' strategic skills and mathematics achievement.* Paper presented at the annual meeting of the American Educational Research Association, Washington, DC.

Cleary, T. J., & Zimmerman, B. J. (2001). Self-regulation differences during athletic practice by experts, non-experts, and novices. *Journal of Applied Sport Psychology, 13,* 61–82.

Cleary, T. J., & Zimmerman, B. J. (2004). Self-regulation Empowerment Program: A school-based program to enhance self-regulated and self-motivated cycles of student learning. *Psychology in the Schools, 41,* 537–550.

Cleary, T. J., & Zimmerman, B. J. (2006). Teachers' perceived usefulness of strategy microanalyic assessment information. *Psychology in the Schools, 43,* 149–155.

Deci, E., & Ryan, R. M. (1985). *Intrinsic motivation and self-determination in human behavior.* New York: Plenum Press.

DiBenedetto, M. K., & Bembenutty, H. (2013). Within the science pipeline: Self-regulated learning and academic achievement among college students in science classes. *Learning and Individual Differences, 2,* 218–224.

DiBenedetto, M. K., & Zimmerman, B. J. (2010). Differences in self-regulatory processes among students studying science: A microanalytic investigation. *International Journal of Educational and Psychological Assessment, 5*(1), 2–24.

DiBenedetto, M. K., & Zimmerman, B. J. (2013). Construct and predictive validity of microanalytic measures of students' self-regulation of science learning. *Learning and Individual Differences, 26,* 30–41.

Dweck, C., & Leggett, E. (1988), A social-cognitive approach to motivation and personality. *Psychological Review, 95,* 256–273.

Fast, L. A., Lewis, J. L., Bryant, M. J., Bocian, K. A., Cardullo, R. A., Rettig, M., et al. (2010). Does math self-efficacy mediate the effect of the perceived classroom environment on standardized math test performance? *Journal of Educational Psychology, 102,* 729–740.

Ghatala, E. S., Levin, J. R., Foorman, B. R., & Pressley, M. (1989). Improving children's regulation of their reading PREP time. *Contemporary Educational Psychology, 14,* 49–66.

Graham, S., & Williams, C. (2009). An attributional approach to motivation in school. In K. R. Wentzel & A. Wigfield (Eds.), *Handbook of motivation at school* (pp. 11–33). New York: Routledge.

Hacker, D. J., & Bol, L. (2004). Metacognitive theory: Considering the social-cognitive influences. In D. M. McInerney & S. V. Etten (Eds.), *Big theories revisited* (pp. 275–297). Greenwich, CT: Information Age.

Hattie, J., & Timperley, H. (2007). The power of feedback. *Review of Educational Research, 77,* 81–112.

Hidi, S., & Renninger, K. A. (2006). The four-phase model of interest development. *Educational Psychologist, 41,* 111–127.

Joët, G., Usher, E. L., & Bressoux, P. (2011). Sources of self-efficacy: An investigation of elementary school students in France. *Journal of Educational Psychology, 103,* 649–663.

Karabenick, S. A. (2011). Methodological and assessment issues in research on help seeking. In B. J. Zimmerman & D. H. Schunk (Eds.), *Handbook of self-regulation of learning and performance* (pp. 267–281). New York: Routledge.

Kitsantas, A., Reiser, B., & Doster, J. (2004). Goal setting, cues, and evaluation during acquisition of procedural skills: Empowering students' learning during independent practice. *Journal of Experimental Education, 72,* 269–287.

Kitsantas, A., & Zimmerman, B. J. (2002). Comparing self-regulatory processes among novice, non-expert, and expert volleyball players: A microanalytic study. *Journal of Applied Sport Psychology, 14,* 91–105.

Klassen, R. M. (2002). A question of calibration: A review of the self-efficacy beliefs of students with learning disabilities. *Learning Disability Quarterly, 25,* 88–102.

Kruger, J., & Dunning, D. (1999). Unskilled and unaware of it: How difficulties in recognizing one's own incompetences led to inflated self-assessments. *Journal of Personality and Social Psychology, 77,* 1121–1134.

Locke, E. A., & Latham, G. P. (1990). *A theory of goal setting and task performance.* Upper Saddle River, NJ: Prentice Hall.

Moos, D. C., & Azevedo, R. (2009). Learning with computer-based learning environments: A literature review of computer self-efficacy. *Review of Educational Research, 79,* 576–600.

Pajares, F. (1996). Self-efficacy beliefs in academic settings. *Review of Educational Research, 66,* 543–578.

Pajares, F., & Kranzler, J. (1995). Self-efficacy beliefs and general mental ability in mathematical problem-solving. *Contemporary Educational Psychology, 20,* 426–443.

Pajares, F., & Miller, M. D. (1994). Role of self-efficacy and self-concept beliefs in mathematical problem solving: A path analysis. *Journal of Educational Psychology, 86,* 193–203.

Patall, E. A. (2012). The motivational complexity of choosing: A review of theory and research. In R. M. Ryan (Ed.), *The Oxford handbook of human motivation* (pp. 248–279). Oxford, UK: Oxford University Press.

Pelham, B. W. (1995). Self-investment and esteem: Evidence for a Jamesian model of self-worth. *Journal of Personality and Social Psychology, 69,* 1141–1150.

Pintrich, P. R., & De Groot, E. (1990). Motivational and self-regulated learning components of classroom academic performance. *Journal of Educational Psychology, 82,* 33–40.

Pressley, G. M. (1976). Mental imagery helps eight-year-olds remember what they read. *Journal of Educational Psychology, 24,* 355–359.

Ramdass, D. H., Zimmerman, B. J. (2008). Effects of self-correction strategy training on middle school students' self-efficacy, self-evaluation, and mathematics division learning. *Journal of Advanced Academics, 20,* 18–41.

Rubinstein, A. (2008). On practicing. Retrieved from *http://lci.typepad.com/leaders_resourcing_leader/2008/04/on-practicing-b.html.*

Schmitz, B., & Wiese, B. S. (2006). New perspectives for the evaluation of training sessions in self-regulated learning: Time-series analyses of diary data. *Contemporary Educational Psychology, 31,* 64–96.

Schunk, D. H. (1981). Modeling and attributional feedback effects on children's achievement: A self-efficacy analysis. *Journal of Educational Psychology, 74,* 93–105.

Schunk, D. H. (1982). Effects of effort attributional feedback on children's perceived self-efficacy and achievement. *Journal of Educational Psychology, 74,* 548–556.

Schunk, D. H. (1983a). Ability versus effort attributional feedback: Differential effects on self-efficacy and achievement. *Journal of Educational Psychology, 75,* 848–856.

Schunk, D. H. (1983b). Goal difficulty and attainment information: Effects on children's achievement behaviors. *Human Learning, 3,* 107–117.

Schunk, D. H. (1984). Enhancing self-efficacy and achievement through rewards and goals: Motivational and information effects. *Journal of Educational Research, 78,* 29–34.

Schunk, D. H. (1996). Goal and self-evaluative influences during children's cognitive skill learning. *American Educational Research Journal, 33,* 359–382.

Schunk, D. H. (2008). Attributions as motivators of self-regulated learning. In D. H. Schunk & B. J. Zimmerman (Eds.), *Motivation and self-regulated learning: Theory, research, and applications* (pp. 245–266). New York: Taylor & Francis.

Schunk, D. H. (2012). Social cognitive theory. In

K. R. Harris, S. Graham, & T. Urdan (Eds.), *APA educational psychology handbook: Vol. 1. Theories, constructs, and critical issues* (pp. 101–123). Washington, DC: American Psychological Association.

Schunk, D. H., & DiBenedetto, M. K. (2014). Academic self-efficacy. In M. J. Furlong, R. Gillman, & E. S. Huebner (Eds.), *Handbook of positive psychology in the schools* (2nd ed., pp. 115–130). New York: Routledge.

Schunk, D. H., & DiBenedetto, M. K. (2015). Self-efficacy: Educational aspects. In J. D. Wright (Ed.), *International encyclopedia of the social and behavioral sciences* (2nd ed., pp. 515–521). Oxford, UK: Elsevier.

Schunk, D. H., & Ertmer, P. A. (1999). Self-regulatory processes during computer skill acquisition: Goal and self-evaluative influences. *Journal of Educational Psychology, 91,* 251–260.

Schunk, D. H., & Pajares, F. (2004). Self-efficacy in education revisited. Empirical and applied evidence. In D. M. McInerney & S. V. Etten (Eds.), *Big theories revisited* (pp. 115–138). Greenwich, CT: Information Age.

Schunk, D. H., & Rice, J. M. (1987). Enhancing comprehension skill and self-efficacy with strategy valuation information. *Journal of Reading Behavior, 19,* 285–302.

Schunk, D. H., & Rice, J. M. (1993). Strategy fading and progress feedback: Effects on self-efficacy and comprehension among students receiving remedial reading services. *Journal of Special Education, 27,* 257–276.

Schunk, D. H., & Schwartz, C. W. (1993). Goals and progress feedback: Effects on self-efficacy and writing achievement. *Contemporary Educational Psychology, 18,* 337–354.

Schunk, D. H., & Zimmerman, B. J. (Eds.). (2008). *Motivation and self-regulated learning: Theory, research, and applications.* Mahwah, NJ: Erlbaum.

Siegel, R. G., Galassi, J. P., & Ware, W. B. (1985). A comparison of two models for predicting mathematics: Social learning versus math-aptitude anxiety. *Journal of Counseling Psychology, 32,* 531–538.

Stinebrickner, T., & Stinebrickner, R. (2012). Learning about academic ability and the college dropout decision. *Journal of Labor Economics, 30,* 707–718.

Stoeger, H., & Ziegler, A. (2011). Self-regulatory training through elementary-school students' homework completion. In B. J. Zimmerman & D. H. Schunk (Eds.), *Handbook of self-regulation of learning and performance* (pp. 87–101). New York: Routledge.

Usher, E. L. (2009). Sources of middle school students' self-efficacy in mathematics: A qualitative investigation. *American Educational Research Journal, 46,* 275–314.

Weiner, B. (1992). *Human motivation: Metaphors, theories, and research.* Newbury Park, CA: Sage.

Weinstein, C. E., & Mayer, R. E. (1986). The teaching of learning strategies. In M. C. Wittrock (Ed.), *Handbook of research on teaching* (pp. 315–327). New York: Macmillan.

Wigfield, A., Cambria, J., & Eccles, J. S. (2012). Motivation in education. In R. M. Ryan (Ed.), *The Oxford handbook of human motivation* (pp. 463–478). Oxford, UK: Oxford University Press.

Wigfield, A., & Eccles, J. S. (2002). The development of competence beliefs and values from childhood through adolescence. In A. Wigfield & J. S. Eccles (Eds.), *Development of achievement motivation* (pp. 92–120). San Diego, CA: Academic Press.

Winne, P. H., & Hadwin, A. F. (1998). Studying as self-regulated learning. In D. J. Hacker, J. Dunlosky, & A. C. Graesser (Eds.), *Metacognition in educational theory and practice* (pp. 277–304). Hillsdale, NJ: Erlbaum.

Wolters, C. A., Benzon, M. B., & Arroyo-Giner, C. (2011). Assessing strategies for self-regulation of motivation. In B. J. Zimmerman & D. H. Schunk (Eds.), *Handbook of self-regulation of learning and performance* (pp. 298–312). New York: Routledge.

Zimmerman, B. J. (1995). Self-regulation involves more than metacognition: A social cognitive perspective. *Educational Psychologist, 30,* 217–221.

Zimmerman, B. J. (2000). Attaining self-regulation: A social cognitive perspective. In M. Boekaerts, P. Pintrich, & M. Zeidner (Eds.), *Handbook of self-regulation* (pp. 13–39). San Diego, CA: Academic Press.

Zimmerman, B. J. (2008). In search of self-regulated learning: A personal quest. In H. W. Marsh, R. G. Craven, & D. M. McInerney (Eds.), *Self-processes, learning, and enabling human potential: Dynamic new approaches* (pp. 171–191). Greenwich, CT: Information Age.

Zimmerman, B. J., & Bell, J. A. (1972). Observer verbalization and abstraction in vicarious rule learning, generalization, and retention. *Developmental Psychology, 7,* 227–231.

Zimmerman, B. J., & Kitsantas, A. (1996). Self-regulated learning of a motoric skill: The role of goal setting and self-monitoring. *Journal of Applied Sport Psychology, 8,* 69–84.

Zimmerman, B. J., & Kitsantas, A. (1997). Developmental phases in self-regulation: Shifting from process to outcome goals. *Journal of Educational Psychology, 89,* 29–36.

Zimmerman, B. J., & Kitsantas, A. (1999).

Acquiring writing revision skill: Shifting from process to outcome self-regulatory goals. *Journal of Educational Psychology, 91,* 1–10.

Zimmerman, B. J., & Kitsantas, A. (2014). Comparing students' self-discipline and self-regulation measures and their prediction of academic achievement. *Contemporary Educational Psychology, 39,* 145–155.

Zimmerman, B. J., & Martinez-Pons, M. (1986). Development of a structured interview for assessing students' use of self-regulated learning strategies. *American Educational Research Journal, 23,* 614–628.

Zimmerman, B. J., & Martinez-Pons, M. (1990). Student differences in selfregulated learning: Relating grade, sex, and giftedness to selfefficacy and strategy use. *Journal of Educational Psychology, 82,* 51–59.

Zimmerman, B. J., Moylan, A., Hudesman, J., White, N., & Flugman, B. (2011). Enhancing self-reflection and mathematics achievement of at-risk urban technical college students. *Psychological Test and Assessment Modeling, 53,* 108–127.

Zimmerman, B. J., Schunk, D. H., & DiBenedetto, M. K. (2015). A personal agency view of self-regulated learning: The role of goal setting. In F. Guay, H. Marsh, D. M. McInerney, & R. G. Craven (Eds.), *Self-concept, motivation, and identity: Underpinning success with research and practice* (pp. 83–114). Charlotte, NC: Information Age.

CHAPTER 18

Interest
Theory and Application

JUDITH M. HARACKIEWICZ
MAXIMILIAN KNOGLER

While an exact understanding of human motivation continues to evolve, some concepts have proven conducive to our understanding of motivation and the further advancement of motivational models and theories. One of these concepts is intrinsic motivation, which is often related to, and contrasted with, extrinsic motivation. This distinction does not refer to quantitative aspects, such as the amount or intensity of motivation people bring to a task, but to different qualities or kinds of motivation related to why people engage in a certain task or behavior (Ryan & Deci, 2000). The differences relate to different motives, reasons, attitudes, or goals that underlie peoples' behaviors and actions. On the one hand, extrinsically motivated behaviors are governed by the prospect of some instrumental gain or loss. Individuals who are extrinsically motivated engage with tasks because they expect that their engagement will result in desirable outcomes, such as monetary rewards, high grades, or praise, or an avoidance of negative consequences, such as stress or pain. On the other hand, individuals engage in intrinsically motivated behaviors because they seem to be ends in themselves rather than a means to a separate outcome (Cerasoli, Nicklin, & Ford,

2014; Sansone & Harackiewicz, 2000). Intrinsic motivation is based on the natural curiosity people possess (White, 1959) and refers to doing something because it is inherently interesting or enjoyable (Deci & Ryan, 1985). For example, people may freely choose to engage in climbing or birding or regularly visit museums and exhibitions, thereby expressing their passion for sports, nature, art, and history. The positive energy associated with intrinsically motivated activities allows people to expand their knowledge, skills, and competencies related to this motivation fairly effortlessly. Therefore, the concept is highly relevant for this volume, as it connects motivation and competence in a synergistic way.

Historically, intrinsic motivation emerged as a concept only fairly recently to explain the motivation for activities and behaviors for which the only rewards are perceptions of interest or the experience of enjoyment (Ryan & Deci, 2000). Intrinsic motivation was therefore used to explain behaviors for which previous frameworks, such as drive theories or behaviorism, could not account. Today, intrinsic motivation is still a versatile and relevant concept that cuts across several theories of motivation and demands the attention of educators striving to facilitate high-quality learning for their students and the development of their competence in sustainable ways. The experience of intrinsically motivated learning can be supported in environments where people can freely explore and pursue already existing interests, or have the opportunity to explore and appreciate new activities and objects. As theory developed, several frameworks came to include concepts of intrinsic motivation. *Self-determination theory* (Deci & Ryan, 1985) argues that intrinsically motivated behaviors relate to the satisfaction of three innate basic psychological needs for the experience of competence, autonomy, and relatedness. For a high level of intrinsic motivation, people must experience satisfaction of these needs and act on their environment to ensure that those needs are met. According to *flow theory* (Csikszentmihalyi, 2013), people engage in intrinsically motivating activities because they seek experiences that reflect complete involvement with the activity, together with the accompanying loss of awareness of time and space. And according to *interest theory* (Hidi & Renninger, 2006; Krapp, 2002), people engage in intrinsically motivated behaviors because of personal preferences to interact with a particular content (individual interest) or due to stimulating task characteristics that, on average, many people find to be interesting (situational interest).

In this chapter, we focus on interest as a prototypical intrinsic motivational construct. "Interest" is conceptualized as a content-specific, motivational variable that can inform us about why individuals are motivated to engage and to learn specific subject matter (Hidi, 2000). Thus, calling an individual *interested* or *not interested* always requires a description of his or her object of interest. Individuals can be interested in skydiving or in a particular academic topic, but they cannot be generally interested in the same way that they might be considered to be curious (Grossnickle, 2016), open to experience (Goldberg, 1990), or as having a growth mindset (Dweck, 2006). Theories of academic interest have demonstrated the usefulness of the concept first in terms of a theoretical framework for conceptualizing intrinsic motivation and academic motivation, and second, as a framework for the development of educational interventions

to promote interest in particular topics, as well as applications to strengthen the relation between a person and an object (Mitchell, 1993; Renninger & Hidi, 2016). In this chapter, we first describe the fundamental concepts of interest theory, which offers a unique perspective on intrinsic motivation in terms of a dynamic person–object relationship that is consequential for how people learn and develop over time. Motivational theories of interest conceptualize interest in terms of a state-like and a trait-like construct, with a developmental framework connecting the two (Krapp, Hidi, & Renninger, 1992). Interest theory not only provides a descriptive framework for how interest develops, but it also describes ways in which interest can be supported to develop in both a short-term and a sustainable long-term manner (Hidi & Renninger, 2006; Renninger & Hidi, 2016). In the second part of the chapter we consider intervention research examining how to promote and sustain interest in educational contexts.

THEORIES AND CONCEPTS

Interest as a State-Like Construct

Ideally, there are many tasks and activities in our daily lives that we pursue in a state of interest. We may experience interest while reading well-written books, while having good conversations, and while tackling intriguing challenges in our jobs. From an interest theory perspective, being intrinsically motivated can be conceived as being in a state of interest while doing something. In this action-related sense, interest captures the desire to engage in activities in the moment and refers to a temporary experience of interest while being engaged with a task (Krapp et al., 1992; Renninger & Hidi, 2016). This concept of state interest focuses on the experience of the present moment. It acknowledges the fact that our level of interest is malleable and can change from one moment to the next. In order to understand these changes, researchers explore the complexity of momentary circumstances often conceptualized as "situations." Therefore, researchers who investigate state interest are typically looking at person-in-context experiences of interest and the changes that result from short-term engagement with the environment (Ainley, 2006).

According to interest research, the state of interest combines positive affective qualities, such as feelings of enjoyment and curiosity, with cognitive qualities of focused attention, as well as perceptions of value and personal importance (Hidi & Renninger, 2006; Linnenbrink-Garcia et al., 2010). Thus, being in a state of interest means that positive affective reactions and cognitive functioning are intertwined, which makes cognitive engagement and focusing of attention feel relatively effortless. Thus, the state of interest is an ideal state, and one to strive for whenever possible. This is not only because this state of being interested is typically charged with positive feelings and engagement, but also because interest can energize higher levels of performance. Dewey (1913) characterized "interest" as an undivided activity that combines the assessment of personal importance of the activity and positive emotional evaluations of the activity. Accordingly, during interesting activities, there is no conflict between what people think is important for them and what they like to do (Krapp, 2002). Research findings reveal that when this state is activated, learning and attention feel more effortless (Ainley, Hidi, & Berndorff, 2002; Hidi, 2006), that being in a state of interest is positively related to self-regulation and persistence (Thoman, Smith, & Silvia, 2011; Tulis & Fulmer, 2013), and that interest increases task engagement (Ainley, 2006; Sansone & Thoman, 2005), as well as the use of deep learning strategies (Flowerday, Schraw, & Stevens, 2004).

Interest is a phenomenon that emerges from individuals interacting with their environments (Krapp, 2002). The intrinsic quality of interest lies in the positive interaction between a person and a task, which finds its expression in a state of interest and occurs independently of extrinsic outcomes. The intrinsic quality stems from stimulating task characteristics (*task-intrinsic motivation*) that facilitate an individual's motivation to engage in a task for its own sake (Deci & Ryan, 1985; Hidi, 2000), as well as from personal dispositional preferences for the task that the person brings to the situation

(*person-intrinsic motivation*). The study of domain-specific intrinsic motivation therefore covers two broad types of interest: situational and individual interest. In the following section, we highlight situational and individual interest as two different perspectives on the psychological state of interest.

The *situational interest perspective* views state interest as an immediate consequence of the contextual factors present in a situation. These factors or situational cues are assumed to elicit situational interest across individuals. As such, situational interest emerges from the situation and is bound to it. This volatile view of interest implies that every situation has the power not only to support but also to thwart peoples' state of interest. If situations fail to support people's interests, then individuals might lose their interest immediately, even if they came into the situation with some interest. Many researchers have highlighted external influences or environmental triggers as prevailing situational elements that influence states of interest (Durik & Harackiewicz, 2007; Hidi & Harackiewicz, 2000). Features of the environment that stimulate interest have also been referred to as "collative variables" (Berlyne, 1970) or "interestingness of the context" (Krapp et al., 1992; Schunk, Pintrich, & Meece, 2010). Empirically, this has resulted in a substantial body of research investigating content, activities, stimuli, or environmental conditions assumed to generate or discourage interest (Bergin, 1999; Cordova & Lepper, 1996). Various contextual variables or task characteristics embedded in texts, classroom situations, and other contexts have been identified as generating and promoting situational interest (Palmer, 2009; Renninger & Hidi, 2011); these may include factors such as novelty, complexity, challenge, or task conditions that support learners' choice and autonomy, their feelings of competence, and social relatedness (Deci, 1992; Schraw & Lehman, 2001).

At the same time, interest theory offers an *individual interest perspective* on the state of interest. This perspective highlights the influence of individuals' dispositions and stable preferences for specific content as a reason for being in a state of interest in a particular situation. Here, the immediate experience of interest taps into a well-developed personal preference to enjoy or cherish a particular content or activity consistently across situations and contexts. *Individual interest* is conceived as a latent disposition that can be activated in the situation (Ainley, 2006; Ainley & Hidi, 2002). Thus, some researchers use the term *actualized individual interest* to signify that the experience of interest in some situations is primarily elicited by a person's latent disposition rather than environmental features (Krapp, 2002; Schraw & Lehman, 2001). For example, a student may be particularly likely to be in a state of interest during a class that is dealing with one of his or her favorite topics. The individual interest perspective encourages researchers to consider how people enter situations, as well as the situational consistencies in momentary experiences and behaviors. When people enter situations with a high level of interest, for example, they might be protected from losing interest if the situation (without the presence of any other kind of support) matches their interests (Linnenbrink-Garcia, Patall, & Messersmith, 2012; Tsai, Kunter, Lütke, Trautwein, & Ryan, 2008). For example, a student who loves organic chemistry may be able to get through a boring lecture on the topic, whereas other students might lose interest in the same situation. Similarly, other stable personal characteristics can positively influence interest during learning activities, such as higher levels of prior knowledge (Alexander & Jetton, 1996) or mastery goal orientations (Harackiewicz, Barron, Carter, Lehto, & Elliot, 1997; Harackiewicz, Durik, Barron, Linnenbrink-Garcia, & Tauer, 2008; Hulleman, Durik, Schweigert, & Harackiewicz, 2008; Tanaka & Murayama, 2014). This demonstrates that the experience of interest can be influenced by person-level factors, and suggests that interest is not simply a product of situational circumstances.

So far, research has not provided any evidence for a phenomenological difference between a state of interest that has its origins primarily in individual or dispositional interest and a state of interest that stems from stimulating situational conditions (Schiefele, 2009). To the individual, both states feel the same, and there is no other way to experience interest other than being in a state of interest. Current theory therefore assumes that there is only one kind of interest experience, or psychological state of interest, but that this state can originate from two different sources and is therefore associated with different mechanisms (individual vs. situational) (Hidi & Renninger, 2006). In other words, situational interest and individual interest share the same psychological state (Renninger & Hidi, 2016). Thus, if the state of being interested does not feel different as a function of its source, then questions about its origin are difficult to address empirically. Findings have accumulated about person-related variables, situation-related variables, and their mutual relations that influence states of interest (e.g., Durik, Hulleman, & Harackiewicz, 2015; Tanaka & Murayama, 2014; Tsai et al., 2008). Considered together, these studies show that both internal, personal factors and external, environmental factors can shape an individual's experience of interest in any given moment (Renninger & Hidi, 2011).

In a recent study (Knogler, Harackiewicz, Gegenfurtner, & Lewalter, 2015), we used a latent variable approach combined with repeated measures design to disentangle variance in individuals' states of interest that might be attributed to either individual or situational sources. We asked students to rate their interest several times in response to different instructional situations related to the same topic (e.g., inquiry, presentation of results, discussion, and reflection). These data were analyzed with latent state–trait models that were used to parse out cross-situational, stable variance in repeated measures from situation-specific variance (Geiser & Lockhart, 2012). Results indicated that half of the variance was situation-specific and therefore related to particular instructional situations, whereas the other half was consistent or stable across situations. Thus, even though students were dealing with the same topic across a series of lessons, the different instructional arrangements (i.e., the "situations") had a strong impact on students' state interest. These findings therefore offer some indication that situation-specific variance might be truly situational. Students' initial individual interest in the topic, as measured before the instruction began, was correlated with the stable cross-situational part of variance but unrelated to the situation-specific parts. Considered together, these findings offer empirical support that the situational interest perspective and the individual interest perspective are not mutually exclusive ways to look at states of interest. Rather, we found evidence for both types of interest across the learning situations. In line with Krapp's (2002) argument that "any interest has a history," there is often an actualizing mechanism at work that influences interest at any given moment, and over time stabilizes individuals' states of interest. At the same time, there are motivational forces in each and every situation that influence individuals' states of interest irrespective of their previous experiences with the content. Given the magnitude of effects found in this study, both perspectives need to be considered to explain and conceive of interest as a state phenomenon. Moreover, they also need to be considered as representing two different avenues for promoting interest during learning. Interventions can generally focus on harnessing the power of an already existing interest or on harnessing the power of situational cues that can induce situational interest (as discussed in later sections of this chapter).

Just like many other experiences, states of interest are embedded in a flowing stream of situations. And while situational and individual perspectives on these states can be separated conceptually, they are interdependent in the ongoing experience of learners. In order to better understand the experience of interest, future research will have to consider theories and methods that examine the dynamic aspects of situations and situation change. In line with a renewed interest and increasing attention to the general study of situations (e.g., Rauthmann & Sherman, 2015), there are more and more forthcoming studies that treat interest as a state- and situation-dependent phenomenon by applying repeated and *in situ* measurement (e.g., Ainley, 2006; Tanaka & Murayama, 2014). Using data-analytic procedures that allow the study of interest fluctuations at the within-person level, future research may provide an even richer description of the situational nature of interest.

Interest as a Trait-Like Concept

An individual interest approach focuses on individuals' enduring preferences for and a predisposition to reengage in particular activities or domains. Individual interest differs from other motivational concepts because it always refers to a *particular* person–object relation. In other words, one is always interested *in something*. The person–object theory of interest (Krapp, 2002) conceives of individual interest as an object-specific and trait-like variable that varies between persons but is relatively stable across time and across contexts. People differ in their interests, as some are more and some are less interested, for example, in sports, in climbing or birding, or in a particular research topic. If a person holds a particular individual interest, this is usually the outcome of a positive and long-term engagement with this content. Consider, for example, the case of researchers, who often have a long history of reading, writing, discussing, and experimenting with "personal research interests" over the course of months, years, and decades. Since such a deep and repeated engagement is required and longer periods of time are necessary, individuals usually possess a limited number of well-developed interests but always have the potential for more, as circumstances change (Hofer, 2010). Most of the time, but not always, people are reflectively aware of and identified with their individual interests, and are able specify them. Many researchers, for example, highlight their set of interests usually in "personal research interest sections" or additionally in an "other interests or hobby sections" on their websites or curricula vitae (CVs). Such a reflective awareness puts learners in a position to pursue their interests actively by seeking out the best opportunities for further development (Renninger & Su, 2012).

Individual interests are stable, trait-like concepts that do not simply derive from repeated and long-term engagement but are also used to explain people's choices and activities. If people have the opportunity to decide how to spend their time without any constraints, we would expect them to consistently choose activities related to their individual interests over other activities. In several studies with college students (Harackiewicz, Barron, Tauer, Carter, & Elliot, 2000; Harackiewicz, Barron, Tauer, & Elliot, 2002; Harackiewicz et al., 2008), for example, it was found that interest in psychology, developed in introductory psychology courses, predicted subsequent course taking over several years, and students' choice of academic major (i.e., whether they majored in psychology or not). In this sense, individual interest has the power to consistently influence students' behaviors, their learning, as well as their momentary motivational states. Individual interest may also have a cyclic, self-affirming tendency: Initial individual interest can strengthen and deepen subsequent individual interest. For example, individual interest can act as a filter that directs attention toward some subject content that is related to it but not to other types of content. A bird-watcher might travel to different countries and see unusual birds, deepening his or her interest in birding more generally. This increases the likelihood of further engagement with that content, which in turn further develops and deepens that interest (Renninger, 2000). Entering settings and contexts with initial individual interest can predispose individuals to experience more interest during activities, which can then promote the development of subsequent individual interest in terms of a deepened connection between a person and some topic or subject (Harackiewicz et al., 2008; Linnenbrink-Garcia et al., 2012).

In terms of construct content, the robust person–object relationship, which builds the core of the individual interest concept, has been operationalized in several different ways. Here, we present the two most prominent theoretical conceptions in the interest literature: (1) interest as a two-component construct that includes positive affect and value and (2) interest as a two-component construct that includes stored value and accumulated knowledge. The first conceptualization, offered by Schiefele (2001, 2009) and Krapp (2002, 2005), identifies interest as a rather stable set of value beliefs with a close combination of affect- and value-related components. In other words, persons with a strong individual interest consistently evaluate their interest object as both enjoyable and exciting to interact with, and personally significant and therefore as one element of their stored value system. These beliefs and evaluations not only coincide but also are directly related to their interest object and therefore intrinsic in nature. According to Krapp (2002, 2005), affect- and value-related components stem from a dual regulation system, which assumes both cognitive–rational and implicit–affective control mechanisms to operate and manifest in stable beliefs. Empirical studies confirmed that these two sets of beliefs tend to be highly correlated and that their interaction supports positive outcomes such as self-regulation and performance (O'Keefe & Linnenbrink-Garcia, 2014).

Although both components are critical, the model allows individual interests to be more strongly based on either affect-related or value-related beliefs (Schiefele, 2009). For example, Frenzel, Dicke, Pekrun, and Goetz (2012) observed a qualitative temporal shift from a more affect-based notion of interest to a more value-based notion of interest during adolescence. The shift occurred over the course of five school years (grades 5–9) for the students' interest in mathematics. The authors concluded that, "younger students tend to predominantly associate positive emotional experiences with the phenomenon of being interested, whereas older students appear to become increasingly aware that being interested also involves the desire to learn more and autonomously choose to reengage in the respective domain" (p. 1078). The theoretical model is flexible and allows for some differences in the configuration of the construct content in terms of more value-related and more affect-related interests, but this adds psychometric complexity. However, these results suggest that it is critically important to examine the structure of interest through a developmental lens.

The second conceptualization of individual interest was developed by Renninger and Hidi (Hidi & Renninger, 2006; Renninger, 2000, 2009; Renninger & Hidi, 2016). Like Krapp (2002, 2005) and Schiefele (2001, 2009), they conceive of individual interest as a multifaceted construct. In their conception, however, individual interest combines stored value and accumulated discourse knowledge as major components. According to this perspective, people with an individual interest have more stored value and more knowledge accumulated for their domain of interest than for other domains or activities in which they are involved. In particular, Renninger (2000, 2009) emphasized the centrality of high levels of stored domain knowledge as an important quality of individual interest. The "knowledge" component refers to a person's developing understanding of the procedures and discourse knowledge of particular activities or ideas. The individual who is interested in climbing, for example, develops climbing skills over time and learns more about different places to climb. This interest emerges in relation to the kind of questioning a person undertakes with respect to particular subject content. The driving forces for knowledge accumulation are so-called "curiosity questions" that are rooted in already existing knowledge and energize people to further explore content and learn about previously unknown aspects of the domain. This in turn supports the continued development of interest.

Considered together, these two conceptualizations of individual interest highlight the three critical components of positive affect, stored value, and stored knowledge. All of these components play an important role in the development and maintenance of interest (Hidi & Renninger, 2006) and might therefore be considered in the operationalization of the construct. However, it is difficult to include all three components psychometrically because stored knowledge is not typically assessed with self-report measures. In order to avoid complications associated with integrating knowledge measures (see Schiefele, 2009), an operationalization of individual interest can include indicators of content-specific, knowledge-seeking intentions or behaviors that are concerned with deepening knowledge and adding new ideas to one's repertoire (Knogler et al., 2015; Krapp & Prenzel, 2011).

Interest Development: From Situation to Disposition

From very early on, the idea that interest develops, and can be helped to develop, was as important as the positive consequences that were thought to be associated with the experience of interest (Dewey, 1913). Since then, theorists have frequently stressed that interest is a variable with a strong developmental character (e.g., Krapp, 2002; Renninger & Hidi, 2016). Indeed, interest development has become the major focus of current interest research (Renninger & Su, 2012). Models of interest development typically take a positive view on development and describe both the possibilities of people forming new interests and the process of how an interest grows and deepens over time as a result of ongoing engagement with particular content. At the same time, theorists consider the case that, as frequently observed in everyday life, interest development can come to a halt, or that a particular interest might regress or fall off without adequate support (Hidi & Renninger, 2006).

As with any relational variable, the developmental trajectory becomes a question about the extent to which the characteristics of the learning environment fit with the characteristics of the learner (Renninger & Su, 2012). This is true throughout the developmental continuum. Therefore, research on interest development addresses questions about internal and external factors, as well as how their interaction affects the development and deepening of interest. On the one hand, individuals' characteristics and their particular strengths and needs have been identified as important determinants for interest development. Demographic variables such as age (Frenzel et al., 2012), gender (Häussler & Hoffmann, 2000; Gilmartin, Li, & Aschbacher, 2006), and socioeconomic status (Aschbacher, Li, & Roth, 2010; Harackiewicz, Canning, et al., 2014) have been shown to influence interest development, as well as psychological variables such as prior interest (Durik & Harackiewicz, 2007; Harackiewicz et al., 2008), prior knowledge (Alexander & Jetton, 1996) and self-concept (Durik, Schechter, Noh, Rozek, & Harackiewicz, 2015; Marsh, Trautwein, Lüdtke, Köller, & Baumert, 2005). On the other hand, it has been shown that, regardless of how well developed a person's interest may be and however independent learners have become, the interest experience is not exclusively self-sustained, but requires an appropriate environment that supports or at least allows people to pursue their interests (Renninger & Hidi, 2011).

According to Krapp and colleagues (1992), the process of interest development starts with situational interest and a single, situation-specific person–object relationship (e.g., hearing about supernovas for the first time). When people move further in their development of interest, this situational frame is blurred, and over time, this connection gains stability and strength, such that dispositional individual interest refers to a person–object relationship with a high level of stability across situations and contexts (e.g., strong interest in astronomy) (Renninger, 2009). Coinciding with changes in stability, the development from situational interest to dispositional individual interest is also marked by an underlying shift in the locus of control. Whereas a situational interest is primarily caused by factors external to the individual (e.g., a TV show about supernovas), individual interest stems from internal factors. Thus, interest development refers to two fundamental processes: a strengthening of the tendency to reengage content and an increase in the independence from external support.

Hidi and Renninger (2006) have framed this process of a continually evolving person–object relationship in terms of four distinct and sequential phases. In order for interest to develop, it first needs to be elicited by external factors in a given situation. This first phase is referred to as *triggered situational interest*. If tasks and content are perceived to be meaningful and involving, interest development may enter its second phase of *maintained situational interest*. If maintained interest endures beyond the particular situation and is associated with the accumulation of knowledge, it may develop into *emerging individual interest* and thereby enter its third phase (Harackiewicz et al., 2008). Given that knowledge and stored value increase further, learners may eventually enter the fourth phase of *well-developed individual interest*. Hidi and Renninger argued that with this development comes a qualitative change from what may be considered primarily an emotion at the initial triggering of situational interest to a greater emphasis on cognitive components in later phases. Moreover, as interest deepens across these four phases, individuals develop an increasing metacognitive awareness of their own interest (Renninger & Hidi, 2016).

A main contention of the four-phase model of interest development is that interest development is sequential, and that this sequence can be disrupted at any time. This also implies that interest development can go dormant. Whether development continues will depend on not only the person but also on the possibilities and opportunities provided by the environment. Interests that are piqued by situational factors but not supported in subsequent situations may become dormant, and interests can be abandoned at any stage of development if situations do not afford support and continued stimulation. In the following section, we highlight recent research that examines how interest can be promoted in educational contexts.

PROMOTING INTEREST IN EDUCATIONAL CONTEXTS

Educators and policymakers have called on motivational researchers to align the agenda of advancing motivational theories with use of research to make a difference in educational contexts (Harackiewicz, Smith, & Priniski, 2016; Kaplan, Katz, & Flum, 2012; Pintrich, 2003; Turner, 2010). To promote this aim, researchers suggested amplifying efforts to investigate motivation in ecological contexts, as well as developing and testing interventions as a means to address critical challenges in student motivation (Harackiewicz, Tibbetts, Canning, & Hyde, 2014; Tibbetts, Harackiewicz, Priniski, & Canning, 2016; Walton, 2014). The major challenge related to interest and intrinsic motivation pertains to the question of how best to support individuals in developing and solidifying their interests in certain areas, as well as how to help learners to become interested and identify with critical subject content, so that they can harness all the potential benefits of interest as they confront challenging courses.

Interest as an energizer of task-related behavior is relevant in almost every teaching and learning context (Schunk et al., 2010) because students become more engaged and learn more when they are interested in the topic. Yet research may be particularly needed in academic domains that many students do not find interesting or in which they typically lose interest as they progress through formal education. For example, there is considerable evidence documenting a decline of students' academic interest in middle school and high school, particularly in science education and science, technology, engineering, and math (STEM) subjects (e.g., Eccles et al., 1993; Krapp & Prenzel, 2011; Renninger, Nieswandt, & Hidi, 2015). Theorists have highlighted general developmental trends, such as age-related changes, as explanations for this decline, especially during the transitions from primary to secondary levels of education. Moreover, concerns have been voiced about the way that science, technology, and mathematics are taught in school (Tröbst, Kleickmann, Lange-Schubert, Rothkopf, & Möller, 2016). Instructional practices often seem to fail to actively engage students (Seidel & Prenzel, 2006). Most critically, there seems to be a large gap between what schools offer and what students value, prefer, and are interested in (Brophy, 2008; Potvin & Hasni, 2014). Thus, there is a great potential for changes in instructional practices based on insights from interest research to help counteract these downward trends.

In the following sections we consider three general avenues for intervention, all of which are guided by interest theory and target motivational processes and, in turn, educational outcomes. As highlighted earlier, effective support for interest development may also depend on a learner's phase of interest and variability in other learner characteristics. From an interest theory perspective that emphasizes the match between personal preferences and opportunities provided by the environment, we suggest two general and complementary avenues for intervention (see also Pintrich, 2003):

1. Build on existing individual interest: Provide content material and tasks designed to facilitate the connection of academic content to be learned with already existing interests.
2. Generate situational interest: Provide stimulating tasks, activities, and materials that use universal structural features (i.e., problems, challenges) in order to trigger and maintain situational interest for all students.

Build on Existing Individual Interest: Personalized Instruction

The individual interest approach to cultivating interest emphasizes students' individual preferences as a basis for frequent reengagement. To cultivate the development of interest, this approach promotes building on individual learner characteristics, especially the current interests of the student population. Researchers seek to capitalize on the active role of individual interest in the coregulation of person-in-context experiences of interest by increasing the fit between content and learners' individual interests. Of course, efforts in this direction would not seem worthwhile or even necessary if curricula and the content of lessons were already largely aligned with students' interests. However, it has frequently been pointed out that a core problem with today's schools and curricula is that academic content is not often a good fit with students' individual interests (Baram-Tsabari, 2015; Baumert & Köller, 1998; Harackiewicz et al., 2016). Indeed, many students pursue their most cherished individual interests outside of school (Bergin, 1999; Hofer, 2010).

To build learning environments around existing interests could represent an easy fix for educators, as connections to content do not have to be created from scratch, and the positive effects of individual interest on motivation and performance have been amply demonstrated (Renninger & Hidi, 2011). However, this approach may not be practical for instructors of large classes given the unpredictability and heterogeneity of individual interests among diverse students. Indeed, researchers and practitioners alike have noted that it seems rather challenging and time consuming to cater simultaneously to the personal interests of a heterogeneous group of students (e.g., in a classroom), if students differ significantly in terms of their interests and motivational characteristics for various school tasks (Harackiewicz et al., 2016; Hidi, 2000). Furthermore, curricula are standardized and formally restricted, and often provide narrow guidelines regarding content to be studied, which might not support adaptation to students' interests.

However, thanks to the recent shift from input- to output-driven education, which now provides competence-based learning goals instead of precise content for input, teachers are granted more flexibility as to what specific content to choose for competence-based instruction (Organization for Economic Cooperation and Development [OECD], 2007). For example, in current science curricula, the competence of creating a scientifically sound argument is most relevant (Osborne, 2010). Such a competence-based goal, however, does not overly determine particular content. Thus, teachers are free to choose science topics and instructional strategies that can be more aligned with students' interests and their everyday life. Moreover, this increasing flexibility also comes at a time when advanced technology systems and learning technologies can provide feasible and scalable solutions for tailoring instruction to learners' needs and interests (Collins & Halverson, 2009).

A possible way to facilitate connections between learners and content that is based on individual interest is use of adaptive approaches to instruction such as *context personalization*. The practice of context personalization refers to matching instructional tasks or educational content with characters, objects, and themes of students' out-of-school interests (Cordova & Lepper, 1996; Høgheim & Reber, 2015; Walkington & Bernacki, 2014). For example, in a physics class, a learner interested in extreme sports might be given a task that involves parachutes and skydiving to learn about the concept of gravity and air resistance (see Palmer, 2009). The same learner could be given reading assignments based on texts related to extreme sports in English or foreign language classes to extend his or her vocabulary and practice communication skills. Thus, even though there are content constraints about what students are expected to learn, there is flexibility in terms of the choice of context in which this content is embedded. Choosing contexts that relates to students' interests connects new content and tasks to learner's preexisting individual

interests. The positive effects associated with individual interest for learning are hypothesized to transfer onto new content and to foster learners' experience of interest and, in turn, performance.

Evidence from experimental research suggests that context personalization strategies are effective in fostering interest, effort, and performance. In an earlier study (Cordova & Lepper, 1996) with elementary students, individualized information related to students' backgrounds and interests was inserted in a computer game using arithmetic. Compared to students in nonpersonalized conditions, this led to higher gains in students' intrinsic motivation, involvement, and learning. A recent review of studies on context personalization (see Walkington & Bernacki, 2014) confirmed these early findings. Studies in middle and high school mathematics indicated that learners adopt more positive attitudes toward personalized rather than generic material. Students displayed more effort and continued to perform better on personalized tasks compared to a control group, even after personalization had been removed (Walkington, 2013). These positive effects were most pronounced in students struggling with mathematics (Walkington, 2013) and among learners with low individual interest (Høgheim & Reber, 2015; Renninger, Ewen, & Lasher, 2002). In line with Durik and Harackiewicz (2007), these studies suggest that context personalization interventions could be particularly useful in supporting less engaged learners who begin a task with lower levels of interest. Studies also suggested that the provision of task choice could further enhance these positive effects, possibly through further increasing the match between learners' interests and their interest-related choices in the learning environment (Cordova & Lepper, 1996; Høgheim & Reber, 2015; Palmer, 2009; Patall, 2013).

Theoretical mechanisms used to explain these findings are anchored in interest theory. In line with other findings that indicate individual interest in academic content can act as a resource for learning (e.g., Knogler et al., 2015; Tsai et al., 2008), the success of these context manipulations is attributed to the potential of learners' individual interest to influence momentary instructional experiences and, in turn, learning outcomes. More specifically, context personalization can support learner motivation, as well as further knowledge acquisition through mechanisms that build on positive affect, perceived value, and accumulated knowledge as the three core components of individual interest. First, tasks and material that connect to a learner's individual interest are more likely to elicit an immediate positive affective reaction, which may or may not translate into more maintained states of interest. Second, existing amounts of stored value can enhance perceptions of value for the task, which have been shown both to trigger and maintain student's interest (Hulleman, Godes, Hendricks & Harackiewicz, 2010). Third, learners interested in a subject area such as extreme sports or astronomy are likely to have accumulated some prior knowledge that can act as a catalyst for further knowledge development in this content domain. In conclusion, all three of these mechanisms operating in tandem may prove to be a powerful combination to ground new content effectively in existing affective and cognitive structures, so that they become easier to identify with and to grasp. As only a few studies have addressed these issues so far, the field of context personalization awaits further research that also considers different kinds of interventions.

To provide better orientation and to foster systematic research in this area, Walkington and Bernacki (2014) have recently classified context personalization interventions along three dimensions: depth, grain size, and ownership. *Depth* refers to the quality of the connections to learners' existing interests established by the intervention. Here, interventions range from simple insertions of surface-level information about students' interests (e.g., one's favorite movie) to very elaborate contextualized tasks that are deeply embedded in students' interests. *Grain size* refers to the size of the reference group and differentiates between tasks that are tailored to the interest of an individual learner or to certain groups of learners, such as a particular school class or a certain age group. *Ownership* addresses the fact that different people can personalize context and therefore own the process. Although personalization might typically be considered to be the territory of teachers and curriculum designers, learners have also been successfully encouraged to personalize context for themselves by reflecting on content and its relevance to their own lives (Harackiewicz, Canning, Tibbetts, Priniski, & Hyde, 2016; Hulleman & Harackiewicz, 2009; Hulleman et al., 2010; Yeager et al., 2014). Moreover, research suggests that the self-generation of value statements is more powerful than learning about value connections from other individuals (Canning & Harackiewicz, 2015), supporting the ownership idea. We discuss these utility–value interventions below.

Further research on personalization strategies will need to clarify which combinations of these criteria make the most effective interventions that harness the potential of personalization in fostering important learning outcomes. The easy access to modern computer technology, such as intelligent tutoring systems, offers many, perfectly scalable ways both to assess students' individual interests and sophisticated methodologies for personalizing instruction. Thus, digital technology significantly lowers the implementation threshold for effectively personalizing interventions, and this can support them in becoming a standard feature of interest-based STEM education.

Generating Situational Interest

Utility-Value Interventions

Keeping students interested in their courses is crucial to their academic success. One way to develop interest in activities is to help students find meaning and value in those activities (Harackiewicz & Hulleman, 2010; Harackiewicz et al., 2016), and one type of task value that has proven to be a powerful predictor of interest, effort, and performance is *utility value*. People find utility value in a task if they believe it is useful and relevant beyond the immediate situation, for other tasks or aspects of their life (e.g., "This material will be important when I shop for healthy food"). Recent experimental research indicates that it is possible to promote perceived utility value with simple interventions that ask students to write about the relevance of course topics to their own lives or to the life of a family member or close friend.

The utility-value intervention (UVI) is based in expectancy–value and interest theory. According to Eccles's expectancy–value theory, a person chooses to take on a challenging task—such as persisting in a college biology course or choosing to major in biology—if the person (1) values the task, and (2) expects that he or she can succeed at the task (based on self-beliefs). Beliefs about the self and beliefs about the value of the task are both critically important in predicting interest, course choices, persistence, and choice of a major. In Eccles's model, task value has several components, including intrinsic value (the enjoyment an individual experiences from performing a task), attainment value (the personal importance of doing well on a task), and utility value (how useful or relevant the task is in terms of the individual's future plans). Intrinsic value is, of course, closely aligned with situational interest, and there are many interesting overlaps between expectancy–value and interest theories. The UVI focuses on utility value, however, because it is the task value most amenable to external influence and intervention (Harackiewicz & Hulleman, 2010). In other words, educators may be able to influence students' perceptions of utility value (UV) with simple interventions, and these perceptions of utility may in turn promote interest development.

Extensive experimental and longitudinal survey studies have documented the importance of both expectancy (e.g., confidence) and value-related beliefs (perceptions of usefulness and personal relevance). The perceived value of any academic course is influenced by how closely it relates to the student's identity and both short- and long-term goals (Eccles, 2009). When a student says, "I can do science, but I don't want to," such a choice likely reflects a relatively low perceived value of science. When students do perceive value in course topics, however, they develop greater interest in the course, work harder, perform better, persist longer, and are more likely to take additional courses and complete their degree programs (Harackiewicz et al., 2008; Hulleman et al., 2008; Wigfield, 1994). Educators can influence students' perceptions of UV in science

courses using writing activities focused on course content. The UVI works by changing how students think about academic topics. On their own and in their own terms, students generate connections between course topics and their lives—helping them appreciate the value of their coursework and promoting a deeper level of engagement. Thus, the externally administered UVI may help students relate course material to their own interests. As such, the UVI represents a combination of the two approaches to promoting interest: It may spark situational interest in a topic, and it may help students connect that topic to their own interests, which can build on individual interest.

Laboratory studies have demonstrated that self-generated UV information (as produced by the UVI) is much more powerful than externally provided UV information (e.g., as might be produced when teachers tell students that material is important and relevant) in promoting interest and performance (Canning & Harackiewicz, 2015; Durik et al., 2015). The key is having students actively work to find the value for themselves. The efficacy of this approach for promoting perceived UV, interest, and performance has been demonstrated in ninth-grade science and undergraduate introductory psychology, with the strongest benefits for students with low confidence or lower levels of performance (Hulleman & Harackiewicz, 2009; Hulleman et al., 2010). More recently, Harackiewicz, Canning, Tibbetts, Priniski, and Hyde (2016) documented the potential of the UVI to close achievement gaps for first-generation and underrepresented minority students in college biology courses. In addition, Harackiewicz, Rozek, Hulleman, and Hyde (2012) found that a UVI that targeted the parents of high school students led the students to take, on average, an extra semester of math or science in their last 2 years of high school.

According to interest theory, being interested in an activity motivates us to pursue activities and careers. Interest may be triggered by UVIs, then develop further as the individual experiences positive feelings and comes to value an activity. By integrating expectancy–value and interest theories, we propose two ways that UV can influence interest, motivation, and persistence in academic contexts. First, perceiving UV in a course can directly influence interest and subsequent course enrollment choices because of the importance of these courses for future goals. Second, perceiving UV in courses can influence subsequent course choices and career decisions through the process of interest development; that is, perceiving value in courses can promote deeper interest in the topic, and interest may be the more proximal motivator of career decisions. Thus, interest may be a pathway through which UVIs influence motivation and performance (Harackiewicz et al., 2016).

Problem-Based Instruction

A situational approach to cultivating interest views interest as a situated and malleable construct that offers a great potential for change and influence in features of the environment. In educational settings, this view highlights the importance of creating a stimulating learning environment in which students are supported in connecting to content, especially when the content is not related to their preferences and existing interests. The situational approach acknowledges that educators do not have influence over students' incoming individual interest, yet they do have influence over students' situational interest as a short-term response to the learning environment they create, for example, during a particular lesson. Furthermore, if continued situational support is provided, initial situational interest may develop beyond situational confines and support long-term interest development in a domain (Chen et al., 2016).

Situational interest and its antecedents have been extensively studied in the context of text comprehension, which has demonstrated, among other things, that readers are interested in texts that include surprising, novel, or unusual elements and text features such as personal relevance, coherence, and vividness (Ainley et al., 2002; Schraw & Lehman, 2001). Following Mitchell's (1993) seminal study in the mathematics classroom, the focus of this research has broadened recently, and more studies are forthcoming that analyze activities and tasks that generate interest in any learning environment for many individuals (see Renninger &

Hidi, 2011, for a review). Researchers have investigated various instructional practices and their potential role in fostering interest. For the context of STEM education, a recent review (Potvin & Hasni, 2014) identified problem- and inquiry-based approaches to instruction as very effective in fostering interest and learning. Using interest theory as a framework for modeling motivational dynamics, researchers have used problem-based learning environments to analyze the promotion and maintenance of interest (Belland, Kim, & Hannafin, 2013; Palmer, 2009; Rotgans & Schmidt, 2011, 2014; Schmidt, Rotgans, & Yew, 2011; Wijnia, Loyens, & Derous, 2011; Wijnia, Loyens, Derous, & Schmidt, 2014).

Problem-based learning has been defined as "an instructional method that initiates students' learning by creating a need to solve an authentic problem" (Hung, Jonassen, & Liu, 2007, p. 486). From an interest theory perspective, problems are a means to stimulate curiosity questions that in later phases of interest development are activated from within the person and represent a core mechanism for extending and solidifying his or her interests (Renninger & Su, 2012). Compared to the previously discussed individual interest approach, which taps into individual interest and an associated fund of knowledge as a resource, a problem-based approach signals to learners that they *lack* some critical knowledge. This can be an effective trigger for situational interest and stimulate initial engagement with a certain task or domain (Berlyne, 1970; Rotgans & Schmidt, 2014). Since there is no immediate answer for many problems, learners are required to figure out what is unknown to them or to reorganize what they have understood to date. In this sense, situational interest can play an important role in energizing the acquisition of knowledge (Rotgans & Schmidt, 2011).

Recently, Rotgans and Schmidt (2014) suggested that learning materials are effective at eliciting situational interest in all learners when they confront learners with an intriguing problem. In several studies, they used history problems and asked secondary students from Singapore why the Japanese were able to conquer the island during the World War II, despite the fact that they were highly outnumbered by the Allied Forces. This problem initially triggered students' situational interest, and their mean levels of interest were significantly higher after problem presentation than before. Students were then provided reading material that contained relevant information to resolve the problem. After reading the text, students' situational interest decreased again. This pattern was only found if students did not know the solution beforehand and if they were aware of their deficit. Rotgans and Schmidt explained their results with a knowledge deprivation mechanism that construes situational interest as arising from a perceived gap between what students know and what they need or want to know (Schmidt et al., 2011). Initially, problems can create this gap and in turn stimulate situational interest. Subsequently, as students gain relevant knowledge while working to solve the problem, they close the gap, which again reduces their levels of situational interest (Rotgans & Schmidt, 2011, 2014). According to this research, problem-based learning environments appear to be a reliable way to generate situational interest with the presentation of challenging problems. However, the findings also suggest that problems may be a rather temporary stimulus, not necessarily leading to repeated engagement, as students' interest steadily decreases once they start working on and solving the problem. Moreover, these findings may not generalize across all types of problems.

In previous research on problem-based learning, learning outcomes also depended on the type of problem used. In their meta-analysis, Walker and Leary (2009) found complex and ill-structured problems to be more effective with regard to student learning than well-structured problems. As Rotgans and Schmidt had focused their investigations on problems belonging to the latter category (Jonassen, 2011), Knogler, Gröschner, and Lewalter (2016) tested a complex problem and its capacity to foster students' situational interest. In line with the knowledge deprivation hypothesis, they assumed complex problems to be more effective in stimulating situational interest. They argued that even though learners may gain relevant knowledge while investigating a complex problem (e.g., climate change), the problem cannot be solved as straightforwardly as simple problems; instead, complex problems are evolving in nature and gradually reveal additional layers of complexity. These create newly emerging knowledge gaps as learners acquire a deeper understanding while they continue to investigate und develop solutions (Jonassen, 2011).

In their study, Knogler and colleagues (2016) presented to secondary students a problem scenario in which they had to negotiate a solution for the energy supply of a rural district that wanted to shift from nuclear power to renewable sources. The students were then engaged in collaborative problem solving over the course of 15 lessons, exploring and discussing different solutions and their limitations. Repeated measures of situational interest indicated a developmental pattern whereby situational interest was stimulated not just once but repeatedly. In post hoc interviews, students frequently referred to the experience of novelty and the ability to expand their knowledge in the face of novel information as subjective cause for higher levels of situational interest during complex problem solving (see also Palmer, 2009). This confirmed the assumption that a more complex problem structure holds more potential for the continuing perception of knowledge gaps or opportunities to learn compared to well-structured problems with a single gap. In addition to knowledge-based mechanisms, rich and complex problem-based learning environments also feature a rich array of other contextual stimuli, such as perceived autonomy or social relatedness supportive of situational interest (Krapp, 2005). Thus, problem-based learning environments may be particularly well suited to support situational interest as they offer challenging problems and an engaging set of learning activities. Additional research can help to further unleash this potential and identify effective problem structures or scaffolding strategies that optimally support learners in confronting these problems (Belland et al., 2013).

This line of research is relevant for STEM education because science offers many intriguing and complex problems. To leverage their potential for a more interest-based STEM education, teachers and curriculum designers would need to create more learning environments based on problems. Such an effort would also be in line with recent reforms that promote inquiry-based teaching and problem-based learning together with crosscutting themes and core ideas for science education.

CONCLUSION

A careful consideration of the nature of interest, whether conceptualized as an individual-difference variable, a situational process, a developmental trajectory, an educational outcome, or, as we have argued here, all of these combined, affords insight into important motivational processes. The theoretical and empirical progress to date has yielded several promising directions for intervention in educational contexts. By analyzing the malleable and more stable aspects of interest, we can design interventions that spark the development of new interests or support the further development of existing interests that can shape students' academic trajectories.

REFERENCES

Ainley, M. (2006). Connecting with learning: Motivation, affect and cognition in interest processes. *Educational Psychological Review, 18,* 391–405.

Ainley, M., & Hidi, S. (2002). Dynamic measures for studying interest and learning. In P. R. Pintrich & M. L. Maehr (Eds.), *Advances in motivation and achievement: New directions in measures and methods* (Vol. 12, pp. 43–76) Amsterdam, The Netherlands: JAI Press.

Ainley, M., Hidi, S., & Berndorff, D. (2002). Interest, learning, and the psychological processes that mediate their relationship. *Journal of Educational Psychology, 94,* 545–561.

Alexander, P. A., & Jetton, T. L. (1996). The role of importance and interest in the processing of text. *Educational Psychology Review, 8,* 89–121.

Aschbacher, P. R., Li, E., & Roth, E. J. (2010). Is science me?: High school students' identities, participation and aspirations in science, engineering, and medicine. *Journal of Research in Science Teaching, 47,* 564–582.

Baram-Tsabari, A. (2015). Promoting information seeking and questioning in science. In K.

A. Renninger, M. Nieswandt, & S. Hidi (Eds.), *Interest in mathematics and science learning* (pp. 135–152). Washington, DC: American Educational Research Association.

Baumert, J., & Köller, O. (1998). Interest research in secondary level I: An overview. In L. Hoffmann, A. Krapp, K. A. Renninger, & J. Baumert (Eds.), *Interest and learning: Proceedings of the Seeon Conference on Interest and Gender* (pp. 241–256). Kiel, Germany: IPN.

Belland, B. R., Kim, C., & Hannafin, M. J. (2013). A framework for designing scaffolds that improve motivation and cognition. *Educational Psychologist, 48,* 243–270.

Bergin, D. A. (1999). Influences on classroom interest. *Educational Psychologist, 34,* 87–98.

Berlyne, D. E. (1970). Novelty, complexity, and hedonic value. *Perception and Psychophysics, 8,* 279–286.

Brophy, J. (2008). Developing students' appreciation for what is taught in school. *Educational Psychologist, 43,* 132–141.

Canning, E. A., & Harackiewicz, J. M. (2015). Teach it, don't preach it: The differential effects of directly-communicated and self-generated utility value information. *Motivation Science, 1,* 47–71.

Cerasoli, C. P., Nicklin, J. M., & Ford, M. T. (2014). Intrinsic motivation and extrinsic incentives jointly predict performance: A 40-year meta-analysis. *Psychological Bulletin, 140,* 980–1008.

Chen, J. A., Tutwiler, M. S., Metcalf, S. J., Kamarainen, A., Grotzer, T., & Dede, C. (2016). A multi-user virtual environment to support students' self-efficacy and interest in science: A latent growth model analysis. *Learning and Instruction, 41,* 11–22.

Collins, A., & Halverson, R. (2009). *Rethinking education in the age of technology: The digital revolution and schooling in America.* New York: Teachers College Press.

Cordova, D. I., & Lepper, M. R. (1996). Intrinsic motivation and the process of learning: Beneficial effects of contextualization, personalization, and choice. *Journal of Personality and Social Psychology, 88,* 715–730.

Csikszentmihalyi, M. (2013). *Flow: The psychology of happiness.* New York: Random House.

Deci, E., & Ryan, R. (1985). *Intrinsic motivation and self-determination in human behavior.* New York: Pantheon.

Deci, E. L. (1992). The relation of interest to the motivation of behavior: A self-determination theory perspective. In K. A. Renninger, S. Hidi, & A. Krapp (Eds.), *The role of interest in learning and development* (pp. 43–71). Hillsdale, NJ: Erlbaum.

Dewey, J. (1913). *Interest and effort in education.* New York: Houghton Mifflin.

Durik, A. M., & Harackiewicz, J. M. (2007). Different strokes for different folks: How individual interest moderates the effects of situational factors on task interest. *Journal of Educational Psychology, 99,* 597–610.

Durik, A. M., Hulleman, C. S., & Harackiewicz, J. M. (2015). One size fits some: Instructional enhancements to promote interest don't work the same for everyone. In K. A. Renninger, M. Nieswandt, & S. Hidi (Eds.), *Interest in mathematics and science learning* (pp. 49–62). Washington, DC: American Educational Research Association.

Durik, A. M., Shechter, O., Noh, M. S., Rozek, C. S., & Harackiewicz, J. M. (2015). What if I can't?: Perceived competence as a moderator of the effects of utility value information on situational interest and performance. *Motivation and Emotion, 39,* 104–118.

Dweck, C. (2006). *Mindset: The new psychology of success.* New York: Random House.

Eccles, J. S. (2009). Who am I and what am I going to do with my life?: Personal and collective identities as motivators of action. *Educational Psychologist, 44,* 78–89.

Eccles, J. S., Midgley, C., Wigfield, A., Buchanan, C. M., Reuman, D., Flanagan, C., et al. (1993). Development during adolescence: The impact of stage-environment fit on young adolecents' experiences in schools and families. *American Psychologist, 48,* 90–101.

Flowerday, T., Schraw, G., & Stevens, J. (2004). The role of choice and interest in reader engagement. *Journal of Experimental Education, 72,* 93–114.

Frenzel, A. C., Dicke, A. L., Pekrun, R., & Goetz, T. (2012). Beyond quantitative decline: Conceptual shifts in adolescents' development of interest in mathematics. *Developmental Psychology, 48,* 1069–1082.

Geiser, C., & Lockhart, G. (2012). A comparison of four approaches to account for method effects in latent state–trait analyses. *Psychological Methods, 17,* 255–283.

Gilmartin, S. K., Li, E., & Aschbacher, P. (2006). The relationship between interest in physical science/engineering, science class experiences, and family contexts: Variations by gender and race/ethnicity among secondary students. *Journal of Women and Minorities in Science and Engineering, 12,* 179–207.

Goldberg, L. R. (1990). An alternative "description of personality": The big-five factor structure. *Journal of Personality and Social Psychology, 59,* 1216–1229.

Grossnickle, E. M. (2016). Disentangling curiosity: Dimensionality, definitions, and distinctions from interest in educational contexts. *Educational Psychology Review, 28*(1), 23–60.

Harackiewicz, J. M., Barron, K. E., Carter, S. M., Lehto, A. T., & Elliot, A. J. (1997). Predictors and consequences of achievement goals in the college classroom: Maintaining interest and making the grade. *Journal of Personality and Social Psychology, 73,* 1284–1295.

Harackiewicz, J. M., Barron, K. E., Tauer, J. M., Carter, S. M., & Elliot, A. J. (2000). Short-term and long-term consequences of achievement goals: Predicting interest and performance over time. *Journal of Educational Psychology, 92,* 316–330.

Harackiewicz, J. M., Barron, K. E., Tauer, J. M., & Elliot, A. J. (2002). Predicting success in college: A longitudinal study of achievement goals and ability measures as predictors of interest and performance from freshman year through graduation. *Journal of Educational Psychology, 94,* 562–575.

Harackiewicz, J. M., Canning, E. A., Tibbetts, Y., Giffen, C. J., Blair, S. S., Rouse, D. I., et al. (2014). Closing the social class achievement gap for first-generation students in undergraduate biology. *Journal of Educational Psychology, 106,* 375–389.

Harackiewicz, J. M., Canning, E. A., Tibbetts, Y., Priniski, S. J., & Hyde, J. S. (2016). Closing achievement gaps with a utility-value intervention: Disentangling race and social class. *Journal of Personality and Social Psychology, 111,* 745–765.

Harackiewicz, J. M., Durik, A. M., Barron, K. E., Linnenbrink-Garcia, L., & Tauer, J. M. (2008). The role of achievement goals in the development of interest: Reciprocal relations between achievement goals, interest, and performance. *Journal of Educational Psychology, 100,* 105–122.

Harackiewicz, J. M., & Hulleman, C. S. (2010). The importance of interest: The role of achievement goals and task values in promoting the development of interest. *Social and Personality Psychology Compass, 4,* 42–52.

Harackiewicz, J. M., Rozek, C. S., Hulleman, C. S., & Hyde, J. S. (2012). Helping parents to motivate adolescents in mathematics and science: An experimental test of a utility-value intervention. *Psychological Science, 43,* 899–906.

Harackiewicz, J. M., Smith, J. L., & Priniski, S. J. (2016). Interest matters: The importance of promoting interest in education. *Policy Insights from the Behavioral and Brain Sciences, 3,* 220–227.

Harackiewicz, J. M., Tibbetts, Y., Canning, E. A., & Hyde, J. S. (2014). Harnessing values to promote motivation in education. In S. Karabenick & T. Urden (Eds.), *Advances in motivation and achievement: Vol. 18. Motivational interventions* (pp. 71–105). Bingley, UK: Emerald Group.

Häussler, P., & Hoffmann, L. (2000). A curricular frame for physics education: Development, comparison with students' interests, and impact on students' achievement and self-concept. *Science Education, 84,* 689–705.

Hidi, S. (2000). An interest researcher's perspective: The effects of extrinsic and intrinsic factors on motivation. In C. Sansone & J. M. Harackiewicz (Eds.), *Intrinsic and extrinsic motivation: The search for optimal motivation and performance* (pp. 309–339). San Diego, CA: Academic Press.

Hidi, S. (2006). Interest: A unique motivational variable. *Educational Research Review,1*(2), 69–82.

Hidi, S., & Harackiewicz, J. M. (2000). Motivating the academically unmotivated: A critical issue for the 21st century. *Review of Educational Research, 79,* 151–179.

Hidi, S., & Renninger, K. A. (2006). The four-phase model of interest development. *Educational Psychologist, 41,* 111–127.

Hofer, M. (2010). Adolescents' development of individual interests: A product of multiple goal regulation? *Educational Psychologist, 45,* 149–166.

Høgheim, S., & Reber, R. (2015). Supporting interest of middle school students in mathematics through context personalization and example choice. *Contemporary Educational Psychology, 42,* 17–25.

Hulleman, C. S., Durik, A. M., Schweigert, S. B., & Harackiewicz, J. M. (2008). Task values, achievement goals, and interest: An integrative analysis. *Journal of Educational Psychology, 100,* 398–416.

Hulleman, C. S., Godes, O., Hendricks, B. L., & Harackiewicz, J. M. (2010). Enhancing interest and performance with a utility value intervention. *Journal of Educational Psychology, 102,* 880–895.

Hulleman, C. S., & Harackiewicz, J. M. (2009). Promoting interest and performance in high school science classes. *Science, 326,* 1410–1412.

Hung, W., Jonassen, D. H., & Liu, R. (2007). Problem-based learning. In J. M. Spector, M. D. Merrill, J. V. Merrienboer, & M. P. Driscoll (Eds.), *Handbook of research on educational communications and technology* (3rd ed., pp. 485–506). New York: Routledge.

Jonassen, D. H. (2011). *Learning to solve problems: A handbook for designing problem-solving learning environments.* New York: Routledge.

Kaplan, A., Katz, I., & Flum, H. (2012). Motivation theory in educational practice: Knowledge claims, challenges, and future directions. In K. R. Harris, S. Graham, & T. C. Urdan (Eds.), *APA educational psychology handbook: Vol 2. Individual differences and cultural and contextual factors* (pp. 165–194). Washington, DC: American Psychological Association.

Knogler, M., Gröschner, A., & Lewalter, D. (2016, August). *What makes and keeps complex problem-solving interesting?* Paper presented at the International Conference on Motivation (ICM), Thessaloniki, Greece.

Knogler, M., Harackiewicz, J. M., Gegenfurtner, A., & Lewalter, D. (2015). How situational is situational interest?: Investigating the longitudinal structure of situational interest. *Contemporary Educational Psychology, 43,* 39–50.

Krapp, A. (2002). Structural and dynamic aspects of interest development: Theoretical considerations from an ontogenetic perspective. *Learning and Instruction, 13,* 383–409.

Krapp, A. (2005). Basic needs and the development of interest and intrinsic motivational orientations. *Learning and Instruction, 15,* 381–395.

Krapp, A., Hidi, S., & Renninger, K. A. (1992). Interest, learning, and development. In K. A. Renninger, S. Hidi, & A. Krapp (Eds.), *The role of interest in learning and development* (pp. 3–25). Hillsdale, NJ: Erlbaum.

Krapp, A., & Prenzel, M. (2011). Research on interest in science: Theories, methods, and findings. *International Journal of Science Education, 33,* 27–50.

Linnenbrink-Garcia, L., Durik, A. M., Conley, A. M., Barron, K. E., Tauer, J. M., Karabenick, S. A., et al. (2010). Measuring situational interest in academic domains. *Educational and Psychological Measurement, 70,* 647–671.

Linnenbrink-Garcia, L., Patall, E. A., & Messersmith, E. E. (2012). Antecedents and consequences of situational interest. *British Journal of Educational Psychology, 83,* 591–614.

Marsh, H. W., Trautwein, U., Lüdtke, O., Köller, O., & Baumert, J. (2005). Academic self-concept, interest, grades, and standardized test scores: Reciprocal effects models of causal ordering. *Child Development, 76,* 397–416.

Mitchell, M. (1993). Situational interest: Its multifaceted structure in the secondary school mathematics classroom. *Journal of Educational Psychology, 85,* 424–436.

O'Keefe, P. A., & Linnenbrink-Garcia, L. (2014). The role of interest in optimizing performance and self-regulation. *Journal of Experimental Social Psychology, 53,* 70–78.

Organisation for Economic Co-operation & Development. (2007). *PISA 2006: Science competencies for tomorrow's world.* Paris: Author.

Osborne, J. (2010). Arguing to learn in science: The role of collaborative, critical discourse. *Science, 328,* 463–466.

Palmer, D. H. (2009). Student interest generated during an inquiry skills lesson. *Journal of Research in Science Teaching, 46,* 147–165.

Patall, E. A. (2013). Constructing motivation through choice, interest, and interestingness. *Journal of Educational Psychology, 105,* 522–534.

Pintrich, P. R. (2003). A motivational science perspective on the role of student motivation in learning and teaching contexts. *Journal of Educational Psychology, 95,* 667–686.

Potvin, P., & Hasni, A. (2014). Interest, motivation and attitude towards science and technology at K–12 levels: A systematic review of 12 years of educational research. *Studies in Science Education, 50,* 85–129.

Rauthmann, J. F., & Sherman, R. A. (2015). Situation change: Stability and change of situation variables between and within persons. *Frontiers in Psychology, 6,* 1938.

Renninger, K. (2000). Individual interest and its implications for understanding intrinsic motivation. In C. Sansone & J. M. Harackiewicz (Eds.), *Intrinsic and extrinsic motivation* (pp. 373–404). New York: Academic Press.

Renninger, K. A. (2009). Interest and identity development in instruction: An inductive model. *Educational Psychologist, 44,* 105–118.

Renninger, K. A., Ewen, L., & Lasher, A. K. (2002). Individual interest as context in expository text and mathematical word problems. *Learning and Instruction, 12,* 467–490.

Renninger, K. A., & Hidi, S. (2011). Revisiting the conceptualization, measurement, and generation of interest. *Educational Psychologist, 46,* 168–184.

Renninger, K. A., & Hidi, S. (2016). *The power of interest for motivation and engagement.* New York: Routledge.

Renninger, K. A., Nieswandt, M., & Hidi, S. (Eds.). (2015). *Interest in mathematics and science learning.* Washington, DC: American Educational Research Association.

Renninger, K. A., & Su, S. (2012). Interest and its development. In R. Ryan (Ed.), *The Oxford handbook of human motivation* (pp. 167–187). Oxford, UK: Oxford University Press.

Rotgans, J. I., & Schmidt, H. G. (2011). Situational interest and academic achievement in the active-learning classroom. *Learning and Instruction, 21,* 58–67.

Rotgans, J. I., & Schmidt, H. G. (2014). Situational interest and learning: Thirst for knowledge. *Learning and Instruction, 32,* 37–50.

Ryan, R. M., & Deci, E. L. (2000). Self-determination theory and the facilitation of intrinsic motivation, social development, and well-being. *American Psychologist, 55,* 68–78.

Sansone, C., & Harackiewicz, J. M. (Eds.). (2000). *Intrinsic and extrinsic motivation: The search for optimal motivation and performance.* New York: Academic Press.

Sansone, C., & Thoman, D. B. (2005). Interest as the missing motivator in self-regulation. *European Psychologist, 10,* 175–186.

Schiefele, U. (2001). The role of interest in motivation and learning. In J. M. Collis & S. Messick (Eds.), *Intelligence and personality: Bridging the gap in theory and measurement* (pp. 163–194). Mahwah, NJ: Erlbaum.

Schiefele, U. (2009). Situational and individual interest. In K. Wentzel & A. Wigfield (Eds.), *Handbook of motivation at school* (pp. 197–222). New York: Routledge.

Schmidt, H. G., Rotgans, J. I., & Yew, E. H. (2011). The process of problem-based learning: What works and why. *Medical Education, 45,* 792–806.

Schraw, G., & Lehman, S. (2001). Situational interest: A review of literature and directions for further research. *Educational Psychological Review, 13,* 23–52.

Schunk, D. H., Pintrich, P. R., & Meece, J. L. (2010). *Motivation in education: Theory, research and application.* London: Pearson.

Seidel, T., & Prenzel, M. (2006). Stability of teaching patterns in physics instruction: Findings from a video study. *Learning and Instruction, 16,* 228–240.

Tanaka, A., & Murayama, K. (2014). Within-person analyses of situational interest and boredom: Interactions between task-specific perceptions and achievement goals. *Journal of Educational Psychology, 106,* 1122–1134.

Thoman, D. B., Smith, J. L., & Silvia, P. (2011). The resource replenishment function of interest. *Social Psychological and Personality Science, 2,* 592–599.

Tibbetts, Y., Harackiewicz, J. M., Priniski, S. J., & Canning, E. A. (2016). Broadening participation in the life sciences with social–psychological interventions. *CBE-Life Sciences Education, 15*(3), es4.

Tröbst, S., Kleickmann, T., Lange-Schubert, K., Rothkopf, A., & Möller, K. (2016). Instruction and students' declining interest in science: An analysis of German fourth- and sixth-grade classrooms. *American Educational Research Journal, 53,* 162–193.

Tsai, Y.-M., Kunter, M., Lütke, O., Trautwein, U., & Ryan, M. R. (2008). What makes lessons interesting?: The roles of situational and individual factors in three school subjects. *Journal of Educational Psychology, 100,* 460–472.

Tulis, M., & Fulmer, S. M. (2013). Students' motivational and emotional experiences and their relationship to persistence during academic challenge in mathematics and reading. *Learning and Individual Differences, 27,* 35–46.

Turner, J. C. (2010). Unfinished business: Putting motivation theory to the "Classroom Test." In S. Karabenick & T. Urdan (Eds.), *The decade ahead: Applications and contexts of motivation and achievement* (Vol. 16B, pp. 109–138). Bingley, UK: Emerald Group.

Walker, A., & Leary, H. (2009). A problem based learning meta-analysis: Differences across problem types, implementation types, disciplines, and assessment levels. *Interdisciplinary Journal of Problem-Based Learning, 3,* 12–43.

Walkington, C. A. (2013). Using adaptive learning technologies to personalize instruction to student interests: The impact of relevant contexts on performance and learning outcomes. *Journal of Educational Psychology, 105,* 932–945.

Walkington, C., & Bernacki, M. L. (2014). Motivating students by "personalizing" learning around individual interests: A consideration of theory, design, and implementation issues. *Advances in Motivation and Achievement, 18,* 139–176.

Walton, G. M. (2014). The new science of wise interventions. *Current Directions in Psychological Science, 23,* 73–82.

White, R. W. (1959). Motivation reconsidered: the concept of competence. *Psychological Review, 66,* 297–318.

Wigfield, A. (1994). Expectancy–value theory of achievement motivation: A developmental perspective. *Educational Psychology Review, 6,* 49–78.

Wijnia, L., Loyens, S. M., & Derous, E. (2011). Investigating effects of problem-based versus lecture-based learning environments on student motivation. *Contemporary Educational Psychology, 36,* 101–113.

Wijnia, L., Loyens, S. M., Derous, E., & Schmidt, H. G. (2014). Do students' topic interest and tutors' instructional style matter in problem-based learning? *Journal of Educational Psychology, 106,* 919–933.

Yeager, D. S., Henderson, M., Paunesku, D., Walton, G., Spitzer, B., D'Mello, S., et al. (2014). Boring but important: A self-transcendent purpose for learning fosters academic self-regulation. *Journal of Personality and Social Psychology, 107,* 559–580.

CHAPTER 19

On Becoming Creative

Basic Theory with Implications for the Workplace

CARSTEN K. W. DE DREU
BERNARD A. NIJSTAD

Relative to other species, humans stand out for their capacity to create and innovate, both as individuals and as groups. While other animals certainly show signs of creativity—in nest building, in mate attraction, in tool use, and even in basic forms of cultural rites and rituals (Fogarty, Creanza, & Feldman, 2015; Tomasello, Kruger, & Ratner, 1993)—these can hardly be compared to human creative achievements in arts, science, and technology. No other species travels by airplane, communicates through cellular phones, invents mechanistic theories about the entire universe, or marvels at 1,000-year-old paintings exhibited in architecturally unique museums. Clearly, then, there is something special about the human capacity for creativity.

Scientists across disciplines, the psychological sciences included, have made great advances in understanding the conditions and processes accounting for human creativity. Although creativity is sometimes treated as an attribute of a few brilliant minds, psychological science converges on the assumption that creativity is inherent to human cognitive functioning and is therefore a capacity many rather than few possess (Ward, Smith, & Finke, 1999; also see Guilford, 1950). Second, there now is growing consensus

that *creativity* can be best defined as the production of ideas, insights, products, or services that are both novel and original, and potentially useful (e.g., Amabile, 1983; Sternberg & Lubart, 1999). Thus, ideas that are very novel but not useful at all are typically considered "weird," whereas insights that are very useful but commonplace and not at all novel are considered mundane or boring (Nijstad, De Dreu, Rietzschel, & Baas, 2010; Sternberg & Lubart, 1999). As such, it is also commonly accepted that what is creative in one particular context or time may be considered weird or boring in other contexts or times—novelty and usefulness are social evaluations by producers and recipients alike. And finally, scientists agree that creative products, whether ideas, insights, or problem solutions, cannot be generated *ex nihilo* but build on existing knowledge and that, as such, creativity requires some domain-relevant knowledge and skills (Kleibeuker, De Dreu, & Crone, 2013; Nijstad & Stroebe, 2006; Weisberg, 1999).

There is less consensus about what helps or hinders creative performance. Abundant work indicates that creativity benefits from (trait- or state-based) intrinsic motivation, from positive affective states, and from approach orientation. But there is enough work also to argue that creativity benefits also, or even especially, from exogenous stressors, such as time pressure or social conflict, (trait- and state-based) anxiety and frustration, extrinsic rewards, and avoidance motivation. Here we review and integrate these and related literatures in order to achieve a nuanced understanding of what helps or, instead, hinders people in being creative. As starting point we use the dual pathway to creativity model (De Dreu, Baas, & Nijstad, 2008; Nijstad et al., 2010), which proposes that creativity can be achieved by flexibly switching not only through different approaches, categories, and perspectives (cognitive flexibility) but also through focused, systematic, and sustained effort (cognitive persistence). This model further proposes that some situational and dispositional variables affect creativity because they enhance cognitive flexibility, whereas others impact creativity primarily because they impact cognitive persistence. Accordingly, the model allows both benign situations and positive states, as well as more aversive settings and negative states, to promote creative performance.

Our second goal here is to examine the extent to which basic principles and processes identified in this model, and the research base on which it builds, can be used to understand and predict creative performance in work settings. We specifically focus on three aspects of work and organizational behavior that have already received quite a lot of attention in the research literatures, and for which good information is therefore available: employee affect, work-related constraints and opportunities, and cultural norms and practices. Throughout, we explore how workplace design and leadership can assist in reducing barriers to creative performance and/or boost employee creativity.

THE DUAL PATHWAY TO CREATIVITY MODEL

The dual pathway to creativity model (DPCM) builds on, integrates, and expands 40 years of research and theory development around creativity. These different research traditions all converges on the "four P's of creativity": person, press, process, and product (Rhodes, 1961; also see Simonton, 2003). In particular, the DPCM proposes that personality (and other individual differences) and press (situational factors) impact cognitive–motivational processes, and these processes lead to products that vary in creativity. The DPCM is graphically depicted in Figure 19.1.

Products

Creative outputs, or products, are those that are original yet potentially useful. In work settings, for example, a *creative idea or product* is defined as such by employees or supervisors who rate a colleague's idea or product as creative or not (e.g., Binnewies & Wörnlein, 2011; Eisenberger & Aselage, 2009; George & Zhou, 2001; Ohly, Sonnentag, & Pluntke, 2006).

In social and personality psychology, researchers examine creative performance on a variety of tasks. First, there are creative production tasks such as making drawings, musical improvisation, or telling stories. Domain relevant experts judge the originality and usefulness of the resulting product; a product is assumed to be creative when experts agree that is it creative (Amabile, 1982).

Second, there is performance on perceptual and conceptual insight tasks (Harkins, 2006; Kounios & Beeman, 2009). Insight problems have only one correct solution, which is not immediately apparent. An example is the Remote Associates Test (RAT; Mednick, 1962), in which participants, in a number of trials, are given three words (e.g., *club, gown, mare*) and have to find a fourth word that is associated with all of them (e.g., *night*). Another example is the Gestalt Completion Task (GCT; Ekstrom, French, Harman, & Dermen, 1976), in which participants see incompletely drawn pictures of mundane objects, and have to "see" what is depicted. In these tasks, participants need to generate solutions internally that subsequently must be tested for correctness. Finding the solution typically leads to an "a-ha experience" (Schooler & Melcher, 1995).

Third, creative production is studied with idea generation tasks. Participants are asked to generate responses to some problem.

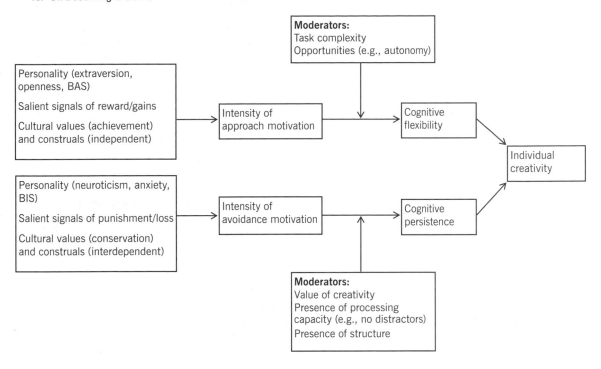

FIGURE 19.1. The DPCM and employee creativity.

Examples include unusual uses tasks (find unusual uses for a common object, such as a brick or a newspaper) or brainstorming tasks, such as generating ideas on how to improve university teaching (Guilford, 1967; Torrance, 1966). Creativity is often scored as the number of ideas generated ("fluency"), or as the statistical infrequency of ideas (ideas that are less often generated are assumed to be more original).

Creative Processes

How people achieve creative insights, original ideas, novel poems, and new products is the subject of many distinct theoretical propositions. Some propose that, similar to biological evolution, creativity involves a process of random (or blind) variation and selective retention (e.g., Campbell, 1960; Simonton, 1999). In this view, the human brain produces variations to known ideas in an essentially random or quasi-random way. This may result in new combinations, some of which are promising and are retained, and others that appear useless and are discarded.

This process of selective retention may occur both within the mind of the inventor and within the society that adopts useful ideas and disregards those that seemingly have no value at that time (Csikszentmihalyi, 1999; Simonton, 1999, 2003).

An alternative, "creative cognition approach" (Finke, 1996) proceeds on the basis of the assumption that (1) creativity is a hallmark of normal human cognitive functioning (i.e., people are inherently creative); (2) the processes leading to creativity are open to rigorous experimental investigation; and (3) creativity results from ordinary mental processes that are in principle observable (Ward et al., 1999, p. 189). These ordinary mental processes include both generative processes—the retrieval of existing structures from memory, the formation of simple associations among these structures, and the mental synthesis and transformation of existing structures—and explorative processes—new ideas being examined and evaluated for new or desired attributes (Finke, Ward, & Smith, 1992; also see Nijstad & Stroebe, 2006).

While most researchers would agree that creativity involves cognitive processes such as retrieval and the formation of new associations, others argue that creative thinking benefits from defocused attention and unsystematic (random) processes (e.g., spreading of activation) that result in the generation of associations that are more remotely related to existing ideas (and therefore more original) (e.g., Eysenck, 1993, 1995; Guilford, 1967; Mednick, 1962; Simonton, 1999, 2003). One (brain) mechanism through which this might work is *latent inhibition*— the capability of the brain to filter out of current attentional focus those stimuli previously experienced as irrelevant. While doing so is highly adaptive in general (Lubow, 1989), creative insights and ideas more likely emerge from seemingly irrelevant stimuli that are allowed to enter attention, which in turn increases the availability of elements to work with during a creative task, leading to more original responses (e.g., Carson, Peterson, & Higgins, 2003; Eysenck, 1993, 1995; Martindale, 1995).

From a bird's-eye perspective, the previously discussed models and propositions on creative processes emphasize either *cognitive flexibility* (the degree to which people switch to a different approach, solution category, and perspective), or *cognitive persistence* (the degree of sustained and focused task-directed effort). Cognitive flexibility is associated with the use of broad and inclusive cognitive categories (Eysenck, 1993), making remote associations (Mednick, 1962), and holistic or global processing (Förster, 2009). Cognitive flexibility is what most people associate with creative processes, such as "out-of-the-box thinking." It involves some randomness in making new associations (Campbell, 1960; Simonton, 1999, 2003), relatively low levels of cognitive control (also see Baird et al., 2012; Dijksterhuis & Meurs, 2006; Martindale, 1995), and may lead to quite sudden and sometimes surprising ideas, insights, and solutions.

Cognitive persistence, on the other hand, is associated with prolonged and motivated effort (Duckworth & Seligman, 2005; Eisenberger & Rhoades, 2001; Rietzschel, De Dreu, & Nijstad, 2007; Rietzschel, Nijstad, & Stroebe, 2007). It involves systematically searching problem space for solutions (Newell & Simon, 1972), high cognitive control and focused attention, and local and narrow processing. Most people do not associate creativity with focused attention and systematic search processes, and, indeed, systematic thinking may at first lead to the generation of ideas and solutions that are unoriginal and readily available (also see Nijstad et al., 2010; Ward, 1994). However, after the most accessible and least original ideas have been tried and abandoned, systematic search will also lead to the generation of solutions and ideas that are truly new and worthwhile (for evidence, see Nijstad et al., 2010; Rietzschel, De Dreu, et al., 2007; Rietzschel, Nijstad, et al., 2007). Because systematic search requires cognitive control, a consequence is that the capacity for cognitive control and focused thinking positively relates to creativity (mainly) through the persistence pathway. This prediction was recently confirmed in a series of studies in which cognitive capacity was operationalized as working memory capacity (WMC; see, e.g., Barrett, Tugade, & Engle, 2004; Unsworth & Engle, 2007), and in which positive effects on creativity were mediated by persistence (De Dreu, Nijstad, Baas, Wolsink, & Roskes, 2012).

Cognitive flexibility and cognitive persistence are to some degree mutually incompatible: One cannot at the same time engage in global and local thinking, or have low and high cognitive control (see, e.g., Cools, 2008; Dreisbach & Goschke, 2004; Fischer & Hommel, 2012). However, over time, people can switch between more flexible and focused types of processing (e.g., Finke, 1996; Leber, Turk-Browne, & Chun, 2008), making flexibility and persistence relatively independent when a longer time frame is considered (for evidence, see Nijstad et al., 2010). An intriguing hypothesis is that creativity in the end is especially dependent on the modulation of cognitive control: engaging in flexible processing when possible, and in persistent thinking when needed.

Press and Person

A key assumption made within the DPCM is that situational and personality antecedents of creativity can be parsimoniously understood in terms of the extent to which they *activate* (vs. deactivate) a general biobehavioral *approach–avoidance* system (Carver, 2006; Davidson, 1998; Elliot, 2006; Elliot & Thrash, 2002, 2010; Gray, 1982). The approach system relies on dopaminergic brain circuitries (Ashby, Isen, & Turken, 1999), and deals with appetitive motivation and approach behavior toward rewarding and novel stimuli (Carver, 2006; Elliot, 2006). It is associated with feelings of elation, cheerfulness, and eagerness when there is good progress toward, and successful attainment of, rewards and desired end states (Baas, De Dreu, & Nijstad, 2011). The approach system is associated with extraversion, positive affectivity, openness to experience, and individual differences in the behavioral activation system (BAS; Baas, Roskes, Sligte, Nijstad, & De Dreu, 2013; Depue & Collins, 1999; Elliot & Thrash, 2002; Watson, Wiese, Vaidya, & Tellegen, 1999). In contrast to this, the avoidance system deals with withdrawal motivation and avoidance behavior, away from aversive stimuli and threatening circumstances (Carver, 2006). It is associated with feelings of fear, tension, and vigilance when people regulate aversive circumstances and stimuli (Baas et al., 2011), and is related to neuroticism, negative affectivity, and individual differences in the behavioral inhibition system (BIS; Carver, 2006; Elliot & Thrash, 2002; Watson et al., 1999).

According to the DPCM, when neither approach nor avoidance is activated, the individual is at rest and creative performance is not expected. When either approach or avoidance is activated, however, creative performance is expected. Specifically, traits and states that activate and intensify approach motivation predict creativity through the flexibility pathway, whereas traits and states that activate and intensify avoidance motivation predict systematic, persistent processing that, under certain conditions, enables creativity (see Baas et al., 2013; Nijstad et al., 2010). That activation of approach motivation predicts creativity through flexibility is consistent with extant research showing that approach motivation is positively related to creativity (e.g., Cretenet & Dru, 2009; Elliot, Maier, Binser, Friedman, & Pekrun, 2009; Friedman & Förster, 2002; Mehta & Zhu, 2009), and that the same is true for

approach-related traits such as extraversion, openness to experience, and positive affectivity (e.g., Baas et al., 2008, 2013; Feist, 1998; McCrae, 1987; also see Elliot & Thrash, 2002). The activation of approach motivation implies a focus on rewards, gains, and advancement, and occurs when a situation is perceived as benign. This leads to a flexible processing style in which alternative courses of action are eagerly explored (e.g., Ashby et al., 1999; Fredrickson, 2001; Friedman & Förster, 2010). The implication is that approach motivation enhances creativity in situations in which flexible processing is facilitated rather than inhibited (for evidence, see De Dreu, Nijstad, & Baas, 2011).

Activation of avoidance motivation implies a focus on losses and punishments, and occurs when a situation is construed as potentially malevolent, leading to a narrower attentional focus and higher persistence. That activation of avoidance motivation can boost creativity because of persistence is consistent with work that indicates activating avoidance motivation stimulates vigilance (Elliot, 2006; Friedman & Förster, 2005), focused attention (Mehta & Zhu, 2009), persistence in problem solving (Friedman & Elliot, 2008), and more effortful and controlled processing (Koch, Holland, & Van Knippenberg, 2008). It also is consistent with work showing that trait anxiety negatively relates to broad, inclusive, and flexible thinking, but not to creativity in itself (Baas, De Dreu, & Nijstad, 2008; but see Byron & Khazanchi, 2011, and below).

Two sets of experimental studies suggest that both approach- and avoidance-motivated individuals can achieve high creativity, but that they do so in different ways (through flexibility vs. persistence, respectively), and that effects strongly depend on cognitive activation. Baas and colleagues (2011) proposed that both approach and avoidance motivation triggers creative performance when and as long as individuals are cognitively activated and mobilize energy to sustain attention and effort toward goal-related activities (see, e.g., Brehm & Self, 1989; Derryberry & Tucker, 1994; Watson et al., 1999). Such activation is more likely when the individual's (approach or avoidance) goals are not fulfilled rather than fulfilled, or are decidedly unattainable. Baas and colleagues tested these ideas in four experiments and obtained solid support for the hypothesis that creative performance is high especially when goals are unfulfilled and concomitant cognitive activation of either the approach or avoidance system is high.

Roskes, De Dreu and Nijstad (2012) replicated and extended these findings by showing that approach- and avoidance-motivated individuals achieve creativity through different cognitive pathways. In five experiments, Roskes and colleagues manipulated whether creative performance was functional for avoiding loss or attaining gains. Approach-motivated individuals displayed high levels of flexibility and were relatively creative regardless of whether performance was functional. Avoidance-motivated individuals engaged in persistent processing and reached high levels of creativity only when creative performance was functional. Presumably, avoidance-oriented individuals were only willing to incur the costs of their more effortful processing style when reaching high creativity was valuable and functional. Interestingly, these individuals also reported highest levels of fatigue upon task completion, and their performance was undermined more by a concurrent load on working memory. Clearly, avoidance-motivated individuals can be as creative as approach-motivated individuals, but the former need to invest more deliberate effort, and their persistent cognitive processing style is relatively depleting. Avoidance-motivated individuals therefore need to be willing (creativity must be valued) and able (have sufficient processing capacity) to engage in systematic and effortful information processing in order to be creative (also see Figure 19.1).

Summary

DPCM captures creative performance in terms of two broad and mutually compatible processes—flexibility and persistence—and incorporates a broad range of states and traits known to help (or hinder) creativity. DPCM builds on four decades of research in social and personality psychology, and while it certainly cannot cover all that has been discovered, we believe it does a fair job in capturing the basic principles and mechanisms underlying human creativity. That being said, DPCM rests on work largely done in research laboratories with undergraduate students. This creates some concern over generality and relevance, issues that we examine further in the next sections when we focus on workplace creativity in general, and in particular on (1) mood and affective states, including job (dis)satisfaction; (2) exogenous constraints, including time pressure, concurrent workload, and more or less salient external threats; and (3) cultural norms and construals.

HAPPY WORKERS AND GRUMPY EMPLOYEES

Emotion researchers have long argued and shown that affective experiences should be distinguished according to their hedonic tone (positive–negative; e.g., happy vs. sad), as well as the degree to which they are activating and arousing (activating–deactivating; e.g., happy vs. relaxed, and angry or anxious vs. sad; Barrett & Russell, 1998; Watson, Clark, & Tellegen, 1988). Moderate levels of arousal, such as that associated with activating (positive and negative) moods, increase motivation and enhance various aspects of human information processing, including memory performance, sustained attention, and switching between tasks (see, e.g., Broadbent, 1972; Flaherty, 2005; Gardner, 1986; Robbins, 1984; Staw, Sandelands, & Dutton, 1981). Furthermore, affective states have been argued to trigger approach and avoidance motivation (e.g., Crawford & Cacioppo, 2002; Tooby & Cosmides, 1992), with, for example, happiness leading to an intensifying approach motivation, and fear and anxiety leading to an intensifying avoidance motivation (also see Baas et al., 2011).

In terms of DPCM, activating mood states more likely stimulate creativity than do deactivating mood states because activating moods are more strongly connected to the activation of the biobehavioral approach–avoidance system. Positive mood states more likely associate with approach motivation and therefore with cognitive flexibility; negative mood states typically associate with avoidance motivation and generally may be linked more to persistence (e.g., Clore, Schwarz, & Conway, 1994; Schwarz & Bless, 1991). Thus, DPCM predicts positive activating moods such as excitement and happiness to make individuals creative because of enhanced cognitive flexibility; negative activating moods such as anger and anxiety make individuals creative because of enhanced cognitive persistence. A series of laboratory experiments provided good empirical support for this core proposition: Whereas positive activating moods (e.g., happy, elated) induced cognitive flexibility and creativity, negative activating mood states (e.g., fear, anger) induced persistence—they generated more ideas *within* semantic categories and spent longer time on their task (De Dreu et al., 2008).

Several studies conducted with employees in organizations reveal effects similar to those in De Dreu and colleagues (2008) and, at the same time, hint at some relevant boundary conditions. To, Fisher, and Ashkanasy (2012), for example, observed that day-to-day variations in mood predict fluctuations in creative process engagement (CPE). Only activating moods had effects. Positive moods only had effects on immediate CPE, negative active moods also had effects on lagged CPE (several hours later), suggesting that creativity came about through persistence. Furthermore, effects of positive moods were stronger when employees had strong learning orientation, and weaker when employees had strong performance motivation. Along similar lines, Madrid, Patterson, and Birdi (2014) found that innovative behavior for people high in openness to experience was mediated by high-activated positive affect, and Madjar, Oldham, and Pratt (2002) showed that social support at work or at home predicts employee creativity because it enhances positive moods, especially in people rated as generally low in creativity.

With regard to negative mood states, such as job dissatisfaction, George and Zhou (2002; also see Zhou & George, 2001) observed positive associations with creativity when perceived recognition for creativity was high and clarity of feelings (a meta-affective experience) was high as well. This finding with employees resonates with the findings by Roskes and colleagues (2012) discussed earlier, which showed that

avoidance motivation promotes persistent thinking and creativity, especially when creativity was useful in avoiding loss. Thus, when creativity is valued—by the individual or his or her environment—negative mood states promote effortful working and lead to creative production.

The evidence therefore suggests that when moods are activating rather than deactivating, individuals are more creative because of flexible processing in the case of positive, and persistent processing, in the case of negative moods. The evidence comes from laboratory experiments (De Dreu et al., 2008; also see Baas et al., 2008, 2011), and fits a variety of organizational field studies (e.g., George & Zhou, 2002; Madrid et al., 2014; To et al., 2012; Zhou & George, 2001). There are two worthwhile implications for managers wishing to have creative employees. First, because employees need to be cognitively activated and aroused for creativity to come about, a first piece of advice is that mood states such as relief, feeling calm and at ease, being relaxed, or being sad and somewhat blue, should be avoided. Rather, managers should stimulate activating emotions and mood states because these potentially drive employees to be creative. In doing so, managers may enhance happiness, excitement, and elation or, alternatively, fear and anger (also see Nifgatkar, Tsui, & Ashford, 2012; Van Kleef, Anastasopoulou, & Nijstad, 2010). When opting for the latter, they should realize that fear and anger drive creative performance because of persistence. Accordingly, up-regulation of fear and anger in employees should be done in conjunction with removing obstacles to persistent processing, such as time pressure or concurrent workload. It is to these exogenous stressors that we now turn.

EXOGENOUS OPPORTUNITIES AND CONSTRAINTS

Work situations offer a variety of opportunities and constraints, including (lack of) autonomy and support, time pressures, and task constraints. These opportunities and constraints may, first of all, activate approach and avoidance tendencies because they signal either a benign situation, in which gains and rewards may be obtained, or a problematic situation, in which losses and punishment may occur (also see Gutnick, Walter, Nijstad, & De Dreu, 2012). Second, opportunities and constraints may either facilitate or inhibit flexible versus persistent processing. For example, the previously discussed work of De Dreu and colleagues (2011) suggests that approach motivation is positively associated with creativity only when the task or situation facilitates rather than impedes flexible processing. Similarly, avoidance motivation may stimulate creativity through persistence, but this is contingent on the value of creativity to the individual and the absence of constraints such as time pressure or concurrent working memory load (Roskes et al., 2012).

Direct evidence for these possibilities comes from a series of studies by Roskes, Elliot, Nijstad, and De Dreu (2013), who experimentally manipulated approach and avoidance motivation, and crossed this with a manipulation of time pressure. Time pressure is distracting because it induces stress and arousal, heightens the need to monitor task progress and time remaining, and taxes cognitive resources (e.g., Bargh, 1992; De Dreu, 2003; Karau & Kelly, 1992; Kruglanski & Freund, 1983). Because cognitive resources are needed especially for focused and persistent processing (De Dreu et al., 2012), and because such processing occurs more under avoidance than approach motivation, Roskes and colleagues (2013) predicted and found that time pressure undermined creative performance, but only for avoidance-motivated individuals, not for those with an approach motivation.

That exogenous stressors undermine creativity especially among avoidance-motivated individuals fits meta-analytic findings from Byron and Khazanchi (2011) on the relation between anxiety and creativity. While effects of anxiety on creativity were generally negative, this relationship was stronger for trait anxiety than for state anxiety, and emerged especially when tasks were complex and exogenous stressors were present rather than absent.

Evidence among employees also indicates that stressors such as time pressure do not always undermine creative performance. In Byron, Khazanchi, and Nazarian's (2010) meta-analysis, for example, social-evaluative stressors showed a curvilinear (inverted U shape) rather than a negative and linear relation with creativity, indicating that some degree of stress may be activating and improve rather than harming creative performance. Effects of other stressors (Byron et al. labeled these "uncontrollable stressors") were negative. Interestingly, however, the meta-analysis also showed that negative effects of stressors were much more pronounced for employees high in trait anxiety than for those low in trait anxiety. Perhaps these employees were more likely to evaluate stressors as a threat and less likely to appraise them as a challenge. Indeed, Baer and Oldham (2006) found a positive relationship between time pressure and creativity among employees high in openness to experience who also experienced high support for creativity. In other cases, creative time pressure was negatively related to creativity. Thus, exogenous stressors and constraints undermine creativity among avoidance-oriented people. In supportive environments, stressors may actually promote creative performance among employees with strong approach orientation (also see Ohly & Fritz, 2010; Sacramento, Fay, & West, 2013).

So far, the evidence suggests that under benevolent situations (e.g., high support), approach-motivated employees achieve high creativity, and that this is more true when tasks are relatively ill-structured and ill-defined, thus allowing for flexible processing. In these situations, and when approach orientation is strong, stressors may even benefit creative performance to the extent that they activate and energize the individual. In contrast, stressors and constraints undermine creative performance under avoidance motivation. To combat this negative effect, leaders may offer structure and guidance. In their meta-analysis, Rosing, Frese, and Bausch (2011) found that *initiating structure*, leadership behavior that consists of structuring tasks and clearly defining goals, was positively related to innovation. Experimental work adds to this by showing that providing structure during a brainstorming task by decomposing a topic into subtopics (Coskun, Paulus, Brown, & Sherwood, 2000) or by more narrowly defining a brainstorming topic (Rietzschel, Nijstad, & Stroebe, 2014) enhances creativity. Offering structure would enhance performance especially for employees who are avoidance motivated, have a low tolerance for ambiguity, or have a tendency to take a structured and systematic approach to creative tasks (also see Rietzschel, De Dreu, et al., 2007). In short, providing structure may benefit those individuals who, because of their avoidance orientation, engage persistent processing as a means to achieve creative production.

Taken together, the DPCM and the research reviewed earlier suggest two main ways to manage creativity at work. First, especially when tasks are complex and heuristic, or when considerable pressure is present, leaders may emphasize positive outcomes and gains and deemphasize potential negative outcomes and losses. For example, transformational leadership, which has been related to a promotion focus and approach motivation (Kark & Van Dijk, 2007), has been found to be especially effective when working on complex and radical innovations (Keller, 1992, 2006), and good leader–follower relations (high leader–member exchange [LMX]) help employees remain creative when under strain (Van Dyne, Jehn, & Cummings, 2002). Second, when the situation is aversive and losses loom, leaders may create the conditions under which employees can be creative through persistence: They should reduce distractors and stressors, and provide guidance and structure.

CULTURAL NORMS AND CONSTRUALS

Work takes place in a social context, and so does creative performance. Differences in social context, whether explicit or implicit and operating outside of awareness, matter a great deal. Thus, the diversity of people one is around (Shin, Kim, & Lee, 2012), whether others can or will monitor (De Vet & De Dreu, 2007; Slijkhuis, Rietzschel, & Van Yperen, 2013), whether rewards for creativity are offered (Eisenberger & Aselage, 2009; Eisenberger & Rhoades, 2001), and whether social context provides psychological safety or instead instills intolerance for errors (Gong, Cheung, & Wang, 2012), all determine the extent to which

people can and will be creative. In short, the organizational climate and broader culture within which employees operate may have a substantial impact on their creativity. In essence, climate and culture activate an approach or avoidance motivation, and provide social constraints and facilitators of flexible and persistent processing. Here we review some of the evidence, focusing in particular on cross-cultural differences in terms of individualism–collectivism.

Cross-cultural studies on (employee) creativity are relatively scarce. Exceptions include Erez and Nouri (2010), who found that cross-cultural differences in creative performance emerge more when individuals work in groups than when they work alone; Zhou and Su (2010), who observed that directive leadership, typically seen as reducing creativity in Western culture, promotes creative performance in Eastern contexts; Mok and Morris (2010), who found that priming one culture rather than the other may either promote or inhibit creative performance among individuals with a dual cultural identification; and Ng (2003), who found that individualism is positively related to an independent self-construal and creative behavior, whereas collectivism is related to an interdependent self-construal and lower creativity (but higher conformity).

One possible explanation for these rather systematic effects is that when it comes to creative performance, Western norms prioritize originality and novelty over usefulness and appropriateness, whereas Eastern norms prioritize usefulness over originality (Morris & Leung, 2010; Zou et al., 2009). To the extent that culturally divergent social norms are salient, individuals with an Eastern background may be more concerned with usefulness than with originality and engage different implicit or explicit standards to downplay or elaborate ideas and insights than their counterparts with a Western background. For example, employees in an Eastern context may be more concerned with producing useful rather than original ideas, expect others to value usefulness more than originality, and through feedback loops, reinforce within their team or organization a focus on usefulness rather than originality. Such a team or organizational culture may sustain over time, as old-timers socialize newcomers up to a point where (expectations of) the culture may entirely explain why individual team members focus on usefulness rather than originality (the same argument holds for a culture valuing originality rather than usefulness) (De Dreu, 2010).

Some direct evidence for these cultural differences in prioritizing usefulness and originality was obtained in a study of three-person groups who brainstormed about ways to improve university teaching (Bechtoldt, De Dreu, Nijstad, & Choi, 2010). In two experiments these groups comprised Dutch (individualistic) students; in one study, these groups were comprised Korean (collectivistic) students. Motivating individualistic group members to do their very best increased originality of ideas but did not affect their usefulness; motivating collectivistic group members to do their very best increased usefulness of ideas but did not affect their originality. A final study confirmed that among Dutch students the default norm is to be original. When, through a priming procedure, the norm was changed to being useful rather than original, individualistic students from the Netherlands behaved like their collectivistic counterparts from Korea.

What emerges from these works is that individualism, and associated independent self-construal, may be more conducive to originality and creativity than collectivism and interdependent self-construal (for direct support, see Bechtoldt, Choi, & Nijstad, 2012; Goncalo & Staw, 2006; Ng, 2003; Rinne, Steel, & Fairweather, 2013). Individualistic cultures value uniqueness, originality, and independence, and standing out is an important motivator. Collectivist cultures value conformity; usefulness; and focus on duties, loyalty, and obligations. Plausibly, collectivist cultures focus more on avoidance goals, whereas in individualistic cultures approach motivation may be more rewarding and valued. Indeed, people from collectivist cultures find situations involving potential losses more important, whereas people from individualistic cultures find situations involving potential gains more important (Lee, Aaker, & Gardner, 2000). Furthermore, a focus on gains and advancement (approach motivation) is related to Western

values such as achievement, whereas a focus on losses, duties, and obligations (avoidance motivation) is associated with Eastern values such as security, conformity, and tradition (Leikas, Lönnqvist, Verkasalo, & Lindeman, 2009). Thus, there seems to be an intimate relation among culture, self-construal, and motivational orientation, and the link between culture and motivational orientation can potentially explain cultural differences in creativity.

It should be noted, though, that Eastern values such as conservation (i.e., valuing tradition, conformity, and security) do not necessarily undermine creativity. For example, Shin and Zhou (2003) observed, in a Korean sample, that conservation is not significantly associated with supervisor-rated creativity, but that this association is positive (rather than negative) when the leader demonstrates a transformational leadership style. Furthermore, Wang and Cheng (2010) found that benevolent leadership, an Eastern type of leadership that is characterized not only by leader support but also by obedience and loyalty, is positively related to research and development (R&D) workers' creativity, and that this is especially the case when employee autonomy is high. In other words, Eastern values that are associated with avoidance motivation may at times benefit creativity, and these effects are potentially mediated by persistence and hard work (rather than flexibility).

If cultural differences in creativity are largely caused by differences in motivational orientation, then this would have major consequences for managing creativity across cultures. Thus, in Western cultures with a stronger approach orientation, creativity may flourish in situations that facilitate flexible processing (e.g., high autonomy and support, heuristic and complex jobs). In Eastern cultures with a stronger emphasis on avoidance, creativity may benefit from situations that enable systematic and persistent processing (e.g., lack of distraction and stressors, structured work and clear directions, explicit valuation of creativity). This seems to fit with the earlier mentioned study by Zhou and Su (2010), who found that directive leadership benefited creativity of Eastern employees.

CONCLUSIONS AND IMPLICATIONS

The DPCM (see Figure 19.1) integrates various earlier models and theories about human creativity into the core proposition that creativity can come about through both flexible and systematic and persistent processing. It adds that flexible processing is a function of the intensity of approach motivation, and that persistence is a function of the intensity of avoidance motivation. Finally, the model suggests that approach motivation mainly leads to creativity through flexibility under conditions in which flexible processing is facilitated and enabled (e.g., complex and heuristic tasks, high autonomy), whereas avoidance motivation only relates to creativity through persistence when creativity is valued and sufficient processing capacity is available (e.g., no distraction, having structured work). This model leads, as we have illustrated, to a reinterpretation of some creativity research among employees and to testable new hypotheses. In this concluding section, we highlight what we think are the most important avenues for future research and the most important conclusions.

Avenues for Future Research

Within the DPCM, motivational orientation (approach vs. avoidance) plays an important role. Although motivational orientation has been found to be an important determinant of creativity in laboratory studies (e.g., Baas et al., 2011; Cretenet & Dru, 2009; Elliot et al., 2009; Friedman & Förster, 2002; Mehta & Zhu, 2009; Roskes et al., 2012, 2013), motivational orientation has not been systematically studied as an antecedent of workplace creativity. This is a particularly important omission because we have argued that effects of (other) contextual variables, such as workplace stressors and leadership, on employee creativity largely depend on employee motivational orientation. New work is needed to capture more fully the role of biobehavioral approach and avoidance in employee creativity.

More closely examining motivational orientation is also important because the DPCM suggests that dispositional and situational variables may impact employee creativity through their effects of motivational orientation (see Figure 19.1). Thus, motivational orientation may mediate effects and serve as an explanatory variable between antecedents and employee creative performance. For example, effects of the cultural dimension of individualism–collectivism on creativity (e.g., Ng, 2003) may potentially be mediated by approach and avoidance motivation. For such mediation effects to be established, researchers need to be able to assess motivational orientation as a state variable that is influenced by other variables rather than as a trait variable. However, although trait measures of motivational orientation are available (e.g., Carver & White's [1994] BAS–BIS measure, and Elliot & Thrash's [2010] measure of approach and avoidance temperament), we are not aware of measures of state motivational orientation. Measures of state regulatory focus are available, however, and some research suggests that regulatory focus mediates effects of leadership on creativity (Neubert, Kacmar, Carlson, Chonko, & Roberts, 2008). Alternatively, measures of workplace challenge (approach) versus threat (avoidance) appraisals may be used to examine the role of motivational orientation (e.g., Ohly & Fritz, 2010; also see Gutnick et al., 2012), or researchers may rely on affective measures that are related to approach (e.g., happiness) and avoidance motivation (e.g., anxiety).

In addition, the DPCM suggests that effects of situational and dispositional variables on employee creativity are mediated by cognitive flexibility (under benign situations) and cognitive persistence (under less benign situations). In laboratory research we have directly assessed cognitive flexibility and persistence (e.g., De Dreu et al., 2008; Roskes et al., 2012), and new research outside of the laboratory is much needed.

The DPCM, and much of the research on which it builds, focuses on individuals being more or less creative. More and more, however, creative performance is the outcome of a group process, and group processes may be a constraint, as well as facilitator, of both flexible and persistent processing at the individual level. Group processes may induce positive moods, highlight threats and opportunities, create noise and cognitive load, and so on. In addition to such top-down influences, however, there may be a host of bottom-up processes whereby individual contributions combine into a more or less creative group product. For example, group composition may be critical, in that groups of approach-motivated individuals may be more flexible, whereas groups of avoidance-motivated individuals may be more persistent. What we do not know, however, is whether heterogeneous groups of both approach- and avoidance-motivated individuals that, in principle, combine both flexible and persistent processing styles, outperform homogeneous groups only approach-, or only avoidance-motivated individuals. It is these types of questions about which the DPCM is silent, and that future work should address.

In summary, individuals at work, as well as other settings in which some more or less ill-defined task needs to be performed, can be equally creative when approach or avoidance motivated, as long as they can pursue their flexible and persistent processing styles, respectively. Avoidance-motivated individuals expend more effort and are more influenced by endogenous constraints such as time pressure and concurrent work load. Removing such constraints, and emphasizing challenges and opportunities are therefore among the most promising interventions that organizational leaders, team managers, mentors, or parents should consider when seeking to promote creative performance in their employees, team members, pupils, or offspring.

ACKNOWLEDGMENTS

Authors are listed alphabetically and contributed equally. Carsten K. W. De Dreu was supported by a Fellowship from the Netherlands Institute for Advanced Study. Bernard A. Nijstad was supported by a Vici grant from the Netherlands Organization for Scientific Research (No. NWO-45 3-1 5-002).

REFERENCES

Amabile, T. M. (1982). Social psychology of creativity: A consensual assessment procedure. *Journal of Personality and Social Psychology, 43,* 997–1013.

Amabile, T. M. (1983). The social psychology of creativity: A componential conceptualization. *Journal of Personality and Social Psychology, 45,* 357–376.

Ashby, F. G., Isen, A. M., & Turken, A. U. (1999). A neuropsychological theory of positive affect and its influence on cognition. *Psychological Review, 106,* 529–550.

Baas, M., De Dreu, C. K. W., & Nijstad, B. A. (2008). A meta-analysis of 25 years of research on mood and creativity: Hedonic tone, activation, or regulatory focus? *Psychological Bulletin, 134,* 779–806.

Baas, M., De Dreu, C. K. W., & Nijstad, B. A. (2011). When prevention promotes creativity: The role of mood, regulatory focus and regulatory closure. *Journal of Personality and Social Psychology, 100,* 794–809.

Baas, M., Roskes, M., Sligte, D., Nijstad, B. A., & De Dreu, C. K. W. (2013). Personality and creativity: The dual pathway to creativity model and a research agenda. *Social Psychology and Personality Compass, 7,* 732–748.

Baer, M., & Oldham, G. R. (2006). The curvilinear relation between experienced creative time pressure and creativity: Moderating effects of openness to experience and support for creativity. *Journal of Applied Psychology, 91,* 963–970.

Baird, B., Smallwood, J., Mrazek, M. D., Kam, J. W. Y., Franklin, M. S., & Schooler, J. W. (2012). Inspired by distraction: Mind wandering facilitates creative incubation. *Psychological Science, 23,* 1117–1122.

Bargh, J. A. (1992). The ecology of automaticity: Toward establishing the conditions needed to produce automatic processing effects. *American Journal of Psychology, 105,* 181–199.

Barrett, L. F., & Russell, J. A. (1998). Independence and bipolarity in the structure of current affect. *Journal of Personality and Social Psychology, 74,* 967–984.

Barrett, L. F., Tugade, M. M., & Engle, R. W. (2004). Individual differences in working memory capacity and dual-process theories of the mind. *Psychological Bulletin, 130,* 553–573.

Bechtoldt, M. N., Choi, H.-S., & Nijstad, B. A. (2012). Individuals in mind, mates by heart: Individualistic self-construal and collective value orientation as predictors of group creativity. *Journal of Experimental Social Psychology, 48,* 838–844.

Bechtoldt, M. N., De Dreu, C. K. W., Nijstad, B. A., & Choi, H.-S. (2010). Motivated information processing, epistemic social tuning, and group creativity. *Journal of Personality and Social Psychology, 99*, 622–637.

Binnewies, C., & Wörnlein, S. C. (2011). What makes a creative day?: A diary study on the interplay between affect, job stressors, and job control. *Journal of Organizational Behavior, 32*, 589–607.

Brehm, J. W., & Self, E. A. (1989). The intensity of motivation. *Annual Review of Psychology, 40*, 109–131.

Broadbent, D. E. (1972). *Decision and stress.* New York: Academic Press.

Byron, K., & Khazanchi, S. (2011). A meta-analytic investigation of the relationship of state and trait anxiety to performance on figural and verbal creative tasks. *Personality and Social Psychology Bulletin, 37*, 269–283.

Byron, K., Khazanchi, S., & Nazarian, D. (2010). The relationship between stressors and creativity: A meta-analysis examining competing theoretical models. *Journal of Applied Psychology, 95*, 201–212.

Campbell, D. T. (1960). Blind variation and selective retention in creative thought as in other knowledge processes. *Psychological Review, 67*, 380–400.

Carson, S. H., Peterson, J. B., & Higgins, D. M. (2003). Decreased latent inhibition is associated with increased creative achievement in high-functioning individuals. *Journal of Personality and Social Psychology, 85*, 499–506.

Carver, C. S. (2006). Approach, avoidance, and the self-regulation of affect and action. *Motivation and Emotion, 30*, 105–110.

Carver, C. S., & White, T. L. (1994). Behavioral inhibition, behavioral activation, and affective responses to impending reward and punishment: The BIS/BAS scales. *Journal of Personality and Social Psychology, 67*, 319–333.

Clore, G. L., Schwarz, N., & Conway, M. (1994). Affective causes and consequences of social information processing. In R. S. Wyer & T. K. Srull (Eds.), *Handbook of social cognition* (Vol. 1, pp. 323–417). Hillsdale, NJ: Erlbaum.

Cools, R. (2008). Role of dopamine in the motivational and cognitive control of behavior. *The Neuroscientist, 4*, 381–395.

Coskun, H., Paulus, P. B., Brown, V., & Sherwood, J. J. (2000). Cognitive stimulation and problem presentation in idea-generating groups. *Group Dynamics: Theory, Research and Practice, 4*, 307–329.

Crawford, L. E., & Cacioppo, J. T. (2002). Learning where to look for danger: Integrating affective and spatial information. *Psychological Science, 13*, 449–453.

Cretenet, J., & Dru, V. (2009). Influence of peripheral and motivational cues on rigid–flexible functioning: Perceptual, behavioral, and cognitive aspects. *Journal of Experimental Psychology: General, 138*, 201–217.

Csikszentmihalyi, M. (1999). Implications of a systems perspective for the study of creativity. In R. J. Sternberg (Ed.), *Handbook of creativity* (pp. 313–335). New York: Cambridge University Press.

Davidson, R. J. (1998). Affective style and affective disorders: Perspectives from affective neuroscience. *Cognition and Emotion, 12*, 307–330.

De Dreu, C. K. W. (2003). Time pressure and closing of the mind in negotiation. *Organizational Behavior and Human Decision Processes, 91*, 280–295.

De Dreu, C. K. W. (2010). Human creativity: Reflections on the role of culture. *Management and Organization Review, 6*, 437–446.

De Dreu, C. K. W., Baas, M., & Nijstad, B. A. (2008). Hedonic tone and activation in the mood–creativity link: Towards a dual pathway to creativity model. *Journal of Personality and Social Psychology, 94*, 739–756.

De Dreu, C. K. W., Nijstad, B. A., & Baas, M. (2011). Behavioral activation links to creativity because it promotes cognitive flexibility. *Social Psychological and Personality Science, 2*, 72–80.

De Dreu, C. K. W., Nijstad, B. A., Baas, M., Wolsink, I., & Roskes, M. (2012). Working memory benefits creative insight, musical improvisation and original ideation through maintained task-focused attention. *Personality and Social Psychology Bulletin, 38*, 656–669.

Depue, R. A., & Collins, P. F. (1999). Neurobiology of the structure of personality: Dopamine, facilitation of incentive motivation, and extraversion. *Behavioral and Brain Sciences, 22*(3), 491–517; discussion 518–569.

Derryberry, D., & Tucker, D. M. (1994). Motivating the focus of attention. In P. M. Niedenthal & S. Kitayama (Eds.), *The heart's eye: Emotional influences in perception and attention* (pp. 167–196). San Diego, CA: Academic Press.

De Vet, A. J., & De Dreu, C. K. W. (2007). The influence of articulation, self-monitoring ability, and sensitivity to others on creativity. *European Journal of Social Psychology, 37*, 747–760.

Dijksterhuis, A., & Meurs, T. (2006). Where creativity resides: The generative power of unconscious thought. *Consciousness and Cognition, 15*, 135–146.

Dreisbach, G., & Goschke, T. (2004). How positive affect modulates cognitive control:

Reduced perseveration at the cost of increased distractibility. *Journal of Experimental Psychology: Learning, Memory, and Cognition, 30*, 343–353.

Duckworth, A. L., & Seligman, M. E. P. (2005). Self-discipline outdoes IQ in predicting academic performance of adolescents. *Psychological Science, 16*, 939–944.

Eisenberger, R., & Aselage, J. (2009). Incremental effects of reward on experienced performance pressure: Positive outcomes for intrinsic interest and creativity, *Journal of Organizational Behavior, 30*, 95–117.

Eisenberger, R., & Rhoades, L. (2001). Incremental effects of reward on creativity. *Journal of Personality and Social Psychology, 81*, 728–741.

Ekstrom, R. B., French, J. W., Harman, H. H., & Dermen, D. (1976). *Manual for kit of factor-referenced cognitive tests*. Princeton, NJ: Educational Testing Service.

Elliot, A. J. (2006). The hierarchical model of approach–avoidance motivation. *Motivation and Emotion, 30*, 111–116.

Elliot, A. J., Maier, M. A., Binser, M. J., Friedman, R., & Pekrun, R. (2009). The effect of red on avoidance behavior in achievement contexts. *Personality and Social Psychology Bulletin, 35*, 365–375.

Elliot, A. J., & Thrash, T. M. (2002). Approach–avoidance motivation in personality: Approach and avoidance temperaments and goals. *Journal of Personality and Social Psychology, 82*, 804–818.

Elliot, A. J., & Thrash, T. M. (2010). Approach and avoidance temperament as basic dimensions of personality. *Journal of Personality, 78*, 865–906.

Erez, M., & Nouri, R. (2010). Creativity: The influence of cultural, social, and work contexts. *Management and Organization Review, 6*, 351–370.

Eysenck, H. J. (1993). Creativity and personality: Suggestions for a theory. *Psychological Inquiry, 4*, 147–178.

Eysenck, H. J. (1995). *Genius: The natural history of creativity*. Cambridge, UK: Cambridge University Press.

Feist, G. J. (1998). A meta-analysis of the impact of personality on scientific and artistic creativity. *Personality and Social Psychology Review, 2*, 290–309.

Finke, R. A. (1996). Imagery, creativity, and emergent structure. *Consciousness and Cognition, 5*, 381–393.

Finke, R. A., Ward, T. B., & Smith, S. M. (1992). *Creative cognition: Theory, research and applications*. Cambridge, MA: MIT Press.

Fischer, R., & Hommel, B. (2012). Deep thinking increases task-set shielding and reduces shifting in dual-task performance. *Cognition, 123*, 303–307.

Flaherty, A. W. (2005). Frontotemporal and dopaminergic control of idea generation and creative drive. *Journal of Comparative Neurology, 493*, 147–153.

Fogarty, L., Creanza, N., & Feldman, M. W. (2015). Cultural evolutionary perspectives on creativity and human innovation. *Trends in Ecology and Evolution, 30*, 736–754.

Förster, J. (2009). Relations between perceptual and conceptual scope: How global versus local processing fits a focus on similarity versus dissimilarity. *Journal of Experimental Psychology: General, 138*, 88–111.

Fredrickson, B. L. (2001). The role of positive emotions in positive psychology: The broaden-and-build theory of positive emotions. *American Psychologist, 56*, 218–226.

Friedman, R., & Elliot, A. J. (2008). The effect of arm crossing on persistence and performance. *European Journal of Social Psychology, 38*, 449–461.

Friedman, R. S., & Förster, J. (2002). The influence of approach and avoidance motor actions on creative cognition. *Journal of Experimental Social Psychology, 38*, 41–55.

Friedman, R. S., & Förster, J. (2005). The influence of approach and avoidance cues on attentional flexibility. *Motivation and Emotion, 29*, 69–81.

Friedman, R. S., & Förster, J. (2010). Implicit affective cues and attentional tuning: An integrative review. *Psychological Bulletin, 136*, 875–893.

Gardner, D. G. (1986). Activation theory and task design—an empirical test of several new predictions. *Journal of Applied Psychology, 71*, 411–418.

George, J. M., & Zhou, J. (2001). When openness to experience and conscientiousness are related to creative behavior: An interactional approach. *Journal of Applied Psychology, 86*, 513–524.

George, J. M., & Zhou, J. (2002). Understanding when bad moods foster creativity and good ones don't: The role of context and clarity of feelings. *Journal of Applied Psychology, 87*, 687–697.

Goncalo, J. A., & Staw, B. M. (2006). Individualism–collectivism and group creativity. *Organizational Behavior and Human Decision Processes, 100*, 96–109.

Gong, Y., Cheung, S.-Y., & Wang, M. (2012). Unfolding the proactive process for creativity: Integration of employee proactivity, information exchange, and psychological safety perspectives. *Journal of Management, 38,* 1611–1633.

Gray, J. A. (1982). The neuropsychology of anxiety: An enquiry into the functions of the septohippocampal system. *Behavioral and Brain Sciences, 5,* 469–534.

Guilford, J. P. (1950). Creativity. *American Psychologist, 5,* 444–454.

Guilford, J. P. (1967). *The nature of human intelligence.* New York: McGraw-Hill.

Gutnick, D., Walter, F., Nijstad, B. A., & De Dreu, C. K. W. (2012). Creative performance under pressure: An integrative conceptual framework. *Organizational Psychology Review, 2,* 189–207.

Harkins, S. G. (2006). Mere effort as the mediator of the evaluation–performance relationship. *Journal of Personality and Social Psychology, 91,* 436–455.

Karau, S. J., & Kelly, J. R. (1992). The effects of time scarcity and time abundance on group performance quality and interaction process. *Journal of Experimental Social Psychology, 28,* 542–571.

Kark, R., & Van Dijk, D. (2007). Motivation to lead, motivation to follow: The role of self-regulatory focus in leadership processes. *Academy of Management Review, 32,* 500–528.

Keller, R. T. (1992). Transformational leadership and the performance of research and development project groups. *Journal of Management, 18,* 489–501.

Keller, R. T. (2006). Transformational leadership, initiating structure, and substitutes for leadership: A longitudinal study of research and development project team performance. *Journal of Applied Psychology, 91,* 202–210.

Kleibeuker, S. W., De Dreu, C. K. W., & Crone, E. A. (2013). The development of creative cognition across adolescence: Distinct trajectories for insight and divergent thinking. *Developmental Science, 16,* 2–12.

Koch, S., Holland, R. W., & Van Knippenberg, A. (2008). Regulating cognitive control through approach–avoidance motor actions. *Cognition, 109,* 133–142.

Kounios, J., & Beeman, M. (2009). The Aha! moment: The cognitive neuroscience of insight. *Current Directions in Psychological Science, 18,* 210–216.

Kruglanski, A. W., & Freund, T. (1983). The freezing and unfreezing of lay-inferences: Effects on impressional primacy, ethnic stereotyping, and numerical anchoring. *Journal of Experimental Social Psychology, 19,* 448–468.

Leber, A. B., Turk-Browne, N. B., & Chun, M. M. (2008). Neural predictor of moment-to-moment fluctuations in cognitive flexibility. *Proceedings of the National Academy of Sciences USA, 105,* 13592–13597.

Lee, A. Y., Aaker, J. L., & Gardner, W. L. (2000). The pleasures and pains of distinct self-construals: The role of interdependence in regulatory focus. *Journal of Personality and Social Psychology, 78,* 1122–1134.

Leikas, S., Lönnqvist, J.-E., Verkasalo, M., & Lindeman, M. (2009). Regulatory focus systems and personal values. *European Journal of Social Psychology, 39,* 415–429.

Lubow, R. E. (1989). *Latent inhibition and conditioned attention theory.* Cambridge, UK: Cambridge University Press.

Madjar, N., Oldham, G. R., & Pratt, M. G. (2002). There's no place like home?: The contributions of work and nonwork creativity support to employees' creative performance. *Academy of Management Journal, 45,* 757–767.

Madrid, H. P., Patterson, M. G., & Birdi, K. S. (2014). The role of weekly high-activated positive mood, context, and personality in innovative work behavior: A multilevel and interactional model. *Journal of Organizational Behavior, 35,* 234–256.

Martindale, C. (1995). Creativity and connectionism. In S. M. Smith, T. B. Ward, & R. A. Finke (Eds.), *The creative cognition approach* (pp. 249–268). Cambridge, MA: MIT Press.

McCrae, R. R. (1987). Creativity, divergent thinking, and openness to experience. *Journal of Personality and Social Psychology, 52,* 1258–1265.

Mednick, S. A. (1962). The associative basis of the creative process. *Psychological Review, 69,* 220–232.

Mehta, R., & Zhu, R. (2009). Blue or red?: Exploring the effect of color on cognitive task performances. *Science, 323,* 1226–1229.

Mok, A., & Morris, M. W. (2010). Asian-Americans' creative styles in Asian and American situations: Assimilative and contrastive responses as a function of bicultural identity integration. *Management and Organization Review, 6,* 371–390.

Morris, M. W., & Leung, K. (2010). Creativity East and West: Perspectives and parallels. *Management and Organization Review, 6,* 313–327.

Neubert, M. J., Kacmar, K. M., Carlson, D. S., Chonko, L. B., & Roberts, J. A. (2008). Regulatory focus as a mediator of the influence of initiating structure and servant leadership on employee behavior. *Journal of Applied Psychology, 93,* 1220–1233.

Newell, A., & Simon, H. A. (1972). *Human problem solving.* Englewood Cliffs, NJ: Prentice Hall.

Ng, A. K. (2003). A cultural model of creative and conforming behavior. *Creativity Research Journal, 15,* 223–233.

Nifadgar, S., Tsui, A. S., & Ashford, B. E. (2012). The way you make me feel and behave: Supervisor-triggered newcomer affect and approach-avoidance behavior. *Academy of Management Journal, 55,* 1146–1168.

Nijstad, B. A., De Dreu, C. K. W., Rietzschel, E. F., & Baas, M. (2010). The dual pathway to creativity model: Creative ideation as a function of flexibility and persistence. In W. Stroebe & M. Hewstone (Eds.), *European review of social psychology* (Vol. 21, pp. 34–77). London: Psychology Press.

Nijstad, B. A., & Stroebe, W. (2006). How the group affects the mind: A cognitive model of idea generation in groups. *Personality and Social Psychology Review, 10,* 186–213.

Ohly, S., & Fritz, C. (2010). Work characteristics, challenge appraisal, creativity, and proactive behavior: A multi-level study. *Journal of Organizational Behavior, 31,* 543–565.

Ohly, S., Sonnentag, S., & Pluntke, F. (2006). Routinization, work characteristics and their relationships with creative and proactive behaviors. *Journal of Organizational Behavior, 27,* 257–279.

Rhodes, M. (1961). An analysis of creativity. *Phi Beta Kappan, 42,* 305–310.

Rietzschel, E. F., De Dreu, C. K. W., & Nijstad, B. A. (2007). Personal need for structure and creative performance: The moderating influence of fear of invalidity. *Personality and Social Psychology Bulletin, 33,* 855–866.

Rietzschel, E. F., Nijstad, B. A., & Stroebe, W. (2007). Relative accessibility of domain knowledge and creativity: The effects of knowledge activation on the quantity and quality of generated ideas. *Journal of Experimental Social Psychology, 43,* 933–946.

Rietzschel, E. F., Nijstad, B. A., & Stroebe, W. (2014). Effects of problem scope and creativity instructions on idea generation and selection. *Creativity Research Journal, 26(2),* 185–191.

Rinne, T., Steel, G. D., & Fairweather, J. (2013). The role of Hofstede's individualism in national-level creativity. *Creativity Research Journal, 25,* 129–136.

Robbins, T. W. (1984). Cortical noradrenaline, attention and arousal. *Psychological Medicine, 14,* 13–21.

Rosing, K., Frese, M., & Bausch, A. (2011). Explaining the heterogeneity of the leadership–innovation relationship: Ambidextrous leadership. *Leadership Quarterly, 22,* 956–974.

Roskes, M., De Dreu, C. K. W., & Nijstad, B. A. (2012). Necessity is the mother of invention: Avoidance motivation stimulates creativity through cognitive effort. *Journal of Personality and Social Psychology, 103,* 242–256.

Roskes, M., Elliot, A., Nijstad, B. A., & De Dreu, C. K. W. (2013). Time pressure undermines performance more under avoidance than approach motivation. *Personality and Social Psychology Bulletin, 39,* 803–813.

Sacramento, C. A., Fay, D., & West, M. A. (2013). Workplace duties or opportunities?: Challenge stressors, regulatory focus, and creativity. *Organizational Behavior and Human Decision Processes, 121,* 141–157.

Schooler, J. W., & Melcher, J. (1995). The ineffability of insight. In S. M. Smith, M. Steven, T. B. Ward, & R. A. Finke (Eds.), *The creative cognition approach* (pp. 97–133). Cambridge, MA: MIT Press.

Schwarz, N., & Bless, H. (1991). Happy and mindless, but sad and smart?: The impact of affective states on analytic reasoning. In J. P. Forgas (Ed.), *Emotion and social judgments* (pp. 55–71). Elmsford, NY: Pergamon Press.

Shin, S. J., Kim, T.-Y., & Lee, J.-Y. (2012). Cognitive team diversity and individual team member creativity: A cross-level interaction. *Academy of Management Journal, 55,* 197–212.

Shin, S. J., & Zhou, J. (2003). Transformational leadership, conservation, and creativity: Evidence from Korea. *Academy of Management Journal, 46,* 703–714.

Simonton, D. K. (1999). *Origins of genius: Darwinian perspectives on creativity.* New York: Oxford University Press.

Simonton, D. K. (2003). Scientific creativity as stochastic behavior: The integration of product, person, and process perspectives. *Psychological Bulletin, 129,* 475–494.

Slijkhuis, J. M., Rietzschel, E. F., & Van Yperen, N. W. (2013). How evaluation and need for structure affect motivation and creativity. *European Journal of Work and Organizational Psychology, 22,* 15–25.

Staw, B. M., Sandelands, L. E., & Dutton, J. E. (1981). Threat-rigidity effects in organizational behavior: A multilevel analysis. *Administrative Science Quarterly, 26,* 501–524.

Sternberg, R. J., & Lubart, T. I. (1999). The concept of creativity: Prospects and paradigms. In R. J. Sternberg (Ed.), *Handbook of creativity* (pp. 3–15). New York: Cambridge University Press.

To, M. L., Fisher, C. D., & Ashkanasy, N. M.

(2012). Within-person relationships between mood and creativity. *Journal of Applied Psychology, 97,* 599–612.

Tomasello, M., Kruger, A. C., & Ratner, H. H. (1993). Cultural learning. *Brain and Behavioral Sciences, 16,* 495–511.

Tooby, J., & Cosmides, L. (1992). The psychological foundations of culture. In J. Barkow, L. Cosmides, & J. Tooby (Eds.), *The adapted mind* (pp. 19–136). New York: Oxford University Press.

Torrance, E. P. (1966). *Torrance tests of creative thinking.* Princeton, NJ: Personnel Press.

Unsworth, N., & Engle, R. W. (2007). The nature of individual differences in working memory capacity: Active maintenance in primary memory and controlled search from secondary memory. *Psychological Review, 114,* 104–132.

Van Dyne, L., Jehn, K. A., & Cummings, A. (2002). Differential effects of strain on two forms of work performance: Individual employee sales and creativity. *Journal of Organizational Behavior, 23,* 57–74.

Van Kleef, G. A., Anastasopoulou, C., & Nijstad, B. A. (2010). Can expressions of anger enhance creativity?: A test of the Emotions as Social Information (EASI) model. *Journal of Experimental Social Psychology, 46,* 1042–1048.

Wang, A.-C., & Cheng, D.-S. (2010). When does benevolent leadership lead to creativity?: The moderating role of creative role identity and job autonomy. *Journal of Organizational Behavior, 31,* 106–121.

Ward, T. B. (1994). Structured imagination: The role of category structure in exemplar generation. *Cognitive Psychology, 27,* 1–40.

Ward, T. B., Smith, S. M., & Finke, R. A. (1999). Creative cognition. In R. J. Sternberg (Ed.), *Handbook of creativity* (pp. 189–212). New York: Cambridge University Press.

Watson, D., Clark, L. A., & Tellegen, A. (1988). Development and validation of brief measures of positive and negative affect: The PANAS scales. *Journal of Personality and Social Psychology, 54,* 1063–1070.

Watson, D., Wiese, D., Vaidya, J., & Tellegen, A. (1999). The two general activation systems of affect: Structural findings, evolutionary considerations, and psychobiological evidence. *Journal of Personality and Social Psychology, 76,* 820–838.

Weisberg, R. W. (1999). Creativity and knowledge: A challenge to theories. In R. J. Sternberg (Ed.), *Handbook of creativity* (pp. 226–250). New York: Cambridge University Press.

Zhou, J., & George, J. M. (2001). When job dissatisfaction leads to creativity: Encouraging the expression of voice. *Academy of Management Journal, 44,* 682–696.

Zhou, J., & Su, Y. (2010). A missing piece of the puzzle: The organizational context in cultural patterns of creativity. *Management and Organization Review, 6,* 391–413.

Zou, X., Tam, K., Morris, M. W., Lee, L., Lau, I., & Chiu, C. Y. (2009). Culture as common sense: Perceived consensus vs. personal beliefs as mechanisms of cultural influence. *Journal of Personality and Social Psychology, 97,* 579–597.

CHAPTER 20

Motivation, Competence, and Job Burnout

MICHAEL P. LEITER
CHRISTINA MASLACH

Burnout has long been recognized as a phenomenon reflecting a crisis in work-related motivation (Maslach, Schaufeli, & Leiter, 2001). The basic narrative begins with new employees displaying keen enthusiasm, continues through their experience of periods of overcommitment and frustration, and ends as they decline into a syndrome of chronic exhaustion, cynicism, and discouragement. This narrative signals that burnout is not simply a lack of motivation but a loss of motivation that was evident in a more idealistic past (Cherniss, 1980). A career crisis arises when employees fail to find fulfillment within their work. As that experience persists, employees may disengage from worklife. Some may find fulfillment in other life domains, but many are stymied in doing so. Work not only consumes much of people's lives, limiting chances for fulfillment in other domains, but it is also a domain in which people establish competence, develop fulfilling relationships, and discover their capacity to make things happen. When thwarted in the work domain, many people lack viable alternatives for seeking fulfillment. Left unaddressed, the frustrations that contribute to burnout lead employees to withdraw their emotional and cognitive engagement with work (Bakker, Albrecht, & Leiter, 2011) and in some instances to

develop depression (Hakanen, Schaufeli, & Ahola, 2008).

CORE NEEDS

This chapter focuses on the motivational implications for job burnout relative to the three core needs of self-determination theory (SDT; Deci & Ryan, 1985): belonging or relatedness, autonomy, and competence. The SDT model contends that these needs are fundamental to human experience. The have implications for job burnout because of their direct relevance to the work context.

1. *Belonging or relatedness*. Contemporary work occurs in a social context. Few people work as independent practitioners (Galegher, Kraut, & Egido, 2014). People work as part of a team. Whether it be a cohesive group of individuals working in immediate proximity to one another or a widely dispersed global network, team structures define interdependencies among the work of its participants. A sense of belonging at work fulfills people's core need to be consequential in the utilitarian sense of furthering careers and in the emotional sense of sharing existence with people of similar interests and background.

2. *Autonomy or agency.* Work settings have authority structures that define employees' prerogatives for making decisions and taking initiative. Opportunities for employees to use highly developed skills and capabilities allow them to exercise agency through their work, thereby fulfilling their need for autonomy.

3. *Competence.* Work settings are the places where most people exercise their most sophisticated skills, with opportunities to witness their impact. Although many jobs fall short of an ideal level of skills use and direct feedback, work settings have a greater potential than most other life domains for fulfilling the core need for competence.

Within the SDT, the critical issue for motivation is the degree of need satisfaction rather than need strength because, regardless of need strength, the gap between need and satisfaction translates most directly into motivation to address that need (Van den Broeck, Vansteenkiste, De Witte, & Lens, 2008). The fulfillment of one need has positive implications for the fulfillment of the other two needs, such that researchers have consolidated assessment of the needs to refer to a composite need fulfillment metric (e. g., Vansteenkiste, Neyrinck, Niemic, Soenens, & De Witte, 2007).

Two Dynamics

Research and theorizing have identified two general dynamics occurring in the process of burnout. One dynamic follows a hydraulic model in which employees allocate a finite store of energy to pursuing their goals and aspirations at work (Schaufeli & Bakker, 2004). Energy is a limited personal resource; people allocate only so much of their individual energy to work. As work demands become more intense, consume more time, or otherwise exceed employees' capacity, employees devote more of their personal energy to work to compensate for the job resource shortfall. Replenishing the work-dedicated portion of energy from nonwork life can diminish the quality of personal life. When excessive demands persist, people exhaust their personal energy, which culminates in the exhaustion, distancing, and

inefficacy of burnout. Demands that result in chronic exhaustion lead to long-term health consequences for employees.

From a job demands/resources perspective, each demand consumes packets of energy. Access to job resources allows employees to spread those energy requirements over workplace as well as personal resources. In a well-resourced work environment, employees can accommodate more job demands through their access to job resources, moderating the effect of demands on their personal energy. Similarly, the biopsychosocial model (Blascovich, Mendes, Hunter, & Salomon, 1999) provided more evidence of distinct physiological responses to challenge situations (in which resources matched demands) than to threat situations (in which demands overwhelmed available resources). The conservation of resources perspective (COR; Hobfoll, 1989) posits a fundamental motivation to conserve, recover, and acquire resources to maintain a capacity to address demands as they arise. The COR posits that employees must acquire, manage, and carefully allocate their personal resources as a prerequisite for pursuing any objectives at work.

Both the COR (Hobfoll, 1989) and job demands–resources model (JD/R; Demerouti, Bakker, Nachreiner, & Schaufeli, 2001) have qualities of limited theory (Dweck, 2012; Job, Dweck, & Walton, 2010), in that they propose that energy is a finite resource that is depleted through use. In contrast, a growth mindset opens the potential for thriving by reinterpreting the nature of a demand or people's capacity to respond effectively to that demand. From a limited mindset perspective, energy depletion presents a problem. COR addresses that problem by proposing that people are motivated to protect and to gather resources: The more resources one gathers, the better one is able to control the rate of inevitable energy depletion. The availability of personal energy provides the necessary infrastructure for pursuing other goals and fulfilling other needs because all goal-oriented activity requires energy.

The JD/R addresses energy depletion through a focus on the availability and accessibility of job resources. People may call on job resources to reduce the load on their personal resources, to augment the potential impact of those personal resources, or to replenish those resources after depletion. Job demands deplete resources, leading to burnout when left unattended; job resources supplement resources, leading to work engagement when sustained.

The JD/R perspective proposes that job resources provide a means for needs satisfaction. In a resource-rich environment, employees are able to thrive more because relevant resources are meeting their core needs. In contrast, demanding environments with sparse resources frustrate employees, causing them to maintain an energy-depleting process that can eventually result in job burnout (Schaufeli & Bakker, 2004). Van den Broeck and colleagues (2008) found support for this proposition in demonstrating that SDT need fulfillment partially mediates relationships of job demands and job resources with both exhaustion and the vigor aspect of work engagement. However, the self-report survey format presents serious challenges to separating job resources from need fulfillment. For example, the sample item for the job resource of task autonomy was "I can choose my way of working," while the sample item for the need satisfaction for autonomy was "I feel like I can pretty much be myself at work." The sample item for the job resource of positive feedback was "I get mainly positive feedback on my work method," while the sample item for the fulfillment of belonging was "People at work care about me." It is difficult to explain how respondents could answer positively to one side of these item pairs without responding similarly to the other side of the pair. Not surprisingly, the path from job resources to need satisfaction was 0.86. The upshot is that some amount of the strong association of need fulfillment with job resources arises from overlapping constructs, not solely a process of job resources contributing to need fulfillment. A more convincing argument would draw on an evaluation of job resources from an independent data source.

Crawford, LePine, and Rich (2010) extended the JD/R theory in applying a differentiation of challenge versus hindrance demands. In their meta-analysis, they found that challenge demands were associated with increased engagement, whereas hindrance demands were associated with decreased engagement and increased burnout. They pointed out that this differentiation requires an extension of the JD/R theory because the differentiation rests on individual appraisal rather than an inherent quality of the demand itself. They speculated that a demand that may be considered a challenge at one point in a career may be experienced as a hindrance at another point as employees experience chronic frustration in addressing the demand. In subsequent research (e.g., Demerouti & Bakker, 2011; Tuckey, Bakker, & Dollard, 2012), JD/R proponents have embraced the differentiation of challenge from hindrance demands. However, these authors have not fully appreciated the implications of this development as a shift away from limited to growth perspectives on employees' energy at work.

The second dynamic concerns value congruence (Maslach & Leiter, 1997). This perspective proposes that the greater the congruence between employees' preferred manner of working and the management environment of their workplaces, the more they engage with their work. Mismatches between employees and important areas of worklife have the capacity to deplete energy, introduce cynical distancing, and undermine employees' sense of efficacy. This dynamic suggests a perpetual motion machine, in that exerting energy within the context of value congruence is energizing in itself. But energy does not spontaneously appear; rather, working in a value-congruent context allows people to develop creative responses to their work. This proposition has been supported by Duffy, Dik, and Steger (2011), who reported that people who experienced their work as a calling have better work outcomes. The essence of a calling arises from an alignment of strong work values with work contexts that support those values. An important part of this dynamic rests on the following: "Intrinsically motivated behaviors, which are performed out of interest and satisfy the innate psychological needs for competence and autonomy are the prototype of self-determined behavior" (Ryan & Deci, 2000, p. 65). That is, intrinsically motivated behaviors implicitly fulfill core needs, such that these actions are energizing in themselves and also have the benefit of absolving employees of expending energy to fulfill these needs elsewhere.

Areas of Worklife

The areas of worklife model (AW; Leiter & Maslach, 2004; Maslach & Leiter, 1997) focuses on congruence between employees' approach to work and the management environment of their workplaces. The AW model encompasses six areas with specific reference to job burnout: manageable workload, control, reward, community, fairness, and values. To some extent, the values area of worklife has the broadest relevance in its focus on the alignment of organizational values in action (Argyris & Schön, 1974) with employees' personal and professional values.

Employees' positions on the other five areas of worklife concern their values pertaining to the management of their time at work. The extent to which *workload* is manageable concerns not only employees' preferences as to how much they wish to exert themselves but also their values concerning the relative importance of work activities. For example, human service providers' incongruity regarding a large caseload may concern primarily the opportunity to reduce the numbers of clients in order to pursue the more time-consuming interactions required for developing a meaningful therapeutic relationship. The providers may be happy to contribute their energy to the goal of meeting client demand but resent the workload structure that excludes meeting that demand in a manner consistent with the providers' values. Rather than fulfilling their motives for autonomy and competence, providers experience their workload as unmanageable, thereby undermining their sense of need satisfaction for both motives.

The *control* area of worklife pertains not only to employees' need to experience a sense of agency in their work but also the value they place on important managerial issues, including the exercise of authority, leader–follower relationships, and qualities of teamwork. For some employees, being fully integrated into a workgroup increases their sense of control, whereas others may prefer their work to the clearly separated from that of others in the workplace. As with reward, community, and fairness, employees' compatibility with the control area of worklife has implications for their needs for belonging, autonomy, and competence. Employees interpret receiving a greater range of control over their work as a vote of confidence from the supervisor regarding their competence. As such, an increase in their autonomy provides fulfillment of their needs for competence and belonging, with its implications for an improved supervisory relationship.

In contrast, job crafting may increase employees' sense of control, independent of the supervisory relationship (Bakker, Demerouti, & Sanz-Vergel, 2014). Although job crafting may occur as part of a collaborative process involving colleagues, its central premise rests on employees identifying ways to modify their individual work activities to increase the proportion of their work time devoted to valued activities at the expense of less valued activities. Wrzesniewski and Dutton (2001) defined job crafting as "the physical and cognitive changes individuals make in the task or relational boundaries of their work" (p. 179). From this definition, individuals act to craft their jobs but recognize that such changes have implications for their relationships at work.

The *reward* area of worklife concerns recognition from people at work. Recognition has its most direct relevance to employees' competence, but such confirmation of competence occurs within the context of relationships that have both a history and future expectations (Høigaard, Giske, & Sundsli, 2012). Employees experience confirmation of their competence, as well as their sense of belonging, when receiving recognition from colleagues and supervisors for the quality of their contribution to the work. Collegial recognition has distinct relevance to competence because coworkers have a realistic understanding of what the job demands entail (Okello & Gilson, 2015). Being recognized as a competent contributor provides a solid foundation for being a valued member of a workgroup.

The *community* area of worklife has the most direct relevance to belonging, in that it reflects employees' standing within their workgroup. The quality of relationships among people in their day-to-day workplace encounters lets people know where they stand. The deep emotional and practical importance of workplace social relationships prompts people to carefully monitor their social encounters for metacommunications about their relationships (Leiter, 2013). Negative social encounters, including the subtlest instances of incivility, may be alarming. Although a negative encounter may lack intensity, the metacomment conveyed verbally or nonverbally thwarts the potential for relatedness. In contrast, civil encounters contribute to fulfilling a need for belonging because civility conveys a metacommunication confirming acceptance within the workplace community.

The *fairness* area of worklife also has implications for employees' sense of belonging because just treatment functions similarly to civility in confirming membership in the workplace community (Estes & Wang, 2008; Mouffe, 1992). The process of justice has implications for other areas of worklife, as it influences employees' workload, decision-making authority, and recognition of their contributions. Injustice has a demotivating quality, in that it has the capacity to interrupt the connection of employees' contributions and the reception of expected intrinsic or extrinsic outcomes. For example, when management ignores an employee's extraordinary contribution, or colleagues take undeserved credit for another's contribution, the attractiveness of making further contributions diminishes.

The most encompassing of the six areas of worklife and the one with the broadest implications for core needs is *values*. The congruence of personal and workplace values opens pathways for employees to pursue goals that are personally fulfilling, while contributing to the workgroup's mission. In situations of value congruence, employees are most likely to experience both intrinsic and extrinsic satisfaction because they are not only furthering their own personal or professional values but also making progress on goals favored by their employers.

In summary, Figure 20.1 displays the relationships of core needs from the SDT model with the six areas of worklife. The chart indicates the primary need for each of area of worklife, with workload and reward relating to competence, control relating to

	Belonging	Autonomy	Competence
Workload			x
Control		x	
Reward			x
Community	x		
Fairness	x		
Values	x	x	x

FIGURE 20.1. Relationship of core needs with areas of worklife.

autonomy, and community and fairness relating to belonging. Value congruence has direct implications for all three core needs. As noted, worklife areas have relevance beyond the primary need noted in Figure 20.1.

Two Processes of the AW Model

The AW model contains two distinct processes. The energy process begins with the direct path from manageable workload to exhaustion that mediates workload's relationships with cynicism and inefficacy. The values process begins with direct paths from value congruence to all three aspects of burnout. Value congruence mediates the relationships of control, reward, community, and fairness with burnout. Figure 20.2 displays the two-process model.

A survey of Canadian and Spanish nurses found support for a two-process model in which exhaustion mediated the relationship of manageable workload with the other two aspects of burnout, while values maintained direct relationships with exhaustion, cynicism, and inefficacy (Leiter, Gascon, & Martínez-Jarreta, 2008). Values mediated relationships of the other areas of worklife with burnout. The analysis noted variations in the relative importance of the two processes in that the exhaustion process was more salient with the Canadian sample, while the values process was more salient for the Spanish sample. Leiter, Frank, and Matheson (2009) in a survey of 2,536 Canadian physicians, also found support for this

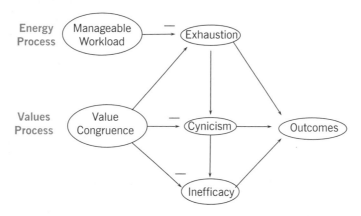

FIGURE 20.2. The two-process model of burnout.

two-process model, with exhaustion more closely related to manageable workload, while all three aspects of burnout had direct relationships with value congruence.

More broadly, in their consideration of a variety of samples for their examination of the AW model, Leiter and Maslach (2004) found that the control area of worklife could work as a starting point for both processes. Regarding the energy process, a positive experience of control implied that employees exercised some degree of discretion over the quality, content, or pacing of their work; that is, the manageability of workload did not just depend on the nature of assigned tasks. Manageability also reflected the extent to which employees had the capacity—in terms of both ability and authority—to make decisions about the tasks they were to undertake. A manageable workload may result from the thoughtful task assignments of a perceptive, accommodating supervisor or a detailed, realistic job analysis that produces job demands that fit comfortably within the capacity, skills, and abilities of employees. Alternatively, manageable workload rests on employees exercising discretion over the extent to which they accommodate job demands. A context resulting from a positive level of control has the advantage of increased flexibility, as employees accommodate their response to job demands according to their available time and energy as it fluctuates across days and situations.

Regarding the values process, control is indicative of employees' capacity to pursue goals they consider important and to pursue those goals in the manner in which they prefer to work. Having some choice of the people with whom they work provides employees with the potential to exercise discretion over the nature of their team participation. Control within the community area of worklife permits employees to avoid occasions for mistreatment from other people at work. Instead, they may concentrate their social encounters at work on people who provide meaningful confirmation of their membership within the workgroup and the efficacy evident in their contributions to the team's work. Control regarding fairness implies that employees have access to procedures to participate in important workplace decisions. An additional issue regarding fairness is access to procedures to appeal decisions with which they take exception. Related to fairness, control in the reward area of worklife implies that employees have opportunities to participate in activities that bring recognition from peers and managers. The fairness with which the organization allocates extrinsic rewards and provides opportunities for intrinsically rewarding work constitute an important dimension of fairness within the organization. In both these areas—reward and fairness—control translates into access to procedures that permit individuals to go beyond passively awaiting reasonable treatment to taking a proactive role in ensuring justice for themselves and for their colleagues. Exercising agency in regard to fair treatment can be a potentially powerful dimension of fulfilling employees' needs for a sense of autonomy. Participating in the important decisions that govern the encounters among members of an organization, regarding both formal and informal dimensions of worklife, makes a significant contribution to employees' engagement with their work (Cohen-Charash, & Spector, 2001).

IMPLICATIONS FOR INTERVENTION

Interventions to address burnout cover a range from primary prevention initiatives to prepare employees for the rigors of worklife through secondary prevention initiatives to assist at-risk individuals to manage their worklife crises, to treatment initiatives to facilitate recovery for people who are experiencing burnout (Conyne, 1991). These initiatives work on two sides of the employment relationship. One side concerns workplace structures and procedures: Managers can improve the extent to which their practices motivate employees to work effectively in pursuit of the organizational mission. These initiatives generally involve increasing flexibility in workplace practices. Increased flexibility opens opportunities for good person–job fit to a wider variety of employees. The other side concerns employees' skills, attitudes, and practices to maintain their motivations to pursue their aspirations and to contribute effectively to the organization's well-being. These approaches are complementary; however, in practice the individual approach has received greater emphasis (Leiter & Maslach, 2014). Motivation is central to both approaches.

Primary Prevention: Occupational Life Skills

As work has become more independent of physical location and time of day, maintaining the work–nonwork boundary has become a core life skill for individuals and an important policy issue for management (Hislop & Axtell, 2011; Kirchmeyer, 1995). The fundamental challenge is that allocating time to either work or personal life is much more a matter of choice: individuals choose when and where to focus on work; management sets both implicit and explicit expectations. Neither the setting nor time of day determines whether employees are engaged in work.

Fluid work–nonwork boundaries hold potential pitfalls. By undercommitting to their jobs, employees run the risk of dismissal or at least poor performance reviews. Although leaders have promoted results-only performance evaluations (Aguinis, Joo, & Gottfredson, 2011), the amount of time employees spend at the job setting contributes strongly to their reputation at work. Considerations of job burnout have emphasized employees' overcommitment to their jobs as a contributing factor (e.g., Moen, Lam, Ammons, & Kelly, 2013). These examinations prompt considerations of employees' capacity to work, reflecting on the number of work hours that people can possibly sustain. That capacity appears to vary with the type of work, the intensity of afterhours interruptions, personal priorities, and the competing demands on employees' lives in terms of family or unpaid commitments (Donahue et al., 2012). A closely related issue is equity. Work that occurs outside of regular business hours at other locations may lack recognition for compensation or performance considerations (Khamisa, Peltzer, & Oldenburg, 2013).

Much of the available advice and training on maintaining work–life balance builds upon individuals reflecting on their priorities, setting goals, and maintaining a consistent schedule through self-discipline aided by insight. For example, Allen (2015) advises avoiding the compelling forces of work addiction and of workplace guilt to construct a reasonable balance of work through careful time management. Morales (2011) advises an approach that resembles mindfulness meditation, in which people free their minds from concentrating on work or other externally imposed structures. The success of these approaches has not been conclusively demonstrated.

Research on organizational initiatives to improve work–life balance have covered policies designed to limit work hours, equity initiatives to provide recognition of nonwork interference, and efforts to embed work–nonwork balance into organizational cultures (Brough & O'Driscoll, 2010). Hammer, Neal, Newsom, Brockwood, and

Colton (2005) found that individuals' use of alternative work arrangements was associated with greater job satisfaction, but that couples' use of these arrangements was not related to their reports of work–family conflict. They further reported that use of alternative work arrangements was positively associated with women's reports of family–work interference. In short, the work–nonwork balance has dynamic qualities that defy simple solutions.

Some have proposed that maintaining a balance between work and nonwork defies the capacity of individual discipline or organizational policies. White, Hill, McGovern, Mills, and Smeaton (2003) noted contradictions between high-performance management policies and practices that maintain work–life balance. Meeting the requirements of high-performance expectations in a competitive global economy requires not only more time than is allowed within a standard work day but also a broader perspective than one can establish within a corporate culture. Fleming (2014) went further, noting that unpaid work has become a feature of contemporary work that exceeds whatever individuals can learn to manage. He differentiated among free work, free self-organization, and free self-development. He proposed that contemporary corporations act as if compelled to go beyond the domain of the work organization to draw on employees' personal time, activities, and cultural perspectives to connect with their markets and to position themselves advantageously in relation to competitors. From this perspective, corporations, as well as public sector organizations, compel employees consistently to contribute time from their personal and social lives, far beyond the occasional demands of additional unpaid work hours. Self-organizing time includes the personal commitment involved in arranging family life around work schedules, commuting, having appropriate clothing, and attending extramural organizational events. Self-development includes not only formal and ongoing informal education and skills development but also employees' awareness of cultural trends that could have implications for marketing or client development initiatives for the employing organizations. Maintaining a balanced life in relation to work is more akin to treading water in a fast-moving current than being the master of one's fate regarding choices of how to spend one's time or contribute one's talents.

Central themes for motivation concern the extent to which frustrations in maintaining a reasonable balance between work and nonwork contribute to burnout. Although work is an important domain for employees to fulfill their aspirations for belonging, autonomy, and competence, it is not the only domain for doing so (Deci & Ryan, 1985). A convincing argument could be made for work being many employees' primary domain for finding fulfillment regarding competence; an even stronger case could be made for family being the primary area for finding fulfillment for belonging. In some ways, a more comprehensive participation in work may further employees' sense of agency regarding their work participation. But in other ways, an expanding involvement in work beyond the time and space of the usual workweek may reflect a serious lack of autonomy.

In light of the challenges inherent in maintaining a viable relationship with work in the 21st century, employees would benefit from thorough preparation in maintaining fulfilling, balanced, and meaningful participation in work. However, the current state of knowledge appears to be lacking. Without systematic evaluations of individual training programs or company policies, it is difficult to construct a valid curriculum for action.

Secondary Prevention: Improving Relationships with Work

Personal Qualities

Employees vary in their vulnerability to burnout. Some aspects of vulnerability may be evident from the beginning of an employment relationship. Personal qualities of employees and structural qualities of workplaces may be indicative of risk.

To a modest extent, personal characteristics are associated with propensity to experience burnout. Burnout correlates negatively with emotional stability, extraversion, and intellect/autonomy (Bakker, Van Der Zee, Lewig, & Dollard, 2006). Exhaustion and cynicism are correlated with anxiety attachment styles; inefficacy is correlated with avoidance attachment (Leiter, Day, & Price, 2015). In addition to these direct effects, analyses have confirmed moderating effects for personal characteristics, such that they strengthen or weaken relationships of workplace qualities with the three aspects of burnout (Bakker et al., 2006). A potential strategy for secondary prevention is to increase the capacity of people with certain personal characteristics to anticipate their vulnerabilities to workplace distress.

To a much greater extent, job burnout reflects strains in the relationships of individuals with the work environment. For example, although some people may be especially sensitive to the strains of work overload, everyone has a limit beyond which work demands become overwhelming. A considerable body of research has defined qualities of worklife that employees experience as aggravating and conducive to job burnout.

Energy Process

The AW model (Leiter & Maslach, 2004; Maslach & Leiter, 1997) points toward six areas of worklife in which mismatches of employees with their work context contribute to burnout. As noted, mismatches in these worklife areas reflect frustrations in employees' efforts to fulfill core needs of belonging, autonomy, and competence. A better alignment can occur through management modifying policies, practices, and structures to better accommodate employees' preferences and aspirations. Improvement may also occur through employees' broadening of their capacity to interact effectively with these areas of worklife. A combination of initiatives from management and from employees provides a means of creating a better alignment of aspirations with conditions.

Figure 20.3 displays an overview of these two strategies regarding the energy process. Management efforts could focus on changing the quantity, content, or process of work assignments. The simplest, but often the least available, approach would be for management to reduce work demands on employees. More complex, but often more available, strategies focus on the content or process of work assignments rather than striving to reduce employees' workload.

Lean management provides a means of redesigning workload to improve its alignment with employees' approach to work (Arnheiter & Maleyeff, 2005). Semmer, Tschan, Meier, Facchin, and Jacobshagen (2010) have provided a valuable perspective on the power of poorly organized work to contribute to workplace distress,

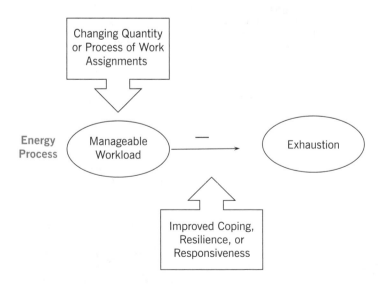

FIGURE 20.3. Intervention approaches: Energy process.

including burnout. Employees experience illegitimate tasks as especially burdensome. Illegitimate tasks share qualities with the hindrance demands discussed previously. They are work expectations that lie beyond what employees consider to be their expertise, responsibility, or professional domain. *Illegitimate tasks* include poorly organized work that requires employees to exert additional effort to bring the task demand to the point at which they can begin constructive action. Such job demands frustrate employees' pursuit of autonomy, in that illegitimate tasks impose work that employees would not have sought on their own initiative. These demands frustrate their sense of efficacy because they are outside of the domain of their expertise or professional responsibility. Even successful completion of illegitimate tasks is unfulfilling because it concerns work employees do not value.

A lean management intervention is focused primarily on eliminating waste as a means of improving organizational performance (Arnheiter & Maleyeff, 2005). Voogd (2009) discussed the potential for lean management to reduce employees' burnout in the context of a lean intervention occurring in a Dutch health care organization. Unfortunately, the project did not proceed to providing data to evaluate its impact on burnout, but it did describe a process through which that impact could occur. This is an area with considerable potential for constructive intervention, by improving organizational performance while alleviating unnecessary pressures on employees' experience of workplace demands.

Job crafting is a complementary approach to improving the energy process contributing to burnout. Employees explore the potential for unilaterally modifying their work activities, with the goal of improving the proportion of effort devoted to preferred activities (Berg, Wrzesniewski, & Dutton, 2010). Crafting may not change the total amount of effort or time that employees devote to work, but it improves the balance of the work activities that they consider to be legitimate tasks. As with a lean management intervention, job crafting holds the potential for contributing to employees' fulfillment of autonomy motives. The very process of crafting confirms that employees' function

with agency in shaping their jobs beyond the direction of management. The job crafting process potentially increases the proportion of employees' workdays devoted to autonomous activities. By emphasizing legitimate tasks, employees are more likely to engage in activities that confirm their sense of competence because they are emphasizing work that aligns with their values.

Values Process

The values process focuses primarily on the alignment of the management environment with employees' personal and professional values. The focus may be on the content of work activities. For example, health care providers may value devoting more of their work time to supportive communication with patients, in contrast to clinical procedures and record keeping. Alternatively, the focus may be on the process of work or the work environment. For example, many health care professionals prefer to exercise discretion in their practice. Doing so not only contributes to fulfilling their core need for autonomy but it also confirms their professional status as people who possess refined expertise, and who manage their contributions with direct reference to the welfare of patients. Figure 20.4 displays the values intervention process.

CREW (Civility, Respect, and Engagement with Work) provides an example of a values process intervention focusing on the social environment of workplaces (Leiter, Day, Oore, & Spence Laschinger, 2012; Leiter, Laschinger, Day, & Oore, 2011; Osatuke, Moore, Ward, Dyrenforth, & Belton, 2009). In the CREW process, facilitators lead conversations about the quality of workplace interactions. The primary focus in on the contrast of civility with incivility. Rather than reference an abstract set of etiquette rules, facilitators elicit from participants their understanding of what constitutes civility and respect in their workgroup. Group conversations contrast these behaviors and statements with those reflecting incivility. Through an ongoing series of meetings—usually over the course of 6 months—participants explore initiatives to increase the proportion of civil interactions within their workgroups. The first priority

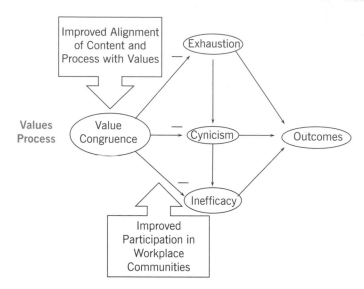

FIGURE 20.4. Intervention approaches: Values process.

for facilitators is establishing a sense of psychological safety among participants in the meetings. In the meetings, rather than being concerned with stamping out incivility, the role plays and conversations are designed to increase civility. This focus on the positive side of social encounters is integral to the CREW approach.

CREW constitutes a values process intervention because it strives to encourage behavior that is more consistent with employees' ideals for work (Leiter, 2013). The core motive for belonging or relatedness does not include finding fulfillment in the mere proximity of people. Negative social encounters actively thwart that motive. Recent research on workplace incivility has highlighted the importance of civil social exchanges (Cortina, 2008). This work has demonstrated that incivility, as low-intensity social interactions, creates distress out of proportion with the severity of the behavior. A passing moment in which a colleague rolls his or her eyes in response to an employee's comment, or neglects to respond to a greeting, can have a major impact on an employee.

Leiter (2013) proposed risk perception as a dynamic that contributes to the power of incivility. Uncivil behavior conveys a meta-communication that excludes the recipient of that behavior from the community of the instigator. In addition, anyone witnessing

the interaction would know that the behavior is meant to exclude the recipient. Being excluded from a community constitutes a serious threat to people who are fundamentally social creatures. The need for belonging is basic and powerful because it is important. Group membership was certainly essential in primitive times, but it remains essential in the very social world of contemporary work.

Civil social exchanges are consistent with the values of the large majority of people at work (Hershcovis, 2011; Lim, Cortina, & Magley, 2008), although exceptions exist. Central to the definition of incivility is its ambiguous intent: People may take offense at behavior whose instigator had not intended to cause offense. For example, an employee may engage in a pleasant conversation in the hallway without realizing that a coworker reading a complex document nearby finds that conversation to be annoying. The experienced incivility arises from a momentary lack of consideration or a flaw in workplace design, rather than a coworker's callous disregard for others.

Leiter and colleagues (2011, 2012) found that CREW was effective at improving employees' experiences of civility within their workgroups and that this improvement mediated improvements in job burnout, commitment, and trust. They identified the behavioral design of CREW as essential to its success. The role plays, conversations, and assignments to enact new behaviors within the work setting move values from thoughts or words into action. That is, people do not simply voice a preference for civil social relationships; they develop behavioral repertoires that put that commitment into action. The 1-year follow-up assessment (Leiter et al., 2012) found that most of the improvements were sustained. The robustness of these improvements was attributed to the design of CREW as a workgroup intervention. Instead of employees learning social skills or improved emotional intelligence as individuals, members of the workgroup collaborated on develop a new social dynamic. Not only did people strive to initiate more civil interactions but their colleagues also committed to reacting accordingly. By working on both ends of social encounters, the intervention gained momentum that was sustained over time.

The CREW intervention furthered employees' potential for fulfilling needs for belonging, autonomy, and competence. Increased civility provides a more inviting social environment at work, facilitating employees' interactions with one another. Much of contemporary work occurs within the context of teamwork. It is through collaborative work that people confirm their competence and gain the collegial respect necessary to support autonomous participation in worklife.

Secondary prevention initiatives increase employees' resilience at work by both improving employees' individual capacities and designing work to be more humane, responsive, and sensitive. An important theme is that well-designed workplaces inspire motivation by providing more opportunities for employees to fulfill their core needs. Improving workplaces combines the removal of demotivating qualities from work and an increase of motivating opportunities that confirm employees' belonging, autonomy, and competence.

TREATMENT: RECOVERY STRATEGIES

A sustained period of burnout presents major challenges for recovery that are inherent in the three aspects of the syndrome.

First, when exhausted, people face difficulties in experiencing motives and lack the capacity to translate motivation into effective action. For example, teachers experiencing exhaustion from the highly social work of instructing may feel averse to contact with other people because it brings social demands. Even if they feel motivated through loneliness to seek out other people, they lack the energy to arrange social contact or to attend an event. Second, the cynical, depersonalized quality of burnout reflects indifference to anything associated with work. The process of distancing oneself from work decreases the energy and attention that people bring to motives pertaining to work. Third, the low sense of efficacy that defines burnout reflects an inability through work to fulfill the core need of competence.

One method for alleviating serious burnout is cognitive-behavioral therapy (CBT). Lloyd, Bond, and Flaxman (2013) reported success of CBT, in contrast to a waiting-list control group. They proposed that an important underlying dynamic of this treatment was the increase in cognitive flexibility that participants achieved through CBT. The improvement was especially evident with regard to exhaustion and depersonalization, suggesting that the increase in flexibility allowed participants to access their energy and their interest. Another research group (Van Dam, Keijsers, Eling, & Becker, 2012) found that "perceived job competence, involvement in work and responsiveness to rewards had returned to normal levels" (p. 333). These findings confirmed that burnout symptoms persisted for many months, and that a return of previously suppressed motivation was an integral part of the recovery process.

CONCLUSION

This overview of motivation, competence, and burnout has focused on burnout as a crisis in both motivation and competence for employees. The core aspects of burnout—exhaustion, cynicism, and inefficacy—reflect a state in which employees are less likely not only to feel motivated but also to translate motivations into action. A primary theme in burnout intervention is to increase employees' capacity to find fulfillment of core motives through their work participation. Improving both employees' capacity to cope and the management environment of work results in an environment in which people can better pursue their core values through their work. These issues pertain to the full range, from primary intervention to secondary intervention and treatment.

REFERENCES

Aguinis, H., Joo, H., & Gottfredson, R. K. (2011). Why we hate performance management—And why we should love it. *Business Horizons, 54,* 503–507.

Allen, M. (2015). Top 10 tips: Getting a work–life balance. Retrieved from *www.jobs.ac.uk/careers-advice/careers-advice/1339/top-10-tips-getting-a-work-life-balance.*

Argyris, C., & Schön, D. (1974). *Theory in practice: Increasing professional effectiveness.* San Francisco: Jossey-Bass.

Arnheiter, E. D., & Maleyeff, J. (2005). The integration of lean management and Six Sigma. *The TQM Journal, 17,* 5–18.

Bakker, A. B., Albrecht, S. L., & Leiter, M. P. (2011). Key questions regarding work engagement. *European Journal of Work and Organizational Psychology, 20,* 4–28.

Bakker, A. B., Demerouti, E., & Sanz-Vergel, I. (2014). Burnout and work engagement: The JD–R approach. *Annual Review of Organizational Psychology and Organizational Behavior, 1,* 389–411.

Bakker, A. B., Van Der Zee, K. I., Lewig, K. A., & Dollard, M. F. (2006). The relationship between the Big Five personality factors and burnout: A study among volunteer counselors. *Journal of Social Psychology, 146,* 31–50.

Berg, J. M., Wrzesniewski, A., & Dutton, J. E. (2010). Perceiving and responding to challenges in job crafting at different ranks: When proactivity requires adaptivity. *Journal of Organizational Behavior, 31,* 158–186.

Blascovich, J., Mendes, W. B., Hunter, S. B., & Salomon, K. (1999). Social "facilitation" as challenge and threat. *Journal of Personality and Social Psychology, 77,* 68–77.

Brough, P., & O'Driscoll, M. P. (2010). Organizational interventions for balancing work and home demands: An overview. *Work and Stress, 24*(3), 280–297.

Cherniss, C. (1980). *Professional burnout in human service organizations.* New York: Praeger.

Cohen-Charash, Y., & Spector, P. E. (2001). The role of justice in organizations: A meta-analysis. *Organizational Behavior and Human Decision Processes, 86,* 278–321.

Conyne, R. K. (1991). Gains in primary prevention: Implications for the counseling profession. *Journal of Counseling and Development, 69,* 277–279.

Cortina, L. M. (2008). Unseen injustice: Incivility as modern discrimination in organizations. *Academy of Management Review, 33,* 55–75.

Crawford, E. R., LePine, J. A., & Rich, B. L. (2010). Linking job demands and resources to employee engagement and burnout: A theoretical extension and meta-analytic test. *Journal of Applied Psychology, 95,* 834–848.

Deci, E. L., & Ryan, R. M. (1985). *Intrinsic motivation and self-determination in human behavior.* New York: Plenum Press.

Demerouti, E., & Bakker, A. B. (2011). The job demands–resources model: Challenges for future research. *SA Journal of Industrial Psychology, 37,* Article 974.

Demerouti, E., Bakker, A. B., Nachreiner, F., & Schaufeli, W. B. (2001). The job demands–resources model of burnout. *Journal of Applied Psychology, 86,* 499–512.

Donahue, E. G., Forest, J., Vallerand, R. J., Lemyre, P. N., Crevier-Braud, L., & Bergeron, É. (2012). Passion for work and emotional exhaustion: The mediating role of rumination and recovery. *Applied Psychology: Health and Well-Being, 4,* 341–368.

Duffy, R. D., Dik, B. J., & Steger, M. F. (2011). Calling and work-related outcomes: Career commitment as a mediator. *Journal of Vocational Behavior, 78,* 210–218.

Dweck, C. S. (2012). Mindsets and human nature: Promoting change in the Middle East, the schoolyard, the racial divide, and willpower. *American Psychologist, 67,* 614–622.

Estes, B., & Wang, J. (2008). Workplace incivility: Impacts on individual and organizational performance. *Human Resource Development Review, 7,* 218–240.

Fleming, P. (2014). *Resisting work: The corporatization of life and its discontents.* Philadelphia: Temple University Press.

Galegher, J., Kraut, R. E., & Egido, C. (2014). *Intellectual teamwork: Social and technological foundations of cooperative work.* Hove, UK: Psychology Press.

Hakanen, J. J., Schaufeli, W. B., & Ahola, K. (2008). The job demands–resources model: A three-year cross-lagged study of burnout, depression, commitment, and work engagement. *Work and Stress, 22,* 224–241.

Hammer, L. B., Neal, M. B., Newsom, J. T., Brockwood, K. J., & Colton, C. L. (2005). A longitudinal study of the effects of dual-earner couples' utilization of family-friendly workplace supports on work and family outcomes. *Journal of Applied Psychology, 90,* 799–810.

Hershcovis, M. S. (2011). "Incivility, social undermining, bullying . . . oh my!": A call to reconcile constructs within workplace aggression research. *Journal of Organizational Behavior, 32,* 499–519.

Hislop, D., & Axtell, C. (2011). Mobile phones during work and non-work time: A case study of mobile, non-managerial workers. *Information and Organization, 21,* 41–56.

Hobfoll, S. E. (1989). Conservation of resources: A new attempt at conceptualizing stress. *American Psychologist, 44,* 513–524.

Høigaard, R., Giske, R., & Sundsli, K. (2012). Newly qualified teachers' work engagement and teacher efficacy influences on job satisfaction, burnout, and the intention to quit. *European Journal of Teacher Education, 35,* 347–357.

Job, V., Dweck, C. S., & Walton, G. M. (2010). Ego depletion—Is it all in your head?: Implicit theories about willpower affect self-regulation. *Psychological Science, 21,* 1686–1693.

Khamisa, N., Peltzer, K., & Oldenburg, B. (2013). Burnout in relation to specific contributing factors and health outcomes among nurses: A systematic review. *International Journal of Environmental Research and Public Health, 10*(6), 2214–2240.

Kirchmeyer, C. (1995). Managing the work-nonwork boundary: An assessment of organizational responses. *Human Relations, 48,* 515–536.

Leiter, M. P. (2013). *Analyzing and theorizing the dynamics of the workplace incivility crisis.* Amsterdam, The Netherlands: Springer.

Leiter, M. P., Day, A., Oore, D. G., & Spence Laschinger, H. K. (2012). Getting better and staying better: Assessing civility, incivility, distress and job attitudes one year after a civility intervention. *Journal of Occupational Health Psychology 17*(4), 425–434.

Leiter, M. P., Day, A., & Price, L. (2015). Attachment styles at work: Measurement, collegial relationships, and burnout. *Burnout Research, 2,* 25–35.

Leiter, M. P., Frank, E., & Matheson, T. J. (2009). Demands, values, and burnout: Their relevance for physicians. *Canadian Family Physician, 55,* 1224–1225.

Leiter, M. P., Gascón, S., & Martínez-Jarreta, B. (2008). A two process model of burnout: Their relevance to Spanish and Canadian nurses. *Psychology in Spain, 12,* 37–45.

Leiter, M. P., Laschinger, H. K., Day, A., & Oore, D. G. (2011). The impact of civility interventions on employee social behavior, distress, and attitudes. *Journal of Applied Psychology, 96*(6), 1258–1275.

Leiter, M. P., & Maslach, C. (2004). Areas of worklife: A structured approach to organizational predictors of job burnout. In P. Perrewé & D. C. Ganster (Eds.), *Research in occupational stress and well-being: Vol. 3. Emotional and physiological processes and positive intervention strategies* (pp. 91–134). Oxford, UK: JAI Press/Elsevier.

Leiter, M. P., & Maslach, C. (2014). Interventions to prevent and alleviate burnout. In M. P. Leiter, A. B. Bakker, & C. Maslach (Eds.), *Burnout at work: A psychological perspective* (pp. 145–167). Hove, UK: Psychology Press.

Lim, S., Cortina, L., M., & Magley, V. J. (2008). Personal and workgroup incivility. Impact on work and health outcomes. *Journal of Applied Psychology, 93,* 95–107.

Lloyd, J., Bond, F. W., & Flaxman, P. E. (2013). The value of psychological flexibility: Examining psychological mechanisms underpinning a cognitive behavioral therapy intervention for burnout. *Work and Stress, 27,* 181–199.

Maslach, C., & Leiter, M. P. (1997). *The truth about burnout.* San Francisco: Jossey-Bass.

Maslach, C., Schaufeli, W. B., & Leiter, M. P. (2001). Job burnout. *Annual Review of Psychology, 52,* 397–422.

Moen, P., Lam, J., Ammons, S., & Kelly, E. L. (2013). Time work by overworked professionals: Strategies in response to the stress of higher status. *Work and Occupations, 40,* 79–114.

Morales, S. (2011). 7 steps to bring balance to your life. Retrieved from *www.huffingtonpost.com/susan-morales-msw/life-balancing-advice-_b_997408.html.*

Mouffe, C. (1992). Democratic citizenship and the political community. In C. Mouffe (Ed.), *Dimensions of radical democracy: Pluralism, citizenship, community* (pp. 225–239). London: Routledge.

Okello, D. R., & Gilson, L. (2015). Exploring the influence of trust relationships on motivation in the health sector: A systematic review *Human Resources for Health, 13,* 16–34.

Osatuke, K., Moore, S. C., Ward, C., Dyrenforth, S., & Belton, L. (2009). Civility, Respect, Engagement in the Workplace (CREW): Nationwide organization development intervention at Veteran's Health Administration. *Journal of Applied Behavioral Science, 45,* 384–410.

Ryan, R. M., & Deci, E. L. (2000). Intrinsic and extrinsic motivations: Classic definitions and new directions. *Contemporary Educational Psychology, 25,* 54–67.

Schaufeli, W. B., & Bakker, A. B. (2004). Job demands, job resources, and their relationship with burnout and engagement: A multi-sample study. *Journal of Organizational Behavior, 25*, 293–315.

Semmer, N. K., Tschan, F., Meier, L. L., Facchin, S., & Jacobshagen, N. (2010). Illegitimate tasks and counterproductive work behavior. *Applied Psychology, 59*, 70–96.

Tuckey, M. R., Bakker, A. B., & Dollard, M. F. (2012). Empowering leaders optimize working conditions for engagement: A multilevel study. *Journal of Occupational Health Psychology, 17*, 15–27.

van Dam, A., Keijsers, G. P., Eling, P. A., & Becker, E. S. (2012). Impaired cognitive performance and responsiveness to reward in burnout patients: Two years later. *Work and Stress, 26*, 333–346.

Van den Broeck, A., Vansteenkiste, M., De Witte, H., & Lens, W. (2008). Explaining the relationships between job characteristics, burnout, and engagement: The role of basic psychological need satisfaction. *Work and Stress, 22*, 277–294.

Vansteenkiste, M., Neyrinck, B., Niemic, C., Soenens, B., & De Witte, H. (2007). Examining the relations among extrinsic versus intrinsic work value orientations, basic need satisfaction, and job experience: A self-determination theory approach. *Journal of Occupational and Organizational Psychology, 80*, 251–277.

Voogd, E. (2009). *Process reengineering in the Dutch health care.* Groningen, The Netherlands: Studentenbureau Publicaties.

White, M., Hill, S., McGovern, P., Mills, C., & Smeaton, D. (2003). "High-performance" management practices, working hours and work–life balance. *British Journal of Industrial Relations, 41*(2), 175–195.

Wrzesniewski, A., & Dutton, J. E. (2001). Crafting a job: Revisioning employees as active crafters of their work. *Academy of Management Review, 26*, 179–201.

PART IV

DEVELOPMENT

CHAPTER 21

Early Reasoning about Competence
Is Not Irrationally Optimistic, Nor Does It Stem
from Inadequate Cognitive Representations

ANDREI CIMPIAN

Young children's reasoning about compe-tence and achievement often seems out of step with reality. For instance, after failing to solve four puzzles in a row, most 3- and 4-year-olds are nevertheless "very sure" that they will be able to solve a similar fifth puz-zle (Parsons & Ruble, 1977). Along the same lines, after getting only about 15 points out of 100 on the first few rounds of a game, preschoolers generally expect that they will get more than 90 points on the next round (Stipek & Hoffman, 1980). Young children's judgments about competence are puzzling across a variety of contexts and tasks: Con-sider also that 5-year-olds often judge a per-son who breezed through a test to be *less* smart than a person who had to work really hard to get the same grade (Nicholls, 1978). Beyond these specific examples, classic work on this topic in the 1970s and 1980s iden-tified dramatic developmental differences in reasoning about competence. Relative to older children and adults, young chil-dren were often found to display irrational-seeming judgments and inflated assessments of their abilities and chances of success.

These differences inspired a general per-spective on children's early reasoning about competence that is considered largely correct to this day. According to this canonical per-spective, the differences between younger and older children's competence judgments are due to qualitative differences in the con-cepts with which they are operating (e.g., their concepts of ability, causation, quan-tity). In other words, the apparent irratio-nality of young children's reasoning about achievement was assumed to stem from structural flaws in their mental represen-tations. My main goal in this chapter is to challenge this long-held assumption.

Although once it may have been reason-able to assume that development brings about dramatic, qualitative changes in chil-dren's concepts, the contemporary literature on cognitive development no longer sup-ports such a view. In fact, as I outline later in this chapter, most of the concepts involved in reasoning about competence seem to be present in relatively mature form in chil-dren as young as age 3—and sometimes even in infants (e.g., Baillargeon, Scott, & Bian, 2016; Izard, Sann, Spelke, & Streri, 2009). Thus, we must look elsewhere—not to young children's conceptual shortcom-ings—to understand why their competence judgments in many laboratory tasks seem out of step with reality.

This chapter proceeds as follows. After some introductory remarks, I go on to summarize several of the major claims making up the canonical view that there are qualitative differences between younger and older children's competence-related concepts. I then present evidence that contradicts this canonical view and instead suggests continuity in the underlying concepts. Finally, I reconcile the continuity claim with the observed discontinuity in judgments: If younger and older children have access to a similar set of concepts, why does their reasoning about competence often look so different?

Throughout, I highlight the implications of this debate about discontinuity versus continuity in mental representations for children's motivation. According to the canonical view, children's conceptual shortcomings make them optimistic about their abilities, which in turn is thought to have adaptive consequences for children's motivation, allowing them to remain engaged with a task even in the face of failure (e.g., Harter, 2012; Nicholls & Miller, 1984a; Stipek, 1984). However, if young children's concepts do not actually limit them to clueless optimism, their motivation may not be as resilient to failure as previous theories have supposed. Instead, the same sorts of experiences and beliefs that demotivate older children are likely to take a toll on young children's motivation as well (e.g., Heyman, Dweck, & Cain, 1992).

Finally, I should point out that I do not attempt to be comprehensive in my review of the competing claims (discontinuity vs. continuity); the literatures relevant to these issues are vast. Thus, I discuss the evidence that I think best illustrates the two views and highlights the contrast between them. Also note that the argument I am making here is not new. Others have challenged aspects of the canonical view on similar grounds (e.g., Butler, 2005; Dweck, 1998, 1999), and much of what I say here echoes these other scholars' comments.

INTRODUCTORY REMARKS

In this section, I provide some of the background that is needed to understand the canonical view. While doing so, I also outline the reasons why one should be skeptical of this view.

The assumption of qualitative shifts in children's competence-related concepts is best understood in its historical context. This assumption is in line with the style of developmental theorizing that was popular when the canonical perspective emerged (in the 1970s and 1980s). Theories at the time tended to portray development as a series of step-like transitions between stages that differed dramatically in their representational capacities. In particular, Piaget's stage theory of cognitive development (e.g., Piaget, 1952; Piaget & Inhelder, 1969) was still influential—and was probably a source of inspiration—despite the fact that many of Piaget's specific claims were already beginning to be overturned (e.g., Baillargeon, Spelke, & Wasserman, 1985; McGarrigle & Donaldson, 1974). According to Piaget, before the age of 6 or 7 (i.e., during what he termed the *preoperational* stage of cognitive development), children's thinking exhibits serious structural flaws (e.g., an inability to think logically and abstractly) that impose a hard limit on how accurately they can represent reality. If this is right, then, of course, it is plausible to assume that young children's reasoning about competence is necessarily flawed as well, which provides a ready-made explanation for their puzzling behaviors in achievement contexts.

The problem, however, is that very few of Piaget's claims about the representational deficits of preoperational thought are left standing in the contemporary literature on cognitive development. In fact, most of the post-Piagetian work on cognitive development can be summarized with a simple phrase: "more capacity than meets the eye" (Gelman & Gallistel, 1986). On task after task, young children's wrong answers turned out to be less due to their cognitive ineptitude and more to our own shortsightedness as researchers. Irrational judgments that were initially taken as evidence for immature, undifferentiated concepts were later revealed to be reasonable extrapolations from children's everyday experiences—a conclusion that, as I argue later, applies to their irrational-seeming judgments about competence as well.

To understand the interpretive problems that arose with many Piagetian tasks, consider a classic test of children's understanding of number (Piaget, 1941): The experimenter lays out two rows containing the same number of coins and asks the child if these rows have the same number. (Children almost always get this question right.) The experimenter then deliberately lengthens one of the two rows by stretching the coins father apart and asks the child, for a second time, whether the two rows have the same number of coins in them. At this point, the vast majority of preschoolers say "no," incorrectly choosing the longer row as having more coins. For Piaget, this typical mistake signaled an inability to represent number as distinct from spatial extent—the two concepts were assumed to be undifferentiated in children's minds. Others, however, pointed out a plausible alternative explanation for children's answers. In everyday conversation, adults' actions typically direct children's attention to information of relevance to the ongoing conversation (quite unlike the experimenter's lengthening of the row; e.g., McGarrigle & Donaldson, 1974). In addition, adults do not usually repeat a question unless the first answer is no longer valid (e.g., Rose & Blank, 1974). Might children's mistakes have been due to the simple fact that they did not realize that the rules of everyday conversation are suspended when talking with an experimenter? Indeed, when the conversationally odd elements are removed from the task (e.g., the row is lengthened by accident rather than on purpose), children's performance improves dramatically (McGarrigle & Donaldson, 1974; Rose & Blank, 1974)—"more capacity than meets the eye." Thus, what was initially interpreted as a representational deficit instead turned out to be a sophisticated pragmatic inference about the communicative intentions of the experimenter (see also Clark, 1987; Diesendruck, 2005; Horowitz & Frank, 2016). Countless variations of this scenario have played themselves out over the past 40 years of research in cognitive development, to the point that the influence of Piaget is nowadays felt mostly at the level of the broad questions cognitive developmentalists tend to pursue (e.g., How do children represent number? How do they understand

mental states?) and in their general approach to pursuing these questions (e.g., investigating the normative course of development), not at the level of specific claims about what young children can and cannot represent (e.g., Baillargeon et al., 2016; Spelke & Kinzler, 2007).

In contrast, Piaget-inspired claims about qualitative differences between the representational capacities of younger and older children still dominate the literature on children's reasoning about competence and achievement. Of course, in principle, it is possible that the competence domain, unlike those that have been studied by cognitive developmentalists, relies on mental representations that undergo radical transformations. More likely, however, reasoning about competence invokes the same basic representations that children use to navigate the world more generally (e.g., concepts of cause and effect, quantity, mental states, traits and dispositions) and that are now understood to be largely continuous across development (e.g., Baillargeon, 2004; Baillargeon et al., 2016; Cimpian, 2016; Schulz, 2012; Spelke & Kinzler, 2007). Most developmental changes seem to be quantitative in nature and to occur in the control processes that operate over these representations (e.g., working memory, inhibitory control, metacognitive monitoring; Carlozzi, Tulsky, Kail, & Beaumont, 2013; Cowan, 2005; Kuhn, 2000; Williams, Ponesse, Schachar, Logan, & Tannock, 1999), as well as in children's knowledge about how these basic concepts are instantiated in the world. Correspondingly, as was the case with the supposed conceptual confusions of the preoperational child, the puzzling behaviors documented in the classic work on achievement may be better explained by nonconceptual factors such as young children's inexperience with laboratory testing situations, where many everyday rules no longer apply.

Thus, the central claim of this chapter is as follows: The nature of the mental representations underlying early reasoning about competence has long been mischaracterized. For the past 40 years, young children's optimistic predictions in achievement contexts have been used to argue for deficits in their mental representations. In contrast, the vast contemporary literature on cognitive development—from which the work on competence cognitions has remained isolated—suggests far more continuity than change in the basic representations children use to understand reality. In light of this new evidence, differences in the competence-related judgments of younger and older children are more plausibly explained as reflecting a rational process of extrapolation from children's typical schooling/achievement environments, which change dramatically over the course of childhood (e.g., Butler, 2005; Eccles, Midgeley, & Adler, 1984; Rosenholtz & Simpson, 1984), than stage-like transitions in the underlying concepts. Setting aside gradual improvements in resources such as working memory and inhibitory control, younger and older children have access to largely similar ways of thinking about competence and achievement. Which one dominates their reasoning at any one point in development is a function of, among other things, the typical contexts in which they spend their time. To the extent that the ways of thinking and talking about competence that are salient in these contexts present a mismatch to the ones children are expected to adopt when talking to an experimenter, their answers will seem irrational. But being naive about the "appropriate" way to conceptualize competence in an unfamiliar context is not evidence for the absence of the relevant concepts, and is a far cry from being irrational.

Moreover, to the extent that optimism about one's abilities and future performance is a source of sustained motivation in the face of failure, showing that young children's optimism is not an unavoidable by-product of their cognitive immaturity (as I intend to do here) has clear implications for motivation science. Specifically, the present argument suggests that young children's ability to remain engaged with a task that they find difficult is far more fragile than previously assumed. This point underscores the substantial real-world implications of investigating early reasoning about achievement. Adequate theories on this topic are essential in determining how to optimize motivation and achievement in early childhood. If young children's optimism about their abilities is not due to their inescapable

cognitive shortcomings, as the canonical view assumes, we cannot take it for granted that children will remain motivated regardless of the outcome. In addition, if their optimistic outlook is in part a function of their typical achievement environments, changes in these environments could bring about systematic changes in children's attitudes toward learning as well, potentially for the worse.

Consider that, over the last decade or so, the early childhood education system in the United States has seen ever greater regimentation and emphasis on testing, and less of the self-directed activity that used to be the norm in preschools and kindergartens. For example, a recent study that compared nationally representative samples of kindergartens in 1998 and 2010 found that the percentage of teachers who thought that most children should learn how to read in kindergarten jumped from 31 to 80% in this relatively brief interval (Bassok, Latham, & Rorem, 2016). Similarly, use of textbooks, teacher-directed whole-class instruction, and standardized tests in kindergarten saw considerable increases over this period, whereas resources for child-selected and directed activities (e.g., sand and water tables, dramatic play areas) decreased by a similarly wide margin. If young children have access to multiple ways of conceptualizing competence, then a shift toward more formal, evaluative, and competitive early schooling environments might induce a corresponding activation of conceptions of ability as a stable capacity that one possesses more or less of than others—a perspective that has been shown to bring about negative self-assessments, lowered persistence, and maladaptive achievement outcomes in many older children (e.g., Dweck, 1999, 2006; Nicholls, 1990; Nicholls & Miller, 1984a). Thus, a more accurate understanding of young children's reasoning about competence is essential for predicting the effects of these secular trends in the education system, and more generally for fostering a positive, constructive attitude toward learning in early childhood.

Returning to the issue of continuity versus discontinuity in mental representations, one may wonder why theories regarding young children's reasoning about competence (which posit discontinuities in the underlying concepts) have remained isolated from the contemporary literature on cognitive development (most of which reveals continuity instead). Part of the reason may simply be that research on early achievement cognitions slowed to a trickle after the early 1990s. This slowdown might have been caused in part by the success of the canonical view itself. Persuaded by the claim that young children's conceptual deficiencies make them irrational optimists whose motivation is invulnerable to failure (e.g., Nicholls & Miller, 1984a), many achievement researchers may have chosen to focus on older children instead, whose presumed conceptual sophistication put them at greater risk for maladaptive thoughts (e.g., low self-esteem, helplessness). Due to the scarcity of contemporary work on early reasoning about competence, I will occasionally rely on research from outside the competence domain to illustrate young children's greater-than-anticipated facility with relevant concepts. It is encouraging, however, that this line of research has recently seen something of a resurgence, with several important contributions to our understanding of early competence beliefs coming out just in the last 5 years or so (e.g., Beilock, Gunderson, Ramirez, & Levine, 2010; Cimpian, Mu, & Erickson, 2012; Gunderson et al., 2013; Haimovitz & Dweck, 2016; Pomerantz & Kempner, 2013). I highlight some of these contributions in the relevant sections below.

THE CANONICAL VIEW: CONCEPTUAL DISCONTINUITIES BETWEEN YOUNGER AND OLDER CHILDREN

In what follows, I summarize three key claims concerning children's supposed conceptual shortcomings in the competence domain. It is hard to overstate the influence these claims still have on the contemporary literature investigating the development of achievement cognitions. As a simple search will reveal, most work published on this topic in recent years references at least one of them as an established fact about young children's reasoning about competence.

An Undifferentiated Concept of Ability

As adults, we have multiple ways of thinking about success and failure. Sometimes we see achievement outcomes as reflecting a dynamic process (e.g., putting in effort, applying strategies); other times, we see them as reflecting a static underlying entity (e.g., capacity, talent) or a combination of the two (e.g., effort matters, but only up to the limit imposed by capacity) (Dweck, 1999, 2006; Nicholls, 1978, 1984, 1990). In contrast, a major claim of the canonical view is that young children have access to only one of these perspectives. According to Nicholls (1978; for reviews, see Nicholls, 1984, 1990; Nicholls & Miller, 1984a), young children simply cannot conceive of outcomes as being influenced by capacity. For them, effort is the only relevant causal variable. In fact, Nicholls (1978, 1990) went so far as to claim that through the age of 6, children may not even see the relationship between effort and outcome as causal. Rather, they may simply think of effort and outcome as the same thing: "Effort and outcome are not distinguished as cause and effect. . . . Ability, effort, and outcome are not distinguished as separate dimensions" (Nicholls, 1978, p. 812). According to Nicholls, even when children become able to differentiate effort as cause and outcome as effect (at around age 7), they still cannot grasp that any factors beyond effort might affect performance. The concept of capacity as a causal influence on achievement outcomes is argued not to be reliably present until children are 12 or 13 years old.

The most direct evidence for these claims came from children's reasoning about vignettes in which one student works harder than another yet performs either as well or less well (e.g., Nicholls, 1978; Nicholls & Miller, 1984b). After being presented with these vignettes, children were asked to judge, for example, which child is smarter or "how come they got the same when one worked hard and one didn't work hard" (Nicholls, 1978, p. 803). Their answers to a number of these questions were considered holistically and used to assign children to a particular stage of reasoning about ability; the first two stages (in a sequence of four) are characterized by major conceptual short-comings, as just described.

According to this perspective, young children's conceptual immaturity explains many of their strangely optimistic judgments in the competence domain. For instance, if children initially conflate effort and outcome (or, at best, think that effort completely determines the outcome), there is no reason *not* to be optimistic in the face of failure. Past failure is more or less meaningless—with more effort, one can always succeed in the future. Thus, the flawed conceptual framework young children use to reason about competence serves an important protective role, whereas more mature concepts automatically expose older children to maladaptive thoughts and outcomes: "Ironically, a more mature understanding of ability can have unfortunate consequences for competence motivation and, thereby, for continued intellectual development. Development has its discontents. These discontents stem [in part] from the 'natural' process of cognitive and affective development" (Nicholls & Miller, 1984a, p. 186).

Once children's concepts mature to the point where they can understand that performance can reflect one's capacity or talent, failure becomes more aversive. Failure (especially on tasks that others can accomplish) signals that one is somehow deficient, which in turn can undermine one's motivation to pursue the tasks in question.[1]

Young children's inability to understand that one's performance depends in part on one's talent or capacity, and not just on effort, was argued to contribute to another facet of their optimism as well: their curious disinterest in social comparison (i.e., figuring out how their performance stacks up against that of others). Young children's self-evaluations seem unaffected by information about others' performance: Whether their performance is better or worse than that of other children, kindergartners and first graders remain equally optimistic about their abilities (e.g., Ruble, Boggiano, Feldman, & Loebl, 1980). This is as expected, of course, if young children cannot understand others' performance to reveal anything beyond the amount of effort expended. This limitation, along with other supposed

shortcomings of preoperational thought (e.g., centration, inability to seriate), was also invoked to explain why children in the early elementary grades are clueless about their relative standing among their peers, which they often grossly overestimate (e.g., Nicholls, 1978; Stipek, 1984).

In summary, Nicholls's view posits structural limitations on the concepts young children use to understand achievement. In turn, these limitations are used to account for the optimistic character of children's early competence-related reasoning.

Overly Concrete and Positive Representations of Self

Harter's influential theory on the development of children's representations of the self is another pillar of the canonical view (e.g., Harter, 1982; Harter & Pike, 1984; for recent reviews, see Harter, 2001, 2012). Harter argues that young children's immature mental representations impose a fundamental limit on their ability to reason about the self, with downstream consequences for their reasoning about competence as well. Below, I describe several of these hypothesized cognitive limitations and their implications for children's thinking about achievement, as well as their motivation.

First, Harter (2012) argues that young children are unable to conceive of themselves as possessing general capacities or traits. Instead, young children "can only construct very concrete cognitive representations of observable behaviors or features of the self (e.g., 'I'm a boy,' 'I have a television in my room,' 'I have a kitty that is orange')" (p. 30). Because children cannot abstract any broader commonalities across such concrete features, their self-representations are "isolated from one another," "compartmentalized," "disjointed," and lacking in coherence (p. 30). Even when children mention abstract-sounding trait terms in their self-descriptions (e.g., "I'm smart"), these should not be taken at face value, since their semantic content may not be the same as for older children and adults:

Although children may describe themselves in such terminology as good or bad, nice or mean, smart or dumb, these characteristics do not represent "traits," given their typical psychological meanings. . . . At this age, the use of such terms are more likely to reflect the use of self-labels that have been modeled by others (e.g., parents or teachers). (Harter, 2012, p. 52)

In other words, whenever trait terms appear in young children's self-descriptions, it is likely that children are simply mimicking adults' use of trait terms (e.g., mom saying they are smart), without truly understanding their meaning.[2] This claim was consistent with several prominent studies from the same period (e.g., Rholes & Ruble, 1984; Rotenberg, 1980), which appeared to show that children are unable to interpret others' behaviors in terms of general dispositions (traits, capacities, etc.) until they are 9 or 10 years of age (for a review, see Rholes, Newman, & Ruble, 1990).

So far, I have described the claim that young children's concrete thinking prevents them from forming more sophisticated types of self-representations (e.g., traits, abilities). Several other cognitive deficits are invoked to account for the irrational-seeming positivity of young children's self-representations. For instance, young children are claimed to be unable to compare abstract quantities, such as their performance versus another's (Harter, 2012), which means that they cannot use social comparison to bring their self-evaluations to more realistic levels. Following Piaget (1960), Harter (2012) also argues that young children are egocentric—that is, unable to understand other people's perspectives, and mental states more generally. Because of this perspective-taking failure, young children do not understand that others can be critical of them and therefore fail to incorporate this information into their self-views. Another representational deficit that was thought to exacerbate the positivity of young children's self-views is their "difficulty distinguishing between their desired and their actual competence" (p. 31). That is, young children have overly positive self-views in part because they confuse *wanting* to be good at many things with *actually* being good at these things (see the next section for an elaboration of this claim).

In summary, Harter's theory accounts for the quirks in children's early reasoning about competence by appealing to a number of fundamental deficits in their concepts. As was the case with Nicholls (e.g., 1978, 1990), these cognitive limitations were also thought to serve important protective functions for their motivation, enabling young children to remain resilient in the face of daunting challenges.

Wishful Thinking

A narrower, but nevertheless influential, element of the canonical view proposes that young children's positivity is due to a single conceptual confusion. Prompted by the observation that children are often more realistic and accurate when they're reasoning about others' competence rather than their own, Stipek (1984; Stipek, Roberts, & Sanborn, 1984) hypothesized that the source of their optimism lies in an immature, egocentric understanding of physical causality (Piaget, 1930). Having frequently experienced the contiguity between their desires (e.g., "I want food") and events in the world (e.g., "I am fed"), young children may develop an exaggerated sense of personal efficacy, believing that their desires have a *direct* causal effect on the world. Perhaps, then, this "wishful thinking" tendency explains why children display inflated expectations of success.

As just mentioned, this claim is supported by self–other asymmetries in competence judgments. When it comes to predicting their own future performance, preschoolers typically expect to do well, regardless of how they did in the past; in contrast, when making predictions about how another person will do, young children reason much like older children and adults, lowering their expectations if the person has failed in the past (e.g., Stipek & Hoffman, 1980). A similar conclusion applies to how young children *evaluate* themselves compared to others: Although kindergartners and first graders overestimate their own standing among their peers, they are as accurate as older children when estimating where others rank in terms of their smarts (Stipek, 1981). In addition, their estimations of others' (but not their own) rank are in agreement with more objective standards, such as teacher ratings. Also consistent with claims of wishful thinking, young children are overoptimistic about another person's future performance when they stand to benefit from this person's success: When 4-year-olds were told that they would receive a bag of marbles if another child did well, the children's expectations for the other child were as inflated as when they predicted their own future performance (Stipek et al., 1984). The influence of self-interest on young children's expectations, whether for their own or for others' performance, seems to support the "wishful thinking" claim that they possess an immature concept of causality (i.e., that they believe their wishes have a direct causal effect on the world).

Interim Summary

Although they differ in their details, the previous views are all instantiations of the same claim—namely, that younger and older children operate with fundamentally different sets of concepts, which is why their competence judgments are so different. This discontinuity claim is assumed to be true in most contemporary research on children's motivation and achievement. There are, however, valid reasons to be skeptical of it.

THE CASE AGAINST DEVELOPMENTAL DISCONTINUITIES

This section contains two arguments against the canonical (discontinuity) view. First, I argue that the developmental differences in competence judgments—which the canonical view seeks to explain—are not nearly as stark as one would expect if they were due to the fundamental, inescapable limitations of young children's concepts. Looking at the sum of the evidence, one finds no real discontinuity in competence judgments. In fact, there are many circumstances in which younger children's reasoning is identical to that of older children. And without a sharp discontinuity in judgments, there is little reason to posit a sharp discontinuity in the concepts underlying these judgments.

Thus, the first argument questions the very existence of the phenomenon that inspired the canonical view. Second, I argue directly against the claim that the concepts underlying reasoning about competence undergo qualitative shifts. Although this claim was at one point in agreement with the state of the art in cognitive development, it no longer is. With increasing use of methodologies that are less taxing on young children's attention, memory, and language, research in this area has shown early concepts to be remarkably sophisticated. This evidence undermines any strong claims of qualitative changes in the mental representations that younger and older children use to understand the world.

Is There a Sharp Discontinuity in Competence Judgments?

If young children are truly incapable of grasping reality in the same way as older children and adults, their judgments about competence should be consistently off-target. To the extent that young children's judgments look rational in some contexts or tasks and irrational in others, it becomes less plausible to argue that they are incapable of rational responses because of their inherent conceptual limitations. Such variability across contexts or tasks would suggest instead that young children might grasp the relevant basic concepts but sometimes fail to demonstrate their grasp because of extraneous factors (e.g., unusual pragmatics, unfamiliar contexts, tasks that exceed their linguistic ability). In what follows, I review evidence revealing substantial variability in the judgments that the canonical view sought to explain.

Insensitivity to Outcomes

Do young children always fail to integrate information about outcomes into their competence judgments? Are they blindly optimistic about their abilities and their chances of success? The answer is "no." In fact, I have already reviewed evidence that preschoolers are perfectly capable of factoring outcome information into their judgments: Past performance is routinely taken into account when evaluating and making predictions about others' performance (Stipek et al., 1984); young children's optimism is restricted mostly to assessments of their *own* competence. In many contexts, however, young children use evidence to adjust their self-evaluations as well. For instance, when 4-year-olds rank themselves and their peers on dimensions that are familiar and meaningful to them (e.g., how fast they can run), their rankings actually correspond with objective measures (Morris & Nemcek, 1982; see also Marsh, Ellis, & Craven, 2002). When their past failures are made salient, such as when their unsolved puzzles are left out in front of them, 4- and 5-year-olds lower their expectations of future success (Hebert & Dweck, 1985, described in Dweck, 1991; see also Stipek et al., 1984). Similarly, many 5- and 6-year-olds display negative self-evaluations and low expectations when their performance is criticized by an adult, which also makes failure salient and relevant to children (Heyman et al., 1992).

More generally, the claim that young children are irrationally optimistic about their abilities is difficult to reconcile with their behavior outside the laboratory (Butler, 2005). In real life, young children's achievement behavior does not seem qualitatively different from that of older children and adults. Even casual observations of a preschool classroom, for example, are likely to reveal that 4-year-olds generally know when they have failed and when they have succeeded, and adjust their behavior accordingly (e.g., asking for help when they run into difficulties). In addition, failure often takes a toll on young children's motivation, much like it does on that of older children. Many preschoolers give up on tasks they cannot master in a few tries; they do not simply breeze past their failed attempts as if nothing happened. Moreover, young children's self-assessments outside the laboratory are not consistently off-base; many children seem to have surprisingly precise insights into their abilities. I remember, for example, talking to a preschooler who explained that she could cross the monkey bars in only one way— by getting both hands onto one bar before reaching for the next. She knew that other children could cross the monkey bars faster, using only one hand per bar, and it was clear to her that she could not. To the extent that these observations capture young children's actual achievement cognitions and behavior, they also raise doubts about the claim that children this age are undaunted optimists who always overestimate their abilities.

Absence of, and Insensitivity to, Social Comparisons

The canonical view is premised in part on the idea that young children are neither motivated nor able to (1) *engage in* social comparisons, and (2) *use* social comparisons to evaluate their abilities. However, these empirical claims may not be valid. Much of the evidence supporting them came from laboratory studies in which the social comparison information was provided to children in unfamiliar, decontextualized ways. For example, a classic study measured whether young children engage in social comparison by counting how often they pressed a button to display an image of another child's work on a video monitor—arguably, quite unlike what children might do outside the laboratory to obtain this sort of information (Ruble, Feldman, & Boggiano, 1976). Similarly, studies investigating whether children make use of social comparison information often presented this information in complex, abstract formats that may not have held much meaning for young children. For example, Nicholls (1978) showed children cards with 18 schematic faces that differed in color (yellow vs. white) depending on whether the individuals depicted could or could not solve a problem. Although adults are familiar with such symbolic means of depicting frequencies or proportions, young children are probably not.

Evidence obtained with simpler, more naturalistic methods contradicts these claims and suggests instead that young children both perform and use social comparisons. Observational studies of classroom contexts, for example, revealed that social comparison behaviors such as looking at other children's work or making comparative statements are common as early as kindergarten (e.g., Pomerantz, Ruble, Frey, & Greulich,

1995) and even preschool (e.g., Mosatche & Bragonier, 1981). Given that young children can accurately estimate their own and others' relative standing on meaningful dimensions (e.g., Morris & Nemcek, 1982; Stipek, 1981), this seems hardly surprising: It is difficult to see how children could rank themselves and their classmates with any degree of accuracy if they were completely uninterested in, or incapable of performing, social comparisons.

Notably, this rank-estimation evidence also suggests that young children *use* social comparisons to inform their evaluations of themselves and others, contradicting earlier claims (e.g., Ruble et al., 1976, 1980). Young children's sensitivity to social comparison information was subsequently documented in experimental work as well, using simpler paradigms that better reflected how young children might compare themselves to others in everyday contexts. For example, Butler (1998) used a drawing task in which children had to trace as much of a winding path as they could in a certain amount of time. Children were then shown the drawing of a child who had clearly traced more or less of the path than they had. In this context, even 4- and 5-year-olds took notice of the comparison: They judged that they did less well—and even that they were less good at tracing tasks in general—when the other child traced more than they had (see also Rhodes & Brickman, 2008). Preschoolers' motivation was also affected by the social comparison information, as was that of older children. Children who experienced relative failure often avoided the tracing activity when allowed to choose between it and another activity.

In summary, there is little evidence of a sharp discontinuity between younger and older children's reasoning about competence. Whether one looks at young children's ability to incorporate outcomes into their evaluations or at their motivation to engage in social comparisons and their use of this information in their subsequent judgments, the same conclusion emerges: In contexts that are familiar and meaningful, young children's competence judgments are much more similar than dissimilar to those of older children, as are their motivational patterns in response to failure. Thus, the irrational judgments that the canonical view was formulated to explain may be, in some measure, an artifact of the methods initially used to investigate young children's thinking.

Are There Sharp Discontinuities in the Concepts Underlying Competence Judgments?

The preceding section suggests that reasoning about competence is relatively continuous across development. In and of itself, this conclusion makes moot any claims of discontinuities in the underlying concepts. However, even when judged on its own merits, the idea that development brings about radical transformations in the concepts involved in reasoning about competence is out of step with contemporary developmental science. Although children's information-processing abilities (e.g., working memory capacity, inhibitory control) and their knowledge undoubtedly grow as they get older, their understanding of the world does not change in fundamental ways. Below, I briefly review recent evidence against the conceptual limitations invoked by the canonical view. Where relevant, I also articulate the implications of this new evidence for children's motivation.

Egocentrism

Is it possible that young children's seemingly inflated self-views arise because they are egocentric—unable to consider other people's perspectives about themselves (e.g., Harter, 2012)? Others' negative views about them should lower their self-assessments, so perhaps children's positivity is due in part to a failure to understand other people's mental states. This claim is implausible. In fact, even infants understand that others' perceptions, preferences, beliefs, and so forth, may be different from their own (e.g., Luo & Johnson, 2009; Onishi & Baillargeon, 2005; Repacholi & Gopnik, 1997; for a review, see Baillargeon et al., 2016). The prior evidence for egocentrism, as well as for other major flaws in young children's "theory of mind" (e.g., Wimmer & Perner, 1983), was largely a methodological artifact. The use of tasks that needlessly taxed young children's information-processing resources made it appear that they had a limited understanding of others' minds, when in fact their understanding was fairly sophisticated (e.g., Baillargeon, Scott, & He, 2010).

Inability to Compare Abstract Quantities

Can it be that young children's seeming insensitivity to (relative) failure is due to their inability to compare abstract quantities, which prevents them from realizing when their performance is inferior to others' (e.g., Harter, 2012)? Contrary to this possibility, it seems that humans are actually born with the ability to perform such abstract quantitative comparisons. For instance, newborns familiarized with strings of four syllables subsequently looked longer at images containing four objects than at images containing 12 objects, and vice versa—newborns familiarized with strings of 12 syllables looked longer at sets containing 12 rather than four objects (Izard et al., 2009; see also Jordan & Brannon, 2006). Newborns' ability to compare numerical quantities across sensory modalities speaks to the abstractness of the numerical and quantitative representations with which our species is endowed (for a review, see Hyde, 2015). Thus, there is no reason to believe that an inability to make abstract quantitative comparisons hinders children's reasoning about competence.

Overly Concrete Mental Representations

The seeming irrationality of young children's reasoning about competence was also attributed to the concreteness of their mental representations, which was argued to prevent them from conceiving of general, abstract abilities (e.g., Harter, 2012). However, as illustrated by the foregoing discussion of numerical concepts, young children's thinking turns out to be surprisingly powerful and abstract. This conclusion is supported by a wide range of studies investigating how infants generalize from experience (e.g., Dewar & Xu, 2010; Yin & Csibra, 2015), how they learn language (e.g., Marcus, Vijayan, Rao, & Vishton, 1999; Smith, Jones, Landau, Gershkoff-Stowe, & Samuelson, 2002), how they reason about the

relations between objects (e.g., Ferry, Hespos, & Gentner, 2015; Walker & Gopnik, 2014), how they reason about living organisms (e.g., Setoh, Wu, Baillargeon, & Gelman, 2013; Simons & Keil, 1995), and so on. Thus, there is no longer any reason to be skeptical of young children's ability to think abstractly about their achievement experiences (in fact, see Cvencek, Greenwald, & Meltzoff, 2016; Marsh et al., 2002).

Immature Reasoning about Physical Causality

Perhaps young children don't understand how the physical world works, believing that their wishes—in and of themselves—have causal effects. This misunderstanding was thought to be part of the reason why young children display overly optimistic performance expectations (e.g., Stipek, 1984). However, none of the subsequent research on early causal reasoning provides any support for this "wishful thinking" claim. On the contrary, humans' basic understanding of physical objects and their causal interactions seems, by and large, to be preserved across development (for reviews, see Baillargeon, 2004; Spelke & Kinzler, 2007) and even across species (e.g., Chiandetti & Vallortigara, 2013; Wood, 2013). Importantly, this initial understanding is unlikely to contain any "wishful" beliefs. Consider, for example, that when 9-month-olds were allowed to reach toward one of two similar-looking boxes that differed in weight, they reached preferentially toward the lighter box, which they had been able to manipulate more easily in the past (Hauf, Paulus, & Baillargeon, 2012). Thus, infants do not disregard past failures—they do not expect that just because they might wish it so, all of a sudden it might be easier to play with the heavier box. This result, and others like it (e.g., Hespos & Baillargeon, 2008), speak against the idea of irrational optimism in early causal reasoning.

All this being said, even if young children did occasionally allow their wishes to color their judgments, they would be in good company: Motives and desires influence reasoning throughout life and across domains, to the point that adults may also be reasonably characterized as "wishful thinkers" (e.g., Hughes & Zaki, 2015; Jost, Glazer,

Kruglanski, & Sulloway, 2003; Mather & Carstensen, 2005). If adults' concepts are not deemed inadequate simply because their reasoning is sometimes motivated, children's concepts should not be either (see also Butler, 2005).

Inability to Understand Ability as a Trait

Arguably, the most influential claim of the canonical view is that young children cannot understand ability as a capacity or trait (e.g., Harter, 2012; Nicholls, 1978, 1984, 1990), partly because they cannot understand behavior in terms of stable traits in the first place (e.g., Rholes et al., 1990). Young children's immature concept of ability (as depending exclusively on effort) was thought to account for their optimistic outlook on achievement. Despite its remarkably persistent influence on the field, this claim does not fare any better than the others when evaluated against the relevant evidence.

Let us consider, first, the broader claim that children do not understand others' behaviors in terms of underlying traits— that is, stable psychological tendencies that predispose people to act a certain way. Several researchers have pointed out that in many of the studies providing evidence for this claim, children's responses were judged against an unreasonably high bar: Children were told about one trait-relevant behavior (e.g., Jill shared part of her lunch with a child who had nothing to eat) and were asked whether the protagonist would exhibit behavior consistent with this trait in a different circumstance (e.g., Will Jill help another child rake the leaves in the yard?; e.g., Rholes & Ruble, 1984; Rotenberg, 1980). To show that they understood traits in such a task, children would need to go through a complicated chain of reasoning (for details of this argument, see Heyman & Gelman, 1999; Liu, Gelman, & Wellman, 2007). Specifically, children would need to (1) infer a stable trait (e.g., generous) on the basis of a single trait-relevant behavior (e.g., sharing one's lunch) (behavior → trait step), then (2) use the inferred trait to predict a different trait-consistent behavior in a different context (e.g., helping with yard work) (trait → behavior step). Not only do such tasks involve a multistep inferential chain,

but they also assume that the influence of traits on behavior is more deterministic than seems warranted; that is, one can fully appreciate that human behavior is guided by traits, yet still be unsure whether the protagonist will spend "all her play time raking leaves" (Rholes & Ruble, 1984, p. 552) just because she shared part of her lunch with someone who had nothing to eat.

Evidence obtained with simpler, less ambiguous tasks suggests that young children do in fact possess the concept of a dispositional trait. Even 3- and 4-year-olds infer traits from relevant behaviors, especially when these behaviors are intentional and frequent (e.g., Boseovski, Chiu, & Marcovitch, 2013; Boseovski & Lee, 2006; Giles & Heyman, 2003; Hermes, Behne, & Rakoczy, 2015; Liu et al., 2007). Moreover, 3- and 4-year-olds reliably use trait information to predict a person's future motives, behaviors, and emotional reactions (e.g., Heyman & Gelman, 1999, 2000; Hermes et al., 2015; Liu et al., 2007; see also Boseovski et al., 2013; Boseovski & Lee, 2006; Cain, Heyman, & Walker, 1997).

Strikingly, even infants seem to have a basic understanding of dispositional traits, consistent with the recent surge of evidence suggesting sophisticated mental-state understanding early in life (e.g., Baillargeon et al., 2016). For example, 15-month-olds expected a person who had repeatedly displayed anger toward an action to continue displaying this emotion on later occasions when similar actions were performed (e.g., Repacholi, Meltzoff, Toub, & Ruba, 2016; see also Kuhlmeier, Wynn, & Bloom, 2003; Repacholi, Meltzoff, Hennings, & Ruba, 2016); 13-month-olds expected a person who had performed an action with several objects (e.g., sliding them back and forth) to continue performing this action with different objects on later occasions (e.g., Song, Baillargeon, & Fisher, 2005); and 5-month-olds expected an unfamiliar agent who had repeatedly reached toward one of two objects to continue reaching toward the preferred object, even when their positions were later switched (Luo & Baillargeon, 2005; see also Luo & Johnson, 2009; Woodward, 1998).

Why did the infants expect behavioral consistency in these studies? In particular, did they actually attribute a disposition to the actor, or were their expectations driven by shallower processes (e.g., a superficial tendency to expect more of the same)? Although this question cannot be conclusively settled with the data available, two considerations favor the richer, trait-based interpretation. First, infants did not display the same expectations of consistency in control conditions that were superficially similar to those described earlier. For instance, the 5-month-olds in Luo and Baillargeon's (2005) experiments did not expect the agent to reach toward the same object on later occasions if that object had been the only one present during the initial phase. It was only when infants saw the agent actively choose between two objects during the initial phase—that is, when they had evidence for a *preference* (a disposition)—that they later expected behavioral consistency. Second, since 3- and 4-year-olds seem to understand traits already (e.g., Heyman & Gelman, 1999, 2000; Liu et al., 2007), it seems uncharitable to interpret infants' trait-like judgments as driven entirely by low-level processes. How likely is it that infants' expectations of behavioral consistency arise from superficial associations when (1) their expectations are nuanced and context-sensitive, (2) there is extensive independent evidence for sophisticated theory-of-mind abilities at this age (e.g., Baillargeon et al., 2016), and (3) the same expectations of consistency seem to stem from a veridical understanding of traits in children who are only slightly older?

In summary, young children interpret others' behaviors in terms of stable underlying traits at least by the age of 3 or 4 years, and perhaps as early as infancy. In and of itself, this evidence casts some doubt on the claim that young children cannot understand *ability* as a trait (e.g., Harter, 2012; Nicholls, 1978, 1984, 1990). Aside from this general reason to be skeptical, there are now many findings that contradict this claim directly. These findings suggest instead that young children are able to interpret competence-related behaviors, just like any other behaviors, as arising from stable underlying dispositions.

First, ability-related traits were featured in some of the previously mentioned studies that documented trait reasoning in young children. For example, 4-year-olds who saw an actor provide accurate, detailed names for a number of objects (e.g., supersonic airplane, fusilli pasta) subsequently judged this actor to be "smarter" (but not "stronger" or "nicer") than an actor whom they had seen successfully lift a number of heavy objects (e.g., a potato sack, a big suitcase; Hermes et al., 2015). Moreover, they expected the "smart" actor to be able to name other, unfamiliar objects, as well as succeed in a number of knowledge-based (but not strength-based) activities. The latter result suggests that children had a relatively abstract understanding of the trait "smart," extending it to an appropriately broad set of activities beyond the ones initially used to infer the trait. The 4-year-olds also accurately labeled the actor who had been able to lift heavy objects as "stronger" (but not "smarter" or "nicer") than the other actor, and they expected this "strong" actor to be able to manipulate unfamiliar objects with ease and succeed in other strength-based (but not knowledge-based) activities. This nuanced pattern of competence judgments and predictions contradicts the view that young children's concept of ability is inadequate. A concept that simply equates ability with effort cannot account for 4-year-olds' domain-differentiated, sensible responses in this and similar studies (e.g., Cain et al., 1997; Marsh et al., 2002).

Second, consistent with the idea that younger and older children have access to similar ability concepts, Heyman and Compton (2006) demonstrated that young children give "mature," ability-as-trait responses with a minimal change to the classic Nicholls (1978) task. Recall that, in this task, children are asked to reason about two actors who get the same score on a test despite spending different amounts of time working on it. The first question children are always asked in this task is, "Was one working harder or were they the same?" (Nicholls, 1978, p. 803; see also Nicholls & Miller, 1984b). The fixed order of the questions in this task raises the following possibility: Perhaps young children's responses to the subsequent questions about ability typically reveal an ability-as-effort conception simply because the first question (about working hard) activates this conception.

If so, asking a question that activates the ability-as-trait conception instead should produce a corresponding shift in children's responses to the later ability questions. For example, we might ask children whether one actor found the test *easier*. Even 2-year-olds recognize that someone who needs to exert less effort to complete a task finds it easier (Jara-Ettinger, Tenenbaum, & Schulz, 2015; see also Heyman & Compton, 2006). Moreover, prompting children to think about differences in the actors' mental states (rather than just their behaviors) may draw their attention to differences in the underlying mental capacities (Heyman, Gee, & Giles, 2003), thereby activating the ability-as-trait conception. In turn, activating this conception might lead children to give more trait-based responses to the subsequent questions about the actors' abilities (assuming, of course, that young children possess the ability-as-trait conception in the first place).

Following this logic, Heyman and Compton (2006) presented Nicholls-style vignettes to kindergartners and simply manipulated which question was asked first: whether the actors tried hard or not on the test (as in the original task), or whether the actors thought the test was easy or difficult. When first asked whether the actors tried hard, children did not subsequently judge the faster actors to be smarter, consistent with the findings of Nicholls (1978) and others. However, when first asked whether the actors found the test easy or difficult, the vast majority of children (82%) *did* judge the faster actors to be smarter and the slower actors to be less smart, as would be expected if this question had prompted children to think of ability as a trait (Heyman & Compton, 2006, Study 2). Also consistent with this possibility, the easy–difficult question led children to predict that the slower actor would do "worse than most of the kids in [the] class" in the future, which suggests that they attributed a stable trait to this person (Study 3). Similarly, a full 65% of the children primed with the easy–difficult question also agreed that "some people . . . could never be really good" (which is a clear expression of the ability-as-trait perspective), compared with only 29% such responses when the effort question was first. In summary, the results of this simple manipulation suggest that young children

have access to the same ways of thinking about ability as older children and adults, and that subtle features of the context determine which of these ways is most salient to children at a particular time.

Third, not only can young children conceive of ability as a trait, but they also display the maladaptive behaviors that often accompany this conception in older children and adults. Experiments on the effects of trait versus nontrait praise provide direct evidence for this point. For example, when 4-year-olds' successes were praised with a trait term (e.g., "You are a good drawer"; see also Gelman & Heyman, 1999), they reacted more negatively to later mistakes than when their successes were praised with a nontrait phrase that was otherwise analogous (e.g., "You did a good job drawing"; Cimpian, Arce, Markman, & Dweck, 2007; Morris & Zentall, 2014; Zentall & Morris, 2010, 2012). Note that, initially, the trait and nontrait praise statements were equally rewarding: Regardless of which praise they got, children felt happy and competent. However, their reactions diverged dramatically the moment they made a mistake. Relative to children who received the nontrait praise, children who had been told they were "good drawers" felt sadder, thought they were less good at drawing, and said more often that they would not want to draw again in the future—in short, they displayed the helpless reaction to failure that is common when people conceive of ability as a fixed trait that is out of their control (for similar results, see Cimpian, 2010; Cimpian et al., 2012; Kamins & Dweck, 1999; Rhodes & Brickman, 2008). These findings underscore that even young children are capable of conceiving of ability as a trait, with all that entails for their self-evaluation, motivation, and achievement. Moreover, these studies highlight how exquisitely sensitive to context children's conceptual frameworks are. A few simple statements from an unfamiliar experimenter were able to shift how children conceptualized their successes and, subsequently, how they reacted to failures.

Interim Summary

The evidence in this section suggests that competence judgments and concepts do not change qualitatively across development. The canonical view, despite its intuitive appeal and continuing influence on the field, is no longer tenable. Young children can make sense of their achievement experiences in all the same ways that older children can, and they are thus vulnerable to the same negative, helpless patterns of cognitions and behaviors.

WHAT EXPLAINS THE GREATER POSITIVITY IN YOUNG CHILDREN'S JUDGMENTS?

This final section is intended to resolve a lingering tension. On the one hand, it is clear that young children's judgments are not *blindly* optimistic. Under certain circumstances, they can be as realistic as older children are—consistent with the argument that they have access to similar competence-related concepts. On the other hand, young children's answers in many studies do have a more optimistic bent than those of older children. What explains this tendency toward positivity, especially if conceptual limitations are not to blame? As anticipated earlier in the chapter, the answer might have to do with the dominant messages in children's environments. What changes across development is not the content of children's ability concepts, but rather which of these concepts or perspectives is emphasized in their daily lives. Many children's early environments (e.g., home, daycare, preschool) are centered around learning and growth (e.g., Butler, 2005; Eccles et al., 1984; Rosenholtz & Simpson, 1984; Stipek & Daniels, 1988). These environments are relatively unstructured, with children having considerable control over the activities in which they engage. Because there are few group activities (at least academic ones), children often cannot compare their performance with same-age peers on the same task. In addition, children's performance is seldom formally evaluated, especially since children this age are expected to acquire only very basic skills (e.g., counting from 1 to 10, reciting the alphabet). In summary, in children's early environments, success is largely a function of paying attention and trying hard; differences between children in their

skills and capacities are of little importance. As children progress through the school system, however, the frequency of challenging, teacher-directed, whole-class activities— which provide ample opportunities for social comparison—increases considerably, and with it the prominence of grades, class ranks, and other formal systems of evaluation. Such environments inevitably draw attention to differences between children's abilities, highlighting the idea that success depends on more than just paying attention.

Thus, young children's responses may be somewhat more positive and effort-focused than older children's because that is the default perspective they bring with them to the laboratory. Young children are perfectly capable of adopting the alternative, ability-as-trait perspective (with its more realistic outlook and its higher risk of helpless reactions to setbacks), but they are unlikely to do so unless somehow prompted. I have already reviewed some evidence that supports this view. For example, despite young children's typical focus on effort, just a few statements or questions from an adult seem sufficient to prompt children to think of ability as a trait (e.g., Cimpian, 2010; Cimpian et al., 2007, 2012; Heyman & Compton, 2006; Morris & Zentall, 2014; Zentall & Morris, 2010, 2012). Also consistent with this view, young children whose home environments differ systematically in whether effort or traits are emphasized seem to adopt different "default" beliefs about ability as well (Gunderson et al., 2013; see also Haimovitz & Dweck, 2016; Pomerantz & Kempner, 2013). The structure of young children's classroom environments (e.g., more vs. less evaluative) is similarly predictive of their competence judgments. For example, in kindergarten classrooms that were more regimented, and in which evaluative feedback was more common and salient, children were significantly more realistic when estimating their class rank (Stipek & Daniels, 1988; see also Butler & Ruzany, 1993). This evidence converges on the idea that young children can flexibly switch between different ways of conceptualizing ability, depending on their experiences; the fact that they are typically optimistic is just a reflection of their typical environments. An implication of this view is that systematic changes in young children's environments, such as those currently under way in the American education system (Bassok et al., 2016), are likely to bring about corresponding shifts in how children reason about ability. In the coming decades, kindergartners' default perspective on achievement may bear little resemblance to that of the resilient kindergartners from 20 or 30 years ago.

The relative positivity of young children's judgments may also be due to the relative appropriateness of *self-congratulatory behaviors* in the first few years of life (e.g., Butler, 2005; Frey & Ruble, 1987; Pomerantz et al., 1995). In many contexts, it is socially acceptable, even desirable, for young children to boast about their abilities and performance, even when their claims are not entirely warranted. Parents of young children (in the United States, at least) may encourage these self-congratulatory behaviors partly as a means of fostering children's self-esteem (e.g., Miller, Wiley, Fung, & Liang, 1997). With age, however, overt behaviors of this sort are increasingly perceived as undesirable, not just by adults but by children themselves. For example, in Pomerantz and colleagues' (1995) study, only about 5% of kindergartners had a negative perception of others' boastful statements (e.g., "My picture is the best"), whereas more than 50% of fourth and fifth graders did. Paralleling this increase in negative perceptions, the frequency of the behaviors themselves (i.e., overt comparison statements) declined sharply. These shifting norms likely explain part of the decrease in children's self-reported optimism about their abilities. To the extent that statements about one's high ability are not frowned upon in young children's everyday lives, such statements may be relatively common in response to an experimenter's questions. (Interestingly, although self-congratulatory behaviors become less socially acceptable with age, the motivation to present oneself in a positive light might actually ramp up, as children are exposed to an increasingly competitive environment in which it is desirable to look more competent than others [e.g., Butler, 1998]. Thus, children need to learn how to balance the desire to enhance their image in others' eyes with the social costs of doing so.)

In summary, the relative positivity of young children's competence judgments is likely to arise not from their conceptual shortcomings but rather from the fact that their typical social environments (1) emphasize effort and downplay individual differences between children, and (2) condone, or even encourage, self-congratulatory judgments and behavior.

CONCLUSIONS

Young children's competence judgments are often portrayed as qualitatively different from those of older children (e.g., grossly inflated, irrationally oblivious to evidence). Moreover, these differences in judgments are often claimed to be due to flaws in the mental representations with which young children reason about competence (e.g., inadequate concepts of ability, traits, causality, quantity). The evidence reviewed here suggests that neither of these claims is valid. In reality, younger and older children interpret their achievement experiences with largely the same set of concepts. And while competence judgments are on average more optimistic in early childhood, this difference is simply the result of contingent facts about the typical environments of young (middle-class American) children that instill a default—but easily revisable—perspective on achievement that is effort-centric and confident.

By portraying young children as irrational optimists, the outmoded ideas that currently dominate the literature have stifled research on early reasoning about achievement. There is much we do not know, but should know, about the achievement beliefs and mindsets (e.g., Dweck, 2006; Yeager, Paunesku, Walton, & Dweck, 2013) of young children: how to measure them, what shapes their content, how to change them, what their long-term effects are, and so on. The early years set a crucial foundation for children's attitudes toward school. Without a better understanding of young children's thinking about competence, we are missing an opportunity to help every child enter school with, and maintain, a productive, learning-focused mindset.

ACKNOWLEDGMENTS

Many thanks to Joe Cimpian, David Yeager, and the members of the Cognitive Development Lab at the University of Illinois for providing feedback on previous drafts of this chapter. The writing of this chapter was supported in part by National Science Foundation Grant Nos. BCS-1530669 and HRD-1561723.

NOTES

1. The view that conceptual maturity, in and of itself, sets the stage for such negative outcomes raises a puzzle, though: Why do many adults persevere through difficulties (rather than giving up the moment they fail)? According to Nicholls (1990), older children and adults can choose whether to use the most sophisticated conceptual framework available to them or instead revert to young children's simpler ways of thinking. Under certain circumstances, then, even adults "can function like little children" (p. 35), taking failure in stride and redoubling their efforts on activities that their more sophisticated concepts would indicate they don't have capacity for.

2. It is worth noting that Harter's (2012) claims about early self-representations are based largely on evidence obtained from children's verbalizations—their responses to explicit prompts to describe and evaluate themselves. The exclusive reliance on such evidence is rooted in Harter's view that the ability to consciously, verbally reflect on a feature is necessary for the feature to truly be part of one's self-representations: "the 'self' is defined as how one consciously reflects upon and evaluates one's characteristics in a manner that he/she can verbalize" (p. 22).

REFERENCES

Baillargeon, R. (2004). Infants' physical world. *Current Directions in Psychological Science, 13*(3), 89–94.

Baillargeon, R., Scott, R. M., & Bian, L. (2016). Psychological reasoning in infancy. *Annual Review of Psychology, 67,* 159–186.

Baillargeon, R., Scott, R. M., & He, Z. (2010). False-belief understanding in infants. *Trends in Cognitive Sciences, 14*(3), 110–118.

Baillargeon, R., Spelke, E. S., & Wasserman, S. (1985). Object permanence in five-month-old infants. *Cognition, 20,* 191–208.

Bassok, D., Latham, S., & Rorem, A. (2016). Is kindergarten the new first grade? *AERA Open, 1*(4), 1–31.

Beilock, S. L., Gunderson, E. A., Ramirez, G., & Levine, S. C. (2010). Female teachers' math anxiety affects girls' math achievement. *Proceedings of the National Academy of Sciences USA, 107*(5), 1860–1863.

Boseovski, J. J., Chiu, K., & Marcovitch, S. (2013). Integration of behavioral frequency and intention information in young children's trait attributions. *Social Development, 22*(1), 38–57.

Boseovski, J. J., & Lee, K. (2006). Children's use of frequency information for trait categorization and behavioral prediction. *Developmental Psychology, 42*(3), 500–513.

Butler, R. (1998). Age trends in the use of social and temporal comparison for self-evaluation: Examination of a novel developmental hypothesis. *Child Development, 69*(4), 1054–1073.

Butler, R. (2005). Competence assessment, competence, and motivation between early and middle childhood. In A. J. Elliott & C. S. Dweck (Eds.), *Handbook of competence and motivation* (pp. 202–221). New York: Guilford Press.

Butler, R., & Ruzany, N. (1993). Age and socialization effects on the development of social comparison motives and normative ability assessment in kibbutz and urban children. *Child Development, 64*(2), 532–543.

Cain, K. M., Heyman, G. D., & Walker, M. E. (1997). Preschoolers' ability to make dispositional predictions within and across domain. *Social Development, 6*(1), 53–75.

Carlozzi, N. E., Tulsky, D. S., Kail, R. V., & Beaumont, J. L. (2013). VI. NIH Toolbox Cognition Battery (CB): Measuring Processing Speed. *Monographs of the Society for Research in Child Development, 78,* 88–102.

Chiandetti, C., & Vallortigara, G. (2013). The origins of physics, number, and space cognition: Insights from a chick's brain. *Human Evolution, 28*(1–2), 1–16.

Cimpian, A. (2010). The impact of generic language about ability on children's achievement motivation. *Developmental Psychology, 46*(5), 1333–1340.

Cimpian, A. (2016). The privileged status of category representations in early development. *Child Development Perspectives, 10*(2), 99–104.

Cimpian, A., Arce, H. C., Markman, E. M., & Dweck, C. S. (2007). Subtle linguistic cues affect children's motivation. *Psychological Science, 18*(4), 314–316.

Cimpian, A., Mu, Y., & Erickson, L. C. (2012).

Who is good at this game?: Linking an activity to a social category undermines children's achievement. *Psychological Science, 23*(5), 533–541.

Clark, E. V. (1987). The principle of contrast: A constraint on language acquisition. In B. MacWhinney (Ed.), *Mechanisms of language acquisition* (pp. 1–33). Hillsdale, NJ: Erlbaum.

Cowan, N. (2005). *Working memory capacity.* New York: Psychology Press.

Cvencek, D., Greenwald, A. G., & Meltzoff, A. N. (2016). Implicit measures for preschool children confirm self-esteem's role in maintaining a balanced identity. *Journal of Experimental Social Psychology, 62,* 50–57.

Dewar, K. M., & Xu, F. (2010). Induction, overhypothesis, and the origin of abstract knowledge: Evidence from 9-month-old infants. *Psychological Science, 21*(12), 1871–1877.

Diesendruck, G. (2005). The principles of conventionality and contrast in word learning: An empirical examination. *Developmental Psychology, 41*(3), 451–463.

Dweck, C. S. (1991). Self-theories and goals: Their role in motivation, personality, and development. *Nebraska Symposium on Motivation, 38,* 199–235.

Dweck, C. S. (1998). The development of early self-conceptions: Their relevance for motivational processes. In J. Heckhausen & C. S. Dweck (Eds.), *Motivation and self-regulation across the life span* (pp. 257–280). New York: Cambridge University Press.

Dweck, C. S. (1999). *Self-theories: Their role in motivation, personality, and development.* Philadelphia: Psychology Press.

Dweck, C. S. (2006). *Mindset: The new psychology of success.* New York: Random House.

Eccles, J., Midgley, C., & Adler, T. F. (1984). Grade-related changes in the school environment: Effects on achievement motivation. In J. G. Nicholls (Ed.), *The development of achievement motivation* (pp. 282–331). Greenwich, CT: JAI Press.

Ferry, A. L., Hespos, S. J., & Gentner, D. (2015). Prelinguistic relational concepts: Investigating analogical processing in infants. *Child Development, 86*(5), 1386–1405.

Frey, K. S., & Ruble, D. N. (1987). What children say about classroom performance: Sex and grade differences in perceived competence. *Child Development, 58*(4), 1066–1078.

Gelman, R., & Gallistel, C. R. (1986). *The child's understanding of number.* Cambridge, MA: Harvard University Press.

Gelman, S. A., & Heyman, G. D. (1999). Carroteaters and creature-believers: The effects of lexicalization on children's inferences about social categories. *Psychological Science, 10*(6), 489–493.

Giles, J. W., & Heyman, G. D. (2003). Preschoolers' beliefs about the stability of antisocial behavior: Implications for navigating social challenges. *Social Development, 12*(2), 182–197.

Gunderson, E. A., Gripshover, S. J., Romero, C., Dweck, C. S., Goldin-Meadow, S., & Levine, S. C. (2013). Parent praise to 1- to 3-year-olds predicts children's motivational frameworks 5 years later. *Child Development, 84*(5), 1526–1541.

Haimovitz, K., & Dweck, C. S. (2016). What predicts children's fixed and growth intelligence mind-sets?: Not their parents' views of intelligence but their parents' views of failure. *Psychological Science.* [Epub ahead of print]

Harter, S. (1982). The perceived competence scale for children. *Child Development, 53,* 87–97.

Harter, S. (2001). Self-development in childhood. In N. J. Smelser & P. B. Baltes (Eds.), *International encyclopedia of the social and behavioral sciences* (Vol. 20, pp. 13807–13812). Oxford, UK: Elsevier.

Harter, S. (2012). *The construction of the self: Developmental and sociocultural foundations* (2nd ed.). New York: Guilford Press.

Harter, S., & Pike, R. (1984). The pictorial scale of perceived competence and social acceptance for young children. *Child Development, 55,* 1969–1982.

Hauf, P., Paulus, M., & Baillargeon, R. (2012). Infants use compression information to infer objects' weights: Examining cognition, exploration, and prospective action in a preferential-reaching task. *Child Development, 83*(6), 1978–1995.

Hebert, C. A., & Dweck, C. S. (1985). *Mediators of persistence in preschoolers: Implications for development.* Unpublished manuscript, Harvard University, Cambridge, MA.

Hermes, J., Behne, T., & Rakoczy, H. (2015). The role of trait reasoning in young children's selective trust. *Developmental Psychology, 51*(11), 1574–1587.

Hespos, S. J., & Baillargeon, R. (2008). Young infants' actions reveal their developing knowledge of support variables: Converging evidence for violation-of-expectation findings. *Cognition, 107*(1), 304–316.

Heyman, G. D., & Compton, B. J. (2006). Context sensitivity in children's reasoning about ability across the elementary school years. *Developmental Science, 9*(6), 616–627.

Heyman, G. D., Dweck, C. S., & Cain, K. M. (1992). Young children's vulnerability to self-blame and helplessness: Relationship to beliefs about goodness. *Child Development, 63,* 401–415.

Heyman, G. D., Gee, C. L., & Giles, J. W. (2003). Preschool children's reasoning about ability. *Child Development, 74*(2), 516–534.

Heyman, G. D., & Gelman, S. A. (1999). The use of trait labels in making psychological inferences. *Child Development, 70*(3), 604–619.

Heyman, G. D., & Gelman, S. A. (2000). Preschool children's use of trait labels to make inductive inferences. *Journal of Experimental Child Psychology, 77*(1), 1–19.

Horowitz, A. C., & Frank, M. C. (2016). Children's pragmatic inferences as a route for learning about the world. *Child Development, 87*(3), 807–819.

Hughes, B. L., & Zaki, J. (2015). The neuroscience of motivated cognition. *Trends in Cognitive Sciences, 19*(2), 62–64.

Hyde, D. C. (2015). Numerosity. In A. W. Toga & R. A. Poldrack (Eds.), *Brain mapping: An encyclopedic reference* (Vol. 3, pp. 559–564). San Diego, CA: Elsevier.

Izard, V., Sann, C., Spelke, E. S., & Streri, A. (2009). Newborn infants perceive abstract numbers. *Proceedings of the National Academy of Sciences USA, 106*(25), 10382–10385.

Jordan, K. E., & Brannon, E. M. (2006). The multisensory representation of number in infancy. *Proceedings of the National Academy of Sciences USA, 103*(9), 3486–3489.

Jost, J. T., Glaser, J., Kruglanski, A. W., & Sulloway, F. J. (2003). Political conservatism as motivated social cognition. *Psychological Bulletin, 129*(3), 339–375.

Kamins, M. L., & Dweck, C. S. (1999). Person versus process praise and criticism: Implications for contingent self-worth and coping. *Developmental Psychology, 35*(3), 835–847.

Kuhlmeier, V., Wynn, K., & Bloom, P. (2003). Attribution of dispositional states by 12-month-olds. *Psychological Science, 14*(5), 402–408.

Kuhn, D. (2000). Metacognitive development. *Current Directions in Psychological Science, 9*(5), 178–181.

Jara-Ettinger, J., Tenenbaum, J. B., & Schulz, L. E. (2015). Not so innocent: Toddlers' inferences about costs and culpability. *Psychological Science, 26*(5), 633–640.

Liu, D., Gelman, S. A., & Wellman, H. M. (2007). Components of young children's trait understanding: Behavior-to-trait inferences and trait-to-behavior predictions. *Child Development, 78*(5), 1543–1558.

Luo, Y., & Baillargeon, R. (2005). Can a self-propelled box have a goal?: Psychological reasoning in 5-month-old infants. *Psychological Science, 16*(8), 601–608.

Luo, Y., & Johnson, S. C. (2009). Recognizing the role of perception in action at 6 months. *Developmental Science, 12*(1), 142–149.

Marcus, G. F., Vijayan, S., Rao, S. B., & Vishton, P. M. (1999). Rule learning by seven-month-old infants. *Science, 283,* 77–80.

Marsh, H. W., Ellis, L. A., & Craven, R. G. (2002). How do preschool children feel about themselves?: Unraveling measurement and multidimensional self-concept structure. *Developmental Psychology, 38*(3), 376–393.

Mather, M., & Carstensen, L. L. (2005). Aging and motivated cognition: The positivity effect in attention and memory. *Trends in Cognitive Sciences, 9*(10), 496–502.

McGarrigle, J., & Donaldson, M. (1974). Conservation accidents. *Cognition, 3*(4), 341–350.

Miller, P. J., Wiley, A. R., Fung, H., & Liang, C.-H. (1997). Personal storytelling as a medium of socialization in Chinese and American families. *Child Development, 68*(3), 557–568.

Morris, B. J., & Zentall, S. R. (2014). High fives motivate: The effects of gestural and ambiguous verbal praise on motivation. *Frontiers in Psychology, 5,* 928.

Morris, W. N., & Nemcek, D. (1982). The development of social comparison motivation among preschoolers: Evidence of a stepwise progression. *Merrill–Palmer Quarterly, 28*(3), 413–425.

Mosatche, H. S., & Bragonier, P. (1981). An observational study of social comparison in preschoolers. *Child Development, 52*(1), 376–378.

Nicholls, J. G. (1978). The development of the concepts of effort and ability, perception of academic attainment, and the understanding that difficult tasks require more ability. *Child Development, 49,* 800–814.

Nicholls, J. G. (1984). Achievement motivation: Conceptions of ability, subjective experience, task choice, and performance. *Psychological Review, 91*(3), 328–346.

Nicholls, J. G. (1990). What is ability and why are we mindful of it?: A developmental perspective. In R. J. Sternberg & J. Kolligian, Jr. (Eds.), *Competence considered* (pp. 11–40). New Haven, CT: Yale University Press.

Nicholls, J. G., & Miller, A. T. (1984a). Development and its discontents: The differentiation of the concept of ability. In J. G. Nicholls (Ed.), *The development of achievement motivation* (pp. 185–218). Greenwich, CT: JAI Press.

Nicholls, J. G., & Miller, A. T. (1984b). Reasoning about the ability of self and others:

A developmental study. *Child Development, 55*(6), 1990–1999.

Onishi, K. H., & Baillargeon, R. (2005). Do 15-month-old infants understand false beliefs? *Science, 308,* 255–258.

Parsons, J. E., & Ruble, D. N. (1977). The development of achievement-related expectancies. *Child Development, 48,* 1075–1079.

Piaget, J. (1930). *The child's conception of physical causality.* London: Routledge & Kegan Paul.

Piaget, J. (1941). *The child's conception of number.* London: Routledge & Kegan Paul.

Piaget, J. (1952). *The origins of intelligence in children.* New York: International Universities Press.

Piaget, J. (1960). *The psychology of intelligence.* Patterson, NJ: Littlefield, Adams.

Piaget, J., & Inhelder, B. (1969). *The psychology of the child.* New York: Basic Books.

Pomerantz, E. M., & Kempner, S. G. (2013). Mothers' daily person and process praise: Implications for children's theory of intelligence and motivation. *Developmental Psychology, 49*(11), 2040–2046.

Pomerantz, E. M., Ruble, D. N., Frey, K. S., & Greulich, F. (1995). Meeting goals and confronting conflict: Children's changing perceptions of social comparison. *Child Development, 66*(3), 723–738.

Repacholi, B. M., & Gopnik, A. (1997). Early reasoning about desires: Evidence from 14- and 18-month-olds. *Developmental Psychology, 33*(1), 12–21.

Repacholi, B. M., Meltzoff, A. N., Hennings, T. M., & Ruba, A. L. (2016). Transfer of social learning across contexts: Exploring infants' attribution of trait-like emotions to adults. *Infancy.* [Epub ahead of print]

Repacholi, B. M., Meltzoff, A. N., Toub, T. S., & Ruba, A. L. (2016). Infants' generalizations about other people's emotions: Foundations for trait-like attributions. *Developmental Psychology, 52*(3), 364–378.

Rhodes, M., & Brickman, D. (2008). Preschoolers' responses to social comparisons involving relative failure. *Psychological Science, 19*(10), 968–972.

Rholes, W. S., Newman, L. S., & Ruble, D. N. (1990). Understanding self and other: Developmental and motivational aspects of perceiving persons in terms of invariant dispositions. In E. T. Higgins & R. M. Sorrentino (Eds.), *Handbook of motivation and cognition: Foundations of social behavior* (Vol. 2, pp. 369–407). New York: Guilford Press.

Rholes, W. S., & Ruble, D. N. (1984). Children's understanding of dispositional characteristics of others. *Child Development, 55,* 550–560.

Rose, S. A., & Blank, M. (1974). The potency of context in children's cognition: An illustration through conservation. *Child Development, 45,* 499–502.

Rosenholtz, S. J., & Simpson, C. (1984). The formation of ability conceptions: Developmental trend or social construction? *Review of Education Research, 54,* 31–63.

Rotenberg, K. J. (1980). Children's use of intentionality in judgments of character and disposition. *Child Development, 51*(1), 282–284.

Ruble, D. N., Boggiano, A. K., Feldman, N. S., & Loebl, J. H. (1980). Developmental analysis of the role of social comparison in self-evaluation. *Developmental Psychology, 16*(2), 105–115.

Ruble, D. N., Feldman, N. S., & Boggiano, A. K. (1976). Social comparison between young children in achievement situations. *Developmental Psychology, 12*(3), 192–197.

Schulz, L. (2012). The origins of inquiry: Inductive inference and exploration in early childhood. *Trends in Cognitive Sciences, 16*(7), 382–389.

Setoh, P., Wu, D., Baillargeon, R., & Gelman, R. (2013). Young infants have biological expectations about animals. *Proceedings of the National Academy of Sciences USA, 110*(40), 15937–15942.

Simons, D. J., & Keil, F. C. (1995). An abstract to concrete shift in the development of biological thought: The insides story. *Cognition, 56,* 129–163.

Smith, L. B., Jones, S. S., Landau, B., Gershkoff-Stowe, L., & Samuelson, L. (2002). Object name learning provides on-the-job training for attention. *Psychological Science, 13*(1), 13–19.

Song, H., Baillargeon, R., & Fisher, C. (2005). Can infants attribute to an agent a disposition to perform a particular action? *Cognition, 98,* B45–B55.

Spelke, E. S., & Kinzler, K. D. (2007). Core knowledge. *Developmental Science, 10*(1), 89–96.

Stipek, D. J. (1981). Children's perceptions of their own and their classmates' ability. *Journal of Educational Psychology, 73*(3), 404–410.

Stipek, D. J. (1984). Young children's performance expectations: Logical analysis or wishful thinking? In J. G. Nicholls (Ed.), *The development of achievement motivation* (pp. 33–56). Greenwich, CT: JAI Press.

Stipek, D. J., & Daniels, D. H. (1988). Declining perceptions of competence: A consequence of changes in the child or in the educational environment? *Journal of Educational Psychology, 80*(3), 352–356.

Stipek, D. J., & Hoffman, J. M. (1980). Development of children's performance-related judgments. *Child Development, 51*(3), 912–914.

Stipek, D. J., Roberts, T. A., & Sanborn, M. E. (1984). Preschool-age children's performance expectations for themselves and another child as a function of the incentive value of success and the salience of past performance. *Child Development, 55*(6), 1983–1989.

Walker, C. M., & Gopnik, A. (2014). Toddlers infer higher-order relational principles in causal learning. *Psychological Science, 25*(1), 161–169.

Williams, B. R., Ponesse, J. S., Schachar, R. J., Logan, G. D., & Tannock, R. (1999). Development of inhibitory control across the life span. *Developmental Psychology, 35*(1), 205–213.

Wimmer, H., & Perner, J. (1983). Beliefs about beliefs: Representation and constraining function of wrong beliefs in young children's understanding of deception. *Cognition, 13*(1), 103–128.

Wood, J. N. (2013). Newborn chickens generate invariant object representations at the onset of visual object experience. *Proceedings of the National Academy of Sciences USA, 110*(34), 14000–14005.

Woodward, A. L. (1998). Infants selectively encode the goal object of an actor's reach. *Cognition, 69*(1), 1–34.

Yeager, D. S., Paunesku, D., Walton, G. M., & Dweck, C. S. (2013). *How can we instill productive mindsets at scale?: A review of the evidence and an initial R&D agenda.* White paper prepared for the White House meeting on "Excellence in Education: The Importance of Academic Mindsets." Retrieved from *http://mindsetscholarsnetwork.org/research_library/how-can-we-instill-productive-mindsets-at-scale-a-review-of-the-evidence-and-an-initial-rd-agenda-a-white-paper-prepared-for-the-white-house-meeting-on-excellence-in-education-the-importa.*

Yin, J., & Csibra, G. (2015). Concept-based word learning in human infants. *Psychological Science, 26*(8), 1316–1324.

Zentall, S. R., & Morris, B. J. (2010). "Good job, you're so smart": The effects of inconsistency of praise type on young children's motivation. *Journal of Experimental Child Psychology, 107*, 155–163.

Zentall, S. R., & Morris, B. J. (2012). A critical eye: Praise directed toward traits increases children's eye fixations on errors and decreases motivation. *Psychonomic Bulletin and Review, 19*(6), 1073–1077.

CHAPTER 22

Self-Regulation in Early Childhood
Implications for Motivation and Achievement

C. CYBELE RAVER
KATHERINE A. ADAMS
CLANCY BLAIR

In much research on adolescents' competence and motivation, students' academic effort and achievement are based on what they know and believe about themselves, the nature of their goals, and their educational environments. In short, an impressive body of research demonstrates that students' cognitions are forceful shapers of belief, mood, effort, and outcome in ways that are empowering and liberating (Dweck, 1999). Yet those models of motivation and achievement, while innovative, are relatively silent on the ways that cognitions may not yet be the behavioral and motivational "driver" for many children, particularly in the earlier grades. Many children in prekindergarten through the early elementary grades often find themselves acting without thinking, reacting rather than reflecting, losing track of larger goals over short-term distractions, and struggling to manage feelings. Other children demonstrate an early capacity to "keep a cool head" in emotionally and cognitively challenging classroom situations, focusing and meeting their goals despite academic and social hurdles. How do developmental scientists understand the trajectory of growth and change that those children navigate across the early elementary years?

In this chapter, we briefly outline several advances in developmental research on self-regulation in early childhood that we hope are informative about larger questions of student competence and motivation. We first discuss higher-order cognitive processes, termed *executive functions,* which underlie young children's self-regulation. In so doing, we point to ways that key components of executive function in early childhood, including constructs of cognitive flexibility versus inflexibility, executive attention, and greater versus lower inhibitory control, have each been found to play important roles in children's achievement of academic goals. We then shift to consider the role of young children's regulation of their emotions as a key, related neuropsychological system that may alternatively support or disrupt children's tendencies to respond to challenging situations in reactive versus reflective ways. Children's executive functions and emotion regulation serve as two interlocking pieces of a comprehensive theoretical and empirical framework for models of self-regulation. In this chapter, we also focus on a third, less thoroughly investigated domain of development, namely, children's increasing capacity to focus and shift their attention. We provide a brief outline for ways that children's attentional regulation can be understood as a pivotal neuropsychological link between emotional regulation and executive function.

After providing this brief overview of these domains of self-regulation in early childhood, we then shift to consider how children's self-regulation is shaped by environmental forces. We consider the role of poverty for young children's self-regulation, in light of overwhelming empirical evidence that socioeconomic disadvantage places children's educational and developmental trajectories in jeopardy. Stated another way, questions of poverty's cost have shifted to focus not on whether poverty is deleterious to young children's learning but how it takes such a negative toll and what can be done to mitigate those negative sequelae. We therefore discuss the extent to which self-regulation processes are not only threatened by poverty-related stressors but also amenable to "repair," examining ways that those processes can be bolstered in the context of school-based intervention. Finally, we draw from that review to consider new directions that our field might take in considering executive functions, attention deployment, and emotion regulation in the preschool period as potent sources of individual differences in students' social cognitions, motivation, and engagement later in development.

WHAT DO WE MEAN BY SELF-REGULATION AND WHY IS IT IMPORTANT?

In simple terms, self-regulation is often thought of as the intentional control of behavior that requires that the individual consciously and intentionally strive to regulate his or her actions (Oettingen & Gollwitzer, 2004). An example of self-regulation would be when a kindergartner exerts mental, emotional, and behavioral effort to read aloud or answer a math problem in front of his or her teacher and peers. That example includes a goal (e.g., completing the read-aloud passage) and the child's management of multiple and often competing thoughts, feelings, and intentions that work in concert to bring that student either closer or further away from that goal. For older children in school settings, intentional self-regulation involves a set of higher-order cognitive processes (or executive functions) that we describe in detail later. Those executive functions allow students to exert "willpower" in ways that have been depicted as "cool" and logical by reflecting on a given situation (e.g., that class speech), setting goals, and monitoring progress toward them, and implementing specific strategies to manage behavior and meet those goals (Mischel, Cantor, & Feldman, 1996; Zelazo & Cunningham, 2007).

Clearly, this reflective exertion of intentional control represents only one part of the theoretical framework needed to understand children's ability to meet goals. A more comprehensive way of thinking about self-regulation can be found in what is known as *dual-processing theory* or *dual-systems theory* (Evans, 2008). While theories of dual processes have been invoked for many systems (including memory, learning, attitudes and evaluation; e.g., Cunningham, Zelazo, Packer, & Van Bavel, 2007; Smith & DeCoster, 2000), those theories share the key insight that in addition to this more reflective, "cool," and logical way of responding to a stimulus, individuals can respond in more reactive, nonconscious, emotionally charged or "quick-and-dirty" fashion. In our use of the dual-process model to unpack key components of children's self-regulation, we emphasize that reflective, volitional processes (as they pertain to setting and achieving goals; e.g., the ability to plan, problem-solve, and monitor goals and actions) are shaped by and in some instances overridden by those nonconscious (automatic) reflexive, reactive, and often emotionally charged aspects of self-regulation. The reflexive, automatic aspects of self-regulation (often referred to as "hot" processes) include very fast systems of emotional responding to highly salient, sometimes frustrating or distressing features of the situation or task at hand (Mischel & Ayduk, 2011). The distinction between affectively "hot" and "cool" is one that we consider to function on a continuum. Rather than distinct neural and behavioral systems underlying "hot" and "cool" emotion regulation and executive function processes, recent evidence from neuroscience suggests that self-regulation is best understood as a set of interrelated neural and behavioral systems for which the affective valence of a given regulatory challenge is highly salient for the functioning of those systems. Advances in neuroscience underscore the intricate, complex ways in which connectivity rather than modularity of function is the way that the brain works in real time (Lewis & Todd, 2007).

We use this heuristic in the following sections to provide a thumbnail sketch of the processes involved in young children's ability to meet academic goals and expectations. To address both the intentional, slower dimensions as well as faster, more automatic dimensions of self-regulation, we anchor our discussion by first focusing on young children's *executive function* (including their working memory, attention, and inhibitory control). We briefly outline processes of *emotion regulation* in conditions of anxiety and threat, and examine implications of emotion and emotion regulation for the deployment of executive function abilities in academic contexts. We then discuss the role of *attention* as a key mechanism linking emotion regulation and higher-order cognitive control.

Executive Functions

As mentioned earlier, *executive functions (EFs)* refer to volitional cognitive abilities generally associated with cognitive flexibility, goal setting, planning, and problem solving; in short, a set of higher-order cognitive processes that are involved in the control and coordination of information in the service of goal-directed actions (Diamond, 2013; Fuster, 1997). Recall the example of the first grader who is asked to read aloud or complete a math problem: He or she must monitor the teacher's request, find the right section of the page to work from, pay attention to and process the competing details of the task, and provide an answer, while not becoming lost or distracted. At a more fine-grained level, EF has come to refer to specific interrelated information-processing abilities that enable the resolution of conflicting information: These include *working memory*, defined as the holding in mind and updating information while performing some operation on it; *inhibitory control*,

defined as the inhibition of prepotent or automatized responding when engaged in task completion; and *attention shifting*, defined as the ability to shift cognitive set among distinct but related dimensions or aspects of a given task (Davidson, Amso, Anderson, & Diamond, 2006; Miyake et al., 2000; Zelazo et al., 2003). EFs are often assessed through easel- or computer-based multitrial tasks that require children to direct their attention and point to competing or conflicting dimensions of visual stimuli based on simple sets of rules. A good example is the "fish flanker task" from the Attentional Network Task (ANT) battery, in which the child being assessed is asked to help "feed the fish" located in the center of a long row of brightly colored fishes, by hitting the computer arrow key that corresponds to the direction that the center fish is facing. The task is easy when all the fish in the row are facing in the same direction, aligned tip to tail, so to speak, to point in a single direction. The cognitive challenge arises when the fish on either side of (or flanking) the center fish are pointing in the opposite direction: The child must remember the rule, focus his or her attention on the center fish only, and inhibit the prepotent tendency to hit the wrong key (corresponding to the flanking fish) (Rueda, Posner, & Rothbart, 2005). Children's performance on these types of tasks is determined by both their accuracy and their reaction time given that children typically take longer to respond to the "incongruent" trials because of their cognitive complexity.

Neurocognitively speaking, EFs are associated with prefrontal cortex (PFC) and the extensive neural connections of PFC with posterior cortex, most notably parietal cortex, and also subcortical structures, including the basal ganglia, amygdala, and hippocampus (Fuster, 1997). By resolving competing or conflicting information through monitoring, set shifting, and inhibitory control, EFs can be understood to regulate activity in lower-level neural systems associated with the regulation of attention, emotional, and physiological responses to stimulation. Connectivity of PFC with other brain regions matures slowly, leaving ample opportunity for experiential shaping of neural networks that underlie EFs and self-regulation. Brain areas responsible for children's EFs, however, undergo rapid growth in the preschool period, and their top-down organizing role enables school readiness and allows young children to focus, plan, and exert inhibitory control in classroom contexts that may become noisy, chaotic, or less organized (Blair & Ursache, 2011; Carlson, 2005; Casey, Giedd, & Thomas, 2000; Espy et al., 2004; Gogtay et al., 2004).

As such, EFs are thinking skills that are clearly important for learning, with EF components such as children's working memory, set shifting, and inhibitory control consistently and reliably predicting academic achievement in early years of schooling (Bull & Scerif, 2001; Espy et al., 2004; McClelland et al., 2007). In the classroom example provided earlier, the first grader must remember simple computational rules, such as how to "borrow" and "carry," must select and use those rules in some cases and not in others (e.g., when adding two numbers that equal more than 10 and when they do not). In our research, we have consistently demonstrated that individual differences in EF as early as the age of 4 or 5 are both concurrently and longitudinally predictive of children's math and literacy ability from preschool through later elementary school, across multiple samples of children from low-income homes (Blair & Raver, 2014; Blair & Razza, 2007; Friedman-Krauss & Raver, 2015; Welsh, Nix, Blair, Bierman, & Nelson, 2010). Importantly, however, alternatively we have also found that young children's EFs can be supported or derailed by their emotional state and by the physiological response to stress that accompanies emotional response to environmental challenge (Blair, Raver, Granger, Mills-Koonce, & Hibel, 2011; Evans & Schamberg, 2009).

Emotion Regulation

Increasingly, research on young children's self-regulation and learning highlights the complementary roles of emotion regulation (ER) and EF for meeting goals in classroom contexts. Theories of emotion underscore the temporal course of how feelings emerge and how we manage them—the process is rooted in initial activation of a positive or negative affective response to a stimulus (through activation of the brain stem, hypothalamus, amygdala, and related subcortical areas of the brain) following initial attention to it (Lewis, 2005). Through the recruitment of the anterior cingulate cortex, as well as dorsolateral and ventromedial prefrontal cortices of the brain, individuals quickly appraise a given stimulus in positively or negatively valenced ways (considered as activated emotions), then are more or less capable of modulating or controlling those emotions through the use of a variety of cognitive and behavioral strategies (considered as ER) (Cole, Martin, & Dennis, 2004; Gross, 2002; Gross & Thompson, 2007; Harris, Hare, & Rangel, 2013).

A classic means of assessing ER at behavioral and neuropsychological levels is to ask children to look at or watch stimuli that are emotionally evocative and moderately stressful, such as watching a sad versus funny movie clip, or to discriminate among happy, sad, angry, and neutral facial expressions from photos or screenshots on a computer screen. Children's accuracy and their latency of response in performing a variety of tasks when presented with emotionally negative versus neutral stimuli serve as behavioral indicators of the ease or difficulty with which they regulate negative emotion (e.g., Tottenham, Hare, & Casey, 2011). Correspondingly, children's brain activity is monitored during those tasks using advanced imaging techniques and, when analyzed, help us to understand the localized brain regions and connectivity associated with emotion processing (Tottenham et al., 2011). Recent event-related potential (ERP) evidence from research with anxious and nonanxious children suggests that fast-acting processes in areas such as the PFC cortex and anterior cingulate cortex play key roles in the emotional regulatory process: Anxious children's tendency to recruit prefrontal cortical regions in response to a wide array of stimuli may account for their behavioral profiles of high vigilance and attentional bias toward threat, placing them on a pathway to more negative responding (Lamm, Decety, & Singer, 2011).

As the "other half" of the dual processes involved in self-regulation, emotions are powerful amplifiers of our cognitive responses to our environments. Emotional arousal sharpens and strengthens children's attention to the details of their environment that are relevant or salient to goals and interests, helping to screen out other, less relevant perceptual details through a filtering process involving activation of the occipital cortex (Mather & Sutherland, 2011; Phillips, Ladoceur, & Drevets, 2008). But emotions can also disrupt higher-order cognitive control: Modulating emotional arousal also involves activity in key cortical areas of the brain (Hare, Tottenham, Davison, Glover, & Casey, 2005). Emotions can direct children's attention to features of their environment that are distracting or anxiety provoking, and can compete with or deplete cognitive resources when trying to meet goals (Mischel & Ayduk, 2011; see also Bar-Haim, Lamy, Pergamin, Bakermans-Kranenburg, & van IJzendoorn, 2007; Lamm et al., 2011; Lewis, Todd, & Honsberg, 2007).

Why is regulating emotion seemingly so hard for some children, and less so for others? Clearly, some children simply develop emotional competence (e.g., stronger vocabularies and higher use of expressive language) earlier than do others. In addition, children differ in their biobehavioral and genetic propensity to become easily distressed, to become more or less intensely distressed, and to recover from distress (key dimensions of child temperament) in the first years of life (Derryberry & Rothbart, 1997; Posner & Rothbart, 1998; Rothbart, 2004; Rothbart & Ahadi, 1994). Individual differences in temperament are understood as the give and take between biologically based tendencies toward emotional and motor reactivity, and the regulation of this reactivity through both approach and withdrawal behavioral strategies, and attention (Posner & Rothbart, 2000). This give and take between emotional reactivity and regulation (i.e., a behavioral repertoire that modifies that initial emotional response) has powerful implications for learning in school contexts. Specifically, the relation between reactivity and regulation is that of an inverted-U-shaped curve (Arnsten, 2009; Diamond, Campbell, Park, Halonen, & Zoladz, 2007). With a moderate increase in emotional and physiological reactivity, children's attention to their environments is increased, and effortful regulation is maximized. At very high levels of reactivity, however, high levels of arousal are registered in the emotional–motivational, alerting, and orienting systems of the brain, and a stress response is activated, stimulating the production of corticotropin-releasing hormone (CRH) from the hypothalamus. CRH initiates the rapid sympathetic adrenal response and production of catecholamines, namely, norepinephrine and dopamine, and also initiates activity in the slower acting hypothalamic–pituitary–adrenal (HPA) axis response and resulting production of the steroid hormone cortisol (Gunnar & Quevedo, 2007).

What does this mean for children's engagement in an academic task? At low levels of task demand, children's HPA axis activity may be correspondingly low. However, as task demands become greater and levels of these neurochemicals rise to moderate levels, neural activity in the PFC is high and EF abilities are maximized; children's performance at the task is likely to be supported. As task demands become too stressful, these neurochemicals continue to rise beyond a moderate level, however; activity in the PFC is reduced, and children's performance is likely to be poorer as a result. Instead, activity in brain areas associated with reactive motoric and emotional–motivational responses to stimulation is increased (Ramos & Arnsten, 2007). In this way, the neurobiology of EFs maps onto the well-known inverted-U-shaped Yerkes–Dodson curve relating anxiety to performance, in which the individual faces an acute stressor at a particular moment in time; at moderate levels of stress, performance is increased, while at very low or very high levels, performance is frequently compromised. As we discuss later in this chapter, recent advances in the study of children's development in the context of prolonged exposure to chronic stressors suggests promising support for this neuropsychologically anchored developmental model of ER and EF.

This model of the relation between ER and cognitive performance also aligns with two decades of behavioral developmental research suggesting that young children become increasingly capable of managing their emotions without adult help, and that young children's ability to regulate their emotions may alternatively fuel or disrupt their inhibitory control and academic performance (Cole et al., 2011; Graziano, Reavis,

Keane, & Calkins, 2007; Howse, Calkins, Anastopoulos, Keane, & Shelton, 2003; Trentacosta & Izard, 2007). From developmentally and neuropsychologically informed perspectives, it is clear that children's regulation of positive and negative affect works in concert with their deployment of attention and higher-order cognitive skills in bidirectional fashion, with EFs reciprocally related to and dependent on bottom-up, less volitional, and more automatic responses to the environment that centrally involve emotion, attention, and stress response processes (Blair, 2002; Blair & Dennis, 2010; Calkins & Marcovitch, 2010). For example, children's patterns of reactivity and regulation in infancy have been found to jointly predict higher levels of EF in early childhood (Ursache, Blair, Granger, Stifter, & Voegtline, 2014). Children who experience high levels of distress (including anxiety) have been found to demonstrate significantly lower performance on EF tasks, as well as both academic and behavioral problems in the classroom (Osterman, 2000). Conversely, children who can regulate distress are able to cognitively disengage from upsetting, frustrating, or anxiety-provoking episodes, and are able to suppress the impulsive responses in favor of more reflective academic engagement (see review by Ursache, Blair, & Raver, 2012). For that first grader working out the math problem at the chalkboard, this would mean keeping feelings of anxiety in check while taking a long look at the problem and persevering to solve it rather than panicking, giving up, and heading back to his or her seat.

Neuroscientific studies of the role of negative emotions in disrupting EFs (including more difficulty with executive attention, working memory, inhibitory control, and planning) are traceable to increased activity in the amygdala and decreased activity in dorsolateral PFC, and support a model characterized by competition between emotional and executive cognitive systems (Dennis & Chen, 2007; Hart, Green, Casp, & Belger, 2010; Pessoa, 2009; Plewnia, Schroeder, Kunze, Faehling, & Wolkenstein, 2015). Importantly, recent research suggests that some children may be more vulnerable than others to the effects of emotionally threatening or frustrating stimuli on higher-order cognitive processes, with children's proneness to negative affectivity "tuning" their attention preferentially to more negative features of their environments (Solomon, O'Toole, Hong, & Dennis, 2014). While prior research has emphasized this vulnerability to be temperamentally or trait-based, children's exposure to environmental risk (including persistently turbulent or threatening environments) may also increase their vulnerability to the disruptive effects of negative emotion on their attention deployment, working memory, inhibitory control, and ability to resolve cognitive conflict (discussed in greater detail below).

EFs are not only affected by emotion but can also aid in controlling emotion in a top-down fashion. Young children's increasing capacity to reign in negative emotion and to exert greater behavioral control are thought to reflect increasing maturation of the medial frontal cortex and greater cognitive control (Dennis, Malone, & Chen, 2009). For example, older children have been found to be able to exercise top-down cognitive control of negative emotions of anxiety and frustration through strategic allocation of executive attention, conscious activation of inhibitory control (McRae, Ciesielski, & Gross, 2012; Ochsner et al., 2004), and coping strategies of suppression and reappraisal (Webb, Miles, & Sheeran, 2012). These studies clearly illustrate the ways that EFs can be consciously recruited to support students in meeting goals and expectations even when they are anxious, sad, or frustrated. Providing older students with concrete top-down support of emotions through cognitive reappraisal, such as arming students with specific strategies to identify and reinterpret distress through writing exercises, is associated with substantial benefit in academic performance (Jamieson, Mendes, Blackstock, & Schmader, 2010; Ramirez & Beilock, 2011). But it is less clear whether younger children can benefit as well from the same mechanisms of top-down cognitive control: Field-based experimental research implementing interventions targeting reappraisal (described below) provides only modest support for this mechanism for preschoolers. Instead, past theory and research suggests that recruitment and allocation of attention, earlier "upstream" in the emotional regulatory process, may be a more advantageous path to pursue in supporting young children's self-regulation.

Attention Regulation: A Bridge Linking Emotion and Cognition

A burgeoning research literature explores the role of attention as a key bridging mechanism linking emotion regulation and higher-order cognitive control (e.g., Blair & Diamond, 2008; Posner & Rothbart, 2000; Rueda, Checa, & Rothbart, 2010; Rueda, Posner, et al., 2005; Ruff & Rothbart, 1996). Even the earliest theoretical accounts of cognition recognize that what we selectively attend to—and what we ignore—shape our experiences and behavior (James, 1890). Early in the systematic study of attention, Broadbent (1959) proposed an influential filter theory that describes selective attention in terms of a bottleneck that limits information processing of sensory input. The wealth of neurocognitive studies that followed showed that attention modulates early perceptual processing, as well as higher, more integrative decision areas (e.g., Colby & Golberg, 1999; Martínez et al., 2001; O'Connor, Fukui, Pinsk, & Kastner, 2002). Importantly, neurocognitive models identify ways that attention can be initially recruited in automatic, stimulus-driven ways through alerting and orienting networks, as well as through a consciously controlled executive network, where attention can be purposively focused and redirected in service of emotion modulation and the attainment of goals (Cole et al., 2004; Norman & Shallice; 1986; Posner & Dehaene, 1994; Posner & Petersen, 1990).

For example, as early as the first year of life, attentional orienting represents a means to regulate internal states such as distress (Harman, Rothbart, & Posner, 1997). The ability to disengage attention from overly arousing stimuli in infancy is associated with toddlers' expressions of lower levels of negative emotions. Later on, in the preschool period, the ability to flexibly deploy and sustain attention is associated with greater emotional control: Children who can marshal their attention away from a tempting but prohibited object during delay of gratification tasks are substantially less likely to exhibit distress than are children who are less skilled in modulating their attention (Cole, 1986; Mischel, Shoda, & Rodriguez, 1989; Raver, Blackburn, Bancroft, & Torp, 1999).

At the neurocognitive level, ERP studies highlight the ways that individual differences in young children's selective attention to emotional stimuli are associated with greater emotional and behavioral control, as rated by parents (Dennis et al., 2009). Additional developmental studies point to the executive attention network as the neural substrate supporting effortful control and higher levels of empathy, as well as lower levels of aggression (Derryberry & Rothbart, 1997). Greater skill in regulating attention is also associated with lower risk of exhibiting dysregulated profiles of aggressive and acting-out behavior, as well as symptoms of anxiety, depression, and withdrawal (NICHD Early Child Care Research Network, 2003; Rothbart, Ziaie, & O'Boyle, 1992; Stifter & Braungart, 1995). In short, the development of alerting, orienting, and executive attention systems facilitates children's regulation of emotions and serves as the foundation for higher-order cognitive processing in the contexts of emotionally challenging situations such as peer conflict and distress.

Individual differences in each of the domains of selective, sustained, and executive attention are also clearly and consistently associated with proficiency in early academic skills. Steele, Karmiloff-Smith, Cornish, and Scerif (2012) found that executive attention predicted concurrent abilities in letter knowledge and basic math, whereas an attention factor that comprised both selective and sustained attention predicted math skills a year later. These findings support robust research connecting executive attention and children's arithmetic performance (Bull & Scerif, 2001; Espy et al., 2004) even when researchers controlled for general intelligence (Blair & Razza, 2007). Recent longitudinal research shows that selective attention skills in kindergarten predict future reading acquisition in first and second grade (Franceschini, Gori, Ruffino, Pedrolli, & Faocetti, 2012).

THE ROLE OF POVERTY-RELATED ADVERSITY IN THE DEVELOPMENT OF SELF-REGULATION

In the previous sections of this chapter, we outlined ways that children's early self-regulatory skills—the skills needed to modulate emotions, attention, and thought processes in service of a goal—are key foundations for academic success. Those sections provided a thumbnail sketch of the complex and very rapid processes occurring inside children's brains as they navigate classroom challenges; they provided little detail, however, on the ways that those self-regulatory skills are shaped by the environment. We now shift our attention to a very different level of analysis and time scale to consider evidence for ways that children's self-regulation is canalized by the larger socioeconomic context of poverty (and the stressors that often accompany insufficient family income) over multiple years in a child's lifetime. This is an important lens through which to examine the foundations of student academic competence given that over 20% of all children in the United States live in households where families struggle to make ends meet on roughly $24,000 a year (the 2015 federal poverty threshold for a family of four; Jiang, Ekono, & Skinner, 2016). We outline clear evidence of the cost of poverty-related stressors for children's self-regulation, drawing recent groundbreaking evidence of poverty's toll on development. We then discuss the potential of supporting low-income children's self-regulation through classroom-based intervention.

The Cost of Poverty to Children's Self-Regulation

Researchers within the area of "poverty, policy, and child development" have found evidence for a wide range of mechanisms through which poverty takes a toll, across levels of analysis ranging from the biomedical (e.g., poor children's greater risk of lower nutrition) to the institutional (e.g., their segregation in less resourced and lower-quality schools) (see Duncan, Magnuson, & Votruba-Drzal, 2015, for a review). For our purposes in this chapter, we focus on unpacking the neuropsychological and behavioral mechanisms that relate to children's self-regulation given unequivocal evidence that young children in low-income households are at higher risk of more emotional, cognitive, and behavioral dysregulation than their more affluent counterparts (Aber, Jones, & Raver, 2007; Blair, 2002, 2010).

First, does poverty play a role in shaping neurocognitive processes related to self-regulation? Recent advances in developmental neuroscience suggest that the answer is "yes": Children in poverty have been found to have lower grey-matter volume in frontal and parietal regions of the cortex, lower hippocampal volume, and slower growth of those areas of the brain in infancy than their more financially well-off counterparts (Hair, Hanson, Wolfe, & Pollak, 2015; Hanson et al., 2015; Hanson, Chandra, Wolfe, & Pollak, 2011). At the behavioral level, children from financially disadvantaged households have been consistentlty found to be at higher risk for lower levels of EF, greater difficulty modulating fear and anger, and less optimal patterns of attention deployment from late infancy through early childhood (Blair, 2010; Briggs-Gowan et al., 2015; Dilworth-Bart, Khurshid, & Vandell, 2007; Micch, Essex, & Goldsmith, 2001; Noble, Tottenham, & Casey, 2005; Raver, Blair, & Willoughby, 2013). Models of those mechanisms highlight the ways that poverty dramatically increases the likelihood that children experience a set of adverse environmental contexts and events (broadly termed *stressors*) that place healthy neuroendocrine, neurocognitive, and behavioral development in greater jeopardy (Blair et al., 2011; Brito & Noble, 2014; Bryck & Fisher, 2012; Hanson et al., 2015). For example, in one recent study, Hanson and colleagues (2015) found clear evidence of the ways that early life stressors, including low income and poverty, are associated with lower hippocampal and amygdala volume, with those structural differences associated, in turn, with greater emotional and behavioral dysregulation (as indicated by more behavior problems). The multiple neural and endocrine mechanisms of those links are more complex than can be covered in this chapter, and are discussed in greater detail elsewhere (see Blair, 2010; Hanson et al., 2015). Three environmentally mediating avenues through which poverty confers higher risk to young children's self-regulation include lack of contingent care by adults early in life, exposure to high levels of instability or turbulence, and chronic exposure to people and places that are threatening or unsafe.

Lack of Contingent Care

The quality of care that children receive from adults from early infancy onward is strongly implicated as a driving force in the ontogeny of EF, ER, and attention regulation (see Blair & Raver, 2012, for review). Adults' warm and contingent behavioral responses to infant distress and their reliable structuring of infants' increasing skills in modulating emotions and attention have consistently been found to predict higher EF and greater emotional control, even after taking into account biobehavioral differences in temperament (Bernier, Beauchamp, Carlson, & Lalonde, 2015; Calkins, 2011). Parents' provision of sensitive, contingent care has been found not only to entrain or scaffold children's competent behavioral strategies for modulating emotion and organizing attention but also to support optimal connectivity at neurobiological levels (see Gee et al., 2014; Tottenham, 2014). Conversely, studies of children who have experienced severe levels of neglectful caregiving indicate clear neurobiological and behavioral consequences, with those children demonstrating both structural and functional compromise in multiple brain regions, including the medial temporal lobe (areas responsible for ER) (DeBellis & Thomas, 2003; Fox, Almas, Degnan, Nelson, & Zeanah, 2011; Maheu et al., 2010). Additional studies of young children's neuroendocrine function have demonstrated that low- quality care from primary caregivers at home (Blair et al., 2008, 2011; Evans, Kim, Ting, Tesher, & Shannis, 2007; Sturge-Apple, Davies, Cicchetti, & Manning, 2012) and caregivers in child care (Dettling, Gunnar, & Donzella, 1999; Watamura, Donzella, Alwin, & Gunnar, 2003) are associated with patterns of HPA activity that are not conducive to executive function and socioemotional well-being. Notably, Blair and colleagues (2008, 2011) have demonstrated across several different analyses that poverty's predictive power in young children's emotional arousal and EF is largely explained by the mediating role of parental caregiving.

Turbulence

Our work in developing and testing theories of self-regulation in the context of poverty-related stressors has led us to look beyond the bounds of parent–child interaction to include larger forces in the lives of low-income families, including unpredictability and instability. Evidence from both animal and human models suggests that chaotic, unpredictable, or unstable conditions may compromise organisms' ability to appropriately regulate their physiological, cognitive, and behavioral responses to stress (Arnsten, 2000; Evans & Wachs, 2010; Lewis, Dozier, Ackerman, & Sepulveda-Kozakowsi, 2007; Sanchez, Ladd, & Plotsky, 2001).

In our own research, we find that children's experiences of high levels of household turbulence (e.g., when adults move in or out of the household or the family needs to relocate multiple times) are associated with lower levels of self-regulation, even after taking families' poverty due to low income into account (McCoy & Raver, 2014). Of course, a single move to a nicer home or a better neighborhood is likely to offer several self-regulatory benefits to children. However, when children must weather multiple household transitions and relocations (e.g., through eviction, moving into and out of a shelter, or "doubling up"), that household instability takes a toll on the stress physiology that underlies healthy development of EF in early childhood (see Blair et al., 2011). The role of high levels of mobility or instability extends beyond early childhood, with moves across multiple residences and switching schools frequently in early childhood predictive of longer-term difficulties with EF in later elementary school, even after accounting for the role of family income (Friedman-Krauss & Raver, 2015; Roy, McCoy, & Raver, 2014).

Threat

Research on attention and ER underscore the ways that humans' brains are evolutionarily hardwired to be especially good at detecting and responding to potentially threatening or dangerous features of our environments (LeDoux, 2003). This sensitivity to threatening or fear-inducing stimuli extends to signals from other conspecifics (including adults or other children), so that children can quickly detect and readily interpret others' expression of fear and anger. Exposure to extreme levels of threat such as physical abuse by a caregiver has been consistently found to significantly alter young children's attention and ER processes, increasing their "perceptual sensitivity" to threat, distorting their cognitive attributions, and altering their emotional response (Pollak & Kistler, 2002; Pollak & Sinha, 2002; Weiss, Dodge, Bates, & Pettit, 1992).

Importantly, our own work, as well as that of our colleagues, suggests that less acute exposure to other forms of environmental threat also have deleterious consequences for children's self-regulation. Specifically, separate traditions of neuroscientific research and research on development and psychopathology have recently converged to elucidate the pernicious role of violence in children's brain development. For example, our own work suggests that exposure to violent crimes in the neighborhood has deleterious consequences for children's attention regulation (McCoy, Roy, & Raver, 2016; Sharkey, Tirado-Strayer, Papachristos, & Raver, 2012). For those analyses, our colleagues Sharkey and colleagues (2012) were able to link our team's neurocognitively oriented assessments of children's attention regulation to Chicago's crime data during the same period or "window" as our data collection effort. This matching process (as well as the use of sophisticated "fixed effects" analyses) allowed the team to compare the performance of children who had been exposed to violent crimes that occurred just a few days prior to our research team's visit to the performance of children exposed to violent crimes just a few days after the assessment. Our analyses (as well as findings by numerous other investigators) demonstrated that children exposed to violent crimes such as homicide showed significant decrements in their attentional control (at age 4) and greater bias to threat (in elementary school). These findings highlight the ways that exposure to violent, traumatic events restructures children's attentional, emotional, and cognitive control networks to be on "high alert." That is, adults and children who have been exposed to traumatic threats have consistently been found to demonstrate biased attention to negative cues, more difficulty switching cognitive "gears" in the face of negatively valenced information, and more negative affect in a wide range of laboratory paradigms (Dennis, O'Toole, & DeCicco, 2013; Kim et al., 2008). Those behavioral effects of exposure to violent events are paralleled by clear evidence of changes in activation and connectivity of brain regions associated with emotion processing, attention, and EF, such as the anterior cingulate and dorsolateral prefrontal cortices (Moser et al., 2015; Stevens et al., 2013). Witnessing or experiencing aggression between adults in the household is associated with significant compromises in children's physiological stress response, their ability to remember and pay attention in the context of emotional stimuli, and their capacity to downregulate negative emotions and exert effortful control (Gustafsson et al., 2013; Hibel, Senguttuvan, & Bauer, 2013; Raver et al., 2013; Sturge-Apple, Skibo, Rogosch, Ignjatovic, & Heinzelman, 2011).

Importantly negative effects of threatening events and experiences extend to children's experiences of violence in school contexts. Recent analyses of the impact of bullying among older children suggests that chronic exposure to threat of violence from peers also negatively biases children's regulation of stress response physiology, attention, emotion, and cognition (Ouillet-Morin et al., 2011; Schippell, Vasey, Cravens-Brown, & Bretveld, 2003; Silk, Davis, McMakin, Dahl, & Forbes, 2012). The resulting biased attention to negative social cues and hypervigilant and reactive cognitive profiles of responding may help children to detect early warning signs of conflict in the short run but may be maladaptive in the long run (Troop-Gordon, Gordon, Vogel-Ciernia, Ewing Lee & Visconti, 2016).

What conclusions can we draw from this bleak evidence of the costs of poverty-related risks for young children's self-regulation? A key implication is that many young children in low-income, unsafe neighborhoods do not come to school with equal neuropsychological positioning as more affluent students who have experienced fewer adverse events, in terms of their ability to remain reflective, calm, and attentionally focused in the context of cognitive or interpersonal challenge. Whether through exposure to greater emotional or residential turmoil at home or school, many students in low-income communities are likely to be on the lookout for negative cues from their environments, and are more likely than their less stressed counterparts in wealthier school districts to react reflexively rather than reflectively to situations that involve feelings of frustration, anxiety, or threat.

We want to be clear: There are many, many children in low-income communities who are doing well in school—exposure to adverse events does not consign a given child to be destined for difficulties in regulating cognition, emotion, and attention. Instead, it raises a given child's probability of facing regulatory difficulty, making it more difficult to navigate the sometimes choppy waters of school demands and expectations. Just as it is important to recognize the toll that poverty takes on children's potential, it is equally important to examine and extend the ways that interventions can support low-income children's self-regulation, providing "more oars in the water" to help them meet their academic potential. We now turn to evidence for the impact of early intervention on young children's self-regulation.

THE ROLE OF EARLY INTERVENTION IN SUPPORTING SELF-REGULATION IN EARLY CHILDHOOD

Interventions Targeting EF

Our recent work suggests that children's EF can be powerfully shaped by implementing classroom interventions in early educational settings. For example, one comprehensive intervention approach, Tools of the Mind, has shown considerable promise across a range of efficacy trials. Building on the fundamental insights of Lev Vygotsky, Alexander Luria, and post-Vygotskian scholars, Tools of the Mind embeds techniques for supporting, or "scaffolding," the development of EF skills in all classroom activities throughout the day, from transitions to classroom routines, classroom management techniques, and the learning of academic content. Implemented in preschool settings, findings from an early efficacy trial suggested clear benefits for children's performance on complex EF tasks such as the flanker task (Diamond et al., 2007). As with many educational interventions in which efficacy and effectiveness are (appropriately) tested through rigorous experimental design, subsequent evidence for the benefits of Tools of the Mind has been mixed (Farran, Lipsey, & Wilson, 2011; Morris et al., 2014). Our recent examination of the efficacy of this comprehensive approach suggests the

importance of looking carefully at both academic skills and children's underlying EF, attentional, and physiological regulation when carrying out an educational evaluation. For example, when implemented with kindergartners in a large number of schools in Massachusetts, our recent randomized controlled trial (RCT) demonstrated that Tools of the Mind significantly improved treatment-assigned children's working memory and executive attention relative to the control group (Blair & Raver, 2014). Furthermore, our analyses suggest that gains were largest for low-income children attending high-poverty schools. This finding offers empirical support for our theoretically grounded hypotheses regarding the plasticity of children's EF in the context of poverty-related stressors. It also highlights the value of this type of intervention for reducing educational inequality at the "starting gate" of early elementary school (Lee & Burkham, 2002) Neurocognitive benefits paralleled impressive gains in children's academic performance, as indicated by their language, vocabulary, and fluid reasoning skills. Preliminary evidence suggests that young children's EF is also supported by educational experiences that require abstract reasoning and "code switching," such as bilingual instruction and math instruction.

Interventions Targeting ER

Changing young children's appraisals of their own and others' emotions as regulable is arguably a key foundation of early social information-processing models of intervention—children are trained through curricula and teachers' instruction to stop, think, and select appropriate responses to interpersonally or emotionally challenging situations—a hallmark approach of what are termed *socioemotional learning (SEL)* models (Oberle, Domitrovich, Meyers, & Weissberg, 2016). These well-designed and tested models for older children have been extended downward for younger children through a range of different curricular approaches (Riggs, Greenberg, Kusché, & Pentz, 2006). A recent adaptation of the Preschool PATHS (Promoting Alternative THinking Strategies) model entitled the Head Start REDI (REsearch-based, Developmentally

Informed) program (Bierman et al., 2008) targets children's self-regulation primarily through curricular lessons focusing on children's understanding and expression of emotions, strengthening their early cognitive representations of proactive strategies for emotional and behavioral self-control, and supporting their social problem-solving skills (Domitrovich, Cortes, & Greenberg, 2007). The REDI program has yielded evidence of modest positive impact on children's emotional regulation and EF, suggesting that children's cognitive attributions may be a nascent developmental domain that can be supported prior to formal school entry.

Alternatively, children's self-regulation has been targeted through the hypothesized mechanisms of emotional and cognitive regulatory support provided by teachers in early educational classrooms (Jones & Bouffard, 2012; Merz, Landry, Johnson, Williams, & Jung, 2016; Raver et al., 2008, 2009). Some interventions, such as the Chicago School Readiness Project, have specifically targeted self-regulation by training teachers to use more proactive and emotionally positive forms of instruction and classroom management, and helping children to use more effective ways to regulate their attention, behavior, and feelings of distress (Raver et al., 2011). By developing increased control over emotions, inhibitory control dimensions of EF, and attention, children receiving these programs were hypothesized to not only show improvements in computerized measures of EF and ER but also to be better equipped to take advantage of learning opportunities in the classroom. Our results (as well as the recent findings reported by our colleagues) suggests clear benefit of this approach for low-income children, with gains yielded across both self-regulation and early academic domains (Merz et al., 2016; Raver et al., 2012). Similar approaches taken by other behaviorally oriented models, such as the Incredible Years Teacher Classroom Management (IY-TCM) program, show significant improvement in teacher behavior, as well as reductions in student conduct problems (e.g., Webster-Stratton, Reid, & Hammond, 2001, 2004; Williford & Shelton, 2008). Importantly, RCT evidence from the IY-TCM program suggests that these services may increase student motivation at school by decreasing levels of disengagement (Webster-Stratton, Reid, & Stoolmiller, 2008) and increasing on-task behavior in intervention classrooms (Hutchings, Martin-Forbes, Daley, & Williams, 2013).

Using a broader, school-based perspective, some school reform initiatives target school climate and students' self-regulation as an empowering means to improve student well-being and academic achievement (Borman, Hewes, Overman, & Brown, 2003; Brackett, Alstr, Wolfe, Katulak, & Fale, 2007; Durlak, Weissberg, Dymnicki, Taylor, & Schellinger, 2011; Wang & Degol, 2015). Interventions that extend beyond the classroom to include playgrounds, cafeterias, hallways, and stairwells have not only transformed classrooms and school buildings in terms of emotional warmth and connectedness, but also have reduced children's risk of exposure to threatening situations, thus promote a setting more conducive to improving children's self-regulation (Bierman et al., 2014; Liew, 2012; Reynolds, Temple, Ou, Arteaga, & White, 2011; Rivers, Brackett, Reyes, Elbertson, & Salovey, 2013). School-Wide Positive Behavioral Interventions and Supports (SWPBIS), for example, a school climate intervention implemented in over 16,000 public elementary schools across the United States, demonstrates the promise of scaling of school climate reform programs to improve student regulatory behaviors (Bradshaw, Waasdorp, & Leaf, 2015). A 4-year randomized controlled effectiveness trial of SWPBIS in 37 elementary schools, representing diverse socioeconomic levels, found that children in SWPBIS schools had lower levels of aggressive and disruptive behaviors, fewer concentration problems, increased prosocial behavior, and better emotion regulation than children in control schools. Our research, as well as research by others, has found that school climate also moderates the impact of a socioemotional learning interventions aimed at supporting children's self-regulation in low-income urban elementary schools (McCormick, Cappella, O'Connor, & McClowry, 2015; Zhai, Raver, & Jones, 2012).

Given that lower income children face a higher propensity for exposure to traumatic events, a number of investigators have extended school-based models to include trauma-informed approaches to supporting children's emotion regulation. For example, the Attachment, Self-Regulation, and Competency (ARC) framework is a widely implemented program that provides support within the caregiving system to help trauma-exposed children build skills in self-regulation and school readiness through development of more emotionally positive, trustworthy, and predictable relationships with caregivers, as well as through structured play. Children who completed clinic-based ARC treatment showed a greater reduction in behavior dysregulation on the Child Behavior Checklist (CBCL) than children who discontinued services. Importantly, the ARC framework engages caregivers such as teachers and school staff in educational settings to strengthen the emotional security that students experience when interacting with adults, and is designed to be flexibly implemented across contexts such as schools (Hodgdon, Kinniburgh, Gabowitz, Blaustein, & Spinazzola, 2013). For older children in low-income neighborhoods, trauma-informed interventions designed for school settings show promise of improving student self-regulation and school engagement. A recent pilot study evaluating the RAP Club, a 12-session, school-based cognitive-behavioral and mindfulness intervention for middle school youth in low-income communities, found positive intervention effects on teacher-rated ER, social and academic competence, classroom behavior, and discipline (Mendelson, Tandon, O'Brennan, Leaf, & Ialongo, 2015; for promising cognitive-behavioral approaches in school settings, see Stein et al., 2003). One potential implication of the research reviewed earlier on the links between ER and higher-order cognitive processes is that trauma-informed, emotion-focused interventions may also affect students' cognitive schemas, or attributions regarding emotions, their modifiability, and controllability—sources that could potentially inform students' attention to emotion cues, as well as their appraisals of their own and others' emotions and intentions.

Interventions Targeting Attention

As outlined earlier, the main function of the executive attention network is to resolve conflict and regulate other brain networks, supporting behavioral self-regulation and effortful control. How modifiable is this network to environmental "input"? Evidence from intervention effort that narrowly targets the training of young children's attention is promising: After several weeks of computerized attention training exercises, 4- to 6-year-old participants showed improved performance on an IQ test and more adult-like brain activity in the anterior cingulate cortex, an area associated with executive attention (Rueda, Rothbart, McCandliss, Saccomanno, & Posner, 2005). A follow-up study found that 5-year-old children were able to activate the executive attention network faster and more efficiently following attention training, and these effects were observed up to 2 months later. Children in the training group showed improvements in measures of fluid cognition and regulation of affect, indicating that attention training generalizes to other domains thought to rely on attentional control skills (Rueda, Checa, & Combita, 2012).

Attention training may be an especially important tool to improve school readiness for children from disadvantaged backgrounds. Children from low-socioeconomic-status (SES) backgrounds demonstrate poorer proficiency in measures of attention neural network efficiency (Mezzacappa, 2004). Moreover, children's ability to sustain attention partially accounts for the relation between family environment and achievement and language outcomes (NICHD Early Child Care Network, 2003). A family-based attention training program targeting low-SES preschoolers found that brain function supporting selective attention, measures of cognition, and child and parent behavior improved more in the treatment group than in the control group (Neville et al., 2013).

Important to our discussion of attention in the context of adversity and threat, several attentional interventions have been designed to target maladaptive attention biases that may result from stress in the home environment. In an experimental manipulation, Eldar, Ricon, and Bar-Haim (2008) demonstrated plasticity in attentional biases by inducing vigilance to threat. Based on this model, a recent RCT indicated that attention training for anxious children to induce bias away from threat effectively facilitated attention disengagement from threatening stimuli and reduced anxiety during a stressor task compared to controls (Bar-Haim, Morag, & Glickman, 2011).

In summary, across these different types of intervention, we have clear evidence of the plasticity of children's attention deployment, emotion regulation, and EFs. While poverty-related risks clearly place children's self-regulation in jeopardy, the evidence from these interventions suggests that gaps in students' early academic performance can be at least partially closed with significant investment across family, classroom, and school contexts.

IMPLICATIONS AND CONCLUSIONS

Unanswered Questions in Early Childhood Self-Regulation and Academic Performance

First, this review has highlighted many productive empirical next steps that can be taken in testing the combined roles of emotion, attention, and higher-order cognitive regulation in young children's academic performance. Models of self-regulation in early childhood may be particularly important in understanding how children deal with difficult material, making errors, or failing a task or test—this area of study on young children's motivation in the face of academic challenge is ripe for empirical exploration and analysis.

For example, we have robust theory but few tests of the ways that "bottom-up" processes of emotional distress (including feelings of fear, anxiety, and frustration) may disrupt attentional control and higher-order cognitive processing. We have well-validated tasks that place children in conditions of social evaluative threat, such as the Trier Social Stress Test, in which children face high performance demands (e.g., when they must make a speech to a set of judges) (Kirschbaum, Pirke, & Hellhammer, 1993). In those tasks, children clearly show increased activation of markers of physiological stress, but the extent to which those neuroendocrine processes may be accompanied by increased difficulty in allocation of cognitive resources to support

higher academic performance is less well established. Similarly, through interventions supporting simple behavioral strategies that children can activate to lower distress (e.g., the "turtle technique") we have only just begun to map the "top-down" pathways that young children can consciously and nonconsciously use to exert cognitive control in conditions of emotional distress (e.g., Preschool PATHS). Similarly, our review of extant research on preschoolers' attention deployment strategies during delay of gratification tasks suggests that young children develop nascent competence in coping through parental socialization, as well as structured educational support. However, our review of SEL interventions with preschoolers suggests that social information-processing and metacognitive coping models may be of limited benefit for young children; alternatively, indirectly routed interventions that build top-down regulatory competence through strengthened EFs show greater promise. We look forward to emerging findings on other approaches, including mindfulness training, as ways to support young children's modulation of feelings of anxiety and fear in academic contexts.

Second, we mentioned how fields of developmental science and neuroscience are on the cusp of major breakthroughs in understanding both early biologically based and environmentally shaped individual differences in young children's ability to regulate emotions, attention, and higher-order cognitive processing. We highlighted these individual differences as important factors to consider for models of motivation and persistence in later childhood and adolescence. We are just beginning to understand the neurobiological substrata through which toxic stressors such as turbulence and family violence "get under the skin" to orient children toward more negative attributions about the world, about their relationships with peers and teachers, and about themselves in deterministic rather than probabilistic fashion. We hypothesize that poverty-related risk may place young children on shaky self-regulatory ground in terms of deploying "cool" cognitive strategies in the face of "hot," emotionally negative situations such the risk of academic failure. This represents an exciting new area for further research.

EF, ER, and Attention Deployment as Potential Moderators and Mediators of Mindset Intervention

In addition, we can use this body of theory and research on young children's self-regulation as a springboard to develop and extend models of cognitive appraisal in the face of learning contexts that are potentially threatening. We draw here from highly promising work on mindset interventions discussed in other chapters of this volume (see also Paunesku et al., 2015; Yeager & Walton, 2011; Yeager et al., 2014). Specifically, in a landmark review, Schmader, Johns, and Forbes (2008) suggest that it is these processes of self-regulation that underlie older students' vulnerability to "high-stakes" situations such as social-evaluative threat, test-taking anxiety, and stereotype threat. Students' encounters with situational cues that highlight expectations of failure not only capture their attention but also trigger emotional dysregulation through threats to students' sense of self. Successful performance in the face of that threat involves greater EF, including resolution of cognitive conflict and higher-order coordination of information processing (Schmader et al., 2008). In addition, a small series of mindset induction studies demonstrates that one mechanism underlying improvement in vulnerable students' performance is through experimental strengthening of students' modulation of negative affect and support for EFs such as error detection and set shifting among competing demands (Schroder, Dawood, Yalch, Donnellan, & Moser, 2014).

These innovative studies lead us to ask about the role of stronger versus weaker self-regulatory skills (including better attention deployment, more competent ER, and stronger EFs) as predictors of (1) children's vulnerability to situational triggers that are characterized by threats to the self and subsequent compromises in academic performance, and (2) the ease or difficulty with which children's mindsets can be shifted. That is, do individuals with nascent flexibility in ways of seeing their own performance develop those implicit biases because they are more able to detect error, respond flexibly, and encode that awareness into more flexible attributional style? Individual differences in EFs may predispose some students to be more likely shift their attention from errors in their performance (and the threat that those errors pose to their self-evaluation) to taking "the next right step" in completing the task and meeting larger goals, such as focusing on answering subsequent test questions without perseverating too greatly on past performance (Mangels, Good, Whiteman, Maniscalco, & Dweck, 2012). Other students with less skill in flexibly deploying their attention and greater propensity toward lower levels of cognitive control may struggle to internalize and use the coping strategies offered by mindset intervention. We look forward to tests of the role of students' EFs from early to middle childhood as an important moderator of interventions that arm students with more positive coping strategies in the future. In addition, changes in children's capacity to use more reflective versus reactive responses in the face of academic and interpersonal challenge may be a key mechanism through which mindset interventions work.

We close with a reminder of the power of self-regulation for students' success: The role of socioemotional, motivational, and behavioral factors in students' academic standing is large relative to their cognitive ability or aptitude. Socioemotionally and motivationally oriented behaviors in later childhood (including being able to complete homework, attend class, and to remain focused and persistent in the context of more challenging work) have been highlighted as predicting 61% of the variance in students' risk of failing a class in ninth grade—far greater than the 12% of variance predicted by prior test scores and background characteristics such as race/ethnicity and gender (Allensworth & Easton, 2007). It is centrally important that we find innovative ways to support the foundations of those motivational and behavioral factors in early childhood, particularly for children who may be both economically and academically vulnerable.

REFERENCES

Aber, J. L., Jones, S. M., & Raver, C. C. (2007). *Poverty and child development: New perspectives on a defining issue.* In L. J. Aber, S. J.

Bishop-Josef, S. M. Jones, K. T. McLearn, & D. A. Phillips (Eds.), *Child development and social policy: Knowledge for action* (pp. 149–166). Washington, DC: American Psychological Association.

Allensworth, E. M., & Easton, J. Q. (2007). *What matters for staying on track and graduating in Chicago Public High Schools*. Chicago: Consortium on Chicago School Research.

Arnsten, A. F. (2000). Through the looking glass: Differential noradenergic modulation of prefrontal cortical function. *Neural Plasticity, 7*(1–2), 133–146.

Arnsten, A. F. (2009). Stress signalling pathways that impair prefrontal cortex structure and function. *Nature Reviews Neuroscience, 10*(6), 410–422.

Bar-Haim, Y., Lamy, D., Pergamin, L., Bakermans-Kranenburg, M. J., & van IJzendoorn, M. H. (2007). Threat-related attentional bias in anxious and nonanxious individuals: A meta-analytic study. *Psychological Bulletin, 133*(1), 1–24.

Bar-Haim, Y., Morag, I., & Glickman, S. (2011). Training anxious children to disengage attention from threat: A randomized controlled trial. *Journal of Child Psychology and Psychiatry, 52*(8), 861–869.

Bernier, A., Beauchamp, M. H., Carlson, S. M., & Lalonde, G. (2015). A secure base from which to regulate: Attachment security in toddlerhood as a predictor of executive functioning at school entry. *Developmental Psychology, 51*(9), 1177–1189.

Bierman, K. L., Domitrovich, C. E., Nix, R. L., Gest, S. D., Welsh, J. A., Greenberg, M. T., et al. (2008). Promoting academic and social–emotional school readiness: The Head Start REDI program. *Child Development, 79*(6), 1802–1817.

Bierman, K. L., Nix, R. L., Heinrichs, B. S., Domitrovich, C. E., Gest, S. D., Welsh, J. A., et al. (2014). Effects of Head Start REDI on children's outcomes 1 year later in different kindergarten contexts. *Child Development, 85*(1), 140–159.

Blair, C. (2002). School readiness: Integrating cognition and emotion in a neurobiological conceptualization of children's functioning at school entry. *American Psychologist, 57*, 111–127.

Blair, C. (2010). Stress and the development of self-regulation in context. *Child Development Perspectives, 4*, 181–188.

Blair, C., & Dennis, T. (2010). An optimal balance: The integration of emotion and cognition in context. In S. D. Calkins & M. A. Bell (Eds.), *Child development at the intersection of emotion and cognition* (pp. 17–35).

Washington, DC: American Psychological Association.

Blair, C., & Diamond, A. (2008). Biological processes in prevention and intervention: The promotion of self-regulation as a means of preventing school failure. *Development and Psychopathology, 20*, 899–911.

Blair, C., Granger, D. A., Kivlighan, K. T., Mills-Koonce, R., Willoughby, M., Greenberg, M. T., et al. (2008). Maternal and child contributions to cortisol response to emotional arousal in young children from low-income, rural communities. *Developmental Psychology, 44*, 1095–1109.

Blair, C., & Raver, C. C. (2012). Child development in the context of adversity: experiential canalization of brain and behavior. *American Psychologist, 67*, 309–318.

Blair, C., & Raver, C. C. (2014). Closing the achievement gap through modification of neurocognitive and neuroendocrine function: Results from a cluster randomized controlled trial of an innovative approach to the education of children in kindergarten. *PLoS ONE, 1*(11), e112393.

Blair, C., Raver, C. C., Granger, D., Mills-Koonce, R., & Hibel, L. (2011). Allostasis and allostatic load in the context of poverty in early childhood. *Development and Psychopathology, 23*(3), 845–857.

Blair, C., & Razza, R. P. (2007). Relating effortful control, executive function, and false belief understanding to emerging math and literacy ability in kindergarten. *Child Development, 78*(2), 647–663.

Blair, C., & Ursache, A. (2011). A bidirectional model of executive functions and self-regulation. In K. D. Vohs & R. F. Baumeister (Eds.), *Handbook of self-regulation: Research, theory, and applications* (2nd ed., pp. 300–320). New York: Guilford Press.

Borman, G. D., Hewes, G. M., Overman, L. T., & Brown, S. (2003). Comprehensive school reform and achievement: A meta-analysis. *Review of Educational Research, 73*(2), 125–230.

Brackett, M. A., Alster, B., Wolfe, C. J., Katulak, N., & Fale, E. (2007). Creating an emotionally intelligent school district: A skill-based approach. In R. Bar-On, J. G. Maree, & M. J. Elias (Eds.), *Educating people to be emotionally intelligent* (pp. 123–137). Westport, CT: Praeger.

Bradshaw, C. P., Waasdorp, T. E., & Leaf, P. J. (2015). Examining variation in the impact of school-wide positive behavioral interventions and supports: Findings from a randomized controlled effectiveness trial. *Journal of Educational Psychology, 107*(2), 546–557.

Briggs-Gowan, M. J., Pollak, S. D., Grasso, D., Voss, J., Mian, N. D., Zobel, E., et al. (2015). Attention bias and anxiety in young children exposed to family violence. *Journal of Child Psychology and Psychiatry, 56*(11), 1194–1201.

Brito, N. H., & Noble, K. G. (2014). Socioeconomic status and structural brain development. *Frontiers in Neuroscience, 8,* 276.

Broadbent, D. E. (1959). *Perception and communication.* Elmsford, NY: Pergamon Press.

Bryck, R. L., & Fisher, P. A. (2012). Training the brain: Practical applications of neural plasticity from the intersection of cognitive neuroscience, developmental psychology, and prevention science. *American Psychologist, 67*(2), 87–100.

Bull, R., & Scerif, G. (2001). Executive functioning as a predictor of children's mathematics ability: Inhibition, switching, and working memory. *Developmental Neuropsychology, 19*(3), 273–293.

Calkins, S. D. (2011). Caregiving as coregulation: Psychobiological processes and child functioning. In A. Booth, S. M. McHale, & N. Landale (Eds.), *Biosocial foundations of family processes* (pp. 49–59). New York: Springer.

Calkins, S. D., & Marcovitch, S. (2010). Emotion regulation and executive functioning in early development: Integrated mechanisms of control supporting adaptive functioning. In S. D. Calkins & M. A. Bell (Eds.), *Child development at the intersection of emotion and cognition* (pp. 37–57). Washington, DC: American Psychological Association.

Carlson, S. M. (2005). Developmentally sensitive measures of executive function in preschool children. *Developmental Neuropsychology, 28*(2), 595–616.

Casey, B. J., Giedd, J. N., & Thomas, K. M. (2000). Structural and functional brain development and its relation to cognitive development. *Biological Psychology, 54*(1), 241–257.

Colby, C. L., & Goldberg, M. E. (1999). Space and attention in parietal cortex. *Annual Review of Neuroscience, 22*(1), 319–349.

Cole, P. M. (1986). Children's spontaneous control of facial expression. *Child Development, 57,* 1309–1321.

Cole, P. M., Martin, S. E., & Dennis, T. A. (2004). Emotion regulation as a scientific construct: Methodological challenges and directions for child development research. *Child Development, 75,* 317–333.

Cole, P. M., Tan, P. Z., Hall, S. E., Zhang, Y., Crnic, K. A., Blair, C. B., et al. (2011). Developmental changes in anger expression and attention focus: Learning to wait. *Developmental Psychology, 47*(4), 1078–1089.

Cunningham, W. A., Zelazo, P. D., Packer, D. J., & Van Bavel, J. J. (2007). The iterative reprocessing model: A multilevel framework for attitudes and evaluation. *Social Cognition, 25*(5), 736–760.

Davidson, M. C., Amso, D., Anderson, L. C., & Diamond, A. (2006). Development of cognitive control and executive functions from 4 to 13 years: Evidence from manipulations of memory, inhibition, and task switching. *Neuropsychologia, 44*(11), 2037–2078.

De Bellis, M. D., & Thomas, L. A. (2003). Biologic findings of post-traumatic stress disorder and child maltreatment. *Current Psychiatry Reports, 5*(2), 108–117.

Dennis, T. A., & Chen, C.-C. (2007). Neurophysiological mechanisms in the emotional modulation of attention: The interplay between threat sensitivity and attentional control. *Biological Psychology, 76*(1), 1–10.

Dennis, T. A., Malone, M. M., & Chen, C.-C. (2009). Emotional face processing and emotion regulation in children: An ERP study. *Developmental Neuropsychology, 34*(1), 85–102.

Dennis, T. A., O'Toole, L. J., & DeCicco, J. M. (2013). Emotion regulation from the perspective of developmental neuroscience: What, where, when and why. In K. C. Barrett, N. A. Fox, D. J. Fidler, & L. A. Daunhaure (Eds.), *Handbook of self-regulatory processes in development: New directions and international perspectives* (pp. 135–172). New York: Psychology Press.

Derryberry, D., & Rothbart, M. K. (1997). Reactive and effortful processes in the organization of temperament. *Development and Psychopathology, 9*(4), 633–652.

Dettling, A. C., Gunnar, M. R., & Donzella, B. (1999). Cortisol levels of young children in full-day childcare centers: Relations with age and temperament. *Psychoneuroendocrinology, 24*(5), 519–536.

Diamond, A. (2013). Executive functions. *Annual Review of Psychology, 64,* 135–168.

Diamond, D. M., Campbell, A. M., Park, C. R., Halonen, J., & Zoladz, P. R. (2007). The temporal dynamics model of emotional memory processing: A synthesis on the neurobiological basis of stress-induced amnesia, flashbulb and traumatic memories, and the Yerkes–Dodson law. *Neural Plasticity, 2007,* 60803.

Dilworth-Bart, J. E., Khurshid, A., & Vandell, D. L. (2007). Do maternal stress and home environment mediate the relation between early income-to-need and 54-months attentional abilities? *Infant and Child Development, 16*(5), 525–552.

Domitrovich, C. E., Cortes, R. C., & Greenberg,

M. T. (2007). Improving young children's social and emotional competence: A randomized trial of the preschool "PATHS" curriculum. *Journal of Primary Prevention, 28*(2), 67–91.

Duncan, G. J., Magnuson, K., & Votruba-Drzal, E. (2015). Children and socioeconomic status. In R. M. Lerner (Ed.-in-Chief) & M. H. Bornstein & T. Leventhal (Vol. Eds.), *Handbook of child psychology and developmental science* (Vol. 4, pp. 534–573). Hoboken, NJ: Wiley.

Durlak, J. A., Weissberg, R. P., Dymnicki, A. B., Taylor, R. D., & Schellinger, K. B. (2011). The impact of enhancing students' social and emotional learning: A meta-analysis of school-based universal interventions. *Child Development, 82*(1), 405–432.

Dweck, C. S. (1999). *Self-theories: Their role in motivation, personality, and development.* Philadelphia: Psychology Press.

Dweck, C. S. (2012). Mindsets and human nature: Promoting change in the Middle East, the schoolyard, the racial divide, and willpower. *American Psychologist, 67*(8), 614–622.

Eldar, S., Ricon, T., & Bar-Haim, Y. (2008). Plasticity in attention: Implications for stress response in children. *Behaviour Research and Therapy, 46*(4), 450–461.

Espy, K. A., McDiarmid, M. M., Cwik, M. F., Stalets, M. M., Hamby, A., & Senn, T. E. (2004). The contribution of executive functions to emergent mathematic skills in preschool children. *Developmental Neuropsychology, 26*(1), 465–486.

Evans, G. W., Kim, P., Ting, A. H., Tesher, H. B., & Shannis, D. (2007). Cumulative risk, maternal responsiveness, and allostatic load among young adolescents. *Developmental Psychology, 43*(2), 341–351.

Evans, G. W., & Schamberg, M. A. (2009). Childhood poverty, chronic stress, and adult working memory. *Proceedings of the National Academy of Sciences, 106*(16), 6545–6549.

Evans, G. W., & Wachs, T. D. (2010). *Chaos and its influence on children's development.* Washington, DC: American Psychological Association.

Evans, J. S. B. (2008). Dual-processing accounts of reasoning, judgment, and social cognition. *Annual Review of Psychology, 59,* 255–278.

Farran, D. C., Lipsey, M. W., & Wilson, S. (2011). *Experimental evaluation of the Tools of the Mind pre-K curriculum* (Technical report, Peabody Research Institute). Nashville, TN: Vanderbilt University.

Fox, N. A., Almas, A. N., Degnan, K. A., Nelson, C. A., & Zeanah, C. H. (2011). The effects of severe psychosocial deprivation and foster care intervention on cognitive development at 8 years of age: Findings from the Bucharest Early Intervention Project. *Journal of Child Psychology and Psychiatry, 52*(9), 919–928.

Franceschini, S., Gori, S., Ruffino, M., Pedrolli, K., & Facoetti, A. (2012). A causal link between visual spatial attention and reading acquisition. *Current Biology, 22*(9), 814–819.

Friedman-Krauss, A. H., & Raver, C. C. (2015). Does school mobility place elementary school children at risk for lower math achievement?: The mediating role of cognitive dysregulation. *Developmental Psychology, 51*(12), 1725.

Fuster, J. M. (1997). *The prefrontal cortex: Anatomy, physiology and neuropsychology of the frontal lobe* (2nd ed.). New York: Raven.

Gee, D. G., Gabard-Durnam, L., Telzer, E. H., Humphreys, K. L., Goff, B., Shapiro, M., et al. (2014). Maternal buffering of human amygdala–prefrontal circuitry during childhood but not during adolescence. *Psychological Science, 25*(11), 2067–2078.

Gogtay, N., Giedd, J. N., Lusk, L., Hayashi, K. M., Greenstein, D., Vaituzis, A. C., et al. (2004). Dynamic mapping of human cortical development during childhood through early adulthood. *Proceedings of the National Academy of Sciences USA, 101*(21), 8174–8179.

Graziano, P. A., Reavis, R. D., Keane, S. P., & Calkins, S. D. (2007). The role of emotion regulation in children's early academic success. *Journal of School Psychology, 45*(1), 3–19.

Gross, J. J. (2002). Emotion regulation: Affective, cognitive, and social consequences. *Psychophysiology, 39*(3), 281–291.

Gross, J. J., & Thompson, R. A. (2007). Emotion regulation: Conceptual foundations. In J. J. Gross (Ed.), *Handbook of emotion regulation* (pp. 3–24). New York: Guilford Press.

Gunnar, M. R., & Quevedo, K. M. (2007). Early care experiences and HPA axis regulation in children: A mechanism for later trauma vulnerability. *Progress in Brain Research, 167,* 137–149.

Gustafsson, H. C., Coffman, J. L., Harris, L. S., Langley, H. A., Ornstein, P. A., & Cox, M. J. (2013). Intimate partner violence and children's memory. *Journal of Family Psychology, 27*(6), 937–944.

Hair, N. L., Hanson, J. L., Wolfe, B. L., & Pollak, S. D. (2015). Association of child poverty, brain development, and academic achievement. *JAMA Pediatrics, 169*(9), 822–829.

Hanson, J. L., Chandra, A., Wolfe, B. L., & Pollak, S. D. (2011). Association between income and the hippocampus. *PLoS ONE, 6*(5), e18712.

Hanson, J. L., Nacewicz, B. M., Sutterer, M. J., Cayo, A. A., Schaefer, S. M., Rudolph, K. D., et al. (2015). Behavioral problems after early life stress: Contributions of the hippocampus and amygdala. *Biological Psychiatry, 77*(4), 314–323.

Hare, T. A., Tottenham, N., Davidson, M. C., Glover, G. H., & Casey, B. J. (2005). Contributions of amygdala and striatal activity in emotion regulation. *Biological Psychiatry, 57*(6), 624–632.

Harman, C., Rothbart, M. K., & Posner, M. I. (1997). Distress and attention interactions in early infancy. *Motivation and Emotion, 21*(1), 27–44.

Harris, A., Hare, T., & Rangel, A. (2013). Temporally dissociable mechanisms of self-control: Early attentional filtering versus late value modulation. *Journal of Neuroscience, 33*(48), 18917–18931.

Hart, S. J., Green, S. R., Casp, M., & Belger, A. (2010). Emotional priming effects during Stroop task performance. *NeuroImage, 49*(3), 2662–2670.

Hibel, L. C., Senguttuvan, U., & Bauer, N. S. (2013). Do state factors moderate the relationship between depressive symptoms and morning cortisol? *Hormones and Behavior, 63*(3), 484–490.

Hodgdon, H. B., Kinniburgh, K., Gabowitz, D., Blaustein, M. E., & Spinazzola, J. (2013). Development and implementation of trauma-informed programming in youth residential treatment centers using the ARC framework. *Journal of Family Violence, 28*(7), 679–692.

Howse, R. B., Calkins, S. D., Anastopoulos, A. D., Keane, S. P., & Shelton, T. L. (2003). Regulatory contributors to children's kindergarten achievement. *Early Education and Development, 14*(1), 101–120.

Hutchings, J., Martin-Forbes, P., Daley, D., & Williams, M. E. (2013). A randomized controlled trial of the impact of a teacher classroom management program on the classroom behavior of children with and without behavior problems. *Journal of School Psychology, 51*(5), 571–585.

James, W. (1890). *The principles of psychology.* New York: Holt.

Jamieson, J. P., Mendes, W. B., Blackstock, E., & Schmader, T. (2010). Turning the knots in your stomach into bows: Reappraising arousal improves performance on the GRE. *Journal of Experimental Social Psychology, 46*(1), 208–212.

Jiang, Y., Ekono, M., & Skinner, C. (2016). *Basic facts about low-income children, 2015.* New York: National Center for Children in Poverty.

Jones, S. M., & Bouffard, S. M. (2012). Social and emotional learning in schools: From programs to strategies. *Social Policy Report, 26*(4), 1–32.

Kim, M. J., Chey, J., Chung, A., Bae, S., Khang, H., Ham, B., et al. (2008). Diminished rostral anterior cingulate activity in response to threat-related events in posttraumatic stress disorder. *Journal of Psychiatric Research, 42*(4), 268–277.

Kirschbaum, C., Pirke, K. M., & Hellhammer, D. H. (1993). The "Trier Social Stress Test"—a tool for investigating psychobiological stress responses in a laboratory setting. *Neuropsychobiology, 28*(1–2), 76–81.

Lamm, C., Decety, J., & Singer, T. (2011). Meta-analytic evidence for common and distinct neural networks associated with directly experienced pain and empathy for pain. *NeuroImage, 54*(3), 2492–2502.

LeDoux, J. (2003). The emotional brain, fear, and the amygdala. *Cellular and Molecular Neurobiology, 23*(4–5), 727–738.

Lee, V. E., & Burkam, D. T. (2002). *Inequality at the starting gate: Social background differences in achievement as children begin school.* Washington, DC: Economic Policy Institute.

Lewis, E. E., Dozier, M., Ackerman, J., & Sepulveda-Kozakowski, S. (2007). The effect of placement instability on adopted children's inhibitory control abilities and oppositional behavior. *Developmental Psychology, 43*(6), 1415–1427.

Lewis, M. D. (2005). Bridging emotion theory and neurobiology through dynamic systems modeling. *Behavioral and Brain Sciences, 28*(2), 169–194.

Lewis, M. D., & Todd, R. M. (2007). The self-regulating brain: Cortical–subcortical feedback and the development of intelligent action. *Cognitive Development, 22*(4), 406–430.

Lewis, M. D., Todd, R. M., & Honsberger, M. J. (2007). Event-related potential measures of emotion regulation in early childhood. *NeuroReport, 18*(1), 61–65.

Liew, J. (2012). Effortful control, executive functions, and education: Bringing self-regulatory and social-emotional competencies to the table: Self-regulation and education. *Child Development Perspectives, 6*(2), 105–111.

Maheu, F. S., Dozier, M., Guyer, A. E., Mandell, D., Peloso, E., Poeth, K., et al. (2010). A preliminary study of medial temporal lobe function in youths with a history of caregiver deprivation and emotional neglect. *Cognitive, Affective, and Behavioral Neuroscience, 10*(1), 34–49.

Mangels, J. A., Good, C., Whiteman, R. C., Maniscalco, B., & Dweck, C. S. (2012). Emotion blocks the path to learning under stereotype threat. *Social Cognitive and Affective Neuroscience, 7*(2), 230–241.

Martínez, A., DiRusso, F., Anllo-Vento, L., Sereno, M. I., Buxton, R. B., & Hillyard, S.

A. (2001). Putting spatial attention on the map: Timing and localization of stimulus selection processes in striate and extrastriate visual areas. *Vision Research, 41*(10–11), 1437–1457.

Mather, M., & Sutherland, M. R. (2011). Arousal-biased competition in perception and memory. *Perspectives on Psychological Science, 6*(2), 114–133.

McClelland, M. M., Cameron, C. E., Connor, C. M., Farris, C. L., Jewkes, A. M., & Morrison, F. J. (2007). Links between behavioral regulation and preschoolers' literacy, vocabulary, and math skills. *Developmental Psychology, 43*(4), 947–959.

McCormick, M. P., Cappella, E., O'Connor, E. E., & McClowry, S. G. (2015). Context matters for social–emotional learning: Examining variation in program impact by dimensions of school climate. *American Journal of Community Psychology, 56*(1–2), 101–119.

McCoy, D. C., & Raver, C. C. (2014). Household instability and self-regulation among poor children. *Journal of Children and Poverty, 20*(2), 131–152.

McCoy, D. C., Roy, A. L., & Raver, C. C. (2016). Neighborhood crime as a predictor of individual differences in emotional processing and regulation. *Developmental Science, 19*(1), 164–174.

McRae, K., Ciesielski, B., & Gross, J. J. (2012). Unpacking cognitive reappraisal: goals, tactics, and outcomes. *Emotion, 12*(2), 250–255.

Mendelson, T., Tandon, S. D., O'Brennan, L., Leaf, P. J., & Ialongo, N. S. (2015). Brief report: Moving prevention into schools: The impact of a trauma-informed school-based intervention. *Journal of Adolescence, 43*, 142–147.

Merz, E. C., Landry, S. H., Johnson, U. Y., Williams, J. M., & Jung, K. (2016). Effects of a responsiveness-focused intervention in family child care homes on children's executive function. *Early Childhood Research Quarterly, 34*, 128–139.

Mezzacappa, E. (2004). Alerting, orienting, and executive attention: Developmental properties and sociodemographic correlates in an epidemiological sample of young, urban children. *Child Development, 75*(5), 1373–1386.

Miech, R., Essex, M. J., & Goldsmith, H. H. (2001). Socioeconomic status and the adjustment to school: The role of self-regulation during early childhood. *Sociology of Education, 74*(2), 102–120.

Mischel, W., & Ayduk, O. (2011). Willpower in a cognitive affect processing system: The dynamics of delay of gratification. In K. D. Vohs & R. F. Baumeister (Eds.), *Handbook of self-regulation: Research, theory, and applications* (2nd ed., pp. 83–105). New York: Guilford Press.

Mischel, W., Cantor, N., & Feldman, S. (1996). Principles of self-regulation: The nature of willpower and self-control. In E. T. Higgins & A. W. Kruglanski (Eds.), *Social psychology: Handbook of basic principles* (pp. 329–360). New York: Guilford Press.

Mischel, W., Shoda, Y., & Rodriguez, M. I. (1989). Delay of gratification in children. *Science, 244*, 933.

Miyake, A., Friedman, N. P., Emerson, M. J., Witzki, A. H., Howerter, A., & Wager, T. D. (2000). The unity and diversity of executive functions and their contributions to complex "frontal lobe" tasks: A latent variable analysis. *Cognitive Psychology, 41*(1), 49–100.

Morris, P., Mattera, S. K., Castells, N., Bangser, M., Bierman, K., & Raver, C. (2014). *Impact findings from the Head Start CARES Demonstration: National evaluation of three approaches to improving preschoolers' social and emotional competence* (Executive Summary, OPRE Report 2014–44). New York: MDRC.

Moser, D. A., Aue, T., Suardi, F., Kutlikova, H., Cordero, M. I., Rossignol, A. S., et al. (2015). Violence-related PTSD and neural activation when seeing emotionally charged male–female interactions. *Social Cognitive and Affective Neuroscience, 10*(5), 643–653.

Nelson, C. A., Fox, N. A., & Zeanah, C. H. (2014). *Romania's abandoned children: Deprivation, brain development, and the struggle for recovery.* Cambridge, MA: Harvard University Press.

Neville, H. J., Stevens, C., Pakulak, E., Bell, T. A., Fanning, J., Klein, S., et al. (2013). Family-based training program improves brain function, cognition, and behavior in lower socioeconomic status preschoolers. *Proceedings of the National Academy of Sciences USA, 110*(29), 12138–12143.

NICHD Early Child Care Research Network. (2003). Do children's attention processes mediate the link between family predictors and school readiness? *Developmental Psychology, 39*(3), 581–593.

Noble, K. G., Tottenham, N., & Casey, B. J. (2005). Neuroscience perspectives on disparities in school readiness and cognitive achievement. *The Future of Children, 15*(1), 71–89.

Norman, D. A., & Shallice, T. (1986). Attention to action. In R. J. Davidson, G. E. Schwartz, & D. Shapiro (Eds.), *Consciousness and self-regulation* (pp. 1–18). Boston: Springer.

Oberle, E., Domitrovich, C. E., Meyers, D. C., & Weissberg, R. P. (2016). Establishing systemic social and emotional learning approaches in schools: A framework for schoolwide implementation. *Cambridge Journal of Education, 46*(3), 277–297.

Ochsner, K. N., Ray, R. D., Cooper, J. C., Robertson, E. R., Chopra, S., Gabrieli, J. D., et al. (2004). For better or for worse: Neural systems supporting the cognitive down- and up-regulation of negative emotion. *NeuroImage, 23*(2), 483–499.

O'Connor, D. H., Fukui, M. M., Pinsk, M. A., & Kastner, S. (2002). Attention modulates responses in the human lateral geniculate nucleus. *Nature Neuroscience, 5*(11), 1203–1209.

Oettingen, G., & Gollwitzer, P. M. (2004). Goal setting and goal striving. In M. B. Brewer & M. Hewstone (Eds.), *Emotion and motivation* (pp. 165–183). Oxford, UK: Blackwell.

Osterman, K. F. (2000). Students' need for belonging in the school community. *Review of Educational Research, 70*(3), 323–367.

Ouellet-Morin, I., Odgers, C. L., Danese, A., Bowes, L., Shakoor, S., Papadopoulos, A. S., et al. (2011). Blunted cortisol responses to stress signal social and behavioral problems among maltreated/bullied 12-year-old children. *Biological Psychiatry, 70*(11), 1016–1023.

Paunesku, D., Walton, G. M., Romero, C., Smith, E. N., Yeager, D. S., & Dweck, C. S. (2015). Mind-set interventions are a scalable treatment for academic underachievement. *Psychological Science.* [Epub ahead of print]

Pessoa, L. (2009). How do emotion and motivation direct executive control? *Trends in Cognitive Sciences, 13*(4), 160–166.

Phillips, M. L., Ladouceur, C. D., & Drevets, W. C. (2008). A neural model of voluntary and automatic emotion regulation: Implications for understanding the pathophysiology and neurodevelopment of bipolar disorder. *Molecular Psychiatry, 13*(9), 829–857.

Plewnia, C., Schroeder, P. A., Kunze, R., Faehling, F., & Wolkenstein, L. (2015). Keep calm and carry on: Improved frustration tolerance and processing speed by transcranial direct current stimulation (tDCS). *PLoS ONE, 10*(4), e0122578.

Pollak, S. D., & Kistler, D. J. (2002). Early experience is associated with the development of categorical representations for facial expressions of emotion. *Proceedings of the National Academy of Sciences USA, 99*(13), 9072–9076.

Pollak, S. D., & Sinha, P. (2002). Effects of early experience on children's recognition of facial displays of emotion. *Developmental Psychology, 38*(5), 784–791.

Posner, M. I., & Dehaene, S. (1994). Attentional networks. *Trends in Neurosciences, 17*(2), 75–79.

Posner, M. I., & Petersen, S. E. (1990). The attention system of the human brain. *Annual Review of Neuroscience, 13*(1), 25–42.

Posner, M. I., & Rothbart, M. K. (1998). Attention, self–regulation and consciousness. *Philosophical Transactions of the Royal Society B: Biological Sciences, 353*, 1915–1927.

Posner, M. I., & Rothbart, M. K. (2000). Developing mechanisms of self-regulation. *Development and Psychopathology, 12*(3), 427–441.

Ramirez, G., & Beilock, S. L. (2011). Writing about testing worries boosts exam performance in the classroom. *Science, 331*, 211–213.

Ramos, B. P., & Arnsten, A. F. (2007). Adrenergic pharmacology and cognition: Focus on the prefrontal cortex. *Pharmacology and Therapeutics, 113*(3), 523–536.

Raver, C. C., Blackburn, E. K., Bancroft, M., & Torp, N. (1999). Relations between effective emotional self-regulation, attentional control, and low-income preschoolers' social competence with peers. *Early Education and Development, 10*, 333–350.

Raver, C. C., Blair, C., & Willoughby, M. (2013). Poverty as a predictor of 4-year-olds' executive function: New perspectives on models of differential susceptibility. *Developmental Psychology, 49*(2), 292–304.

Raver, C. C., Jones, S. M., Li-Grining, C. P., Metzger, M., Champion, K. M., & Sardin, L. (2008). Improving preschool classroom processes: Preliminary findings from a randomized trial implemented in Head Start settings. *Early Childhood Research Quarterly, 23*(1), 10–26.

Raver, C. C., Jones, S. M., Li-Grining, C., Zhai, F., Bub, K., & Pressler, E. (2011). CSRP's impact on low-income preschoolers' preacademic skills: Self-regulation as a mediating mechanism. *Child Development, 82*(1), 362–378.

Raver, C. C., Jones, S. M., Li-Grining, C., Zhai, F., Metzger, M. W., & Solomon, B. (2009). Targeting children's behavior problems in preschool classrooms: A cluster-randomized controlled trial. *Journal of Consulting and Clinical Psychology, 77*(2), 302–316.

Reynolds, A. J., Temple, J. A., Ou, S.-R., Arteaga, I. A., & White, B. A. B. (2011). School-based early childhood education and age-28 well-being: Effects by timing, dosage, and subgroups. *Science, 333*, 360–364.

Riggs, N. R., Greenberg, M. T., Kusché, C. A., & Pentz, M. A. (2006). The mediational role of neurocognition in the behavioral outcomes of a social–emotional prevention program in elementary school students: Effects of the PATHS curriculum. *Prevention Science, 7*(1), 91–102.

Rivers, S. E., Brackett, M. A., Reyes, M. R., Elbertson, N. A., & Salovey, P. (2013). Improving the social and emotional climate of classrooms: A clustered randomized controlled trial testing the RULER approach. *Prevention Science, 14,* 77–87.

Rothbart, M. K., & Ahadi, S. A. (1994). Temperament and the development of personality. *Journal of Abnormal Psychology, 103*(1), 55–56.

Rothbart, M. K., Ziaie, H., & O'Boyle, C. G. (1992). Self-regulation and emotion in infancy. *New Directions for Child and Adolescent Development, Spring*(55), 7–23.

Roy, A. L., McCoy, D. C., & Raver, C. C. (2014). Instability versus quality: Residential mobility, neighborhood poverty, and children's self-regulation. *Developmental Psychology, 50*(7), 1891–1896.

Rueda, M. R., Checa, P., & Combita, L. M. (2012). Enhanced efficiency of the executive attention network after training in preschool children: Immediate changes and effects after two months. *Developmental Cognitive Neuroscience, 2,* S192–S204.

Rueda, M. R., Checa, P., & Rothbart, M. K. (2010). Contributions of attentional control to socioemotional and academic development. *Early Education and Development, 21*(5), 744–764.

Rueda, M. R., Posner, M. I., & Rothbart, M. K. (2005). The development of executive attention: Contributions to the emergence of self-regulation. *Developmental Neuropsychology, 28*(2), 573–594.

Rueda, M. R., Rothbart, M. K., McCandliss, B. D., Saccomanno, L., & Posner, M. I. (2005). Training, maturation, and genetic influences on the development of executive attention. *Proceedings of the National Academy of Sciences USA, 102*(41), 14931–14936.

Ruff, H. A., & Rothbart, M. K. (1996). *Attention in early development: Themes and variations.* New York: Oxford University Press.

Sanchez, M., Ladd, C. O., & Plotsky, P. M. (2001). Early adverse experience as a developmental risk factor for later psychopathology: Evidence from rodent and primate models. *Development and Psychopathology, 13*(3), 419–449.

Schippell, P. L., Vasey, M. W., Cravens-Brown, L. M., & Bretveld, R. A. (2003). Suppressed attention to rejection, ridicule, and failure cues: A unique correlate of reactive but not proactive aggression in youth. *Journal of Clinical Child and Adolescent Psychology, 32,* 40–55.

Schmader, T., Johns, M., & Forbes, C. (2008). An integrated process model of stereotype threat effects on performance. *Psychological Review, 115*(2), 336–356.

Schroder, H. S., Dawood, S., Yalch, M. M., Donnellan, M. B., & Moser, J. S. (2014). The role of implicit theories in mental health symptoms, emotion regulation, and hypothetical treatment choices in college students. *Cognitive Therapy and Research, 39*(2), 120–139.

Sharkey, P. T., Tirado-Strayer, N., Papachristos, A. V., & Raver, C. C. (2012). The effect of local violence on children's attention and impulse control. *American Journal of Public Health, 102,* 2287–2293.

Silk, J. S., Davis, S., McMakin, D. L., Dahl, R. E., & Forbes, E. E. (2012). Why do anxious children become depressed teenagers?: The role of social evaluative threat and reward processing. *Psychological Medicine, 42*(10), 2095–2107.

Smith, E. R., & DeCoster, J. (2000). Dual-process models in social and cognitive psychology: conceptual integration and links to underlying memory systems. *Personality and Social Psychology Review, 4,* 108–131

Solomon, B., O'Toole, L., Hong, M., & Dennis, T. A. (2014). Negative affectivity and EEG asymmetry interact to predict emotional interference on attention in early school-aged children. *Brain and Cognition, 87,* 173–180.

Steele, A., Karmiloff-Smith, A., Cornish, K., & Scerif, G. (2012). The multiple subfunctions of attention: Differential developmental gateways to literacy and numeracy. *Child Development, 83*(6), 2028–2041.

Stein, B. D., Jaycox, L. H., Kataoka, S. H., Wong, M., Tu, W., Elliott, M. N., et al. (2003). A mental health intervention for schoolchildren exposed to violence: A randomized controlled trial. *Journal of the American Medical Association, 290*(5), 603–611.

Stevens, J. S., Jovanovic, T., Fani, N., Ely, T. D., Glover, E. M., Bradley, B., et al. (2013). Disrupted amygdala-prefrontal functional connectivity in civilian women with posttraumatic stress disorder. *Journal of Psychiatric Research, 47,* 1469–1478.

Stifter, C. A., & Braungart, J. M. (1995). The regulation of negative reactivity in infancy: Function and development. *Developmental Psychology, 31*(3), 448–455.

Sturge-Apple, M. L., Davies, P. T., Cicchetti, D., & Manning, L. G. (2012). Interparental violence, maternal emotional unavailability and children's cortisol functioning in family contexts. *Developmental Psychology, 48*(1), 237–249.

Sturge-Apple, M. L., Skibo, M. A., Rogosch, F. A., Ignjatovic, Z., & Heinzelman, W. (2011). The impact of allostatic load on maternal sympathovagal functioning in stressful child contexts: Implications for problematic parenting. *Development and Psychopathology, 23*(3), 831–844.

Tottenham, N. (2014). The importance of early experiences for neuro-affective development. In S. L. Andersen & D. S. Pine (Eds.), *The neurobiology of childhood* (pp. 109–129). New York: Springer.

Tottenham, N., Hare, T. A., & Casey, B. J. (2011). Behavioral assessment of emotion discrimination, emotion regulation and cognitive control in childhood, adolescence and adulthood. *Frontiers in Psychology, 2*, 39.

Trentacosta, C. J., & Izard, C. E. (2007). Kindergarten children's emotion competence as a predictor of their academic competence in first grade. *Emotion, 7*(1), 77–88.

Troop-Gordon, W., Gordon, R. D., Vogel-Ciernia, L., Ewing Lee, E., & Visconti, K. J. (2016). Visual attention to dynamic scenes of ambiguous provocation and children's aggressive behavior. *Journal of Clinical Child and Adolescent Psychology.* [Epub ahead of print]

Ursache, A., Blair, C., Granger, D. A., Stifter, C., & Voegtline, K. (2014). Behavioral reactivity to emotion challenge is associated with cortisol reactivity and regulation at 7, 15, and 24 months of age. *Developmental Psychobiology, 56*(3), 474–488.

Ursache, A., Blair, C., & Raver, C. C. (2012). The promotion of self-regulation as a means of enhancing school readiness and early achievement in children at risk for school failure. *Child Development Perspectives, 6*(2), 122–128.

Wang, M.-T., & Degol, J. L. (2015). School climate: A review of the construct, measurement, and impact on student outcomes. *Educational Psychology Review, 28*(2), 1–38.

Webb, T. L., Miles, E., & Sheeran, P. (2012). Dealing with feeling: A meta-analysis of the effectiveness of strategies derived from the process model of emotion regulation. *Psychological Bulletin, 138*(4), 775–808.

Webster-Stratton, C., Reid, M. J., & Hammond, M. (2001). Preventing conduct problems, promoting social competence: A parent and teacher training partnership in Head Start. *Journal of Clinical Child Psychology, 30*(3), 283–302.

Webster-Stratton, C., Reid, M. J., & Hammond, M. (2004). Treating children with early-onset conduct problems: Intervention outcomes for parent, child, and teacher training. *Journal of Clinical Child and Adolescent Psychology, 33*(1), 105–124.

Webster-Stratton, C., Reid, M. J., & Stoolmiller, M. (2008). Preventing conduct problems and improving school readiness: Evaluation of the incredible years teacher and child training programs in high-risk schools. *Journal of Child Psychology and Psychiatry, 49*(5), 471–488.

Weiss, B., Dodge, K. A., Bates, J. E., & Pettit, G. S. (1992). Some consequences of early harsh discipline: Child aggression and a maladaptive social information processing style. *Child Development, 63*, 1321–1335.

Welsh, J. A., Nix, R. L., Blair, C., Bierman, K. L., & Nelson, K. E. (2010). The development of cognitive skills and gains in academic school readiness for children from low-income families. *Journal of Educational Psychology, 102*(1), 43–53.

Williford, A. P., & Shelton, T. L. (2008). Using mental health consultation to decrease disruptive behaviors in preschoolers: Adapting an empirically-supported intervention. *Journal of Child Psychology and Psychiatry, 49*(2), 191–200.

Yeager, D. S., Johnson, R., Spitzer, B. J., Trzesniewski, K. H., Powers, J., & Dweck, C. S. (2014). The far-reaching effects of believing people can change: Implicit theories of personality shape stress, health, and achievement during adolescence. *Journal of Personality and Social Psychology, 106*(6), 867–884.

Yeager, D. S., & Walton, G. M. (2011). Social-psychological interventions in education: They're not magic. *Review of Educational Research, 81*(2), 267–301.

Zelazo, P. D., & Cunningham, W. A. (2007). Executive function: Mechanisms underlying emotion regulation. In J. J. Gross (Ed.), *Handbook of emotion regulation* (pp. 135–158). New York: Guilford Press.

Zelazo, P. D., Müller, U., Frye, D., Marcovitch, S., Argitis, G., Boseovski, J., et al. (2003). The development of executive function in early childhood. *Monographs of the Society for Research in Child Development, 68*(3), vii–137.

Zhai, F., Raver, C. C., & Jones, S. M. (2012). Academic performance of subsequent schools and impacts of early interventions: Evidence from a randomized controlled trial in Head Start settings. *Children and Youth Services Review, 34*(5), 946–954.

CHAPTER 23

Competence and Motivation during Adolescence

DAVID S. YEAGER
HAE YEON LEE
RONALD E. DAHL

Adolescents in the United States are often characterized as disaffected and disengaged in school (Allen & Allen, 2010; Schwartz, 2015; Steinberg, 2014). Indeed, two independent longitudinal studies (seen in Figure 23.1) showed dramatic declines in intrinsic motivation in math across age, corresponding to over 0.75 *SD* units by the end of high school (Gottfried, Fleming, & Gottfried, 2001; Jacobs, Lanza, Osgood, Eccles, & Wigfield, 2002; for a narrative review, see Benner, 2011).

Yet such developmental trends do not mean that adolescents are globally unmotivated to learn. After all, adolescents seem capable of being highly engaged and ready to learn (Steinberg, 2014; Telzer, 2016). In fact, emerging neuroscientific evidence is

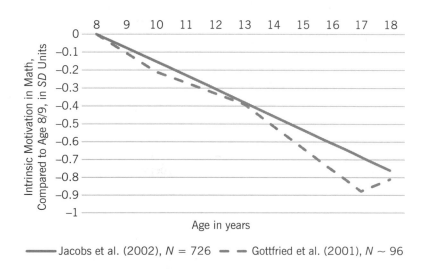

FIGURE 23.1. Intrinsic motivation in math declines precipitously across adolescence. Based on the authors' reanalyses of data from Gottfried et al. (2001) and Jacobs et al. (2002).

431

showing that adolescents are sometimes *better* than adults, at a behavioral and neurological level of analysis, when it comes to learning that involves cognitive flexibility and adaptive decision making (Hauser, Iannaccone, Walitza, Brandeis, & Brem, 2015).

Why is it, then, that adolescence appears to simultaneously be both a stage during which it is difficult to motivate students to learn in school and one in which individuals are highly motivated to rapidly acquire the know-how that allows them to succeed in society (see Steinberg, 2014; Yeager, Dahl, & Dweck, 2016)? Moreover, is it possible to capture adolescents' unique learning sensitivities and channel them into greater motivation in academic settings?

The previous edition of this handbook stated that individuals are motivated when learning allows them to gain, demonstrate, or experience competence (Elliot & Dweck, 2005). If so, then it can be helpful to consider what offers adolescents the feeling of competence, from their perspective.

Since the publication of Coleman's classic text *The Adolescent Society* (1961), studies in sociology, psychology, education, economics, and now neuroscience and behavioral endocrinology have highlighted that adolescents' intellectual goals are not independent of their social ones (Benner, 2011; Crosnoe & Johnson, 2011; Dahl & Vanderschuren, 2011; Telzer, 2016; Wentzel, 1998). Adolescents do not go to school simply because they are motivated to gain knowledge and skills leading to jobs that approximate those of their parents. Rather, motivation and engagement are intertwined with the desire to fit in and to achieve social success both now and in the future (Crosnoe, 2011).

A number of factors lead to adolescents' shifts toward valuing more strongly the feelings that come from *social* competence, such as admiration or respect. These include puberty (and associated neural and endocrine developments), social-cognitive achievements, changes in social relationships, and school transitions. Various authors, at different levels of analysis, have described this "social reorienting" (Blakemore & Mills, 2014; Crosnoe & McNeely, 2008; Eccles, Lord, & Midgley, 1991; Erikson, 1968; Larson & Richards, 1991; Peper

& Dahl, 2013; Wigfield & Wagner, 2005). This chapter adds to this tradition, in particular highlighting research that was not covered (or available) in the corresponding chapter in the previous edition (Wigfield & Wagner, 2005).

Our primary contribution is to review developmental changes that alter what it means to acquire competence during adolescence, and therefore what feels motivating in school. We then highlight how developmental changes create new, stage-enhanced opportunities to motivate adolescents in academic settings—for instance, by latching on to desires to feel autonomous from uninvited adult control (Vansteenkiste, Simons, Lens, Sheldon, & Deci, 2004), to feel related socially to valued peers (Cohen & Prinstein, 2006; Paluck & Shepherd, 2012; Yeager, Johnson, et al., 2014), to avoid the stigmatizing implication of intellectual incompetence (or, sometimes, competence) (Blackwell, Trzesniewski, & Dweck, 2007; Yeager, Purdie-Vaughns, et al., 2014), and to develop an identity as a person who can make a meaningful contribution to the world beyond the self (Yeager, Henderson, et al., 2014).

A secondary contribution is to summarize examples of "developmentally wise" psychological interventions—interventions that work with, rather than against, adolescents' developmentally cued tendencies, and in doing so create motivation (Garcia & Cohen, 2012; Walton, 2014; Wilson, 2011; Yeager et al., 2016; Yeager & Walton, 2011). As we will show, experimental interventions that do not mention schoolwork or academic motivation can nevertheless capture adolescents' beliefs and desires, and bring about improvements in academic competence. Such experiments have the dual purpose of demonstrating causality and supporting the theoretical synthesis presented here.

In doing so, we challenge the notion that adolescents' social motives are inherently in conflict with their intellectual development, or that adolescents are hopelessly peer-focused, to the exclusion of adult advice. For instance, numerous studies illustrate that academic motivation and persistence can be profoundly affected by relationships with thoughtful adults who honor adolescents' desire for status and respect (Allen, Pianta, Gregory, Mikami, & Lun, 2011; Gregory &

Weinstein, 2008; Hurd, Sánchez, Zimmerman, & Caldwell, 2012; Treisman, 1992). Instead, adolescents may often simply be in a predicament in which their intellectual goals conflict with their social ones. Wise educational environments seek to align the two so that they work with, rather than against, each other.

RECENT ADVANCES IN DEVELOPMENTAL SCIENCE HAVE REVISED OUR VIEWS OF ADOLESCENCE

What is Adolescence?

Adolescence begins with the onset of puberty—a set of biological changes that marks the end of childhood. The end of adolescence, however, does not have any clear-cut biological markers. Rather, the transition from adolescence into adulthood is largely determined by social and cultural factors, most notably establishing independence from one's parents and acquiring adult social roles (Blakemore, 2010; Blakemore & Mills, 2014; Crone & Dahl, 2012; Steinberg, 2014).

Adolescence is not a Western social construction; most societies, including preindustrial societies around the world, recognize a developmental stage that is beyond childhood but not yet an adult (see Crone & Dahl, 2012, for a review). What is unique to adolescence in modern Western society (and increasingly in the rest of the world), is that the length of time in this transitional state between childhood and adulthood has expanded significantly. This expansion is due to the fact that whereas puberty has been beginning at earlier ages, the age at which adolescents achieve independent adult status has been occurring later. For example, in the mid-19th century, the average age of menarche was 15–16 years in Europe and the United States, while the average age of marriage was 21; now the average age of menarche is 11.5 years and the average age of taking on independent adult roles is typically later, in the mid-20s (Crone & Dahl, 2012; Steinberg, 2014). That is, adolescents stay in this transition period much longer than ever (Allen & Allen, 2010; Steinberg, 2014). In light of this, one can think of expanded opportunities for learning and change, as well as expanded vulnerabilities to the risks.

Problems with the "All Gas, No Brake" Metaphor

In everyday contexts, adults often characterize adolescents more by their *incompetence* than by their competence. Indeed, adolescence is a period of tremendous increases in preventable deaths—car crashes, other fatal accidents, homicides, and suicides (Kann et al., 2014)—and a strong spike in rates of depression and related internalizing psychopathologies (Thapar, Collishaw, Pine, & Thapar, 2012). Adolescents suffer from high school dropout, substance abuse, unwanted pregnancies, obesity, and more (Steinberg, 2015).

In recent years, a metaphor has been proposed to characterize adolescents' seeming incompetence at making wise decisions: "all gasoline, no brakes, and no steering wheel" (Bell & McBride, 2010, p. 565; also see Dahl, 2001). This refers to the idea that adolescents have a strong, surging desire to experience thrills but a weak self-regulatory mechanism to constrain that desire (see Figure 23.2). According to this model, adolescents engage in riskier behavior than children or adults; whereas children have a weaker desire for thrills, adults may have developed a mature self-control system. This metaphor has proven useful especially in

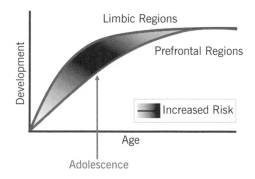

FIGURE 23.2. Adolescents' sensation-seeking urges (limbic regions) are thought to increase faster than their ability to control them (prefrontal regions). From Somerville, Jones, and Casey (2010, p. 126). Copyright © 2010 by Elsevier. Reprinted by permission.

juvenile justice contexts, most prominently to justify shorter sentences for youth offenders on the grounds that youth are not yet mature (Steinberg, 2014; but for a criticism of this, see Johnson, Blum, & Giedd, 2009).

Despite the appeal of the "all gas, no brakes" metaphor—and while acknowledging its important effect on creating more just sentencing guidelines—a growing number of developmental scientists have described the ways in which it may be misleading (Blakemore & Mills, 2014; Crone & Dahl, 2012; also see Casey & Caudle, 2013). They have posed an alternative to the metaphor of adolescents' inability to steer safely and slow down appropriately: Might these behaviors actually reflect another version of adolescents' natural proclivity for *learning through exploration?* That is, might adolescents' inclinations toward risk and experimentation at the outer edge of what they can comfortably control represent a particularly effective way to learn about—and more quickly master—control capacities?

On the one hand, a tendency to explore the edge of control may lead to more errors (and greater real-world risks of tragic accidents); on the other hand, making more errors (and adjusting behavior in response to these errors) may contribute to greater learning. Moving beyond the simplistic metaphor of learning to drive a car, this set of principles is relevant to the challenges of learning the control skills necessary for social competence in adolescence.

Furthermore, the gas-and-brake metaphor underappreciates the strengths of the adolescent brain. The adolescent brain might appear inferior to the adult brain in terms of a proclivity to explore, take risks, and make errors. However, experiments indicate that the adolescent brain is also extremely well adapted to the core task of adolescent development: *learning* how to navigate complex, fast-changing, and emotionally charged social contexts (Hauser et al., 2015; Telzer, 2016). Consider, for instance, findings from Casey and Caudle (2013), showing that by age 15, adolescents are no worse than adults at performing emotionally neutral self-control tasks. Where adolescents' performance suffers (compared to children and adults) is when these neutral, tedious, self-control tasks have to compete with social-emotional stimuli (Casey & Caudle, 2013).

Adolescents find the emotional stimuli highly salient, and fail the tedious, unemotional self-control tasks. Yet making more errors because of emotional stimuli may look like inferior performance even as it is underpinning advantageous learning about social emotions.

An Alternative View of Adolescent Strengths

Research is converging on the notion that adolescents may be uniquely adept at perceiving, learning about, reacting to, and adjusting their behavior to the demands of their social worlds (Blakemore & Mills, 2014; Casey & Caudle, 2013; Crone & Dahl, 2012; Telzer, 2016). Adolescents appear more sensitive than children or adults to social situations in which they may be ashamed or admired, and can shift their preferences, behaviors, and identities in response to those possibilities more rapidly than people at other stages (see, e.g., Cohen & Prinstein, 2006; Helms et al., 2014). This ability may therefore represent a natural shift in a window of sensitivity for social learning—one that could represent an underutilized asset for developing academic competence.

Such a formulation has implications for whether adolescents should be deprived of unsafe opportunities (if they are incompetent; Steinberg, 2015) or the exact opposite—that is, be given *more* opportunities for responsibly exploring their social environment (if they are learning; also see Eccles et al., 1991). This formulation might also affect whether society ought to prefer educational models that withhold versus expand opportunities for discovery, autonomy, or responsibility.

In general, the field is in the midst of a sea change in theories of adolescent behavior (Allen, Moore, & Kuperminc, 1997; Crone & Dahl, 2012; Ellis et al., 2012; Steinberg, 2015; Yeager et al., 2016). More and more, risk-taking, so often seen as a liability, is increasingly being seen as potentially positive under some circumstances. Behaviors such as raising one's hand in class, going out for a sport or a class play, starting a conversation with someone that one finds attractive or popular—all of these are ways of exploring the social environment that can be at once scary and possibly offer respect and admiration from others. These may contribute to competence by helping adolescents develop skills at the frontiers of their abilities. Adolescents' heightened risk taking can be viewed, then, as practice and learning about how to manage high-intensity competing "stop" emotions (fear) with "go" emotions (excitement) (see Spielberg, Olino, Forbes, & Dahl, 2014).

DEVELOPMENTAL CHANGES THAT BEAR ON COMPETENCE AND MOTIVATION IN ADOLESCENCE

Equipped with an understanding of adolescents' underlying natural motives for learning, researchers and practitioners might be able to channel adolescent *strengths* into more educationally beneficial behaviors, such as learning diligently. Specifically, recent developmental science has suggested that adolescents have an appetitive desire to experience positive emotions relevant to status or respect from peers or admired adults, and this can strongly affect their attention, motivation, and learning (Blakemore & Mills, 2014; Crone & Dahl, 2012; Telzer, 2016).

As we have begun to consider a wider set of questions focusing on this adolescent sensitization to some social and affective processing, and the neural systems that underpin these, we suggest a tentative term: the *status-relevant affective learning system.* Regardless of the term, research from multiple levels of analysis supports the conclusion that pubertal maturation is associated with an increase in the motivational salience of self-conscious emotions—ways that make adolescents hungry to experience positive self-conscious emotions (pride, admiration) and avoid negative self-conscious emotions (shame, humiliation).

Status-Relevant Affective Learning System

Pubertal maturation—the biological definition of the onset of adolescence—leads to increases or changes in the functioning of a number of hormones, including testosterone, estradiol, cortisol, oxytocin, and dehydroepiandrosterone sulfate (DHEA-S) (Murray-Close, 2013; Peper & Dahl, 2013). Although all of these hormones are related to the functioning of stress and threat response systems,

as well as attention and behavior, because testosterone has the clearest link with status pursuit and maintenance (and therefore the motivational processes discussed here), we discuss testosterone in greater detail.

In both males and females, pubertal maturation leads to a large surge in the production of testosterone. One rare two-wave cohort-sequential study examined levels of testosterone among adolescents covering a period from 8 to 27 years of age (Braams, van Duijvenvoorde, Peper, & Crone, 2015); see Figure 23.3. Adolescents' testosterone increases from ages 10 to 15 (for females), and from ages 10 to 18 (for males), and individual differences in increases in testosterone (for both males and females) predict individual differences in increases in behavioral and neural indicators of risk taking equally for males and females (Braams et al., 2015).

It is important to clarify that testosterone is not so much an *aggression* hormone as it is a hormone that facilitates conscious and unconscious attention to and striving for competence that may bring about status or respect in one's environment (see Eisenegger, Haushofer, & Fehr, 2011; Terburg & van Honk, 2013). Testosterone effects on behavior are embedded in social context because what counts for social competence varies across contexts. Illustrating this, testosterone predicts aggressive behavior when boys have deviant friends, but leadership when boys do not have deviant friends (Rowe, Maughan, Worthman, Costello, & Angold, 2004). Hence, the pubertal surge in testosterone does not inevitably lead to aggression, but rather leads to a willingness to attend to and align oneself with identities and preferences that might lead to experiences of status and respect. This can be a powerful source of motivation.

Next, we emphasize that learning about social status/respect is not purely cognitive; it is strongly affective. Our view is that adolescents not only want to know about what leads to gaining or maintaining status or reputation, but they also want to *experience,* firsthand, positive affect related to status, then learn how to reproduce those positive emotions while avoiding negative ones.

Indeed, pubertal maturation alters the processing of emotions in adolescents (Goddings, Burnett Heyes, Bird, Viner, & Blakemore, 2012), and this is particularly

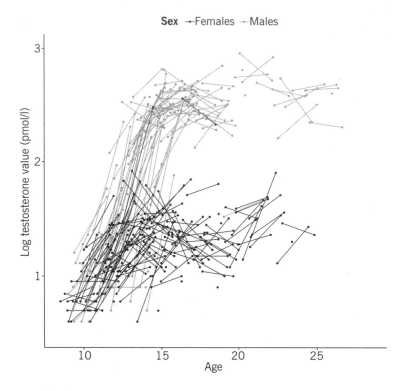

FIGURE 23.3. Testosterone—a hormone that increases attention to social status and respect and drives motivation to acquire it—rises dramatically for both males and females across adolescence, but begins and peaks earlier for females. From Braams, van Duijvenvoorde, Peper, and Crone (2015).

concentrated in the domain of *social,* self-conscious emotions such as humiliation, guilt, or pride, rather than in basic emotions such as fear or disgust (Burnett, Bird, Moll, Frith, & Blakemore, 2009; Klapwijk et al., 2013). In the brain, adolescents show greater reward processing when they experience or have the potential to experience social successes (ventral striatum and orbitofrontal cortex; Chein, Albert, O'Brien, Uckert, & Steinberg, 2011), and greater distress when they experience social failure (subgenual angerior cingulate; Sebastian, Viding, Williams, & Blakemore, 2010). In line with the latter, at a hormonal level of analysis, adolescents show elevated cortisol response to social threats (Gunnar, Wewerka, Frenn, Long, & Griggs, 2009).

Summary and Integration

Taken together, these maturational changes contribute to the following view of competence and motivation in adolescence.

Adolescence may represent an "experience expectant" developmental window for learning how to navigate and succeed in their peer and adult social contexts (Greenough & Black, 1992). When the thrill of social success and the agony of public humiliation feel overwhelming, then adolescents may be on the alert for quickly forming mental representations about how to behave in their social world. As a result, adolescents may be uniquely competent when the task is to perceive rapidly what counts for status, or to learn a skill so that they can acquire status. They may allocate their attention to learning what social behaviors cause it, then rehearse those behaviors until they are routine. Hence, what may look like a disengagement from academic tasks (i.e., loss of school motivation and engagement) may actually represent sustained engagement in learning how to acquire adolescent-specific social competence.

Next, looking back at the shape of the quadratic trends in Figure 23.3, one cannot help but notice the parallels with Figure 23.1. The age at which pubertal levels of testosterone (known to focus attention on status/respect) are the greatest for boys also happen to be the age of lowest interest in and enjoyment of math in school. Also note the parallels between the quadratic slope in levels of testosterone for boys and girls (Figure 23.3) and the levels of sensation seeking ("limbic regions" in Figure 23.2). When testosterone is increasing most, so too is risk taking—a relation that was confirmed directly in analyses of developmental and individual differences (Braams et al., 2015).

These developmental trends might be related. Academic work in school sometimes requires a long wade through drudgery to achieve something that eventually seems to have only low-probability, long-term, self-interested payoffs, while it perhaps affords too few opportunities to experience peer regard and self-respect in the immediate term (Allen & Allen, 2010). Yet instructional methods that allow adolescents to take on meaningful challenges offer them an opportunity to matter in the eyes of valued others. Furthermore, pedagogical practices such as experiential or "discovery" learning may be especially motivating in adolescence because they capitalize on this sensation-seeking tendency—they may create opportunities to experience the thrill of discovery or unexpected success (see Telzer, 2016).

MOTIVATIONAL VARIABLES THAT TAKE ON SPECIAL IMPORTANCE DURING ADOLESCENCE

What implications arise from this view for how to create academic competence and motivation among adolescents? Our theory has been that it is possible for adolescents to capitalize on developmentally cued social learning sensitivity and achieve impressive changes in academic motivation and achievement (see Cohen & Sherman, 2014; Lazowski & Hulleman, 2015; Walton, 2014; Yeager et al., 2016; Yeager & Walton, 2011). We argue that the way to do this is to tap into values or "prestige criteria" that confer status and respect during adolescence—or create the feeling of being respected and having higher status. Self-determination theory (Ryan & Deci, 2000) provides a helpful way

to organize some of these values in terms of the needs for *autonomy, relatedness,* and *(academic) competence.* Following some previous theories (Williams, 2009), to these we add *meaning and purpose* as an intrinsically motivating value for adolescents that signals one's social worth to others and to oneself.

In the next section we briefly summarize several clusters of variables—each well established in its own right in the social-psychological literature—that can have the effect of signaling to an adolescent or to his or her peers that he or she has high status or is respected, capturing strong adolescent motivation. Our goal is not to provide comprehensive reviews—indeed, each value deserves its own chapter. Rather, our goal is to provide a few concrete examples of how these variables have powerfully shaped motivation and competence for adolescents.

Nor do we argue that these variables only have motivational force in adolescence; they clearly matter during other stages. Yet they may take on important motivational salience during adolescence, as we explain for each below.

Autonomy

One clear sign of disrespect and diminishment is to rob a person of his or her autonomy to make choices that he or she should be competent enough to carry out—at least in Western cultures. The implication of such autonomy threat is that one is not a full person—that one is a mere child, not a burgeoning adult. Hence, the developmental changes in the status-relevant affective learning system provide one justification for why feelings of autonomy and autonomy threat may be especially influential for motivation during adolescence (see Table 23.1).

A long tradition of psychological research (Allen, Kuperminc, Philliber, & Herre, 1994; Bandura, 1989; Deci, 1975; Deci & Ryan, 1985; Reis, Sheldon, Gable, Roscoe, & Ryan, 2000; Ryan & Deci, 2000; Steinberg & Silverberg, 1986) has documented that autonomy is a core value for human motivation. The concept of *autonomy* has been defined as psychological states that provide individuals with a sense of *free will, freedom of choice, self-reliance,* and *self-governing* experiences. Therefore, autonomy, by its

TABLE 23.1. Summary of Experiences That Could Threaten versus Capture the Adolescent Status-Relevant Affective Learning System in Academic Settings

Need/value	Developmental differences in relevance of need/value for status/respect	Sample methods to capture the desire for status/respect
Autonomy	• Adolescents may interpret even mundane suggestions to change their behavior as implying a lack of competence to make personal choices. • Depriving adolescents of the ability to author their own learning experiences fails to engage their desire for firsthand affective learning experiences.	• Offer authentic opportunities for choice or change language from "should" to "might" (*autonomy support*) • Create opportunities for a feeling of discovery, as if one is the first to have a certain thought or perspective (*discovery learning*)
Relatedness	• Adolescents may have their attention and motivation more tied to their current feelings of social success in the peer group. • Adolescents may be more willing to self-handicap to avoid losing peer regard.	• Help adolescents view current social struggles as *common* and *improvable* (a *social belonging* or *incremental theory of personality* approach) • Create a climate where peers respect and celebrate effort and learning (*social norms*)
(Academic) competence	• Adolescents may be more motivated to avoid feeling intellectually incompetent in front of peers, or to demonstrate their greater intellectual competence as compared to peers.	• Reduce the potential that one will be seen as lacking intellectual ability (*growth mindset*) • Create relationships with with teachers that respect adolescents' potential (*wise critical feedback*)
Meaning/ purpose	• Adolescents may not value long-term self-interested outcomes (e.g., health) as much as adults.	• Offer adolescents an opportunity to earn immediate eudaimonic reward by having an effect some part of the world beyond the self (a *self-transcendent purpose for learning*)

definition, implies one's felt psychological independence from interpersonal (e.g., parents, peers, or school or organizational authorities; Steinberg & Silverberg, 1986) or situational forces (e.g., rewards, punishments, evaluative pressures, imposed goals, surveillance, or choice constraints; Ryan & Deci, 2000) that may extrinsically influence individuals' behaviors in given settings. *Autonomy threat* occurs when one's agency has been removed or drawn into question.

Among adults and adolescents, support of autonomy has been shown to enhance psychological functioning and well-being—indicated by improved academic performance and persistence (Vansteenkiste et al., 2004, Vansteenkiste, Simons, Lens, Soenens, & Matos, 2005), conceptual learning in school (Furtak & Kunter, 2012; Reeve, 2009), lower high school dropout rates (Vallerand, Fortier, & Guay, 1997), positive

daily moods (Reis et al., 2000), lowered reactance against authorities (Hodgins, Yacko, & Gottlieb, 2006; Hodgins et al., 2010), and even greater adherence to health-promoting behaviors such as smoking cessation, glucose control, medication, and exercise (Williams, Rodin, Ryan, Grolnick, & Deci, 1998; Williams, Niemiec, Patrick, Ryan, & Deci, 2009).

Autonomy threat can be highly demotivating at a basic level. In one study, adolescents who watched video clips of their mothers telling them how they should change their behavior (e.g., clean their room, take their shoes downstairs, be nice to their sister) showed a pattern of neural activity that suggested they were not processing the criticism or planning to alter their behavior (Lee, Siegle, Dahl, Hooley, & Silk, 2014). Specifically, regions of the brain relevant to anger were activated in response to maternal criticism, while regions relevant to processing information and making plans showed blunted activation.

Experimental research shows how autonomy experiences can be changed—and these studies therefore suggest effective methods to capture adolescents' latent motives. Studies have experimentally manipulated the level of autonomy granting, using brief language cues (e.g., "You can/might" vs. "You should/ought to") or semantic priming (e.g., a sentence scramble task with "I usually have choice" vs. "We must do this"; Bargh, Chen, & Burrows, 1996). Individuals' experiences of autonomy then boost intrinsic motivation and feelings of agency, as well as their compliant behavior.

Qualitative observations of expert teachers indicate that these experiences support autonomy—they create in students the feeling that they are seen as having the competence to make choices and influence their personal outcomes (Wallace, Sung, & Williams, 2014). This conveys respect and wins student compliance with classroom procedures.

Some developmentally informed psychological interventions (Allen et al., 1994; Philliber & Allen, 1992) have attempted to honor adolescents' feelings of autonomy and have had success in inspiring and increasing motivation in school—reducing school failure, suspension, and dropout—while also reducing risk behavior such as teenage pregnancy. The Teen Outreach Program combines volunteer service activities with school classroom-based, curriculum-guided group discussions. Allen and colleagues (1994) allowed adolescents to choose different volunteer activities and engage in interactions with adult program facilitators in autonomous ways. Over 7 years of randomized trials with over 6,000 at-risk youth, the Teen Outreach Program (Philliber & Allen, 1992) reduced teenage pregnancy and school failure/dropout rates by 15–50% compared to matched control groups. Evidence for mechanism came from students' perceived sense of autonomy: This was a significant predictor of lower rates of problem behaviors in middle school sites at the program exit year. Furthermore, autonomy-enhancing qualities of volunteer work also promoted a greater reduction in problematic behaviors.

More recently, Allen and colleagues (2011) conducted a teacher training intervention called "My Teaching Partner—Secondary" with 78 secondary school teachers involving over 2,200 students. To prevent student's performance decline and school disengagement in the secondary school, this program intervened with teachers' interaction styles with students. The authors observed improvement in students' academic achievement in the post-intervention year. This was mediated by teacher–student interaction qualities—in particular, the extent to which teachers support students' psychological needs for autonomy during their instructional interactions. Altogether, autonomy support can capture adolescents' desire for status/respect. This can lead to greater treatment effects for intervention programs in schools.

Relatedness

A second developmentally cued motive is a desire to belong and be connected to others. Few outcomes could be more threatening to adolescents than the possibility of "social death"—of being disconnected from peers or valued adults and feeling incapable of demonstrating one's worth to them.

At all ages, a desire to belong and form social connections is fundamental to human motivation (Baumeister & Leary, 1995; Reis, 1994; Ryan & Deci, 2000). Individuals' psychological adjustment, motivation, and well-being tend to thrive when they feel social connectedness and relatedness to others (Leary, 2004; Oudekerk, Allen, Hessel, & Molloy, 2015; Reis et al., 2000; Walton, Cohen, Cwir, & Spencer, 2012). Experiencing threat to social belonging and relatedness has been known to predict a wide array of outcomes, including intellectual underperformance (Baumeister, Twenge, & Nuss, 2002), dampened academic motivation (Cheryan, Plaut, Davies, & Steele, 2009; Murphy, Steele, & Gross, 2007), a global perception of lost meaning in life (Stillman & Baumeister, 2009), health risk behavior, and early death (Cacioppo & Patrick, 2008).

Growing evidence from neuroscience and behavioral studies (Albert, Chein, & Steinberg, 2013; Cohen & Prinstein, 2006; Crone & Dahl, 2012; DeWall, Maner, &

Rouby, 2009; Helms et al., 2014; Sebastian et al., 2010; Somerville, 2013) has converged on the notion that adolescents are particularly sensitive to signs of belonging, social inclusion–exclusion, and positive or negative peer evaluation. Consequently, adolescents' behavioral choices are readily affected by perceived peer social norms, and they are therefore susceptible to exhibiting peer contagion and conformity effects.

For example, Helms and colleagues (2014) demonstrated that adolescents tend to overestimate the frequencies of high-status peers' engagement in risk behaviors (e.g., substance use, vandalism, risky sexual behaviors), then conform to those incorrect estimates. Misperceived behavioral norms of high-status peers in grade 9 significantly predicted increases in adolescents' own adoption of same risk behaviors between grades 9 and 11. Other laboratory researchers who directly manipulated the perceived behaviors of high-status peers found that adolescents conform to those in the immediate term—both good and bad (Cohen & Prinstein, 2006; Paluck & Shepherd, 2012).

One method to honor adolescents' desire for strong social relationships with peers is to decrease the psychological impact of potential threats to peer relationships. That is, adolescents can be buffered from negative social experiences—triggering the thoughts "I am socially worthless," "I am not a likeable person," or "No one wants to be friends with me"—so that those experiences do not elicit strong threats to their social status. If such thoughts could be prevented, then adolescents' attention might not be monopolized by social concerns, and they might be allowed the psychological space to focus on their schoolwork.

One method for doing this is to intervene on adolescents' implicit theories of personality (Dweck, Chiu, & Hong, 1995; Yeager, Johnson, et al., 2014; Yeager, Trzesniewski, Tirri, Nokelainen, & Dweck, 2011). Implicit theories of personality interventions teach students that one's socially relevant characteristics have the potential to change and develop. This is called an "incremental theory of personality," which is known to reduce the feeling that if one is excluded or left out, it means that one will always be a "loser" or "not likable" (Yeager et al.,

2011); by preventing such fixed attributions, the incremental theory can create a feeling that one has the resources to cope with the demands posed by a socially difficult situation (Yeager, Lee, & Jamieson, 2016).

The implicit theories of personality intervention can buffer adolescents from the negative effects of *social* experiences, then spill over into their *academic* performance. First, research shows that adolescents who received incremental theory of personality messages tend to exhibit less hostile attributional styles following peer social exclusion (Yeager et al., 2011), weaker desire for vengeful retaliation in response to peer provocations (Yeager, Trzesniewski, & Dweck, 2013), and reduced global stress and improved physical health (Yeager, Johnson, et al., 2014). That is, it buffers them from social experiences. Next, by promoting lower general threat-type responses to social difficulty, the one-time incremental theory of personality intervention raised academic grades in high school over a year later in three different experiments (Yeager, Johnson, et al., 2014; Yeager et al., 2016)—even though the intervention never mentioned academic motivation. This highlights the importance of the effect of adolescents' ability to cope with social difficulties on their academic performance.

Competence

Much of the rest of this volume focuses on the importance of feelings of academic competence for one's motivation. Here we wish to highlight a simple point: When success in school may potentially reflect on one's gain or loss of social status, then the status-relevant affective learning system may come strongly into play. Hence, adolescence is a developmental period in which academic competence perceptions—and the self-conscious emotions activated in these situations—take on special importance. Deeper understanding of these issues may inform innovations in tapping into these natural sources of motivation for learning in ways that serve rather than interfere with engagement with learning in school.

Take the well-known example of implicit theories of intelligence, which illustrates how the implication that one might be "dumb" could threaten social status and undermine motivation (Aronson, Fried, & Good, 2002; Blackwell et al., 2007; Dweck, 2006; Dweck et al., 1995; Good, Aronson, & Inzlicht, 2003; Yeager & Dweck, 2012). As addressed elsewhere in this volume, Dweck (2006; see also Yeager & Dweck, 2012) has found that individuals may believe that ability is fixed (*entity theory*) or malleable (*incremental theory*). Interventions that have taught adolescents to endorse more of an incremental theory have caused adolescents to interpret their difficulties as obstacles that can be overcome rather than as fixed impediments that condemn them to being viewed as having low ability. Because such changes can facilitate motivation in the face of adversity, these interventions have improved overall grades weeks and months after receiving incremental theory of intelligence messages (Aronson et al., 2002; Blackwell et al., 2007; Good et al., 2003; Paunesku et al., 2015). Incremental theory of intelligence interventions can prevent social emotions such as shame by preventing problematic self-blaming attributions for failures, such as "I'm not smart enough at this" (Mueller & Dweck, 1998).

Also consider concerns about being viewed as incompetent by authorities on the basis of one's social identity. Young children can detect stereotypes against their racial groups, and nearly 100% of minority youth are aware of these stereotypes by sixth grade (McKown & Weinstein, 2003). These stereotypes are disrespectful. Therefore, one method to be sensitive to adolescents' concerns about disrespect is to take the stereotype off the table in one's interactions with students.

Following experimental research by Cohen, Steele, and Ross (1999), Yeager, Purdie-Vaughns, and colleagues (2014) tested the efficacy of a "wise feedback" approach to creating feelings of respect among negatively stereotyped racial-minority seventh-grade adolescents. *Wise feedback* refers to an approach that conveys teachers *high standards* for the student's performance, as well as a belief in the student's *potential* to reach the performance standard. It follows directly from survey research showing that the *combination* of both high academic expectations and strong

relationships—but not one or the other—is a powerful way to create trust among negatively stereotyped students (Gregory & Ripski, 2008) and reduce the achievement gaps of entire schools (Shouse, 1996).

In Yeager, Purdie-Vaughns, and colleagues' (2014) field experiments, receiving a wise feedback note ("I'm giving you these comments because I have very high expectations and I know that you can reach them") let to adolescents' greater willingness to revise essays after critical feedback. This effect was especially great for African American students, increasing rates of essay revisions from 17 to 72% (Yeager, Purdie-Vaughns, et al., 2014, Study 1). Moreover, the critical moderator of these effects was the feeling of respect: Students of color who had chronically felt disrespected by teachers benefited the most when an adult took them seriously and treated them as though they had intellectual promise.

The case of the wise feedback intervention suggests effective ways to boost academic motivation and competence by making disrespectful negative stereotypes about one's group an implausible reason for the teacher's interpersonal treatment (Cohen & Steele, 2002; Steele, 2011). By taking the potential for social disrespect off the table, the wise feedback approach allowed students to engage in behavior that developed their intellectual competence.

Meaning/Purpose

Adolescents are often characterized as selfish and primarily concerned with short-term gains. Yet adolescents are also highly motivated to contribute to some part of the world beyond the self (Damon, Menon, & Bronk, 2003)—to "matter" in the eyes of valued others, or in one's own evaluation (Marshall, 2001; Yeager, Henderson, et al., 2014). In brain neural sensitivity studies, adolescents appear to derive so-called "eudemonic rewards" from contributing to the world beyond the self (Telzer, Fuligni, Lieberman, & Galván, 2014). This phenomenon is captured by adolescents' precocious attraction to social movements (see Robinson, 2010). Furthermore, at a neurobiological level, there is evidence that testosterone—a key pubertal hormone—can heighten attention to unfairness (Eisenegger, Naef, Snozzi, Heinrichs, & Fehr, 2010), a precursor to the desire to remediate unfairness through social action.

Typical schoolwork seems at odds with adolescents' desire to matter, however, because it often involves rote exercises, boring practice, and the underlying long-term, self-oriented rationale "it will be good for you later"—a societal argument that has been dubbed "the big wait" (Allen & Allen, 2010). It is a bit like eating one's vegetables, only worse; indeed, over half of middle school students in the United States would rather eat broccoli than do their math homework, according to a survey by the Raytheon Company (Research Now, 2012).

It would seem, then, that the importance of finding meaning/purpose would work against motivation in school. Yet recent research indicates that it is possible to harness adolescents' desire to experience meaning and self-transcendent purpose in life, and align it with the goal of learning in school (Yeager, Henderson, et al., 2014). This research examines a *self-transcendent purpose for learning*, defined as a motive for learning in school that has both long-term benefit to the self and a positive effect on some component of the world beyond the self (Yeager & Bundick, 2009; Yeager, Henderson, et al., 2014).

Importantly, a purpose for learning appears most beneficial for students who are the *most* disengaged—who chronically were uninterested in school, or who were feeling the most bored (Paunesku et al., 2015; Yeager, Henderson, et al., 2014). In correlational research, Yeager, Henderson, and colleagues (2014) have found that adolescents who say that they are learning in school so that they can make a positive difference in the world—but not adolescents who say that they are pursuing an interesting and enjoyable life—showed greater grit and self-control, greater behavioral persistence on a tedious task, and even greater persistence in college many months later. Below we explain how experimental research has manipulated adolescents' purposes for learning and observed effects on consequential behavior over time.

How can a treatment promote a self-transcendent purpose for learning? Yeager,

Henderson, and colleagues (2014) developed a "purpose for learning" intervention that has been evaluated in a series of double-blind, randomized experimental trials in high schools and universities (Paunesku et al., 2015). To create rapid internalization of the message, it borrows elements of "wise" interventions, well documented in past research, analogous to the incremental theory intervention described earlier (Walton, 2014; Yeager & Walton, 2011).

The purpose for learning intervention begins by asking adolescents to reflect on social issues that matter most to them or on people about whom they care. Next, the purpose for learning intervention seeks to channel this social-justice reactance into a desire to learn deeply from schoolwork on a daily basis. It presents survey statistics to adolescents, explaining to them that many students like themselves desire to learn, so that they can make a difference—not just so that they can achieve self-oriented ends. Second, the intervention presents stories from upperclassmen who describe their mixture of self-oriented and self-transcendent motives for learning. Finally, adolescents engage in self-persuasion writing exercises.

In an initial study conducted with over 400 ninth-grade students at one high school, a one-time exposure to the purpose for learning intervention in the spring semester improved grade point averages for all students at the end of the semester by approximately .10 grade points; for students who had previously earned low grades, the benefit was twice as large (Yeager, Henderson, et al., 2014). In another study conducted with over 1,500 students in a number of high schools across the country (Paunesku et al., 2015), these effects were replicated. The purpose for learning intervention's effect sizes were comparable to the growth mindset of intelligence effect sizes (Paunesku et al., 2015).

PULLING IT ALL TOGETHER: LEARNING FROM "BRIGHT SPOTS"

Is it possible to create environments that honor *all* of adolescents' developmental sensitivities simultaneously? Research has not directly addressed this. Yet psychologists may begin to learn how to do this from an analysis of "bright spots" (Heath & Heath, 2010). Some educational settings demonstrate the existence of a rare possibility: places where adolescents channel their status-relevant affective learning system into a desire to diligently improve their academic skills.

One such bright spot is EL Education schools (formerly, Expeditionary Learning). EL is a network that provides professional development and support to public schools in low-income neighborhoods in the United States. These schools are successful at creating a rare desire for learning that also translates into higher test scores and graduation rates when compared to analogous schools that serve similar student populations (UMASS Donahue Institute, 2011).

EL schools do not typically ask adolescents to participate in "the big wait" (Allen & Allen, 2010). Assignments in school are frequently connected to a thematic unit—an "expedition"—that has as its core the possibility of learning something that can make a difference in the world beyond the self right away. Students are members of meaningful social groups or "crews" that engage in these expeditions together. Students then acquire the intellectual skills they need to discover new insights, so that they can address these meaningful topics. Expeditions end in public presentations—to the school, to family, and ultimately to local government officials or other leaders. The principles of this education model very clearly reflect the adolescent developmental needs summarized earlier: "real-world curriculum," "respectful culture," "self-discovery," "responsibility for learning," "solitude and reflection," and "service and compassion" (*www.eleducation.org*). These kinds of changes—which represent much of what appears in the right column in Table 23.1—may well ward off the trends observed in Figure 23.1.

Consistent with the idea that this model honors adolescents' desire to be respected—and that doing so can improve motivation—EL schools improve the academic achievement and intrinsic motivation of students who have the most reason to feel disrespected: Students who face harmful racial/ethnic or socioeconomic stereotypes about their group. Hence, EL reduces achievement gaps at scale (UMASS Donahue Institute, 2011). Although EL has not isolated the precise psychological variables that account for its success, this "bright spot" (and perhaps many others) may well provide source material for psychology to advance theory and improve practice.

CONCLUSION

Recent advances in developmental science—at neural, endocrine, cognitive, behavioral, and contextual levels of analysis—have led the field to a new set of conceptualizations of what it means to be competent during adolescence. This research has demonstrated contexts in which adolescents appear to be deficient such as when they fail at basic self-control tasks that children can do well, and instead attend to social-emotional stimuli (Casey & Caudle, 2013), or when they endorse riskier choices and greater reward sensitivity following those risky choices (Braams et al., 2015). Yet these same patterns can also be interpreted in another light: that adolescents outperform children and adults in terms of attending to cues that will help them achieve social competence in the their local hierarchies and contexts (Blakemore & Mills, 2014; Crone & Dahl, 2012; Telzer, 2016).

Viewed from the latter perspective, it can be helpful to align long-term outcomes with the very real, immediate social rewards of developing adolescent-specific competence. Experimental manipulations and educational settings that *both* afford the opportunity to win peer or valued adult admiration *and* prepare oneself for the future may show the greatest benefit.

This goes far beyond simple "gamification" of learning. We are not suggesting that boring math programs simply need to provide a way to share one's scores with peers or to dominate an opponent. Instead, we propose that there are deeply human and developmentally sensitized needs for meaningful social relationships. Feelings of respect that go to the heart of what it means to be an adolescent (and an adult, for that matter). We do not believe that superficially triggering social motivation will create the kind of sustained commitment required to develop true intellectual competence. The problems that underlie the trends in Figure 23.1 are much more substantial than that.

But honoring this desire for respect on an authentic level—with respectful relationships and opportunities to earn social status, as in the EL schools model described earlier—may come as a surprising breath of fresh air for adolescents. In that light, in this review we have presented a set of principles that, we hope, may be practically useful for the design of motivating instructional environments. With time, it may be possible to slow or even reverse the declines in motivation typically seen across adolescence.

ACKNOWLEDGMENT

Support for this research comes from a scholars award provided by the William T. Grant Foundation.

REFERENCES

Albert, D., Chein, J., & Steinberg, L. (2013). The teenage brain: Peer influences on adolescent decision making. *Current Directions in Psychological Science, 22*(2), 114–120.

Allen, J. P., & Allen, C. W. (2010). The big wait. *Educational Leadership, 68*(1), 22–26.

Allen, J. P., Kuperminc, G., Philliber, S., & Herre, K. (1994). Programmatic prevention of adolescent problem behaviors: The role of autonomy, relatedness, and volunteer service in the Teen Outreach Program. *American Journal of Community Psychology, 22*(5), 595–615.

Allen, J. P., Moore, C. M., & Kuperminc, G. P. (1997). Developmental approaches to understanding adolescent deviance. In S. Luther, J. A. Burack, & D. Cicchetti (Eds.), *Developmental psychopathology: Perspectives on adjustment, risk, and disorder* (pp. 548–567). New York: Cambridge University Press.

Allen, J. P., Pianta, R. C., Gregory, A., Mikami, A. Y., & Lun, J. (2011). An interaction-based approach to enhancing secondary school instruction and student achievement. *Science, 333*, 1034–1037.

Aronson, J. M., Fried, C. B., & Good, C. (2002). Reducing the effects of stereotype threat on African American college students by shaping theories of intelligence. *Journal of Experimental Social Psychology, 38*(2), 113–125.

Bandura, A. (1989). Human agency in social cognitive theory. *American Psychologist, 44*, 1175–1184.

Bargh, J. A., Chen, M., & Burrows, L. (1996). Automaticity of social behavior: Direct effects of trait construct and stereotype activation on action. *Journal of Personality and Social Psychology, 71*(2), 230–244.

Baumeister, R. F., & Leary, M. R. (1995). The need to belong: Desire for interpersonal attachments as a fundamental human motivation. *Psychological Bulletin, 117*(3), 497–529.

Baumeister, R. F., Twenge, J. M., & Nuss, C. K. (2002). Effects of social exclusion on cognitive processes: Anticipated aloneness reduces intelligent thought. *Journal of Personality and Social Psychology, 83*(4), 817–827.

Bell, C. C., & McBride, D. F. (2010). Affect regulation and prevention of risky behaviors. *Journal of the American Medical Association, 304*(5), 565–566.

Benner, A. D. (2011). The transition to high school: Current knowledge, future directions. *Educational Psychology Review, 23*(3), 299–328.

Blackwell, L. S., Trzesniewski, K. H., & Dweck, C. S. (2007). Implicit theories of intelligence predict achievement across an adolescent transition: A longitudinal study and an intervention. *Child Development, 78*(1), 246–263.

Blakemore, S.-J. (2010). The developing social brain: Implications for education. *Neuron, 65*(6), 744–747.

Blakemore, S.-J., & Mills, K. L. (2014). Is adolescence a sensitive period for sociocultural processing? *Annual Review of Psychology, 65*, 187–207.

Braams, B. R., van Duijvenvoorde, A. C. K., Peper, J. S., & Crone, E. A. (2015). Longitudinal changes in adolescent risk-taking: A comprehensive study of neural responses to rewards, pubertal development, and risk-taking behavior. *Journal of Neuroscience, 35*(18), 7226–7238.

Burnett, S., Bird, G., Moll, J., Frith, C., & Blakemore, S.-J. (2009). Development during adolescence of the neural processing of social emotion. *Journal of Cognitive Neuroscience, 21*(9), 1736–1750.

Cacioppo, J. T., & Patrick, B. (2008). *Loneliness: Human nature and the need for social connection.* New York: Norton.

Casey, B. J., & Caudle, K. (2013). The teenage brain: Self control. *Current Directions in Psychological Science, 22*(2), 82–87.

Casey, B. J., Jones, R. M., & Somerville, L. H. (2011). Braking and accelerating of the adolescent brain. *Journal of Research on Adolescence, 21*(1), 21–33.

Chein, J., Albert, D., O'Brien, L., Uckert, K., & Steinberg, L. (2011). Peers increase adolescent risk taking by enhancing activity in the brain's reward circuitry. *Developmental Science, 14*(2), 1–10.

Cheryan, S., Plaut, V. C., Davies, P. G., & Steele, C. M. (2009). Ambient belonging: how stereotypical cues impact gender participation in computer science. *Journal of Personality and Social Psychology, 97*(6), 1045–1060.

Cohen, G. L., & Prinstein, M. J. (2006). Peer contagion of aggression and health risk behavior among adolescent males: An experimental investigation of effects on public conduct and private attitudes. *Child Development, 77*(4), 967–983.

Cohen, G. L., & Sherman, D. K. (2014). The psychology of change: Self-affirmation and social psychological intervention. *Annual Review of Psychology, 65*(1), 333–371.

Cohen, G. L., & Steele, C. M. (2002). A barrier of mistrust: How negative stereotypes affect cross-race mentoring. In J. M. Aronson (Ed.), *Improving academic achievement: Impact of psychological factors on education* (pp. 303–327). Bingley, UK: Emerald Group.

Cohen, G. L., Steele, C. M., & Ross, L. D. (1999). The mentor's dilemma: Providing critical feedback across the racial divide. *Personality and Social Psychology Bulletin, 25*(10), 1302–1318.

Coleman, J. S. (1961). *The adolescent society.* New York: Free Press of Glencoe.

Crone, E. A., & Dahl, R. E. (2012). Understanding adolescence as a period of social–affective engagement and goal flexibility. *Nature Reviews Neuroscience, 13*(9), 636–650.

Crosnoe, R. (2011). *Fitting in, standing out: Navigating the social challenges of high school to get an education.* New York: Cambridge University Press.

Crosnoe, R., & Johnson, M. K. (2011). Research on adolescence in the twenty-first century. *Annual Review of Sociology, 37*(1), 439–460.

Crosnoe, R., & McNeely, C. (2008). Peer relations, adolescent behavior, and public health research and practice. *Family and Community Health, 31*(18), 71–80.

Dahl, R. E. (2001). Affect regulation, brain development, and behavioral/emotional health in adolescence. *CNS Spectrums, 6*(1), 60–72.

Dahl, R. E., & Vanderschuren, L. J. (2011). The feeling of motivation in the developing brain. *Developmental Cognitive Neuroscience, 1*(4), 361–363.

Damon, W., Menon, J., & Bronk, K. C. (2003). The development of purpose during adolescence. *Applied Developmental Science, 7*(3), 119–128.

Deci, E. L. (1975). *Intrinsic motivation.* New York: Plenum Press.

Deci, E. L., & Ryan, R. M. (1985). The general causality orientations scale: Self-determination in personality. *Journal of Research in Personality, 19*(2), 109–134.

DeWall, C. N., Maner, J. K., & Rouby, D. A. (2009). Social exclusion and early-stage interpersonal perception: Selective attention to signs of acceptance. *Journal of Personality and Social Psychology, 96*(4), 729–741.

Dweck, C. S. (2006). *Mindset: The new psychology of success.* New York: Random House.

Dweck, C. S., Chiu, C., & Hong, Y. (1995). Implicit theories and their role in judgments and reactions: A world from two perspectives. *Psychological Inquiry, 6*(4), 267–285.

Eccles, J. S., Lord, S., & Midgley, C. (1991). What are we doing to early adolescents?: The impact of educational contexts on early adolescents. *American Journal of Education, 99*(4), 521–521.

Eisenegger, C., Haushofer, J., & Fehr, E. (2011). The role of testosterone in social interaction. *Trends in Cognitive Sciences, 15*(6), 263–271.

Eisenegger, C., Naef, M., Snozzi, R., Heinrichs, M., & Fehr, E. (2010). Prejudice and truth about the effect of testosterone on human bargaining behaviour. *Nature, 463*, 356–359.

Elliot, A. J., & Dweck, C. S. (Eds.). (2005). *Handbook of competence and motivation.* New York: Guilford Press.

Ellis, B. J., Del Giudice, M., Dishion, T. J., Figueredo, A. J., Gray, P., Griskevicius, V., et al. (2012). The evolutionary basis of risky adolescent behavior: Implications for science, policy, and practice. *Developmental Psychology, 48*(3), 598–623.

Erikson, E. (1968). *Identity: Youth and crisis.* Oxford, UK: Norton.

Furtak, E. M., & Kunter, M. (2012). Effects of autonomy-supportive teaching on student learning and motivation. *Journal of Experimental Education, 80*(3), 284–316.

Garcia, J., & Cohen, G. L. (2012). A social psychological perspective to educational intervention. In E. Shafir (Ed.), *Behavioral foundations of public policy* (pp. 329–347). Princeton, NJ: Princeton University Press.

Goddings, A., Burnett Heyes, S., Bird, G., Viner, R. M., & Blakemore, S. (2012). The relationship between puberty and social emotion processing. *Developmental Science, 15*(6), 801–811.

Good, C., Aronson, J., & Inzlicht, M. (2003). Improving adolescents' standardized test performance: An intervention to reduce the effects of stereotype threat. *Journal of Applied Developmental Psychology, 24*(6), 645–662.

Gottfried, A. E., Fleming, J. S., & Gottfried, A. W. (2001). Continuity of academic intrinsic motivation from childhood through late adolescence: A longitudinal study. *Journal of Educational Psychology, 93*(1), 3–13.

Greenough, W. T., & Black, J. E. (1992). Induction of brain structure by experience:

Substrates for cognitive development. In M. R. Gunnar & C. A. Nelson (Eds.), *Developmental behavioral neuroscience* (Vol. 24, pp. 155–200). Hillsdale, NJ: Erlbaum.

Gregory, A., & Ripski, M. B. (2008). Adolescent trust in teachers: Implications for behavior in the high school classroom. *School Psychology Review, 37*(3), 337–353.

Gregory, A., & Weinstein, R. S. (2008). The discipline gap and African Americans: Defiance or cooperation in the high school classroom. *Journal of School Psychology, 46*(4), 455–475.

Gunnar, M. R., Wewerka, S., Frenn, K., Long, J. D., & Griggs, C. (2009). Developmental changes in hypothalamus–pituitary–adrenal activity over the transition to adolescence: Normative changes and associations with puberty. *Development and Psychopathology, 21*(1), 69–85.

Hauser, T. U., Iannaccone, R., Walitza, S., Brandeis, D., & Brem, S. (2015). Cognitive flexibility in adolescence: Neural and behavioral mechanisms of reward prediction error processing in adaptive decision making during development. *NeuroImage, 104*, 347–354.

Heath, C., & Heath, D. (2010). *Switch: How to change things when change is hard*. New York: Broadway Books.

Helms, S. W., Choukas-Bradley, S., Widman, L., Giletta, M., Cohen, G. L., & Prinstein, M. J. (2014). Adolescents misperceive and are influenced by high-status peers' health risk, deviant, and adaptive behavior. *Developmental Psychology, 50*(12), 2697–2714.

Hodgins, H. S., Weibust, K. S., Weinstein, N., Shiffman, S., Miller, A., Coombs, G., et al. (2010). The cost of self-protection: Threat response and performance as a function of autonomous and controlled motivations. *Personality and Social Psychology Bulletin, 36*(8), 1101–1114.

Hodgins, H. S., Yacko, H. A., & Gottlieb, E. (2006). Autonomy and nondefensiveness. *Motivation and Emotion, 30*(4), 283–293.

Hurd, N. M., Sánchez, B., Zimmerman, M. A., & Caldwell, C. H. (2012). Natural mentors, racial identity, and educational attainment among African American adolescents: Exploring pathways to success. *Child Development, 83*(4), 1196–1212.

Jacobs, J. E., Lanza, S., Osgood, D. W., Eccles, J. S., & Wigfield, A. (2002). Changes in children's self-competence and values: Gender and domain differences across grades one through twelve. *Child Development, 73*(2), 509–527.

Johnson, S. B., Blum, R. W., & Giedd, J. N. (2009). Adolescent maturity and the brain: The promise and pitfalls of neuroscience research in adolescent health policy. *Journal of Adolescent Health, 45*(3), 216–221.

Kann, L., Kinchen, S., Shanklin, S. L., Flint, K. H., Kawkins, J., Harris, W. A., et al. (2014). Youth risk behavior surveillance—United States, 2013. *Morbidity and Mortality Weekly Report, 63*(4), 1–168.

Klapwijk, E. T., Goddings, A.-L., Heyes, S. B., Bird, G., Viner, R. M., & Blakemore, S.-J. (2013). Increased functional connectivity with puberty in the mentalising network involved in social emotion processing. *Hormones and Behavior, 64*(2), 314–322.

Larson, R., & Richards, M. H. (1991). Daily companionship in late childhood and early adolescence: Changing developmental contexts. *Child Development, 62*(2), 284–300.

Lazowski, R. A., & Hulleman, C. S. (2015). Motivation interventions in education: A meta-analytic review. *Review of Educational Research*. [Epub ahead of print]

Leary, M. R. (2004). The function of self-esteem in terror management theory and sociometer theory: Comment on Pyszczynski et al. (2004). *Psychological Bulletin, 130*, 478–482.

Lee, K. H., Siegle, G. J., Dahl, R. E., Hooley, J. M., & Silk, J. S. (2014). Neural responses to maternal criticism in healthy youth. *Social Cognitive and Affective Neuroscience, 10*(7), 902–912.

Marshall, S. K. (2001). Do I matter?: Construct validation of adolescents' perceived mattering to parents and friends. *Journal of Adolescence, 24*(4), 473–490.

McKown, C., & Weinstein, R. S. (2003). The development and consequences of stereotype consciousness in middle childhood. *Child Development, 74*(2), 498–515.

Mueller, C. M., & Dweck, C. S. (1998). Praise for intelligence can undermine children's motivation and performance. *Journal of Personality and Social Psychology, 75*(1), 33–52.

Murphy, M. C., Steele, C. M., & Gross, J. J. (2007). Signaling threat how situational cues affect women in math, science, and engineering settings. *Psychological Science, 18*(10), 879–885.

Murray-Close, D. (2013). Psychophysiology of adolescent peer relations: I. Theory and research findings. *Journal of Research on Adolescence, 23*(2), 236–259.

Oudekerk, B. A., Allen, J. P., Hessel, E. T., & Molloy, L. E. (2015). The cascading development of autonomy and relatedness from adolescence to adulthood. *Child Development, 86*(2), 472–485.

Paluck, E. L., & Shepherd, H. (2012). The salience of social referents: A field experiment on collective norms and harassment behavior in a school social network. *Journal of Personality and Social Psychology, 103*(6), 899–915.

Paunesku, D., Walton, G. M., Romero, C., Smith, E. N., Yeager, D. S., & Dweck, C. S. (2015). Mindset interventions are a scalable treatment for academic underachievement. *Psychological Science, 26*(6), 284–293.

Peper, J. S., & Dahl, R. E. (2013). The teenage brain: Surging hormones—brain–behavior interactions during puberty. *Current Directions in Psychological Science, 22*(2), 134–139.

Philliber, S., & Allen, J. P. (1992). Life options and community service: Teen Outreach Program. In B. C. Miller, J. J. Card, R. L. Paikoff, & J. L. Peterson (Eds.), *Preventing adolescent pregnancy: Model programs and evaluations* (pp. 139–155). Newbury Park, CA: Sage.

Reeve, J. (2009). Why teachers adopt a controlling motivating style toward students and how they can become more autonomy supportive. *Educational Psychologist, 44*(3), 159–175.

Reis, H. T. (1994). Domains of experience: Investigating relationship processes from three perspectives. In R. Erber & R. Gilmour (Eds.), *Theoretical frameworks for personal relationships* (pp. 87–110). Hillsdale, NJ: Erlbaum.

Reis, H. T., Sheldon, K. M., Gable, S. L., Roscoe, J., & Ryan, R. M. (2000). Daily well-being: The role of autonomy, competence, and relatedness. *Personality and Social Psychology Bulletin, 26*(4), 419–435.

Research Now. (2012). *Math relevance to U.S. middle school students: A survey commissioned by Raytheon Company*. New York: Author.

Robinson, T. N. (2010). Save the world, prevent obesity: Piggybacking on existing social and ideological movements. *Obesity, 18*(S1), 17–22.

Rowe, R., Maughan, B., Worthman, C. M., Costello, E. J., & Angold, A. (2004). Testosterone, antisocial behavior, and social dominance in boys: Pubertal development and biosocial interaction. *Biological Psychiatry, 55*(5), 546–552.

Ryan, R. M., & Deci, E. L. (2000). Self-determination theory and the facilitation of intrinsic motivation, social development, and well-being. *American Psychologist, 55*(1), 68–78.

Schwartz, K. (2015, December 21). Harnessing the incredible learning potential of the adolescent brain. Retrieved December 30, 2015, from *http://ww2.kqed.org/mindshift/2015/12/21/harnessing-the-incredible-learning-potential-of-the-adolescent-brain*.

Sebastian, C., Viding, E., Williams, K. D., & Blakemore, S.-J. (2010). Social brain development and the affective consequences of ostracism in adolescence. *Brain and Cognition, 72*(1), 134–145.

Shouse, R. C. (1996). Academic press and sense of community: Conflict, congruence, and implications for student achievement. *Social Psychology of Education, 1*(1), 47–68.

Somerville, L. H. (2013). The teenage brain: Sensitivity to social evaluation. *Current Directions in Psychological Science, 22*(2), 121–127.

Spielberg, J. M., Olino, T. M., Forbes, E. E., & Dahl, R. E. (2014). Exciting fear in adolescence: Does pubertal development alter threat processing? *Developmental Cognitive Neuroscience, 8*, 86–95.

Steele, C. M. (2011). *Whistling Vivaldi: How stereotypes affect us and what we can do*. New York: Norton.

Steinberg, L. (2014). *Age of opportunity: Lessons from the new science of adolescence*. Boston: Houghton Mifflin Harcourt.

Steinberg, L. (2015). How to improve the health of American adolescents. *Perspectives on Psychological Science, 10*(6), 711–715.

Steinberg, L., & Silverberg, S. B. (1986). The vicissitudes of autonomy in early adolescence. *Child Development, 57*(4), 841–851.

Stillman, T. F., & Baumeister, R. F. (2009). Uncertainty, belongingness, and four needs for meaning. *Psychological Inquiry, 20*(4), 249–251.

Telzer, E. H. (2016). Dopaminergic reward sensitivity can promote adolescent health: A new perspective on the mechanism of ventral striatum activation. *Developmental Cognitive Neuroscience, 17*, 57–67.

Telzer, E. H., Fuligni, A. J., Lieberman, M. D., & Galván, A. (2014). Neural sensitivity to eudaimonic and hedonic rewards differentially predict adolescent depressive symptoms over time. *Proceedings of the National Academy of Sciences USA, 111*(18), 6600–6605.

Terburg, D., & van Honk, J. (2013). Approach–avoidance versus dominance–submissiveness: A multilevel neural framework on how testosterone promotes social status. *Emotion Review, 5*(3), 296–302.

Thapar, A., Collishaw, S., Pine, D. S., & Thapar, A. K. (2012). Depression in adolescence. *The Lancet, 379*, 1056–1067.

Treisman, U. (1992). Studying students studying calculus: A look at the lives of minority mathematics students in college. *College Mathematics Journal, 23*(5), 362–372.

UMASS Donahue Institute. (2011). *Expeditionary learning: Analysis of impact on achievement gaps*. Hadley, MA: Author.

Vallerand, R. J., Fortier, M. S., & Guay, F. (1997). Self-determination and persistence in a real-life setting: Toward a motivational model of high school dropout. *Journal of Personality and Social Psychology, 72*(5), 1161–1176.

Vansteenkiste, M., Simons, J., Lens, W., Sheldon, K. M., & Deci, E. L. (2004). Motivating learning, performance, and persistence: The synergistic effects of intrinsic goal contents and autonomy-supportive contexts. *Journal of Personality and Social Psychology, 87*(2), 246–260.

Vansteenkiste, M., Simons, J., Lens, W., Soenens, B., & Matos, L. (2005). Examining the motivational impact of intrinsic versus extrinsic goal framing and autonomy-supportive versus internally controlling communication style on early adolescents' academic achievement. *Child Development, 76*(2), 483–501.

Wallace, T. L., Sung, H. C., & Williams, J. D. (2014). The defining features of teacher talk within autonomy-supportive classroom management. *Teaching and Teacher Education, 42*, 34–46.

Walton, G. M. (2014). The new science of wise psychological interventions. *Current Directions in Psychological Science, 23*(1), 73–82.

Walton, G. M., Cohen, G. L., Cwir, D., & Spencer, S. J. (2012). Mere belonging: The power of social connections. *Journal of Personality and Social Psychology, 102*(3), 513–532.

Wentzel, K. R. (1998). Social relationships and motivation in middle school: The role of parents, teachers, and peers. *Journal of Educational Psychology, 90*(2), 202–209.

Wigfield, A., & Wagner, L. A. (2005). Competence, motivation, and identity development during adolescence. In A. J. Elliot & C. S. Dweck (Eds.), *Handbook of competence and motivation* (pp. 222–239). New York: Guilford Press.

Williams, G. C., Minicucci, D. S., Kouides, R. W., Levesque, C. S., Chirkov, V. I., Ryan, R. M., et al. (2002). Self-determination, smoking, diet and health. *Health Education Research, 17*(5), 512–521.

Williams, G. C., Niemiec, C. P., Patrick, H., Ryan, R. M., & Deci, E. L. (2009). The importance of supporting autonomy and perceived competence in facilitating long-term tobacco abstinence. *Annals of Behavioral Medicine, 37*(3), 315–324.

Williams, G. C., Rodin, G. C., Ryan, R. M., Grolnick, W. S., & Deci, E. L. (1998). Autonomous regulation and long-term medication adherence in adult outpatients. *Health Psychology, 17*(3), 269–276.

Williams, K. D. (2009). Ostracism: A temporal need-threat model. In M. P. Zanna (Ed.), *Advances in experimental social psychology* (Vol. 41, pp. 275–314). San Diego, CA: Academic Press.

Wilson, T. D. (2011). *Redirect: The surprising new science of psychological change.* London: Penguin.

Yeager, D. S., & Bundick, M. J. (2009). The role of purposeful work goals in promoting meaning in life and in schoolwork. *Journal of Adolescent Research, 24*(4), 423–452.

Yeager, D. S., Dahl, R., & Dweck, C. S. (2016). *The adolescent paradox: Is adolescence the best time or the worst time for creating behavior change?* Manuscript submitted for publication.

Yeager, D. S., & Dweck, C. S. (2012). Mindsets that promote resilience: When students believe that personal characteristics can be developed. *Educational Psychologist, 47*(4), 302–314.

Yeager, D. S., Henderson, M. D., Paunesku, D., Walton, G. M., D'Mello, S., Spitzer, B. J., et al. (2014). Boring but important: A self-transcendent purpose for learning fosters academic self-regulation. *Journal of Personality and Social Psychology, 107*(4), 559–580.

Yeager, D. S., Johnson, R., Spitzer, B. J., Trzesniewski, K. H., Powers, J., & Dweck, C. S. (2014). The far-reaching effects of believing people can change: Implicit theories of personality shape stress, health, and achievement during adolescence. *Journal of Personality and Social Psychology, 106*(6), 867–884.

Yeager, D. S., Lee, H. Y., & Jamieson, J. P. (2016). How to improve adolescent stress responses: Insights from integrating implicit theories of personality and biopsychosocial models. *Psychological Science, 27*(8), 1078–1091.

Yeager, D. S., Purdie-Vaughns, V., Garcia, J., Apfel, N., Brzustoski, P., Master, A., et al. (2014). Breaking the cycle of mistrust: Wise interventions to provide critical feedback across the racial divide. *Journal of Experimental Psychology: General, 143*(2), 804–824.

Yeager, D. S., Trzesniewski, K. H., & Dweck, C. S. (2013). An implicit theories of personality intervention reduces adolescent aggression in response to victimization and exclusion. *Child Development, 84*(3), 970–988.

Yeager, D. S., Trzesniewski, K. H., Tirri, K., Nokelainen, P., & Dweck, C. S. (2011). Adolescents' implicit theories predict desire for vengeance after peer conflicts: Correlational and experimental evidence. *Developmental Psychology, 47*(4), 1090–1107.

Yeager, D. S., & Walton, G. M. (2011). Social-psychological interventions in education: They're not magic. *Review of Educational Research, 81*(2), 267–301.

CHAPTER 24

Competence and Motivation at Work throughout Adulthood
Making the Most of Changing Capacities and Opportunities

JUTTA HECKHAUSEN
JACOB SHANE
RUTH KANFER

This chapter integrates existing theoretical and empirical work, and proposes a model of lifespan changes in individuals' work lives, their motivational challenges, and how individuals can master these challenges. In the first edition of the *Handbook of Competence and Motivation,* the chapter "Competence and Motivation in Adulthood and Old Age" addressed competence development and motivation during adulthood generally, and applied the motivational theory of lifespan development to conceptualize the motivational challenges and adaptive responses to age-related changes in competence (Heckhausen, 2005). This new chapter has a similar agenda but focuses more closely on what this means for competence development and motivation in the work domain. Throughout the chapter we pay greater attention to the challenges people encounter at different ages and stages of their careers, and how they master these challenges, than to trait-based individual differences in motivational processes involved in work (e.g., interests in work area, implicit achievement motive; for trait-based research, see Kanfer & Ackerman, 2005).

The importance of competence in one's worklife for human adjustment and well-being is widely recognized. Most humans spend a large part of their waking hours at work for most of their adult lifespan. Thriving versus floundering in one's worklife has both proximal and long-term consequences for economic well-being (Halpern-Manners, Warren, Raymo, & Nicholson, 2015), social status (McFadyen, 1998), work–family conflict (Michel, Kotrba, Mitchelson, Clark, & Baltes, 2011), family members (Lim & Sng, 2006; Zhao, Lim, & Teo, 2012), physical and mental health (Burgard, Brand, & House, 2009; McKee-Ryan, Song, Wanberg, & Kinicki, 2005), and even personality (Boyce, Wood, Daly, & Sedikides, 2015).

We suggest that competence and motivation in worklife across the adult lifespan can be best understood in terms of an individual's career progress and success in accomplishing career goals. Objective measures of career success typically refer to achievements across a series of related jobs within a specific industry, sector, or organization. While measures of objective career success typically include elements such as salary progression, pay raises, or promotions, subjective indices of career success refer to satisfaction with career advancement, salary increases, or career development. In this chapter we examine the relationship between competence and motivation in the pursuit of work and career goals that unfold over adulthood and may span anywhere from a few years to multiple decades of adult life.

We use the *motivational theory of lifespan development* (MTD; Heckhausen, Wrosch, & Schulz, 2010), as a conceptual framework to address the following questions:

1. What are the changes in work-related competencies (i.e., skills and abilities) across adulthood and in old age?
2. How do societies and its institutions set up age-graded action fields (i.e., opportunities for and constraints to individual agency) for career promotions, plateaus, and declines?
3. Under which conditions are motivation and competence congruent or incongruent?
4. How can individuals assess the opportunities and constraints and select career goals accordingly?
5. Which strategies of motivation and self-regulation are most effective for goal attainment and in response to mismatches between work competence and the demands and opportunities at work?
6. Under which conditions do individual differences in the motivation to enhance one's competence development (e.g., by additional training or education) make a difference in career development and employment?

We discuss these phenomena as challenges to the individual's developmental regulation, and we provide specific examples of these challenges by using a broad range of careers and career trajectories across adulthood into old age.

AGE-RELATED CHANGE IN CONTROL POTENTIAL ACROSS ADULTHOOD

Growth or decline in one's worklife is a function of two partly interrelated life-course trajectories: the maturation, growth, peaking, and decline of an individual's skills, knowledge, and capabilities on the one hand (see section on competence change in adulthood and old age), and the social structuring of age-graded opportunities and constraints in occupational or professional careers across the adult lifespan on the other (see section on societal opportunities and constraints at different career stages). In other words, it is about what an individual *can do* (i.e., competence) and what the public or private institutions employing the individual will *let him or her do* (i.e., opportunities) at different times of life. Combined, these components set the stage for the individual's career and competence development, and pose specific challenges for individual motivation and self-regulation, depending on the congruence between individual capacities and institutional expectations, opportunities, and constraints.

Change in Ability-Related Competencies across Adulthood

Work activities in different careers are composed of various cognitive and physical domains of competence. Physical and cognitive performance generally follows a trajectory of first exponential growth, then exponential decline, with age of peak function varying across domains (Berthelot et al., 2011). Occupations that rely on high-level physical functioning typically follow competence-trajectories with steep increases, steep decreases, and narrow and relatively early peaks. Coinciding with this, physical work capacity declines by about 20% between ages 40 and 60 years, mosty due to decreases in musculoskeletal and aerobic capacity (Kenny Yarley, Martineau, & Jay, 2008). Examples of careers that require exteme physical fitness are athletic excellence and world-class performances (Ericsson, 1990; Schulz & Curnow, 1988), which have performance peaks at early ages that typically only last for a narrow age window.

Age trajectories of such extremely high competencies reflect early benchmarks for constraints due to biological changes associated with aging. These early declines do not impair performances in most common everyday activities in work, family, and leisure. Older workers can perform as well as younger workers in most common work activities, especially if they are allowed to use their own strategies and resources, and are given ample time to complete the activity (Jeske, & Stamov Roßnagel, 2015; Ng & Feldman, 2012; Salthouse, 2012).

With regard to regular cognitive functioning (e.g., intelligence tests), decline in performance is typically restricted to fluid intellectual skills (e.g., memorizing nouns, mental rotation) that have fallen out of practice, whereas crystallized abilities (i.e., factual and procedural knowledge) remain stable into old age. Recent research in cognitive aging has uncovered a more complex picture of multiple competence dimensions and multiple trajectories reminiscent of what Paul Baltes (1987) and other lifespan scholars refer to as *multidimensionality* and *multidirectionality*. Hartshorne and Germine (2015), using reanalyses of published test data and very large online-based studies comprising some 44,000 participants, showed that age-timing of growth and decline in cognitive subcompetencies varies widely between competence peaks in late adolescence (e.g., recalling word pairs) and the mid-50s (e.g., vocabulary). The authors conclude that "not only is there no age at which humans are performing at peak on all cognitive tasks, there may not be an age at which humans' performance peak on *most* cognitive tasks" (p. 440, original emphasis).

However, age-differences in fluid cognitive abilities do become noticeable in two types of challenging situations. The first such situation is the acquisition of new skills that require strong fluid capacities (e.g., learning computer code, online mental tracking of complex processes, financial analysts, reading music), especially under time constraints. Meta-analytic studies indicate that although middle-age and older workers do as well as younger workers on most relevant facets of job performance, older workers perform less well in structured training and development programs, learn less new knowledge, particularly when it involves new technology, and take longer to reach criterion levels of performance (Kubeck, Delp, Haslett, & McDaniel, 1996; Ng & Feldman, 2012, 2013). Part of this decline in capacity for learning new and complex information and processes is likely due to the well-documented decrease in working memory capacity in older adults (Oberauer, Wendland, & Kliegl, 2003; Salthouse, 2004).

Cognitive aging also has negative effects on competence when new learning and more complex and coordinated cognitive processing relying on high-capacity information processing are required (Kliegl, Smith, & Baltes, 1989; Salthouse, 2004). Some researchers have called this the age × complexity hypothesis (McDaniel, Pesta, & Banks, 2012; Salthouse, 2004), with complexity denoting the speed of processing and working memory capacity. An example of the latter is any kind of multiple cognitive demand, such as driving while speaking on the phone or monitoring multiple processes or people simultaneously. Age-related competence detriments can be expected in these complex professions that involve a high level of developed expertise only achieved by those who invest extensively in deliberate practice over long periods of time (Ericsson, 2004).

The second situation in which age-differences in fluid cognitive abilities become noticeable is during multitasking. Research in cognitive aging using dual-task paradigms has uncovered drastic declines in multitask performance during early midlife (Li, Lindenberger, Freund, & Baltes, 2001; Lindenberger, Marsiske, & Baltes, 2000), but also uncovered specific strategies used by younger and older adults when trying to maintain reasonable performance levels in either task (Kemper, Herman, & Lian, 2003). These aging-related declines in multitasking are influenced by coinciding decreases in working memory capacity (Oberauer et al., 2003). Examples of work activities that are reliant on multitasking include driving and talking (e.g., taxi driver), monitoring multiple moving objects (e.g., air traffic controller, cook), and directing or responding to groups of diversely acting individuals (e.g., teacher, nurse, waiter, front-line supervisor). Air traffic controllers face unique challenges with monitoring and directing multiple moving aircraft under continuously and interdependently changing conditions that require complex imagery and prediction of interrelated processes. Reviewing an extensive literature on age differences in air traffic controllers, Salthouse (2012) concludes that the cognitive abilities involved in this profession exhibit strong normative, age-related decline prior to the mandatory retirement at age 56.

Training and practice effects can further mitigate the effect of individuals' fluid cognitive decline on their work capacity. Up to very old age, fluid skills can be reactivated to levels comparable to those of younger adults through instruction and minimal practice (Baltes, Dittman-Kohli, & Kliegl, 1986; Baltes, Sowarka, & Kliegl, 1989). Moreover, older adults can acquire new fluid skills (e.g., memory for nouns, names) and attain levels of performance comparable to those of young adults (Baltes et al., 1986; Baltes & Kliegl, 1992; Baltes & Lindenberger, 1988). For instance, research on memory performance using the method of loci (i.e., associating memory items with locations on a preset route by forming vivid mental images) indicates that after some practice, older adults' memory performance becomes comparable to that of their younger adult counterparts. It is only when time constraints (i.e., shortened presentation interval) and cognitive load (i.e., interference from previous lists) are pushed to the limit that older adults' performance falls short of younger adults' performance (Mayr & Kliegl, 1993; Mayr, Kliegl, & Krampe, 1996). However, in adults age 80 years and older, memory training using the method of loci produced only modest performance gains immediately after training that were not further enhanced by practice (Singer, Lindenberger, & Baltes, 2003). These decreases in experimentally induced cognitive plasticity mirrors declines in perceptual speed, memory and fluency found in a population of German older adults, with the old-old segment of this sample showing the steepest decline (Singer, Verhaeghen, Ghisletta, Lindenberger, & Baltes, 2003). Moreover, even factual knowledge, a stable and age-resilient crystallized intellectual ability, showed decline in participants older than 90 years of age. Thus, cognitive decline is more general and the plasticity of fluid skills appears to fade away in very advanced old age.

For most practical purposes, older adults do not experience a decline in cognitive functioning until very advanced old age. Older adults can use their extensive factual and procedural knowledge effectively in situations that require expertise-relevant and/or overlearned responses (see Kliegl, Krampe, & Mayr, 2003), allowing them to compensate for process-dependent losses in the effectiveness of episodic and working memory. Basic general cognitive processes show relatively few aging effects, and those can be compensated for by increased time investment and focus (see, e.g., research on aging, high-level experts; Charness & Tuffiash, 2008; Horton, Baker, & Shorer, 2008).

These findings are mirrored in the literature on age differences in work performance (Salthouse, 2012). While this literature is limited by the dearth of studies on older adults, the inherent selectivity effects in older workers and professionals, and weaknesses regarding performance indicators (e.g., supervisor ratings), several meta-analyses have shown no significant associations between age and job performance (e.g., Davies & Sparrow, 1988; McEvoy & Cascio, 1989; Sturman, 2003). Salthouse (2012) provides four explanations for this lack of age differences in job performance studies: (1) individual workers and professionals seldom having to perform at their maximum capacity; (2) the shift from novel problem solving to reliance on known solutions; (3) the growth of other factors besides cognition with age (e.g., conscientiousness, motivation); and (4) the use of accommodation strategies, such as avoiding high-speed and multitask situations by shifting to other activities, positions, or jobs. We elaborate on potential factors regarding the second, third, and fourth explanations in the section "Application of the MTD to Changing Career-Related Challenges across Adulthood and into Old Age."

Job-relevant domain knowledge can also offset age-related decline in fluid intellectual abilities (Ackerman, 1996, 2014; Ackerman & Rolfhus, 1999; Beier & Ackerman, 2003, 2005). According to PPIK (Intelligence as Process, Personality, Interests and Knowledge) theory (Ackerman, 1996), individuals build domain knowledge during adolescence and early adulthood as a function of personality, interest, and motivational factors that form trait complexes supporting domain-specific learning. Four such trait complexes have been identified in numerous studies (Ackerman, 2000; Ackerman, Bowen, Beier,

& Kanfer, 2001; Ackerman & Rolfhus, 1999; Beier & Ackerman, 2001, 2003; see review in Kanfer & Ackerman, 2005): (1) *social trait complex* (e.g., enterprising, possessing social interests, extraversion, social potency, and well-being, but neutral relation to intelligence); (2) *clerical/conventional trait complex* (e.g., conscientiousness, traditionalism, perceptual speed, preference for high level of structure in environment, personal organization); (3) *science/math trait complex* (e.g., investigative and realistic interests, self-concept in science, technology, math, high fluid intelligence ability, but no relation to personality traits); (4) *intellectual/cultural trait complex* (e.g., investigative interests, crystallized intelligence, educational/experiential knowledge, artistic interests, preference for cultural/educational activities, personality trait of openness to experience). Consistent with the notion that novel problem solving is more difficult than recall of previously learned knowledge, older workers who have developed deep and broad relevant knowledge in their preferred domain can be expected to maintain work competencies similar to those of younger adults.

In summary, age-related declines in job competencies are rarely found in studies comparing younger and older employees, although such declines in select competencies that place high demands on age-sensitive fluid intellectual short-term memory and reasoning abilities can be observed within individual workers or professionals over time (e.g., Jeske & Stamov Roßnagel, 2015; Ng & Feldman, 2012; Salthouse, 2012). This is due to the large number of individual and institution-based factors that can compensate for age-related decline in specific work-related capacities. Among them are age-related increases in certain maturity-related personality and motive characteristics (e.g., conscientiousness, agreeableness; Caspi, Roberts, & Shiner, 2005; Kooij, De Lange, Jansen, Kanfer, & Dikkers, 2011), compensation by investment in the development of domain knowledge, expertise and automatized skills (Ackerman, 1996), age-sensitive training formats (Carter & Beier, 2010), increased effort and time investment, and reassigning older workers to responsibilities better matched to their strengths

(De Lange, Kooij, & Van der Heijden, 2015; Kooij, Tims, & Kanfer, 2015).

At the beginning of careers, demand–competence gaps can be expected to be largest for those occupations that benefit most from experience and extensive expertise. In these occupations, new employees (usually younger adults) may initially feel overwhelmed, but their competence should improve with training and experience. Those with the steepest learning curves are likely to gain respect from their supervisors and be first in line for career advancements. For older employees at the tail end of career trajectories, demand–competence gaps are most likely to arise under the following conditions: (1) occupations that make strong demands on fluid intellectual abilities and sensory activities, especially under severe time constraints; (2) occupations requiring multitasking that cannot be resolved (automatized) based on job experience; and (3) occupations that involve rapid technology-driven change and require frequent retraining.

Changes in Non-Ability-Related Characteristics across Adulthood

Financial need, improved health, and changing retirement program policies have led many individuals to work later in life, by either delaying retirement from their primary career or seeking work in a similar or less demanding career following retirement (Kanfer, Beier, & Ackerman, 2013). As the number of older workers grows and age-related workforce diversity increases, organizational psychologists have focused on age-related changes in non-ability-related worker attributes as they affect work motivation and competence (Kanfer & Ackerman, 2004; Kanfer et al., 2013; Super, 1980; Vondracek, Lerner, & Schulenberg, 1983). One area that has received substantial study pertains to age-related changes in work motives. Meta-analytic research findings by Kooij and colleagues (2011) indicate that growth-related work goals (e.g., new learning, promotions) decline with age, but that intrinsic (e.g., performing interesting work, utilizing skills, helping others) and security work goals increased in salience with age. These findings are consistent with lifespan theory and findings that show an age-related decline in gain-oriented goals and an increase in loss-prevention-oriented goals over the lifespan (Ebner, Freund, & Baltes, 2006; Heckhausen, 1997). From a practical perspective, these results suggest that older workers (presumably in later stages of their careers) are more strongly motivated by work opportunities that preserve prior career gains and promote existing skills utilization than are younger adults in earlier stages of their career who are more oriented toward future growth potential.

SOCIETAL AND OCCUPATIONAL OPPORTUNITIES AND CONSTRAINTS AT DIFFERENT CAREER STAGES

Jobs and careers differ in the extent to which they hold developmental and promotional potential, and the degree to which explicit information about these opportunities is provided. Additional differences include the demands of a particular job, the specific role demands, tasks and goals a job entails, and the culture and climate of the given organization in which the work is being performed (for a review, see Kanfer & Ackerman, 2005). Collectively, these opportunities and demands convey to individuals when and for which outcome engagement is warranted, when a deadline for the next promotion is coming closer and what is required to achieve it, how to meet or outperform expectations, and how to counteract or sidestep skill obsolescence by training or changing one's responsibilities. Ideally, individuals' age- and experience-related changes in competence will coincide with their work-related opportunities and demands. However, this convergence can be promoted or undermined by career-specific and workforce-general factors operative during career entry, progression, and exit. A glimpse into these factors can be found in the U.S. Department of Labor classification system, which details the amount of education, experience, and on-the-job training required for career entry and progression in various vocations (National Center for O*NET Development, 2008).

For careers in Job Zone 1 (e.g., cashiers, waiters, cooks, store clerks, cleaners), there are no specific career entry requirements. Promotion prospects in these jobs are largely due to work experience, but opportunities for further advancement past front-line supervisor and management positions are severely limited without additional education or certification. Entry into Job Zone 2 careers (e.g., factory workers, customer service representatives, salespersons) often requires a secondary school degree, in addition to relevant work experience, with competence achieved within a year's worth of on-the-job experience. Similar to Job Zone 1, promotion in Job Zone 2 is generally determined by job tenure and capped at front-line management and supervisor positions. Thus, individuals employed in Job Zones 1 and 2 enjoy a rapid assent to career competence but quickly reach a career plateau. As a result, an individual likely experiences few opportunities to fulfill further competence-related goals at work, necessitating either a career change, or seeking competence growth and fulfillment of the achievement motive through other domains of life.

Many Job Zone 3 occupations are entry-level positions obtained through education, training, and licensing (e.g., electrician, nurse). These vocation-credentialed jobs prolong the time before individuals reach a career plateau; however, opportunities for career advancement typically stagnate well before career exit unless further education is attained. For example, an individual can become a certified nursing assistant (CNA) after as little as 1 month of postsecondary education, and a licensed practical nurse (LPN) after 1 year of postsecondary education. However, at least an associate degree is needed to qualify as a registered nurse (RN), and a master's degree is needed to qualify as an advanced practice registered nurse (APRN). Thus, nursing careers are complementary but bounded from one another by the amount of education and type of licensure needed.

A broad range of careers become available after completing at least a 4-year postsecondary degree, and are generally not directly obtainable from positions in Job Zones 1, 2, or 3 through work experience alone. Teaching, engineering, and many business careers are prominent examples of these Job Zone 4 positions, which delay career entry but allow individuals to continue structured and domain-specific career progressions through middle adulthood. Collectively, Job Zone 4 positions provide opportunities for career advancement well through middle adulthood; however, these opportunities are highly dependent on an individual's own agency for attaining additional education, adapting to changing job demands, and performing well in his or her current position.

For example, teachers' tenure-derived job stability may diminish their motivation for further work-specific competence development. However, the demands of adapting to changing performance measures, students, and new teaching technologies provide opportunities for teachers' continual competence development. In engineering and other jobs that are heavily intertwined with technology, individuals' must adapt to technological changes or risk having their skills and knowledge become obsolete. This is pronounced when the job is dependent on high levels of technical knowledge as opposed to more general knowledge (de Grip & Smits, 2012). Many engineers respond to this pressure to keep up with technological changes by attaining graduate degrees in management as opposed to seeking further technical specializations (Srour, Abdul-Malak, Itani, Bakshan, & Sidani, 2013) in order to facilitate the switch to management careers, especially when changes in technology require extensive retooling (Yeh, 2008). In many business careers, attaining advanced educational degrees (e.g., Master of Business Administration [MBA] degree) and passing licensure exams may facilitate individuals' movement from entry-level to management positions. Reflecting the prevailing belief that advanced business degree attainment will open up further doors of career advancement, business is now the most common field for individuals to pursue a master's degree in the United States (National Center for Education Statistics, U.S. Department of Education, 2014), and their attainment tends to have a positive impact on individuals' career progression (Graduate Management Admission Council, 2015).

Other professional careers become available after individuals attain graduate-level education (Job Zone 5 jobs; e.g., lawyer, doctor, or professor). Career entry is often further delayed through additional training, such as the residency requirements for a medical doctor, or the postdoctoral positions common among academics. Even after competence has been established, individuals in these jobs may be required to continue professional development through recertification procedures, such as the continuing education requirements psychologists, physicians, and lawyers must meet for license renewal. These expertise-focused professions also provide informal opportunities for competence development beyond midlife, well into old age (e.g., learn a new procedure, method, or area of study). However, outside of recertification requirements, whether individuals capitalize on their opportunities for further competence development is more dependent on their own motivation than the demands of their job.

Additional opportunities and constraints for competence development exist in all jobs. For example, learning and adapting to the implicit and explicit work demands, day-to-day-tasks, and organizational culture of a new work setting or position are challenging. Other major classes of challenges include (1) learning new technologies and techniques; (2) interacting with different people; (3) potential loss of or reduction in employment; and (4) inability to find a job in one's chosen field. Many of these challenges are increasingly difficult with advancing age. For instance, switching career fields places high demands on individuals' age-diminishing fluid intelligence skills to learn new information and limits their ability to compensate for this added pressure with domain-specific crystalized intelligence (see the earlier section "Age-Related Change in Control Potential across Adulthood and Old Age").

MOTIVATIONAL THEORY OF LIFESPAN DEVELOPMENT

As individuals move into and through adulthood, their competencies undergo changes that are not necessarily coordinated. Individuals typically are not just passive witnesses to their competence changes, but take an active role in them by trying to control their environment and their own development. Here are the major propositions of our MTD framework (Heckhausen et al., 2010), which have important implications for the way in which individuals deal with changes in competence, and in opportunities and constraints in their worklives.

Primacy of Primary Control Striving

Striving to control one's environment is fundamental to human functioning and the prime motivator of human behavior (Heckhausen & Schulz, 1995, 1999; Heckhausen et al., 2010). In order to be most effective in their striving for control, individuals use both behavioral means of goal engagement, by directly addressing the environment (i.e., *primary control*), and cognitive, self-regulatory means of influencing their own emotional responses and motivation (i.e., *secondary control*). These two means of striving for control work hand in hand, but the overall capacity for primary control across domains and the lifespan holds functional primacy. Worklife and career are at the core of many individual's well-being and are a major resource in striving for control itself because they provide access to a wide range of critical resources for effective functioning, such as food, shelter, health care, education, and skills development, and also determine the kinds of activities that occupy the individual's daily life and prospects for improving his or her circumstances.

Lifespan Trajectories of Control Capacity and Control Striving

The MTD proposes that primary control striving is a constant force across the life course (see solid line in Figure 24.1), reflecting individuals' constant attempts to influence their environment and their own development for the better. However, individuals' capacity for primary control changes with changing competencies and opportunities across the life course. This typically means that from childhood through young adulthood, individuals experience a growth in capacity (see rising section of dashed line in Figure 24.1). In contrast, during later phases of life, capacities and opportunities for control become less plentiful and start to decline (see descending section of dashed

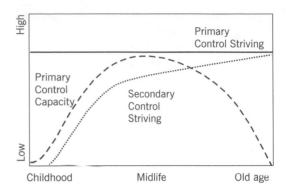

FIGURE 24.1. Hypothetical lifespan trajectories for primary control capacity, and primary and secondary control striving. From J. Heckhausen (1999). Copyright © 1999 Cambridge University Press. Adapted by permission.

line in Figure 24.1). As individuals develop more sophisticated strategies to influence their own emotions, goal engagements and disengagements, and also have to confront more challenges of overburdening or declining control capacities (energy, vitality) in later life, they rely increasingly on secondary control strategies (see dotted line in Figure 24.1). This increase in secondary control strategies helps to offset the individual's declining primary control capacity.

Congruence between Control Striving and Control Opportunities

Individuals' striving to control their own development can be effective only if they take into account the current and expected opportunities in a given domain of life. As capacities and opportunities increase, goals should become more ambitious. Conversely, as primary control potential declines, individuals should downgrade their aspirations and be content with less ambitious goal attainments. Given the multitude of life domains and the complex pattern of changes in competencies and opportunities for increasing primary control across the lifespan, individuals need to manage their control resources carefully to maximize their primary control across domains and across their life course. This involves a simultaneous and orchestrated engagement and disengagement with multiple goals, so that times of optimal opportunities are utilized for goal engagement, and times of declining or deficient opportunities and competencies are avoided.

In the domain of work, societies and their institutions differ in the segregation of career paths and the timing of increase, peak, plateau, and decrease of opportunities of career advancement in various vocational and professional careers. For example, a civil engineer might seek out challenges in his or her professional field during the earlier stages of his or her career, then as younger engineers with more up-to-date skill sets enter the workplace, the mature engineer might seek leadership opportunities for mentoring and management to prove his or her competence in this area, so that he or she can gradually shift into a management position.

Action Phases of Goal Engagement and Disengagement

In order to develop specific predictions about the use of control strategies for engaging with and disengaging from goals at different times of the lifespan and in different life domains, we developed the *action-phase model of developmental regulation* (Heckhausen, 1999; Heckhausen et al., 2010).

As shown in Figure 24.2, during the phase of *optimized goal selection,* people first evaluate their present control opportunities for a given goal and how these control opportunities are likely to change in the foreseeable future, how investing in a given goal might effect other goal pursuits, and whether selecting the given goal will lead to an overly narrow reliance on that goal pursuit. These considerations of optimized goal choice are highly relevant for the domain of work and career striving. For instance, a midcareer senior analyst in a consultant agency might have to decide whether it makes more sense to invest time, energy, and a potential disruption of his or her career in learning the newest developments in the field of big data analytics or to seek out challenges in managing complex projects with highly demanding clients to prove him- or herself competent for a move into a managerial position.

Once an individual has decided on a goal, he or she needs to invest in *goal engagement.* This shift into goal engagement typically involves switching from a deliberative mindset of realistically weighing pros and cons to the implemental mindset of being biased in favor of the chosen goal, with enhanced perceptions of its value and controllability (Achtziger & Gollwitzer, 2010; Heckhausen, 1991; Heckhausen & Gollwitzer, 1987). The *volitional mindset phenomenon,* wherein individuals optimistically bias their control perceptions in order to keep

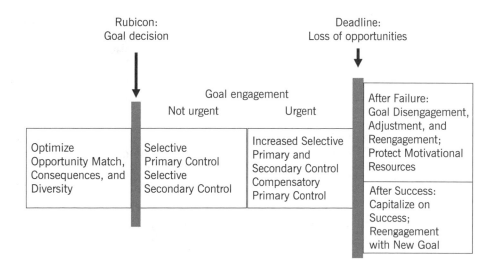

FIGURE 24.2. Action-phase model of developmental regulation. From J. Heckhausen (1999). Copyright © 1999 Cambridge University Press. Adapted by permission.

themselves mobilized toward goal attainment (Gollwitzer & Kinney, 1989), has ramifications for long-term career goals that rely on sustained engagement over extended periods of time. In particular, the volitional mindset leads individuals into believing that they are more competent than may actually be the case. Support comes from previous research, which indicates that young adults who were highly career-goal-engaged (i.e., implemental mindset) reported increased beliefs 1 year later that they had the requisite ability, effort, and social connections to reach their career goals (Shane, Heckhausen, Lessard, Chen, & Greenberger, 2012).

Pursuing career goals requires that an individual manage behavioral investments on a long-term basis. This includes focusing on other short-term needs when required, while being able to return behavioral investment toward these long-term career goals once he or she has taken care of urgent day-to-day matters. This process of delaying and then returning to effortful striving for a long-term goal requires considerable volitional management. Many career changes require that employees master these challenges, particularly when financial pressures require them to maintain their current position during job training or job search. For example, a law school graduate with substantial student loan debt who does not get hired as a lawyer and has to take a temporary job for financial reasons, has to cycle between meeting the demands of his or her current job and maintaining long-term behavioral investment toward finding employment as a lawyer.

As individuals move into the action phase of goal engagement, opportunities for goal pursuit may change. For example, a certain career move may be best done shortly after acquiring a qualification or else the promotion opportunity may disappear (e.g., get new position after earning an MBA, start an apprenticeship after graduating from high school). Other career status changes are tied to certain age periods. These kinds of timing-based changes set up what we refer to as *developmental deadlines*. Not all developmental goals have such deadlines, and many are not clearly delineated in terms of age or months after an event, but most goal pursuits in the life course involve waxing and waning opportunities over time.

Adaptive developmental regulation involves individuals' response to such deadlines with *urgent goal pursuit* before opportunities become scarce and the goal becomes obsolete. Such urgent goal pursuit would typically involve selective primary control and metavolitional strategies (*selective secondary control*), seeking help from others or using additional means previously not tried (*compensatory primary control*). For example, someone who is aiming to become a senior manager might first try to obtain the position without getting additional help from already successful colleagues in that position. However, if he or she struggles in finding employment and senses that the window of opportunity threatens to close, he or she might consider hiring a job hunter or obtaining additional industry-relevant training in order to land the desired position. While most careers do not have firm deadlines, the mounting responsibilities of adulthood, the continual waves of new and perhaps more qualified job seekers, and the changing technology and other rapidly evolving skill sets needed for a career make it increasingly difficult for older individuals to secure employment in fields in which they are not already established (see Wanberg, Kanfer, Hamann, & Zhang, 2016).

Finally, when the window of opportunity closes, individuals must shift from fervent goal engagement to disengagement from the goal. This highly challenging self-regulatory process involves both behavioral deactivation and breaking the motivational commitment. Moreover, given that developmental goals are often long term and their pursuit has required extensive resource investments, disengagement from these goals may entail a blow to a person's self-esteem and purpose in life. Postdeadline developmental regulation therefore needs to involve self-protective strategies, such as avoiding self-blame by attributing failure to reach the goal to others and to circumstances. For example, an individual in pursuit of a career that requires specialized training but does not have abundant job openings (e.g., the career of a lawyer) may need to disengage from this career goal after failing to find a job. Doing so in a self-protective manner (i.e., blaming failure to find a job on the job market rather than on a lack of competence) mitigates the negative consequences of goal disengagement and protects the individual's emotional and motivational resources that are needed for future goal engagement.

Disengagement becomes easier if the individual can already anticipate an alternative goal with which to reengage (see evidence for optimists in Aspinwall & Richter, 1999). For example, the individual who is not able to find a job as a lawyer may find that his or her Juris Doctor (JD) opens up alternate employment opportunities, such as in the business, government, and nonprofit sectors. Being able to identify these alternate career goals should allow an individual to swiftly and efficiently disengage from the previous career goal and feel confident and positive about directing his or her energy toward obtaining the alternate, yet still highly regarded, career goal.

Another key proposition of our theory regarding the model of action phases is that the transitions between the three major action phases (i.e., optimized goal choice, engagement, and disengagement–reengagement) should be discrete and organized rather than continuous and disjointed. The various control strategies and elements of the cognitive–motivational mindset are ideally orchestrated in a coherent manner, support each other, and are goal–phase congruent. For example, an individual who likes building and fixing things may be drawn to a career as an engineer. After choosing this career, the individual should devote his or her time and effort toward identifying and gaining admittance to a postsecondary institution, where he or she can study engineering. If the individual is successful in his or her studies, he or she should springboard into finding an engineering job in his or her chosen specialty. If the individual struggles with his or her classes, he or she can redouble his or her commitment toward the classwork, switch majors, or drop out of school altogether. Ideally, the choice between these options will be made without a period of floundering, wherein he or she continues to take and to fail engineering classes. If disengagement is chosen, the individual will

be better able to adaptively disengage from the engineering career goal if he or she can avoid blaming him- or herself and identify an alternative, feasible, and attractive goal pursuit (e.g., mechanic, electrician).

APPLICATION OF THE MTD TO CHANGING CAREER-RELATED CHALLENGES ACROSS ADULTHOOD

Self-regulatory motivational challenges in careers across the adult lifespan include (1) identifying opportunities and constraints in one's career to allow optimized goal choice; (2) effectively engaging with work activities and career goals; (3) disengaging from work activities and career goals when they are obsolete; and (4) reengaging with activities and goals within or outside work that are accessible for the individual.

Before we discuss these four types of self-regulatory challenges in greater detail, we should consider the types of goals people pursue in their worklives. Individual career-related goals can be grouped into three broad categories: (1) producing certain *outcomes, products, or consequences* for their own sake (e.g., helping others who are sick); (2) *developing one's own competence* (e.g., becoming better at solving engineering problems); and (3) attaining *higher career positions* (e.g., moving up from sales to managerial rank in a department store). In the ideal case, these three go hand in hand; but when they are different, their institutional/societal and individual developmental causation and setup is distinct, and they involve different motivational processes. For example, individuals who care more about autonomy in activity selection and continuous challenge in their work (e.g., artists, academics) are often willing to sacrifice predictability and income in order to maximize opportunities to optimize their autonomous competence development over the course of a career. Many others deem the external rewards more important and therefore pay most attention to salary, job security, and opportunities for promotion. To add to the complexity, across the lifespan of a given career, an individual's motivational focus can shift from a focus on activity and competence growth to a focus on work outcomes or consequences, or to a preference for enhancing one's position and status, or vice versa (see Kanfer & Ackerman, 2004, for a review). Even the meaning of career success differs across jobs, social contexts, cultures, time periods, and an individual's own lifespan (Dries, 2011; Gunz & Mayrhofer, 2011; Hennequin, 2007; Heslin, 2005).

Identifying Opportunities and Constraints (Optimization)

Opportunities and constraints are set at the individual (capacity, talent, maturation, aging) and institutional/societal (career entry, advancement) levels. To be most adaptive, individuals need to optimize their career goals and the paths they choose to attain them before embarking on paths of career goal engagement. Research on this area is scarce, although initial studies show that a focus on career opportunities at work declines with a foreshortened future time perspective (Zacher & Frese, 2009) and increasing age (Zacher & Frese, 2011).

At the Beginning of Careers

After evaluating the match between his or her capacities and skills and the demands of the job, a competence–demand gap should prompt the individual to generate expectations about whether or not, in what time frame, and with what kind of effort the gap can be narrowed. In order to master this challenge, the individual needs to integrate knowledge about his or her own previous capacities and strategies to bridge competence–demand gaps, and gather any available information from others who have experienced and mastered this entry phase themselves. Competence–demand gaps at career entry will be greater for those occupations that rely on extensive and specialized education, training, and experience.

The possibility for advancement is also part of an individual's initial assessments of personal fit with a career. Careers in the U.S. used to have great permeability (Hamilton, 1990), but career entry and promotion prospects are increasingly differentiated by educational requirements (Carnevale, Smith, & Strohl, 2010). Educational attainment continues to increase year after year in the United States (U.S. Census Bureau, 2015), reflecting the role that education and formal training play in job attainment (Bills, 2003), career promotions (Spilerman & Lunde, 1991) and pay (Bureau of Labor Statistics, U.S. Department of Labor, 2015). Laypersons' views of upward mobility possibilities have typically not kept pace with this development, with U.S. citizens' generally overestimating upward social mobility prospects (Kraus & Tan, 2015) despite unequal access to education across socioeconomic backgrounds (Haveman & Smeeding, 2006). While believing that upward social mobility is attainable and dependent on one's merit promotes goal engagement (Shane & Heckhausen, 2013, 2016), these beliefs can lead to disappointment and discouragement soon after career entry if they prove unrealistic.

It is important for individuals to assess how well their capacities and resources match the opportunity structure in a new career. For example, promotion prospects in retail depend on job performance for the initial steps to sales and first-line managerial positions, but beyond that, postsecondary education is required. So someone who is not going to be content with a first-line managerial position in the long run will need to plan on expanding his or her educational resume, with all the consequences this may have for other domains of life, such as the time commitment of going to college while working, and the economic sacrifice of going to college without working (McDowell, 1982).

Within-Career Promotion and Competence Development

As we discussed in the section "Societal and Occupational Opportunities and Constraints at Different Career Stages," careers offer a wide variety of promotion prospects that typically come with increases in responsibility, autonomy, influence on others, status, and pay. So, for promotions, the three types of work-related goals (outcome-, competence-, and position-focused) are typically convergent. In some cases, however, they may not converge, and those instances generate important tradeoffs to be considered when making decisions to strive for or forego a promotion. Moreover, as we discussed before, career paths in the United States have become increasingly dependent on formal education requirements, particularly with regard to professional degrees (master's programs in many areas), far beyond the traditional fields of medicine, law, and academia.

Nursing is a fascinating career area for investigating the motivational implications of structural differences in related but educationally segregated careers. Entry-level nursing positions can be obtained within a few months (CNA) or a year (LPN), while the path based on more formal education requires a 2-year associate's degree (RN), or for the more advanced careers in nursing, a specialized master's degree or a Doctor of Nursing Practice (DNP) is required. Making a decision to apply for and enter advanced degree programs involves long-term planning and goal pursuit spanning several years, in combination with the economic stress of lost income and the considerable cost of a professional degree program.

Plateau and Decline

An important aspect of identifying promotion opportunities and constraints is timing. Does a given career involve normative timing for first and last promotion, and how much can individuals depart from, push ahead, or fall behind this timing pattern? The more variability, the greater the individual's potential to take control and advance promotions or push age constraints beyond their upper limits. Most careers have an implicit notion of deadline for reaching the top position available in a given career path. These notions are generally not directly associated with actual decline in work performance given that in most careers individuals can compensate for age-related declines in fluid intelligence functioning and multitasking (see prior section "Change in Ability-Related Competencies across Adulthood"). However, some jobs (e.g., air traffic controller, neurosurgeon, fighter pilot) require functioning at high levels of complexity and with relentless time pressure. As Kanfer and Ackerman (2005) noted, such work is often viewed as "young adult jobs," with the expectation that individuals hold

these jobs early in their careers but are subsequently promoted to supervisory, administrative, or training positions that make fewer demands on age-sensitive abilities. To enforce this career progression, several of these jobs have institutionally regulated retirement requirements that push individuals toward disengagement and new goal engagement.

In knowledge-based careers, such as lawyer or physician, the high initial investment in domain-specific knowledge permits new learning with less investment of time and effort, and provides an opportunity for continued career development through midlife. If, however, there is substantial change in the technology or knowledge base, career progress and competence may be thwarted by the high demands associated with new learning (Kanfer & Ackerman, 2005). For example, programmers who fail to update their skills for a decade or more may find it more difficult to find employment following a job layoff than programmers who engage in continuous skill learning while employed.

Engaging

Once someone has made a decision to pursue a certain career-related goal, he or she needs to mobilize motivational and behavioral resources to engage with and pursue the goal. Goal decisions do not automatically lead to goal engagement and implementation of action (Gollwitzer, Heckhausen, & Ratajczak, 1990). The nature of the goal plays a key role in the direction of action and the demands that the goal places on self-regulation (Kanfer, 2012). For example, consider two individuals who seek career advancement; one within her work unit and the other by getting a degree that qualifies him for a higher position within and outside his current employing organization. The former goal requires continuously sustained engagement and ambitious volunteering for challenging projects, whereas the latter goal is more structured, requiring a decision to apply to an educational program, then follow through with its requirements. The promotion-based advancement goal will work best for workers with a matching implicit motive (e.g., achievement motive for an engineer, power motive for a teacher or manager), who find their work intrinsically motivating and have the capacity to expand their responsibility effectively. However, if either the implicit or the intrinsic motivation is insufficient, the individual will need superior self-regulatory skills to sustain goal engagement (Kehr, 2004). Education-based advancement goals also require engagement, but the educational institution will typically provide a scaffold for the day-to-day behavioral investment, with self-regulation skills needed to sustain learning within the program.

Engaging with career-related goals is most important for performance at work and for career development when individual agency and autonomy are enhanced relative to societal and organizational structure. On a macro level, the modern social and economic climate emphasizes individual agency in career progression and social mobility pursuit (see Heckhausen, 2010; Heckhausen & Shane, 2015). This is further captured by the concepts of a protean (Hall, 1996) and boundaryless (Arthur & Rousseau, 1996) career, which outline the increased demands on individuals to self-direct their career development in the wake of the disruption of traditional and highly structured within-organization career progressions. Typically, higher-level careers also provide the greatest degree of autonomy to the individual, both in career development and in day-to-day work activities. Given such autonomy, it falls to the individual to generate the motivational and volitional self-regulation to stay appropriately engaged. For example, individuals in academic careers have relatively little structure in their day-to-day activities, and after job stability has been secured via tenure, often have reduced extrinsic incentives for motivational engagement with work. Individuals who maintain engagement and high levels of productivity in such a situation likely find their work intrinsically motivating and use their work as a vehicle through which they can satisfy their implicit and explicit motives.

Situations in which an employee might become discouraged or even feel threatened in his or her occupational self-confidence are important testing grounds for career-related motivational engagement. Under these conditions, individual differences in self-regulation become influential (Heckhausen & Wrosch, 2016). In order to stay on track with challenging goals, the individual needs to use metavolitional strategies to boost his or her perceived control over goal attainment, enhance the anticipated affective consequences of goal attainment, down-regulate the value of alternative goals, and avoid distractions (Heckhausen et al., 2010). In previous work on college students' pursuit in academic goals and youth's striving for apprenticeship positions, we found that such metavolitional skills (referred to as *selective secondary control* in the MTD) are effective for maintaining goal-engaged activities, especially under adverse conditions of low control (Hamm et al., 2013) or highly distracting negative life events (Poulin & Heckhausen, 2007). Moreover, certain personality differences may work to facilitate such self-regulatory strategy use (Heckhausen & Wrosch, 2016; Kanfer & Heggestad, 1997). For example, differences in dispositional optimism have major consequences for the regulation of behavior, persistence, and problem-focused coping in controllable but challenging situations (Carver & Scheier, 2014; Rasmussen, Wrosch, Scheier, & Carver, 2006; Scheier & Carver, 1985). Action versus state orientation is another important individual difference variable for action-phase consistent behavior, such as strong volitional commitment when goal-engaged (Beckmann & Kuhl, 1984; Kuhl, 1981). Volitional self-regulation is especially needed when sustained effort is required for a certain career goal but the implicit motive and intrinsic motivation are insufficient to support such long-term and continuous goal engagement.

Another highly relevant issue for sustaining career engagement pertains to participation in continued education during advanced career stages. In some professions, such as clinical psychology, law, and medicine, continued education is required to maintain one's formal standing in the profession. In other careers, such as in academia, taking steps to enhance or maintain one's skill level and keep up with innovations in one's field of expertise is largely left up to the individual. Here, individual differences in achievement motivation for growing one's competence are critical. Learning new skills and acquiring further knowledge in a profession can also, in and of itself, enhance the activity-inherent enjoyment of a job.

Disengaging and Reengaging

Engagement with work-related goals is adaptive only as long as these goals are attainable. Previous research indicates that individuals who were highly engaged with goals that offered little control reported a compromised ability to sustain high levels of engagement, and negative job-related mental and physical health across a 9-year interval (Shane & Heckhausen, 2012). Thus, the most adaptive course of action in some cases is to disengage from fruitless goals and reengage with more promising career goals. With goals as important and lifetime encompassing as work and career goals, disengagement, reorientation, and commitment to new goals can be quite difficult because life circumstances (financial obligations, family responsibility), an individual's identity and self-worth, and future prospects (economic independence, resources for retirement) are wrapped up in one's current work life.

At the Beginning of Careers

When starting out in a given career, a certain readiness for goal disengagement and goal adjustment may be as useful as the ability to engage strongly and persistently with one's career goals. At the career-entry stage, the costs of disengaging from a suboptimal career and reengaging with a better matching career are low because one has yet to invest lots of time and resources. So it is essential to determine whether the currently entered career is a good fit for oneself; see the section "Identifying Opportunities and Constraints (Optimization)." Many careers are actually set up to provide the opportunity to try out an employee–employer fit in a semiserious and not-yet binding way, in the form of internships. Switching one's career preferences after an internship is an expected and welcome move if the fit is not right, and the threshold for disengagement is therefore lowered.

Moreover, moving away from a current goal is a lot easier if one has an alternative goal in mind, effectively turning disengagement

into reengagement with a new goal (Wrosch, Scheier, Carver, & Schulz, 2003). Indeed, as proposed by the MTD, disengagement from unattainable goals is primarily adaptive because it allows the individual to become reengaged with more promising control pursuits (Heckhausen et al., 2010) and improves the subjective well-being of individuals. For example, an individual who is struggling to attain his or her original career goal of becoming a physician may disengage from this goal more quickly if he or she is able to identify related and valued careers, such as nursing, emergency medical technician, or medical researcher.

Midcareer

At later career stages, the costs of changing course are greater; therefore, individuals are more inclined to stay in a suboptimal career, with the possible calamitous development of motivational entrapment or escalated commitment (Brockner, 1992; Staw, 1997). However, sustained engagement with low-opportunity goals can have serious mental and physical health consequences (Nesse, 2000; Shane & Heckhausen, 2012; Wrosch et al., 2003). Thus, in spite of the great costs of midcareer disengagement, there are a number of scenarios that can make career reorientation a worthwhile yet challenging life-course maneuver.

Individuals may initially entertain high-flying ambitions only to run into serious obstacles that may ultimately make these ambitions impossible to obtain and/or too costly to pursue (e.g., too much overtime to keep up with responsibilities as a parent). Career ambitions may fail for several reasons, including, but not limited to, a lack of available positions at the aspired rank, discriminatory barriers impeding rank attainment, or a lack of competence to move up to the aspired rank. Of course, the emotional and motivational implications of these scenarios are quite different given that in the former two the institution takes the blame, whereas in the latter it is the individual who is accepting the blame for insufficient competence. While repeated failure to obtain a job is likely to cause almost all individuals to disengage, we can expect that individuals who were denied employment due to external causes are more likely to continue pursuing their goal longer than do individuals who were denied employment because of a lack of competence.

Disengagement from one's long-term career goal may be particularly difficult when individuals have developed a strong identity based on the pursuit or envisioned attainment of the career goal. As people become increasingly dissatisfied with their current position and discouraged about ever being able to achieve their cherished career goal, they may experience an "action crisis" (Brandstätter, Hermann, & Schüler, 2013; Brandstätter & Schüler, 2013). Such an action crisis may be more easily resolved if the individual has another area of potential goal engagement that corresponds well to the motives associated with the primary career goal.

Plateau and Decline

Career plateaus bring with them the challenge of stunted opportunities for further competence and motive fulfillment, and/or feeling inconsequential and bored. Career plateaus happen particularly early in careers of Job Zones 1 and 2, and may therefore prompt individuals to retrain for a different vocation or to seek further educational qualifications to reenter work life for Job Zone 3 or 4 careers. However, due to financial, familial, or other constraints that preclude a return to postsecondary education (e.g., McDowell, 1982), many people never take such steps to enter a new career. Some institutions and employers may provide new avenues of engagement by encouraging senior employees to function as mentors and instructors for younger employees, or move into management positions in which they supervise a few employees. For example, service-oriented organizations with high employee turnover may ask their senior employees to train new hires. Regardless of whether the senior employee receives a new title or increased pay, the opportunity for training and mentoring new colleagues may provide an avenue for further competence development and motive satisfaction.

Another strategy for dealing with a mismatch between opportunity and motivation is to find alternative mastery or social activities outside of one's worklife, such as in leisure activities, family involvement, volunteering, and other community engagements. Such strategies would involve a combined disengagement from work-related ambitions and engagement with non-work-related ambitions. With such a reallocation of goal engagement, work activities may suffer unless they are supplanted by self-regulatory efforts or extrinsic rewards.

CONCLUSION AND FUTURE RESEARCH

There is considerable potential for productive research in the area of motivational processes involved in career-related behavior. Careers vary widely in how structured and predictable they are, and how much autonomy they allow for and demand of the individual agent. At the same time, individuals differ in how well they determine opportunities, tradeoffs, and consequences involved in optimized choice; how long their future time expectations extend; and how well they can sustain and maximize goal engagement, manage goal disengagement, and self-protection, and adjust their career goals. Such individual differences can be assessed using measurement instruments developed within the motivational theory of lifespan development (Heckhausen et al., 2010) and other related conceptual approaches, such as career adaptability and career entrenchment (Savickas & Porfeli, 2012; Zacher, Ambiel, & Noronha, 2015) and implicit motives and trait-complexes (Kanfer & Ackerman, 2005).

The overall trend in modern industrial societies has moved toward the individual exerting greater influence and responsibility for his or her own career trajectory (see Arthur & Rousseau, 1996; Hall, 1996; Heckhausen, 2010; Heckhausen & Shane, 2015). Especially in relatively unstructured professional careers, individuals need to be planful and proactive in seeking opportunities within and between employers, and to match their choices of goals and striving for the next career step to the opportunity structure. At the same time, individuals should be aware of their own skills, knowledge, and motivational orientations when making decisions about entering, leaving, or shifting careers. Cognitive and socioemotional characteristics that promote such valid opportunity assessment, planfulness in anticipating long-term and interdomain consequences, and motivational self-awareness are invaluable assets for individuals.

Unstructured careers that require an all-out continuous investment of effort and talent, without much opportunity for strategic career moves within or outside one's current employment, are likely to be mastered best by individuals who have a high capacity for goal engagement, a low readiness to disengage from a goal once it has been chosen, and a high implicit motive and intrinsic motivation matching the predominant career activity. On the other hand, structured careers that follow a set sequence of education, training, and work experience, may be best mastered by individuals with exceptionally high goal-engagement capacity and a great ability for metavolitional control (avoid distractions, imagine the joy of attaining one's goal, etc.). For highly structured careers, individual planning skills are less needed.

Career progress is often slow and a long-term endeavor, and boundary conditions in society may change. Intense, long-term, and uninterrupted engagement in a career may render a person blind to potential drawbacks or disadvantages that have crept up over time. Therefore, it may be advantageous to regularly take stock and reevaluate one's career path, and to occasionally step out of the strong metavolitional commitment to the current career.

In addition to these combinations of individual motivational/self-regulatory dispositions and career challenges, we identify several topics in work and career-related behavior that provide particularly promising avenues for future research.

1. *Managing career delay.* How do individuals self-regulate when opportunities for taking on career-relevant tasks and challenges are delayed due to institution or employer constraints (e.g., promotion is not possible until someone currently in the position retires)?

2. *Involuntary job loss at midcareer.* There is increasing evidence of the importance of self-regulatory and motivational

processes following job loss (Kanfer, Wanberg, & Kantrowitz, 2001). However, the role of goal engagement, adjustment, or disengagement strategies for individuals seeking to find employment in the same career path following an involuntary job loss remains an area in need of further research.

3. *Motivational career scarring.* Prolonged inability to find employment during the early phase of career development may reset thresholds for disengaging from career goals, change career values, and challenge endorsement of societal institutions and norms. How individuals adjust to these socioeconomic barriers to career entry, and the resulting implications for individuals and societies, is a fascinating topic for future research.

4. *Career retirement.* Cahill, Giandrea, and Quinn (2006) report that many older workers in career jobs make a gradual exit from the workforce. Societal and institutional factors also influence the nature of this exit in terms of taking "bridge jobs" and suggest that economic and psychological factors may have different effects on the pattern of career disengagement and reengagement. Continued research is needed to understand more fully the factors that influence how individuals approach and respond to the retirement transition.

Researchers have much to gain from integrating lifespan developmental, motivational, and industrial and organizational psychology approaches to career development across the lifespan. Societal, institutional, and workplace contexts set up age-graded structures of career opportunities and constraints for individual workers and professionals. Many careers hold little potential for growth, but those that do are most beneficial for individuals who have the cognitive, motivational, and self-regulatory characteristics that enable them to take advantage of the career opportunities with and beyond their current employer.

REFERENCES

Achtziger, A., & Gollwitzer, P. M. (2010). Motivation and volition in the course of action. In

J. Heckhausen & H. Heckhausen (Eds.), *Motivation and action* (pp. 272–295). Cambridge, UK: Cambridge University Press.

Ackerman, P. L. (1996). A theory of adult intellectual development: Process, personality, interests, and knowledge. *Intelligence, 22,* 229–259.

Ackerman, P. L. (2000). Domain-specific knowledge as the "dark matter" of adult intelligence Gf/Gc, personality and interest correlates. *Journals of Gerontology B: Psychological Sciences, 55*(2), P69–P84.

Ackerman, P. L. (2014). Adolescent and adult intellectual development. *Current Directions in Psychological Science, 23,* 246–251.

Ackerman, P. L., Bowen, K. R., Beier, M., & Kanfer, R. (2001). Determinants of individual differences and gender differences in knowledge. *Journal of Educational Psychology, 93,* 797–825.

Ackerman, P. L., & Rolfhus, E. L. (1999). The locus of adult intelligence: Knowledge, abilities, and non-ability traits. *Psychology and Aging, 14,* 314–330.

Arthur, M. B., & Rousseau, D. M. (1996). *The boundaryless career: A new employment principle for a new organizational era.* Oxford, UK: Oxford University Press.

Aspinwall, L. G., & Richter, L. (1999). Optimism and self-mastery predict more rapid disengagement from unsolvable tasks in the presence of alternatives. *Motivation and Emotion, 23,* 221–245.

Baltes, P. B. (1987). Theoretical propositions of life-span developmental psychology: On the dynamics between growth and decline. *Developmental Psychology, 23,* 611–626.

Baltes, P. B., Dittman-Kohli, F., & Kliegl, R. (1986). Reserve capacity of the elderly in aging-sensitive tests of fluid intelligence: Replication and extension. *Psychology and Aging, 1,* 172–177.

Baltes, P. B., & Kliegl, R. (1992). Negative age differences in cognitive plasticity of a memory skill during adulthood: Further testing the limits. *Developmental Psychology, 28,* 121–125.

Baltes, P. B., & Lindenberger, U. (1988). On the range of cognitive plasticity in old age as a function of experience: 15 years of intervention research. *Behavior Therapy, 19,* 283–300.

Baltes, P. B., Sowarka, D., & Kliegl, R. (1989). Cognitive training research on fluid intelligence in old age: What can older adults achieve by themselves? *Psychology and Aging, 4,* 217–221.

Beckmann, J., & Kuhl, J. (1984). Altering information to gain action control: Functional aspects of human information processing in decision making. *Journal of Research in Personality, 18,* 224–237.

Beier, M. E., & Ackerman, P. L. (2001). Current-events knowledge in adults: An investigation of age, intelligence, and nonability determinants. *Psychology and Aging, 16*(4), 615–628.

Beier, M. E., & Ackerman, P. L. (2003). Determinants of health knowledge: An investigation of age, gender, abilities, personality, and interests. *Journal of Personality and Social Psychology, 84*(2), 439–448.

Beier, M. E., & Ackerman, P. L. (2005). Age, ability and the role of prior knowledge on theacquisition of new domain knowledge. *Psychology and Aging, 20,* 341–355.

Berthelot, G., Len, S., Hellard, P., Tafflet, M., Guillaume, M., Vollmer, J. C., et al. (2011). Exponential growth combined with exponential decline explains lifetime performance evolution in individual and human species. *Age, 34,* 1001–1009.

Bills, D. B. (2003). Credentials, signals, and screens: Explaining the relationship between schooling and job assignment. *Review of Educational Research, 73,* 441–449.

Boyce, C. J., Wood, A. M., Daly, M., & Sedikides, C. (2015). Personality change following unemployment. *Journal of Applied Psychology, 100,* 991–1011.

Brandstätter, V., Hermann, M., & Schüler, J. (2013). The struggle of giving up personal goals: Affective, physiological, and cognitive consequences of an action crisis. *Personality and Social Psychology Bulletin, 20,* 1–15.

Brandstätter, V. & Schüler, J. (2013). Action crisis and cost–benefit thinking: A cognitive analysis of a goal-disengagement phase. *Journal of Experimental Psychology, 49,* 543–553.

Brockner, J. (1992). The escalation of commitment to a failing course of action: Toward theoretical progress. *Academy of Management Review, 17,* 39–61.

Bureau of Labor Statistics, U.S. Department of Labor (2015). The Economics Daily: Median weekly earnings by educational attainment in 2014. Retrieved from *www.bls.gov/opub/ted/2015/median-weekly-earnings-by-education-gender-race-and-ethnicity-in-2014.htm.*

Burgard, S. A., Brand, J. E., & House, J. S. (2009). Perceived job insecurity and worker health in the United States. *Social Science and Medicine, 69,* 777–785.

Cahill, K. E., Giandrea, M. D., & Quinn, J. F. (2006). Retirement patterns from career employment. *The Gerontologist, 46,* 514–523.

Carnevale, A. P., Smith, N., & Strohl, J. (2010). *Help wanted: Projections of job and education requirements through 2018.* Washington, DC: Center on Education and the Workforce.

Carter, M., & Beier, M. E. (2010). The effectiveness of error management training with working-aged adults. *Personnel Psychology, 63,* 641–675.

Carver, C. S., & Scheier, M. F. (2014). Dispositional optimism. *Trends in Cognitive Sciences, 18,* 293–299.

Caspi, A., Roberts, B. W., Shiner, R. L. (2005). Personality development: Stability and change. *Annual Review of Psychology, 56,* 453–484.

Charness, N., & Tuffiash, M. (2008). The role of expertise research and human factors in capturing, explaining, and producing superior performance. *Human Factors, 50,* 427–432.

Davies, D. R., & Sparrow, P. R. (1988). Effects of age, tenure, training, and job complexity on job performance. *Psychology and Aging, 3,* 307–314.

de Grip, A., & Smits, W. (2012). What affects lifelong learning of scientists and engineers? *International Journal of Manpower, 33,* 583–597.

De Lange, A. H., Kooij, D. T. A. M., & van der Heijden, B. I. J. M. (2015) Human resource management and sustainability at work across the life-span: An integrative perspective. In L. Finkelstein, D. Truxillo, F. Fraccaroli, & R. Kanfer (Eds.), *Facing the challenges of a multi-age workforce* (pp. 50–80). New York: Routledge.

Dries, N. (2011). The meaning of career success: Avoiding reification through a closer inspection of historical, cultural, and ideological contexts. *Career Development International, 16,* 364–384.

Ebner, N. C., Freund, A. M., & Baltes, P. B. (2006). Developmental changes in personal goal orientation from young to late adulthood: From striving for gains to maintenance and prevention of losses. *Psychology and Aging, 21,* 664–678.

Ericsson, K. A. (1990). Peak performance and age: An examination of peak performance in sports. In P. B. Baltes & M. M. Baltes (Eds.), *Successful aging: Perspectives from the behavioral sciences* (pp. 164–196). New York: Cambridge University Press.

Ericsson, K. A. (2004). Deliberate practice and the acquisition and maintenance of expert performance in medicine and related domains. *Academic Medicine, 79,* S70–S81.

Gollwitzer, P., Heckhausen, H., & Ratajczak, H. (1990). From weighing to willing: Approaching a change decision through pre-or postdecisional mentation. *Organizational Behavior and Human Decision Processes, 45,* 41–65.

Gollwitzer, P., & Kinney, R. F. (1989). Effects of deliberative and implemental mind-sets on illusion of control. *Journal of Personality and Social Psychology, 50,* 531–542.

Graduate Management Admission Council. (2015). 2015 alumni perspectives survey report. Retrieved from *www.gmac.com/market-intelligence-and-research/research-library/measuring-program-roi/2015-alumni-perspectives-survey-report.aspx.*

Gunz, H., & Mayrhofer, W. (2011). Reconceptualizing career success: A contextual approach. *Zeitschrift Für ArbeitsmarktForschung, 43,* 251–260.

Hall, D. T. (1996). Protean careers of the 21st century. *Academy of Management Executive, 10,* 8–16.

Halpern-Manners, A., Warren, J. R., Raymo, J. M., & Nicholson, D. A. (2015). The impact of work and family life histories on economic well-being at older ages. *Social Forces, 93,* 1369–1396.

Hamilton, S. F. (1990). *Apprenticeship for adulthood: Preparing youth for the future.* New York: Free Press.

Hamm, J. M., Stewart, T. L., Perry, R. P., Clifton, R. A., Chipperfield, J. G., & Heckhausen, J. (2013). Sustaining primary control striving for achievement goals during challenging transitions: The role of secondary control strategies. *Basic and Applied Social Psychology, 35,* 286–297.

Hartshorne, J. K., & Germine, L. T. (2015). When does cognitive functioning peak?: The asynchronous rise and fall of different cognitive abilities across the life span. *Psychological Science, 26,* 433–443.

Haveman, R. H., & Smeeding, T. M. (2006). The role of higher education in social mobility. *The Future of Children, 16,* 125–150.

Heckhausen, H. (1991). *Motivation and action.* New York: Springer-Verlag.

Heckhausen, H., & Gollwitzer, P. M. (1987). Thought contents and cognitive functioning in motivational and volitional states of mind. *Motivation and Emotion, 11,* 101–120.

Heckhausen, J. (1997). Developmental regulation across adulthood: Primary and secondary control of age-related challenges. *Developmental Psychology, 33,* 176–187.

Heckhausen, J. (1999). *Developmental regulation in adulthood: Age-normative and socio-structural constraints as adaptive challenges.* Cambridge, UK: Cambridge University Press.

Heckhausen, J. (2005). Competence and motivation in adulthood and old age: Making the most of changing capacities and resources. In A. J. Elliot & C. S. Dweck (Eds.), *Handbook of competence and motivation* (pp. 240–256). New York: Guilford Press.

Heckhausen, J. (2010). Globalization, social inequality, and individual agency in human development: Social change for better or worse? In R. K. Silbereisen & X. Chen (Eds.), *Social change and human development: Concept and results* (pp. 148–163). London: Sage.

Heckhausen, J., & Schulz, R. (1995). A life-span theory of control. *Psychological Review, 102,* 284–304.

Heckhausen, J., & Schulz, R. (1999). The primacy of primary control is a human universal: A reply to Gould's critique of the life-span theory of control. *Psychological Review, 106,* 605–609.

Heckhausen, J., & Shane, J. (2015). Social mobility in the transition to adulthood: Educational systems, career entry, and individual agency. In L. A. Jensen (Ed.), *The Oxford handbook of human development and culture* (pp. 535–553). New York: Oxford University Press.

Heckhausen, J., & Wrosch, C. (2016). Challenges to developmental regulation across the life course: What are they and which individual differences matter? *International Journal of Behavioral Development, 40*(2),145–150.

Heckhausen, J., Wrosch, C., & Schulz, R. (2010). A motivational theory of life-span development. *Psychological Review, 117,* 32–60.

Hennequin, E. (2007). What "career success" means to blue-collar workers. *Career Development International, 12,* 565–581.

Heslin, P. A. (2005). Conceptualizing and evaluating career success. *Journal of Organizational Behavior, 26*(2), 113–136.

Horton, S., Baker, J., & Shorer, J. (2008). Expertise and aging: Maintaining skills throughout the lifespan. *European Review of Aging and Physical Activity, 5,* 89–96.

Jeske, D., & Stamov Roßnagel, C. (2015). Learning capability and performance in later working life: Towards a contextual view. *Education + Training, 57,* 378–391.

Kanfer, R. (2012). Work motivation: Theory, practice, and future directions. In S. W. J. Kozlowski (Ed.), *The Oxford handbook of industrial and organizational psychology* (pp. 455–495). Oxford, UK: Blackwell.

Kanfer, R., & Ackerman, P. L. (2004). Aging, adult development, and work motivation. *Academy of Management Review, 29*(3), 440–458.

Kanfer, R., & Ackerman, P. L. (2005). Work competence: A person-oriented perspective. In A. J. Elliott & C. S. Dweck (Eds.), *Handbook of competence and motivation* (pp. 336–353). New York: Guilford Press.

Kanfer, R., Beier, M. E., & Ackerman, P. L.

(2013). Goals and motivation related to work in later adulthood: An organizing framework. *European Journal of Work and Organizational Psychology, 22*(3), 253–264.

Kanfer, R., & Heggestad, E. (1997). Motivational traits and skills: A person-centered approach to work motivation. *Research in Organizational Behavior, 18,* 1–57.

Kanfer, R., Wanberg, C. R., & Kantrowitz, T. M. (2001). Job search and employment: A personality–motivational analysis and meta-analytic review. *Journal of Applied Psychology, 86,* 837–855.

Kehr, H. (2004). Implicit/explicit motive discrepancies and volitional depletion among managers. *Personality and Social Psychology Bulletin, 30,* 315–327.

Kemper, S., Herman, R. E., & Lian, C. H. T. (2003). The costs of doing two things at once for young and older adults: Talking while walking, finger tapping, and ignoring speech or noise. *Psychology and Aging, 18,* 181–192.

Kenny, G. P., Yardley, J. E., Martineau, L., & Jay, O. (2008). Physical work capacity in older adults: Implications for the aging worker. *American Journal of Industrial Medicine, 51,* 610–625.

Kliegl, R., Krampe, R. T. & Mayr, U. (2003). Formal models of age differences in task-complexity effects. In U. M. Staudinger & U. Lindenberger (Eds.), *Understanding human development: Dialogues with lifespan psychology* (pp. 289–313). Boston: Kluwer Academic.

Kliegl, R., Smith, J., & Baltes, P. (1989). Testing-the-limits and the study of adult age differences in cognitive plasticity of a mnemonic skill. *Developmental Psychology, 25,* 247–256.

Kooij, D. T., De Lange, A. H., Jansen, P. G., Kanfer, R., & Dikkers, J. S. (2011). Age and work-related motives: Results of a meta-analysis. *Journal of Organizational Behavior, 32,* 197–225.

Kooij, D. T., Tims, M., & Kanfer, R. (2015). Successful aging at work: The role of job crafting. In B. P. Matthjs, D. T. A. M. Kooij, & D. M. Rousseau (Eds.), *Aging workers and the employee–employer relationship* (pp. 145–161). Cham, Switzerland: Springer International.

Kraus, M. W., & Tan, J. J. X. (2015). Americans overestimate social class mobility. *Journal of Experimental Social Psychology, 58,* 101–111.

Kubeck, J. E., Delp, N. D., Haslett, T. K., & McDaniel, M. A. (1996). Does job-related training performance decline with age? *Psychology and Aging, 11,* 92–107.

Kuhl, J. (1981). Motivational and functional

helplessness: The moderating effect of state versus action orientation. *Journal of Personality and Social Psychology, 40,* 155–170.

Li, K. Z. H., Lindenberger, U., Freund, A. M., & Baltes, P. B. (2001). Walking while memorizing: Age-related differences in compensatory behavior. *Psychological Science, 12,* 230–237.

Lim, V. K. G., & Sng, Q. S. (2006). Does parental job insecurity matter?: Money anxiety, money motives, and work motivation. *Journal of Applied Psychology, 91,* 1078–1087.

Lindenberger, U., Marsiske, M., & Baltes, P. B. (2000). Memorizing while walking: Increase in dual-task costs from young adulthood to old age. *Psychology and Aging, 15*(3), 417–436.

Mayr, U., & Kliegl, R. (1993). Sequential and coordinative complexity: Age-based processing limitations in figural transformations. *Journal of Experimental Psychology: Learning, Memory, and Cognition, 19,* 1297–1320.

Mayr, U., Kliegl, R., & Krampe, R. T. (1996). Sequential and coordinative processing dynamics across the life span. *Cognition, 59,* 61–90.

McDaniel, M., Pesta, B., & Banks, G. (2012). Job performance and the aging worker. In J. W. Hedge & W. C. Borman (Eds.), *The Oxford handbook of work and aging* (pp. 280–297). Oxford, UK: Oxford University Press.

McDowell, J. M. (1982). Obsolescence of knowledge and career publication profiles: Some evidence of differences among fields in costs of interrupted careers. *American Economic Review, 72,* 752–768.

McEvoy, G. M., & Cascio, W. F. (1989). Cumulative evidence of the relationship between employee age and job performance. *Journal of Applied Psychology, 74,* 11–17.

McFadyen, R. G. (1998). Attitudes toward the unemployed. *Human Relations, 51,* 179–199.

McKee-Ryan, F. M., Song, Z., Wanberg, C. R., & Kinicki, A. J. (2005). Psychological and physical well-being during unemployment: A meta-analytic study. *Journal of Applied Psychology, 90,* 53–76.

Michel, J. S., Kotrba, L. M., Mitchelson, J. K., Clark, M. A., & Baltes, B. B. (2011). Antecedents of work–family conflict: A meta-analytic review. *Journal of Organizational Behavior, 32,* 689–725.

National Center for Education Statistics, U.S. Department of Education. (2014). Higher Education General Information Survey (HEGIS), Degrees and Other Formal Awards Conferred surveys, 1970–71 through 1985–86; Integrated Postsecondary Education Data System (IPEDS), Completions Survey (IPEDS-C:91–99); and IPEDS Fall 2000 through Fall 2013, Completions Component. Retrieved from *http://nces.ed.gov/programs/digest/d14/tables/dt14_323.10.asp*.

National Center for O*NET Development. (2008). Procedures for O*NET Job Zone Assignment. Retrieved from *www.onetcenter.org/dl_files/jobzoneprocedure.pdf*.

Nesse, R. M. (2000). Is depression an adaptation? *Archives of General Psychiatry, 57,* 14–20.

Ng, T. W. H., & Feldman, D. C. (2012). Evaluating six common stereotypes about older workers with meta-analytical data. *Personnel Psychology, 65,* 821–858.

Ng, T. W. H., & Feldman, D. C. (2013). How do within-person changes due to aging affect job performance? *Journal of Vocational Behavior, 83,* 500–513.

Oberauer, K., Wendland, M., & Kliegl, R. (2003). Age differences in working memory: The roles of storage and selective access. *Memory and Cognition, 31,* 563–569.

Poulin, M. J., & Heckhausen, J. (2007). Stressful events compromise control strivings during a major life transition. *Motivation and Emotion, 31,* 300–311.

Rasmussen, H. N., Wrosch, C., Scheier, M. F., & Carver, C. S. (2006). Self-regulation processes and health: The importance of optimism and goal adjustment. *Journal of Personality, 74,* 1721–1747.

Salthouse, T. A. (2004). What and when of cognitive aging. *Current Directions in Psychological Science, 13,* 140–144.

Salthouse, T. (2012). Consequences of age-related cognitive declines. *Annual Review of Psychology, 63,* 201–226.

Savickas, M. L., & Porfeli, E. J. (2012). Career-Adapt-Abilities Scale: Construction, reliability, and measurement equivalence across 13 countries. *Journal of Vocational Behavior, 80,* 661–673.

Scheier, M. F., & Carver, C. S. (1985). Optimism, coping, and health: Assessment and implications of generalized outcome expectancies. *Health Psychology, 4,* 219–247.

Schulz, R., & Curnow, C. (1988). Peak performance and age among superathletes: Track and field, swimming, baseball, tennis, and golf. *Journals of Gerontology B: Psychological Sciences, 43,* 113–120.

Shane, J., & Heckhausen, J. (2012). Motivational self-regulation in the work domain: Congruence of individuals' control striving and the control potential in their developmental ecologies. *Research in Human Development, 9,* 337–357.

Shane, J., & Heckhausen, J. (2013). University students' causal conceptions about social mobility: Diverging pathways for believers in personal merit and luck. *Journal of Vocational Behavior, 82,* 10–19.

Shane, J., & Heckhausen, J. (2016). For better or worse: Young adults' opportunity beliefs and motivational self-regulation during career entry. *International Journal of Behavioral Development, 42*(2), 107–116.

Shane, J., Heckhausen, J., Lessard, J., Chen, C., & Greenberger, E. (2012). Career-related goal pursuit among post-high school youth: Relations between personal control beliefs and control strivings. *Motivation and Emotion, 36,* 159–169.

Singer, T., Lindenberger, U., & Baltes, P. B. (2003). Plasticity of memory for new learning in very old age: A story of major loss? *Psychology and Aging, 18,* 306–317.

Singer, T., Verhaeghen, P., Ghirsletta, P., Lindenberger, U., & Baltes, P. B. (2003). The fate of cognition in very old age: Six-year longitudinal findings in the Berlin Aging Study (BASE). *Psychology and Aging, 18,* 318–331.

Spilerman, S., & Lunde, T. (1991). Features of educational attainment and job promotion prospects. *American Journal of Sociology, 97,* 689–720.

Srour, I., Abdul-Malak, M. A., Itani, M., Bakshan, A., & Sidani, Y. (2013). Career planning and progression for engineering management graduates: An exploratory study. *Engineering Management Journal, 25,* 85–98.

Staw, B. M. (1997). The escalation of commitment: An update and appraisal. In Z. Shapira (Ed.), *Organizational decision making* (pp. 191–215). New York: Cambridge University Press.

Sturman, M. C. (2003). Searching for the inverted U-shaped relationship between time and performance: Meta-analyses of the experience/performance, tenure/performance, and age/performance relationships. *Journal of Management, 29,* 609–640.

Super, D. E. (1980). A life-span, life-space approach to career development. *Journal of Vocational Behavior, 16,* 282–298.

U.S. Census Bureau. (2015). Educational attainment: CPS historical time series tables. Retrieved from *www.census.gov/hhes/socdemo/education/data/cps/historical.*

Veroff, J., Reuman, D., & Feld, S. (1984). Motives in American men and women across the adult life span. *Developmental Psychology, 20,* 1142–1158.

Vondracek, F. W., Lerner, R. M., & Schulenberg, J. E. (1983). The concept of development in vocational theory and intervention. *Journal of Vocational Behavior, 23,* 179–202.

Wanberg, C. R., Kanfer, R., Hamann, D. J., & Zhang, Z. (2016). Age and reemployment success after job loss: An integrative model and meta-analysis. *Psychological Bulletin, 142*(4), 400–426.

Wrosch, C., Scheier, M. F., Carver, C. S., & Schulz, R. (2003). The importance of goal disengagement in adaptive self-regulation: When giving up is beneficial. *Self and Identity, 2,* 1–20.

Yeh, Q. J. (2008). Exploring career stages of midcareer and older engineers: When managerial transition matters. *IEEE Transactions on Engineering Management, 55,* 82–93.

Zacher, H., Ambiel, R. A. M., & Noronha, A. P. P. (2015). Career adaptability and career entrenchment. *Journal of Vocational Behavior, 88,* 164–173.

Zacher, H., & Frese, M. (2009). Remaining time and opportunities at work: Relationships between age, work characteristics, and occupational future time perspective. *Psychology and Aging, 24,* 487–493.

Zacher, H., & Frese, M. (2011). Maintaining a focus on opportunities at work: The interplay between age, job complexity, and the use of selection, optimization, and compensation strategies. *Journal of Organizational Behavior, 32,* 291–318.

Zhao, X., Lim, V. K. G., & Teo, T. S. H. (2012). The long arm of job insecurity: Its impact on career-specific parenting behaviors and youths' career self-efficacy. *Journal of Vocational Behavior, 80,* 619–628.

CHAPTER 25

Motivational Factors as Mechanisms of Gene–Environment Transactions in Cognitive Development and Academic Achievement

ELLIOT M. TUCKER-DROB

Genetic differences between people are statistically associated with differences in their cognitive development and academic achievement (Plomin & Deary, 2015; Rietveld et al., 2013; Shakeshaft et al., 2013). Differences in the types and the quality of environments experienced are also associated with differences in cognitive development and academic achievement (Duncan & Murnane, 2011; Huston & Bentley, 2010). While these simple observations have historically been viewed as incompatible with one another, the contemporary scientist and, indeed, even the educated layperson will be quick to point out the fallacy in this apparent paradox: Rather than competing with one another, genetic and environmental influences act synergistically to affect human development. The recent mainstream acceptance of *interactionism* (Tabery, 2014), however, still leaves open many scientific questions regarding mechanism. What are the specific biological, social, and developmental processes through which genetic and environmental factors work together to influence human development?

In this chapter I describe a set of theoretical models that posit dynamic developmental mechanisms through which genetic and environmental factors *transact*, leading children to become nonrandomly matched to educationally relevant environmental experiences that foster academic achievement. I pay particular attention the role of motivational factors as driving forces in these dynamic transactions, and I describe how these processes may give rise to gene × environment interactions. First, I begin with an overview of how the basic behavioral genetic paradigm is used to estimate the statistical contributions of genetic and environmental factors to individual differences in psychological outcomes such as achievement test scores, grade-point average (GPA), and achievement motivation.

A SHORT PRIMER ON BEHAVIORAL GENETIC METHODOLOGY

Classical behavioral genetic methodology capitalizes on data from samples of sets of individuals that vary in their degrees of genetic relatedness (e.g., identical vs. fraternal twins, close-in-age biological siblings vs. close-in-age adoptive siblings) and/or shared rearing environment (e.g., siblings raised together vs. siblings raised apart) to build statistical models that estimate genetic and environmental contributions to variation in one or more outcomes of interest (e.g., motivational factors, personality traits, achievement test scores or GPA). Typically, total variation in an outcome is decomposed into three components: a genetic component, a shared environmental component, and a nonshared environmental component. The magnitude of variance in an outcome attributable to the genetic component is inferred from the extent to which, holding the amount of objectively shared rearing environment constant, more genetically similar individuals (e.g., identical twins raised together) resemble one another on that outcome more than do less genetically similar individuals (e.g., fraternal twins raised together). The magnitude of variance in an outcome attributable to the shared environmental component is inferred from the extent to which, holding genetic relatedness constant, individuals reared together (e.g., genetically unrelated adoptive siblings) resemble one another on that outcome more than do individuals reared apart (e.g., random pairs of individuals). It can also be inferred from the extent to which genetically related individuals reared together (e.g., identical twins reared together and fraternal twins reared together) resemble one another on the outcome to a greater extent than can be attributed to genetic relatedness alone. Finally, the magnitude of variance in an outcome attributable to the nonshared environmental component is inferred from the extent to which individuals are even more dissimilar on an outcome than would be expected from differences in their rearing environment and genetic makeup. For instance, the extent to which identical twins raised together (who have nearly identical genetic makeup and are raised in the same homes by the same parents and often attend the same school) differ on an outcome (to a greater extent than would be expected on the basis of measurement error alone) is attributable to the nonshared environment.

It is important to keep in mind that behavioral genetic methods are only useful for studying variation that exists in the population sampled. Behavioral genetic methods are able to provide insight into the extent to which between-person differences in genetic sequence are statistically associated with individual differences in their outcomes, but they are unable to provide direct insight into the extent to which portions of genetic sequence that are invariant across individuals give rise to universals shared by all humans. For instance, behavioral genetic methods cannot be used to determine the role of genetics in the fact that (nearly) all humans have 10 fingers and 10 toes, or in the fact that (nearly) all human adults are capable of producing and understanding complex language. Similarly, behavioral genetic methods are able to provide insight into the extent to which variation in environmental experiences that naturally exists in the population sampled is statistically related to individual differences in the outcomes under investigation, but they are (like all observational methods in the social sciences) not able to provide direct insight into the extent to which environments not experienced by participants in the sample (including interventions or policies that have yet to be implemented), or environments that are universally experienced by all participants in the sample (e.g., going to school) are related to the outcomes under investigation. This is an important and oftentimes underappreciated point: High estimates of heritability on an outcome *do not* place constraints on whether a new intervention or policy can be effective in influencing that outcome. Behavioral genetic methods can, of course, be informative about the effects of existing interventions or policies that vary (either naturally, or as a result of experimental control) in the population sampled. Indeed, as I discuss in the final section of this chapter, the application of behavioral genetic designs to randomized experiments is a potentially fruitful avenue for understanding how individuals might differentially respond to interventions (Plomin & Haworth, 2010; Tucker-Drob, 2011) and how interventions might change not only mean levels of an outcome (e.g., academic achievement) but also the distribution of levels of that outcome across individuals and families.

The merits, assumptions, and limitations of various behavioral genetic aipproaches have been discussed at length elsewhere (McGue, Elkins, Walden, & Iacono, 2005;

Turkheimer, 2015) and I will not repeat them here. However, the reader should be aware that evidence for genetic influences on cognitive and educational outcomes does not derive from one particular paradigm, but rather from an assortment of different approaches, including twin, extended family, adoption and, most recently, molecular genetic studies. Because each method relies on somewhat different assumptions, violations of which have different implications for model estimates, and because the general pattern of results regarding genetic influences on cognitive and educational outcomes has been robust to the particular method employed, the general body of behavioral genetic work rests of very solid ground (for an accessible overview, see Munafo, 2016). Arguments about whether there are statistical associations between genotype and cognitive and educational outcomes are outdated. The associations exist and, on average, are moderate in magnitude. An important question remains: What are the mechanisms that give rise to these associations? Thus, in the remainder of this chapter I focus on a class of theoretical models that propose dynamic developmental processes through which genetic influences on cognitive and educational outcomes come to be realized.

TRANSACTIONAL MODELS OF COGNITIVE DEVELOPMENT AND ACADEMIC ACHIEVEMENT

According to transactional models of cognitive development and academic achievement, individuals differ in the experiences that they select, evoke, and attend to, on the basis of their genetically influenced interests, goals, aptitudes, and motivations. These environments, in turn, have causal effects on their cognitive development and academic achievement. Because environments are nonrandomly experienced on the basis of genetically influenced psychological and behavioral tendencies, the causal effects of environmental experience on learning result in the differentiation of individuals' educational outcomes by genotype. Thus, in contrast to the lay view that genetic influences compete with experiential influences, transactional models hold that genetic influences

on cognition and achievement occur, at least in part, by way of environmental experience.

One of the first explicit proposals of the transactional hypothesis was by Hayes (1962), who made the following four-point argument:

> (a) Differences in motivation may be genetically determined. (b) These motivational differences, along with differences in environment, cause differences in experience. (c) Differences in experience lead to differences in ability. (d) The differences commonly referred to as intellectual are nothing more than differences in acquired abilities. (p. 303)

In other words, according to Hayes, genetically influenced motivational factors, what he referred to as *experience producing drives,* play instrumental roles in what environments are experienced by individuals, and variation in experience leads to variation in intellectual development, such that genetic influences in motivational factors give rise to individual differences in intellectual development.

Transactional models also build on Scarr and McCartney's (1983) developmental theory of genotype–environment correlation (rGE), which itself builds on the work of Plomin, DeFries, and Loehlin (1977). rGE refers to the correlations that arise between genetic differences between people and differences in the environments that they experience. Plomin and colleagues developed a tripartite taxonomy of rGE. *Passive rGE* arises when children who are reared by their biological parents inherit genes from the same individuals who provide them with their rearing environment. For example, children raised by more educationally motivated parents not only inherit a disposition toward educational motivation but are also raised in a family environment in which high academic achievement is valued and promoted. *Active rGE* occurs when children actively choose experiences from their environment on the basis of their genetically influenced traits. For example, children who are disposed toward high academic motivation may enroll in more rigorous coursework and seek out extracurricular activities that promote positive academic skills. *Evocative rGE* (originally termed *reactive rGE*) arises when children evoke different experiences from individuals and institutions within their broader environmental contexts on the basis of their genetically influenced traits. For example, children disposed toward high motivation may be more likely to respond positively to attention from teachers, thus positively reinforcing teachers' tendency to provide them with further time and attention. Both active and evocative forms of rGE are hypothesized to have central roles in transactional processes between children and their environments. As proposed by Scarr and McCartney (1983), "the degree to which experience is influenced by individual genotypes increases with development and with the shift from passive to active genotype → environment effects, as individuals select their own experiences" (p. 427) . . . "and build niches that are correlated with their talents, interests, and personality characteristics" (p. 433) with age.

Other notable contributions to the development of the transactional perspective come from the work of Sameroff (1975), who wrote that "the constants in development are not some set of traits but rather the processes by which these traits are maintained in the transactions between organism and environment" (p. 281). More recently Sameroff and McKenzie (2003, p. 614) wrote that

> the development of the child is a product of the continuous dynamic interactions of the child and the experience provided by his or her family and social context. What is central to the transactional model is the equal emphasis placed on the bidirectional effects of the child and of the environment. Experiences provided by the environment are not viewed as independent of the child.

Like the theory of Scarr and McCartney (1983), Sameroff's (1975) transactional perspective is a more general framework of psychological development that was not specifically developed with cognition or academic achievement in mind. Unlike the theory of Scarr and McCartney, however, Sameroff's perspective does not directly address the role of genotype in the transactional process. It does, however, consider "constitution."

In their bioecological model, Bronfrenbrenner and Ceci (1994) further expanded on the concept of reciprocal causation between the child and his or her immediate environment, explicitly hypothesizing that such transactions are a primary basis for genetic effects on adaptive psychological outcomes, including intelligence. They wrote:

> Human development takes place through processes of progressively more complex reciprocal interaction between an active, evolving biopsychological human organism and the persons, objects, and symbols in its immediate environment. To be effective, the interaction must occur on a fairly regular basis over extended periods of time. Such enduring forms of interaction in the immediate environment are referred to henceforth as *proximal processes*. . . . Proximal processes serve as a mechanism for actualizing genetic potential for effective psychological development. (p. 572)

Importantly, as indicated by the previous quotation, Bronfrenbrenner and Ceci (1994) hypothesized that proximal processes must recur over prolonged periods of time, and that their effects on psychological development accumulate progressively over time.

Recently, transactional models have been mathematically formalized. Dickens and Flynn (2001), for instance developed a simulation model of "strong reciprocal causation between phenotypic IQ and environment" (p. 346) in which initial genetically influenced individual differences in cognitive ability lead to more cognitively stimulating environments, which in turn lead to higher cognitive ability, leading to "a positive correlation between environment and genotype that masks the potency of environment" (p. 346). Beam, Turkheimer, Dickens, and Davis (2015) adapted the Dickens and Flynn (2001) model as a structural equation model, which they fit to longitudinal IQ data from the Louisville Twin Study. They concluded that the transactional model (which allows latent genetic factors to predict subsequent latent environmental factors via phenotypic IQ) provides a better fit to the data than a conventional autoregressive simplex model (which models time-point-to-time-point stability of IQ as the simple result of time point to time point stability of genetic and environmental factors, but does not allow associations between genetic and later environmental factors).

Fundamental to the Dickens and Flynn (2001) model is the postulation (also found in Bronfrenbrenner and Ceci's [1994] bioecological model) that, in order for environmental experiences to have meaningful effects on cognitive development, they must systematically recur over extended periods of time. Experiences that are systematic and recurring, Dickens and Flynn have argued, stem from socially entrenched and institutionalized processes (e.g., social class, race, historical period, and culture) and from gene–environment transactions. On this latter point, Dickens and Flynn have reasoned that experiences selected on the basis of relatively stable and enduring genetically influenced tendencies tend to recur systematically over time. Apart from experiences that result from macrosocietal forces in which individuals are deeply embedded, those that result from nongenetic factors, Dickens and Flynn argued, have a stronger tendency to be arbitrary, tend not to recur, and therefore tend to have unappreciable and ephemeral effects on psychological development. This postulation is crucial to the prediction that transactional processes lead to the differentiation of individuals by genotype, rather than simply by initial states, over time (Tucker-Drob & Harden, 2012a).

MOTIVATIONAL FACTORS AS PROPULSIVE FORCES IN ACADEMICALLY RELEVANT GENE–ENVIRONMENT TRANSACTIONS

What are the specific genetically influenced factors that lead individuals to differentially select and evoke achievement-relevant environments? Some authors (e.g., Dickens & Flynn, 2001; Beam et al., 2015) have suggested that early, genetically influenced individual differences in cognitive ability lead to differentiation of environmental experience, which in turn further differentiates individuals by cognitive ability. Other research, including the early work of Hayes (1962) and the influential work of Scarr and McCartney (1983), has placed strong emphasis on genetically influenced variation in motivations, interests, and personality as propelling individuals to differentially select and evoke environmental niches. High levels of motivational factors such as intellectual interest and achievement motivation may lead children to actively choose more intellectually stimulating peer groups, coursework, and extracurricular experiences from the ecologies in which they are embedded. At the same time, behaviors stemming from such motivational factors, when observed by others, may evoke from them more stimulating interactions, attract more achievement-oriented friendship networks, and lead teachers and parents to provide individuals with greater and/or higher-quality experiences. Motivational factors are also likely to be related to the extent to which different children attend to, deeply process, and expend effort even in the same educational setting. On the whole, differences in the amount and quality of environments experienced, and differences in the extent to which these environments are attended to and processed, lead to differences in both the cognitive development and academic achievement and the motivational traits that lead to the different experiences in the first place (Tucker-Drob & Harden, 2012b; see Figure 25.1).

Tucker-Drob and Harden (in press) recently reviewed the evidence relevant to the roles of a broad constellation of motivational factors in the processes by which individuals come to nonrandomly experience different academically relevant environments as functions of their genotypes. These included Openness, Conscientiousness, Intellectual Interest, Academic Interest, Self-Perceived Ability, Grit, Self-Control, Achievement Goal Orientations, Intelligence Mindsets, Expectancies, and Values. We suggested six general criteria that should be fulfilled in order for a motivational factor to be implicated in academically relevant gene–environment transactions:

1. The motivational factor should be correlated with academic achievement in observational data because a correlation is typically a necessary, though not sufficient, condition of causality within a naturally occurring system.
2. The motivational factor should statistically predict achievement above and beyond both cognitive ability (2a) and the Big Five personality factors (2b), as

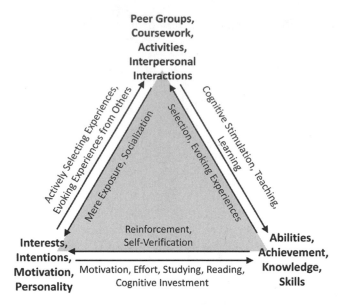

Peer Groups,
Coursework,
Activities,
Interpersonal
Interactions

Actively Selecting Experiences,
Evoking Experiences from Others

Mere Exposure, Socialization

Selection, Evoking Experiences

Cognitive Stimulation, Teaching,
Learning

Reinforcement,
Self-Verification

Interests,
Intentions,
Motivation,
Personality

Motivation, Effort, Studying, Reading,
Cognitive Investment

Abilities,
Achievement,
Knowledge,
Skills

FIGURE 25.1. A conceptual model for the mutual relations between motivational factors, proximal environments, and achievement. From Tucker-Drob and Harden (2012b). Copyright © 2012 Society for Research in Child Development. Reprinted by permission.

incremental prediction is necessary to rule out simple third variable (and "jangle") confounds attributable to overlap with the most well-studied psychological dimensions of individual differences.

3. In order to serve as a mechanism by which genotypes become matched to experiences, the motivational factor must be heritable.

4. In order for the motivational factor to mediate genetic effects on achievement, achievement must be influenced by some of the same genes that influence the motivational factor (i.e., there should be a nonzero genetic correlation between the motivational factor and achievement.

5. The direction of causation within the naturally occurring system, as tested using longitudinal methods such as cross-lagged panel analysis, should at least partially be from the motivational factor to achievement.

6. As a direct test of the role of gene–environment correlation in the motivation–achievement association, measured academically relevant environments should at least partially mediate genetic links between the motivational factor and achievement.

Based on our literature review (Tucker-Drob & Harden, in press), we were able to verify that nearly all of the motivational factors considered are correlated with academic achievement at nontrivial levels (Criterion 1), and in many cases such associations were robust to controls for intelligence (Criterion 2a). We found that many motivational factors, however, were not well studied using behavioral genetic methods. Notable exceptions include Openness, Conscientiousness, which, as major dimensions of personality, have been highly studied in genetically informed samples, as well as—but to a much lesser extent—Intellectual and Academic Interest, Self-Perceived Ability, and Self-Control, all of which have been found to be moderately heritable (Criterion 3). We found that there has been very little, if any, behavioral genetic work on Grit, Achievement Goal Orientations, Mindsets, or Expectancies and Values. In the cases of Conscientiousness, Openness, Intellectual Interest, and Self Perceived Ability, there was also evidence that genetic factors at least partially mediate associations with academic achievement (Criterion 4). There was emerging evidence that many of the motivational factors longitudinally predict achievement, even when researchers controlled for past achievement, indicating that the direction of causation may at least partially originate from the motivational factors (Criterion 5). Finally, with the exception of Expectancies and Values, we were unable to identify strong longitudinal research testing for mediation of the motivational factor–achievement association by measured environments. Nor did we find any work that tested such mediation using genetically informed methods (Criterion 6). We suggested that measuring environmental factors that children are able to dynamically select and evoke, and that are relevant to achievement, may indeed be one of the biggest ongoing challenges in empirical tests of transactional models. Finally, we found that the extent to which motivational factors relate to one another and to the Big Five personality traits had not been well studied, and it was therefore unclear whether many of the commonly studied factors represent the same, independent, or partially overlapping dimensions of individual differences (Criterion 2b).

Recently, my colleagues and I published an article reporting results of a project that has attempted to fill many of the previously identified gaps in the literature (Tucker-Drob, Briley, Engelhardt, Mann, & Harden, 2016). Using data that we collected from a racially, ethnically, and socioeconomically diverse population-based sample of 811 third- through eighth-grade twins and triplets from the Texas Twin Project (Harden, Tucker-Drob, & Tackett, 2013), we examined how seven popular character traits (*Grit, Intellectual Curiosity, Intellectual Self-Concept, Mastery Orientation, Educational Value, Intelligence Mindset,* and *Test Motivation*) (1) relate to measures of the Big Five personality traits; (2) relate to one another; (3) are associated with genetic and environmental variance components, and whether such effects operate through common dimensions of individual differences; and (4) are related to verbal knowledge and academic achievement through genetic and environmental pathways, both before and after we controlled for fluid intelligence. We found that the character measures correlated moderately with one another and with measures of Openness and Conscientiousness from the Big Five Inventory (BFI; John, Naumann, & Soto, 2008). When these measures

were included in a factor analysis, two latent factors emerged: (1) a latent factor that we named Openness, upon which Intellectual Self-Concept, Intellectual Curiosity (Need for Cognition), and BFI Openness loaded appreciably, and (2) a latent factor that we named Conscientiousness, upon which Grit, Intellectual Curiosity, Mastery Orientation, Educational Value, Intelligence Mindset, and BFI Conscientiousness loaded appreciably. Both latent factors (which were correlated at $r = .44$) were influenced approximately 50% by genetic factors and 50% by nonshared environmental factors. For nearly all of the individual measures, there were also residual genetic and nonshared environmental influences that were not accounted for by the latent Openness and Conscientiousness factors. There was no indication of shared environmental influence at either factor- or the measure-specific levels. Both when character was examined at the level of the Openness and Conscientiousness factors, and when it was examined at the level of the individual measures (Figure 25.2), relations with verbal knowledge and academic achievement were positive, and persisted after we controlled for fluid intelligence. Consistent with the predictions of transactional models, genetic factors primarily mediated these associations. Nonshared environmental mediation was generally trivial and inconsistent across variables.

The sum of the paired light gray (i.e., genetically mediated contribution) and dark gray (i.e., environmentally mediated contribution) bars in Figure 25.2 represents the net model-implied correlation between each individual character/personality measure and a knowledge/achievement factor. The cross-hatched portion of the gray and dark gray bars represents genetic and environmental contributions to associations between character/personality and knowledge/achievement shared with fluid intelligence. The solid portion of the gray and dark gray bars represents genetic and environmental contributions to associations between character/personality and knowledge/achievement incremental to fluid intelligence. Shared and incremental effects sum to the total genetic and environmental effects. For instances in which the shared and incremental effects were in opposite directions, the aggregated effect is displayed.

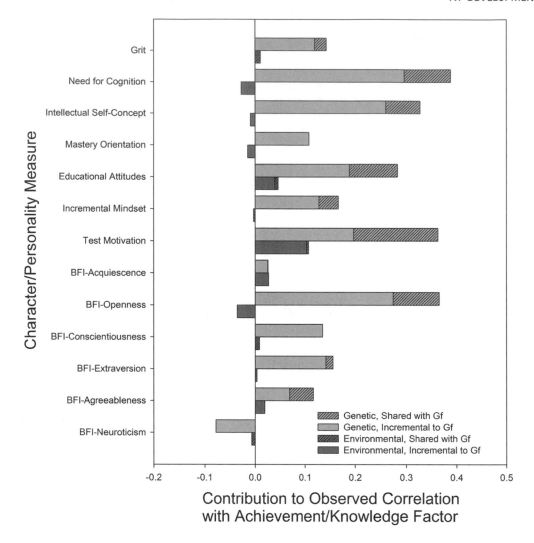

FIGURE 25.2. Barplot representing correlations between the character/Big Five Inventory scores and a latent achievement/knowledge factor. Gf, fluid intelligence. From Tucker-Drob et al. (2016). Copyright 2016 by the American Psychological Association. Reprinted by permission.

TRANSACTIONAL PROCESSES AS MECHANISMS OF DEVELOPMENTAL INCREASES IN HERITABILITY

A highly robust and counterintuitive finding from the past quarter-century of behavioral genetic research is that of developmental changes in the heritability of cognitive abilities. Some researchers (e.g., Fryer & Levitt, 2006; Spelke, 2005) have speculated that genetic influences on psychological outcomes should be strongest in early life and decrease with age, as the effects of environmental influences accumulate and account for a larger and larger share of the individual-differences pie. However, the empirical pattern of developmental changes in in the heritability of cognitive abilities is exactly the reverse. Genetic influences on cognitive abilities account for very small proportions of variance during infancy, with proportions increasing continuously over the course of child development, such that by late adolescence, genetic influences on cognitive abilities are between approximately 60 and 70% (Briley & Tucker-Drob, 2015; Haworth et al.,

2010; McCartney, Harris, & Bernieri, 1990; Tucker-Drob, Briley, & Harden, 2013).

Two general classes of mechanisms have the potential to account for this pattern (Briley & Tucker-Drob, 2013; Plomin, 1986). *Innovation* refers to a circumstance in which novel genetic factors, not previously relevant for cognitive abilities in early development, become relevant for cognitive abilities at later ages. This can occur because portions of genetic code are not transcribed until later in development, at which point they become epigenetically activated (Bocklandt et al., 2011; Hannum et al., 2013; Horvath, 2013; Reik, 2007). Innovation can also occur when genetic factors that are expressed early in life influence noncognitive but not cognitive abilities, and become increasingly relevant for cognitive abilities over the course of development. *Amplification* refers to a circumstance in which the same genetic factors relevant for cognitive abilities in early life have increasingly large effects on those abilities with age, such that their effects are amplified over development.

In a series of articles, Daniel Briley and I (Briley & Tucker-Drob, 2013, 2015; Tucker-Drob & Briley, 2014) meta-analyzed longitudinal behavioral genetic studies to examine the extent to which genetic influences on cognitive abilities persist forward and the extent to which novel genetic influences arise over time. We found that over the first decade of life, increasing heritability is driven by innovation processes, in which genetic factors not previously relevant for cognitive abilities become relevant at later ages. In the second decade of life, amplification process become the predominant drivers of increasing heritability: Heritability of cognitive abilities continues increasing during middle childhood and adolescence by way of amplifying the effects of genetic factors relevant for cognitive abilities beginning at approximately age 10 years.

Transactional models provide a plausible explanation for both the innovation pattern observed in infancy and early childhood and the amplification pattern observed in middle childhood and adolescence. Under transactional models, genetically influenced motivational factors are initially irrelevant for cognitive development. As time passes, and as children have increasing autonomy to select their experiences, they differentially accrue different environmental experiences as a function of their genetically influenced motivational factors. Genetic influences on motivational factors that were originally irrelevant for cognitive abilities are expected to become relevant for cognitive abilities over time (i.e., innovation). Once genetic influences on motivational factors become coupled to cognitive abilities, transactional processes are expected to continue, further differentiating children's experiences, and hence their cognitive abilities, by genotype (i.e., amplification). Consistent with more conventional wisdom, such a transactional perspective postulates that the effects of environmental experience on cognitive abilities accrue over time. However, because environments are nonrandomly experienced on the basis of genetically influenced factors, the result is increasing heritability of cognitive abilities over development.

TRANSACTIONAL PROCESSES AS MECHANISMS OF GENE-BY-ENVIRONMENT INTERACTIONS

Thus far in this chapter, I have discussed *gene–environment transactions*, which are dynamic processes in which individuals come to be differentially exposed to environmental experiences on the basis of genetically influenced dispositional factors, *and* these environments in turn affect their cognitive development and academic achievement. *Gene × environment interactions* are conceptually and mathematically distinct phenomena whereby genetic differences between people are associated with differences in effects of an environmental input on their psychological development, *and* the magnitude of genetic effect on an outcome is stronger is some environmental contexts than in others (Plomin et al., 1977). Interestingly, macroenvironmental contexts may modulate the magnitude of heritability by way of constraining or facilitating transactional processes. In other words, gene–environment transactions may serve as a basis for gene × environment interactions. This hypothesis has been stated by a number of separate authors over the past two decades, as exemplified by the following quotes:

The entire theory [of gene–environment correlation] depends on people having a varied environment from which to choose and construct experiences. The theory does not apply, therefore, to people with few choices or few opportunities for experiences that match their genotypes. (Scarr, 1992, p. 9)

Heritability (assessed by h^2) varies markedly and systematically as a function of levels of proximal process. (Bronfrenbrenner & Ceci, 1994, p. 570)

Under a transactional model of cognitive development, children are expected to select and evoke their environmental experiences on the basis of genetically influenced dispositions, but this process depends on the existence of adequate opportunities for such experiences. (Tucker-Drob et al., 2013, pp. 351–352)

Genes without sufficient match to suitable environments lose influence on development. (Beam et al., 2015, p. 625)

One of the most commonly mentioned macroenvironmental dimensions hypothesized to be associated with differences in the efficiency of academically and intellectually relevant transactional processes is childhood socioeconomic status (SES). Children living in lower SES settings are provided with fewer opportunities to seek out high-quality educational experiences, and live under conditions of hardship that may limit the ability of those around them to be attentive to and supportive of their interests, talents, and goals. Consistent with this hypothesis, a number of studies (Bates, Lewis, & Weiss, 2013; Harden, Turkheimer, & Loehlin, 2007; Rowe, Jacobson, & Van den Oord, 1999; Scarr-Salapatek, 1971; Tucker-Drob, Rhemtulla, Harden, Turkheimer, & Fask, 2011; Turkheimer, Haley, D'Onofrio, Waldron, & Gottesman, 2003) have reported that genetic influences on cognitive ability and academic achievement are suppressed under conditions of socioeconomic privation. A recent meta-analysis (Tucker-Drob & Bates, 2016) confirms this gene × childhood SES interaction in the United States (Figure 25.3): at 2 standard deviations below the mean SES, model-implied heritability of cognitive ability and academic achievement is approximately 24%, with progressive increases in heritability throughout the range of SES, such that at 2 standard deviations above the mean SES, model-implied heritability is approximately 61%. Interestingly, our meta-analysis indicated that such an interaction is not apparent in in samples from Western Europe and Australia, with the difference between U.S. and Western European/Australian interaction effects sizes itself being statistically significant. Sensitivity analyses indicated robustness of this cross-national pattern to other hypothesized moderators, and there was no significant evidence of p-hacking or publication bias that could have biased or distorted estimates (Simonsohn, Nelson, & Simmons, 2014). One provocative interpretation, then, of these cross-national differences is that opportunities for cognitively and academically relevant gene–environment transaction are far less stratified by SES in Western Europe and Australia than they are in the United States.

My colleagues and I have conducted series of studies probing whether SES moderates the role of motivational factors on academic achievement. In one study (Tucker-Drob & Briley, 2012) of $N = 375,000$ U.S. high school students, we investigated whether family SES moderated the relation between domain-specific interests and domain-specific knowledge in 11 academic, vocational/professional, and recreational domains, including art, literature, music, biological sciences, physical sciences, and sports. Consistent with our hypothesis that higher SES contexts afford children greater opportunities to pursue learning experiences on the basis of their interests, we found that interest was appreciably more related to knowledge at higher levels of SES for all domains except for farming. In another study (Tucker-Drob, Cheung, & Briley, 2014) of approximately 400,000 high school students from 57 countries, we investigated moderation of science interest–science achievement associations by family SES, school SES, and national gross domestic product (GDP). Again, consistent with the hypothesis that higher SES contexts allow children to select and evoke learning opportunities on the basis of their interests, we found that family SES positively moderated interest–achievement associations, such that science interest was a stronger predictor of science achievement test scores at higher levels of family and school SES. Importantly, however, the magnitude of

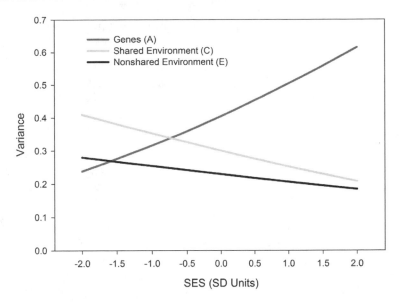

FIGURE 25.3. Meta-analytic results for gene-by-socioeconomic status (SES) interaction on intelligence and achievement in the United States. The *x*-axis represents family SES and the *y*-axis represents variance in intelligence and achievement that is explained by genetic, shared environmental, and nonshared environmental factors. For further explanation of the meaning of genetic, shared environmental, and nonshared environmental variance components, see the section "A Short Primer on Behavioral Genetic Methodology." From Tucker-Drob and Bates (2016). Copyright © 2016 Association for Psychological Science. Reprinted by permission.

moderation varied by country, with one of the largest interaction estimates obtained in the U.S. subsample. We also found strong moderation of the within-country science interest–achievement association by national GDP: In the richest countries, the standardized association between interest in achievement was over .30, but in the poorest countries, the association was essentially 0. The correlation between log-transformed national GDP and the country-specific effect size representing the science interest–science achievement association was 0.753, 95% confidence interval = .639, .867).

In two separate behavioral genetic studies of U.S. children, we have found that this SES × interest interaction mediates the gene × childhood SES interaction on achievement discussed earlier. Tucker-Drob and Harden (2012b) used a sample of 777 pairs of U.S. high school twins (i.e., *N* = 1,554 individuals). We fit bivariate gene × environment interaction models to examine the association between intellectual interest and an academic achievement composite measure that comprised English Usage, Mathematics

Usage, Social Science Reading, Natural Science Reading, and Word Usage. Results indicated that for low-SES students, genetic variance in intellectual interest was unrelated to academic achievement, but that for high-SES students, genetic variance in intellectual interest accounted for approximately 30% of the variance in academic achievement. This interaction with genes for intellectual interest accounted for the previously identified gene × childhood SES interaction on achievement. In a separate sample of 650 pairs of preschool-age twins, we (Tucker-Drob & Harden, 2012c) similarly found that genetic influences on learning motivation were unrelated to early mathematics skills in low-SES children, but accounted for approximately 30% of the variance in early mathematics skills in higher SES children. This interaction with genes for motivation accounted for the previously identified gene × childhood SES interaction on mathematics skills. Together these results are consistent with the hypothesis that, in the United States, higher SES affords greater opportunities for children to engage in transactional processes in which they select and evoke learning experiences on the basis of their genetically influenced interests and motivations to learn.

Some comments are warranted. First, it is important to note that not all motivational factors may interact with SES in the same way. Our previous research has largely focused on interest, but other motivational factors, such as self-concept or self-control, may interact with SES in different ways. For instance, it is possible that in high-SES environments, where external support systems help children to structure their time and follow through on their goals, individual differences in self-regulatory factors may be less important for achievement.

Second, while this section has focused on interactions involving SES, there are many other environmental factors that may interact with motivational factors to influence achievement. For instance, specific aspects of the school environment, such as teacher quality, have been reported to interact with genetic influences on achievement (Taylor, Roehrig, Hensler, Connor, & Schatschneider, 2010), and it is possible that motivational factors may play a role in this interaction.

Third, motivational factors may interact with one another in the prediction of student achievement. A recent series of studies has provided evidence for expectancy × value interactions in both engagement in educational activities (Nagengast et al., 2011) and academic achievement (Trautwein et al., 2012; Tucker-Drob et al., 2014). Although I am aware of no genetically informed work on this topic, an exciting area for future research may be to examine whether genetic and/or environmental components of expectancies and values serve as the basis of these interaction. Expectancy–value interactions may constitute gene × environment interactions, environment × environment interactions, gene × gene interactions, or some combination of the aforementioned.

CONSIDERING INTERVENTIONS

What are the implications of transactional models, and of behavioral genetic research on motivation and achievement more generally, for policy and intervention? It is important to make clear that current knowledge regarding the developmental–genetic mechanisms of motivation and achievement is based almost exclusively on observational research, and that it would therefore be inappropriate to rely on such research to make recommendations for the enactment of specific policies or interventions within society. Rather, this research is at a point in which it can be used to generate hypotheses about how new interventions or policies might be designed, and to make probabilistic statements about what sorts of policies or interventions might be more or less likely to be effective in the context of a carefully designed program evaluation. Rigorous approaches to treatment and policy evaluation, ideally approaches that rely on randomized controlled designs, would be necessary before recommendations could be made regarding implementation outside of a research context.

It is also useful to make explicit what insights from behavioral genetics do *not* mean in terms of implications for intervention and policy research. Simply because an outcome is genetically influenced does not mean that the environment does not matter. Genetic influences on outcomes rarely, if ever, account for all of the variation in psychological outcomes. Thus, even acceptance of the fallacious view that the genetic portion of the variance pie reflects an immutable component, still leaves plenty of room for a plastic component of the pie.

Moreover, genetically influenced variation in psychological outcomes are likely to often occur via environmental mechanisms. For instance, genetic influences on musical expertise occur, in part, by way of genetically influenced variation in the propensity to practice a musical instrument, and it is the environmental experience of consistently playing the musical instrument that results in the development of musical expertise (Hambrick & Tucker-Drob, 2015). Similarly, transactional models predict that genetically influenced variation in cognitive ability and academic achievement occur, in part, by way of variation in time, effort, and attention dedicated to learning experiences on the basis of genetically influenced motivational traits. Thus, one potentially fruitful avenue for policy and intervention research would be to first empirically trace the specific learning-relevant behaviors and experiences that motivated children to engage in and then develop programs and curricula that foster these behaviors, either through changing the motivational factors themselves or changing the behaviors that are downstream from the motivational factors. Another potentially fruitful avenue for such research would be to examine how modulating the contextual supports for person-driven selection and evocation of learning experiences might shift both overall average levels of achievement and heterogeneity in achievement outcomes. It may also be advantageous to develop and test interventions that increase opportunities for highly motivated children to select and evoke environments, and at the same time restrict opportunities for children who are low in motivation to select suboptimal learning experiences. Indeed, work described earlier on gene × environment interaction highlights the potential utility of a dual emphasis on both personal and contextual factors in the development of policy and intervention hypotheses.

The finding that shared environmental influences on motivational factors are low, if not entirely absent, does call into question the common wisdom that the socializing effects of between-family variation in environmental experiences are a primary mechanism of naturally existing variation in these factors. Trivial estimates of shared environmental influence on measures of motivational outcomes imply that (1) family environments have differential effects on the motivational outcomes of individuals within the same family and/or (2) environmental experiences that naturally vary (at nontrivial prevalence rates) in the general population are not very potent causes of motivational outcomes. The implication of trivial shared environmental influences on motivational factors for intervention research is that in order to be successful in producing a nontrivial average causal effect on motivational factors, an intervention would likely need to implement a treatment that is not already varying at the family-level within the general population. As my colleagues and I (Tucker-Drob et al., 2016) have previously stated,

the lack of evidence for shared environmental influence on the character measures examined does "not inform the question of whether interventions or policies that have yet to be implemented, did not naturally occur for children in the current sample, or were universally experienced by all children in the sample could potentially make children raised together more similar in their character" (p. 19).

Finally, it is important to keep in mind that treatment effects, as they are typically estimated in the context of a randomized controlled experiment, are estimates of average causal effects of the treatment across individuals. Treatment effects, however, may not be the same for all individuals within the population sampled. Methods for the estimating variability in, and correlates of, individual causal effects exist (Tucker-Drob, 2011), but such approaches are rarely (or inappropriately) implemented. Studying heterogeneity in treatment effects, however, can be tremendously valuable. Such knowledge could be used to (1) choose the most appropriate intervention for an individual student or subpopulation of students; (2) produce the best informed a priori estimate of how much of an effect to expect for a particular student or subpopulation of students, and of the potential range of magnitude of effect to be expected; and (3) identify subpopulations of students that are most likely to benefit from a policy or intervention, and those that are likely to not benefit or to even react adversely. In fact, the incorporation of randomized experimental approaches and behavioral genetic approaches can be used to test whether the treatment under study magnifies and/or constricts genetic and environmental influences on the outcomes of interest. One potential goal of an intervention might be to increase overall average levels of achievement and reduce between-family (shared environmental) variation in achievement (i.e., reduce achievement gaps). One underappreciated consequence of such a result is that, all else being equal, a greater proportion of remaining variation in achievement will be associated with genetic factors. As my colleagues and I (Tucker-Drob et al., 2013) have previously hypothesized, "a social, educational, and economic opportunities increase in a society, genetic differences will account for increasing variation in cognition—and perhaps ultimately in educational and economic attainment" (p. 353). Effective interventions that boost overall achievement and narrow socioeconomic inequalities in achievement outcomes may also increase the relative salience of genetic influences on those outcomes. This, however, is not a necessary consequence of all interventions that boost mean achievement; some interventions may boost achievement while increasing between-family disparities. Ceci and Papierno (2005, p. 149) have described such a situation as being one in which "the 'have-nots' gain but the 'haves' gain even more." Whether such an outcome is, on balance, desirable from a policy or social justice perspective is a matter of values. Regardless, the question of hetereogeneity in treatment effect is an important scientific question that can be used to inform policy decisions.

CONCLUSIONS

In this chapter, I have described a set of theoretical models that posit dynamic developmental mechanisms through which individuals become nonrandomly matched to environmental experiences on the basis of their genetically influenced traits, and these experiences in turn have causal effects on their cognitive development and academic achievement. While early genetically influenced levels of cognitive ability and scholastic aptitude may themselves be propulsive factors in such transactional processes, there is a growing body of both theoretical and empirical evidence implicating genetically influenced motivational factors as themselves being propulsive. In other words, genetically influenced individual differences in personality, interests, goals, and other motivational factors lead to differences in the types and qualities of academically relevant environments that children select, evoke, and attend to, leading to the differentiation of individuals' cognitive and educational outcomes by genotype over time. If macroenvironmental factors, such as SES, are related to the efficiencies of such dynamic processes, genetic influences on cognitive and educational outcomes are expected to differ as systematic functions of macroenvironmental measures (i.e., a gene × environment interaction). Future work will be necessary to identify and test the specific motivational factors responsible for gene–environment transactions, to identify the specific educationally relevant environments that come to be correlated with genotypes over time, and to further delineate the macroenvironmental conditions under which transactional processes are modulated. Suck work may ultimately help to inform the design of policies and interventions that would then need to be evaluated using rigorous randomized controlled methods before being implemented in society at large.

ACKNOWLEDGMENTS

During the time that I was preparing this chapter, I was supported as a Visiting Scholar at the Russell Sage Foundation, and my research was supported by Grant Nos. HD083613, HD081437, and AA023322 from the National Institutes of Health. I am also a member of the Population Research Center at the University of Texas at Austin, which is supported by Grant No. HD042849 from the National Institutes of Health.

REFERENCES

Bates, T. C., Lewis, G. J., & Weiss, A. (2013). Childhood socioeconomic status amplifies genetic effects on adult intelligence. *Psychological Science*, 24(10), 2111–2116.

Beam, C. R., Turkheimer, E., Dickens, W. T., & Davis, D. W. (2015). Twin differentiation of cognitive ability through phenotype to environment transmission: The Louisville Twin Study. *Behavior Genetics*, 45(6), 622–634.

Bocklandt, S., Lin, W., Sehl, M. E., Sánchez, F. J., Sinsheimer, J. S., Horvath, S., et al. (2011). Epigenetic predictor of age. *PLoS ONE*, 6, e14821.

Briley, D. A., & Tucker-Drob, E. M. (2013). Explaining the increasing heritability of cognition over development: A meta-analysis of longitudinal twin and adoption studies. *Psychological Science*, 24, 1704–1713.

Briley, D. A., & Tucker-Drob, E. M. (2015). Comparing the developmental genetics of cognition and personality over the life span [Special issue]. *Journal of Personality*. [Epub ahead of print]

Bronfenbrenner, U., & Ceci, S. J. (1994).

Nature–nuture reconceptualized in developmental perspective: A bioecological model. *Psychological Review, 101,* 568–586.

Ceci, S. J., & Papierno, P. B. (2005). The rhetoric and reality of gap closing: When the "have-nots" gain but the "haves" gain even more. *American Psychologist, 60,* 149–160.

Dickens, W. T., & Flynn, J. R. (2001). Heritability estimates versus large environmental effects: The IQ paradox resolved. *Psychological Review, 108,* 346–369.

Duncan, G. J., & Murnane, R. J. (Eds.). (2011). *Whither opportunity?: Rising inequality, schools, and children's life chances.* New York: Russell Sage Foundation.

Fryer, R. G., & Levitt, S. (2006). *Testing for racial differences in the mental ability of young children* (NBER Working Paper No. 12066). Cambridge, MA: National Bureau of Economic Research.

Hambrick, D. Z., & Tucker-Drob, E. M. (2015). The genetics of music accomplishment; Evidence for gene–environment interaction and correlation. *Psychonomic Bulletin and Review, 22,* 112–120.

Hannum, G., Guinney, J., Zhao, L., Zhang, L., Hughes, G., Sadda, S., et al. (2013). Genome-wide methylation profiles reveal quantitative views of human aging rates. *Molecular Cell, 49*(2), 359–367.

Harden, K. P., Tucker-Drob, E. M., & Tackett, J. L. (2013). The Texas Twin Project [Special issue]. *Twin Research and Human Genetics, 16,* 385–390.

Harden, K. P., Turkheimer, E., & Loehlin, J. C. (2007). Genotype-by-environment interaction in adolescents' cognitive ability. *Behavior Genetics, 37,* 273–283.

Haworth, C. M. A., Wright, M. J., Luciano, M., Martin, N. G., De Geus, E. J. C., Van Beijsterveldt, C. E. M., et al. (2010). The heritability of general cognitive ability increases linearly from childhood to young adulthood. *Molecular Psychiatry, 15*(11), 1112–1120.

Hayes, K. J. (1962). Genes, drives, and intellect. *Psychological Reports, 10,* 299–342.

Horvath, S. (2013). DNA methylation age of human tissues and cell types. *Genome Biology, 14*(10), 1–20.

Huston, A. C., & Bentley, A. C. (2010). Human development in societal context. *Annual Review of Psychology, 61,* 411–437.

John, O. P., Naumann, L. P., & Soto, C. J. (2008). Paradigm shift to the integrative Big Five trait taxonomy: History: measurement, and conceptual issues. In O. P. John, R. W. Robins, & L. A. Pervin (Eds.), *Handbook of personality: Theory and research* (3rd ed., pp. 114–158). New York: Guilford Press.

McCartney, K., Harris, M. J., & Bernieri, F. (1990). Growing up and growing apart: A developmental meta-analysis of twin studies. *Psychological Bulletin, 107*(2), 226–237.

McGue, M., Elkins, I., Walden, B., & Iacono, W. G. (2005). The essential role of behavioral genetics in developmental psychology: Reply to Partridge (2005) and Greenberg (2005). *Developmental Psychology, 14,* 993–997.

Munafo, M. (2016). Genetic denialism is unhelpful—genes play a role in who we are. *The Guardian.* Retrieved March 11, 2016, from *www.theguardian.com/science/sifting-the-evidence/2016/mar/04/genetic-denialism-is-unhelpful-genes-play-a-role-in-who-we-are.*

Nagengast, B., Marsh, H. W., Scalas, L. F., Xu, M. K., Hau, K. T., & Trautwein, U. (2011). Who took the "×" out of expectancy–value theory?: A psychological mystery, a substantive–methodological synergy, and a cross-national generalization. *Psychological Science, 22,* 1058–1066.

Plomin, R. (1986). Multivariate analysis and developmental behavioral genetics: Developmental change as well as continuity. *Behavior Genetics, 16,* 25–43.

Plomin, R., & Deary, I. J. (2015). Genetics and intelligence differences: Five special findings. *Molecular Psychiatry, 20,* 98–108.

Plomin, R., DeFries, J. C., & Loehlin, J. C. (1977). Genotype–environment interaction and correlation in the analysis of human behavior. *Psychological Bulletin, 84*(2), 309–322.

Plomin, R., & Haworth, C. M. (2010). Genetics and intervention research. *Perspectives on Psychological Science, 5,* 557–563.

Reik, W. (2007). Stability and flexibility of epigenetic gene regulation in mammalian development. *Nature, 447,* 425–432.

Rietveld, C. A., Medland, S. E., Derringer, J., Yang, J., Esko, T., Martin, N. W., et al. (2013). GWAS of 126,559 individuals identifies genetic variants associated with educational attainment. *Science, 340,* 1467–1471.

Rowe, D. C., Jacobson, K. C., & Van den Oord, E. J. (1999). Genetic and environmental influences on vocabulary IQ: Parental education level as moderator. *Child Development, 70*(5), 1151–1162.

Sameroff, A. (1975). Transactional models in early social relations. *Human Development, 18*(1–2), 65–79.

Sameroff, A. J., & MacKenzie, M. J. (2003). Research strategies for capturing transactional models of development: The limits of the possible. *Development and Psychopathology, 15*(3), 613–640.

Scarr, S. (1992). Developmental theories for the 1990s: Development and individual differences. *Child Development, 63*(1), 1–19.

Scarr, S., & McCartney, K. (1983). How people make their own environments: A theory of genotype → environment effects. *Child Development, 54*(2), 424–435.

Scarr-Salapatek, S. (1971). Race, social class, and IQ. *Science, 174,* 1285–1295.

Shakeshaft, N. G., Trzaskowski, M., McMillan, A., Rimfeld, K., Krapohl, E., Haworth, C. M., et al. (2013). Strong genetic influence on a UK nationwide test of educational achievement at the end of compulsory education at age 16. *PLoS ONE, 8*(12), e80341.

Simonsohn, U., Nelson, L. D., & Simmons, J. P. (2014). P-curve: A key to the file-drawer. *Journal of Experimental Psychology: General, 143,* 534–547.

Spelke, E. S. (2005). Sex differences in intrinsic aptitude for mathematics and science?: A critical review. *American Psychologist, 60,* 950–958.

Tabery, J. (2014). *Beyond versus: The struggle to understand the interaction of nature and nurture.* Cambridge, MA: MIT Press.

Taylor, J., Roehrig, A. D., Hensler, B. S., Connor, C. M., & Schatschneider, C. (2010). Teacher quality moderates the genetic effects on early reading. *Science, 328,* 512–514.

Trautwein, U., Marsh, H. W., Nagengast, B., Lüdtke, O., Nagy, G., & Jonkmann, K. (2012). Probing for the multiplicative term in modern expectancy–value theory: A latent interaction modeling study. *Journal of Educational Psychology, 104,* 763–777.

Tucker-Drob, E. M. (2011). Individual differences methods for randomized experiments. *Psychological Methods, 16,* 298–318.

Tucker-Drob, E. M., & Bates, T. C. (2016). Large cross-national differences in gene × socioeconomic status interaction on intelligence. *Psychological Science, 27,* 138–149.

Tucker-Drob, E. M., & Briley, D. A. (2012). Socioeconomic status modifies interest–knowledge associations among adolescents. *Personality and Individual Differences, 53,* 9–15.

Tucker-Drob, E. M., & Briley, D. A. (2014). Continuity of genetic and environmental influences on cognition across the life span: A meta-analysis of longitudinal twin and adoption studies. *Psychological Bulletin, 140,* 949–979.

Tucker-Drob, E. M., Briley, D. A., Engelhardt, L. E., Mann, F. D. & Harden, K. P. (2016). Genetically-mediated associations between measures of childhood character and academic achievement. *Journal of Personality and Social Psychology, 111,* 790–815.

Tucker-Drob, E. M., Briley, D. A., & Harden, K. P. (2013). Genetic and environmental influences on cognition across development and context. *Current Directions in Psychological Science, 22,* 349–355.

Tucker-Drob, E. M., Cheung, A. K., & Briley, D. A. (2014). Gross domestic product, science interest, and science achievement: A person × nation interaction. *Psychological Science, 25,* 2047–2057.

Tucker-Drob, E. M., & Harden, K. P. (2012a). Early childhood cognitive development and parental cognitive stimulation: Evidence for reciprocal gene–environment transactions. *Developmental Science, 15,* 250–259.

Tucker-Drob, E. M., & Harden, K. P. (2012b). Intellectual interest mediates gene-by-socioeconomic status interaction on adolescent academic achievement. *Child Development, 83,* 743–757.

Tucker-Drob, E. M., & Harden, K. P. (2012c). Learning motivation mediates gene-by-socioeconomic status interaction on early mathematics achievement. *Learning and Individual Differences, 22,* 37–45.

Tucker-Drob, E. M., & Harden, K. P. (in press). A behavioral genetic perspective on noncognitive factors and academic achievement. In S. Bouregy, E. Grigorenko, S. Latham, & M. Tan (Eds.), *Current perspective in psychology: Genetics, ethics, and education.* New York: Cambridge University Press.

Tucker-Drob, E. M., Rhemtulla, M., Harden, K. P., Turkheimer, E., & Fask, D. (2011). Emergence of a gene-by-socioeconomic status interaction on infant mental ability between 10 months to 2 years. *Psychological Science, 22,* 125–133.

Turkheimer, E. (2015). Arsonists at the cathedral. *PsycCRITIQUES, 60*(40).

Turkheimer, E., Haley, A., D'Onofrio, B., Waldron, M., & Gottesman, I. I. (2003). Socioeconomic status modifies heritability of IQ in young children. *Psychological Science, 14,* 623–628.

PART V

SOCIAL GROUPS AND SOCIAL INFLUENCES

CHAPTER 26

Gender and Competence Motivation

RUTH BUTLER
LIAT HASENFRATZ

Since the turn of the century, the United States has already seen two major federal educational reform initiatives: No Child Left Behind and Race to the Top. Neither targeted gender as a major cause for concern and therefore as a focus for intervention. One possibility is that gender no longer matters, in the sense of meaningfully influencing educational and achievement outcomes. This is not the case in the United States, as it is around the world. On the one hand, girls receive higher grades than do boys from elementary school through college; boys are more likely than girls to drop out of school and are less likely to continue to further education (Organisation for Economic Cooperation and Development [OECD], 2013; National Center for Education Statistics [NCES], 2013; Voyer & Voyer, 2014). On the other hand, women are still underrepresented in science, technology, engineering, and math (STEM)-related degrees and occupations, and men continue to earn and achieve more in later life than do women in many fields. Even in academia, women continue to be underrepresented in most fields in almost every country; they also publish less than their male counterparts (Larivière, Ni, Gingras, Cronin & Sugimoto 2013). In 2010, 80% of the books reviewed in *The New York Review of Books*, which

emphasizes the humanities, were written by men (*www.vidaweb.org/the-count-2010*).

In this chapter we discuss whether and how gender continues to influence competence motivation in ways that contribute to these different patterns of achievement. The emergence of systematic interest in gender influences on achievement motivation coincided, not surprisingly, with second-wave feminism and concerns about the relatively lower occupational achievement of women. By and large, this was the focus also of Hyde and Durik's (2005) chapter on gender, competence, and motivation in the first edition of this handbook. Recently, much discussion has taken a "boy-turn" (Weaver-Hightower, 2003), characterized by concerns about the relatively lower academic achievement of boys. We therefore ask whether and how gender impacts motivation, task engagement, self-regulation, and educational aspirations, choices, and outcomes among both females and males.

Recently, Butler (2014) proposed that gendered tendencies for males are relatively more motivated toward proving their abilities and maintaining and protecting favorable perceptions their competence, while females tend more toward doubting their abilities and working hard. We continue this theme, paying particular attention to pervasive beliefs among socializers, students, and even some researchers that males are smarter, especially at higher levels of ability, and that females need to try harder to succeed. We discuss the benefits and costs of "proving and protecting" and of "doubting and trying," and how these contribute to spur high-achieving boys to succeed more in later life than similarly able girls, and to put low-achieving boys at particular risk for academic disengagement. Any discussion of gendered tendencies raises the specter of essentialist claims of innate differences between the sexes. We consider such claims, but our emphasis is on the ways boys and girls construct and maintain motivating and motivated competence beliefs and strategies within the social and educational contexts of their lives. Thus, we refer throughout to "gender" rather "sex." We also discuss how gender intersects with other categories of social membership and identity, and with gendered patterns of socialization, values, and behaviors in achievement and other, especially relational arenas. In the final section of this chapter we ask whether and how different kinds of educational interventions and programs address the benefits and costs of gendered motivational tendencies.

Some preliminary clarifications and cautions are in order. First, gender influences can be expressed in differences in the mean level of a motivational construct (e.g., self-concept), in the distribution of a construct, or in the associations among variables (e.g., between self-concept and persistence or academic choices). In many articles, researchers do not analyze gender, however. Some do not mention gender at all, or they do so only when describing the sample (e.g., 48% female). In other studies, researchers control for gender, masking any potential role of gender in moderating associations among variables. As a result, it can be difficult to evaluate whether gender differences have changed over time, as one might expect given advances in social attitudes and affordances. In a similar vein, although we have tried to prioritize research published in the last decade, we sometimes had to rely on earlier results that may or may not still maintain today. Second, variance within gender in motivational variables is invariably far larger than that between genders;

any mean differences are typically small and not always significant. Thus, there is a real risk of exaggerating gender differences and failing to consider no less informative gender similarities (Hyde, 2014). But even small differences in theoretically related variables can have cumulative and reciprocal effects that can yield meaningful gendered motivational styles and consequences.

CLEVER BOYS, CONSCIENTIOUS GIRLS

Alone among the "big" theories of competence motivation discussed in this volume, the expectancy–value (E-V) model was initially developed to consider gender differences in educational and career choices, and especially the underrepresentation of women in STEM fields (Eccles et al., 1983). This approach continues to guide much of the research on gender and motivation. In keeping with other social-cognitive approaches, E-V theory emphasizes the role of subjective beliefs, positing that motivation to invest in and pursue a particular domain depends on the degree to which individuals both expect to succeed and value success. Expectancies are typically assessed in terms of self-concepts and values in terms of a composite of students' reports of their interest, desire to succeed, and the perceived utility of success for future plans. Students form expectancies and values via processes of social learning and social construction, based on their outcomes and the expectancies, values, and gender role beliefs of parents, teachers, peers, and the cultural milieu. Studies have consistently confirmed the motivational role of expectancies and values (see Wigfield et al., Chapter 7, this volume). Academic self-concepts and values predict school achievement and educational and vocational choices in generally similar ways among males and females. Thus, any gender differences in expectancies and values will have important consequences for the achievement and continuing motivation of boys and girls.

Expectancies and Values

Studies continue to show small but robust gender differences in academic self-concepts. Researchers have typically focused on math because of concerns about the underrepresentation of women in STEM fields, but some have examined language, both for purposes of comparison and because of concerns about boys' relatively poorer achievement in this domain. Results from recent large-scale international assessments are consistent with those of earlier studies. In most countries, boys on average had more positive self-concepts than girls in math and science, while girls had more positive self-concepts than boys in language (OECD, 2010, 2013). In a recent meta-analysis, Huang (2013) found an overall difference favoring males in academic self-efficacy that derived mainly but not solely from a marked male advantage in STEM domains such as math and computer science; females reported higher self-efficacy than males only in language arts.

Overall, boys tend to value success in math more than do girls, while girls value success in language more than do boys (Hyde, 2014), but differences vary for different kinds of values. In contrast with the generally small differences in other motivational variables, studies continue to show marked gender differences in interests. Far more young boys than girls had a strong interest in science and construction, while more girls than boys had an interest in reading and writing, sociodramatic play, and arts and crafts (Alexander, Johnson, Leibham, & Kelley, 2008). Gender differences in interest in systems versus people, in math and science versus language-related school subjects, and in STEM versus social and artistic occupations continue from childhood through adulthood (e.g., Frenzel, Goetz, Pekrun, & Watt, 2010; Su, Rounds, & Armstrong, 2009; Weisgram, Bigler, & Liben, 2010). Early interests build later ones. When students are interested in a topic or domain, they tend to engage in it more intensively, to understand it better, and therefore to develop competence, confidence, and a sustained personal interest (Hidi & Renninger, 2006). In a longitudinal study of students in grades 5–8, Tracey (2002) confirmed reciprocal influences whereby interest promoted competence beliefs, which then enhanced interest.

However, gender differences in self-concepts and interest do not solely either reflect or result in differences in the achievements of boys and girls. Girls achieve higher grades than boys in language-related subjects throughout the school years, but this tends to be the case in all subjects, including math and science (Voyer & Voyer, 2014). In international assessments of school-based competencies (OECD, 2010, 2013), girls outperformed boys in reading in every country. Results for math and science were more variable. In many countries, boys performed better than girls, but in others there was no difference, and in still others some girls did better. In her review of research on tests of cognitive abilities Hyde (2014) concluded that recent studies do not show a meaningful overall gender difference in either math or verbal abilities.

Interpretations of gender differences in motivational beliefs often emphasize the role of sociocultural beliefs and expectations that orient students to be more confident and to value success more in stereotypically gender-appropriate domains (Eccles & Wigfield, 2002). As early as second grade, and continuing through adulthood, participants implicitly associated math and science with male (Cvencek, Meltzoff, & Greenwald, 2011; Nosek, Banaji, & Greenwald, 2002; Nosek et al., 2009). As we discuss at greater length later in this chapter, to the extent that parents, teachers, and students endorse explicit gender stereotypes, they tend to believe that males are more talented in math and females in language (Frome & Eccles, 1998; Plante, Théorêt, & Favreau, 2009; Retelsdorf, Schwartz, & Asbrock, 2015). Many studies have documented the influence of parents', teachers', and students' math-related gender stereotypes on the self-concepts and educational choices of boys and girls (for reviews, see Gunderson, Ramirez, Levine, & Beilock, 2012; Leaper & Brown, 2014). In studies of gender-based stereotype threat, priming gender undermined the math performance of girls to a modest but significant extent throughout the school years (for a review, see Picho, Rodriguez, & Finnie, 2013). There has been less research on language, but elementary school teachers' beliefs that boys are less competent readers predicted declines in boys' reading self-concepts over the school year (Retelsdorf et al., 2015).

In general, people tend more to positive and positively biased self-appraisals in valued domains (Crocker & Park, 2004). When researchers examined self-evaluative bias for math, boys showed more positive bias relative to school grades or teacher ratings than girls; more girls than boys showed negative bias, whereby perceived competence in math was lower than expected on the basis of achievements (Dupeyrat, Escribe, Huet, & Regner, 2011; Gonida & Leondari, 2011; Kurman, 2004). Importantly, in these and other studies, girls and women did not show more positive and boys and men more negative self-evaluative bias in stereotypically female domains. Controlling for achievement eliminated gender differences in self-efficacy in language (Pajares & Valiante, 1999). Boys were also more likely to overestimate and girls to underestimate their general academic competence (Cole, Martin, Peeke, Seroczynski, & Fier, 1999). In a similar vein, most people believe that they are "better than average" (BTA), but in a study of some 15,000 adolescents in the Netherlands, the BTA effect was stronger among boys than among girls for self-ratings of general academic ability (Kuyper, Dijkstra, Buunk, & van der Werf, 2011). Boys showed a greater BTA effect than girls not only for math, but also for history and geography; girls did not show a greater BTA effect than boys for either Dutch or English (Kuyper & Dijkstra, 2009). In a recent study, girls did not have more positive reading self-concepts than boys, despite teachers' beliefs that girls are better at reading and girls' superior performance on reading tests (Retelsdorf et al., 2015).

Similar patterns emerge for perceptions of intelligence. In a meta-analysis of some 50 studies in four continents, Syzmanowicz and Furnham (2011) found substantial differences favoring males in self-estimates of numerical intelligence that are considerably larger than those for tested abilities. Estimates of general and, to some extent, verbal intelligence also favored males, even though there is no gender difference in mean general IQ and the albeit slight difference in tested verbal abilities favors females (Hyde, 2014). In keeping with findings for academic self-concepts, males overestimated and females underestimated their quantitative IQ, but females did not overestimate their verbal IQ more than did males (Steinmayr &

Spinath, 2009). Boys might value success and self-aggrandize more in STEM than in the humanities not only because the former are typed as masculine, but also because of beliefs that they require higher intelligence. In support, Leslie, Cimpian, Meyer, and Freeland (2015) found that academics rated "brilliance" as more crucial to becoming a top scholar in most STEM fields than in most of the humanities and social sciences.

Thus, stereotypical beliefs about gender-appropriate domains do not tell the whole story. Boys and men are more likely to overestimate their abilities, especially but not only in "masculine" domains. Girls and women tend to more realistic self-views, even in "feminine" domains. They are also more likely than boys and men to underestimate their competence, especially but not only in domains believed to require high ability. These tendencies emerge early. In several longitudinal studies, gender differences in math, language, general academic self-concepts, and in positive bias emerged in the early school grades, intensified during elementary school, and remained stable during adolescence, despite the generally higher achievement of girls throughout the school years (Cole et al., 1999; Jacobs, Lanza, Osgood, Eccles, & Wigfield, 2002; Measelle, Ablow, Cowan, & Cowan, 1998; Nagy, Watt, Eccles, Trautwein, Lüdtke, & Baumert, 2010; Wigfield et al., 1997). Experimental studies show similar patterns (Butler, 1998a; Ruble, Eisenberg, & Higgins, 1994). Given the same outcome, there were no gender differences in ratings of performance, ability, or expectations among children in preschool. Beginning at ages 6–7, boys evaluated themselves more favorably than did girls.

It is clearly important if, on average, males tend to be more confident in their abilities than females, especially since there do not seem to be gender differences in perceptions of the role of ability. Men and women did not differ in their ratings of the importance of natural ability for success in a field (Leslie et al., 2015). Males might tend more than females to believe that they are not only more intelligent but also that they can become more intelligent. In a recent study with a large sample of adolescents Diseth, Meland, and Breidablik (2014) examined implicit beliefs about intelligence (Dweck, 1999). While there was no gender difference in entity beliefs that intelligence is a fixed, innate trait, boys scored higher than girls on incremental beliefs that intelligence is a malleable capacity that can be acquired. Given the motivational role of perceived competence, it is pertinent to ask how and why girls do better in school. Given that academic outcomes are the major determinant of perceived competence and that, on average, boys do less well in school, one can also ask how and why boys maintain greater positive illusions than do girls. We begin to address these questions in the following sections.

Prioritizing Effort versus Prioritizing Ability

A common explanation for girls' superior grades is that they try harder. Across different countries, social backgrounds, and ages, according to parent, teacher, and self-reports, girls invest more in schoolwork than do boys (e.g., Duckworth & Seligman, 2006; Mullola et al., 2012; Oyserman, Johnson, & James; 2011; Rogers & Hallam, 2006; Yeung, 2011). On average, girls spend more time on homework and test revision, are more likely to complete assignments, and they try harder to master difficult material. In a recent study, boys were far more likely than girls to report that their goal in school is to avoid work and minimize effort (Dekker et al., 2013). Girls, more than boys, use effective self-regulation and learning strategies such as goal setting, planning, paying attention and taking notes in class, resisting distractions, and asking for help if they need it (e.g., Butler, 2008; Denton et al., 2015; Dresel & Haugwitz, 2005; Duckworth & Seligman, 2006).

But why do girls try harder? In part, because they believe they need to, especially in math and science. From elementary school through college, females tend to perceive effort to be a more important and ability to be a less important determinant of success than do males (for extended discussions, see Butler, 2014; Hyde & Durik, 2005). In a study of some 5,000 gifted students, this difference was marked already in grade 3 (Assouline, Colangelo, Ihrig, & Forstadt, 2006). Girls and women tend to

rate inadequate ability as a more important determinant of failure in math and science, while boys and men tend to give greater weight to causes that do not reflect on their ability—incompetent or hostile teachers, or low interest and motivation (see Butler, 2014). Thus, in stereotypically masculine domains, males and females tend more to high versus low expectancy attributional styles that both reflect and reinforce differences in perceived competence. In keeping with results from the self-concept literature, females typically are not more likely than males to show a high expectancy attributional style in feminine or neutral academic domains (e.g., Beyer, 1999; Kurman, 2004). A meta-analysis of experimental studies showed that males displayed greater self-serving bias to accept more responsibility for success than for failure (Campbell & Sedikides, 1999).

Differences in additional self-evaluative preferences and strategies contribute to maintaining boys' greater illusions of competence and girls' more modest and realistic beliefs. From childhood through college, girls and women base self-appraisals and self-efficacy beliefs on both positive and negative feedback from parents, teachers, and peers far more than do boys and men. Boys and men rely more on internal standards and on social comparison (for reviews, see Butler, 2014; Usher & Pajares, 2008). In keeping with the onset of gender differences in other self-evaluative biases, beginning at ages 6–7, boys, but not girls, relied on downward more than upward comparisons (Butler, 2014). When given conflicting success and failure information, more girls considered both, while more boys attended selectively to that which was more favorable. Thus, it is not surprising that females are more likely than males to lower their evaluations and expectancies after receiving negative evaluations (Roberts, 1991). In her review of this literature, Roberts proposed that men tend to treat evaluative settings as competitive arenas that call on them to prove their capacities, to stand by their own self-views, and therefore to discount negative evaluations. Women are more inclined to treat evaluative settings as opportunities to learn about their abilities and therefore treat negative feedback as diagnostic for both evaluating and developing their capacities. More generally, gendered patterns of competence beliefs, attributions, and approaches to evaluation are reminiscent of those associated with self-enhancement versus veridical and self-improvement motives for self-evaluation (Butler, 2014).

IMPLICATIONS FOR COMPETENCE MOTIVATION

Proving and Protecting versus Doubting and Trying

The self-evaluative motives, beliefs, strategies, and judgments more typical of males and females can be described in terms of tendencies toward "proving and protecting" and toward "doubting and trying" that have both motivational benefits and motivational costs. Prioritizing effort, as girls tend to do, is adaptive for maintaining motivation, orienting students to continue to work hard when they are doing well, and to keep trying rather than giving up when they encounter difficulty. On average, teachers perceive girls to be better motivated than boys (e.g., Mullola et al., 2012). Sustained application is crucial for doing well in school, especially when, as is often the case, the material is difficult, the subject is unappealing, the teacher is boring, the class is disruptive, or social media and other attractive alternatives beckon. Gender differences in student and teacher reports of academic self-discipline partially mediated the difference favoring girls in grades (Duckworth & Seligman, 2006).

Sensitivity to negative feedback also carries with it the risk of losing confidence and devaluing one's capacities. Trying hard can be a low-ability cue that signals the need for compensatory investment and invites concerns that at some point effort might not suffice. When children in grades 3 and 6 responded to vignettes about a same-sex child who answered wrong in class, girls agreed less than boys that greater effort would ensure correct answers in the future, and that the child would volunteer to answer when the teacher asked another question (Butler, 1994). Girls also inferred, more than boys, that the child would feel shame. In keeping with the generally higher tendency of females toward internalizing

problems, girls worry more than boys about schoolwork, even when they are doing well in school (Pomerantz, Altermatt, & Saxon, 2002). Already during elementary school, gender differences in anxiety and depression significantly accounted for gender differences in under- versus overestimations of academic competence (Cole et al., 1999).

The combination of less confidence, greater anxiety, and beliefs that one must invest sustained effort to succeed, together with self-discipline and constructive learning strategies, is adaptive for maintaining motivation for required assignments and courses. But it may also influence girls and women to set their sights lower than necessary when making educational and career choices. If women tend to doubt and discount their capacities in fields believed to require high ability, they might well be reluctant to enter them. Academics' ratings of the importance of brilliance for success in their field strongly predicted the underrepresentation of women among PhD recipients in STEM fields and their greater representation in fields in which sustained application was perceived as relatively more important (Leslie et al., 2015). Dweck (1986) reasoned that bright girls may be more vulnerable to developing maladaptive patterns of self-denigration and challenge-avoidance in math than similarly able boys because the girls are more likely to experience difficulty as reflecting inadequate ability, and the boys, as a challenge they are capable of meeting. Gender differences in motivational beliefs for math are more marked at high levels of ability (Butler, 2008; OECD, 2013; Preckel, Goetz, Pekrun, & Kleine, 2008).

Attributing success to ability, favoring not only effort but also external factors and lack of interest to account for failure, and favoring positive over negative feedback, as is more typical of males, has clear benefits for maintaining confidence. If boys are more likely to believe that they have the ability to succeed in a challenging domain if they want to, they might well be more likely to choose to pursue it than will similarly able girls. The greater overestimation of math performance by male as compared with female college students accounted for men's greater intentions to pursue math-related fields (Bench et al., 2015). Prioritizing ability carries the risk of focusing on maintaining self-esteem at the expense of investing in learning and developing competence, however. Males tend more than females to construe effort as a double-edged sword whereby the perceived benefits of investing effort are undermined by beliefs that high effort implies low ability and detracts from the value of success (Covington & Omelich, 1979). In samples of college students, women agreed more than men that they valued effortful accomplishment, while men agreed more than women that they valued and admired success achieved with little effort, a clear marker of high ability (Hirt & McCrea, 2009). When concerned about potentially negative outcomes, males are more likely than females to preempt inferences of low ability by themselves and others by withdrawing effort, refraining from drawing attention to difficulty by asking for help, and cheating (e.g., Butler, 1998b; Urdan & Midgley, 2001).

For high-achieving boys who generally succeed, investing the effort necessary to ensure that they continue to prove their ability has benefits for both self-esteem and learning. Male proving and protecting should render low-achieving boys particularly susceptible to defensively withdrawing effort, disengaging from schooling, and seeking other arenas in which they can prove themselves. In samples of African American, Latino, and low-income youth in the United States, who, on average, do less well in school, boys reported higher perceived competence in math and science than girls, and girls reported higher academic motivation and effort, and more positive attitudes toward school than did boys (Else-Quest, Mineo, & Higgins, 2013; Oyserman et al., 2011). On the one hand, these patterns parallel those among middle-class and majority groups. On the other hand, disparities favoring girls in academic identification, aspirations, and achievement are greatest among low achievers and students from low-income and some minority groups (Else-Quest et al., 2013; NCES, 2013; Oyserman et al., 2011).

Achievement Goals

According to Nicholls (1989), valuing effortful versus effortless success is at the heart of different achievement goals.

Achievement goal theory (Dweck, 1986; Elliot, 1999; Nicholls, 1989) is discussed extensively by Elliot and Hulleman (Chapter 4, this volume). Here we focus mainly on approach forms of performance or ego goals to demonstrate superior ability and attainment versus mastery, task, or learning goals to acquire and develop competence. Performance goals orient students to prioritize ability as the main determinant of achievement outcomes. Thus, they also evoke self-enhancing and self-protective tendencies to accept more responsibility for success than for failure, and to avoid attributions of failure to ability, for example, by self-handicapping and help avoidance. Mastery goals orient students to value effortful learning and accomplishment, and to seek and attend to information relevant to accurately assessing their abilities and identifying and trying to improve any weaknesses (for a review, see Butler, 2000).

In this case, one might expect males to tend more to performance goals and females to mastery goals. We know of no systematic meta-analyses, perhaps because gender has not been a major focus of achievement goal research. Researchers do not always test for gender effects; when they do, some find significant differences in both goals, others find a difference in only one goal, and still others do not find a difference in either, especially among college students. As a result, Hyde and Durik (2005) concluded that gender does not reliably impact achievement goals. Students' achievement goals are influenced by the degree to which they perceive the classroom context as placing greater emphasis on deep learning and individual progress and effort (mastery classroom goal structure) or on the level of students' ability and attainment compared with that of their peers (performance classroom goal structure). Thus, contextual emphases might override any differential tendencies among girls and boys to favor mastery or performance goals (Meece, Glienke, & Burg, 2006). It is suggestive, however, that when some recent studies showed gender differences in school-age samples, boys typically scored higher on performance-approach goals and girls on mastery goals (Butler, 2008; Dicke, Lüdtke, Trautwein, Nagy, & Nagy, 2012; Dupeyrat et al., 2011; Gonida

& Leondari, 2011; Kenney-Benson, Pomer-antz, Ryan, & Patrick, 2006; Luo, Hogan, & Paris, 2011).

Mastery goals and contexts are associated with positive patterns of academic engagement—with greater persistence and more constructive self-regulation, especially in the event of setbacks, and with interest in learning and satisfaction with schooling. Results for performance goals and contexts are less consistent. In some studies, they are associated with negative kinds of student engagement, including anxiety, disruptive behavior, avoidant responses to setbacks, and dissatisfaction with schooling, while in others they are associated with positive processes and outcomes, including graded achievement. In yet other studies, performance goals and contexts do not predict either positive or negative engagement and learning outcomes (for reviews, see Linnenbrink-Garcia, Tyson, & Patall, 2008; Midgely, Kaplan, & Middleton, 2001; Rolland, 2012; Senko, Hulleman, & Harackiewicz, 2011).

One possibility is that while mastery-oriented goals and classrooms seem to be beneficial for most students, performance-oriented goals and classrooms may influence different students differently. Males enjoy competing and often perform better in competitive settings, whereas females tend to respond to competition with discomfort, anxiety, and decrements in performance (for a review, see Croson & Gneezy, 2009). In this case, performance goals and contexts might be more beneficial for boys and mastery goals and contexts more beneficial for girls. It is difficult to evaluate this proposal because in many studies researchers either ignored or controlled for gender rather than testing for possible moderation. In some experimental studies, performance contexts were indeed associated with higher interest, confidence, and performance among boys than among girls, but mastery contexts were equally beneficial for both boys and girls (Butler, 1992, 1993). In their review of associations between personal goals and achievement, Linnenbrink-Garcia and colleagues (2008) concluded that while a few studies showed that performance goals were more beneficial for boys than girls, most did not show significant moderation.

Students perceive the classroom goal structure in part through the lens of their own achievement goals, however. If boys and girls tend to construe evaluative settings as competitive arenas and learning opportunities, respectively, this might be the case for their perceptions of the classroom goal structure as well. Researchers have rarely tested for gender differences, but in several instances, boys scored higher on perceived performance goal structure than did girls (e.g., Butler, 2012; Friedel, Cortina, Turner, & Midgley, 2007; Luo et al., 2011; Urdan, Midgley, & Anderman, 1998). Only Butler (2012) also reported a significant gender difference in perceived mastery classroom goal structure. More studies are needed, but if boys tend to perceive the classroom as more competitive, such perceptions should further exacerbate their tendencies toward proving and protecting modes of self-appraisal and self-regulation. Later in this chapter, we raise the possibility that teachers may also interact with male and female students in ways that might create a more performance-oriented classroom environment for boys. In any event, the findings reviewed here are an important reminder of gender similarities, of the benefits of mastery goals and contexts for both boys and girls, and of the malleability of motivational approaches. In a similar vein, in her review of experimental studies, Butler (2000) concluded that mastery and performance goal conditions tend to override gender differences in self-evaluative motives, strategies, and judgments, orienting boys to behave more like girls in mastery goal conditions, orienting girls to behave more like boys in performance goal conditions, and by and large orienting both to show more positive patterns of motivation and self-regulation in mastery conditions.

SOCIOCULTURAL INFLUENCES

Early gender differences in social dominance and deference and in effortful control (Else-Quest, Hyde, Goldsmith, & Van Hulle, 2006) might imply that biological predispositions play some role in orienting males more than females to prove their abilities and females more than males to sustain investment in schoolwork. Some researchers have speculated that biological predispositions toward different interests drive gender differences in achievement motivations and choices (Valla & Ceci, 2011). But there is far stronger evidence of the role of sociocultural influences as transmitted by parents, peers, and teachers.

Parents

Particularly relevant in the present context, when studies showed differential parental beliefs about their sons and daughters, these paralleled gender differences in students' beliefs. Parents tend to have higher expectations for boys than for girls in math, especially if they endorse more gender-typed beliefs (for a review, see Gunderson et al., 2012). Even in recent studies, parents rated sons as more talented than daughters in math, overestimated the math competence of sons, attributed the math success of sons more to ability and that of daughters more to hard work and good study habits, and perceived math as more difficult for daughters than for sons (Lindberg, Hyde, & Hirsch, 2008; Räty, Vänskä, Kasanen, & Kärkkäinen, 2002; Simpkins, Fredricks, & Eccles, 2012). Parents perceived daughters as more competent than sons in language, but their ratings were realistic rather than inflated (Frome & Eccles, 1998). Parents' beliefs about the academic competence of their children predict their sons' and daughters' concurrent and later motivational beliefs and choices in similar rather than different ways (e.g., Simpkins et al., 2012). Parents also perceived sons as more intelligent (Furnham, Reeves, & Budhani, 2002). Parents overestimated the quantitative intelligence of their sons, and underestimated that of their daughters, but did not show a complementary bias favoring daughters for verbal intelligence (Steinmayr & Spinath, 2009).

Parents encourage sex-typed interests and discourage cross-sex ones directly, for example, by buying young sons and daughters different toys (Lytton & Romney, 1991) and steering adolescents in gender-typed academic and vocational directions (Chhin, Bleeker, & Jacobs, 2008) and less directly. For example, parents used more numeric speech with sons (Chang, Sandhofer, & Brown, 2011) and provided young sons with more opportunities than daughters to learn about science (Alexander, Johnson, & Kelley, 2102; Crowley, Callanan, Tenenbaum, & Allen, 2001). Given that parents tend to perceive daughters as better in language, Tennenbaum (2009) recorded parent–child conversations about course selections in the expectation that parents would convey greater confidence in the ability of sons to succeed in math and science and of daughters to succeed in language. As one would expect, parents favored math and science courses for boys and language courses for girls. In contrast to predictions, however, parents used far more discouraging, ability-related language with daughters than with sons in both domains. Parents of boys in grade 1 rated ability as a more important determinant of their child's success not only in math but also in reading than did parents of daughters, who attributed greater importance to effort and study habits (Räty et al., 2002). Kenney-Benson and colleagues (2006) reviewed evidence that parents monitor the academic progress of girls more closely than that of boys and give girls more unsolicited help. These behaviors serve as low-ability cues that convey the need for compensatory effort. Parental tendencies to socialize girls more than boys to please and avoid disappointing adults also orient girls to invest in and worry about schoolwork (Pomerantz et al., 2002).

Studies therefore suggest patterns of differential perceptions and treatment among some parents that not only provide boys with more math and science knowledge but also convey greater confidence in the ability of sons than that of daughters and convey to girls more than boys that they need to try hard to succeed. They also suggest that parents might be more invested in maintaining favorable beliefs about their sons' academic abilities. In this case, they may convey the importance of proving abilities to sons more than daughters. In support, boys perceived parents as placing greater emphasis on performance goals than did girls (Friedel et al., 2007). The patterns reported here do not maintain in all social groups, however. African American parents perceived sons as less academically competent than daughters and had lower academic expectations for sons

(Wood, Kurtz-Costes, Rowley, & Okeke-Adeyanju, 2010).

Peers

Peers and peer groups play a major role in gender socialization (for reviews, see Maccoby, 1998; Martin, Fabes, & Hanish, 2014; Rose & Rudolph, 2006). From an early age, boys engage more than girls in competitive games and sports that invite social comparison and strivings for self-assertion and social dominance. Girls engage more in sociodramatic play that invites coordination and cooperation. In their review of discourse in same-sex peer groups, Maltz and Borker (1982) distinguished between the competitive, adversarial orientation typical of boys who speak to assert themselves, and the collaborative, affiliative orientation of girls who speak to maintain closeness and equality. Beginning in elementary school, boys are more likely to report that it is important for them to influence peers, promote their own interests, and demonstrate social status. Girls, more than boys, report that it is important for them to try to develop social competence and intimate friendships, and to avoid hurting others (Rose & Rudolph, 2006). In a relatively recent study with adolescents, social demonstration goals were quite highly correlated with performance approach, and social development goals with mastery approach academic achievement goals (Shim & Finch, 2014).

Given that gendered tendencies toward different activities, social goals, and interactions develop before school entry, they may play an important role in the development and maintenance of motivational approaches to schoolwork among boys and girls. However, just as mastery versus performance goal contexts tend to override gender differences in achievement goals and behaviors, Martin and colleagues (2104) reviewed evidence that gender differences in aggression and cooperativeness were marked in gender-segregated peer groups and educational settings, and decreased as a function of children's exposure to and experience with other-sex interactions.

Peers and peer groups exert pressure to conform to gender roles by reinforcing gender typicality and sanctioning atypicality and gender role violations (Leaper & Brown, 2014; Maccoby, 1998). Adolescent boys were more likely than girls to perceive their friendship group as supporting STEM interests and achievement, while the reverse was the case for language (Robnett & Leaper, 2013). Some one-third of girls in one study reported hearing disparaging remarks about their STEM abilities from both male and female peers (Leaper & Brown, 2008). There is some evidence that boys respond more negatively than girls to boys who display gender-atypical academic interests (Leaper & Brown, 2014).

The relational socialization and goals that orient girls to please, affiliate, and comply with others incline them to assimilate school and teacher demands more than do boys. But they can also weigh against presenting as clever. Although earlier analyses targeted adolescence as the period in which girls begin to experience conflicts between female roles and academic achievement (Horner, 1972), already in kindergarten girls were more likely than boys both to praise others' work in class and to denigrate their own work (Frey & Ruble, 1987). Concerns about femininity and relationships led women, but not men, to self-denigrate more in public than in private after succeeding on an achievement task (Heatherington et al., 1993). Gifted girls in grades 3–5 in the United States expressed concerns about hurting other students' feelings and appearing boastful and aggressive if they did too well or volunteered to answer many questions in class (Bell, 1989). More recently, in an ethnographic study in grade 5 classrooms in the United Kingdom, Renold (2001b) showed how high-achieving girls concealed, downplayed, and on occasion even denied their superior grades in both math and English. Average-achieving girls described bright girls as unfeminine and believed that they themselves would be less popular if they were in the top rather than the middle math and English ability groups. Thus, girls may still experience conflicts related to excelling academically, femininity, and social acceptance.

While girls tend to be influenced by both girls and boys, boys are influenced mainly by other boys (Maccoby, 1998). Because adult and peer norms of desirable behavior often conflict for boys, but tend to correspond for girls, one path to peer acceptance for boys, more than for girls, is to oppose adult authority. Much discussion, both before and during the current "boy-turn," has focused on the misfit between academic motivation and engagement, and male peer norms and constructions of masculinity (for a review, see Kessels, Heyder, Latsch, & Hannover, 2014). High-achieving boys in the schools studied by Renold (2001a) were indeed taunted by other boys, but for being studious and well behaved rather than clever. Bright boys tried to prove their masculinity by displaying an interest in sports or provoking the teacher, not by downplaying their ability. In contrast with the results for girls, high achieving boys boasted about their achievements, while lower achievers reported getting higher grades than they did. Adolescent boys interviewed by Jackson (2002b) reported that in interactions with peers the pretended they had not studied for tests, bragged about high grades, but kept quiet if they got a low grade. In keeping with results from quantitative studies, they also reported self-handicapping when concerned that they might do poorly on an exam or assignment. Boys who were seen as investing in and worrying about schoolwork, and who deferred to teachers, were perceived as effeminate, but boys perceived as succeeding without studying were admired for being "brainy."

Adherence to hypermasculine norms of toughness and defiance, and perceptions that identification with school demands and academic aspirations violates gender roles and peer norms are more marked among adolescents from lower-income and some ethnic-minority backgrounds (Xie, Dawes, Wurster, & Shi, 2013). As many have pointed out, such norms and perceptions can serve to maintain self-esteem and a sense of identity in the face of not only discrimination and negative cultural stereotypes but also poor academic achievement (Rowley et al., 2014). Indeed, African American adolescents score significantly higher than do white adolescents in the United States on general self-esteem (Bachman, O'Malley, Freedman-Doan, Trzesniewski, & Donnellan, 2011). But they also contribute to the greater academic alienation of boys as compared with girls. In a study of African American and Latino students, Taylor and Graham (2007) found that in grades 2 and 4, most students chose a high-achieving classmate as someone they respected and aspired to be like. In grade 7, more boys than girls chose a low-achieving peer, especially when they perceived more rather than fewer barriers to educational and occupational achievement. In present terms it makes sense that boys who struggle to prove themselves in school will disengage and seek alternative areas in which they can impress their peers, to the possible benefit of their self-worth, but with real costs for their learning and future trajectories.

Thus, for boys, the misfit seems to be less between social acceptance and academic achievement and more between presenting as masculine and as diligent and well behaved on the one hand, and between male proving and low achievement on the other. One implication is that same-sex peers can be a greater impediment to boys' academic engagement than any "feminization" of schooling. Boys dominate classroom environments (Beaman, Wheldall, & Kemp, 2006), to the possible detriment of students of both sexes. For instance, from first grade through high school, the achievement of both girls and boys increased as a function of the number of girls in the class because both boys and girls evidenced more enjoyment, better self-control, less disruptive behavior, and better interpersonal relationships in classes with a higher proportion of girls (Lavy & Schlosser, 2011; Pahlke, Cooper, & Fabes, 2013).

Teachers

The idea that schools are feminine arenas that serve girls well and undermine the academic motivation of boys is very common. Girls are indeed more likely to fit teacher images of the ideal student (Beaman et al., 2006). Teachers perceive girls as more attentive, cooperative, teachable, motivated, hardworking, self-regulated, well behaved, and persistent (Duckworth & Seligman, 2006; Mullola et al., 2012). But teachers, like parents and students also tend to perceive boys as having greater math ability than girls, believe that girls need to try harder in order to succeed and that greater effort will thus be more efficacious for boys, and are more likely to overestimate the ability of boys (Gunderson et al., 2012). For example, teachers in a nationally representative U.S. sample believed that math was easier for their male students, even when they evaluated boys and girls matched for grades and standardized test scores in advanced placement classes (Riegle-Crumb & Humphries, 2012). As we have already noted, teachers perceive girls as better in language. After controlling for their more positive ratings of girls' conduct and approaches to schoolwork, kindergarten teachers rated boys' math competence higher than that of similarly achieving girls, but did not show a complementary bias to underrate the reading competence of boys relative to girls. Teachers' underrating of girls' math proficiency predicted subsequent declines in girls' achievement (Robinson-Cimpian, Lubienski, Ganley, & Copur-Gencturk, 2014).

As do parents, teachers on average tend to interact with boys and girls in ways that convey differential expectations. In an influential early study Dweck, Davidson, Nelson, and Enna (1978) found that elementary school teachers were more likely to praise boys for their achievement and girls for conduct, while criticizing boys mainly for poor conduct and girls for poor achievement. Subsequent studies have confirmed that, on average, teachers both reprimand boys more about their conduct and attention and give boys more academic feedback. They also direct more high-level questions to boys and more low-level questions to girls, especially in math and science classes (for reviews, see Beaman et al., 2006; Sadker, Sadker, & Zittleman, 2009).

While stereotypical perceptions play a role, teachers interact differently with boys and girls in large part because boys demand more attention. Boys dominate classroom interactions because they are more likely to call out answers, especially if they are high achievers, and because they are more disruptive and less cooperative than girls, especially if they are low achievers. Because girls tend to be more disciplined, less confident, and less self-promoting than boys, they demand and receive less attention from teachers. Thus, teachers are more likely to encourage able boys than girls to demonstrate their knowledge and abilities. As a result, they may tend

to create a more performance-oriented climate for boys than for girls (Butler, 2014). Teachers tend to engage in escalating cycles of aversive interactions with low-achieving boys that likely contribute to their greater academic disaffection and alienation relative to low-achieving girls.

IMPLICATIONS AND CONCLUSIONS

Implications for Understanding Academic Motivation among Boys and Girls

There is still so much I want and need to learn. Every sentence I write raises questions that send me back to the literature. How can I submit a manuscript until I'm sure I've understood the full complexity and have something new and worthwhile to say?

—S, a gifted female postdoctoral student (cited by Butler, 2014)

Thinking in terms of gendered tendencies toward proving and protecting versus doubting and trying is only one, and certainly not an exhaustive, way of considering how and why gender continues to impact competence motivation. It has proven useful, however, for understanding how the motivational strengths and vulnerabilities more typical of girls and boys work together to enable girls, on average, to do better in school than boys; to spur high-achieving boys to succeed more, on average, in later life than similarly able girls; and to put low-achieving boys at particular risk for academic disengagement. These approaches emerge early and continue through college. We have discussed how gender stereotypes and socialization in both achievement and relational areas work together in reciprocally reinforcing ways. Experiences and communications in the family, the peer group, and the classroom incline boys more than girls to prove their abilities, especially in male-typed domains, to value effortless accomplishment, and therefore to pursue self-esteem, sometimes at the cost of engaging and investing effort in school. They incline girls more than boys not only to question their ability and downplay their successes, but also to try harder, to acknowledge and try to address difficulties, to value effortful accomplishment, and to accommodate to teachers and school demands. They also steer boys and girls, but boys more than girls, toward stereotypically gender-appropriate interests, academic domains, and occupations.

During the school years, girls' strengths tend to prevail. There is broad agreement among researchers, parents, teachers, and students themselves that girls, on average, show more adaptive patterns of academic motivation than do boys. Girls do better in school, tend to value school more than do boys, and have higher aspirations to continue to higher education. Girls' motivational strengths go hand in hand with their vulnerabilities, however. Already in elementary school girls are more prone to self-doubts, anxiety, and concerns that trying and persisting may not suffice to ensure success, especially in STEM domains. As we have already discussed, these concerns can be costly when girls need to make academic and occupational choices, to the particular detriment of high-achieving girls relative to their male counterparts. Discussion has focused mainly on STEM domains and careers. But returning to the postdoctoral student cited at the beginning of this section, who did not pursue the academic career in psychology to which she was very suited, female motivational strengths and vulnerabilities can converge in constraining women's occupational achievements in other domains as well.

What are the implications of male proving and protecting for boys' academic motivation? We have discussed throughout the benefits of proving and protecting for boys' confidence and the attendant risks of prioritizing ability over sustained application. According to achievement goal theory, boys' greater tendency toward performance goals is less adaptive than girls' tendency toward mastery goals. Boys' social goals also tend to undermine their academic engagement by pushing them to resist school rules and demands. One clear conclusion, however, is that the consequences of male proving are quite different for higher and lower achievers. Boys who do well tend to reap the benefits. Their positive illusions presumably do not require much protection, and their competitive strivings spur them to put in the effort needed to excel. Even in socially diverse schools, the social costs of high achievement can be mitigated by hiding effort and performing as masculine while maintaining high grades. These boys' self-confidence, their greater tendency toward realistic interests and proving values and motives, together with continuing social pressures and gender expectations, incline them to aspire to prestigious, remunerative, typically STEM careers. Overall, however, men are less likely than women to choose majors and careers in fields traditionally associated with the other sex (U.S. Department of Education and National Center for Education Statistics, 2007). Thus, internal and social pressures may prevent some boys from pursuing interests in less prestigious and male-typed courses, degrees, and careers.

In contrast, as we have discussed quite extensively, for lower achieving boys, who typically also belong to less advantaged social groups, "proving and protecting" has few benefits and many costs for their academic motivation and achievement in later life. On the one hand, many such boys continue to maintain high self-esteem, despite failing to prove themselves in school. On the other hand, maintaining self-esteem often involves academic disengagement, alienation, and affiliation with similarly disaffected peers. It is, however, critical to note that while we have focused on psychological processes, negative social stereotypes, social barriers, and outright discrimination play a far more important role in disadvantaging boys in many minority groups (e.g., Rowley et al., 2014).

Before turning to some applied interventions and implications we briefly comment on two general issues. Most important, we have focused on showing how studies guided by different theoretical frameworks that assessed different motivational constructs among diverse social groups show patterns of rather consistent sex differences that can be conceptualized in terms of gendered motivational approaches. But we have also emphasized throughout that mean gender differences tend to be small. Thus, the overlap between the genders is far larger than any differences between them; many girls are more inclined to prove and protect, and many boys, to doubt and to try. No less important, studies guided by expectancy–value theory have shown that associations between expectancies and values and motivational outcomes and choices are very similar for boys and girls.

Overall, we have the impression that this is the case for the correlates of mastery and performance goals and contexts as well. This brings us to our second general comment. Achievement goal theory pointed us in the direction of male proving and female trying, but most researchers who work in this tradition do not share our interest in gender. Of all the many studies we read, those guided by achievement goal theory were most likely to ignore or at best control for gender. Thus, although there is fairly coherent evidence that mastery goals and contexts seem to be similarly beneficial for boys and girls, it is not clear whether and how gender moderates the effects of performance goals and contexts, and whether any such effects differ for low versus high achievers.

Applied Implications

Educational interventions that address gender differ widely in their theoretical rationales, and therefore in their methods and desired outcomes. Most target individuals, mostly students, sometimes teachers, and occasionally parents. Others target contexts, from schools through to educational policies. Interventions differ as to whether they are predicated on an essentialist assumption of categorical, largely innate sex differences or on a view of gendered tendencies as socially learned and constructed, and thus malleable. Interventions of both kinds are often implicitly or explicitly based on the assumption that the path to change lies in influencing motivation, typically, of girls to pursue STEM fields, and in fewer cases of boys in general to engage with language arts, and of low-achieving boys to identify with school and schoolwork.

The effectiveness of interventions is typically assessed in terms of changes in achievement, rather than motivation, however (Liben & Coyle, 2014). It is beyond the scope of this chapter to provide a comprehensive review of gender-based interventions, even of those that directly targeted and assessed motivational outcomes. We also do not review interventions that target skills

training, for example, spatial skills among girls and literacy among boys, though the influence of greater competence on interest and continuing motivation has been well established. Instead, we briefly present and on occasion critique some broad classes of interventions that bear on the motivational strengths and vulnerabilities we reviewed.

Evidence that girls and boys tend toward somewhat different motivational beliefs and approaches suggests three broad kinds of intervention strategies. One is to intervene at the individual level to modify the less adaptive motivational beliefs more common among girls or boys. Another is to capitalize on gender (Bigler, Hayes, & Liben, 2014) by adapting learning contexts to the motivational styles of boys and girls, on the assumption that students are better motivated when contexts match their interests and approaches to learning. But we have also reviewed evidence that gender differences tend to be small, and that certain kinds of beliefs and learning contexts, by and large, influence the motivation of girls and boys in similar ways. Thus, a third strategy would be to learn from the respective benefits and costs of each approach to develop learning environments that better support the competence motivation of most students, regardless of gender.

Changing Beliefs of Individuals

By definition, interventions in this group are predicated on the view that motivational beliefs are malleable. Given that girls' lesser confidence is maintained in part by their greater tendency to attribute negative outcomes to inadequate ability, especially in STEM fields, one strategy might be train them to attribute setbacks to controllable factors, such as effort or strategies. Attribution retraining interventions enhanced the perceived competence and achievement of academically successful girls in an advanced secondary school chemistry course (Zeigler & Stoeger, 2004) and of average-achieving girls in elementary school (Craske, 1985). Interventions of this kind do not address the possibly no less problematic tendency more common tendency among girls to continue to doubt their ability when they succeed, in part because they prioritize effort instead.

Given that girls tend to be quite conscientious and hardworking, emphasizing effort might even be counterproductive in the long term and exacerbate girls' tendencies to worry about their schoolwork. One possibility might be to simultaneously train girls to attribute success to ability, as well as effort. We know of no such systematic interventions, possibly because emphasizing ability can lead to motivational decrements when students encounter setbacks (Dweck, 1999). They might also carry the risk of setting more girls on the path to proving and protecting.

Promoting a growth mindset by teaching students that ability itself is not inborn and fixed, but a malleable capacity that develops and can be increased through learning and practice, seems a more promising direction both for bolstering girls' confidence by promoting beliefs that they can get smarter, and for moderating boys' prioritization of ability over effort by modifying beliefs that greater investment implies lesser ability. Believing that one can acquire ability might also help mitigate the need for low-achieving boys to maintain and protect self-esteem by disengaging from schoolwork. Mindset interventions have resulted in modest but significant positive effects for both girls and boys on achievement, challenge seeking, investment in schoolwork, and effort valuation among middle and high school students, and especially among low achievers (Blackwell, Trzesniewski, & Dweck, 2007; Good, Aronson, & Inzlicht, 2003; Yeager et al., 2016). In support of Dweck's (2007) suggestion that this kind of intervention might be particularly effective in bolstering the STEM confidence of girls, girls profited more than did boys from a mindset intervention relative to a condition that focused on study skills in math (Good et al., 2003).

Values affirmation interventions, during which students write about values that are important to them, have been suggested as a way of enhancing the sense of belonging, academic engagement, and achievement of students from negatively stereotyped groups. One such intervention reduced the male advantage in a college physics class by enhancing the achievement of women (Miyake et al., 2010). Benefits were strongest for women who tended to endorse the stereotype that men are better than women in physics. Another arrested the downward achievement trajectory of Latino middle school male and female students (Sherman et al., 2013).

Another group of relevant interventions focuses on enhancing girls' interest in STEM by highlighting the importance and value that a science career could have for them (see Liben & Coyle, 2014, for a review). Importantly, including lessons about gender-based discrimination in science was more effective than focusing only on career values (Weisgram & Bigler, 2007). On theoretical grounds, teaching students to recognize sexist (and racist) attitudes and exposing them to more gender-egalitarian beliefs should be motivationally beneficial for both girls and boys, making it possible to attribute others' discouraging or disparaging comments to external factors rather than to inadequate ability, and to modify narrow and constraining constructions of gender roles. Typically, interventions of this kind have focused only on girls, however. This is a real lacuna given the role of boys in perpetuating stereotypical beliefs about girls and the negative influence of male peer norms and constructions of masculinity on some boys' motivation, academic engagement, and choices.

Adapting Contexts to Girls' and Boys' Motivational Styles

The major "intervention" in this category is the creation of single-sex schools and classes. As long as discussions emphasized possible benefits for girls, they had little impact on educational policy. Recently, as part of the "boy turn," the establishment of single-sex schools, and especially classes, has been increasing dramatically, in large part as a strategy for enhancing the achievement of boys (Bigler et al., 2014). One kind of motivational rationale discussed by Bigler and colleagues is predicated on an essentialist view of sex differences. Single-sex classes will enhance the motivation of both boys and girls across domains by providing learning materials and assignments that match their different interests, and enabling the creation of a quiet, cooperative, mastery-oriented learning climate for girls, and a rambunctious, competitive, and performance-oriented climate for boys (e.g., Sax, 2005). A very different rationale is that single-sex classes empower girls. Girls will be more confident, less exposed to stereotypes about female abilities and interests, and enjoy more stimulating interactions with teachers than they do in male-dominated coeducational frameworks; they will also be protected from denigration and sexual harassment by boys. Other claims are that the presence of other-gender classmates enhances gender salience and stereotypes, and distracts both boys and girls from schoolwork, especially during adolescence (for an extended discussion, see Bigler et al., 2014).

In present terms, there might be grounds for anticipating that single-sex frameworks may benefit girls by building on their motivational strengths and mitigating their vulnerabilities. But the research reviewed here suggests that single-sex classrooms might exacerbate boys' motivational weaknesses and undermine rather than sustain their academic confidence, especially if they are low achievers. Specifically, single-sex frameworks might reinforce, rather than mitigate, tendencies to pursue performance over mastery goals, to value ability over effort, and to respond to difficulty with attempts to protect and salvage self-esteem, rather than by working harder. As we have already discussed, boys seem to be motivated to prove and protect before male more than female peers. In support, there is some evidence that boy-only classes tend to be characterized by rather high levels of macho displays and defiance of teachers (Jackson, 2002a). Boys also had more positive perceptions of the learning climate and their own engagement in classes with more rather than fewer girls.

Systematic evaluations have focused mainly on achievement. A meta-analysis of studies that controlled for background and selection effects showed no meaningful effects of single-sex versus coeducational frameworks apart from a modest benefit of the former for girls' achievement in science (Pahlke, Hyde, & Allison, 2014). These authors identified few controlled studies that assessed motivation, but these, too, did not show meaningful effects for either boys or girls. The only exception was that girls in single-sex frameworks had higher career

aspirations. They also expressed less gender-stereotyped attitudes. These are potentially important outcomes, but results were based on very few studies. Thus, Pahlke and her colleagues (2014) concluded that, overall, the evidence to date does not show that single-sex frameworks are more beneficial than coeducational ones for either girls or boys.

Creating Equitable Motivational Environments in Coeducational Classrooms

We have shown throughout how gendered motivational styles, strengths, and vulnerabilities are constructed in social interactions. Just as co-educational classrooms play a role in creating gender differences in competence motivation, so can they provide arenas in which both boys and girls can learn to question stereotypical beliefs and constraining gender roles, can develop interests and competence in diverse domains, can experience learning as worthwhile and meaningful achievement as possible, and learn to interact with one another as equals. We briefly note some promising directions. First, training programs designed to raise teachers' awareness of gender biases in their own behavior, in teaching materials, and in classroom discourse have been shown to be effective in changing teachers' often unintended differential treatment of boys and girls, and its attendant motivational consequences (Sadker et al., 2009). In a similar vein, in coeducational classrooms, both boys and girls can learn how gender stereotypes and gender roles both influence their own motivation and lead them to undermine that of their male and female classmates.

Second, rather than matching learning materials to the presumed interests and inclinations of boys and girls, teachers can both provide a range of traditionally masculine, feminine, and gender-neutral activities and assignments, and take an active role in ensuring that students do not gravitate too early and narrowly to gender-typed domains and therefore perpetuate rather than reduce gender differences in motivation for STEM versus language arts (see also Bigler et al., 2014). Third, there is strong evidence that mastery goal classroom structures promote positive patterns of competence motivation among boys and girls of diverse abilities and ethnicities. One feature of such classrooms is that difficulty and mistakes are framed as challenging learning opportunities. Presenting potential difficulties as a challenge orients students away from dwelling on their ability or the lack thereof. Thus, it has also been shown to be helpful in overcoming the negative consequences of stereotype threat (Alter, Aronson, Darley, Rodriguez, & Ruble, 2010). Promoting a growth mindset in the classroom is beneficial in part because believing that ability can be acquired promotes mastery goals (Dweck, 1999).

Mastery, growth-oriented classrooms have the promise of promoting what Nicholls (1989) called "equality of motivational opportunity." Girls can experience the benefits of trying, while being less vulnerable to doubting. For boys, and especially low achievers, classrooms that value effortful accomplishment can mitigate the need to invest resources in protecting self-esteem rather than developing competence. But might such classrooms also lead competent boys to lose some of the drive that spurs them to high achievement? And might girls not also benefit from opportunities to prove and display their abilities? In this context, Butler (2014) suggested that integrating practices of critical peer argumentation (e.g., Asterhan & Schwarz, 2007) in mastery-oriented classrooms may be a fruitful direction. Such practices can provide boys and girls, and lower and higher achievers, with the skills, confidence, and motivation to develop, present, and defend a position, to stand up to criticism, to critically evaluate arguments and solutions, and also to develop understanding and competence.

To conclude, thinking in terms of "proving and protecting" and "doubting and trying" can contribute to understanding how and why gender still matters for the competence motivation of boys and girls, women and men. We believe our approach has promise also for developing more engaging and gender-fair educational environments. It is important to reiterate, however, that competence beliefs and motivation are learned and constructed in social and societal contexts that are still tainted with sexist (and racist) attitudes and gender- and race-based discrimination. Understanding the social context of competence motivation necessitates more comprehensive analysis of social affordances and barriers than we have offered here. Similarly, promoting greater equality of motivational opportunity for both genders in educational contexts is important, but so is the promotion of fairer, more egalitarian societies.

REFERENCES

Alexander, J. M., Johnson, K. E., & Kelley, K. (2012). Longitudinal analysis of the relations between opportunities to learn about science and the development of interests related to science. *Science Education, 96,* 763–786.

Alexander, J. M., Johnson, K. E., Leibham, M. E., & Kelley, K. (2008). The development of conceptual interests in young children. *Cognitive Development, 23,* 324–334.

Alter, A. L., Aronson, J., Darley, J. M., Rodriguez, C., & Ruble, D. N. (2010). Rising to the threat: Reducing *stereotype threat* by reframing the *threat* as a *challenge. Journal of Experimental Social Psychology, 46,* 166–171.

Assouline, S. G., Colangelo, N., Ihrig, D., & Forstadt, L. (2006). Attributional choices for academic success and failure by intellectually gifted students. *Gifted Child Quarterly, 50,* 283–294.

Asterhan, C. S., & Schwarz, B. B. (2007). The effects of monological and dialogical argumentation on concept learning in evolutionary theory. *Journal of Educational Psychology, 99,* 626–639.

Bachman, J. G., O'Malley, P. M., Freedman-Doan, P., Trzesniewski, K. H., & Donnellan, M. B. (2011). Adolescent self-esteem: Differences by race/ethnicity, gender, and age. *Self and Identity, 10,* 445–473.

Beaman, R., Wheldall, K., & Kemp, C. (2006). Differential teacher attention to boys and girls in the classroom. *Educational Review, 58,* 339–366.

Bell, L. A. (1989). Something's wrong here and it's not me: Challenging the dilemmas that block girls' success. *Journal for the Education of the Gifted, 12,* 118–130.

Bench, S. W., Lench, H. C., Liew, J., Miner, K., & Flores, S. A. (2015). Gender gaps in overestimation of math performance. *Sex Roles, 72,* 536–546.

Beyer, S. (1999). Gender differences in causal attributions by college students of performance on course examinations. *Current Psychology, 17,* 346–358.

Bigler, R. S., Hayes, A. R., & Liben, L. S. (2014).

Analysis and evaluation of the rationales for single-sex schooling. In L. S. Liben & R. S. Bigler (Vol. Eds.), The role of gender in educational contexts and outcomes. In J. B. Benson (Series Ed.), *Advances in child development and behavior* (Vol. 47, pp. 225–260). London: Elsevier.

Blackwell, L., Trzesniewski, K., & Dweck, C. S. (2007). Implicit theories of intelligence predict achievement across an adolescent transition: A longitudinal study and an intervention. *Child Development, 78,* 246–263.

Butler, R. (1992). What young people want to know when: Effects of mastery and ability goals on preferences for different kinds of social comparisons. *Journal of Personality and Social Psychology, 62,* 934–943.

Butler, R. (1993). Effects of task and ego achievement goals on information-seeking during task engagement. *Journal of Personality and Social Psychology, 65,* 18–31.

Butler, R. (1994). Teacher communications and student interpretations: Effects of teacher responses to failing students on attributional inferences in two age groups. *British Journal of Educational Psychology, 64,* 277–294.

Butler, R. (1998a). Age trends in the use of social and temporal comparison for self-evaluation: Examination of a novel developmental hypothesis. *Child Development, 69,* 1054–1073.

Butler, R. (1998b). Determinants of help-seeking: Relations between perceived reasons for classroom help-avoidance and help-seeking behaviors in an experimental context. *Journal of Educational Psychology, 90,* 630–643.

Butler, R. (2000). What learners want to know: The role of achievement goals in shaping information-seeking, performance and interest. In C. Sansone & J. Harackiewicz (Eds.), *Intrinsic and extrinsic motivation: The search for optimal motivation and performance* (pp. 161–194). New York: Academic Press.

Butler, R. (2008). Ego-involving and frame of reference effects of tracking on elementary school students' motivational orientations and help seeking in math class. *Social Psychology of Education, 11,* 5–23.

Butler, R. (2012). Striving to connect: Extending an achievement goal approach to teacher motivation to include relational goals for teaching. *Journal of Educational Psychology, 104,* 726–742.

Butler, R. (2014). Motivation in educational contexts: Does gender matter? In L. S. Liben & R. S. Bigler (Vol. Eds.), The role of gender in educational contexts and outcomes. In J. B. Benson (Series Ed.), *Advances in child development and behavior* (Vol. 47, pp. 1–42). London: Elsevier.

Campbell, W. K., & Sedikides, C. (1999). Self-threat magnifies the self-serving bias: A meta-analytic integration. *Review of General Psychology, 3,* 23–43.

Chang, A., Sandhofer, C. M., & Brown, C. S. (2011). Gender biases in early number exposure to preschool-aged children. *Journal of Language and Social Psychology, 30,* 440–450.

Chhin, C. S., Bleeker, M. M., & Jacobs, J. E. (2008). Gender-typed occupational choices: The long-term impact of parents' beliefs and expectations. In H. M. G. Watt & J. S. Eccles (Eds.), *Gender and occupational outcomes: Longitudinal assessments of individual, social, and cultural influences* (pp. 215–234). Washington, DC: American Psychological Association.

Cole, D. A., Martin, J. M., Peeke, L. A., Seroczynski, A. D., & Fier, J. (1999). Children's over- and underestimation of academic competence: A longitudinal study of gender differences, depression, and anxiety. *Child Development, 70,* 459–473.

Covington, M. V., & Omelich, C. L. (1979). Effort: The double-edged sword in school achievement. *Journal of Educational Psychology, 71,* 169–182.

Craske, M. L. (1985). Improving persistence through observational learning and attribution retraining. *British Journal of Educational Psychology, 55,* 138–147.

Crocker, J., & Park, L. E. (2004). The costly pursuit of self-esteem. *Psychological Bulletin, 130,* 392–414.

Croson, R., & Gneezy, U. (2009). Gender differences in preferences. *Journal of Economic Literature, 47,* 448–474.

Crowley, K., Callanan, M. A., Tenenbaum, H. R., & Allen, E. (2001). Parents explain more often to boys than to girls during shared scientific thinking. *Psychological Science, 12,* 258–261.

Cvencek, A., Meltzoff, A. N., & Greenwald, A. G. (2011). Math-gender stereotypes in elementary school children. *Child Development, 82,* 766–779.

Dekker, S., Krabbendam, L., Lee, N. C., Boschloo, A., de Groot, R., & Jolles, J. (2013). Sex differences in goal orientation in adolescents aged 10–19: The older boys adopt work-avoidant goals twice as often as girls. *Learning and Individual Differences, 26,* 196–200.

Denton, C., Wolters, C. A., York, M. J., Swanson, E., Kulesz, P. A., & Francis, D. J. (2015). Adolescents' use of reading comprehension strategies: Differences related to reading proficiency, grade level, and gender. *Learning and Individual Differences, 37,* 81–95.

Dicke, A., Lüdtke, O., Trautwein, U., Nagy, G., & Nagy, N. (2102). Judging students' achievement goal orientations: Are teacher ratings accurate? *Learning and Individual Differences, 22*, 844–849.

Diseth, A., Meland, E., & Breidablik, H. J. (2014). Self-beliefs among students: Grade level and gender differences in self-esteem, self-efficacy and implicit theories of intelligence. *Learning and Individual Differences, 35*, 1–8.

Dresel, M., & Haugwitz, M. (2005). The relationship between cognitive abilities and self-regulated learning: Evidence for interactions with academic self-concept and gender. *High Ability Studies, 16*, 201–218.

Duckworth, A. L., & Seligman, M. E. P. (2006). Self-discipline gives girls the edge: Gender in self-discipline, grades, and achievement test scores. *Journal of Educational Psychology, 98*, 198–208.

Dupeyrat, C., Escribe, C., Huet, N., & Regner, I. (2011). Positive biases in self-assessment of mathematics competence, achievement goals, and mathematics performance. *International Journal of Educational Research, 50*, 241–250.

Dweck, C. S. (1986). Motivational processes affecting learning. *American Psychologist, 41*, 1040–1048.

Dweck, C. S. (1999). *Self-theories: Their role in motivation, personality and development.* Philadelphia: Taylor & Francis/Psychology Press.

Dweck, C. S. (2007). Is math a gift?: Beliefs that put females at risk. In S. J. Ceci & W. M. Williams (Eds.), *Why aren't more women in science?: Top researchers debate the evidence* (pp. 47–55). Washington, DC: American Psychological Association.

Dweck, C. S., Davidson, W., Nelson, S., & Enna, B. (1978). Sex differences in learned helplessness: II. The contingencies of evaluative feedback in the classroom and III. An experimental analysis. *Developmental Psychology, 14*, 268–276.

Eccles, J., Adler, T. F., Futterman, R., Goff, S. B., Kaczala, C. M., Meece, J. L., et al. (1983). Expectations, values and academic behaviors. In J. T. Spence (Ed.), *Perspective on achievement and achievement motivation* (pp. 75–146). San Francisco: Freeman.

Eccles, J. S., & Wigfield, A. (2002). Motivational beliefs, values, and goals. *Annual Review of Psychology, 53*, 109–132.

Elliot, A. J. (1999). Approach and avoidance motivation and achievement goals. *Educational Psychologist, 34*, 169–189.

Else-Quest, N. M., Hyde, J. S., Goldsmith, H. H., & Van Hulle, C. (2006). Sex differences in temperament: A meta-analysis. *Psychological Bulletin, 132*, 33–72.

Else-Quest, N. M., Mineo, C. C., & Higgins, A. (2013). Math and science attitudes and achievement at the intersection of gender and ethnicity. *Psychology of Women Quarterly, 37*, 293–309.

Frenzel, A. C., Goetz, T., Pekrun, R., & Watt, H. M. G. (2010). Development of mathematics interest in adolescence: Influences of gender, family, and school context. *Journal of Research on Adolescence, 20*, 507–537.

Frey, K. S., & Ruble, D. N. (1987). What children say about classroom performance: Sex and grade differences in perceived competence. *Child Development, 58*, 1066–1078.

Friedel, J. M., Cortina, K. S., Turner, J. C., & Midgley, C. (2007). Achievement goals, efficacy beliefs and coping strategies in mathematics: The roles of perceived parent and teacher goal emphases. *Contemporary Educational Psychology, 32*, 434–458.

Frome, P. M., & Eccles, J. S. (1998). Parents' influence on children's achievement-related perceptions. *Journal of Personality and Social Psychology, 74*, 435–452.

Furnham, A., Reeves, E., & Budhani, S. (2002). Parents think their sons are brighter than their daughters: Sex differences in parental self-estimations and estimations of their children's multiple intelligences. *Journal of Genetic Psychology, 163*, 24–39.

Gonida, E. N., & Leondari, A. (2011). Patterns of motivation among adolescents with biased and accurate self-efficacy beliefs. *International Journal of Educational Research, 50*, 209–220.

Good, C., Aronson, J., & Inzlicht, M. (2003). Improving adolescents' standardized test performance: An intervention to reduce the effects of stereotype threat. *Journal of Applied Developmental Psychology, 24*, 645–662.

Gunderson, E. A., Ramirez, G., Levine, S. C., & Beilock, S. L. (2012). The role of parents and teachers in the development of gender-related math attitudes. *Sex Roles, 66*, 153–166.

Heatherington, L., Daubman, K. A., Bates, C., Ahn, A., Brown, H., & Preston, C. (1993). Two investigations of "female modesty" in achievement situations. *Sex Roles, 29*, 739–754.

Hidi, S., & Renninger, K. A. (2006). The four-phase model of interest development. *Educational Psychologist, 41*, 111–127.

Hirt, E. R., & McCrea, S. M. (2009). Man smart, woman smarter?: Getting to the root of gender differences in self-handicapping. *Social and Personality Psychology Compass, 3*, 260–274.

Horner, M. S. (1972). Toward an understanding of achievement-related conflicts in women. *Journal of Social Issues, 28,* 157–175.

Huang, C. (2103). Gender differences in academic self-efficacy: A meta-analysis. *European Journal of Psychology of Education, 28,* 1–35.

Hyde, J. S. (2014). Gender similarities and differences. *Annual Review of Psychology, 65,* 373–398.

Hyde, J. S., & Durik, A. M. (2005). Gender, competence, and motivation. In A. J. Elliot & C. S. Dweck (Eds.), *Handbook of competence and motivation* (pp. 375–391). New York: Guilford Press.

Jackson, C. (2002a). Can single-sex classes in co-educational schools enhance the learning experiences of girls and/or boys?: An exploration of pupils' perceptions. *British Educational Research Journal, 28,* 37–48.

Jackson, C. (2002b). "Laddishness" as a self-worth protection strategy. *Gender and Education, 14,* 37–51.

Jacobs, J. E., Lanza, S., Osgood, D. W., Eccles, J. S., & Wigfield, A. (2002). Changes in children's self-competence and values: Gender and domain differences across grades one through twelve. *Child Development, 73,* 509–527.

Kenney-Benson, G. A., Pomerantz, E. M., Ryan, A. M., & Patrick, H. (2006). Sex differences in math performance: The role of children's approach to schoolwork. *Developmental Psychology, 42,* 11–26.

Kessels, U., Heyder, A., Latsch, M., & Hannover, B. (2014). How gender differences in academic engagement relate to students' gender identity. *Educational Research, 56,* 220–229.

Kurman, J. (2004). Gender, self-enhancement, and self-regulation of learning behaviors in junior high school. *Sex Roles, 50,* 725–735.

Kuyper, H., & Dijkstra, P. (2009). Better-than-average effects in secondary education: A 3-year follow-up. *Educational Research and Evaluation, 15,* 167–184.

Kuyper, H., Dijkstra, P., Buunk, A. P., & van der Werf, M. (2011). Social comparisons in the classroom: An investigation of the better than average effect among secondary school children. *Journal of School Psychology, 49,* 25–53.

Larivière, V., Ni, C., Gingras, Y., Cronin, B., & Sugimoto, C. R. (2013). Global disparities in science. *Nature, 504,* 2011–2013.

Lavy, V., & Schlosser, A. (2011). Mechanisms and impacts of gender peer effects at school. *American Economic Journal: Applied Economics, 3,* 1–33.

Leaper, C., & Brown, C. S. (2008). Perceived experiences with sexism among adolescent girls. *Child Development, 79,* 685–704.

Leaper, C., & Brown, C. S. (2014). Sexism in schools. In L. S. Liben & R. S. Bigler (Vol. Eds.), The role of gender in educational contexts and outcomes. In J. B. Benson (Series Ed.), *Advances in child development and behavior* (Vol. 47, pp. 189–223). London: Elsevier.

Leslie, S. J., Cimpian, A., Meyer, M., & Freeland, E. (2015). Expectations of brilliance underlie gender distributions across academic disciplines. *Science, 347,* 262–265.

Liben, L. S., & Coyle, E. F. (2014). Developmental interventions to address the STEM gender gap: Exploring intended and unintended consequences. In L. S. Liben & R. S. Bigler (Vol. Eds.), The role of gender in educational contexts and outcomes. In J. B. Benson (Series Ed.), *Advances in child development and behavior* (Vol. 47, pp. 77–116). London: Elsevier.

Lindberg, S. M., Hyde, J. S., & Hirsch, L. M. (2008). Gender and mother–child interactions during mathematics homework: The importance of individual differences. *Merrill–Palmer Quarterly, 54,* 232–255.

Linnenbrink-Garcia, L., Tyson, D. F., & Patall, E. A. (2008). When are achievement goal orientations beneficial for academic achievement?: A closer look at main effects and moderating factors. *Revue Internationale de Psychologie Sociale, 21,* 19–70.

Luo, W., Hogan, D., & Paris, S. G. (2011). Predicting Singapore students' achievement goals in their English study: Self-construal and classroom goal structure. *Learning and Individual Differences, 21,* 526–535.

Lytton, H., & Romney, D. M. (1991). Parents' differential socialization of boys and girls: A meta-analysis. *Psychological Bulletin, 109,* 267–296.

Maccoby, E. E. (1998). *The two sexes: Growing up apart, coming together.* Cambridge, MA: Harvard University Press.

Maltz, D. N., & Borker, R. A. (1982). A cultural approach to male–female miscommunication. In J. J. Gumperz (Ed.), *Language and social identity* (pp. 195–216). Cambridge, UK: Cambridge University Press.

Martin, C. L., Fabes, R. A., & Hanish, L. D. (2014). Gendered-peer relationships in educational contexts. In L. S. Liben & R. S. Bigler (Vol. Eds.), The role of gender in educational contexts and outcomes. In J. B. Benson (Series Ed.), *Advances in child development and behavior* (Vol. 47, pp. 151–187). London: Elsevier.

Measelle, J., Ablow, J. C., Cowan, P. A., & Cowan, C. P. (1998). Assessing young children's views of their academic, social, and emotional lives: An evaluation of the self-perception scales of the Berkeley Puppet Interview. *Child Development, 69,* 1556–1576.

Meece, J. L., Glienke, B. B., & Burg, S. (2006). Gender and motivation. *Journal of School Psychology, 44,* 351–373.

Midgley, C., Kaplan, A., & Middleton, M. (2001). Performance-approach goals: Good for what, for whom, under what circumstances, and at what cost? *Journal of Educational Psychology, 93,* 77–86.

Miyake, A., Kost-Smith, L. E., Finkelstein, N. D., Pollock, S. J., Cohen, G. L., & Ito, T. A. (2010). Reducing the gender achievement gap in college science: A classroom study of values affirmation. *Science, 330,* 1234–1237.

Mullola, S., Ravaja, N., Lipsanen, J., Alatupa, S., Hintsanen, M., Jokela, M., et al. (2012). Gender differences in teachers' perceptions of students' temperament, educational competence, and teachability. *British Journal of Educational Psychology, 82,* 185–206.

Nagy, G., Watt, H. M. G., Eccles, J. S., Trautwein, U., Lüdtke, O., & Baumert, J. (2010). The development of students' mathematics self-concept in relation to gender: Different countries, different trajectories? *Journal of Research on Adolescence, 20,* 482–506.

National Center for Education Statistics. (2013). *The condition of education.* Washington, DC: U.S. Department of Education. Retrieved from *http://nces.ed.gov/pubsearch.*

Nicholls, J. G. (1989). *The competitive ethos and democratic education.* Cambridge, MA: Harvard University Press.

Nosek, B., Banaji, M., & Greenwald, A. (2002). Math = male, me = female, therefore math not = me. *Journal of Personality and Social Psychology, 83,* 44–59.

Nosek, B. A., Smyth, F. L., Sriram, N., Lindner, N. M., Devos, T., Ayala, A., et al. (2009). National differences in gender–science stereotypes predict national sex differences in science and math achievement. *Proceedings of the National Academy of Sciences USA, 106,* 10593–10597.

Organisation for Economic Co-operation and Development (OECD). (2010). PISA 2009 Results: What students know and can do—student performance in reading, mathematics and science. Retrieved from *http://dx.doi.org/10.1787/9789264091450-en.*

Organisation for Economic Co-operation and Development (OECD). (2013). Education at a glance 2013: OECD indicators. Retrieved from *http://dx.doi.org/10.1787/eag-2013-en.*

Oyserman, D., Johnson, E., & James, L. (2011). Seeing the destination but not the path: Effects of socioeconomic disadvantage on school-focused possible self content and linked behavioral strategies. *Self and Identity, 10,* 474–492.

Pahlke, E., Cooper, C. E., & Fabes, R. A. (2013). Classroom sex composition and first-grade school outcomes: The role of classroom behavior. *Social Science Research, 42,* 1650–1658.

Pahlke, E., Hyde, J. S., & Allison, C. M. (2014). The effects of single-sex compared with coeducational schooling on students' performance and attitudes: A meta-analysis. *Psychological Bulletin, 140,* 1042–1072.

Pajares, F., & Valiante, G. (1999). Grade level and gender differences in the writing self-beliefs of middle school students. *Contemporary Educational Psychology, 24,* 390–405.

Picho, K., Rodriguez, A., & Finnie, L. (2103). Exploring the moderating role of context on the mathematics performance of females under stereotype threat: A meta-analysis. *Journal of Social Psychology, 153,* 299–333.

Plante, I., Théorêt, M., & Favreau, O. E. (2009). Student gender stereotypes: Contrasting the perceived maleness and femaleness of mathematics and language. *Educational Psychology, 29,* 385–405.

Pomerantz, E., Altermatt, E. R., & Saxon, J. L. (2002). Making the grade but feeling distressed: Gender differences in academic performance and internal distress. *Journal of Educational Psychology, 94,* 396–404.

Preckel, F., Goetz, T., Pekrun, R., & Kleine, M. (2008). Gender differences in gifted and average-ability students: Comparing girls' and boys' achievement, self-concept, interest, and motivation in mathematics. *Gifted Child Quarterly, 52,* 146–159.

Räty, H., Vänskä, J., Kasanen, K., & Kärkkäinen, R. (2002). Parents' explanations of their child's performance in mathematics and reading: A replication and extension of Yee and Eccles. *Sex Roles, 46,* 121–128.

Renold, E. (2001a). Learning the "hard" way: Boys, hegemonic masculinity and the negotiation of learner identities in the primary school. *British Journal of Sociology of Education, 22,* 369–385.

Renold, E. (2001b). "Square-girls," femininity and the negotiation of academic success in the primary school. *British Educational Research Journal, 27,* 577–587.

Retelsdorf, J., Schwartz, K., & Asbrock, F. (2015). "Michael can't read!": Teachers' gender stereotypes and boys' reading self-concept. *Journal of Educational Psychology, 107,* 186–194.

Riegle-Crumb, C., & Humphries, M. (2012). Exploring bias in math teachers' perceptions of students' ability by gender and race/ethnicity. *Gender and Society, 26,* 290–322.

Roberts, T. (1991). Gender and the influence of evaluations on self-assessments in achievement settings. *Psychological Bulletin, 109,* 297–308.

Robinson-Cimpian, J. P., Lubienski, S. T., Ganley, C. M., & Copur-Gencturk, Y. (2014). Teachers' perceptions of students' mathematics proficiency may exacerbate early gender gaps in achievement. *Developmental Psychology, 50,* 1262–1281.

Robnett, R. D., & Leaper, C. (2013). Friendship groups, personal motivation, and gender in relation to high school students' STEM career interest. *Journal of Research on Adolescence, 23,* 652–664.

Rogers, L., & Hallam, S. (2006). Gender differences in approaches to studying for the GCSE among high-achieving pupils. *Educational Studies, 32,* 59–71.

Rolland, R. G. (2012). Synthesizing the evidence on classroom goal structures in middle and secondary schools: A meta-analysis and narrative review. *Review of Educational Research, 82,* 396–435.

Rose, A. J., & Rudolph, K. D. (2006). A review of sex differences in peer relationship processes: Potential trade-offs for the emotional and behavioral development of girls and boys. *Psychological Bulletin, 132,* 98–131.

Rowley, S. J., Ross, L., Lozada, F., Williams, A., Gale, A., & Kurtz-Costes, B. (2014). Framing black boys: Parent, teacher, and student narratives of the academic lives of black boys. In L. S. Liben & R. S. Bigler (Vol. Eds.), The role of gender in educational contexts and outcomes. In J. B. Benson (Series Ed.), *Advances in child development and behavior* (Vol. 47, pp. 301–332). London: Elsevier.

Ruble, D. N., Eisenberg, R., & Higgins, E. T. (1994). Developmental changes in achievement evaluation: Motivational implications of self–other differences. *Child Development, 65,* 1091–1106.

Sadker, D., Sadker, M., & Zittleman, K. R. (2009). *Still failing at fairness: How gender bias cheats girls and boys in school and what we can do about it.* New York: Simon & Schuster.

Sax, L. (2005). *Why gender matters.* New York: Doubleday.

Senko, C., Hulleman, C. S., & Harackiewicz, J. M. (2011). Achievement goal theory at the crossroads: Old controversies, current challenges, and new directions. *Educational Psychologist, 46,* 26–47.

Sherman, D. K., Hartson, K. A., Binning, K.

R., Purdie-Vaughns, V., Garcia, J., Taborsky-Barba, S., et al. (2013). Deflecting the trajectory and changing the narrative: How self-affirmation affects academic performance and motivation under identity threat. *Journal of Personality and Social Psychology, 104,* 591–618.

Shim, S., & Finch, W. H. (2014). Academic and social achievement goals and early adolescents' adjustment: A latent class approach. *Learning and Individual Differences, 30,* 98–105.

Simpkins, S. D., Fredricks, J. A., & Eccles, J. S. (2012). Charting the Eccles' expectancy–value model from mothers' beliefs in childhood to youths' activities in adolescence. *Developmental Psychology, 48,* 1019–1032.

Steinmayr, R., & Spinath, B. (2009). What explains boys' stronger confidence in their intelligence? *Sex Roles, 61,* 736–749.

Su, R., Rounds, J., & Armstrong, P. I. (2009). Men and things, women and people: A meta-analysis of sex differences in interests. *Psychological Bulletin, 135,* 859–884.

Syzmanowicz, A., & Furnham, A. (2011). Gender differences in self-estimates of general, mathematical, spatial and verbal intelligence: Four meta analyses. *Learning and Individual Differences, 21,* 493–504.

Taylor, A. Z., & Graham, S. (2007). An examination of the relationship between achievement values and perceptions of barriers among low-SES African American and Latino students. *Journal of Educational Psychology, 99,* 52–64.

Tenenbaum, H. R. (2009). "You'd be good at that": Gender patterns in parent–child talk about courses. *Social Development, 18,* 447–463.

Tracey, T. J. G. (2002). Development of interests and competency beliefs: A one-year longitudinal study of fifth to eighth grade students using the ICA-R and structural equation modeling. *Journal of Counseling Psychology, 49,* 148–163.

Urdan, T., & Midgley, C. (2001). Academic self-handicapping: What we know, what more there is to learn. *Educational Psychology Review, 13,* 115–138.

Urdan, T., Midgley, C., & Anderman, E. M. (1998). The role of classroom goal structure in students' use of self-handicapping strategies. *American Educational Research Journal, 35,* 101–122.

U.S. Department of Education & National Center for Education Statistics. (2007). Digest of education statistics. Retrieved from *http://nces.ed.gov/index.asp.*

Usher, E. L., & Pajares, F. (2008). Sources of

self-efficacy in school: Critical review of the literature and future directions. *Review of Educational Research, 78,* 751–796.

Valla, J., & Ceci, S. J. (2011). Can sex differences in science be tied to the long reach of prenatal hormones?: Brain organization theory, digit ratio (2D/4D), and sex differences in preferences and cognition. *Perspectives on Psychological Science, 6,* 134–146.

Voyer, D., & Voyer, S. D. (2014). Gender differences in scholastic achievement: A meta-analysis. *Psychological Bulletin, 140,* 1174–1204.

Weaver-Hightower, M. (2003). The "boy turn" in research on gender and education. *Review of Educational Research, 73,* 471–498.

Weisgram, E. S., & Bigler, R. S. (2007). Effects of learning about gender discrimination on adolescent girls' attitudes toward and interest in science. *Psychology of Women Quarterly, 31,* 262–269.

Weisgram, E. S., Bigler, R. S., & Liben, L. S. (2010). Gender, values, and occupational interests among children, adolescents, and adults. *Child Development, 81,* 778–796.

Wigfield, A., Eccles, J. S., Yoon, K. S., Harold, R. D., Arbreton, A. J. A., Freedman-Doan, C., et al. (1997). Change in children's competence beliefs and subjective task values across the elementary school years: A 3-year study. *Journal of Educational Psychology, 89,* 451–469.

Wood, D., Kurtz-Costes, B., Rowley, S. J., & Okeke-Adeyanju, N. (2010). Mothers' academic gender stereotypes and education-related beliefs about sons and daughters in African American families. *Journal of Educational Psychology, 102,* 521–530.

Xie, H., Dawes, M., Wurster, T. J., & Shi, B. (2013). Aggression, academic behaviors, and popularity perceptions among boys of color during the transition to middle school. *American Journal of Orthopsychiatry, 83,* 265–277.

Yeager, D. S., Romero, C., Paunesku, D., Hulleman, C. S., Schneider, B., Hinojosa, C., et al. (2016). Using design thinking to improve psychological interventions: The case of the growth mindset during the transition to high school. *Journal of Educational Psychology, 108,* 374–391.

Yeung, A. S. (2011). Student self-concept and effort: Gender and grade differences. *Educational Psychology, 31,* 749–772.

Ziegler, A., & Stoeger, H. (2004). Evaluation of an attributional retraining (modeling technique) to reduce gender differences in chemistry instruction. *High Ability Studies, 15,* 63–83.

CHAPTER 27

Social Class and Models of Competence
How Gateway Institutions Disadvantage Working-Class Americans and How to Intervene

NICOLE M. STEPHENS
ANDREA G. DITTMANN
SARAH S. M. TOWNSEND

Brittany Bronson occupies an unusual space between social classes: university professor by day, Las Vegas waitress by night. In the pursuit of her middle-class academic aspirations she takes on a working-class[1] position, a "survival job" as she calls it, to make ends meet.

At times she finds herself in situations in which her two worlds collide: She encounters her middle- and upper-class students and their parents while at her waitressing job. She reflects on such encounters in this way:

> Why do I still experience a great feeling of shame when clearing a student's dirty plate? Embarrassment is not an adequate term to describe what I felt when those parents looked at me, clearly stupefied, thinking, "This waitress teaches my child?" It is a shame I share with many of my blue-collar colleagues, a belief that society deems our work inferior, that we have settled on or chosen these paths because we do not have the skills necessary to acquire something better. (Bronson, 2014, p. A35)

According to Bronson (2014), these meetings risk "destroying the facade of success" that she presents to her students in the classroom. Even though Bronson and her restaurant colleagues know that their occupations are "skilled" and require a range of specific competencies to be effective, mainstream American society considers blue-collar work such as waitressing "unskilled" and inferior. As Bronson (2015) explains, although this type of work "requires a constant interaction with people, because of its low-paying status it is deemed a dead end, rather than a testament to an individual's ability to acquire, adapt, and specialize" (p. A31). In other words, mainstream American society does not recognize the skills involved in Bronson's waitressing role as competence. Faced with this realization, she reports experiencing a sense of shame.

Bronson's encounters with her students and their parents reveal an important but rarely recognized assumption about what types of skills count as competent in mainstream American society. Specifically, middle-class ways of being competent (e.g., the behaviors required by her role as a professor) are often seen as the only "right" way to be competent. Yet, as Bronson's story suggests, there is more than one way to be competent. And, as we argue in this chapter, success in different social class contexts requires different ways of being competent. For example, to be competent in her working-class role as a waitress, Bronson must respond to the needs of her customers, adjust to changing situations, and rely on and provide support to her coworkers to get the job done. Alternatively, to be competent in her middle-class role as a university professor, Bronson must display confidence, take charge of the classroom, and express her opinions to her students.

In this chapter, we document and describe how social class shapes competence in four sections. Considering the context-contingent nature of competence, we adopt Elliot and Dweck's (2005) definition of competence as "a fundamental motivation that serves the evolutionary role of helping people develop and adapt to their environment" (p. 6). First, we examine how different social class contexts promote divergent understandings of how to be competent, which we refer to as *models of competence* (see Markus, Ryff, Curhan, & Palmersheim, 2004). Second, we provide evidence that the middle-class model of competence is institutionalized in American society, while the working-class model of competence is often excluded. We do so by focusing on schools and workplaces—two institutions that evaluate individuals' competence and serve as gateways to upward mobility. In the third section, we show how this institutionalization of the middle-class model of competence can disadvantage working-class individuals by limiting access to opportunities, undermining their performance, and leading them to be evaluated as less competent. Finally, we propose interventions at both individual and institutional levels that have the potential to reduce some of the social class inequalities perpetuated by this reliance on the middle-class model of competence.

SOCIAL CLASS PROMOTES DIFFERENT MODELS OF COMPETENCE

Social class contexts provide an important source of variation in models of competence.

These models of competence derive from culture-specific understandings of what it means to be a good or appropriate person in the world—what previous research has referred to as *models of self* (Cross & Madson, 1997; Markus & Kitayama, 1991, 2010). Research conducted in a variety of cultural contexts has identified two common models of self that provide different blueprints for how people should relate to others and to the social world, and, specifically, how to be competent (Adams, Anderson, & Adonu, 2004; Markus & Kitayama, 1991; Plaut & Markus, 2005). An *independent* model of self assumes that a normatively appropriate person should influence the context, be separate from other people, and act freely based on personal motives, goals, and preferences (Markus & Kitayama, 2003). An *interdependent* model of self, in contrast, assumes that a normatively appropriate person should adjust to the conditions of the context, connect to others, and respond to the needs, preferences, and interests of others.

As outlined in Figure 27.1, understanding how different social class contexts promote these models of self and competence requires an analysis of available material resources (e.g., income, access to high-quality education) and social resources (e.g., relationships with family and friends). These conditions are important because they shape the possible patterns of thinking, feeling, and acting in the world, as well as the ways of being that are most likely to be effective in different social class contexts. How people are able to act over time will shape the ways of being a person that are likely to become normative and preferred.

Middle-class American contexts promote an independent model of self and competence (see Figure 27.1). People in middle-class contexts have greater economic capital, fewer environmental constraints, higher power and status, and more opportunities for choice, influence, and control than do people in working-class contexts (Day & Newburger, 2002; Kohn, 1969; Pattillo-McCoy, 1999; Terenzini & Pascarella, 1991). They also tend to have higher levels of geographic mobility, given the need to move away from home to attend college and to pursue subsequent career opportunities

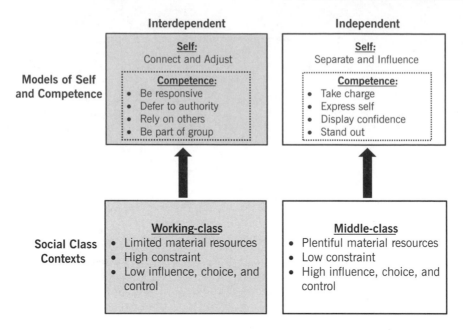

FIGURE 27.1. Social class contexts shape models of self and competence.

(Argyle, 1994). These material realities promote socialization practices that convey to children a sense of self-importance and individual entitlement (Miller, Cho, & Bracey, 2005). For example, parents often engage in *concerted cultivation,* or efforts to identify and encourage their children's personal preferences, ideas, and opinions (Lareau, 2003). Through these interactions, parents convey to children the message that "the world is your oyster" and "your voice matters."

In response to these material and social conditions, middle-class individuals have ample opportunities to influence the situation, to make choices according to their own personal preferences, to develop confidence and a sense of optimism, and to express their ideas and opinions. Over time, these ways of being foster a sense of self as autonomous or separate from others and as able to influence the world according to personal preferences. As shown in Figure 27.1, an independent model of competence stresses that individuals should take charge of their environments, express what they think and feel, show confidence, and stand out from the group. Thus, when Bronson operates in her role as a university professor, she enacts an independent model of competence and is

therefore seen as competent by her middle-class students and peers.

Working-class contexts, on the other hand, promote an interdependent model of self and competence (see Figure 27.1). People in working-class contexts have less access to economic capital, confront more environmental constraints, are exposed to greater risks and uncertainty, and have fewer opportunities for choice, influence, and control than do people in middle-class contexts (Chen & Matthews, 2001; Lachman & Weaver, 1998; Reay, Davies, David, & Ball, 2001). Working-class individuals do not typically move away to attend college, so they often stay in the same geographic location for their entire lives, frequently interact with family members, and tend to be embedded in densely structured social networks (Argyle, 1994; Lamont, 2000; Markus et al., 2004). These material realities often promote socialization practices that encourage children to recognize their place in the social hierarchy, to follow rules and social norms, and to be responsive to others' needs (Fiske & Markus, 2012; Kohn, 1969; Kusserow, 1999; Lamont, 2000; Piff, Kraus, Côté, Cheng, & Keltner, 2010; Stephens, Fryberg, & Markus, 2011). For example, parents in working-class contexts often emphasize to their children that "it's not just about you" and "you can't always get what you want" (Miller et al., 2005; Snibbe & Markus, 2005).

In response to these material and social conditions, working-class individuals must adjust themselves to the social context, be tough and strong, and rely on close others (e.g., family, friends) for support (Stephens, Markus, & Phillips, 2014). Over time, these ways of being foster a sense of self as connected to others and as adjusting to one's environment (Markus & Kitayama, 2003). As shown in Figure 27.1, an interdependent model of competence assumes that individuals should be responsive to the social context, show deference to authority, rely on and support others, and be part of the group. Thus, when Bronson and her restaurant coworkers engage in such behaviors, they enact an interdependent model of competence and will be seen as competent in the eyes of other working-class individuals. Yet from the perspective of middle-class colleagues or students, their ways of being competent will go unseen or be devalued.

THE INSTITUTIONALIZATION OF THE INDEPENDENT MODEL OF COMPETENCE

Although both independent and interdependent models of competence are viable ways of being a person, U.S. institutions tend primarily to endorse and value the independent model. Indeed, U.S. institutions ranging from the media to politics reflect an independent model (e.g., Adams, Biernat, Branscombe, Crandall, & Wrightsman, 2008; Bellah, Madsen, Sullivan, Swidler, & Tipton, 1985; Iyengar, 2010; Markus & Conner, 2013). We focus here on how the independent model organizes two critical gateway institutions: schools and workplaces (Ridgeway & Fisk, 2012). Schools and workplaces play crucial roles in providing access to valued life opportunities (e.g., influential social networks) and upward social mobility. The ideas, practices, and standards of evaluation that are prevalent in these key gateway institutions are not neutral; rather, they reflect an independent model of how to be a competent student

or employee. Importantly, institutions that focus exclusively on the independent model miss out on some of the individual and organizational benefits of interdependence (Hambrick, 1995). For example, institutions are less likely to engage effectively in activities that are necessary to maximize their performance, such as encouraging collaboration and working toward shared goals (Duhigg, 2016; Woolley, Chabris, Pentland, Hashmi, & Malone, 2010).

U.S. institutions of higher education reflect and promote an independent model of competence as the cultural ideal. In a survey of administrators at a diverse range of research universities and liberal arts colleges, the vast majority reported that their institutions expect students to enact an independent model of competence—to pave their own paths, to challenge norms and rules, to express their personal preferences, and to work independently (Fryberg & Markus, 2007; Stephens, Markus, & Fryberg, 2012). Indeed, institutions of higher education tend to focus on the importance of exploring and developing personal interests, and offer students the opportunity to structure their coursework and activities in a way that aligns with their preferences. Thus, an independent model of competence guides administrators' and educators' assumptions about how students should be motivated, learn, and interact with peers and professors. By setting up particular expectations about how good students should behave, an independent model serves as the standard against which educators are likely to interpret and evaluate students' behavior.

Universities promote this standard by encouraging and rewarding students for the development of specialized skills and patterns of behavior (Bowles & Gintis, 1976; Oakes, 1982). In many university classrooms, for example, class participation is a significant part of students' final grades and also contributes to how professors evaluate students' potential more generally. This widespread practice reveals how an independent model of competence—in this case, the act of expressing one's own thoughts, ideas, and opinions—is institutionalized in U.S. higher education and dictates what it means to be a good or competent student (Kim, 2002).

The standard is communicated not only by interactions inside the classroom with peers and professors but also by messages contained in cultural products such as university guidebooks, brochures, and application materials. For example, Yale University's admissions website advises applicants to "pursue what you love and tell us about that. Be yourself." Dartmouth College's site stresses, "What will impress us is YOU. You, letting your application express some aspect of your own story. You've established a great track record. Let your application clearly reflect your interests and motivation." The advice that these universities offer to applicants is guided by the assumption that "qualified" or "competent" students will have the skills to identify and communicate their personal interests—behaviors that are socialized largely in middle-class contexts. By contrast, the interdependent competencies fostered by many working-class contexts (e.g., working together, building community) are largely absent from these university materials. Promoting independent behaviors as the cultural ideal can indeed encourage the development of skills that are important for success in U.S. society. However, focusing exclusively on independence can hinder the development of interdependent competencies—working together on research and class projects, building relationships in extracurricular activities, and supporting one's classmates—that have the potential to enhance students' relational and achievement outcomes (Hackman & Katz, 2010; Hilk, 2013).

An independent model of competence informs not only higher education but also middle-class, professional workplaces that may provide a path to upward mobility in U.S. society for working-class individuals. Managers and other employees in professional firms tend to value employees who take charge and influence the situation, confidently express their ideas and opinions, and promote themselves (Anderson, Brion, Moore, & Kennedy, 2012; Anderson, John, Keltner, & Kring, 2001; Anderson & Kilduff, 2009; Kennedy, Anderson, & Moore, 2013; Van Kleef, Homan, Finkenauer, Gündemir, & Stamkou, 2011). These settings often focus on the importance of personal autonomy and offer employees the opportunity to craft their job (i.e., to shape it in a way that aligns with their individual needs and interests; Berg, Wrzesniewski, & Dutton, 2010; Wrzesniewski & Dutton, 2001). For example, on the website of the investment bank Morgan Stanley, an employee described the type of person who would be effective in the company: "This is a great environment for the self-starter, someone who relishes a lot of autonomy, and seeks to do things the way they think is best. If you have initiative, you can take it and run. The firm will support that and reward that quality." This independent model of competence also guides managers' assumptions about how employees should be motivated, develop skills, and interact with colleagues. By setting up particular expectations about how good employees should behave, an independent model serves as the standard against which managers are likely to interpret and evaluate employees' behavior.

Workplaces tend to promote this standard by encouraging and rewarding workers for the independent competencies they seek to cultivate (Bacon & Storey, 1996; Cooke & Rousseau, 1988; Friedlander, 1965; Hyman, 1994; Lamont, 2000; Urtasun & Núñez, 2012). Even before individuals join an organization, managers and employees expect job applicants to enact an independent model of competence: to ask questions, to express their preferences, and to take risks. Once applicants are hired, these expectations of independence are reinforced further. For example, all team members at Amazon are ranked annually, and those at the bottom are eliminated (Kantor & Streitfeld, 2015). Reflecting an independent model of competence, this system encourages all employees to focus primarily on their individual performance—rather than on the needs of their team or the organization—and to direct their efforts toward outperforming one another. Similarly, Microsoft employees are encouraged to compete with each other. As one employee recounted, "If you were on a team of 10 people, you walked in the first day knowing that, no matter how good everyone was, two people were going to get a great review, seven were going to get mediocre reviews, and one was going to get a terrible review. . . . It leads to employees focusing on competing with each other rather than competing with other companies" (Eichenwald, 2012, para. 162). This employee review practice, which is known as the "bell curve," focuses on zero-sum individual performance rather than on teams working toward a common goal. Notably, this practice eventually played a role in undermining Microsoft's ability to keep up with its competitors (Evans & Dion, 1991; Guzzo & Dickson, 1996).

This independent standard can also be conveyed through cultural products such as company websites or recruiting and hiring practices. Company websites, for example, are saturated with messages that competent applicants or employees must display independence to be successful in the future. The recruiting homepage of Deloitte states: "What's great about the people? . . . Each person is unique and valued for that, among the best and brightest in the business, and takes pride in his or her achievements." Similarly, an employee on Goldman Sachs's website declares that managers "pride themselves on empowering their employees to be creative and to develop solutions to problems at any level." The employee then goes on to say, "This is a place where I can select the opportunities I'm interested in, instead of waiting for the organization to decide for me." In both of these examples, the organizations portray a competent employee as one who has the skills to stand out from others, showcase personal achievements, and take charge of the workplace by making decisions. Largely absent from these messages is an interdependent model of competence, even though harnessing employees' interdependent competencies (e.g., collaborating in teams, having shared goals, supporting one's colleagues) has great potential to add value to organizations.

RELIANCE ON AN INDEPENDENT MODEL OF COMPETENCE DISADVANTAGES WORKING-CLASS AMERICANS

Schools' and workplaces' reliance on an independent model of competence can reduce upward mobility and perpetuate social class inequality by creating a *cultural mismatch* for working-class individuals, who are more often guided by an interdependent model

of competence (Stephens, Markus, et al., 2014). The exclusion of an interdependent model can inadvertently signal to working-class individuals that gateway institutions are not places for people "like them." This perceived lack of fit can in turn undermine working-class individuals' opportunity to succeed in those settings.

In this section, we suggest that working-class individuals experience a cultural mismatch in these gateway institutions in three important domains: (1) *access,* (2) *performance,* and (3) *evaluation.* The disadvantages that these institutions produce can build on one another and create a cycle that perpetuates inequality.

Access

The experience of cultural mismatch may lead individuals from working-class backgrounds to be less motivated to take actions needed to gain access (e.g., apply) to gateway institutions. This mismatch could lead working-class individuals to (1) recognize less often the potential contributions of their own skills in these settings, and (2) feel that they are not welcome or that they do not fit in these settings. Both of these experiences could lead working-class individuals to conclude that they are unlikely to be admitted or hired if they apply, and that even if they were hired, they would be unlikely to benefit from the experience.

Lack of Recognition of Potential Contribution

A cultural mismatch may demotivate working-class individuals from gaining access to gateway institutions by signaling that their interdependent competencies are unlikely to be effective there. In the context of higher education, working-class high school students who do not see their model of competence included in the college setting may infer that they do not have the skills necessary to succeed. They may surmise this from perusing college websites that describe the "type" of (middle-class) student who is likely to be admitted (e.g., one who "has pride in individual accomplishments"). Similarly, successful college graduates from working-class backgrounds who do not see their model of competence included in a workplace may conclude that they do not have the skills to pursue a position in that company. Notably, the most lucrative, high-status occupations are most likely to reflect and promote an independent model of competence (Acker, 2006; Sutton & Hargadon, 1996; Williams, 2012; Wojcicki, 2011).

Anticipated Lack of Fit

A cultural mismatch may also demotivate working-class individuals from gaining access to gateway institutions by leading them to believe that people "like them" are unlikely to fit in the setting. Highlighting the relevance of this concern in higher education, Michael Gove, the United Kingdom's former education secretary, notes that working-class students' "worries about 'not fitting in' will be one reason why [they will be] less likely to apply to the most selective universities" (Graham, 2014, para. 15). These concerns persist beyond college and can impact people's interest in various occupations. Rather than strive to gain admission into certain high-status, lucrative occupations, working-class individuals may instead choose to withdraw from "the game" (e.g., Gray & Kish-Gephart, 2013). These individuals may conclude that there is no point in applying for such opportunities if they imagine that they will never truly belong.

Performance

A cultural mismatch can even undermine the performance of working-class individuals who defy the odds and gain access to higher education and white-collar workplaces. As we explain below, this mismatch may undermine their performance in two ways: (1) They have less experience enacting the skills associated with an independent model, and (2) they lack a sense of comfort and fit in the setting.

Less Experience Enacting an Independent Model of Competence

A cultural mismatch can undermine working-class individuals' performance by encouraging them to enact an independent model of competence with which they are likely to have less experience. Upon gaining entry to key gateway institutions, the prevalence of an independent model likely communicates that enacting independent norms is the only right way to be competent. Working-class students tend to have less exposure to and experience with cultural norms of independence. They also tend to know less about the often-implicit "rules of the game" for these independent norms (cf. Bourdieu, 1984; Ridgeway, 2014). Thus, working-class students may find enacting these cultural norms especially difficult. For example, many college students from working-class backgrounds report difficulty choosing a major, developing and expressing their own ideas in class, and planning out their schedules to manage multiple and often competing demands on their time (e.g., papers and exams). As one working-class student put it, "While my college had done an excellent job recruiting me, I had no road map for what I was supposed to do once I made it to campus" (Capó Crucet, 2015, p. SR6). Even though this student successfully gained access to higher education, her lack of previous experience enacting independence left her unsure of what she needed to do to become a "good" college student.

Often, the experience of not knowing the right way to act does not end with college graduation. Rather, the impact of one's social class background persists far beyond college, even for those who have successfully navigated their way through college and into a middle-class profession (cf. Kish-Gephart & Campbell, 2014). Consider the "outsider" experience of Della Mae Justice, a successful Kentucky lawyer who was raised in poverty in Appalachia. Justice continues to experience difficulty in middle-class settings, and explains how she still spends time "wondering if I'm wearing the right thing, if I'll know what to do. I'm always thinking: How does everybody else know that? How do they know how to act? Why do they all seem so at ease?" (Lewin, 2005, para. 64). Despite her middle-class success, Justice continues to question whether she has the skills or cultural capital necessary to be accepted.

Lack of Fit

A cultural mismatch may also undermine working-class individuals' performance by reducing their comfort and sense of fit with the setting. In the context of higher education, students who feel that their ways of being competent are not valued by their college or university are likely to experience less fit and question whether they can be successful there (e.g., Johnson, Richeson, & Finkel, 2011; Ostrove & Long, 2007). These feelings of discomfort can prevent students from performing up to their potential. Stephens and colleagues (2012) illustrated this process in a laboratory experiment in which they exposed working-class students to a welcome letter that framed their university's expectations in terms of either independence (cultural mismatch) or interdependence (cultural match), and examined the consequences for students' experience and performance (Stephens, Fryberg, Markus, Johnson, & Covarrubias, 2012; Stephens, Townsend, Markus, & Phillips, 2012). Stephens and colleagues found that the independent framing decreased working-class students' academic comfort, as indexed by self-reported difficulty of the task, compared with the interdependent framing. Furthermore, their lower levels of comfort hindered their performance on academic tasks (e.g., anagrams). Moreover, in a longitudinal study in which they followed students throughout their 4 years in college, the authors found that the experience of cultural mismatch reduced working-class students' sense of fit not only at the beginning of college but also throughout college until graduation (Phillips, Stephens, Townsend, & Goudeau 2016). Their reduced fit, in turn, predicted lower grades at the end of college. Together, these studies suggest that one way a cultural mismatch can undermine working-class students' performance is by undermining their sense of fit.

This lack of fit often persists after graduation and can undermine employees' performance as they transition into the workplace. For example, Andrea Todd, a former magazine writer from a working-class background, explains, "I finally just dropped out. . . . It was too many years of *not belonging*. I never made a real, true friend, someone to count on. I was from a different class and they never wanted to know the real me" (cited in Lubrano, 2004, p. 155, emphasis added). Even though Todd was able to gain

access to a middle-class job, over time, her lack of belonging likely hindered her ability to perform up to her potential and led her to leave.

Evaluation

Finally, even if individuals from working-class backgrounds gain access and perform well on the job, the evaluation process may further disadvantage them. Middle-class evaluators' reliance on an independent model of competence may make it difficult to recognize the skills and potential contributions of working-class individuals, whom they may evaluate as incompetent (cf. Fiske, Cuddy, Glick, & Xu, 2002). As we describe below, this may occur even when working-class individuals perform as well as their middle-class counterparts on objective measures of performance.

When evaluating the competence and achievements of working-class individuals, an independent model of competence is likely to shape the views of middle-class observers. Accordingly, when middle-class individuals observe people enacting an independent model of competence (e.g., taking charge), they are likely to value these behaviors. In contrast, they are likely to devalue behaviors that instead reflect an interdependent model of competence (e.g., being socially responsive; cf. Ridgeway & Fisk, 2012; Stephens, Hamedani, Markus, Bergsieker, & Eloul, 2009). For example, colleges and universities recognize students for independent research projects and studying abroad but "don't recognize, in the same way, if you work at the neighborhood 7-Eleven to support your family," notes Anthony Marx, former president of Amherst College (Leonhardt, 2011, p. B1). Similarly, employees in professional work contexts such as law or banking who enact interdependence (e.g., mentor their colleagues or act as team players) may not have their contributions and skills recognized.

Evaluators' failure to recognize the interdependent competencies common among many working-class individuals may further bias their overall assessment of these individuals' abilities and their future potential. For example, even when working-class students perform as well as their middle-class counterparts on standard performance measures (e.g., exams), they may still be evaluated as less competent overall (e.g., on their final grade in a class; cf. Darley & Gross, 1983). Likewise, working-class employees who enact interdependence may appear less qualified for a promotion or future opportunities compared with equally qualified employees who primarily enact independence (Stephens, Markus, et al., 2014; see also Lamont, Beljean, & Clair, 2014). Consistent with this suggestion, Rudman and Glick (1999) found that hypothetical job applicants who endorsed an interdependent orientation (e.g., helping others as a source of accomplishment) were evaluated more poorly and were seen as less hirable than those who endorsed an independent orientation (e.g., wanting to be in charge and to make decisions).

In summary, cultural mismatch effects are likely to disadvantage working-class individuals in three important domains—access, performance, and evaluation—that fuel and perpetuate a cycle of social class inequality.

IMPLICATIONS FOR INTERVENTIONS AIMED AT REDUCING SOCIAL CLASS INEQUALITY IN GATEWAY INSTITUTIONS

To overcome this cycle of inequality that disadvantages working-class individuals, interventions should focus on reducing the mismatch between the independent model of competence that is normative in gateway institutions and the interdependent model of competence that tends to guide the behavior of working-class individuals. The divergence in cultural norms at individual and institutional levels produces this mismatch; therefore, we propose interventions at each of the following levels: (1) individual-level interventions aimed at developing an independent model of competence, and (2) institutional-level interventions aimed at helping institutions to create a more inclusive culture of competence. These individual and institutional interventions should reduce cultural mismatch, thereby increasing working-class individuals' sense of fit in gateway institutions and also empowering them with the skills that they need to be successful (cf. Stephens, Brannon, Markus, & Nelson, 2015).

While we focus here on the importance of increasing fit and providing individuals with skills to better navigate gateway institutions, these psychological changes will undoubtedly have a variety of other downstream consequences for working-class individuals' opportunity to succeed. For example, just as these interventions will encourage working-class individuals to recognize their own potential contribution, so too will they enable evaluators to recognize competence in working-class individuals.

To the best of our knowledge, there are no interventions that perfectly address the cultural mismatch in models of competence that individuals experience in gateway institutions. However, several existing interventions provide useful frameworks for the development of such interventions. We first describe examples of effective interventions at the individual and institutional levels. We then draw on the insights offered by these interventions in proposing specific intervention strategies that could be harnessed to address the mismatch in models of competence and thereby reduce social class inequality.

Individual-Level Interventions

Because working-class individuals are less familiar with and have less experience enacting an independent model of competence, targeted interventions could help working-class individuals become bicultural—that is, teach them to enact an independent model in situations that demand it (LaFromboise, Coleman, & Gerton, 1993). Such efforts can equip students and employees with the skills they need to be successful in gateway institutions. At the same time, knowing the right skills and how to enact them will foster a greater sense of belonging in gateway institutions. Strategies to develop an independent model might include raising awareness about how social class shapes models of competence, and helping working-class individuals develop an independent model of competence (e.g., by giving them opportunities to practice these behaviors). *Difference-education* is one approach that could be adapted for these purposes (Stephens, Hamedani, & Destin, 2014; Stephens, Townsend, Hamedani, Destin, & Manzo, 2015).

Example: The Difference-Education Approach

In an intervention conducted during the college transition, incoming working-class and middle-class students attended a 1-hour student panel in which junior and senior students discussed the ways in which their social class backgrounds impacted their college experience. Specifically, they described the obstacles they encountered, as well as the strengths and strategies they leveraged to be successful during their time in college (see Stephens, Markus, et al., 2014). Afterward, intervention participants completed a brief video testimonial that gave them the opportunity to process what they had learned at the panel. At the end of their first year, working-class students who attended this panel reported a greater sense of fit with their university. They also enacted more of the independent behaviors (e.g., took charge of their experience by taking advantage of college resources) that were required to reach their academic potential. As a result of these behavioral changes, they earned significantly better grades than working-class students who did not attend the panel, which effectively eliminated the social class achievement gap between students. By highlighting how social class background mattered for the college experience, the intervention increased working-class students' awareness of the university's expectations of them and helped them begin to develop the skills and strategies they needed to be most effective in middle-class university settings.

Raising Awareness

As revealed in the difference-education intervention approach, one viable strategy to develop an independent model of competence among working-class individuals is to focus on raising awareness. To address the mismatch in models of competence, working-class individuals entering gateway institutions could be made aware of how social class influences models of competence; that is, they could benefit from learning that there is more than one effective model of competence, and that different social class contexts afford different models. Because the independent model is often taken for granted, working-class individuals may not

understand what assumptions the model includes. To make these "rules of the game" visible, individuals should talk openly about expectations and requirements for success in schools and workplaces. Efforts to raise awareness of this independent model of competence will help working-class individuals understand that their interdependent model is not a sign of deficiency and is normal for those who come from a working-class background. This understanding should help them experience a greater sense of fit in their schools and workplaces, and also recognize the additional skills that they need to develop to succeed in middle-class settings.

Formal and informal channels could be utilized to increase awareness. For example, college advisors could be trained to better understand the shared needs of working-class students and to provide them with the structured mentoring they need to become more familiar with the "rules of the game." Advisors could also be trained to share insights about behaviors that are expected and associated with achievement and future opportunities. Alternatively, students could become more aware of the rules from their peers. Upon entering college, working-class students could be paired up with liaisons or buddies who have been trained to give students the inside story on what college is about and how to be successful there. These liaisons could have either working-class or middle-class backgrounds. Stanford University's First-Generation Low Income Partnership (FLIP) program, for example, pairs current FLIP members with incoming students. The more advanced students mentor the incoming students, answering questions and providing information. Similarly, in workplaces, onboarding practices could be tailored to help people from working-class backgrounds better understand what is expected of them. For example, at Clear Channel Communications, new hires are paired with a "peer coach," who is available to answer questions before their official start date. These peer coaches could be trained to help new hires from working-class backgrounds understand the environment and culture of the company, and what types of behaviors are rewarded and viewed as competent.

Enacting an Independent Model of Competence

As the difference-education approach illustrates, a viable strategy to promote an independent model of competence is to help working-class individuals enact the strategies they need to be effective in middle-class settings. Just as the difference-education intervention provided students with strategies that helped them succeed at their university, future interventions should go one step further: They could give working-class individuals a chance to practice the skills associated with an independent model of competence. Doing so will not only equip working-class students and employees with these skills but also help them to become more comfortable with the independent model.

Workplaces and schools could offer workshops or training sessions, in which working-class individuals can enact the independent model and obtain feedback on their performance. An example of this can be seen in One Goal, a college preparatory program that employs role-playing exercises that allow students to practice strategies that will help them be more effective in college. Such an experience could teach students how to express an opinion in class, talk to professors about possible research opportunities, and seek help from a teaching assistant. Similarly, training programs in the workplace could offer employees practice enacting independent behaviors and give them feedback on their efforts. For example, in their investigation of assertiveness training, Smith-Jentsch, Salas, and Baker (1996) found that both practice and feedback were critical for enhancing assertive behavior. Thus, rather than simply giving working-class individuals written materials or lectures on desired behaviors, interventions should provide them with the opportunity actually to engage in and receive feedback on the independent behaviors they must enact to be perceived as competent.

Institutional-Level Interventions

Because gateway institutions contribute to the mismatch by promoting the independent model of competence as the norm, interventions targeted at an institutional level could also create a more inclusive culture of competence. Doing so will increase working-class individuals' sense of fit and inclusion in gateway institutions. At the same time, this more inclusive culture may lead middle-class evaluators to recognize the interdependent behaviors enacted by working-class individuals as a form of competence. This recognition of interdependent skills such as working together and adjusting to others, in turn, could benefit institutions by fostering group as well as individual performance (Hambrick, 1995). Organizations can create a more inclusive culture by broadening their understandings of competence to include the interdependent model and incentivizing interdependent behaviors. One institutional-level intervention that could be tailored to accomplish this goal is the *relational design* approach (Grant et al., 2007).

Example: The Relational Design Approach

In this intervention, a university call center sought to improve employee persistence and job performance by changing the cultural norms for how organizations motivate employees. While call centers typically motivate their employees using an individual-focused perspective (e.g., setting individual goals to maximize donations), in this intervention the call center gave employees a relational, prosocial reason for their work. Specifically, they offered employees the opportunity to interact in person with a student beneficiary of their fund-raising calling efforts. Employees were called into a break room for a 10-minute session and asked to read a letter from a student beneficiary about how receiving the scholarship had made a difference in his or her life. Then the student beneficiary was invited into the room to answer callers' questions about the student's background and future plans. Before being excused, supervisors remarked to the callers: "Remember this when you're on the phone—this is someone you're supporting." One month later, callers in the intervention condition spent significantly more time on the phone and raised more money than individuals who did not interact with a beneficiary in person. By focusing on relational motives (e.g., working together) rather than on purely individual goals (e.g., outperforming one another), the intervention conveyed that the interdependent model of competence would be respected and included in the workplace. This approach could be similarly employed in more elite professions such as law, consulting, or investment banking. For example, lawyers or investment bankers could be reminded of the benefits to their clients. And, even if employees are not helping individuals directly, they might be reminded of the ways in which their efforts would benefit their communities or society more broadly, perhaps via incentive structures such as prosocial bonuses, in which organizations award money to others rather than to the employees themselves (Anik, Aknin, Norton, Dunn, & Quoidbach, 2013).

Change Incentive Structure

As revealed in the relational design intervention, one strategy to create a more inclusive organizational culture is to change the incentives that are used to motivate students or employees. Traditional incentive approaches, which provide rewards at an individual level (e.g., a bonus for individual performance), could be altered to encourage and reward interdependent behaviors (e.g., working together, helping others) that are often productive in schools and workplaces.

As shown in the Amazon and Microsoft examples, individual-level incentives tend to promote individual-focused behaviors and encourage people to focus exclusively on their own interests.

However, alternative incentives could communicate the importance of behaviors linked to an interdependent model of competence. For example, in the restaurant industry, there are two prevalent models of tip distribution among waitstaff: (1) the typical individual approach, in which each individual keeps all the tips that she earns each shift, or (2) a team-based approach, in which all tips earned by all staff on a given night are pooled and distributed evenly among all workers. The fact that outcomes are jointly determined in the team-based approach encourages waitstaff to work together and to rely on and support one another in the shared goal of improving customers' experience and satisfaction. Similarly, research

on top management teams (TMTs) showcases how interdependence can benefit both employees and organizations (Hambrick, 1995). One CEO decided to make the incentive compensation of all team members uniform, explaining, "The performance of every one of these executives depends heavily on the others. If I want them to work collaboratively, as a team, it creates severe problems to try to reward them differentially" (p. 123). Three years after this change, the team members exhibited great success in their collaborative efforts and in the marketplace more generally. Incentivizing employees at a team level signals that the interdependent model of competence is valued, and can thereby increase working-class individuals' sense of fit in the workplace.

Changing Evaluation Standards to Include Interdependence

The relational design approach illustrates another strategy to create a more inclusive organizational culture: Change the evaluation process so that the criteria are more inclusive of interdependence. Interviewers in many U.S. organizations, for instance, do not have clear standards for evaluating abstract qualities such as motivation or ability. Instead, they often draw heavily from their own personal experiences to determine who is likely to be the "best" hire (Rivera, 2012). The largely middle-class evaluators in gateway institutions naturally draw from an independent model of what it means to be competent to make these judgments. Thus, including more specific and interdependent indicators of competence can counteract the inclination to rely exclusively on the independent model.

Interviewers could implement this practice when deciding whom to admit or hire, and when evaluating students and employees. Instead of asking vague questions (e.g., "How competent is this individual?"), evaluators could consider specific behaviors that reflect not only independent but also interdependent ways of being competent. For example, in addition to asking, "How effective is this individual at taking charge of projects?" evaluators could ask, "How skilled is this individual at collaborating with others?" or "How effective is this employee at supporting other employees?" Indeed, research suggests that instituting more formal policies (e.g., creating standardized, specific criteria for evaluation) can reduce bias in important decisions in the context of organizations' hiring (Reskin & McBrier, 2000) and compensation (Elvira & Graham, 2002). By evaluating individuals in a way that acknowledges the value of interdependence, this strategy should communicate to students and employees from working-class backgrounds that they are likely to fit and perform well in these gateway settings. Additionally, these changes will likely enable middle-class evaluators to recognize more fully the talents and range of skills of their future students or employees from both working- and middle-class backgrounds.

In summary, interventions that help working-class individuals develop an independent model of competence and create more inclusive cultures should increase their comfort and fit in these institutions, and equip them with the skills necessary to better navigate these settings.

SUMMARY AND CONCLUSION

The American Dream stresses that any individual who wants to work hard in pursuit of a better life can succeed by effectively navigating school and the workplace. Yet, as we have documented throughout this chapter, these gateway institutions have "become a powerful force for reinforcing advantage and passing it on through generations" (Pérez-Peña, 2014, p. A1). These institutions produce intergenerational inequality by relying primarily on an independent model of competence, while excluding the interdependent model of competence more common among the working class. As described earlier, this cultural mismatch in models of competence can disadvantage working-class Americans and perpetuate inequality in three key ways that reinforce one other. First, a mismatch can reduce working-class individuals' motivation to gain access to these settings. Second, among the working-class individuals who defy the odds and gain access to higher education or professional workplaces, a

cultural mismatch can hinder their ability to perform up to their potential in these settings. Third, a cultural mismatch can make it more difficult for evaluators (e.g., admissions officers, human resource professionals) to recognize the interdependent competencies of working-class individuals (e.g., their ability to work together).

Changes in mainstream American society's definitions and evaluations of competence will not happen overnight, but both individuals and institutions can take concrete steps to reduce the cultural mismatch in models of competence that fuels inequality. Future interventions should aim to help working-class individuals understand and enact the independent model of competence that institutions frequently take for granted. At the same time, interventions can expand institutional definitions of competence to include interdependence, thereby creating a more comfortable and welcoming environment in which working-class individuals will be more likely to thrive. By changing the ways in which institutions define and evaluate competence (e.g., by including the interdependent model), perhaps mainstream American society will consider the possibility that there is more than one way to be a competent student or employee, and that both independent and interdependent approaches carry advantages in all contexts. Guided by this insight, perhaps Bronson and her working-class colleagues will no longer experience shame for being seen as incompetent in the eyes of others, and instead begin to feel valued for their contribution—both in working-class settings and beyond.

NOTE

1. To incorporate diverse interdisciplinary literatures that define social class differently, we use the term *working-class* to refer to individuals in contexts on the bottom half of the social class divide, including people who have attained less than a 4-year college degree or who have relatively low incomes or lower-status occupations. *Middle-class* refers to individuals in contexts on the top half of the social class divide, including people who have attained at least a 4-year college degree or who have relatively high incomes or higher-status occupations.

REFERENCES

Acker, J. (2006). Inequality regimes: Gender, class, and race in organizations. *Gender and Society, 20*(4), 441–464.

Adams, G., Anderson, S. L., & Adonu, J. K. (2004). The cultural grounding of closeness and intimacy. In D. J. Mashek & A. Aron (Eds.), *Handbook of closeness and intimacy* (pp. 321–339). Mahwah, NJ: Erlbaum.

Adams, G., Biernat, M., Branscombe, N. R., Crandall, C. S., & Wrightsman, L. S. (Eds.). (2008). *Commemorating Brown: The social psychology of racism and discrimination.* Washington, DC: American Psychological Association.

Anderson, C., Brion, S., Moore, D. A., & Kennedy, J. A. (2012). A status-enhancement account of overconfidence. *Journal of Personality and Social Psychology, 103*(4), 718–735.

Anderson, C., John, O. P., Keltner, D., & Kring, A. M. (2001). Who attains social status?: Effects of personality and physical attractiveness in social groups. *Journal of Personality and Social Psychology, 81*(1), 116–132.

Anderson, C., & Kilduff, G. J. (2009). Why do dominant personalities attain influence in face-to-face groups?: The competence-signaling effects of trait dominance. *Journal of Personality and Social Psychology, 96*(2), 491–503.

Anik, L., Aknin, L. B., Norton, M. I., Dunn, E. W., & Quoidbach, J. (2013). Prosocial bonuses increase employee satisfaction and team performance. *PLoS ONE, 8*(9), e75509.

Argyle, M. (1994). *The psychology of social class.* London: Routledge.

Bacon, N., & Storey, J. (1996). Individualism and collectivism and the changing role of trade unions. In P. Ackers, C. Smith, & P. Smith (Eds.), *The new workplace and trade unionism* (pp. 41–76). London: Routledge.

Bellah, R. N., Madsen, R., Sullivan, W. M., Swidler, A., & Tipton, S. M. (1985). *Habits of the heart: Individualism and commitment in American life.* Berkeley: University of California Press.

Berg, J. M., Wrzesniewski, A., & Dutton, J. E. (2010). Perceiving and responding to challenges in job crafting at different ranks: When proactivity requires adaptivity. *Journal of Organizational Behavior, 31*(2–3), 158–186.

Bourdieu, P. (1984). *Distinction: A social critique of the judgement of taste.* Cambridge, MA: Harvard University Press.

Bowles, S., & Gintis, H. (1976). *Schooling in capitalist America* (Vol. 57). New York: Basic Books.

Bronson, B. (2014, December 19). Your waitress, your professor. Retrieved from *www.nytimes.com/2014/12/19/opinion/your-waitress-your-professor.html.*

Bronson, B. (2015, October 1). Do we value low-skilled work? Retrieved from *www.nytimes.com/2015/10/01/opinion/do-we-value-low-skilled-work.html.*

Capó Crucet, J. (2015, August 23). Taking my parents to college. Retrieved from *www.nytimes.com/2015/08/23/opinion/sunday/taking-my-parents-to-college.html.*

Chen, E., & Matthews, K. A. (2001). Cognitive appraisal biases: An approach to understanding the relation between socioeconomic status and cardiovascular reactivity in children. *Annals of Behavioral Medicine, 23*(2), 101–111.

Cooke, R. A., & Rousseau, D. M. (1988). Behavioral norms and expectations: A quantitative approach to the assessment of organizational culture. *Group and Organization Studies, 13*(3), 245–273.

Cross, S. E., & Madson, L. (1997). Models of the self: Self-construals and gender. *Psychological Bulletin, 122*(1), 5–37.

Darley, J. M., & Gross, P. H. (1983). A hypothesis-confirming bias in labeling effects. *Journal of Personality and Social Psychology, 44*(1), 20–33.

Day, J. C., & Newburger, E. C. (2002). The big payoff: Educational attainment and synthetic estimates of work-life earnings. Retrieved from *www.census.gov/prod/2002pubs/p23-210.pdf.*

Duhigg, C. (2016). *Smarter faster better: The secrets of being productive in life and business.* New York: Random House.

Eichenwald, K. (2012, August). Microsoft's lost decade. Retrieved from *www.vanityfair.com/news/business/2012/08/microsoft-lost-mojo-steve-ballmer.*

Elliot, A. J., & Dweck, C. S. (2005). Competence and motivation: Competence as the core of achievement motivation. In A. J. Elliot & C. S. Dweck (Eds.), *Handbook of competence and motivation* (pp. 3–12). New York: Guilford Press.

Elvira, M. M., & Graham, M. E. (2002). Not just a formality: Pay system formalization and sex-related earnings effects. *Organization Science, 13*(6), 601–617.

Evans, C. R., & Dion, K. L. (1991). Group cohesion and performance: A meta-analysis. *Small Group Research, 22*(2), 175–186.

Fiske, S. T., Cuddy, A. J., Glick, P., & Xu, J. (2002). A model of (often mixed) stereotype content: Competence and warmth respectively follow from perceived status and competition.

Journal of Personality and Social Psychology, 82(6), 878–902.

Fiske, S. T., & Markus, H. R. (2012). A wide angle lens on the psychology of social class. In S. T. Fiske & H. R. Markus (Eds.), *Facing social class: Social psychology of social class* (pp. 1–11). New York: Russell Sage Foundation.

Friedlander, F. (1965). Comparative work value systems. *Personnel Psychology, 18*(1), 1–20.

Fryberg, S. A., & Markus, H. R. (2007). Cultural models of education in American Indian, Asian American and European American contexts. *Social Psychology of Education, 10*(2), 213–246.

Graham, G. (2014, March 3). Working class children must learn to be middle class to get on in life, government advisor says. Retrieved from *www.telegraph.co.uk/education/10671048/working-class-children-must-learn-to-be-middle-class-to-get-on-in-life-government-advisor-says.html.*

Grant, A. M., Campbell, E. M., Chen, G., Cottone, K., Lapedis, D., & Lee, K. (2007). Impact and the art of motivation maintenance: The effects of contact with beneficiaries on persistence behavior. *Organizational Behavior and Human Decision Processes, 103*(1), 53–67.

Gray, B., & Kish-Gephart, J. J. (2013). Encountering social class differences at work: How "class work" perpetuates inequality. *Academy of Management Review, 38*(4), 670–699.

Guzzo, R. A., & Dickson, M. W. (1996). Teams in organizations: Recent research on performance and effectiveness. *Annual Review of Psychology, 47,* 307–338.

Hackman, J. R., & Katz, N. (2010). Group behavior and performance. In S. T. Fiske, D. T. Gilbert, & G. Lindzey (Eds.), *Handbook of social psychology* (pp. 1208–1251). Hoboken, NJ: Wiley.

Hambrick, D. C. (1995). Fragmentation and the other problems CEOs have with their top management teams. *California Management Review, 37*(3), 110–127.

Hilk, C. L. (2013). Effects of cooperative, competitive, and individualistic learning structures on college student achievement and peer relationships: A series of meta-analyses. Unpublished doctoral dissertation. Retrieved from *http://conservancy.umn.edu/handle/11299//155783.*

Hyman, R. (1994). Anomaly or artifact?: Comments on Bem and Honorton. *Psychological Bulletin, 115*(1), 19–24.

Iyengar, S. (2010). *The art of choosing.* New York: Twelve.

Johnson, S. E., Richeson, J. A., & Finkel, E. J. (2011). Middle class and marginal?: Socioeconomic status, stigma, and self-regulation at an elite university. *Journal of Personality and Social Psychology, 100*(5), 838–852.

Kantor, J., & Streitfeld, D. (2015, August 15). Inside Amazon: Wrestling big ideas in a bruising workplace. Retrieved from *www.nytimes.com/2015/08/16/technology/inside-amazon-wrestling-big-ideas-in-a-bruising-workplace.html?_r=0.*

Kennedy, J. A., Anderson, C., & Moore, D. A. (2013). When overconfidence is revealed to others: Testing the status-enhancement theory of overconfidence. *Organizational Behavior and Human Decision Processes, 122*(2), 266–279.

Kim, H. S. (2002). We talk, therefore we think?: A cultural analysis of the effect of talking on thinking. *Journal of Personality and Social Psychology, 83*(4), 828–842.

Kish-Gephart, J. J., & Campbell, J. T. (2014). You don't forget your roots: The influence of CEO social class background on strategic risk taking. *Academy of Management Journal, 58*(6), 1614–1636.

Kohn, M. L. (1969). *Class and conformity: A study in values.* Homewood, IL: Dorsey Press.

Kusserow, A. S. (1999). De-homogenizing American individualism: Socializing hard and soft individualism in Manhattan and Queens. *Ethos, 27*(2), 210–234.

Lachman, M. E., & Weaver, S. L. (1998). The sense of control as a moderator of social class differences in health and well-being. *Journal of Personality and Social Psychology, 74*(3), 763–773.

LaFromboise, T., Coleman, H. L. K., & Gerton, J. (1993). Psychological impact of biculturalism: Evidence and theory. *Psychological Bulletin, 114*(3), 395–412.

Lamont, M. (2000). *The dignity of working men: Morality and the boundaries of race, class, and immigration.* New York: Russell Sage Foundation.

Lamont, M., Beljean, S., & Clair, M. (2014). What is missing?: Cultural processes and causal pathways to inequality. *Socio-Economic Review, 12*(3), 573–608.

Lareau, A. (2003). *Unequal childhoods: Class, race and family life.* Berkeley: University of California Press.

Leonhardt, D. (2011, May 25). Top colleges, largely for the elite. Retrieved from *www.nytimes.com/2011/05/25/business/economy/25leonhardt.html.*

Lewin, T. (2005, May 19). Up from the holler: Living in two worlds, at home in neither. Retrieved from *www.nytimes.com/2005/05/19/us/class/up-from-the-holler-living-in-two-worlds-at-home-in-neither.html.*

Lubrano, A. (2004). *Limbo: Blue collar roots, white collar dreams*. Hoboken, NJ: Wiley.

Markus, H. R., & Conner, A. (2013). *Clash!: 8 cultural conflicts that make us who we are*. New York: Hudson Street Press.

Markus, H. R., & Kitayama, S. (1991). Culture and the self: Implications for cognition, emotion, and motivation. *Psychological Review, 98*(2), 224–253.

Markus, H. R., & Kitayama, S. (2003). Models of agency: Sociocultural diversity in the construction of action. In V. Murphy-Berman & J. J. Berman (Eds.), *Cross-cultural differences in perspectives on the self* (Vol. 49, pp. 1–57). Lincoln: University of Nebraska Press.

Markus, H. R., & Kitayama, S. (2010). Cultures and selves: A cycle of mutual constitution. *Perspectives on Psychological Science, 5*(4), 420–430.

Markus, H. R., Ryff, C. D., Curhan, K. B., & Palmersheim, K. A. (2004). In their own words: Well-being at midlife among high school-educated and college-educated adults. In O. G. Brim, C. D. Ryff, & R. C. Kessler (Eds.), *How healthy are we?: A national study of well-being at midlife* (pp. 273–319). Chicago: University of Chicago Press.

Miller, P. J., Cho, G. E., & Bracey, J. R. (2005). Working-class children's experience through the prism of personal storytelling. *Human Development, 48*(3), 115–135.

Oakes, J. (1982). Classroom social relationships: Exploring the Bowles and Gintis hypothesis. *Sociology of Education, 55*(4), 197–212.

Ostrove, J. M., & Long, S. M. (2007). Social class and belonging: Implications for college adjustment. *Review of Higher Education, 30*(4), 363–389.

Pattillo-McCoy, M. (1999). *Black picket fences: Privilege and peril among the black middle class*. Chicago: University of Chicago Press.

Pérez-Peña, R. (2014, August 25). Generation later, poor are still rare at elite colleges. Retrieved from *www.nytimes.com/2014/08/26/education/despite-promises-little-progress-in-drawing-poor-to-elite-colleges.html*.

Phillips, L. T., Stephens, N. M., Townsend, S. S. M., & Goudeau, S. (2016). *Access is not enough: Cultural mismatch persists to limit first-generation students' opportunities for achievement throughout college*. Manuscript submitted for publication.

Piff, P. K., Kraus, M. W., Côté, S., Cheng, B. H., & Keltner, D. (2010). Having less, giving more: The influence of social class on prosocial behavior. *Journal of Personality and Social Psychology, 99*(5), 771–784.

Plaut, V. C., & Markus, H. R. (2005). The "inside" story: A cultural–historical analysis of being smart and motivated, American style. In A. J. Elliot & C. S. Dweck (Eds.), *Handbook of competence and motivation* (pp. 457–488). New York: Guilford Press.

Reay, D., Davies, J., David, M., & Ball, S. J. (2001). Choices of degree or degrees of choice?: Class, "race," and the higher education choice process. *Sociology, 35*(4), 855–874.

Reskin, B. F., & McBrier, D. B. (2000). Why not ascription?: Organizations' employment of male and female managers. *American Sociological Review, 65*(2), 210–233.

Ridgeway, C. L. (2014). Why status matters for inequality. *American Sociological Review, 79*(1), 1–16.

Ridgeway, C. L., & Fisk, S. R. (2012). Class rules, status dynamics, and "gateway" interactions. In S. T. Fiske & H. R. Markus (Eds.), *Facing social class: How societal rank influences interaction* (pp. 131–151). New York: Russell Sage Foundation.

Rivera, L. A. (2012). Hiring as cultural matching: The case of elite professional service firms. *American Sociological Review, 77*(6), 999–1022.

Rudman, L. A., & Glick, P. (1999). Feminized management and backlash toward agentic women: The hidden costs to women of a kinder, gentler image of middle managers. *Journal of Personality and Social Psychology, 77*(5), 1004–1010.

Smith-Jentsch, K. A., Salas, E., & Baker, D. P. (1996). Training team performance-related assertiveness. *Personnel Psychology, 49*(4), 909–936.

Snibbe, A. C., & Markus, H. R. (2005). You can't always get what you want: Educational attainment, agency, and choice. *Journal of Personality and Social Psychology, 88*(4), 703–720.

Stephens, N. M., Brannon, T. N., Markus, H. R., & Nelson, J. E. (2015). Feeling at home in college: Fortifying school-relevant selves to reduce social class disparities in higher education. *Social Issues and Policy Review, 9*(1), 1–24.

Stephens, N. M., Fryberg, S. A., & Markus, H. R. (2011). When choice does not equal freedom: A sociocultural analysis of agency in working-class American contexts. *Social Psychological and Personality Science, 2*(1), 33–41.

Stephens, N. M., Fryberg, S. A., Markus, H. R., Johnson, C. S., & Covarrubias, R. (2012). Unseen disadvantage: How American universities' focus on independence undermines the academic performance of first-generation college students. *Journal of Personality and Social Psychology, 102*(6), 1178–1197.

Stephens, N. M., Hamedani, M. G., & Destin, M. (2014). Closing the social-class achievement gap: A difference-education intervention improves first-generation students' academic performance and all students' college transition. *Psychological Science, 25*(4), 943–953.

Stephens, N. M., Hamedani, M. G., Markus, H. R., Bergsieker, H. B., & Eloul, L. (2009). Why did they "choose" to stay?: Perspectives of Hurricane Katrina observers and survivors. *Psychological Science, 20*(7), 878–886.

Stephens, N. M., Markus, H. R., & Fryberg, S. A. (2012). Social class disparities in health and education: Reducing inequality by applying a sociocultural self model of behavior. *Psychological Review, 119*(4), 723–744.

Stephens, N. M., Markus, H. R., & Phillips, L. T. (2014). Social class culture cycles: How three gateway contexts shape selves and fuel inequality. *Annual Review of Psychology, 65,* 611–634.

Stephens, N. M., Townsend, S. S. M., Hamedani, M. G., Destin, M., & Manzo, V. (2015). A difference-education intervention equips first-generation college students to thrive in the face of stressful college situations. *Psychological Science, 26*(10), 1556–1566.

Stephens, N. M., Townsend, S. S. M., Markus, H. R., & Phillips, T. (2012). A cultural mismatch: Independent cultural norms produce greater increases in cortisol and more negative emotions among first-generation college students. *Journal of Experimental Social Psychology, 48*(6), 1389–1393.

Sutton, R. I., & Hargadon, A. (1996). Brainstorming groups in context: Effectiveness in a product design firm. *Administrative Science Quarterly, 41*(4), 685–718.

Terenzini, P. T., & Pascarella, E. T. (1991). Twenty years of research on college students: Lessons for future research. *Research in Higher Education, 32*(1), 83–92.

Urtasun, A., & Núñez, I. (2012). Work-based competences and careers prospects: A study of Spanish employees. *Personnel Review, 41*(4), 428–449.

Van Kleef, G. A., Homan, A. C., Finkenauer, C., Gündemir, S., & Stamkou, E. (2011). Breaking the rules to rise to power: How norm violators gain power in the eyes of others. *Social Psychological and Personality Science, 2*(5), 500–507.

Williams, J. C. (2012). The class culture gap. In S. T. Fiske & H. R. Markus (Eds.), *Facing social class: How societal rank influences interaction* (pp. 39–57). New York: Russell Sage Foundation.

Wojcicki, S. (2011, July). The eight pillars of innovation. Retrieved from *www.thinkwith-google.com/articles/8-pillars-of-innovation.html*.

Woolley, A. W., Chabris, C. F., Pentland, A., Hashmi, N., & Malone, T. W. (2010). Evidence for a collective intelligence factor in the performance of human groups. *Science, 330,* 686–688.

Wrzesniewski, A., & Dutton, J. E. (2001). Crafting a job: Revisioning employees as active crafters of their work. *Academy of Management Review, 26*(2), 179–201.

CHAPTER 28

Race and Ethnicity in the Study of Competence Motivation

BETH E. KURTZ-COSTES
TANIESHA A. WOODS

As Americans continue to strive for racial and ethnic equity in the 21st century, the fostering of competence motivation in youth of all backgrounds continues to be an important goal for educators. In addition to long-standing historical circumstances that place members of racial/ethnic-minority groups in positions of disadvantage, immigration continues to change the racial/ethnic landscape of the United States. Thus, the roles of race, ethnicity, and culture are a critical component of understanding competence motivation in U.S. youth.

In this chapter, we consider five ways in which race and ethnicity shape children's educational experiences in this country, and thus, their competence motivation. Within each of these sections, we provide examples of educational policy and programs addressing challenges and building on opportunities. First, we briefly consider traditional approaches to the study of motivation and their implications for students of color. In the next section we explore the barriers and benefits that accompany immigration, including linguistic, cultural, and legal barriers, as well as the enhanced motivation that characterizes many immigrants. Third, we discuss structural racism and associated racial and ethnic differences in access to resources. The impact of racial and ethnic stereotypes and individual discrimination on the competence motivation of youth are topics of the fourth section. We focus in the fifth section on role models and mentors, then conclude with recommendations for researchers, educators, and policymakers.

TRADITIONAL MOTIVATION THEORIES AND RACIAL/ETHNIC-MINORITY YOUTH

As aptly elucidated in other chapters in this volume, prominent theories of motivation emphasize competence and self-efficacy (i.e., the belief that effortful behavior in a domain will lead to success), values (e.g., interest, utility), causal attributions, and related-ness/belonging as important factors that predict sustained effort (Conroy, Chapter 3; Elliot & Hulleman, Chapter 4; Marsh et al., Chapter 6; Perry & Hamm, Chapter 5; and Wigfield, Rosenzweig, & Eccles, Chapter 7, all this volume). For example, according to self-determination theory, the needs for competence, autonomy (i.e., perceiving that one is choosing to seek a goal rather than it being imposed), and relatedness (i.e., connection to others with similar goals, or personal connection to a goal) drive goal-directed behavior (Deci & Ryan, 1985; Ryan & Moller, Chapter 12, this volume). Expectancy–value theory posits the importance of self-efficacy and values (attainment value, interest, utility, and cost) in shaping achievement striving of youth (Wigfield et al., Chapter 7, this volume).

Although many aspects of theories of competence motivation have not been tested robustly within racial/ethnic-minority groups, when such research has been conducted, results show greater similarity than differences in motivational processes across groups. For example, self-efficacy and perceptions of competence predict academic motivation and success in white,[1] black, American Indian, and Hispanic students (Awad, 2007; Cham, Hughes, West, & Im, 2014; Gloria & Robinson Kurpius, 2001; Kurtz-Costes & Schneider, 1994). Few group differences were found in the causal attributions of white, black, Hispanic, and American Indian community college students (Powers & Rossman, 1984), and the beliefs of white, black, Hispanic, and Asian youth about the causes of their academic successes and failures predict subsequent motivation in theoretically predicted ways (Bempechat, Nakkula, Wu, & Ginsburg, 1996; Swinton, Kurtz-Costes, Rowley, & Adeyanju, 2011). Similarly, interest, educational utility beliefs, and other aspects of values predict subsequent motivation and success in black, Hispanic, and white youth (Cham et al., 2014; Wood, Kurtz-Costes, & Copping, 2011). Black and white youth have similar affect toward school and are equally likely to have peers who value academic success (Harris, 2006).

In spite of these similarities across racial/ethnic groups, these processes that would lead to healthy competence motivation are disrupted for many racial/ethnic-minority youth because of the challenges associated with immigration; structural racism that places youth in inadequate school environments; racial and ethnic stereotypes that negatively bias the expectations held by teachers, parents, and the youth themselves; personal experiences of discrimination by youth that undermine their perceptions of autonomy and fairness; and—because of

the history of racial/ethnic inequities in this country—a lack of mentors and role models. In the subsequent sections of this chapter we consider each of these topics.

THE IMMIGRANT EXPERIENCE

Approximately 80 million individuals living in the United States—one-fourth of the total population—are either immigrants or children of immigrants (Zong & Batalova, 2015). Immigrants in the United States are highly diverse; some move quickly into the middle class and professional success, but others live in poverty and rely on menial, low-wage jobs. As Portes and MacLeod (1996) have shown, the educational progress of second-generation immigrants is heavily linked to family socioeconomic status and to country of origin.

Most immigrants leave their countries of origin because they believe that moving to a different country will improve their quality of life. Some immigrants are fleeing war or other forms of violence; others are simply seeking better opportunities for themselves and their families. Thus, immigrants frequently arrive in their host country with heightened achievement motivation for themselves and family members (Perez, Espinoza, Ramos, Coronado, & Cortes, 2009). Because the sacrifice of leaving their homeland is justified by expectations for future well-being, they therefore have heightened motivation compared to nonimmigrants (Portes, 1999).

The high achievement motivation of many immigrants is countered by several barriers, one of which is language proficiency. According to 2007 Census data, 68.9% of Hispanics and 64.3% of Asians speak a language other than English at home (Aud, Fox, & KewalRamani, 2010). More than one-fourth of American Indian fourth and eighth graders use a non-English language at least half the time when communicating with family members (DeVoe & Darling-Churchill, 2008).

Lack of English proficiency in students and their parents creates a number of obstacles for these children's achievement striving and academic success (Kurtz-Costes & Pungello, 2000). Children who are not proficient English readers by third grade are at risk of failing to keep up with peers across academic content areas. Lack of English proficiency can lead to decreased motivation in immigrant youth because of their difficulty in understanding academic content, or because of negative attitudes and low expectations of teachers and peers. In an ethnographic study of Latina/o immigrant fifth graders, Monzó and Rueda (2009) found that youth who were not English proficient pretended to understand class material in order to avoid the stigma associated with not understanding. Their attempts to "pass" as English proficient put them at greater risk of academic failure because their teachers were unaware that they frequently failed to understand class materials or instructions.

In addition to struggling to keep up with English-proficient peers in their school assignments, English language learners often do not have the family and home supports that foster competence motivation. For example, in homes where parents are not fluent in English, it is less likely that children will be exposed to English-language books and other print materials. Parents who are not fluent in English are less likely to volunteer at school, to be in contact with their children's teachers, and to be advocates for their children in the educational setting (Kurtz-Costes, Swinton, & Skinner, 2014). Not only do these youth lack the advantages taken for granted by language-proficient peers, but many of these youth also have additional responsibilities such as translating for parents or assuming "adult" roles within the family because of their language proficiency (Roche, Lambert, Ghazarian, & Little, 2015).

The language barriers faced by immigrant youth are often interwoven with cultural barriers (Kurtz-Costes & Pungello, 2000). For example, extracurricular activities are an integral aspect of schooling in the United States, with numerous opportunities for children and adolescents in the arts, athletics, school government, and various clubs (Holloway, 2002). Youth involvement in such activities serves the important functions not only of increasing skills and knowledge within those domains, but also of providing the opportunity for social connections with peers that are likely to lead to a greater sense

of belonging (Eccles, Barber, Stone, & Hunt, 2003; Holloway, 2002). Immigrant youth who come from cultures where such activities are not the norm—and whose parents therefore do not value such activities—miss many opportunities to become connected to peers and to see teachers in a more relaxed setting.

For many immigrant youth, language and cultural barriers are further exacerbated by their legal status as undocumented residents. According to the Pew Hispanic Center (Passel & Cohn, 2010), in 2009, more than 1 million children in the United States were undocumented, and about 4 million had undocumented parents. Besides facing the ubiquitous fear associated with possible detection, separation of family members, and other consequences, undocumented youth must deal with numerous challenges that impede their healthy development and educational progress, particularly as they reach adolescence. Undocumented adolescents cannot go on school trips for which identification is required, cannot legally take part-time employment, cannot obtain drivers licenses, and are usually ineligible for public financial aid for higher education (Abrego, 2006; Gonzáles, 2011). Even if these students have excellent grades and are admitted to colleges and universities, many undocumented youth will not be able to accept admission because of their ineligible status for many types of financial aid. Thus, legal status can have a particularly powerful influence on competence motivation when undocumented youth reach adolescence and face enormous barriers to the upward mobility afforded by higher education (Abrego, 2006). In the following section, we discuss public policy and educational practice aimed at promoting academic achievement and educational attainment among immigrant youth to help them overcome some of these barriers.

IMMIGRANT YOUTH: SCHOOL-BASED INTERVENTIONS AND FEDERAL AND STATE POLICIES

As we mentioned earlier, one disadvantage that many immigrant youth face is lack of English proficiency. An area that has been particularly potent in shaping the teaching and learning practices of English language learning (ELL) students are state-level policies aimed at the K–12 system. Arizona, California, and Massachusetts have passed initiatives requiring that most ELL students be taught in English-only settings (e.g., students with special needs other than a lack of English proficiency may be excluded). Arizona, in particular, requires that subject matter be taught in English, and children learn to read and write in English only (Mackinney & Rios-Aguilar, 2012). These state-level policies are contrary to research showing that bilingual instruction for ELL students in their first language as well as English is a strength-based approach that builds on what students already know and is more likely to improve both their achievement and their social and emotional outcomes (García, 2011; Gil & Bardack, 2010; Hughes, Im, Kwok, Cham, & West, 2015).

González (2011) and others suggest that ELL instruction should build on students' "funds of knowledge" or their everyday experiences, which are connected to their cultural and community identities (González, Moll, & Amanti, 2013; Mackinney & Rios-Aguilar, 2012). Linking ELL students' educational experiences to their cultural and community identities may be especially important for promoting achievement competence because this connection legitimizes their informal or nonacademic knowledge and helps them to identify and engage in family and local resources that foster their academic success (García, 2011; Kurtz-Costes & Pungello, 2000).

Teachers of ELL students are most successful when they receive ongoing professional development that enhances their knowledge of culturally relevant content/curricula, culturally responsive instructional practices, and low-stakes assessment in the service of understanding what students know (Gil & Bardack, 2010; Hogg, 2011). Additionally, preservice teachers need hands-on experience working with children from diverse backgrounds. It is especially important that future teachers of ELL students have opportunities to apply their pedagogical knowledge to the dynamic educational settings they will enter prior to becoming the teacher of record (Téllez & Waxman, 2006).

We now turn to a discussion of federal policies and how they shape the formal education of immigrant youth. The Deferred Action for Childhood Arrivals (DACA) executive order allows undocumented individuals who meet certain criteria (e.g., arrive in the United States before age 16, are under age 31 as of June 15, 2012, pass a background check) to obtain work permits and be exempt from deportation for a 2-year period. Individuals may apply for renewed DACA status if they continue to meet the qualifications. Because DACA recipients can obtain work authorization but are not eligible for federal financial aid and usually do not qualify for in-state tuition rates, DACA probably encourages many young immigrant adults to work rather than pursue higher education. The U.S. Department of Education provides a Resource Guide, "Supporting Undocumented Youth," for educators, counselors, and school leaders so that they are better equipped to support undocumented youth in identifying resources to achieve educational success—a link for this document is included in the reference section of this chapter (U.S. Department of Education, 2015).

Access to and attainment of postsecondary education improves immigrant students' chances of upward economic mobility and enables them to contribute more fully to the economy. Moreover, proposed public policies often require that undocumented students use postsecondary educational attainment as a means to work toward citizenship. For example, the Development, Relief, and Education for Alien Minors (DREAM) Act of 2013, which was introduced in Congress beginning in 2001 but has not passed, creates a pathway for undocumented students to become permanent residents with postsecondary education or military service as part of the requirements (S. 744, Section 2103; U.S. Senate, 2013). Recently introduced legislation, Investing in States to Achieve Tuition Equality for Dreamers (IN-STATE) Act of 2015 (U.S. Senate, 2015), has requirements that are similar to those of the DREAM Act, but instead of a pathway to citizenship, this legislation focuses on undocumented students' eligibility for in-state tuition and financial aid, along with repealing Section 505 of the Illegal Immigration Reform and Immigrant Responsibility (IIRIR) Act of 1996 (U.S. Congress, 1996). As of the writing of this chapter, the IN-STATE Act of 2015 has not been passed in the Senate.

Although federal policies have not been enacted to address postsecondary educational access for undocumented students, some state policies have been developed. As a result of IIRIR Act section 505, states that have enacted laws granting in-state tuition to students regardless of their immigration status typically have done so on the basis of students' attendance at and graduation from a high school in the state rather than legal residency (T. Broder, National Immigration Law Center, personal communication, October 2015). Currently, about 20 states have policies aimed at increasing access to financial aid or scholarships and providing in-state tuition regardless of students' immigration status, if those students completed high school within the state (National Immigration Law Center, 2015).

English language proficiency and immigration status are often correlated with a family's economic stability, which in turn is often related to access to resources, including high-quality schools. In the next section we discuss structural racism and the role of resources in shaping the competence motivation and achievement of students of color.

STRUCTURAL RACISM AND DIFFERENCES IN RESOURCES

In a society in which school funding is often linked to local property taxes, and racial/ethnic differences in household wealth are notable across different school districts, it is not surprising that white students are more likely than students from other racial-ethnic groups to be enrolled in high-quality schools (Kurtz-Costes et al., 2014). At one extreme of the scale are urban public schools serving low-income households in which a majority of students are black or Hispanic, and in which failure rates are high (Payne, 2008). In addition to eroding tax bases, urban schools frequently face challenges infrequently encountered in suburban and rural

areas, such as more mobile populations, high percentages of ELLs, high crime rates, and deteriorating physical structures (Jacob, 2007). Many urban families have experienced the closure of neighborhood schools associated with gentrification of their neighborhoods and the growth of charter schools (Lipman, 2013).

Even when not including the nations' largest, poorest school districts in comparisons, the large stratification in household wealth leads to substantial differences in school quality on various indicators. One such index is teacher training. In high schools with an enrollment of at least 50% black students, 25% of teachers have a primary teaching assignment in a subject in which they have neither a college major nor standard certification. In contrast, in high schools in which 50% or more of the student body is white, 8% of teachers are teaching subjects in which they do not have that academic preparation (Aud et al., 2010).

Compared to schools that serve wealthier families, schools in low-income districts have fewer resources such as computers, science laboratory equipment, art supplies, and books (Eccles & Roeser, 2011). Lower SES high schools offer fewer Advanced Placement courses, SAT preparatory courses, and other opportunities for students to become more competitive for college admission and success (Orfield & Lee, 2006). In 2013 National Center for Education Statistics (NCES) data, only 8% of white students, in contrast to 36% of American Indian students, 45% of black students, and 45% of Hispanic students attended schools in which at least 75% of youth were eligible for free or reduced lunch (Kena et al., 2015). These differences in school poverty rates lead to noted racial/ethnic differences in markers of academic success. Moreover, because tracking occurs along racial/ethnic lines, even within schools, Asians and whites are more likely than blacks and Hispanics to have challenging curricula and opportunities that promote postsecondary educational success (Rowley, Kurtz-Costes, & Cooper, 2010).

The substantial racial/ethnic differences in household wealth that are linked to school quality also shape children's opportunities and therefore their achievement motivation outside of the classroom. Using data from two nationally representative samples, Bouffard and colleagues (2006) reported that youth from economically disadvantaged backgrounds are involved in fewer extracurricular activities than more affluent peers. Schools with fewer resources are not able to provide as many enrichment opportunities for youth as schools with more resources (Stearns & Glennie, 2010). Moreover, because of economic hardship and/or everyday stressors, low-income families are less able than higher-income families to provide the supports necessary (e.g., transportation, fees) for program participation when such programs are available.

Involvement of youth in extracurricular activities, particularly during the adolescent years, is positively related to many indices of competence motivation and academic achievement (Farb & Matjasko, 2012; Stearns & Glennie, 2010). Although there is some evidence that Hispanic youth participate in extracurricular activities at lower rates than other groups, the benefits of extracurricular activities are found for black and Hispanic samples (Darling, 2005; Fredricks & Eccles, 2008). Involvement in activities such as school-based athletics, school clubs, and fine arts increases feelings of competence and school belonging, which in turn increase a youth's competence motivation (Fredricks & Eccles, 2008).

Another example of how differential access to resources leads to racial/ethnic differences in academic outcomes is in the area of college preparation. Students' completion of honors and Advanced Placement (AP) courses in high school is increasingly predictive of college matriculation and success (Long, Iatarola, & Conger, 2009). Yet racial/ethnic differences persist in advanced course-taking patterns in high school. For example, according to 2004 NCES data, 69% of Asians and 54% of whites took advanced mathematics courses in high school, in comparison to just 22% of American Indians (DeVoe & Darling-Churchill, 2008). Differences in course-taking patterns are partly related to availability, with better-funded schools offering more honors and AP courses. Group differences in course-taking patterns within schools are further accentuated by teachers' perceptions and students'

choices, as discussed below in the section on stereotypes and discrimination.

The substantial range in academic preparation at the primary and secondary levels leads to noted racial/ethnic differences in college participation rates. In 2008, 58% of Asians and 44% of whites between ages 18 and 24 were enrolled in a college or university, in comparison to 32% of blacks, 26% of Hispanics, and just 22% of American Indians (Aud et al., 2010). Racial/ethnic group enrollment in higher education also differs substantially across types of schools, with higher percentages of whites and Asians attending private, elite schools, and higher percentages of blacks, Hispanics, and American Indians enrolling in 2-year community colleges and public, 4-year universities (NCES, 2015a). Blacks, Hispanics, and American Indians are also more likely than whites to attend school part-time, which is linked to racial/ethnic differences in graduation rates (NCES, 2015a). To reduce such disparities, particularly those that are driven by family income, some colleges and universities have instituted "need blind" admission procedures and provide full need-based financial support for admitted students through grants, scholarships, work study, and loans (Alon, 2011). In the next section we discuss federal policies and other interventions aimed at decreasing racial/ethnic inequities associated with poverty and school quality.

FEDERAL POLICIES AND STRUCTURAL INTERVENTIONS TO INCREASE ACCESS TO RESOURCES

The Elementary and Secondary Education Act, originally passed by the Johnson administration in 1965 and reauthorized many times since, provides Title I funding to state and local educational agencies to enhance learning opportunities in public and private schools with high percentages of low-income children. Title I funds, which are allocated through statutory formulas based on census poverty estimates and the cost of education in the state, support academic programming (e.g., extra instruction in reading and math, summer school, afterschool programs) aimed at improving learning outcomes (U.S.

Department of Education, Office of State Support, 2015).[2] Depending on the percentage of low-income children in the school, Title I programming targets low-achieving students or is used to support schoolwide programming. A primary goal of Title I funding is to help students, at a minimum, meet state standards in their core academic subjects (NCES, 2015b).

Teachers are an essential resource significantly influencing student achievement; however, urban schools serving high percentages of low-income children often have difficulty recruiting and retaining experienced teachers (Jacob, 2007). One way schools serving high percentages of low-income children have tried to address this issue is through placement of alternative certification teachers. For example, Teach for America (TFA), an alternative certification program, includes a competitive application process to recruit college graduates, provides summer training prior to corps members' entry into the classroom, then places corps members in schools that typically serve low-income students. In a study of North Carolina teachers, Henry and colleagues (2014) found that TFA members were more effective than in-state, public university, undergraduate-prepared teachers with a BA degree in teaching elementary school math; middle school math and science; and high school math, English I, science, and social studies. However, alternative certification teachers from other programs were *less* effective in high school math, science, and social studies than traditionally prepared teachers, even though many alternative certification programs focus on preparing secondary teachers in the areas of math and science (Henry et al., 2014).

A criticism of alternative certification programs is that teaching is a profession that requires training in the science of learning, in addition to content knowledge about a particular subject, and alternative certification programs do not fully take pedagogical training into account. The results of Henry and colleagues (2014) show the diversity of efficaciousness of alternative certification programs, which might be due to selection effects (i.e., TFA is highly selective and may have better-qualified applicants than other programs). Alternative certification

programs can benefit from the science of learning literature and use it to inform their teacher training curricula and practicum experiences. In order to structure teacher preparation programs so educators are best equipped to teach all students, and especially those from low-income backgrounds, insight can be gleaned from the early childhood mathematics education literature. This literature shows that high-quality instruction requires teacher training that includes a focus on child development, the content teachers will teach, effective pedagogy for the content, appropriate assessment techniques, and practicum experiences under the guidance of a master teacher (Ginsburg, Woods, & Hyson, 2014).

Another educational intervention in recent years is "school choice," or the availability of charter schools. Charter schools are promoted by education reformers as a way to meet students' academic needs if their district-assigned public school has low achievement scores. Charter schools receive public funding but operate separately from local public school system policies. Many charter schools require that student applicants enter a lottery, with students randomly selected for admission to the school.

In a quasi-experimental study comparing two methods to assess charter school effectiveness, Davis and Raymond (2012) evaluated the performance of students attending charter schools in 15 states and two urban school districts. A virtual-control record design enabled the researchers to match charter school students and public school students on factors such as demographic attributes, grade in school, eligibility for special programs, and prior achievement test scores. Results showed that charter schools were more effective than public schools in only 19% of comparisons, and the results varied according to student demographics, with ELLs, low-income students, and special education students more likely than others to show benefits from charter school enrollment.

Chingos and West (2015) compared achievement gains of charter school students to those of public school students in the state of Arizona, which tops the nation in the percentage of youth enrolled in charter schools. They found wide variability in results, with averages indicating that at each grade level, public schools were slightly more successful than charter schools in improving student achievement. However, during the period of the study, low-performing charter schools were more likely to close than low-performing public schools, leading Chingos and West to conclude that charter schools might be more responsive or accountable than public schools for student outcomes.

Mathematica researchers evaluated the effectiveness of middle school charter schools, drawing data from 36 schools across 15 states (Gleason, Clark Tuttle, & Dwoyer, 2010). Academic gains of students who were admitted to charter middle schools through a lottery procedure were compared to students who applied for the lottery and were not admitted. Results showed no differences between charter schools and traditional public schools in increasing student achievement or improving student behavior. However, results were highly variable across schools and varied according to student demographics. Charter middle schools that primarily enrolled youth from low-income backgrounds or who were low achieving showed positive math gains, compared to the gains of peers in public middle schools. In contrast, charter middle schools that primarily served students with higher income and higher prior achievement compared negatively to public middle school students (Gleason et al., 2010). Taken together, the results of these studies provide only weak evidence of benefits of charter schools, but indicate that where there are benefits, they are experienced by youth who are in greatest need.

Racial and ethnic disparities in wealth and its perquisites constitute one constellation of factors leading to racial/ethnic achievement gaps. Another significant family of causes is based in cultural stereotypes. We turn next to that topic.

RACIAL/ETHNIC STEREOTYPES AND INDIVIDUAL DISCRIMINATION

Racial/ethnic stereotypes and discrimination promote racial and ethnic differences in competence motivation through several mechanisms. We discuss three of those mechanisms: stereotype threat; students' stereotype endorsement; and differential treatment from teachers, peers, and parents.

Claude Steele's (1997) classic research on stereotype threat has spawned a wealth of studies that demonstrate the deleterious effects of stereotype activation on students' performance. As that research shows, when an individual is aware of a negative stereotype about a social group to which he or she belongs and the stereotype is activated (e.g., by asking the student to indicate his or her race or gender before beginning a skills assessment), performance is negatively affected. Performance is believed to suffer because of three mechanisms: a physiological stress response that impairs cognitive functioning, resources devoted to monitoring performance, and efforts to suppress negative thoughts (Schmader, Johns, & Forbes, 2008).

Steele (1997) argued that if stereotype threat experiences are chronic, they can also influence motivation. An individual who is repeatedly placed in achievement situations in which the negative stereotype is salient may experience disidentification: Self-identity and personal values are altered so that success in the domain is no longer important to the individual (Guyll, Madon, Prieto, & Scherr, 2010; Steele, 1997). Thus, regardless of whether youth endorse negative academic stereotypes about their racial or ethnic group, such stereotypes can lead to decreased competence motivation. Because of the nature of this hypothesized phenomenon (i.e., repeated experiences over long periods of time), few research studies have addressed the disidentification hypothesis. An exception is a recent study using a nationally representative sample of high-achieving science students who, at the time of recruitment, were all expecting to pursue doctoral studies in a science field (Woodcock, Hernandez, Estrada, & Schultz, 2013). Across a 3-year period, Hispanic college students who reported frequent stereotype threat experiences were more likely than peers to show declines in their intention to pursue a science career. Although African Americans in the sample reported higher levels of stereotype threat encounters than did Hispanics, threat experiences did not predict subsequent declines in their motivation.

Woodcock and colleagues (2013) suggested that these racial/ethnic differences might have emerged because of the tendency of many capable African American students to discount negative performance feedback, or because attendance at majority-black institutions buffered black students from potential negative effects of chronic stereotype threat.

Stereotype threat research has shown robustly that racial/ethnic stereotypes can lead to performance decrements. Another mechanism by which stereotypes can hamper motivation is by directly influencing students' beliefs about their self-efficacy within a domain. When youth endorse stereotypes about a social group to which they belong—in this case, their racial/ethnic group—those beliefs may be internalized to shape beliefs about the self. With school achievement controlled, African American middle school youth who endorsed stereotypes about race differences in achievement and who were high in "racial centrality" (i.e., race was important to their individual identity) had lower perceptions of their own academic abilities than youth who did not endorse race stereotypes (Okeke, Howard, Kurtz-Costes, & Rowley, 2009).

Academic stereotypes linked to race and ethnicity may be more important for personal identity beliefs of boys than of girls. Hudley and Graham (2001) asked African American, Hispanic, and white youth to read hypothetical scenarios depicting youth who were high or low in school engagement, and to select a photo matching each hypothetical description. Students were more likely to choose photos of black and Hispanic boys for scenarios of academic disengagement, whereas girls of all racial/ethnic groups were selected for academic engagement scenarios (Hudley & Graham, 2001). In an investigation of links between endorsement of gender and racial academic stereotypes and academic self-concept, endorsement of gender stereotypes was related to black girls' perceptions of their own verbal abilities, whereas endorsement of both gender and race stereotypes predicted black boys' perceptions of their own verbal and math abilities (Evans, Copping, Rowley, & Kurtz-Costes, 2011). Endorsement of stereotypes by youth might influence their self-efficacy/

competence beliefs and interests by pulling them toward some domains (e.g., sports for black boys) and away from other domains (Evans et al., 2011).

A third mechanism by which stereotypes lead to differences in competence motivation is through their links to differential expectations and treatment from teachers, parents, and peers. In a meta-analysis, Tenenbaum and Ruck (2007) showed that, on average, teachers held higher expectations for Asian and white students than for Hispanic and black students. Consistent with these racial/ethnic differences in expectations, teachers engaged in more positive and neutral speech with white students than with Hispanic or black students (Tenenbaum & Ruck, 2007). It is likely that such differential treatment might influence students' motivation. Indeed, there is evidence that by adolescence, students perceive differential treatment from teachers based on race, and that such awareness has negative influences on motivation (Cogburn, Chavous, & Griffin, 2011; Wong, Eccles, & Sameroff, 2003). In longitudinal data from the Maryland Adolescent Development in Context Study (MADICS), African American youth's reports of racial discrimination from teachers and peers in seventh grade were related to drops over the next school year in grades, academic values, and perceptions of academic competence (Wong et al., 2003). MADICS data from later waves also showed that youth reports of discrimination in grades 8 and 9 predicted lower school importance ratings in grade 11 (Chavous, Rivas-Drake, Smalls, Griffin, & Cogburn, 2008).

These detrimental effects of racial discrimination were found in early and late adolescence. In addition, children who are not yet aware of discrimination may nonetheless have lowered competence motivation because of low expectations of teachers and peers. Although the degree to which biased teacher expectations influence student outcomes has been controversial (Jussim & Harber, 2005), there is evidence that teacher expectation effects are stronger among ethnic/racial-minority youth than among whites (Guyll et al., 2010; Riley & Ungerleider, 2012).

One example of ways that biased teacher perceptions are likely to operate is through disciplinary practices. School disciplinary actions, such as being sent to the principal's office, or being suspended or expelled from school, have a disproportionate impact on students of color and have been particularly harmful for black boys and girls (Smith & Harper, 2015). In a review of discipline records from over 350 elementary and middle schools, Skiba and colleagues (2011) found that black elementary school students were more than twice as likely as white peers to be sent to the principal's office for a disciplinary infraction, and the ratio rose to 3.78 in middle school. These numbers are similar to those collected nationally by the U.S. Department of Education: In NCES data from 2007, almost one-half of black boys (49.5%) and one-third of black girls (34.7%) had been suspended from school at least once. A full 16.1% of black boys had been expelled, in contrast to only 1.3% of their white male peers. Skiba and colleagues found that Hispanic and black students are more likely than whites to be expelled or suspended from school when performing similar misbehaviors.

These racial/ethnic differences in disciplinary sanctions promote differences in academic competence and motivation: Students who are suspended or expelled from school are more likely to be held back a grade and to drop out than students who are not suspended or expelled. Moreover, these students are more likely to come into contact with the criminal justice system (Fenning & Rose, 2007; Smith & Harper, 2015). We believe the unequal implementation of school discipline policies is, in part, rooted in racism—both conscious and unconscious, and these discriminatory practices contribute to racial/ethnic differences in competence motivation.

CULTURAL COMPETENCE: BEST PRACTICES AND INTERVENTIONS

Racial/ethnic stereotypes and discrimination pose significant threats to student motivation, learning, and educational attainment. In spite of being well intentioned, many teachers are unprepared to support students of color, who often attend poorly resourced schools, where teachers face numerous challenges, such as needing to meet individual students' learning needs, manage behavior, and still deliver rigorous instruction in spite of a lack of resources. Many teachers may hold unconscious biases about the intentions and abilities of students of color. Other teachers may hold conscious biases but believe the biases are warranted, and therefore perpetuate inequitable educational opportunities (Rowley et al., 2014). In this section, we provide recommendations for reducing discrimination through interventions targeting schools and child welfare systems. By reducing discrimination in these settings, a significant barrier to educational opportunity will be diminished or removed.

The development of cultural competence—the ability to deal effectively with individuals from diverse cultures—is an ongoing process that relies on self-reflection, self-awareness, acceptance of cultural differences, and greater cultural knowledge (Webb & Sergison, 2003). Essential ingredients for successful programs include opportunities for individuals from diverse groups to interact meaningfully with each other over extended periods of time, engagement in collaborative activities that work toward common goals, and learning about the history and practices of other groups (Buhin & Vera, 2009).

An intervention used with those connected to child welfare systems, including school personnel, social service personnel, law enforcement, and community members, is the Undoing Racism workshop by the People's Institute for Survival and Beyond (PISB; *www.pisab.org*). A primary goal of the workshop is to educate workers about race, racism, privilege, and oppression, and how these constructs may operate in decision making across various levels of systems concerned with the welfare of children (Johnson, Antle, & Barbee, 2009). The Undoing Racism workshop lasts 2.5 days, and participants complete pre- and post-training evaluation questionnaires. In Johnson and colleagues' evaluation, about 80% of workshop participants were women, 60% of participants were white, and about 40% identified as black. Almost 85% of participants had a bachelor's degree or higher. Findings revealed significant improvement in participants' racial awareness attitudes and increased awareness of racial privilege and institutional discrimination (Johnson et al., 2009). Educating teachers, school leadership, and other personnel about issues of race, racism, privilege, and how these topics may shape instructional practices and interactions with students, is an important step in increasing equitable educational opportunities. Moreover, additional research on existing interventions can show which programs or practices are most effective in reducing discrimination and promoting cultural competence.

Stereotypes and discrimination in the school setting can also be reduced by working with youth. London, Tierney, Buhin, Greco, and Cooper (2002) implemented a 6-week summer camp multicultural awareness program with 113 students between ages 11 and 14 years. In groups that comprised racially and ethnically diverse peers, these students participated in educational activities through which they learned about other cultures, worked on cooperative projects together, and participated in facilitated, small-group discussions focused on issues of race, racism, and discrimination. Children's prejudice scores significantly decreased, and global self-esteem increased in measures taken before and after the intervention (London et al., 2002).

School-based policies can also reduce discrimination, thereby increasing students' competence motivation. Effective and nondiscriminatory school disciplinary practices can be developed by establishing in each school a proactive discipline team. Each team should include faculty and staff members from diverse racial/ethnic and cultural backgrounds who review and reach consensus on discipline policies prior to implementation (Fenning & Rose, 2007). Additionally, faculty and staff need ongoing opportunities to participate in professional development that promotes cultural competence (Fenning & Rose, 2007). Smith and Harper (2015) provide several useful resources for such professional development. They also discuss the role that schools of education can play in reducing disproportionality of school discipline policies. Preservice teachers and future school leaders need opportunities to examine their unconscious biases and racism, and they should receive instructional tools to support positive discipline and student

learning. Well-trained educators can serve as mentors for students, which is the topic of the next section.

ROLE MODELS AND MENTORS

Role models and mentors who share a racial/ethnic identity with the mentee are important because of the strong influence of social group membership on individual identity: Close to a century of research in social psychology has illustrated that perceptions of the groups to which we belong (e.g., race, gender, religion) influence our perceptions of ourselves, our values, and goals (Brewer & Hewstone, 2004). Thus, role models are important in shaping stduents' views of their abilities, their interests, and their personal goals. Unfortunately, a consequence of longstanding racial and ethnic differences in academic and economic achievement is the smaller numbers of successful black, Hispanic, and American Indian role models available to youth. The dearth of role models is particularly strong in the physical sciences and engineering. For example, according to data from the National Science Foundation (NSF; 2014), in 2013 just 1.7% of PhD degrees in physics were awarded to blacks, and only 0.1% were awarded to American Indians.

The presence of role models and mentors who share a racial/ethnic background with students can reduce stereotype threat effects (Marx, Ko, & Friedman, 2009), influence educational attainment plans and selection of career paths (Karunanayake & Nauta, 2004), and increase students' perceptions of school belonging (Walton & Cohen, 2007). Successful adult mentors can also provide mentees with strategies to cope effectively with discrimination (Thomas & Hollenshead, 2001).

Although the presence of positive role models is important to all youth, within the educational setting, role models are particularly important to members of racial/ethnic groups who are negatively stereotyped (Walton & Cohen, 2007). As Walton and Cohen (2007) argued, youth of underrepresented groups may develop "belonging uncertainty" with regard to higher education and many professional careers, expecting that they will not "fit in" within those settings. Thus, the dearth of black, Hispanic, and American Indian role models poses a significant risk factor for the competence motivation of children, adolescents, and young adults from those groups.

The lack of successful role models might be especially critical for minority boys and young men (Kurtz-Costes et al., 2014; Rowley et al., 2014). Although white girls outperform white boys academically throughout childhood and adolescence, gender gaps favoring girls are greater among black, Hispanic, and American Indian youth than among whites (Aud et al., 2010). Furthermore, these gender gaps increase with development. For example, according to NCES data, women of all races/ethnicities are more likely to matriculate to a college or university than men, and among all black students who entered a college or university in 2007, 43.6% of black women and only 35.2% of black men obtained a degree within 6 years (NCES, 2015a). The corresponding numbers for American Indians were 42.4 and 37.2%, respectively.

Although same-race mentors and role models are particularly beneficial, knowledgeable and nurturing mentors can support youth's competence motivation regardless of the race/ethnicity of the mentor. In Gloria and Robinson Kurpius's (2001) study of American Indian students at a predominantly white university, support from a mentor was one of the strongest predictors of students' persistence in their educational pursuits. Stable mentoring was also identified as one of the keys to success of American Indian college students in a qualitative study (Jackson, Smith, & Hill, 2003).

INTERVENTIONS WITH ROLE MODELS AND MENTORS: SUPPORTS IN K–12 SCHOOLING AND BEYOND

Mentor relationships offer youth support and guidance that can enhance their competence motivation, as well as their social behaviors (Rhodes, Grossman, & Resch, 2000). Important components for mentoring relationships are trust and consistency, which seem to matter more than specific goals (Styles & Morrow, 1995). Needless to

say, this is an area that deserves attention given the numerous effects mentors have on positive youth development.

One mentor intervention program, Big Brothers Big Sisters, has been shown to enhance students' academic competence and school attendance (Rhodes et al., 2000). In Big Brothers Big Sisters, a national program for children ages 5–18, mentor–mentee dyads engage in career-oriented and leisure activities aimed to support positive youth development. Using a national sample in which approximately half of the sample comprised of children of color and over half were boys, Rhodes and colleagues (2000) found that mentor–mentee relationships were linked to youth's improved academic motivation. Mentors positively influenced adolescents' beliefs about the value of school, their school attendance, and their relationships with their parents.

Many mentoring programs target high school and/or college students. These programs are often geared toward supporting students who come from underrepresented groups (e.g., first-generation college students, economically disadvantaged students, students of color), who may not have family members with college experience. The federal TRIO Program, Summer Bridge, and Gaining Early Awareness and Readiness for Undergraduate Program (GEAR UP) are examples of initiatives launched to increase the rates at which underrepresented students complete high school and are prepared to enter and be successful in the postsecondary education system. At the high school level (e.g., Upward Bound, a TRIO program), these programs provide supports such as tutoring; guidance about high school classes required for college admission; and assistance with college applications, college visits, and the completion of college and financial aid applications (Glennie, Dalton, & Knapp, 2015). At the postsecondary level, programs provide contact with student and faculty mentors, study skills training, research experience, and other sorts of academic and professional enrichment.

Although evaluation of these programs is complicated because of their many components and the diversity of students they serve, in general, results show strong benefits. For example, in a large-scale evaluation of Upward Bound Math–Science, program participants, compared to nonparticipants, showed (1) higher high school grades, (2) greater likelihood of taking chemistry and physics in high school, (3) higher rates of enrollment in selective postsecondary institutions, (4) higher frequencies of majoring in math or a science field in college, and (5) higher college graduation rates (U.S. Department of Education, Office of Planning, Evaluation, and Policy Development, Policy and Program Studies Service, 2007).

In addition to these large-scale programs, many colleges and universities have launched programs to support underrepresented students, and most research universities offer summer programs in which undergraduates from underrepresented groups can obtain research experience to prepare them for graduate school. In addition to providing access to supportive mentors and role models, such programs often include opportunities for students to improve their writing and oral presentation skills, preparation for the Graduate Record Exam, and professional development opportunities. Such programs—both local and federal—are undoubtedly in part responsible for improved success rates of students of color in recent decades: Nationwide, the 6-year graduation rate for Hispanic students increased from 45.7 to 51.9% between 1996 and 2006 (NCES, 2015a), and the number of black students awarded doctoral degrees in science or engineering increased from 689 in 2002 to 983 in 2012 (NSF, 2015).

CONCLUSIONS: SUGGESTIONS FOR RESEARCHERS, POLICYMAKERS, AND EDUCATORS

Although we have focused primarily on the challenges facing racial/ethnic-minority youth in the United States, we are optimistic as we look to the future. Conscientious members of Congress continue to attempt to develop and fund programs that will increase educational quality and access for all youth. Although issues of diversity in this country, especially within the current political environment, still need improvement, a celebration and affirmation of racial, ethnic, gender, and other sorts of diversity is also

occurring nationwide. Young adults are awakening to the need for social change, and thanks to social media, social-justice movements such as Black Lives Matter have swept the country. As we look to the future, here are a few suggestions for researchers, educators, and policymakers.

Research on African American and Hispanic youth has increased greatly in recent decades. In contrast, little research has examined competence motivation in American Indian or multiracial youth. Arab Americans, another ethnic group whose healthy development is hampered by negative stereotypes and discrimination, have also been neglected by researchers. Research is needed to identify the specific challenges and strengths of each of these groups, with attention to developmental mechanisms and cascading effects that shape youth's motivation and competence.

At the federal policy level, additional efforts are needed to reduce the enormous inequities in school quality and access to higher education. Federal and state policies could also address the challenges of ELLs. Where sufficient numbers of students share a non-English language (e.g., Spanish, Mandarin, or some American Indian languages), bilingual instruction will help youth achieve their full potential.

At the local and/or school district level, excellent preservice education and ongoing inservice training for teachers and school leaders can be highly effective in improving the experiences of racial/ethnic-minority youth in the classroom. Educators who are exposed to information about racism and white privilege will be more culturally sensitive and effective in promoting competence motivation in students of color. Such preparation is most effective when facilitated by culturally sensitive professional development providers who have expertise in issues of diversity and cultural competence within the context of educational and social service systems.

Cultural sensitivity of educators is critical in all educational areas, one of which is discipline. Behavior management and discipline policies are important for maintaining educational environments that are suited for teaching and learning. However, zero-tolerance disciplinary policies have a tendency to separate students from learning opportunities. Educators who understand their unconscious biases and privilege will be better equipped to interact with students when challenging behaviors arise. If all key stakeholders are involved in setting expectations about and adhering to standards for how students and educators interact with each other, methods are likely to be more culturally sensitive, supported by all, and successful.

Another important resource available to educators is families. School leadership and teachers who solicit meaningful engagement of families can build supportive communities that build on cultural strengths and foster children's competence motivation. Families have funds of knowledge that can be instrumental in understanding and supporting children's learning goals, and building trusting and supportive learning environments. Rigorous research can identify the most effective ways to build on the strengths offered by families from diverse cultural backgrounds.

In addition to family engagement, students of color benefit from nonfamilial mentors and role models who reflect their cultural background and have shared experiences. The opportunity to learn from and be supported by such individuals exposes students of color to the vast opportunities before them.

Finally, a critical step for researchers, policymakers, and practitioners is to pursue collaborative efforts such as this book. Working together, we have enormous potential to positively shape the policies and practices that influence competence motivation and educational outcomes in all students, regardless of race, ethnicity, or cultural background.

ACKNOWLEDGMENTS

We thank Heidi Vuletich and Marketa Burnett for assistance with literature search and editing.

NOTES

1. For the sake of brevity, we have chosen to use the U.S. Bureau of the Census category labels of white, Hispanic, black or African American, Asian, and American Indians. Although we recognize the limitations of those labels (e.g., the labels do not distinguish among subgroups such as Chinese and Korean Americans; the category of "white" represents non-Hispanic whites), most extant research also uses those labels.

2. As this chapter was being written, the Every Student Succeeds Act (ESSA) was under consideration in Congress as the most recent version of legislation guiding Title I funding.

REFERENCES

Abrego, L. J. (2006). "I can't go to college because I don't have papers": Incorporation patterns of Latino undocumented youth. *Latino Studies, 4*(3), 212–231.

Alon, S. (2011). The diversity dividends of a need-blind and color-blind affirmative action policy. *Social Science Research, 40*(6), 1494–1505.

Aud, S., Fox, M. A., & KewalRamani, A. (2010). Status and trends in the education of racial and ethnic groups (NCES 2010–015). Washington, DC: National Center for Education Statistics.

Awad, G. H. (2007). The role of racial identity, academic self-concept, and self-esteem in the prediction of academic outcomes for African American students. *Journal of Black Psychology, 33*(2), 188–207.

Bempechat, J., Nakkula, M. J., Wu, J. T., & Ginsburg, H. P. (1996). Attributions as predictors of mathematics achievement: A comparative study. *Journal of Research and Development in Education, 29,* 53–59.

Bouffard, S. M., Wimer, C., Caronongon, P., Little, P., Dearing, E., & Simpkins, S. D. (2006). Demographic differences in patterns of youth out-of-school time activity participation. *Journal of Youth Development, 1,* 1–15.

Brewer, M. B., & Hewstone, M. E. (2004). *Self and social identity.* Blackwell.

Buhin, L., & Vera, E. M. (2009). Preventing racism and promoting social justice: Person-centered and environment-centered interventions. *Journal of Primary Prevention, 30*(1), 43–59.

Cham, H., Hughes, J. N., West, S. G., & Im, M. H. (2014). Assessment of adolescents' motivation for educational attainment. *Psychological Assessment, 26*(2), 642–659.

Chavous, T. M., Rivas-Drake, D., Smalls, C., Griffin, T., & Cogburn, C. (2008). Gender matters, too: The influences of school racial discrimination and racial identity on academic engagement outcomes among African American adolescents. *Developmental Psychology, 44*(3), 637–654.

Chingos, M. M., & West, M. R. (2015). The uneven performance of Arizona's charter schools. *Educational Evaluation and Policy Analysis, 37,* 120S–134S.

Cogburn, C. D., Chavous, T. M., & Griffin, T. M. (2011). School-based racial and gender discrimination among African American adolescents: Exploring gender variation in frequency and implications for adjustment. *Race and Social Problems, 3*(1), 25–37.

Darling, N. (2005). Participation in extracurricular activities and adolescent adjustment: Cross-sectional and longitudinal findings. *Journal of Youth and Adolescence, 34*(5), 493–505.

Davis, D. H., & Raymond, M. E. (2012). Choices for studying choice: Assessing charter school effectiveness using two quasi-experimental methods. *Economics of Education Review, 31,* 225–236.

Deci, E. L., & Ryan, R. M. (1985). *Intrinsic motivation and self-determination in human behaviour.* New York: Plenum Press.

DeVoe, J. F., & Darling-Churchill, K. E. (2008). *Status and trends in the education of American Indians and Alaska Natives: 2008* (NCES 2008-084, National Center for Education Statistics, Institute of Education Sciences). Washington, DC: U.S. Department of Education.

Eccles, J. S., Barber, B. L., Stone, M., & Hunt, J. (2003). Extracurricular activities and adolescent development. *Journal of Social Issues, 59*(4), 865–889.

Eccles, J. S., & Roeser, R. W. (2011). Schools as developmental contexts during adolescence. *Journal of Research on Adolescence, 21,* 225–241.

Evans, A. B., Copping, K. E., Rowley, S. J., & Kurtz-Costes, B. (2011). Self-concept in black adolescents: Do race and gender stereotypes matter? *Self and Identity, 10,* 263–277.

Farb, A. F., & Matjasko, J. L. (2012). Recent advances in research on school-based extracurricular activities and adolescent development. *Developmental Review, 32,* 1–48.

Fenning, P., & Rose, J. (2007). Overrepresentation of African American students in exclusionary discipline: The role of school policy. *Urban Education, 42*(6), 536–559.

Fredricks, J. A., & Eccles, J. S. (2008). Participation in extracurricular activities in the middle school years: Are there developmental benefits for African American and European American youth? *Journal of Youth and Adolescence, 37*(9), 1029–1043.

García, O. (2011). *Bilingual education in the 21st century: A global perspective.* New York: Wiley.

Gil, L., & Bardack, S. (2010). Common assumptions vs. the evidence: English language learners in the United States (Report for the American Institutes for Research). Retrieved from *www.air.org/sites/default/files/downloads/report/ell_assumptions_and_evidence_0.pdf.*

Ginsburg, H. P., Woods, T. A., & Hyson, M. (2014). The future. In H. P. Ginsburg, M. Hyson, & T. A. Woods (Eds.), *Preparing early childhood educators to teach math: Professional development that works* (pp. 199–210). Baltimore: Brookes.

Gleason, P., Clark Tuttle, C., & Dwoyer, E. (2010). *The evaluation of charter school impacts: Final report* (NCEE 2010-4029). Washington, DC: National Center for Education Evaluation and Regional Assistance, Institute of Education Sciences, U.S. Department of Education.

Glennie, E. J., Dalton, B. W., & Knapp, L. G. (2015). The influence of precollege access programs on postsecondary enrollment and persistence. *Educational Policy, 29*(7), 963–983.

Gloria, A. M., & Robinson Kurpius, S. E. (2001). Influences of self-beliefs, social support, and comfort in the university environment on the academic nonpersistence decisions of American Indian undergraduates. *Cultural Diversity and Ethnic Minority Psychology, 7,* 88–102.

Gonzáles, R. G. (2011). Learning to be illegal: Undocumented youth and shifting legal contexts in the transition to adulthood. *American Sociological Review, 76*(4), 602–619.

González, N., Moll, L. C., & Amanti, C. (Eds.). (2013). *Funds of knowledge: Theorizing practices in households, communities, and classrooms.* New York: Taylor & Francis.

Guyll, M., Madon, S., Prieto, L., & Scherr, K. C. (2010). The potential roles of self-fulfilling prophecies, stigma consciousness, and stereotype threat in linking Latino/a ethnicity and educational outcomes. *Journal of Social Issues, 66*(1), 113–130.

Harris, A. L. (2006). I (don't) hate school: Revisiting oppositional culture theory of blacks' resistance to schooling. *Social Forces, 85*(2), 797–834.

Henry, G. T., Purtell, K. M., Bastian, K. C., Fortner, C. K., Thompson, C. L., Campbell, S. L., et al. (2014). The effects of teacher entry portals on student achievement. *Journal of Teacher Education, 65*(1), 7–23.

Hogg, L. (2011). Funds of knowledge: An investigation of coherence within the literature. *Teaching and Teacher Education, 27,* 666–677.

Holloway, J. H. (2002). Extracurricular activities

and student motivation. *Educational Leadership, 60*(1), 80–81.

Hudley, C., & Graham, S. (2001). Stereotypes of achievement striving among early adolescents. *Social Psychology of Education, 5*(2), 201–224.

Hughes, J. N., Im, M., Kwok, O., Cham, H., & West, S. G. (2015). Latino students' transition to middle school: Role of bilingual education and school ethnic context. *Journal of Research on Adolescence, 25*, 443–458.

Jackson, A. P., Smith, S. A., & Hill, C. L. (2003). Academic persistence among Native American college students. *Journal of College Student Development, 44*(4), 548–565.

Jacob, B. A. (2007). The challenges of staffing urban schools with effective teachers. *The Future of Children, 17*(1), 129–153.

Johnson, L. M., Antle, B. F., & Barbee, A. P. (2009). Addressing disproportionality and disparity in child welfare: Evaluation of an antiracism training for community service providers. *Children and Youth Services Review, 31*, 688–696.

Jussim, L., & Harber, K. D. (2005). Teacher expectations and self-fulfilling prophecies: Knowns and unknowns, resolved and unresolved controversies. *Personality and Social Psychology Review, 9*(2), 131–155.

Karunanayake, D., & Nauta, M. M. (2004). The relationship between race and students' identified career role models and perceived role model influence. *Career Development Quarterly, 52*(3), 225–234.

Kena, G., Musu-Gillette, L., Robinson, J., Wang, X., Rathbun, A., Zhang, J., et al. (2015). *The condition of education 2015* (NCES 2015-144). Washington DC: National Center for Education Statistics.

Kurtz-Costes, B., & Pungello, E. (2000). The acculturation of immigrant children. *Social Education, 64*, 121–125.

Kurtz-Costes, B., Swinton, A. D., & Skinner, O. D. (2014). Race and ethnic gaps in the school performance of Latino, African American, and white students. In F. T. L. Leong, L. Comas-Diaz, G. N. Hall, V. C. McLoyd, & J. Trimble (Eds.), *APA handbook of multicultural psychology: Vol. 1. Theory and research* (pp. 231–246). Washington, DC: American Psychological Association.

Kurtz-Costes, B. E., & Schneider, W. (1994). Self-concept, attributional beliefs, and school achievement: A longitudinal analysis. *Contemporary Educational Psychology, 19*, 199–216.

Lipman, P. (2013). *The new political economy of urban education: Neoliberalism, race, and the right to the city.* New York: Taylor & Francis.

London, L. H., Tierney, G., Buhin, L., Greco, D. M., & Cooper, C. J. (2002). Kids' College: Enhancing children's appreciation and acceptance of cultural diversity. *Journal of Prevention and Intervention in the Community, 24*, 63–78.

Long, M. C., Iatarola, P., & Conger, D. (2009). Explaining gaps in readiness for college-level math: The role of high school courses. *Education, 4*(1), 1–33.

Mackinney, E., & Rios-Aguilar, C. (2012). Negotiating between restrictive language policies and complex teaching conditions: A case study of Arizona's teachers of English learners. *Bilingual Research Journal, 35*, 350–367.

Marx, D. M., Ko, S. J., & Friedman, R. A. (2009). The "Obama effect": How a salient role model reduces race-based performance differences. *Journal of Experimental Social Psychology, 45*(4), 953–956.

Monzó, L. D., & Rueda, R. (2009). Passing for English fluent: Latino immigrant children masking language proficiency. *Anthropology and Education Quarterly, 40*, 20–40.

National Center for Education Statistics (NCES). (2015a). *Digest of education statistics: 2013* (NCES 2015–011). Washington, DC: U.S. Department of Education.

National Center for Education Statistics (NCES). (2015b). *Fast facts: Title 1.* Washington DC: U.S. Department of Education.

National Immigration Law Center. (2015). State bills on access to education for immigrants: 2015. Retrieved from *http://nilc.org/statebillsedu.html*.

National Science Foundation (NSF). (2014). *Doctorate recipients from U.S. universities: 2013* (NSF 15-304). Arlington, VA: Author.

National Science Foundation (NSF). (2015). *Science and engineering degrees by race/ethnicity of recipients: 2002–2012* (NSF 15-321). Arlington, VA: National Science Foundation.

Okeke, N. A., Howard, L. C., Kurtz-Costes, B., & Rowley, S. J. (2009). Academic race stereotypes, academic self-concept, and racial centrality in African American youth. *Journal of Black Psychology, 35*, 366–387.

Orfield, G., & Lee, C. (2006). *Racial transformation and the changing nature of segregation.* Cambridge, MA: Civil Rights Project at Harvard University.

Passel, J. S., & Cohn, D. (2010). *U.S. unauthorized immigration flows are down sharply since mid-decade.* Washington, DC: Pew Hispanic Center.

Payne, C. M. (2008). *So much reform, so little change: The persistence of failure in urban schools.* Cambridge, MA: Harvard Education Press.

Perez, W., Espinoza, R., Ramos, K., Coronado, H. M., & Cortes, R. (2009). Academic resilience among undocumented Latino students. *Hispanic Journal of Behavioral Sciences, 31,* 149–181.

Portes, A., & MacLeod, D. (1996). Educational progress of children of immigrants: The roles of class, ethnicity, and school context. *Sociology of Education, 69,* 255–275.

Portes, P. R. (1999). Social and psychological factors in the academic achievement of children of immigrants. *American Educational Research Journal, 36,* 489–507.

Powers, S., & Rossman, M. H. (1984). Attributions for success and failure among Anglo, black, Hispanic, and Native American community college students. *Journal of Psychology, 117,* 27–31.

Rhodes, J. E., Grossman, J. B., & Resch, N. L. (2000). Agents of change: Pathways through which mentoring relationships influence adolescents' academic adjustment. *Child Development, 71*(6), 1662–1671.

Riley, T., & Ungerleider, C. (2012). Self-fulfilling prophecy: How teachers' attributions, expectations, and stereotypes influence the learning opportunities afforded aboriginal students. *Canadian Journal of Education, 35*(2), 303–333.

Roche, K. M., Lambert, S. F., Ghazarian, S. R., & Little, T. D. (2015). Adolescent language brokering in diverse contexts: Associations with parenting and parent–youth relationships in a new immigrant destination area. *Journal of Youth and Adolescence, 44,* 77–89.

Rowley, S. J., Kurtz-Costes, B., & Cooper, S. (2010). The schooling of African American children. In J. Meece & J. Eccles (Eds.), *Handbook of research on schools, schooling, and human development* (pp. 275–292). Hillsdale, NJ: Erlbaum.

Rowley, S. J., Ross, L., Lozada, F., Williams, A., Gale, A., & Kurtz-Costes, B. (2014). Framing black boys: Parent, teacher, and student narratives of the academic lives of black boys. In L. S. Liben & R. S. Bigler (Eds.), *The role of gender in educational contexts and outcomes* (pp. 301–332). Philadelphia: Elsevier.

Schmader, T., Johns, M., & Forbes, C. (2008). An integrated process model of stereotype threat effects on performance. *Psychological Review, 115*(2), 336–356.

Skiba, R. J., Horner, R. H., Chung, C. G., Karega Rausch, M., May, S. L., & Tobin, T. (2011). Race is not neutral: A national investigation of African American and Latino

disproportionality in school discipline. *School Psychology Review, 40*(1), 85–107.

Smith, E. J., & Harper, S. R. (2015). *Disproportionate impact of K–12 school suspension and expulsion on black students in southern states.* Philadelphia: University of Pennsylvania, Center for the Study of Race and Equity in Education.

Stearns, E., & Glennie, E. J. (2010). Opportunities to participate: Extracurricular activities' distribution across and academic correlates in high schools. *Social Science Research, 39*(2), 296–309.

Steele, C. M. (1997). A threat in the air: How stereotypes shape intellectual identity and performance. *American Psychologist, 52,* 613–629.

Styles, M. B., & Morrow, K. V. (1995). *Understanding how youth and elders form relationships: A study of four linking lifetimes programs.* Philadelphia: Public/Private Ventures.

Swinton, A. D., Kurtz-Costes, B., Rowley, S. J., & Adeyanju, N. O. (2011). A longitudinal examination of African American adolescents' attributions about achievement outcomes. *Child Development, 82,* 1486–1500.

Tenenbaum, H. R., & Ruck, M. D. (2007). Are teachers' expectations different for racial minority than for European American students?: A meta-analysis. *Journal of Educational Psychology, 99*(2), 253–273.

Téllez, K., & Waxman, H. C. (Eds.). (2006). *Preparing quality educators for English language learners: Research, policy, and practice.* Mahwah, NJ: Erlbaum.

Thomas, G. D., & Hollenshead, C. (2001). Resisting from the margins: The coping strategies of black women and other women of color faculty members at a research university. *Journal of Negro Education, 70*(3), 166–175.

U.S. Congress. (1996). Public Law 104–208, Section 505. Illegal Immigration Reform and Immigrant Responsibility (IIRIR) Act of 1996. Retrieved from *www.congress.gov/104/plaws/publ208/plaw-104publ208.pdf.*

U.S. Department of Education. (2015). Resource guide: Supporting undocumented youth: A guide for success in secondary and postsecondary settings. Retrieved from *www2.ed.gov/about/overview/focus/supporting-undocumented-youth.pdf.*

U.S. Department of Education, Office of Planning, Evaluation and Policy Development, Policy and Program Studies Service. (2007). *Upward Bound Math–Science: Program description and interim impact estimates.* Washington, DC: Author.

U.S. Department of Education, Office of State Support. (2015). Improving basic programs operated by local educational agencies (CFDA No. 84.010). Retrieved from *www2.ed.gov/programs/titleiparta/index.html*.

U.S. Senate. (2013). S. 744, Section 2103. Development, Relief, and Education for Alien Minors (DREAM) Act of 2013. Retrieved from *www.congress.gov/113/bills/s744/bills-113s744es.pdf*.

U.S. Senate. (2015). S. 796. Investing in States to Achieve Tuition Equality for Dreamers (IN-STATE) Act of 2015. Retrieved from *www.congress.gov/114/bills/s796/bills-114s796is.pdf*.

Walton, G. M., & Cohen, G. L. (2007). A question of belonging: Race, social fit, and achievement. *Journal of Personality and Social Psychology, 92*(1), 82–96.

Webb, E., & Sergison, M. (2003). Evaluation of cultural competence and anti-racism in child health services. *Archives of Disease in Childhood, 88*(4), 291–294.

Wong, C. A., Eccles, J. S., & Sameroff, A. (2003). The influence of ethnic discrimination and ethnic identification on African American adolescents' school and socioemotional adjustment. *Journal of Personality, 71*(6), 1197–1232.

Wood, D. A., Kurtz-Costes, B., & Copping, K. E. (2011). Motivational pathways to college for African American youth: A test of expectancy–value theory. *Developmental Psychology, 47*, 961–968.

Woodcock, A., Hernandez, P. R., Estrada, M., & Schultz, P. (2012). The consequences of chronic stereotype threat: Domain disidentification and abandonment. *Journal of Personality and Social Psychology, 103*(4), 635–646.

Zong, J., & Batalova, J. (2015). Frequently requested statistics on immigrants and immigration in the United States (ISSN 1946–4037). Retrieved from *www.migrationpolicy.org/article/frequently-requested-statistics-immigrants-and-immigration-united-states*.

CHAPTER 29

Social Striving

*Social Group Membership
and Children's Motivations and Competencies*

REBECCA S. BIGLER
AMY ROBERSON HAYES
MEAGAN M. PATTERSON

One of the hallmarks of humankind is sociality. Humans evolved in the context of group living, and there is nearly universal agreement that we are psychologically adapted to life in groups. Groups are so central to human survival and quality of life that we are likely to have an evolved tendency to tie our sense of self to those social groups in which we are members. Rather than thinking of ourselves exclusively in terms of our particular traits, we universally think of ourselves as group members, at least within some contexts (Deaux, Reid, Mizrahi, & Ethier, 1995; Dunning, 2003). The invariable embedding of the self within social groups means that the developmental process of acquiring motivations and competencies is far more complicated than the maturational unfolding of individuals' biologically based drives and capabilities.

Decades of psychological research document that social group memberships (e.g., categories of belonging based on one's gender, race, ethnicity, nationality, religion, or class) have powerful consequences for development, including children's socioemotional, cognitive, and physical outcomes. Gender, race, and class, for example, are significant forces in shaping children's personal qualities (see Blakemore, Berenbaum, & Liben, 2009; McLoyd, 1998; Quintana et al., 2006). The personal qualities that are the particular focus of this volume—motivations and competencies—are linked to social groups. Motivations and competencies are frequently perceived to vary across social groups and, in some instances, do in fact vary across social groups (e.g., Butler, 2014). For example, at the group level, males and females differ in their motivations for and competencies in cheerleading and wrestling. Although distinguishing between veridical and illusory group differences is sometimes contentious (see Jussim, Cain, Crawford, Harber, & Cohen, 2009), both types of social group differences are likely to be highly consequential for individual and societal outcomes. For example, group differences in motivations and competencies undoubtedly contribute to the group differences that characterize the U.S. workforce, including gender-, racial-, ethnic-, and class-related variations in occupational status and financial compensation. Differences in occupational pursuits in turn predict physical health, mental health, happiness, and life satisfaction (Diener & Biswas-Diener, 2002; Hagerty, 2000; Marmot et al., 1998; Myers,

2000; Ostrove, Adler, Kuppermann, & Washington, 2000; Williams, Yu, Jackson, & Anderson, 1997).

OVERVIEW OF RESEARCH CHALLENGES AND CHAPTER GOALS

An important challenge facing developmental scientists is to explain the causal mechanisms by which social group membership shapes motivations (i.e., desires, drives, and preferences) and competencies (i.e., knowledge and skills) across childhood, adolescence, and adulthood. Returning to our earlier example, scientists must explain *how* being female generally favors the development of interest and competence in cheerleading and lack of interest and competence in wrestling (and how the inverse pattern comes to emerge in most males). In some cases, the identification of such causal mechanisms has been made a national priority, as in the call to understand and then intervene in the mechanisms that produce sex differences in interest, persistence, and accomplishment in science, technology, engineering, and math (STEM) fields (see Ceci, Williams, & Barnett, 2009, for a review).

Explaining the complete set of pathways of influence between social category memberships and children's personal qualities (e.g., traits, knowledge, skills, preferences) is a daunting and as yet unaccomplished task. Consider, for example, the knowledge base required for a complete account of such pathways. As discussed in greater detail below, the potential roles of group-differentiated biological factors (genes, hormones, etc.) and environmental factors (media messages, parental treatment, etc.) need to be catalogued. Inherent in the challenge is also the need to understand the emergence and roles of two cognitive constructs: the child's developing conceptions of social groups and developing conceptions of self. Finally, the causal mechanisms that link children's schemas of social groups to the self need to be identified, as do the variables that mediate and moderate such relations.

There are also serious methodological challenges inherent in identifying the mechanisms of influence between social group membership and developmental outcomes.

Such mechanisms are difficult (albeit not impossible) to identify from studies of actual social groups, such as those based on race, ethnicity, and gender. In part this is true because it is typically impractical or unethical to manipulate an individual's membership in existing social categories; thus, the rich, complex, and interconnecting sets of variables that constitute the "nature" (e.g., genes, hormones) and "nurture" (e.g., environments, experiences) components of social group membership are conflated.

The causal mechanisms involved in linking children's social group memberships and their personal attributes are also difficult to identify, in part, because children are exposed to myriad messages about social groups in the first years of life. That is, children's experiences as members and observers of social groups (e.g., operant, associative, and vicarious learning) begin at birth and are therefore impossible to document exhaustively. For these reasons, we argue that novel group paradigms (see Bigler, 1995; Bigler, Jones, & Lobliner, 1997) are useful in the study of the reciprocal causal processes that link children's views of social groups and the self.

Our primary goal in this chapter is to describe theoretical and methodological advances and limitations in our understanding of the links between children's social group memberships and children's motivations and competencies. We have organized our chapter into five sections. In the following section, we describe major theoretical views of the causal processes linking children's social group membership on the one hand, to their motivation and competence on the other. To do so, we highlight two contemporary models: Liben and Bigler's (2002) dual pathway model and Greenwald and colleagues' (2002) balanced identity model. We then describe empirical studies, including those that make use of novel group paradigms, aimed at understanding the links between children's social groups and personal attributes, including motivations and competencies. In the next section, we outline two contentious issues that have emerged with respect to the practical implications of research on social group membership and individuals' motivations and competencies. In the final section, we offer general conclusions and suggest key directions for future research.

THEORETICAL MODELS OF CAUSAL PATHWAYS LINKING SOCIAL GROUPS AND THE SELF

Numerous models of causal pathways linking children's social group membership with their motivations and competencies have been proposed across the last century. Such models have appeared within the literatures on specific (often stigmatized) social groups, including women (Denmark & Paludi, 2007), African Americans (Neville, Tynes, & Utsey, 2009), and sexual minorities (Poteat, Scheer, & Mereish, 2014). Models have also appeared within literatures focused on specific outcomes, including academic motivation and achievement (Ogbu & Simmons, 1988; Poteat et al., 2014; Wigfield & Eccles, 2000), career interests and attainment (Hughes & Bigler, 2007; Lent, Brown, & Hackett, 1994), and athletic skills and participation (Stone, Lynch, Sjomeling, & Darley, 1999). Rather than provide an exhaustive review, we instead provide a brief classification scheme of three families of approaches relevant to the link between social group membership and self—essentialist, environmentalist, and constructivist—that were first identified by Liben and Bigler (2002) in their discussion of gender development; we then focus in more depth on two contemporary accounts that address causal links between social groups and the self.

Essentialist Models

One broad category of causal models linking children's social group membership and personal attributes might be termed *essentialist*. Such models argue that social groups (e.g., males and females, African Americans and European Americans) differ with respect to motivations and competencies as the result of biological factors (e.g., genes, hormones). Because group differences are viewed as biologically based, they are also typically viewed as natural and inevitable (see Liben, 2015). Essentialist accounts were pervasive and popular during the early and mid-20th century, when they were applied to wide variety of social groups, offering biologically based explanations for differences in academic motivation and competencies between boys and girls (Hyde, 1906), wealthy and poor individuals (Davenport, 1911), and U.S.-born and immigrant individuals (Bingham, 1908). Liben (2015) provides a highly engaging description of Hyde's (1906) writings concerning innate differences between males' and females' intellectual motivations and competencies.

Although less prevalent than in past eras, essentialist approaches continue to appear in the scientific and popular literatures on social group differences. Contemporary writers have attributed boys' and girls' differing academic motivations and competencies to their differing biological makeups (Gurian, 2001; Sax, 2005). Other writers continue to argue that black–white differences in cognitive skills are, in large part, due to heredity (Hernstein & Murray, 2010; Rushton & Jensen, 2005). Additionally, the field of epigenetics (i.e., the study of processes that modify patterns of gene expression without changing the nucleotide sequences of the DNA; Jenuwein & Allis, 2001) has given rise to renewed interests in biological bases of racial and economic differences in physical and mental health. Epigenetics suggests, for example, that racial discrimination may induce changes to the expression of particular genes linked to biological development and disease (Sullivan, 2013). Although epigenetic approaches acknowledge the importance of environmental experience, insofar as effects can potentially be transmitted to offspring biologically, social-group-based variations in a host of affective and cognitive outcomes may be interpreted as having a foundation in biology (Kuzawa & Sweet, 2009).

Environmentalist Models

The next broad class of theories might be termed *environmentalist*, in that group differences in children's qualities, including motivations and competencies, are viewed as the product of environmental agents (Liben & Bigler, 2002). Traditional learning theorists (Skinner, 1938) posited classical and operant conditioning as causal mechanisms that produced social group differences in motivations and competencies; social learning theorists added a causal role for modeling (Bandura, 1977). Such accounts formed the basis of much research across the latter half of the 20th century and continue to provide the theoretical foundation for research on social group differences (e.g., Tenenbaum & Leaper, 2003).

Illustrative of contemporary empirical research grounded in environmentalist theories is a set of studies by Robinson-Cimpian, Lubienski, Ganley, and Copur-Gencturk (2014) examining gender differences in mathematical competence using data from the Early Childhood Longitudinal Study. In their first study, Robinson-Cimpian and colleagues demonstrated that teachers rate boys' mathematics proficiency higher than that of girls' after accounting for other student characteristics, such as problem behavior, approaches to learning, past and current test scores, and demographic factors. In their second study, they found that teachers' tendency to rate boys as mathematically more proficient than girls when they act and behave similarly was linked to the widening gender gap in mathematics performance in elementary school. As the authors note, these data do not identify the mechanisms that link teachers' ratings to children's performance, but they nonetheless suggest that environmental factors are at play. It is possible, for example, that teachers' feedback to male and female students (e.g., praise for performance) may differ as a result of their gender-biased views and, in turn, affect children's proficiencies. Additionally, it is possible that teachers' gender-biased views stem from their own mathematics anxiety, and that female teachers' modeling of math anxiety influences girls' mathematics achievement (Beilock, Gunderson, Ramirez, & Levine, 2010).

Constructivist Models

The third broad class of theories, and the focus of the remainder of this section, has been labeled *constructivist* (Liben & Bigler, 2002). These accounts posit that group differences emerge as the result of a relational interplay of children's characteristics and their social contexts, and unlike other theories, highlight the role of children's creation and construal of their own environments in shaping developmental outcomes. In such accounts, the child is viewed not as a passive recipient of messages that are conveyed by socializing agents, but rather as an active creator of meaning. The child is active first, in the process of constructing knowledge and beliefs about social groups and the self (thereby constructing group and self *schema*), and second, in the process of applying those schemas to new environmental encounters. The active nature of the child's role in determining developmental outcomes is reflected in the term *self-socialization*. Such models are also interactionist in the sense that child qualities and environmental contexts act in dynamic, nonadditive ways to produce outcomes. These models assume that children's developing personal qualities (e.g., their traits, knowledge, and skills) shape the salience, value, and meaning of social groups; thus, exposure to the same environments can produce differing developmental outcomes across children (see Liben, 2014).

At the core of constructivists' theoretical and empirical work (including our own collaborative and individual research programs) are questions concerning the self (e.g., "What am I like?"), social groups (e.g., "What are [members of some group] like?"), and children's conceptions of themselves as members of social groups (e.g., "To which groups do I belong?" and "Am I a typical group member?"). The last of the three concepts is perhaps the least well understood. One reason for the slow progress concerns the wide variety of terms and definitions of the construct. For example, a child's knowledge and beliefs about him- or herself as a group member have been labeled by general terms such as *self-identity, social identity, collective identity,* and, with respect to domain-specific membership, by terms such as *gender identity, racial identity,* and *ethnic identity.* Furthermore, researchers who study one form of identity sometimes neglect to read and cite the work of those studying other forms of identities. As a consequence, the construct has been defined quite differently across scholars and domains (see Tobin, Menon, Menon, Spatta, Hodges, & Perry, 2010).

Several constructivist theories outlining causal pathways that link social group membership and personal attributes originated within the literature on gender role development (Bem, 1981; Liben & Bigler, 2002; Martin & Halverson, 1981). These models highlight the role of the child's cognitions about gender in shaping his or her own preferences and behaviors. Illustratively, Bem (1981) argued about gender development that

> the child also learns to evaluate his or her adequacy as a person in terms of the gender schema, to match his or her preferences, attitudes, behaviors, and personal attributes against the prototypes stored within it. The gender schema becomes a prescriptive standard or guide (Kagan, 1964; Kohlberg, 1966), and self-esteem becomes its hostage. (p. 355)

Rooted in earlier constructivist accounts of gender development (Bem, 1981; Kohlberg, 1966; Martin & Halverson, 1981), Liben and Bigler (2002) proposed a model aimed at explaining the process of gender differentiation across childhood that emphasized three neglected aspects of individual variation across children: individual differences in the extent to which children (1) attend to gender as a social category, (2) use gender to prescribe and proscribe traits and roles, and (3) show interests in particular domains for reasons independent of gender-related attitudes.

Liben and Bigler's Dual-Pathway Model

Liben and Bigler (2002) specified the importance of two pathways by which gender differentiation is produced, leading the model to be referred to as a dual-pathway model (DPM). One of these—the attitudinal pathway—holds that a child's tendency to attend to gender (*gender salience filter*) and beliefs about what is culturally acceptable for girls versus boys (*gender schema filter*) drives the child's own personal preferences and actions (see Figure 29.1). Extrapolating to social groups more generally, the attitudinal pathway posits that existing schemas about social groups guide children's interests, behaviors, and beliefs about the self. This half of the model is rooted in classic theories of intergroup attitude development, including social identity theory (Tajfel & Turner, 1986) and gender schematic processing models of sex typing (Liben & Signorella, 1980; Martin & Halverson, 1981).

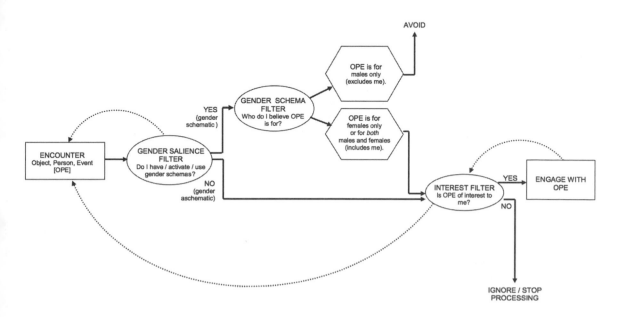

FIGURE 29.1. Attitudinal pathway model from Liben and Bigler (2002). Copyright © 2002 Society for Research in Child Development. Reprinted with permission from authors.

There is much empirical support for the attitudinal pathway. For example, children express greater interest in unfamiliar toys said to be preferred by members of their gender ingroup, labeled as "for" their gender group, or depicted in photographs with an ingroup member (Liben & Hillard, 2010; Martin, Eisenbud, & Rose, 1995).

The other pathway—the personal pathway—identifies an inverse route in which the child's personal interests (*interest filter*) and routine attention to gender (again, the gender salience filter) are thought to drive the further development and modification of their gender attitudes (see Figure 29.2). In the personal pathway, an individual's self-concept and identity shape his or her views of the social group. This half of the model is congruent with social projection models of identity (Krueger, 2007), and posits that a child's own interests, traits, and abilities shape his or her behaviors and subsequent views of the group. Sometimes called a "self-anchoring" effect (Cadinu & Rothbart, 1996), this pathway suggests that children often project views of themselves onto their own ingroups. For example, data on concurrent associations between children's views of self and others were reported by Martin and colleagues (1995),

who found that children expected that their own toy preferences would be shared by members of their gender ingroup but not by members of their outgroup. Longitudinal evidence of the impact of children's views of themselves on their views of others was provided by a study of middle school students (Liben & Bigler, 2002). Among boys, greater endorsement of traditionally feminine personality traits at the start of sixth grade predicted egalitarian gender role attitudes at the end of seventh grade; that is, boys who earlier ascribed a greater number of culturally feminine traits to themselves than did their peers later appeared to have developed more egalitarian gender attitudes than their peers.

Greenwald and Colleagues' Balanced Identity Model

Working within the social-psychological literature on implicit attitudes, Greenwald and colleagues (2002) developed a theoretical model of the relations among adults' social cognitions concerning the self and social groups. The model, which appears in Figure 29.3, distinguishes three types of cognitive associations: (1) links between one's group (top left vertex) and one's self (bottom center

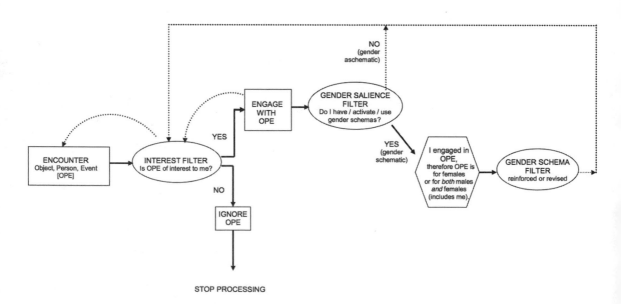

FIGURE 29.2. Personal pathway model from Liben and Bigler (2002). Copyright © 2002 Society for Research in Child Development. Reprinted with permission from authors.

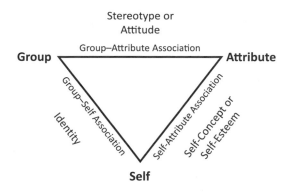

FIGURE 29.3. Greenwald et al.'s (2002) balanced identity model. Copyright © 2002 by the American Psychological Association. Reprinted with permission of the authors.

vertex), termed *identity*; (2) links between one's group (top left vertex) and an attribute (top right vertex), termed *attitude*; and (3) links between one's self (bottom center vertex) and an attribute (top right vertex), termed *self-concept*. That is, people make mental associations among (1) a salient social group, such as a gender or race, and the self (identity; e.g., "I am a typical boy"); (2) a social group and particular attributes (attitudes; e.g., "Boys are good at math"); and (3) the self and particular attributes (self-concept; e.g., "I am good at math"). Each association can vary in strength. Specifically, Greenwald and colleagues proposed that each type of cognitive association is a function of the others, such that the cognitive consistency among the constructs is achieved.

Greenwald and colleagues (2002) reviewed studies that generated findings consistent with their proposed model of the links among individuals' social group identities, attitudes (e.g., stereotypes), and beliefs about their own competence in a given domain. For example, Nosek, Banaji, and Greenwald (2002) demonstrated that, among college students, the strength of an individual's stereotypical association of math with men rather than women, as well as the strength of the individual's identification with his or her own gender, predicted the valence of the individual's math attitudes. Much is left to learn, however, about the relations of these constructs during

childhood (see Tobin et al., 2010). Furthermore, a complete developmental account of the causal relations among social group membership and children's developing motivations and competencies will require identifying the exogenous sources that influence the three core constructs of the model (identities, attitudes, and self-concepts) across the lifespan. In the next section, we highlight some empirical findings from constructivist approaches to understanding the pathways of influence among children's developing identities, attitudes, and self-concepts.

EMPIRICAL STUDIES OF CHILDREN'S VIEWS OF GROUPS AND THE SELF

Although few studies have directly tested the full causal models outlined by Liben and Bigler (2002) and Greenwald and colleagues (2002), several literatures within developmental psychology bear indirectly on these questions of whether, when, and how children coordinate their views of social groups with their self-views. One body of work concerns the consequences of one's sense of belonging (Baumeister & Leary, 1995). Individuals' sense of belonging in a given academic domain appears key to their motivation in that domain (Good, Rattan, & Dweck, 2012). This pathway between an individual's identity and a given trait or domain is analogous to the self-attribute pathway in the Greenwald and colleagues model. According to Good and colleagues (2012), belongingness stems from the perception of oneself as a typical member of an academic community. Within the domain of math, for example, Good and colleagues found that sense of belonging within the math domain was predictive of intent to pursue math as a subject in the future; however, the relation was moderated for women (but not men) by the belief that math ability is a fixed trait (see Yeager & Dweck, 2012).

In contrast to those researchers who have argued that associating social groups with academic domains or tasks facilitates motivation and performance for ingroup members (e.g., Master & Walton, 2013; Moè, 2009; Pajares & Valiante, 2001), Cimpian and colleagues (Cimpian, 2010; Cimpian & Markman, 2011; Cimpian, Mu, & Erickson,

2012) posit that such associations are likely to undermine children's motivation s. In a series of studies, Cimpian and colleagues have found that associating social group membership with performance on a particular task (e.g., "Girls are really good at this game") leads to poorer subsequent performance on the task than associating an individual with performance on the task (e.g., "I know a girl named Sarah who is really good at this game"). Cimpian and colleagues posit that the reason for this effect is that linking performance to social category membership promotes the view that performance in that domain is driven by innate ability rather than effort or practice (Cimpian & Markman, 2011; Cimpian et al., 2012). Such beliefs have been associated with poor domain-specific performance across a range of studies (for reviews, see Burnette, O'Boyle, VanEpps, Pollack, & Finkel, 2013; Dweck, 2000).

A second area of work that is relevant for understanding the pathways that link social group membership and individuals' motivations and competencies concerns children's gender role development. As noted earlier, children who express greater interest in cross-sex-typed toys, activities, and occupations also tend to be more flexible or egalitarian in their gender stereotyping (Liben & Bigler, 2002; Martin & Dinella, 2011; Patterson, 2012). At the same time, however, the literature contains reports of cognitive inconsistency between children's views of gender groups and the self. Examples of such inconsistency come from studies in which children's gender-stereotypical attitudes have been modified as a result of experimental lessons. For example, children have been induced to endorse greater numbers of egalitarian beliefs as a result of classroom instruction concerning occupations (Bigler & Liben, 1990; Weisgram & Bigler, 2006) and sexism (Lamb, Bigler, Liben, & Green, 2009). Overall, these studies report no changes in children's own interest in occupations, activities, or traits, even among children developed more egalitarian attitudes as a result of the lessons. It is possible, of course, that changes to group views produce subsequent changes to self-views gradually over time, and effects are therefore undetectable in studies that span only weeks or months.

Cognitive inconsistency has, however, also been reported in descriptive (nonintervention) studies of gender attitudes and at the level of specific items. For example, Liben and Bigler (2002) reported:

> Eight girls in the longitudinal sample reported that "only men" should be doctors, but six of these same girls reported that they themselves were interested in becoming a doctor. In a parallel example drawn from the personal pathway contingent analysis, 22 girls reported themselves to be "strong," but nearly a third of these same girls (7) stated that "only boys" should be strong. (p. 101)

These findings suggest that children are capable of holding group and self-views that are logically inconsistent.

Although the work of Cimpian and others (e.g., Bigler, 1995; Hilliard & Liben, 2010; Martin et al., 1995) indicates that children's views of existing social groups can be experimentally manipulated, the interpretation of findings about actual social groups is often clouded by children's prior knowledge, beliefs, and experiences with the groups (Bigler & Liben, 1993; Liben & Signorella, 1980). Thus, in some cases, researchers have opted to use experimentally created groups to examine the formation and consequences of children's intergroup attitudes.

Novel Group Studies of Children's Views of Groups and the Self

As noted earlier, children are exposed to myriad messages about the importance and meaning of social groups, such as those based on age, gender, political views, race, and religion (Pahlke, Bigler, & Suizzo, 2012; Patterson & Bigler, 2006). Such messages are embedded in media directed at both children and adults (e.g., television, movies, billboards, magazines), as well as familiar (e.g., parents, siblings, peers) and unfamiliar (strangers) others' verbal and nonverbal behavior. Consider, for example, the exceedingly rich set of messages about gender available to children in a single day. A typical child might hear many dozens of gendered nouns and adjectives ("Good morning, boys and girls," "Please thank him for his help"), experience multiple instances of people sorted by gender (while using public restrooms or shopping in "girls" and "boys" sections of clothing or toy stores), and watch dozens of men and women systematically model different behaviors (e.g., attending a school in which women perform instructional duties and men perform janitorial duties, watching a football game in which women cheer and men play). Given the pervasiveness of such inputs, it is difficult, if not impossible, to identify the causal role of environmental messages about social groups in shaping children's cognition, affect, and behavior.

As a consequence of this complexity, researchers' understanding of the reciprocal causal links between children's social group membership and personal attributes is likely to be advanced via the use of experimental studies of novel groups (see Messick & Mackie, 1989; Olson & Dweck, 2008). Such experiments, referred to as "minimal" or "novel" group studies, typically involve assigning participants to experimentally created social groups on the basis of trivial or random characteristics. Using an experimental novel group paradigm, the meaning and characteristics of the novel groups can be manipulated, providing information about the role of social groups in shaping individuals' motivation and competence (Bigler, 1995; Bigler et al., 1997).

Novel group paradigms have been used in the social sciences for decades (see Messick & Mackie, 1989, for a review). In the classic Robbers Cave study, Sherif, Harvey, White, Hood, and Sherif (1961) induced intergroup prejudice and competition among boys at a summer camp by separating them into two teams. Although the boys were largely similar across dimensions typically associated with stereotypes (e.g., gender, race, religion), their separation into teams (the Eagles and the Rattlers) and provision of opportunities for competition led to strong intragroup affiliation and intergroup animosity. In the decades since the Robbers Cave study, variations on the novel group paradigm have provided information about the mechanisms that affect the formation of stereotyping and prejudice. A benefit of the

novel group approach is that it allows for a test of the *causal* role of various factors in the development of social identities and attitudes. So, for example, the characteristics of social groups, such as their size, perceptual salience, and norms, can be manipulated, and the consequent effects on individuals' attitudes and behaviors examined.

Experimental studies of the formation of intergroup biases (in both children and adults) traditionally examine the effects of "mere categorization" of individuals on intergroup attitudes (Messick & Mackie, 1989, p. 59). Most of these studies involve assigning participants to social groups on the basis of trivial characteristics. For example, in one of the first experimental manipulations of social categorization, Tajfel (1970) asked participants to estimate the number of dots projected onto a screen, and then classified them into "overestimator" and "underestimator" groups. Minimal group studies typically involve a very brief assignment to group membership (i.e., an hour or less); participants know nothing about the novel groups and have no opportunities to interact with group members. In contrast, in novel social group situations (e.g., those reported in Bigler, 1995; Patterson & Bigler, 2006; Sherif et al., 1961), individuals have opportunities to observe and interact with other group members and may receive a variety of messages regarding groups, either experimentally controlled (e.g., messages regarding group characteristics; Bigler, Brown, & Markell, 2001) or not (e.g., messages about group membership from other participants, such as those reported by Sherif et al. [1961] in the Robbers Cave experiment).

From extant novel group research, it is clear that children show a preference for novel ingroups to which they are assigned. When placed into experimentally created groups, children view the ingroup as having more positive characteristics than the outgroup (Bigler et al., 1997; Dunham, Baron, & Carey, 2011; Hayes, 2014; Patterson & Bigler, 2006, 2011). They also demonstrate a preference for unfamiliar peers who are labeled as ingroup members and for toys associated with the novel ingroup (e.g., labeled as "the blue group's favorite"; Patterson & Bigler, 2006). In addition, children are generally more willing to help or share with an ingroup member than with an outgroup member (Dunham et al., 2011; Plötner, Over, Carpenter, & Tomasello, 2015). This preference for experimentally assigned ingroups emerges relatively early in life and is consistently evident in 4- to 6-year-old children (Dunham et al., 2011; Dunham & Emory, 2014; Patterson & Bigler, 2006).

There is also evidence that children expect others to demonstrate an ingroup preference as well; for example, they expect ingroup members to be more willing than outgroup members to share with them (Dunham et al., 2011). Similarly, children expect individuals to be loyal to their groups, and show negative views of group members who are disloyal (e.g., by expressing desire to join another group; Abrams, Rutland, Ferrell, & Pelletier, 2008; Misch, Over, & Carpenter, 2014). Perhaps due to this awareness of these group norms, children are more invested in maintaining a positive reputation among novel ingroup members than among outgroup members (Engelmann, Over, Herrmann, & Tomasello, 2013).

Bigler and colleagues (Bigler, 1995; Bigler et al., 1997, 2001; Brown & Bigler, 2002; Patterson & Bigler, 2006) have made extensive use of novel group designs to examine the formation of intergroup attitudes. In these studies, children's experiences of novel groups are more broadly consequential than those seen in traditional minimal group studies (e.g., Dunham et al., 2011; Tajfel, 1970). In a typical study, participants are 6- to 11-year-old summer school students who are unacquainted with each other when school begins. They are initially given tasks measuring factors (e.g., cognitive-developmental level, self-esteem, self-perceived competence) hypothesized to affect group views. Novel groups are then created, usually by assigning children to wear different colored T-shirts. Characteristics of the groups (e.g., proportional size, purported traits) and their treatment within the classroom (e.g., labeling, segregation) are then manipulated. For example, teachers and other authority figures might use the social groups to organize school activities over a period of weeks. At the conclusion of the summer school program, children's group and self-views are (re)assessed.

Relatively few studies have used novel group paradigms to examine the links between children's group memberships and their motivation or self-perceived competence. Those studies that do exist indicate mixed results. One of the first studies to examine group-level competency messages was conducted by Yee and Brown (1992), who reported that membership in a novel group affected children's perception of their own competence in the classifying domain, in this case, speed in an egg and spoon race. Children who were placed in the "fast" group rated themselves as significantly faster at racing than children placed in the "slow" group, despite the fact that their assignment to groups was arbitrary. Similarly, Nesdale and Flesser (2001) found that children who were placed in a group of "excellent drawers" rated their own drawing ability significantly higher than children who were placed in a group of "good drawers." These two studies suggest that group membership can positively affect children's views of their own competencies. However, the conclusions that can be drawn from these studies are limited by their designs. In both studies, children had no experience with the novel group, and no information about the group other than the domain-specific classifications. Thus, it is unclear how, for example, being placed in the "excellent drawers" group differs meaningfully from being told that one excels at drawing.

Subsequent novel group research has placed greater emphasis on the role of group membership per se, in addition to group-related competence feedback, in shaping self-conceptions. For example, Master and Walton (2013) posit that associating a group with a particular domain can increase children's motivation and persistence within that domain. In their study, preschool-aged children (4–5 years of age) were assigned to group, individual, or control conditions. In the group condition, children were told that they were members of a social group and that the group was associated with a particular domain (i.e., "The blue group does puzzles"; Master & Walton, 2013, p. 740). Children assigned to the group condition persisted significantly longer on the task (i.e., spent more time working on a challenging jigsaw puzzle) compared to children assigned to the control or individual conditions. Master and Walton (2013, Experiment 2) found that this persistence effect was due to the group–domain link, not simply a general positive effect of group membership or belonging. Thus, Master and Walton argued that associating a social group with a domain may serve to promote persistence and motivation for children who are members of that group.

There are several possible explanations for the discrepancy in findings between the work of Master and Walton (2013) and Cimpian and colleagues (Cimpian, 2010; Cimpian & Markman, 2011; Cimpian et al., 2012). The first is that the language used in making group–domain associations was meaningfully different across the studies; that is, the language used by Master and Walton was merely associative (i.e., "The blue group does puzzles"), whereas the language used by Cimpian and colleagues (2012) was both associative and evaluative (i.e., "Girls are good at this game"). It is possible that it is the evaluative nature of the group–domain association used by Cimpian and colleagues promoted a fixed view of ability in that domain, which in turn negatively impacted motivation and persistence.

An alternative possibility has to do with the nature of the groups used in these studies. Master and Walton (2013) used an experimentally created novel group, whereas Cimpian and colleagues (2012) used an established social category (i.e., gender). Children may be more likely to generalize from group to self with established groups than with novel groups (see Robbins & Krueger, 2005; van Veelen, Otten, Cadinu, & Hansen, 2016). Individuals may be more inclined to view established social categories as having stable, innate qualities than to view experimentally created groups as having such characteristics. Cimpian and Markman (2011) addressed this possibility in their research and found that, indeed, children are more likely to generalize about characteristics that refer to broad social categories (e.g., boys and girls in general) rather than narrower social categories (e.g., boys and girls within a particular school).

Patterson and her colleagues (Patterson & Bigler, 2011; Patterson, Bigler, & Swann, 2010) conducted two studies examining the ways in which children coordinate information about self- and group competencies, with a particular interest in instances in which self- and group competencies are in conflict (e.g., "I am good at math, but my group is not"). In both studies, participants were students attending a summer school program and assigned to novel groups within the context of this program. All students wore colored T-shirts to indicate their group membership, and teachers used the novel color groups to label students and organize the classroom environment.

The first study (Patterson et al., 2010) examined the impact of assignments to novel groups that were portrayed as excelling in either academics or athletics. Messages about group competence were conveyed through classroom posters, a means of presenting information about group characteristics that had been shown to be effective in earlier novel group studies (see Bigler et al., 2001; Brown & Bigler, 2002). For example, in a classroom containing red and blue group members, the red group would be depicted as winning all the academic contests (e.g., spelling bees and math contests), whereas the blue group would be depicted as winning all the athletic contests.

Participants' views of the academic and athletic capabilities of the experimental groups were examined both before and after the poster manipulation. Results showed that prior to having been exposed to the posters, children projected their personal identities onto their ingroups (e.g., students who viewed themselves as more competent in the athletic domain also viewed their ingroup as more competent in the athletic domain). There was little evidence for the inverse effect: Messages about group competence had no significant effect on children's self-views in either academic or athletic domains.

One limitation of Patterson and colleagues' (2010) study was that children held established self-views in the relevant domains (academics and athletics) prior to entering the study. Under these conditions, it may be unsurprising that exposure to experimentally manipulated feedback about group performance did little to shift students' self-perceptions. To explore this possibility, Patterson and Bigler (2011) conducted a follow-up study that examined the effects of personal and group feedback on a series of novel tasks (described as "puzzles"). Over the course of the summer school program, children completed three novel tasks and received feedback about their personal performance and their ingroup's performance. Feedback varied across participants in two ways. First, valence of feedback varied: Performance was described as either "excellent" or "OK." Second, consistency of feedback varied: Valence of feedback was either consistent for the individual child and the child's ingroup or it was inconsistent. Thus, in the consistent feedback conditions, children were told that their own performance and their ingroup's performance were either both "excellent" or both "OK." In the inconsistent feedback conditions, the performance of the two targets (individual child and the child's ingroup) were unmatched (i.e., one was said to be "excellent" and the other "OK"). Children completed a battery of measures concerning their views of (1) the novel tasks, (2) the self, and (3) the novel groups. Overall, results indicated few effects of condition (i.e., whether newly acquired views concerning the self and ingroup were consistent or inconsistent). For example, participants who were told that they excelled at the novel task indicated greater engagement with the task than participants who were told that they were mediocre at the task, regardless of whether the children believed their ingroup excelled (or not) at the task. In other words, children showed little in the way of a tendency to integrate information about the self and the group.

It is obviously impossible to draw firm conclusions about the reciprocal causal relations between social group membership on the one hand, and children's motivations and competencies on the other, from these few novel group studies. A few tentative conclusions seem possible, however. First, conceptions of social groups and the self (i.e., identities, attitudes, and self-concepts) may be more independent in children than they are in adults. It is likely that children's developing cognitive skills affect the degree to which their views of social groups and the self are causally related. Liben and Bigler (2002) posited that children's limited logical reasoning and classification skills allow for

inconsistencies in their beliefs concerning identities, attitudes, and self-concepts. For example, Nosek and colleagues (2002) published an article titled, "Math = Male, Me = Female, Therefore Math ≠ Me." Given that young children typically fail to adhere to demands of such logical operations (Piaget, 1970), they may be able to hold inconsistent beliefs about gender (e.g., a girl may believe that math is for boys, that she is a girl, and that math is for her). It is also possible, however, that greater independence of the self- and group views during childhood is a product of greater measurement variability among children than adults (see Liben & Bigler, 2002).

Second, individual, as well as developmental, differences are likely to moderate the degree to which children, first, internalize (attend to and personally endorse) messages about social groups and the self that are present within the environment, and second, adjust the associations among identities, attitudes, and the self-concept in response to such information. With respect to the former, previous research indicates that children frequently distort new information to be consistent with their existing attitudes (Bigler & Liben, 1993; Liben & Signorella, 1980). Children's beliefs about the malleability versus fixity of individual characteristics may also impact their willingness to stereotype individuals or groups (Levy & Dweck, 1999).

As outlined by Liben and Bigler (2002) and Greenwald and colleagues (2002), children may vary in how much they prioritize group membership (i.e., "schematicity") or how much they consider themselves to be a typical group member. Feelings of ingroup typicality may moderate the process of applying group-relevant beliefs or stereotypes to the self (Greenwald et al., 2002; Patterson, 2012; Tobin et al., 2010). In addition, individuals' inclination to conform to others (Ryan, 2001) and their desire for high status (Newheiser, Dunham, Merrill, Hoosain, & Olson, 2014) may moderate the influence of group–attribute associations on a given child's motivation in a particular domain. For example, upon learning that girls are viewed as less talented than boys at math, girls who are high (but not low) in conformity would be expected to view themselves as less competent at math. Additionally, girls who are low in gender typicality or high in status seeking might be more inclined than their peers to distance themselves from their gender group in response to this negative stereotype.

PRACTICAL IMPLICATIONS AND CONTENTIOUS ISSUES

What practical policy implications arise from the notion that social group memberships and individuals' motivations and competences are sometimes causally related? Potential answers to this question raise a host of difficult issues. We highlight two such issues that have been contentious aspects of our own work. The first concerns conflicting views of whether social group membership and social group differences are viewed as beneficial to society or individuals. The second concerns conflicting views of whether interventions that seek to minimize the constraints of social group membership on individuals' outcomes should explicitly acknowledge and address the role of social groups in the domain.

"Viva la Différence" or "Vanquish la Différence"?

Individuals vary in the degree to which they view social group memberships generally—and various social groups in particular (e.g., race, class, caste, religion)—as exerting beneficial effects on development. In the case of gender, for example, there are individuals who feel that the establishment and maintenance of differing areas of accomplishment for males and females promotes societal stability and individual well-being (for discussion of the prevalence of such views, see Bastian & Haslam, 2006; Crompton & Lyonette, 2005; Liben, 2006, 2015, 2016). Such a stance might lead one to promote children's attention to particular social groups, knowledge of particular social groups, their development of a sense of self that is linked to particular social group memberships (e.g., strengthen gender identity), and others' use of a particular social group as a basis of treatment (e.g., encouraging parents and

teachers to provide girls and boys differing opportunities for skill development).

Some theorists, in contrast, view social group memberships as carrying more negative than positive consequences. For example, some theorists have argued that gender differences are largely socially constructed, and that a decreased emphasis on gender would promote optimal human development (Liben & Bigler, 2015). Bem (1993) proposed "a utopia in which gender polarization . . . has been so completely dismantled that—except in narrowly biological contexts like reproduction—the distinction between male and female no longer organizes either the culture or the psyche" (p. 192). Bem's views influenced and are supported by later researchers who found that increasing the environmental salience of social categories promoted stereotype endorsement and intergroup bias (e.g., Bigler, 1995; Hilliard & Liben, 2010).

In previous work, Liben and Bigler (2015) and Patterson and Bigler (2007) argued that the best practice for teachers and others who wish to facilitate motivation among students is to avoid associating social groups with particular domains. We stand by this recommendation. We believe that the preponderance of evidence suggests that emphasizing social groups within educational contexts has more negative than positive impacts on children's attitudes and motivation. Most notably, routine emphasis on social group membership is likely to lead to increased intergroup bias among students (see Bigler & Liben, 2007; Liben & Coyle, 2014; Patterson & Bigler, 2006). There is also the potential that emphasizing group–domain links promotes a fixed view of intelligence, which in turn can undermine academic motivation and achievement, as well as promote stereotyping (see Cimpian, 2010; Cimpian et al., 2012; Levy & Dweck, 1999).

Group-Blind versus Group-Conscious Policies?

If one accepts the position that social group memberships sometimes negatively constrain children's developmental outcomes, one might wish to intervene to disassociate children's thinking about their social group membership on the one hand, and their self-views on the other. Rather than detailing the many ways in which researchers have sought to do so, we note one controversial feature of intervention approaches. Some approaches engage the mechanisms that link groups to the self without explicitly acknowledging the existence of actual or perceived social group differences. Many belongingness interventions operate by making individuals feel more included, without acknowledging social group membership (Walton & Cohen, 2011; Yeager & Walton, 2011). One example comes from a program designed by the University of Texas (UT) in an effort to reduce racial and class disparities in graduation rates. The program, called the University Leadership Network (ULN), targets students who are statistically unlikely to graduate on time (based on a calculation tool called "Dashboard" that makes use of indicators such as family income and parents' educational background). The program provides participants with small classes, tutoring, mentoring, and activities intended to create leadership skills (Tough, 2014). Although the program has seen some success in closing the gap in graduation rates, it does not explicitly engage students in a discussion of group differences. Rather, the program deliberately downplays the students' membership in an "at-risk" group and does not reveal the (true) reason for their selection. In a piece published in the *New York Times,* Tough (2014) noted:

> Perhaps the most striking fact about the success programs is that the selection criteria are never disclosed to students. "From a numbers perspective, the students in these programs are all in the bottom quartile," Laude [UT Senior Vice Provost for Enrollment and Graduation Management] explained. "But here's the key— none of them know that they're in the bottom quartile." The first rule of the Dashboard, in other words, is that you never talk about the Dashboard. (p. 31)

Other intervention programs, in contrast, explicitly address the role of social groups in shaping individuals' outcomes. Some such programs aim to increase youths' consciousness of, and knowledge about, the links between social group memberships and individuals' outcomes. For example, Pahlke, Bigler, and Green (2010) examined the effects of learning about the role of gender discrimination in the careers of female historical figures (e.g., Sandra Day O'Connor) on adolescents' gender attitudes and occupational goals. In the study, adolescents were randomly assigned to receive either standard biographical lessons about historical figures (control condition) or nearly identical lessons that included information about the gender discrimination experienced by the female figures (discrimination condition). Pahlke and colleagues reported that girls who received the discrimination lesson were more likely to detect gender discrimination, and expressed greater commitment to working to end gender discrimination, than those girls who received standard lessons. Adolescents' occupational aspirations were unaffected by either type of lesson.

Although awareness and detection of discrimination and prejudice are not harmless (see Bigler & Wright, 2014), the advantage of group-conscious interventions, in our view, is that they frame the target problem (e.g., the racial gap in achievement, the class gap in graduation rates, the gender gap in STEM) not only as personal challenges to be overcome, but also as societal-level problems that are often systematically produced by institutional and interpersonal forces that include discrimination. In other words, youth who are ignorant of the fact that they are a member of a social group that has been, and—without societal change—will continue to be, undermotivated or underachieving within some domain will be unlikely to contest the situational forces (e.g., discrimination, segregation) that contribute to social group differences. Similarly, youth who are members of high-status groups and ignorant about the systematic privileges afforded them on the basis of their group membership are unlikely to work for social justice and equality.

FUTURE DIRECTIONS AND CONCLUSION

There is a great deal left to learn about the role of social group membership in shaping children's motivations and competencies, and the reciprocal role of children's motivations and competencies in shaping their conceptions of social groups. Each of the core concerns of constructivist theorists (e.g., children's conceptions of themselves, their ingroups and outgroups, and themselves as members of social groups) requires additional study. Among the remaining challenges is the need to better understand why some children but not others develop a strong, stable tendency to think of themselves as members of particular social groups (e.g., develop high gender salience or racial centrality). Also understudied are children's conceptions of the basis for social groups (e.g., the properties that lead one to belong to one or another group) and the consequences of such views for their attitudes, preferences, and behavior.

Answers to questions about the relations of children's self- and group views are likely to have important policy implications. Consider, for example, children who perceive themselves to be atypical of their gender. Should such children be encouraged to alter the self to conform to their views of the genders, either by changing their group membership (e.g., sex/gender reassignment) or by changing their personal interests and preferences? Or should children be encouraged to alter their views of social groups? Furthermore, how best might such changes be facilitated? Developmentalists have the additional challenge of documenting the exogenous and endogenous factors that influence changes over time in children's views of the self, ingroups, and their intersection.

In summary, an important challenge for developmentalists is to expand our knowledge of the mechanisms via which self and group identities influence each other, and to produce an integrated account of the dynamic processes by which individuals' motivations and competencies emerge and change over the lifespan. To do so, it will be important to integrate the relevant intergroup theories and data from both the social and developmental psychology literatures and to devise methodologies capable of detecting bidirectional causal effects. We suggest that novel group paradigms may be useful in this regard. Finally, persons intent upon identifying the applications of intergroup research findings will need to grapple with the values that underlie individuals' views of social groups to design home, school, and work settings that maximize all youths' skills, abilities, and well-being.

REFERENCES

Abrams, D., Rutland, A., Ferrell, J. M., & Pelletier, J. (2008). Children's judgments of disloyal and immoral peer behavior: Subjective group dynamics in minimal intergroup contexts. *Child Development, 79,* 444–461.

Bandura, A. (1977). *Social learning theory.* Englewood Cliffs, NJ: Prentice Hall.

Bastian, B., & Haslam, N. (2006). Psychological essentialism and stereotype endorsement. *Journal of Experimental Social Psychology, 42,* 228–235.

Baumeister, R. F., & Leary, M. R. (1995). The need to belong: Desire for interpersonal attachments as a fundamental human motivation. *Psychological Bulletin, 117,* 497–529.

Beilock, S. L., Gunderson, E. A., Ramirez, G., & Levine, S. C. (2010). Female teachers' math anxiety affects girls' math achievement. *Proceedings of the National Academy of Sciences USA, 107,* 1860–1863.

Bem, S. L. (1981). Gender schema theory: A cognitive account of sex typing. *Psychological Review, 88,* 354–364.

Bem, S. L. (1993). *The lenses of gender: Transforming the debate on sexual inequality.* New Haven, CT: Yale University Press.

Bigler, R. S. (1995). The role of classification skill in moderating environmental influences on children's gender stereotyping: A study of the functional use of gender in the classroom. *Child Development, 66,* 1072–1087.

Bigler, R. S., Brown, C. S., & Markell, M. (2001). When groups are not created equal: Effects of group status on the formation of intergroup attitudes in children. *Child Development, 63,* 1351–1363.

Bigler, R. S., Jones, L. C., & Lobliner, D. B. (1997). Social categorization and the formation of intergroup attitudes in children. *Child Development, 68,* 530–543.

Bigler, R. S., & Liben, L. S. (1990). The role of attitudes and intervention in gender-schematic processing. *Child Development, 61,* 1440–1452.

Bigler, R. S., & Liben, L. S. (1993). A cognitive-developmental approach to racial stereotyping and reconstructive memory in Euro-American children. *Child Development, 64,* 1507–1518.

Bigler, R. S., & Liben, L. S. (2007). Developmental intergroup theory: Explaining and reducing children's social stereotyping and prejudice. *Current Directions in Psychological Science, 16,* 162–171.

Bigler, R. S., & Wright, Y. F. (2014). Reading, writing, arithmetic, and racism?: Risks and benefits to teaching children about intergroup biases. *Child Development Perspectives, 8,* 18–23.

Bingham, T. A. (1908). Foreign criminals in New York. *North American Review, 188*, 383–394.

Blakemore, J. E. O., Berenbaum, S. A., & Liben, L. S. (2009). *Gender development*. New York: Taylor & Francis.

Brown, C. S., & Bigler, R. S. (2002). Effects of minority status in the classroom on children's intergroup attitudes. *Journal of Experimental Child Psychology, 83*, 77–110.

Burnette, J. L., O'Boyle, E. H., VanEpps, E. M., Pollack, J. M., & Finkel, E. J. (2013). Mindsets matter: A meta-analytic review of implicit theories and self-regulation. *Psychological Bulletin, 139*, 655–701.

Butler, R. (2014). Motivation in educational contexts: Does gender matter? In L. S. Liben & R. S. Bigler (Eds.), *Advances in child development and behavior: Vol. 47. The role of gender in educational contexts and outcomes* (pp. 1–41). San Diego, CA: Elsevier.

Cadinu, M. R., & Rothbart, M. (1996). Self-anchoring and differentiation processes in the minimal group setting. *Journal of Personality and Social Psychology, 70*, 661–677.

Ceci, S. J., Williams, W. M., & Barnett, S. M. (2009). Women's underrepresentation in science: Sociocultural and biological considerations. *Psychological Bulletin, 135*, 218–261.

Cho, J. C., & Knowles, E. D. (2013). I'm like you and you're like me: Social projections and self-stereotyping both help explain self-other correspondence. *Journal of Personality and Social Psychology, 104*, 444–456.

Cimpian, A. (2010). The impact of generic language about ability on children's achievement motivation. *Developmental Psychology, 46*, 1333–1340.

Cimpian, A., & Markman, E. M. (2011). The generic/nongeneric distinction influences how children interpret new information about social others. *Child Development, 82*, 471–492.

Cimpian, A., Mu, Y., & Erickson, L. C. (2012). Who is good at this game?: Linking an activity to a social category undermines children's achievement. *Psychological Science, 23*, 533–541.

Crompton, R., & Lyonette, C. (2005). The new gender essentialism–domestic and family "choices" and their relation to attitudes. *British Journal of Sociology, 56*, 601–620.

Davenport, C. B. (1911). *Heredity in relation to eugenics*. New York: Holt.

Deaux, K., Reid, A., Mizrahi, K., & Ethier, K. (1995). Parameters of social identity. *Journal of Personality and Social Psychology, 68*, 280–291.

Denmark, F., & Paludi, M. (Eds.). (2007). *Psychology of women: A handbook of issues and theories* (2nd ed.). Westport, CT: Praeger.

Diener, E., & Biswas-Diener, R. (2002). Will money increase subjective well-being? *Social Indicators Research, 57*, 119–169.

Dunham, Y., Baron, A. S., & Carey, S. (2011). Consequences of "minimal" group affiliations in children. *Child Development, 82*, 793–811.

Dunham, Y., & Emory, J. (2014). Of affect and ambiguity: The emergence of preference for arbitrary ingroups. *Journal of Social Issues, 70*, 81–98.

Dunning, D. (2003). The relation of self to social perception. In M. R. Leary & J. P. Tangney (Eds.), *Handbook of self and identity* (pp. 421–441). New York: Guilford Press.

Dweck, C. S. (2000). *Self-theories: Their role in motivation, personality, and development*. London: Psychology Press.

Engelmann, J. M., Over, H., Herrmann, E., & Tomasello, M. (2013). Young children care more about their reputation with ingroup members and potential reciprocators. *Developmental Science, 16*, 952–958.

Good, C., Rattan, A., & Dweck, C. S. (2012). Why do women opt out?: Sense of belonging and women's representation in mathematics. *Journal of Personality and Social Psychology, 102*, 700–717.

Greenwald, A. G., Banaji, M. R., Rudman, L. A., Farnham, S. D., Nosek, B. A., & Mellott, D. S. (2002). A unified theory of implicit attitudes, stereotypes, self-esteem, and self-concept. *Psychological Review, 109*, 3–25.

Gurian, M. (2001). *Boys and girls learn differently: A guide for teachers and parents*. San Francisco: Jossey-Bass.

Hagerty, M. R. (2000). Social comparisons of income in one's community: Evidence from national surveys of income and happiness. *Journal of Personality and Social Psychology, 78*, 764–771.

Hayes, A. R. (2014). *Transparent versus opaque explanations for social groups and the development of intergroup attitudes and behaviors*. Unpublished doctoral dissertation, University of Texas at Austin, TX.

Hernstein, R. J., & Murray, C. (2010). *Bell curve: Intelligence and class structure in American life*. New York: Simon & Schuster.

Hilliard, L. J., & Liben, L. S. (2010). Differing levels of gender salience in preschool classrooms: Effects on children's gender attitudes and intergroup bias. *Child Development, 81*, 1787–1798.

Hughes, J. M., & Bigler, R. S. (2007). The impact of race on children's occupational aspirations.

In S. M. Quintana & C. McKown (Eds.), *The handbook of race, racism, and the developing child* (pp. 397–423). Hoboken, NJ: Wiley.

Hyde, W. D. (1906). *The college man and the college woman*. Boston: Houghton Mifflin.

Jenuwein, T., & Allis, C. D. (2001). Translating the histone code. *Science, 29,* 1074–1080.

Jussim, L., Cain, T. R., Crawford, J. T., Harber, K., & Cohen, F. (2009). The unbearable accuracy of stereotypes. In T. D. Nelson (Ed.), *Handbook of prejudice, stereotyping, and discrimination* (pp. 199–227). New York: Psychology Press.

Kagan, J. (1964). The child's sex role classification of school objects. *Child Development, 35,* 1051–1056.

Kohlberg, L. A. (1966). A cognitive-developmental analysis of children's sex role concepts and attitudes. In E. E. Maccoby (Ed.), *The development of sex differences* (pp. 82–173). Stanford, CA: Stanford University Press.

Krueger, J. I. (2007). From social projection to social behavior. *European Review of Social Psychology, 18,* 1–35.

Kuzawa, C. W., & Sweet, E. (2009). Epigenetics and the embodiment of race: Developmental origins of US racial disparities in cardiovascular health. *American Journal of Human Biology, 21,* 2–15.

Lamb, L., Bigler, R. S., Liben, L. S., & Green, V. A. (2009). Teaching children to confront peers' sexist remarks: Implications for theories of gender development and educational practice. *Sex Roles, 61,* 361–382.

Lent, R. W., Brown, S. D., & Hackett, G. (1994). Toward a unifying social cognitive theory of career and academic interest, choice, and performance. *Journal of Vocational Behavior, 45,* 79–122.

Levy, S. R., & Dweck, C. S. (1999). The impact of children's static versus dynamic conceptions of people on stereotype formation. *Child Development, 70,* 1163–1180.

Liben, L. S. (2006, April). *"Viva la différence" or "vanquish la différence"?: Setting the historical and political context for debating gender interventions*. Paper presented at the Plenary Symposium at the Gender Development Conference, San Francisco, CA.

Liben, L. S. (2014). The individual ↔ context nexus in developmental intergroup theory: Within and beyond the ivory tower. *Research in Human Development, 11,* 273–290.

Liben, L. S. (2015). Probability values and human values in evaluating single-sex education. *Sex Roles, 72,* 401–426.

Liben, L. S. (2016). We've come a long way, baby (but we're not there yet): Gender past, present, and future. *Child Development, 87,* 5–28.

Liben, L. S., & Bigler, R. S. (2002). The developmental course of gender differentiation: Conceptualizing, measuring, and evaluating constructs and pathways. *Monographs of the Society for Research in Child Development, 67*(2, Serial No. 269), i–viii, 1–147, discussion 148–183.

Liben, L. S., & Bigler, R. S. (2006). A developmental intergroup theory of social stereotypes and prejudice. In R. Kail (Ed.), *Advances in child development and behavior* (Vol. 34, pp. 40–89). San Diego, CA: Academic Press.

Liben, L. S., & Bigler, R. S. (2015). Understanding and undermining the development of gender dichotomies: The legacy of Sandra Lipsitz Bem. *Sex Roles*. [Epub ahead of print]

Liben, L. S., & Coyle, E. J. (2014). Developmental interventions to address the STEM gender gap: Exploring intended and unintended consequences. In L. S. Liben & R. S. Bigler (Eds.), *Advances in child development and behavior: Vol. 47. The role of gender in educational contexts and outcomes* (pp. 77–115). San Diego, CA: Elsevier.

Liben, L. S., & Hilliard, L. J. (2010, April). *Preschoolers' gender vigilance: Effects of classroom organization*. Poster presented at the Gender Development Research Conference, San Francisco, CA.

Liben, L. S., & Signorella, M. L. (1980). Gender-related schemata and constructive memory in children. *Child Development, 51,* 11–18.

Marmot, M. G., Fuhrer, R., Ettner, S. L., Marks, N. F., Bumpass, L. L., & Ryff, C. D. (1998). Contribution of psychosocial factors to socioeconomic differences in health. *Milbank Quarterly, 76,* 403–448.

Martin, C. L., & Dinella, L. M. (2012). Congruence between gender stereotypes and activity preference in self-identified tomboys and nontomboys. *Archives of Sexual Behavior, 41,* 599–610.

Martin, C. L., Eisenbud, L., & Rose, H. (1995). Children's gender-based reasoning about toys. *Child Development, 66,* 1453–1471.

Martin, C. L., & Halverson, C. F. (1981). A schematic professing model of sex typing and stereotyping in children. *Child Development, 52,* 1119–1134.

Master, A., & Walton, G. M. (2013). Minimal groups increase young children's motivation and learning on group-relevant tasks. *Child Development, 84,* 737–751.

McLoyd, V. (1998). Socioeconomic disadvantage and child development. *American Psychologist, 53,* 185–204.

Messick, D. M., & Mackie, D. M. (1989). Intergroup relations. *Annual Review of Psychology, 40*, 45–81.

Misch, A., Over, H., & Carpenter, M. (2014). Stick with your group: Young children's attitudes about group loyalty. *Journal of Experimental Child Psychology, 126*, 19–36.

Moè, A. (2009). Are males always better than females in mental rotation?: Exploring a gender belief explanation. *Learning and Individual Differences, 19*, 21–27.

Myers, D. G. (2000). The funds, friends, and faith of happy people. *American Psychologist, 55*, 56–67.

Nesdale, D., & Flesser, D. (2001). Social identity and the development of children's group attitudes. *Child Development, 72*, 506–517.

Neville, H., Tynes, B. M., & Utsey, S. O. (Eds.). (2009). *Handbook of African American psychology.* Thousand Oaks, CA: Sage.

Newheiser, A.-K., Dunham, Y., Merrill, A., Hoosain, L., & Olson, K. R. (2014). Preference for high status predicts implicit outgroup bias among children from low-status groups. *Developmental Psychology, 50*, 1081–1090.

Nosek, B., Banaji, M. R., & Greenwald, A. G. (2002). Math = male, me = female, therefore math ≠ me. *Journal of Personality and Social Psychology, 83*, 44–59.

Ogbu, J. U., & Simmons, H. D. (1998). Voluntary and involuntary minorities: A cultural–ecological theory of school performance with some implications for education. *Anthropology and Education Quarterly, 29*, 155–188.

Olson, K. R., & Dweck, C. S. (2008). A blueprint for social cognitive development. *Perspectives on Psychological Science, 3*, 193–202.

Ostrove, J. M., Adler, N. E., Kuppermann, M., & Washington, A. E. (2000). Objective and subjective assessments of socioeconomic status and their relationship to self-rated health in an ethnically diverse sample of pregnant women. *Health Psychology, 19*, 613–618.

Pahlke, E., Bigler, R. S., & Green, V. A. (2010). Effects of learning about historical gender discrimination on early adolescents' occupational judgments and aspirations. *Journal of Early Adolescence, 30*, 854–894.

Pahlke, E. E., Bigler, R. S., & Suizzo, M. A. (2012). Relations between colorblind socialization and children's racial bias: Evidence from European American mothers and their preschool children. *Child Development, 83*, 1164–1179.

Pajares, F., & Valiante, G. (2001). Gender differences in writing motivation and achievement of middle school students: A function of gender orientation? *Contemporary Educational Psychology, 26*, 366–381.

Patterson, M. M. (2012). Self-perceived gender typicality, gender-typed attributes, and gender stereotype endorsement in elementary-school-aged children. *Sex Roles, 67*, 422–434.

Patterson, M. M., & Bigler, R. S. (2006). Preschool children's attention to environmental messages about groups: Social categorization and the origins of intergroup bias. *Child Development, 77*, 847–860.

Patterson, M. M., & Bigler, R. S. (2007). Relations among social identities, intergroup attitudes, and schooling: Perspectives from intergroup theory and research. In A. Fuligni (Ed.), *Contesting stereotypes and creating identities: Social categories, social identities and educational participation* (pp. 66–87). New York: Russell Sage Foundation.

Patterson, M. M., & Bigler, R. S. (2011, April). *Negotiating (non) normality: Effects of consistency of feedback regarding the self and the social group.* Poster presented at the biennial meeting of the Society for Research in Child Development, Montreal, Canada.

Patterson, M. M., Bigler, R. S., & Swann, W. B. (2010). When personal identities confirm versus conflict with group identities: Evidence from an intergroup paradigm. *European Journal of Social Psychology, 40*, 652–670.

Piaget, J. (1970). Piaget's theory. In P. H. Mussen (Ed.), *Carmichael's manual of child psychology* (pp. 703–732). New York: Wiley.

Plötner, M., Over, H., Carpenter, M., & Tomasello, M. (2015). The effects of collaboration and minimal-group membership on children's prosocial behavior, liking, affiliation, and trust. *Journal of Experimental Child Psychology, 139*, 161–173.

Poteat, V. P., Scheer, J. R., & Mereish, E. H. (2014). Factors affecting academic achievement among sexual minority and gender-variant youth. *Advances in Child Development and Behavior, 47*, 225–260.

Quintana, S. M., Aboud, F. E., Chao, R. K., Contreras-Grau, J., Cross, W. E., Hudley, C., et al. (2006). Race, ethnicity, and culture in child development: Contemporary research and future directions. *Child Development, 77*, 1129–1141.

Robbins, J. M., & Krueger, J. I. (2005). Social projection to ingroups and outgroups: A review and meta-analysis. *Personality and Social Psychology Review, 9*, 32–47.

Robinson-Cimpian, J. P., Lubienski, S. T., Ganley, C. M., & Copur-Gencturk, Y. (2014). Teachers' perceptions of students' mathematics proficiency may exacerbate early gender gaps in achievement. *Developmental Psychology, 50*, 1262–1281.

Rushton, J. P., & Jensen, A. R. (2005). Thirty

years of research on race differences in cognitive ability. *Psychology, Public Policy, and Law, 11,* 235–294.

Ryan, A. M. (2001). The peer group as a context for the development of young adolescent motivation and achievement. *Child Development, 72,* 1135–1150.

Sax, L. (2005). *Why gender matters.* New York: Doubleday.

Sherif, M., Harvey, O. J., White, B. J., Hood, W. R., & Sherif, C. W. (1961). *Intergroup conflict and cooperation: The Robbers Cave experiment.* Norman, OK: University Book Exchange.

Skinner, B. F. (1938). *The behavior of organisms: An experimental analysis.* Oxford, UK: Appleton-Century.

Stone, J., Lynch, C., Sjomeling, M., & Darley, J. M. (1999). Stereotype threat effects on Black and White athletic performance. *Journal of Personality and Social Psychology, 77,* 1213–1227.

Sullivan, S. (2013). Inheriting racist disparities in health: Epigenetics and the transgenerational effects of white racism. *Critical Philosophy of Race, 1,* 190–218.

Tajfel, H. (1970). Experiments in intergroup discrimination. *Scientific American, 223,* 96–102.

Tajfel, H., & Turner, J. C. (1986). The social identity theory of intergroup behavior. In S. Worschel & W. G. Austin (Eds.), *The social psychology of intergroup relations* (pp. 7–24). Chicago: Nelson-Hall.

Tenenbaum, H. R., & Leaper, C. (2003). Parent–child conversations about science: The socialization of gender inequities? *Developmental Psychology, 39,* 34–47.

Tobin, D. D., Menon, M., Menon, M., Spatta, B. C., Hodges, E. V., & Perry, D. G. (2010). The intrapsychics of gender: A model of self-socialization. *Psychological Review, 117,* 601–622.

Tough, P. (2014, May 18). Who gets to graduate? Retrieved from *www.nytimes.com/2014/05/18/magazine/who-gets-to-graduate.html?_r=0.*

van Veelen, R., Otten, S., Cadinu, M., & Hansen, N. (2016). An integrative model of social identification: Self-stereotyping and self-anchoring as two cognitive pathways. *Personality and Social Psychology Review, 20,* 3–26.

Walton, G. M., & Cohen, G. L. (2011). A brief social-belonging intervention improves academic and health outcomes among minority students. *Science, 331,* 1447–1451.

Weisgram, E. S., & Bigler, R. S. (2006). The role of attitudes and intervention in high school girls' interest in computer science. *Journal of Women and Minorities in Science and Engineering, 12,* 325–336.

Wigfield, A., & Eccles, J. S. (2000). Expectancy–value theory of achievement motivation. *Contemporary Educational Psychology, 25,* 68–81.

Williams, D. R., Yu, Y., Jackson, J. S., & Anderson, N. B. (1997). Racial differences in physical and mental health socio-economic status, stress and discrimination. *Journal of Health Psychology, 2,* 335–351.

Yeager, D. S., & Dweck, C. S. (2012). Mindsets that promote resilience: When students believe that personal characteristics can be developed. *Educational Psychologist, 47,* 302–314.

Yeager, D. S., & Walton, G. M. (2011). Social-psychological interventions in education: They're not magic. *Review of Educational Research, 81,* 267–301.

Yee, M. D., & Brown, R. (1992). Self-evaluation and intergroup attitudes in children aged three to nine. *Child Development, 63,* 619–629.

CHAPTER 30

The Role of Parenting in Children's Motivation and Competence
What Underlies Facilitative Parenting?

EVA M. POMERANTZ
WENDY S. GROLNICK

As American children's achievement in critical areas such as math and literacy falls behind that of their counterparts in other industrialized nations (e.g., Program for International Student Assessment [PISA], 2013), there has been much concern in the United States with how to promote children's learning. To this end, major efforts have been made to understand what can be done on the school front to enhance children's motivation, so that children are effectively engaged in school and, ultimately, develop optimal competence. In this vein, considerable attention has been directed to the classroom environment created by teachers (for a review, see Pianta, Hamre, & Allen, 2012). Although such efforts are essential, fully facilitating children's motivation and competence requires understanding how to support children's learning on the home front as well. Indeed, efforts to foster children's motivation and competence are unlikely to be successful if they fail to include parents.

It is clear that parents contribute to children's motivation and competence in school through their involvement in children's learning (for reviews, see Grolnick, 2016; Pomerantz, Kim, & Cheung, 2012). Consequently, much recent research has been directed at elucidating what shapes parents' involvement given the significance of this issue in designing interventions to optimize children's learning via parents. In this chapter, we begin with an overview of how parents can facilitate or undermine children's motivation and competence. Second, we review the burgeoning theory and research on what drives the quantity and quality of parents' involvement in children's learning. Third, we discuss interventions to enhance parenting that supports children's motivation and competence, with particular attention to the importance of using knowledge about what drives parents' involvement.

HOW DO PARENTS FACILITATE CHILDREN'S MOTIVATION AND COMPETENCE?

Motivational frameworks have guided much of the research on parents' involvement in children's learning. In this vein, Grolnick, Deci, and Ryan (1997) drew on self-determination theory (e.g., Deci & Ryan, 1985) to make the case that parents can set the foundation for children's success in school by supporting children in building the motivational resources necessary for the development of competence. According to self-determination theory, humans have basic psychological needs for competence, autonomy, and relatedness. Fulfillment of these needs allows for the development of motivational resources related to competence (i.e., perceptions of competence and control), autonomy (i.e., experiences of self-determination) and relatedness (i.e., feeling of connectedness to significant others). Grolnick and colleagues (1997) suggest that through their socialization practices (e.g., autonomy support vs. control), parents can either facilitate or undermine children's fulfillment of these needs and therefore children's motivational resources.

Other motivational frameworks focus on parents' role in a variety of different types of motivation (e.g., a concern with developing rather than demonstrating competence) through mechanisms other than need fulfillment (e.g., Gottfried, Fleming, & Gottfried, 1994; Hokoda & Fincham, 1995; Pomerantz, Ng, & Wang, 2006). For example, by emphasizing the process of learning (e.g., effort), parents may lead children to view ability as malleable, thereby fostering a mastery orientation in children, such that children's central concern is with developing their competencies. Conversely, when parents emphasize children's stable attributes (e.g., ability) or performance, they may lead children to develop a performance orientation in which the focus is on demonstrating competencies (e.g., Gunderson et al., 2013; Pomerantz & Kempner, 2013).

In a skills framework in which parents are viewed as directly fostering children's competence (e.g., LeFevre et al., 2009; Senechal & LeFevre, 2002), parents provide a context for children to develop their math and literacy skills via their provision of instruction and exposure to important concepts (for a review, see Rowe, Ramani, & Pomerantz, in press).

Research driven by motivational and skills frameworks repeatedly finds that parents' involvement in children's learning predicts children's achievement (e.g., scores on standardized tests and grades in school) over time, adjusting for a variety of potential confounds (for reviews, see Grolnick, 2016; Pomerantz et al., 2012). Moreover, much evidence points to children's motivation (e.g., autonomous vs. controlled motivation) and skills (e.g., literacy skills) as the mechanisms through which involvement exerts its effects on their achievement (e.g., Cheung & Pomerantz, 2012; Senechal & LeFevre, 2002). However, it is not only the quantity of parents' involvement that matters, but also the quality (Pomerantz, Grolnick, & Price, 2005; Pomerantz, Moorman, & Litwack, 2007). In particular, the benefits of parents' involvement are amplified when it supports children's autonomy rather than intrudes on children, provides children with structure instead of being chaotic, is affectively positive versus negative, and is focused on the process of learning rather than on the stable attributes or performance of the child.

The Quantity of Parents' Involvement in Children's Learning

Although there are a variety of definitions of parents' involvement in children's learning, they all largely reflect Grolnick and Slowiaczek's (1994) idea of parents' commitment to children's academic lives as manifest in parents' time, energy, or other means (e.g., financial). Parents can be involved at school via activities such as attending school events (e.g., open houses or parent–teacher conferences), communicating with teachers about issues relevant to children's learning, and volunteering in the classroom. At home, parents' involvement is often evident in their engaging in learning activities (e.g., reading or math), helping children with homework, and discussing school (e.g., what children are learning or the utility of education). Parents' involvement in children's learning has largely been assessed with parents' and children's retrospective reports, in which they estimate the frequency of a variety of practices reflecting involvement (e.g., Fantuzzo, Tighe, & Childs, 2000; Kohl, Lengua, McMahon, & Conduct Problems Prevention Research Group, 2000). Teachers also serve as reporters (e.g., Kohl et al., 2000), particularly when it comes to involvement at school. Daily assessments, in which parents report on their practices each day for 1–2 weeks, have been used (e.g., Pomerantz, Wang, &

Ng, 2005a; Silinskas, Kiuru, Aunola, Lerkkanen, & Nurmi, 2015), but fairly infrequently (for a discussion of the strengths and weakness of the different types of assessments, see Pomerantz & Monti, 2015).

Parents' involvement in children's learning at school and at home has been argued to benefit children via a variety of mechanisms (for a review, see Pomerantz et al., 2012). For example, drawing from motivational frameworks, parents' involvement emphasizes the value of school to children through parents' commitment of resources to this area (e.g., Cheung & Pomerantz, 2012; Epstein, 1988; Hill et al., 2004). Because parents' involvement often provides support for children in their academic endeavors, parents may also convey to children that they care about them; the ensuing trust and support may foster children's internalization of the value of school, so that children are ultimately more autonomously motivated in the learning context (Cheung & Pomerantz, 2015; Grolnick et al., 1997). Consistent with the skills framework, the instruction and exposure to important concepts that parents' involvement at home provides helps children to develop important skills (e.g., Ramani & Siegler, 2014; Senechal & LeFevre, 2002). Parents' involvement at school may also be beneficial in this vein because it may provide parents with information about what and how children are learning at school, which may enhance parents' involvement at home (e.g., Baker & Stevenson, 1986; Epstein, 1987)—for example, parents may target the skills children are learning at school by quizzing them on relevant math facts.

Quantitative syntheses (i.e., meta-analyses) of studies with concurrent measures of parents' involvement and children's achievement reveal positive associations between a variety of types of parent involvement and children's achievement, with effects in the small to medium range (e.g., Fan & Chen, 2001; Hill & Tyson, 2009; Jeynes, 2003). These associations are not due simply to demographics such as parents' educational attainment (e.g., Jeynes, 2005, 2007). In longitudinal studies, parents' involvement in children's learning predicts children's later motivation and competence, accounting for their earlier motivation and competence (e.g., Izzo, Weissberg, Kasprow,

& Fendrich, 1999; Wang & Sheikh-Khalil, 2014), as well as other potential confounds, such as aspects of parenting that often accompany parents' involvement (e.g., Cheung & Pomerantz, 2011; Steinberg, Lamborn, Dornbusch, & Darling, 1992). Studies using within-person designs also rule out the possibility that the effects are driven by other differences between families (e.g., Dearing, Kreider, Simpkins, & Weiss, 2006). For example, Wang, Hill, and Hofkens (2014) found that when parents' involvement varies from their average level of involvement, children's grades similarly vary.

The effects of parents' assistance with children's homework are less consistent than those of other forms of parents' involvement. Some syntheses of concurrent research yield negative associations between parents' assistance and children's achievement (Hill & Tyson, 2009; Jeynes, 2005). However, in Patall, Cooper, and Robinson's (2008) synthesis, there was a small, albeit significant, positive association, with substantial heterogeneity across studies. Consistent with research on other forms of parents' involvement (e.g., Dearing et al., 2006; Wang & Sheikh-Khalil, 2014), the association was strongest among children from socioeconomically disadvantaged backgrounds. In addition, the association was positive in elementary and high school but negative in middle school (see also Hill & Tyson, 2009), perhaps due to children seeking independence from parents as they enter adolescence, which may lead them to see parents' assistance as intrusive. The heterogeneity may also reflect how and why parents provide assistance. For example, parents appear to increase their assistance with homework when children are having difficulty in school (e.g., Pomerantz et al., 2005a, 2006). Hence, negative associations may reflect child-to-parent influences.

The Quality of Parents' Involvement in Children's Learning

The quality of parents' involvement in children's learning matters, as it may shape the experiences and messages conferred by such involvement (e.g., Pomerantz et al., 2005). Over two decades ago, Steinberg and colleagues (1992) showed that parents' involvement in children's learning during the high school years was more predictive of enhanced subsequent achievement among children with more authoritative (vs. authoritarian) parents. Since then, substantial evidence has accumulated to suggest that the benefits of parents' involvement are amplified when it is characterized by four key qualities: (1) autonomy support (vs. control), (2) structure (vs. chaos), (3) positive (vs. negative) affect, and (4) a focus on the process (vs. person). These qualities satisfy children's needs for competence, autonomy, and relatedness. For example, when parents are involved in a manner supporting children's autonomy, they facilitate children's feelings of self-determination. In addition, involvement that is focused on the process of learning rather than stable attributes of the child may convey to children that ability is malleable, leading them to focus on developing, rather than demonstrating, their competence.

Autonomy-Supportive versus Controlling Involvement

Optimal involvement is autonomy-supportive in that parents provide children with the opportunity to take an active role in solving problems in the learning context and allow, or even encourage, children to take initiative (e.g., Grolnick, Deci, et al., 1997; Grolnick & Pomerantz, 2009). Autonomy-supportive involvement also includes parents taking children's perspectives (e.g., understanding why children may dislike math) and demonstrating their understanding through empathy. Controlling involvement, in contrast, is characterized by parents' attempts to motivate children through commands, directives, love withdrawal, or other methods, without considering children's perspective. A quantitative synthesis of concurrent studies revealed small to medium positive associations between autonomy-supportive parenting and children's motivation and competence (Vasquez, Patall, Fong, Corrigan, & Pine, 2016). Significantly, longitudinal studies find that autonomy-supportive parenting is predictive of enhanced motivation and competence from 6 months to 15 years later, even after adjusting for children's earlier motivation and competence, as well

as other potential confounds, such as parents' educational attainment (e.g., Bindman, Pomerantz, & Roisman, 2015; Wang & Pomerantz, 2009). Moreover, when parents' assistance with children's homework is controlling (e.g., parents sit next to children and immediately correct their mistakes), it has negative effects on children's subsequent motivation and achievement (e.g., Dumont, Trautwein, Nagy, & Nagengast, 2014; Patall et al., 2008).

Structured versus Chaotic Involvement

Structure—that is, parents' organization of the environment so that it facilitates children's competence (Grolnick, Deci, et al., 1997; Grolnick & Pomerantz, 2009)—is a key quality of parent involvement in children's learning as well. Structured involvement includes providing clear and consistent guidelines, expectations, and rules for children in regard to the academic area, with communication of predictable consequences for children's actions (e.g., withdrawal of screen time if children do not complete homework). In contrast, parents' involvement can be chaotic, in that guidelines, expectations, and rules for children are unclear and inconsistent, as well as arbitrary (Skinner, Johnson, & Snyder, 2005). Parents' provision of structure is associated with enhanced motivation and competence among children (e.g., Dumont et al., 2014; Grolnick & Ryan, 1989; Skinner et al., 2005). For example, assessing parents' provision of structure in the academic context with in-depth interviews with children, Grolnick and colleagues (2014) found that parents' structure when children were in sixth grade predicted children's perceptions of their competence, engagement, and grades when in seventh grade, adjusting for children's motivation and performance in sixth grade. Children's perceptions of their competence in school mediated the effect of parents' structure on children's grades.

Affectively Positive versus Negative Involvement

As Dix (1991) emphasized, parenting is an inherently affective endeavor. This may be particularly true of parents' involvement in children's learning given that it may be an opportunity for connection between parents and children. Unfortunately, parents' interactions with children may sometimes be characterized by negative affect because children often experience distress and frustration in the context of academic activities such as homework (e.g., Leone & Richards, 1989), leading parents to become irritated and even critical (Pomerantz et al., 2005a; Silinskas et al., 2015). Several studies support the idea that parents' affect in the context of their involvement matters for children's motivation and competence (e.g., Hokoda & Fincham, 1995; Nolen-Hoeksema, Wolfson, Mumme, & Guskin, 1995). For example, when mothers have a difficult time regulating their affect when assisting children with homework, such that they display dampened positive and heightened negative affect, children's motivation suffers over time (Pomerantz et al., 2005a).

Person- versus Process-Focused Involvement

Parents' focus on the process of learning, rather than children's stable attributes or performance, is also an important quality of their involvement in children's learning (e.g., Gottfried et al., 1994; Hokoda & Fincham, 1995; Pomerantz et al., 2006). A process focus emphasizes the importance and pleasure of effort and learning (e.g., Gottfried et al., 1994; Mueller & Dweck, 1998; Pomerantz et al., 2006); for example, parents may react to children's success by praising their effort. A person focus, in contrast, prioritizes stable attributes (e.g., intelligence) and outcomes (e.g., performance); parents may, for instance, highlight how smart children are when they do well on a test in school. Parents' process- versus person-focused involvement is associated with enhanced motivation and competence among children (e.g., Gottfried et al., 1994; Gottfried, Marcoulides, Gottfried, & Oliver, 2009; Pomerantz et al., 2006). For example, Hokoda and Fincham (1995) found that when mothers react to their children's performance-oriented behavior in a process-focused manner, children are particularly likely to be motivated to develop rather than demonstrate their competence. Pomerantz and Kempner's (2013) had mothers report daily on their responses to their children's successes in school. They found that when mothers refrained from using person-focused praise (e.g., "You are so smart"), children's motivation benefited over time, adjusting for their earlier motivation as well as mothers' educational attainment (see also Gunderson et al., 2013).

WHAT CONTRIBUTES TO PARENTS' INVOLVEMENT IN CHILDREN'S LEARNING?

There is much evidence in line with the idea that parents' involvement in children's learning benefits children's motivation and competence, particularly when parents are autonomy-supportive (vs. controlling), provide structure (vs. chaos), are affectively positive (vs. negative), and process- (vs. person-) focused. Knowledge of what drives parents' involvement is crucial to the success of efforts aimed at fostering it. The antecedents of parents' involvement have received a fair amount of theoretical and empirical attention (e.g., Eccles & Harold, 1996; Grolnick, Benjet, Kurowski, & Apostoleris, 1997; Hoover-Dempsey & Sandler, 1997), but less than the consequences. Consistent with Belsky's (1984) model of the determinants of parenting, there are three central sources of variation among parents in terms of their involvement in children's learning (see also Eccles & Harold, 1996; Grolnick, Benjet, et al., 1997; Hoover-Dempsey & Sandler, 1997; Pomerantz et al., 2012): (1) children (e.g., competence); (2) parents (e.g., beliefs); (3) the environment in which the family resides (e.g., schools).

The Role of Children

Children are active agents in the socialization process, such that they shape parents' practices, which in turn contribute to children's development (e.g., Sameroff, 1975; Sameroff & Mackenzie, 2003). The most salient example of this is in the area of children's aggression. For example, heightened aggression among children appears to elicit more coercive parenting, which in turn appears to elevate children's aggression further (e.g., Patterson, 1982). The question of whether children shape parents' involvement in their learning has also received attention, with evidence suggesting that both the quantity and quality of parents' involvement are driven in part by children. Parents respond to cues indicating that children are having difficulty in school (i.e., competence cues), as well as cues indicating that children want their parents to be engaged in their academic lives (i.e., desire cues). Both these cues may change as children progress through school (e.g., children's desire for parents' engagement declines as children get older).

Competence Cues

Many children are prone to negative competence experiences in the academic area. Such experiences include difficulty meeting standards in school, which can lead to poor achievement, perceiving themselves as lacking competence or control in the academic area, or becoming easily frustrated and helpless in the face of challenge (Pomerantz, Wang, & Ng, 2005b). Pomerantz and colleagues (2005b) made the case that children's negative competence experiences serve as cues to parents that their intervention in the academic area is needed, thereby leading parents to increase their involvement in children's learning. For example, when children are having difficulty in school, parents may contact teachers to talk about children. In line with this idea, Izzo and colleagues (1999) found that the more disengaged children are from school, the more contact parents have with teachers to discuss children's performance and behavior at school.

When children are struggling, parents also intervene by increasing their assistance with homework. Using daily reports, Pomerantz and colleagues (2005a) found that on days mothers felt children were frustrated with homework, they were particularly likely to provide assistance. Children's competence experiences appear to shape parents' assistance over the longer term as well; the more poorly children do in school, the more likely parents are to assist them with homework 6 months to 1 year later (e.g., Pomerantz & Eaton, 2001; Silinskas et al., 2015). However, the quality of such involvement in children's learning can undermine children's motivation and competence (Dumont et al., 2014; Pomerantz et al., 2005a; Silinskas et al., 2015). When children have

difficulty, parents may become frustrated in their efforts to support children, due in part to children's frustration (Pomerantz et al., 2005a). Parents may also become anxious (e.g., because they are worried about children's future or their own ability to help; Pomerantz & Eaton, 2001), which may create additional anxiety in children, thereby disrupting their achievement (Maloney, Ramirez, Gunderson, Levine, & Beilock, 2015).

Parents' frustration and anxiety may lead them to become involved in children's learning in a manner that is controlling (vs. autonomy-supportive), affectively negative (vs. positive), and chaotic (vs. structuring). Indeed, the more children have negative competence experiences, the more parents' assistance with homework is characterized by such qualities (e.g., Pomerantz et al., 2005a; Silinskas et al., 2015). For example, Dumont and colleagues (2014) found that lower academic functioning among children when they were in fifth grade foreshadowed more controlling and chaotic assistance with homework among parents 2 years later, when children were in seventh grade, adjusting for the quality of parents' assistance when children were in fifth grade. Hence, although cues that children are having difficulty may serve to elicit parents' intervention, such intervention does not always alleviate children's difficulty; in fact, it may undermine children's competence further (but see Pomerantz & Eaton, 2001).

Desire Cues

Hoover-Dempsey and Sandler (1997) made the case that children's explicit invitations (e.g., requests for parents to help with homework or talk with teachers about an issue) foster parents' involvement in children's learning. Such invitations may reflect children's negative competence experiences to some extent, but they are only made when children desire parents' support. Some children may invite parents to be involved (e.g., by starting a discussion about what they learned in school or asking parents to volunteer in their classroom) because they want parents to be engaged in an important area of their lives. Children's invitations may also be prompted by school personnel (e.g., instructions to children to have their parents quiz them on math facts or read a book with them) (Green, Walker, Hoover-Dempsey, & Sandler, 2007; Walker, Wilkins, Dallaire, Sandler, & Hoover-Dempsey, 2006).

Children's invitations appear to be one of the most powerful cues in triggering parents' involvement in children's learning, likely because they are the most proximal cues for parents. Parents' perceptions of children's invitations are more strongly associated with their involvement at home than a variety of other potential antecedents (e.g., parents' feelings of efficacy in supporting children and perceptions of their time and energy); parents' perceptions of children's and teachers' invitations are the strongest predictors of parents' involvement at school when compared to other potential antecedents (Anderson & Minke, 2007; Green et al., 2007), although not among Latino parents in the United States (Walker, Ice, Hoover-Dempsey, & Sandler, 2011). Unfortunately, there has not been attention to how children's invitations affect the quality of parents' involvement. However, unlike negative competence experiences, such invitations may lead to constructive involvement given that children desire parents' involvement and they may not be frustrated when they issue their invitations.

Development

As children progress through the school system, parents reduce their involvement in children's learning. This decline is evident over the elementary school years and into the middle and high school years across a variety of types of involvement both at school and at home (e.g., National Center for Education Statistics, 2015). There are likely several interconnected reasons tied to competence and desire cues among children. In regards to competence cues, with age, children become more familiar with the demands of school and develop the skills for meeting such demands, which may heighten their confidence. Consequently, parents may step back. In addition, as children get older, particularly as they make their way into adolescence, they want greater independence (for a review, see Collins & Steinberg, 2006), which may mean that they have less

desire for parents' involvement. Thus, children may issue fewer invitations to parents. In fact, once children reach adolescence, they may even see parents' involvement as intrusive. However, parents' involvement—with the exception of their assistance with homework—benefits children during adolescence, with decreases over this phase predictive of decreases in motivation and competence (e.g., Cheung & Pomerantz, 2011; Wang et al., 2014).

School personnel may also contribute to the tendency for parents to reduce their involvement in children's learning. In an attempt to foster children's developing independence, school personnel may be less likely to encourage parents' involvement as children progress through the school system. It may also be the case that the structure of middle and high schools, which is quite different from that of elementary schools, in that children have different teachers for every subject, decreases communications between teachers and parents that may foster parents' involvement. Indeed, school personnel's communication with parents declines, in that notes, newsletters, and telephone calls to parents from the school become less common as children get older; communications about how to help with children's homework, why particular placements are made for children, and parents' expected role in children's learning also become less frequent (National Center for Education Statistics, 2015). In addition, parents may reduce their involvement in activities such as homework over middle and high school because they do not feel capable of assisting children given how advanced the material becomes (Eccles & Harold, 1996).

The Role of Parents

Because there are socioeconomic disparities in American children's achievement (for a review, see Sirin, 2005), there has been substantial attention to socioeconomically disadvantaged parents' involvement in children's learning (e.g., Cooper & Crosnoe, 2007; Dearing et al., 2006). In the United States, socioeconomically disadvantaged parents are less involved at school than are their more advantaged counterparts (National Center for Education Statistics,

2015). For example, disadvantaged parents are less likely to attend school events (e.g., open houses and general school meetings), volunteer at school, and take part in school fund-raising. At home, there is also less shared reading with children before they start school (Child Trends Databank, 2015). However, socioeconomically disadvantaged (vs. advantaged) parents are just as likely to set aside a place for children to do homework and to check over children's homework (National Center for Education Statistics, 2015).

It is likely that the tendency for socioeconomically disadvantaged parents' to be less involved at school is tied, at least in part, to the lack of material resources and the stress that accompanies such disadvantage. Grolnick, Benjet, and colleagues (1997) explored this possibility by examining families' material resources, including both basic (e.g., food and shelter) and less basic (e.g., money for travel) resources, and parents' exposure to negative life events. The fewer resources mothers report, the less knowledge they had about children's academic lives, and the less they displayed their interest through practices such as asking children about school (see also Benner, Graham, & Mistry, 2008). Similarly, Waanders, Mendez, and Downder (2007) found that the more economic and neighborhood stress parents reported, the more teachers reported having a poor relationship with parents, which may have undermined parents' involvement at school. These results emphasize the importance of opportunities for parents to be involved in children's schooling in a variety of ways, some of which may accommodate families' difficult circumstances in that they, for example, demand relatively little in commitment of energy and time but yield concentrated benefits (e.g., homework instructions that ask children to explain to parents how they did a math problem, which can be brief but give parents information about what children are learning and whether they are having difficulty).

Understanding how parents' involvement varies with their socioeconomic circumstances is important in elucidating the mechanisms behind disparities in children's achievement due to such circumstances. However, there is substantial variability in involvement among parents with similar socioeconomic circumstances; thus, attention should also be directed to other attributes of parents that drive their involvement in children's learning (e.g., Cooper & Crosnoe, 2007; McKay, Atkins, Hawkins, Brown, & Lynn, 2003). In this vein, the implications of parents' beliefs (e.g., about their role in children's learning) and motivation (e.g., the extent to which their involvement is autonomous vs. controlled) for involvement have been studied. Elucidating the role of parents' beliefs and motivation is key because such attributes can be targets of interventions to enhance parents' involvement.

Parents' Beliefs

Parents' beliefs are central drivers of their practices with children (e.g., Darling & Steinberg, 1993; Goodnow & Collins, 1990). Parents' beliefs have been argued to "generate, organize, and shape" their parenting practices (Bornstein, Hahn, & Haynes, 2011, p. 659). Hence, there has been attention to a variety of beliefs that may contribute to parents' involvement in children's learning. In their model of the antecedents of parents' involvement, Hoover-Dempsey and Sandler (1997) identified parents' construction of their role in children's learning and their sense of efficacy for supporting children's learning as the most proximal beliefs contributing to parents' involvement. Since these investigators presented their model, there has been substantial research on the role of these two beliefs in parents' involvement. Theory and research have also been directed to the role of parents' beliefs about ability, as well as parents' expectations and aspirations for children.

CONSTRUCTION OF THE PARENTAL ROLE

Parents ideas about what their roles should be in children's learning develop from their own experiences (e.g., the role that their parents took in their learning), as well as social influences, such as cultural prescriptions. The more parents believe they should be active with regard to children's education—that is, the more they hold an active role construction—the more involved they are in children's learning (e.g., Anderson & Minke,

2007; Green et al., 2007; Grolnick, Benjet, et al., 1997). Walker and colleagues (2011) suggest there are different types of constructions when it comes to parents' role in children's education: (1) A parent-focused role construction reflects the belief that parents have primary responsibility for children's learning; (2) a partnership-focused role construction reflects the idea that responsibility for children's education is shared by families and schools; and (3) a school-focused role construction reflects the view that the responsibility belongs to schools. Studying Latino parents in the United States, Walker and colleagues found that both parent-focused (i.e., a belief in parental responsibility) and partnership-focused (i.e., a belief in shared responsibility) role constructions, but not school-focused role constructions (i.e., a belief in school responsibility), were associated with heightened involvement of parents both at home and at school. However, partnership-focused role constructions were the most powerful predictors of parents' involvement when the three constructions were examined as simultaneous predictors—perhaps because such constructions enhance relationships between parents and teachers.

EFFICACY BELIEFS

Even if parents see it as their role to be involved in children's learning, they may not be able to act on this belief if they lack a sense of efficacy for supporting children's learning. Indeed, parents who feel they are capable of making a difference through their involvement are more involved, particularly at home (e.g., Anderson & Minke, 2007; Grolnick, Benjet, et al., 1997). For example, both Green and colleagues (2007) and Walker and colleagues (2011) examined parents' self-efficacy for helping children in the learning context. They found that parents who felt more efficacious were more involved at home but not necessarily at school. Feelings of efficacy may be more important for involvement at home (vs. school) because such involvement may require knowledge of what children are learning and how to help children learn. Involvement at school, however, often does not require such knowledge. In fact, involvement at school may generate

it (e.g., via the information provided by teachers at parent–teacher conferences).

BELIEFS ABOUT THE MALLEABILITY OF ABILITY

In line with Dweck's (e.g., Dweck, 1999; Dweck & Leggett, 1988) idea that people vary in the extent to which they view ability as an entity that cannot be changed (i.e., a fixed mindset) versus malleable (i.e., a growth mindset), there is variation among parents in the extent to which they hold a fixed (vs. growth) mindset about children's ability in the United States (Pomerantz & Dong, 2006) as well as New Zealand, China, and Japan (Jose & Bellamy, 2012) not only for academic abilities in general but also for math and reading abilities specifically (Muenks, Miele, Ramani, Stapleton, & Rowe, 2015). This variability appears to contribute to children's motivation and competence: Mothers' perceptions of children's academic competencies are more likely to act as self-fulfilling prophecies when they hold a fixed (vs. growth) mindset; for example, when mothers hold a fixed mindset, their perceptions of their children's competence are more predictive of children's subsequent achievement than if they hold a growth mindset (Pomerantz & Dong, 2006; but for evidence that parents' mindsets may not shape children's mindsets, see Haimovitz & Dweck, 2016).

Because parents with a fixed mindset view children's performance as reflecting children's innate competence, a key goal for such parents is ensuring that children demonstrate their competence by performing well, which may make failure threatening. Thus, children's difficulty in school may lead to unconstructive (e.g., controlling and affectively negative) involvement in children's learning. In contrast, when parents hold a growth mindset, they see children's performance as a reflection of their learning. Hence, children's poor performance is something that can be turned around with effort. Such a view may lead parents to be constructively (e.g., autonomy-supportive and affectively positive) involved in children's learning, regardless of whether children experience difficulty. Indeed, Moorman and Pomerantz (2010) found that when mothers were induced to hold a fixed mindset (i.e., they were told that the tasks on which children were working assessed innate ability, with little change in ability over time) versus a growth mindset (i.e., they were told that the tasks on which children were working assessed intellectual potential, with studying helping to develop abilities over time), their involvement was unconstructive (e.g., controlling and affectively negative), particularly when children were having difficulty. A similar pattern is evident when mothers' naturally occurring mindsets are examined (e.g., Jose & Bellamy, 2012; Muenks et al., 2015; but see Haimovitz & Dweck, 2016).

ASPIRATIONS AND EXPECTATIONS FOR CHILDREN

Parents' aspirations and expectations for children in regard to their education have been given much theoretical and empirical attention. However, although some theoretical perspectives identify such beliefs as distinct from parents' involvement in children's learning (e.g., Eccles, 1983), they are often treated as a form of involvement (e.g., Fan & Chen, 2001; Hill & Tyson, 2009). In fact, in quantitative syntheses, parents' expectations and aspirations for their children's school performance and attainment—sometimes referred to as parents' *academic socialization*—are more strongly associated with children's achievement than involvement at school or home (Hill & Tyson, 2009; Jeynes, 2007). However, parents' aspirations and expectations themselves do not necessarily require a commitment of resources to children's academic lives and may not necessarily be conveyed to children. In line with Eccles's (1983) expectancy–value model, parents' aspirations and expectations may instead function as antecedents of parents' involvement (e.g., parents communicate their aspirations and expectations to children and support children in attaining them). Consistent with this idea, the higher parents' expectations for children, the more involved parents are at school over time (e.g., Englund, Luckner, Whaley, & Egeland, 2004; Simpkins, Fredricks, & Eccles, 2012). However, parents' aspirations and expectations may not foster their involvement if they are not

accompanied by other beliefs that are instrumental in being involved (e.g., parents see their role as supporting children's learning and feel efficacious in doing so).

Parents' Motivation

Even when parents hold beliefs that facilitate their involvement in children's learning, they may not get involved, or they may do so in an unconstructive manner, because they feel pressured. Pressure can arise from sources outside of parents (e.g., teachers convey that "good" parents volunteer in the classroom) as well as within parents (e.g., parents feel that part of being a good parent is helping with homework). Drawing from self-determination theory, Grolnick (2015) made the case that parents may be more involved when they do so out of choice rather than feeling pressured or coerced, which can disrupt persistence. Grolnick distinguished four types of motivation, varying along a continuum from autonomous to controlled, that parents may have for their involvement: (1) intrinsic (e.g., parents feel it is fun to go to school events), (2) identified (e.g., parents feel it is important for children's learning to talk with teachers); (3) introjected (e.g., parents feel guilty if they are not involved); and (4) external (e.g., parents feel they are supposed to be involved). Autonomous motivation, as manifest in more identified motives for being involved, was associated with higher involvement among mothers. Moreover, mothers with more autonomous motivation (i.e., intrinsic and identified motives) had more positive affect when they were involved, whereas mothers with more controlled motivation (i.e., introjected and external motives) had more negative affect. These findings underscore the significance of parents believing in the importance of their involvement. Pressuring parents to be involved may facilitate some initial involvement but ultimately may backfire as parents find it unpleasant or push back against the pressure.

A key source of internal pressure may be parents' tendency to base their own worth on children's performance in school. Many people base their worth on some area of their lives—for example, their achievements at work, the support of their family, or their physical appearance (e.g., Crocker, Luhtanen, Cooper, & Bouvrette, 2003). Crocker and colleagues (Crocker & Park, 2004; Crocker & Wolfe, 2001) suggested that the areas on which people's sense of worth hinges often play a central role in their lives as they seek to validate their worth through their accomplishments in such areas. Research with parents in several countries indicates that a significant source of their self-worth is frequently children's school performance (e.g., Grolnick, Price, Beiswenger, & Sauck, 2007; Ng, Pomerantz, & Deng, 2014; Wuyts, Vansteenkiste, Soenens, & Assor, 2015), in part because parents may feel accountable to others for ensuring that children perform up to standards (e.g., Wuyts et al., 2015).

When parents' sense of worth is caught up in children's performance, children's failure may be threatening to parents. When people's feelings of worth are contingent on an area of their lives, their focus on performance in that area may be such that they are insensitive to the needs of others (Crocker & Park, 2004). In the context of their involvement in children's learning, parents may be controlling (vs. autonomy-supportive), affectively negative (vs. positive), and person (vs. process) oriented as they attempt to push children to succeed, without attending to children's needs. Indeed, several studies indicate that the more parents' worth is caught up in children's performance, the more controlling parents are (e.g., Grolnick et al., 2007; Ng et al., 2014). For example, Wuyts and colleagues (2015) found that the more mothers base their worth on children's performance, the more intrusive they are when it comes to children's achievement. Using daily diary and experimental methods to examine children's performance in the academic area, Ng, Pomerantz, Lam, and Deng (2016) documented that the more mothers' sense of worth hinges on children's performance, the more negative their affect when children fail. A key implication of this work is that just as schools should not pressure parents to be involved, they should not link parents' worth to children's performance, which may occur when too much accountability is placed on parents for children's achievement.

The Role of the Environment

The environment in which children and parents reside can shape parents' involvement in children's learning both directly (e.g., teachers' inclusion of parents in children's homework assignments fosters parents' involvement) and indirectly through, for example, parents' beliefs (e.g., school norms shape parents' beliefs about their role in children's learning, which fosters parents' involvement). As Bronfenbrenner (1986) highlights, families reside in a series of nested environments that may interact with one another to affect children. Perhaps most central among such environments when it comes to parents' involvement are the schools that children attend. Schools are a key point of intervention for enhancing both the quantity and quality of parents' involvement. However, schools are not the only environment likely to shape parents' involvement—there is substantial evidence that the culture to which families belong is also of import, with implications for how schools may best foster parents' involvement.

Schools

Schools can be instrumental in fostering parents' involvement in children's learning via practices implemented by teachers and other school personnel. Crucial for schools is outreach to parents via efforts such as educating parents about the transition to elementary school; creating homework that includes parents; and inviting parents to volunteer, attend school events, or be part of school governance. When teachers incorporate parents' involvement into their teaching activities, they may help parents to feel more efficacious, thereby fostering their involvement (Epstein, 1986). Indeed, the more teachers invite parents to be involved, the more parents are involved (e.g., Anderson & Minke, 2007; Dauber & Epstein, 1983; Green et al., 2007). More general school practices also appear to contribute to parents' involvement (e.g., Sheldon, 2005). For example, Galindo and Sheldon (2012) found that school outreach efforts such as hosting school events (e.g., book nights or class plays) and home visits for one-on-one parent education during kindergarten predicted enhanced achievement at the end of kindergarten by heightening parents' involvement at school, adjusting for children's earlier achievement as well as other potential confounds. Such outreach efforts can be particularly beneficial for economically and educationally disadvantaged families (Schulting, Malone, & Dodge, 2005).

Care must be taken, however, to ensure that outreach to parents by school personnel is not too demanding and is tailored to parents' circumstances. Indeed, Grolnick, Benjet, and colleagues (1997) found that elementary school teachers' positive attitudes toward parents' involvement and frequent use of activities to encourage it were only predictive of higher involvement in families who had more resources—specifically, two-parent families, families with less difficult circumstances, and families in which parents felt efficacious in supporting children's learning. It may be that teachers in this study encouraged involvement that was demanding or did not fit with parents' ideas about their roles. Hence, it is critical to identify activities that are not too taxing for parents (see earlier discussion) and that may be scaffolded, so that parents' circumstances and feelings of efficacy do not interfere with their implementation.

School personnel may also need to ensure that their outreach efforts do not put pressure on parents. As highlighted earlier, when parents feel pressured (e.g., because they feel they are supposed to be involved or come to base their worth on their children's performance), their involvement can be unconstructive. Given the increasing emphasis placed on schools to meet achievement standards, school personnel may feel pressure for children to perform well, which may color their interactions with parents. Using experimental methods, Grolnick, Gurland, DeCourcey, and Jacob (2002) manipulated how pressuring the environment was for mothers. In the high-pressure condition, mothers were told that after working with children on a set of tasks, children would be tested to ensure that children "performed well enough." In the low-pressure condition, mothers were told that children would be asked questions related to the tasks, but there were no performance expectations. Grolnick and colleagues reasoned that the

pressuring induction would heighten mothers' investment in children's performance, making them feel that their self-worth was on the line. Mothers in the high- (vs. low-) pressure condition were more controlling during the tasks, particularly if they were already predisposed to use control. It may be that parents who have strongly held beliefs about the importance of supporting children's autonomy are able to resist pressure better.

There have also been calls for attention to the quality of outreach attempts by schools in regard to the extent to which they take a collaborative approach to working with parents (e.g., Christenson & Sheridan, 2001). Central in this line of thinking is the importance of building trusting relationships between school personnel and parents that are characterized by mutual respect, jointly agreed-upon goals, give-and-take communication, and shared decision making. Vickers, Minke, and Anderson (2002) suggested that in their communications with parents, particularly in the context of parent–teacher conferences, teachers use practices (e.g., empathetic listening and collaborative planning) that cultivate such relationships. Unfortunately, to date, there has been no research on whether communications with such qualities enhance parents' involvement. Relationship building may be particularly important in cultivating involvement of parents who do not feel efficacious in supporting children's learning; when such parents feel they have positive relationships with school personnel, it may enable them to request advice and assistance. As we highlight below, positive parent–teacher relationships may also be key in supporting the involvement of parents from diverse cultures, who may feel less comfortable interacting with school personnel because of issues such as societal racism or poor English skills.

Culture

Given sizable ethnic disparities in children's achievement, with African American and Latino children at particular risk (Hemphill & Vanneman, 2010; Vanneman, Hamilton, Baldwin Anderson, & Rahman, 2009), there has been growing attention to how schools can better foster parents' involvement in children's learning among African American and Latino parents (e.g., Hill, 2011; Hill & Torres, 2010). With the exception of attending parent–teacher conferences, African American and Latino parents tend to be less involved at school (e.g., attending school events or volunteering at school) than their European American counterparts (National Center for Education Statistics, 2015). However, African American and Latino parents support their children in doing their homework (e.g., checking over children's homework) just as much—if not more—than do European American parents (National Center for Education Statistics, 2015). Adjusting for socioeconomic status, Wang and colleagues (2014) found that although African (vs. European) American parents engage in less preventive communication with teachers (e.g., asking about homework assignments), they provide more structure around learning (e.g., enforce rules about studying) and emphasize the importance and utility of education to children more.

Parents' involvement at school contributes to children's achievement over and above their involvement at home (e.g., Wang et al., 2014). Moreover, Hill (2011) suggests that for ethnic minorities about which there may be negative stereotypes in regards to achievement, parents' involvement at school may be particularly important because it may serve to break down such stereotypes, leading to better relationships between teachers and parents, as well as more positive perceptions of children among teachers. Hence, a key endeavor is to understand why African American and Latino parents are less involved at school than are their European American counterparts. Minority parents, particularly those who are African American and Latino, often trust teachers less than do European American parents, feel less welcome in schools, and have poorer relationships with teachers (e.g., Beard & Brown, 2008; Hughes & Kwok, 2007; Kohl et al., 2000). Notably, feeling welcome via teachers' invitations is one of the major predictors of African American and Latino parents' involvement at school and home (e.g., Marinez-Lora & Quintana, 2009; McKay et al., 2003). In fact, teachers' invitations trump African American and Latino parents' beliefs about their role in children's

education and their feelings of efficacy in supporting their children (Marinez-Lora & Quintana, 2009).

A variety of forces may contribute to African American and Latino parents not feeling welcome at school. For one, African American parents' perceptions of racism may lead them to be less involved at school (McKay et al., 2003). African American parents may also think they lack the knowledge to be usefully involved and may feel intimidated by school personnel (Hill, 2011). In addition, because African Americans often live in difficult circumstances with inflexible job schedules, attending school events at times scheduled by school personnel may be challenging (Hill, 2011). Latino parents may face similar issues, which are further compounded when parents are recent immigrants and their English is limited, which may hinder their interactions with school personnel, who often speak only English (e.g., Ceballo, Maurizi, Suarez, & Aretakis, 2014; Ramirez, 2003). Latino immigrant parents' involvement may also be restricted by a lack of knowledge about how American schools work and a concern with respecting school personnel so as not to disrupt their relationships with them (e.g., Hill & Torres, 2010; Ramirez, 2003). There has been some speculation that Latino cultural beliefs contribute to dampened involvement as well. Education is seen as including learning in not only the academic area but also other areas (e.g., learning to be moral, respectful, and responsible), with teachers responsible for the academic area and parents responsible for other areas (Auerbach, 2007; Hill & Torres, 2010).

How Can We Promote Parents' Facilitation of Children's Motivation and Competence?

Given the benefits of parents' involvement in children's learning, a number of interventions have focused on fostering parents' involvement. Unfortunately, many of these have been unsuccessful (for a review, see Mattingly, Prislin, McKenzie, Rodriguez, & Kayzar, 2002). One possible conclusion is that more intensive intervention is necessary, but just the opposite may be the case. First, interventions targeting parents' involvement should capitalize on bridges between home and school that already exist (e.g., homework assignments or parent–teacher conferences). Such an approach has the benefit of reaching a far larger proportion of families than intensive interventions. Parents who are most in need of intervention may be the ones who can least afford the time and energy to attend intensive sessions. Second, theory and research on brief interventions (Walton, 2014; Yeager & Walton, 2011) suggest that if interventions precisely target critical psychological mechanisms (e.g., parents' beliefs or motivation) that drive parents' involvement and offer opportunities for them to be involved constructively (e.g., homework assignments that scaffold parents' involvement), they are likely to be successful.

Existing-Bridges Interventions

Epstein, Salinas, and Jackson's (1995) Teachers Involve Parents in Schoolwork (TIPS) program exploits an existing bridge between home and school to promote involvement in children's learning among parents from a variety of backgrounds. TIPS helps teachers to support parents in becoming involved in children's learning via homework assignments, accompanied by a brief orientation for parents about the program that can easily be held at a school open house or other highly attended events. At the core of the TIPS program are homework assignments that guide children in interacting with parents (e.g., asking about parents' memories of an event or showing parents a math skill the student has learned in class). The assignments are designed for parents to play a supportive, rather than instructional, role. Research using quasi-experimental designs to evaluate TIPS yields mixed results (Epstein & Van Voorhis, 2001). Because TIPS targets parents' practices without also targeting their beliefs (e.g., role construction or ability mindsets), it may not create lasting improvement in the quantity and quality of parents' involvement. Hence, in line with the brief intervention approach, a key innovation may be to add a belief component to the TIPS program that draws on existing knowledge about the beliefs that optimize parents' involvement.

Another existing home–school bridge that may prove fruitful in fostering parents' involvement in children's learning is the parent–teacher conference (Vickers et al., 2002). The large majority (89%) of parents of elementary school children in the United States attend parent–teacher conferences, with only minor variation due to socioeconomics or ethnicity (National Center for Education Statistics, 2015). Teachers can provide information at parent–teacher conferences that may foster parents' involvement either directly (e.g., via suggestions for useful practices or invitations to volunteer at school) or indirectly by cultivating beliefs that foster parents' involvement (e.g., via language conveying that ability is malleable or information about what children are learning) in a constructive motivational context (e.g., helping parents to develop personally important reasons for being involved). Parent–teacher conferences are also an excellent opportunity for teachers to build positive relationships with parents through practices such as empathetic listening and collaborative planning to address children's needs (Vickers et al., 2002). There is much advice available about how teachers can optimally communicate with parents during parent–teacher conferences (e.g., Gelfer & Perkins, 1987; Harvard Family Research Project, 2010). However, best practices among teachers have not been empirically verified. Doing so would be useful given that parent–teacher conferences may be an ideal context for efficiently promoting parents' involvement using knowledge about what drives parents to become involved.

Brief Interventions

The brief intervention approach has generally been absent in efforts to enhance parents' involvement in children's learning. However, drawing from Eccles's (1983) expectancy–value model, Harackiewicz, Rozek, Hulleman, and Hyde (2012) used such an approach in their intervention targeting the value parents place on math and science. There is not much evidence for Eccles's (1983) idea that parents' values around education drive their involvement (e.g., Jodl, Michael, Malanchuk, Eccles, & Sameroff, 2001; Simpkins et al., 2012). However, it may be that even when parents see education as valuable, they may not feel it is their role to foster children's learning, or they may not feel efficacious in doing so. Hence, Harackiewicz and colleagues' (2012) brief intervention targeted the utility value (i.e., the usefulness) of math and science for parents (i.e., with a brochure providing information on the importance of math and science for daily lives, as well as a number of careers), while *also* providing parents with resources to build their own and their children's knowledge (e.g., guidance about how to talk to children about the relevance of math and science to their daily lives). Parents who received the utility value intervention along with the resources discussed the importance of math and science, as well as plans for which courses to take in the future, more with children than did parents not receiving the intervention or resources. Parents' heightened discussion mediated the positive effects of the intervention on children's perceptions of the utility value of math and science.

CONCLUSIONS

It is clear that parents' involvement in children's learning can facilitate children's motivation and competence, particularly when parents are involved in an autonomy-supportive (vs. controlling), structured (vs. chaotic), affectively positive (vs. negative), and process- (vs. person-oriented) manner. The emerging body of theory and research on what underlies such facilitative parenting indicates that attributes of children, parents, and the environment are all of significance. Knowledge of the drivers (e.g., parents' beliefs and motivation) of parents' involvement is critical in designing interventions to foster parents' constructive involvement. If interventions attempt to change such antecedents, they may have a lasting impact on parents' involvement, thereby allowing parents to support children's motivation and competence over the school years. Given socioeconomic and ethnic achievement disparities, interventions should be attuned to the forces that hinder involvement among socioeconomically disadvantaged and minority parents (e.g., the time and energy commitment parents can make given difficult circumstances or parents' poor English

skills). Interventions may be able to reach families from diverse backgrounds if they take advantage of existing home–school bridges using brief intervention techniques.

REFERENCES

Anderson, K. J., & Minke, K. M. (2007). Parent involvement in education: Toward an understanding of parents' decision making. *Journal of Educational Research, 100,* 311–323.

Auerbach, S. (2007). From moral supports to struggling advocates: Reconceptualizing parents roles in education through the experience of working-class families of color. *Urban Education, 42,* 250–283.

Baker, D. P., & Stevenson, H. W. (1986). Mothers' strategies for children's school achievement: Managing the transition to high school. *Sociology of Education, 59,* 156–166.

Beard, K. S., & Brown, K. M. (2008). Trusting' schools to meet the academic needs of African-American students?: Suburban mothers' perspectives. *International Journal of Qualitative Studies in Education, 21,* 471–485.

Belsky, J. (1984). The determinants of parenting: A process model. *Child Development, 55,* 83–96.

Benner, A. D., Graham, S., & Mistry, R. S. (2008). Discerning direct and mediated effects of ecological structures and processes on adolescents' educational outcomes. *Developmental Psychology, 44,* 840–854.

Bindman, S. W., Pomerantz, E. M., & Roisman, G. I. (2015). Children's executive functions account for associations between early autonomy-supportive parenting and children's achievement through high school. *Journal of Educational Psychology, 107,* 756–770.

Bornstein, M. H., Hahn, C.-S., & Haynes, O. M. (2011). Maternal personality, parenting cognitions, and parenting practices. *Developmental Psychology, 47,* 658–675.

Bronfenbrenner, U. (1986). Ecology of the family as a context for human development: Research perspectives. *Developmental Psychology, 22,* 723–742.

Ceballo, R., Maurizi, L. K., Suarez, G. A., & Aretakis, M. T. (2014). Gift and sacrifice: Parental involvement in Latino adolescents' education. *Cultural Diversity and Ethnic Minority Psychology, 20,* 126–127.

Cheung, C. S., & Pomerantz, E. M. (2011). Parents' involvement in children's academic lives in the United States and China: Implications for children's academic and emotional adjustment. *Child Development, 82,* 932–950.

Cheung, C. S., & Pomerantz, E. M. (2012). Why does parents' involvement in children's learning enhance children's achievement?: The role of parent-oriented motivation. *Journal of Educational Psychology, 104,* 820–832.

Cheung, C. S., & Pomerantz, E. M. (2015). Value development underlies the benefits of parents' involvement in children's learning: A longitudinal investigation in the United States and China. *Journal of Educational Psychology, 107,* 309–320.

Child Trends Databank. (2015). Reading to young children. Retrieved from *http://childtrends.org/?indicators=reading-to-young-children.*

Christenson, S. L., & Sheridan, S. M. (2001). *Schools and families: Creating essential connections for learning.* New York: Guilford Press.

Collins, W. A., & Steinberg, L. (2006). Adolescent development in interpersonal context. In N. Eisenberg (Ed.), *Handbook of child development: Vol. 3. Social, emotional, and personality development* (6th ed., pp. 1003–1067). Hoboken, NJ: Wiley.

Cooper, C. E., & Crosnoe, R. (2007). The engagement in schooling of economically disadvantaged parents and children. *Youth and Society, 38,* 372–391.

Crocker, J., Luhtanen, R. K., Cooper, M. L., & Bouvrette, A. (2003). Contingencies of self-worth in college students: Theory and measurement. *Journal of Personality and Social Psychology, 85,* 894–908.

Crocker, J., & Park, L. E. (2004). The costly pursuit of self-esteem. *Psychological Bulletin, 130,* 392–414.

Crocker, J., & Wolfe, C. T. (2001). Contingencies of self-worth. *Psychological Review, 108,* 593–623.

Darling, N., & Steinberg, L. (1993). Parenting style as context: An integrative model. *Psychological Bulletin, 113,* 487–496.

Dauber, S. L., & Epstein, J. L. (1983). Parents' attitudes and practices of involvement in inner-city elementary and middle schools. In N. Chavkin (Ed.), *Families and schools in a pluralistic society* (pp. 53–72). Albany: State University of New York Press.

Dearing, E., Kreider, H., Simpkins, S., & Weiss, H. B. (2006). Family involvement in school and low-income children's literacy: Longitudinal associations between and within families. *Journal of Educational Psychology, 98,* 653–664.

Deci, E. L., & Ryan, R. M. (1985). *Intrinsic motivation and self-determination in human behavior.* New York: Plenum Press.

Dix, T. (1991). The affective organization of parenting: Adaptive and maladaptive processes. *Psychological Bulletin, 110,* 3–25.

Dumont, H., Trautwein, U., Nagy, G., & Nagengast, B. (2014). Quality of parental homework involvement: Predictors and reciprocal relations with academic functioning in the reading domain. *Journal of Educational Psychology, 106,* 144–161.

Dweck, C. S. (1999). *Self-theories: Their role in motivation, personality, and development.* New York: Psychology Press.

Dweck, C. S., & Leggett, E. L. (1988). A social-cognitive approach to motivation and personality. *Psychological Review, 95,* 256–273.

Eccles, J. S. (1983). Expectancies, values and academic behaviors. In J. T. Spence (Ed.), *Achievement and achievement motives* (pp. 75–146). San Francisco: Freeman.

Eccles, J. S., & Harold, R. D. (1996). Family involvement in children's and adolescents' schooling. In A. Booth & J. F. Dunn (Eds.), *Family–school links: How do they affect educational outcomes* (pp. 3–34). Mahwah, NJ: Erlbaum.

Englund, M. M., Luckner, A. E., Whaley, G. J. L., & Egeland, B. (2004). Children's achievement in early elementary school: Longitudinal effects of parental involvement, expectations, and quality of assistance. *Journal of Educational Psychology, 96,* 723–730.

Epstein, J. L. (1986). Parents' reactions to teacher practices of parent involvement. *Elementary School Journal, 86,* 277–294.

Epstein, J. L. (1987). What principals should know about parent involvement. *Principal, 66,* 6–9.

Epstein, J. L. (1988). How do we improve programs for parental involvement? *Educational Horizons, 66,* 58–59.

Epstein, J. L., Salinas, K. C., & Jackson, V. E. (1995). *Manual for teachers and prototype activities: Teachers Involve Parents in Schoolwork (TIPS) language arts, science/health, and math interactive homework in the middle grades.* Baltimore: Johns Hopkins University, Center on School, Family, and Community Partnerships.

Epstein, J. L., & Van Voorhis, F. L. (2001). More than minutes: Teachers' roles in designing homework. *Educational Psychologist, 36,* 181–193.

Fan, X., & Chen, M. (2001). Parental involvement and students' academic achievement: A meta-analysis. *Educational Psychology Review, 13,* 1–22.

Fantuzzo, J. W., Tighe, E., & Childs, S. (2000). Family involvement questionnaire: A multivariate assessment of family participation in early childhood education. *Journal of Educational Psychology, 92,* 367–376.

Galindo, C., & Sheldon, S. B. (2012). School and home connections and children's kindergarten achievement gains: The mediating role of family involvement. *Early Childhood Research Quarterly, 27,* 90–103.

Gelfer, J. I., & Perkins, P. G. (1987). Effective communication with parents: A process for parent/teacher conferences. *Childhood Education, 64,* 19–22.

Goodnow, J. J., & Collins, W. A. (1990). *Development according to parents: The nature, sources and consequences of parents' ideas.* Hillsdale, NJ: Erlbaum.

Gottfried, A. E., Fleming, J. S., & Gottfried, A. W. (1994). Role of parental motivational practices in children's academic intrinsic motivation and achievement. *Journal of Educational Psychology, 86,* 104–113.

Gottfried, A. E., Marcoulides, G. A., Gottfried, A. W., & Oliver, P. H. (2009). A latent curve model of parental motivational practices and developmental decline in math and science academic intrinsic motivation. *Journal of Educational Psychology, 101,* 729–739.

Green, C. L., Walker, J. M. T., Hoover-Dempsey, K. V., & Sandler, H. M. (2007). Parents' motivations for involvement in children's education: An empirical test of a theoretical model of parental involvement. *Journal of Educational Psychology, 99,* 532–544.

Grolnick, W. S. (2015). Mothers' motivation for involvement in their children's schooling: Mechanisms and outcomes. *Motivation and Emotion, 39,* 63–73.

Grolnick, W. S. (2016). Parental involvement and children's academic motivation and achievement. In W. C. Liu, J. C. K. Wang, & R. M. Ryan (Eds.), *Building autonomous learners: Perspectives from research and practice using self-determination theory* (pp. 169–183). Singapore: Springer.

Grolnick, W. S., Benjet, C., Kurowski, C. O., & Apostoleris, N. H. (1997). Predictors of parent involvement in children's schooling. *Journal of Educational Psychology, 89,* 538–548.

Grolnick, W. S., Deci, E. L., & Ryan, R. M. (1997). Internalization within the family: The self-determination theory perspective. In J. Grusec & L. Kuczynski (Eds.), *Parenting and children's internalization of values* (pp. 135–161). New York: Wiley.

Grolnick, W. S., Gurland, S. T., DeCourcey, W., & Jacob, K. (2002). Antecedents and consequences of mothers' autonomy support: An experimental investigation. *Developmental Psychology, 38,* 143–154.

Grolnick, W. S., & Pomerantz, E. M. (2009). Issues and challenges in studying parental control: Toward a new conceptualization. *Child Development Perspectives, 3,* 165–170.

Grolnick, W. S., Price, C. E., Beiswenger, K. L., & Sauck, C. C. (2007). Evaluative pressure in mothers: Effects of situation, maternal, and child characteristics on autonomy supportive versus controlling behavior. *Developmental Psychology, 43,* 991–1002.

Grolnick, W. S., Raftery-Helmer, J. N., Marbell, K. N., Flamm, E. S., Cardemil, E. V., & Sanchez, M. (2014). Parental provision of structure: Implementation and correlates in three domains. *Merrill–Palmer Quarterly, 60,* 355–384.

Grolnick, W. S., & Ryan, R. M. (1989). Parent styles associated with children's self-regulation and competence in school. *Journal of Educational Psychology, 81,* 143–154.

Grolnick, W. S., & Slowiaczek, M. L. (1994). Parents' involvement in children's schooling: A multidimensional conceptualization and motivational model. *Child Development, 64,* 237–252.

Gunderson, E. A., Gripshover, S. J., Romero, C., Dweck, C. S., Goldin-Meadow, S., & Levine, S. C. (2013). Parent praise to 1- to 3-year-olds predicts children's motivational frameworks 5 years later. *Child Development, 84,* 1526–1541.

Haimovitz, H., & Dweck, C. S. (2016). What predicts children's fixed and growth intelligence mind-sets?: Not their parents' views of intelligence but their parents' views of failure. *Psychological Science.* [Epub ahead of print]

Harackiewicz, J. M., Rozek, C. S., Hulleman, C. S., & Hyde, J. S. (2012). Helping parents to motivate adolescents in mathematics and science: An experimental test of a utility-value intervention. *Psychological Science, 23,* 899–906.

Harvard Family Research Project. (2010). *Parent–teacher conference tip sheets for principals, teachers, and parents.* Cambridge, MA: Harvard University Press.

Hemphill, F. C., & Vanneman, A. (2010). *Achievement gaps: How Hispanic and White students in public schools perform in mathematics and reading on the National Assessment of Educational Progress* (NCES 2011–459). Washington, DC: National Center for Education Statistics.

Hill, N. E. (2011). Undermining partnerships between African American families and schools: Legacies of discrimination and inequalities. In N. E. Hill, T. L. Mann, & H. E. Fitzgerald (Eds.), *African American* children and mental health: Vol. 1. Development and context (pp. 199–230). Santa Barbara, CA: Praeger.

Hill, N. E., Castellino, D. R., Lansford, J. E., Nowlin, P., Dodge, K. A., Bates, J. E., et al. (2004). Parent–academic involvement as related to school behavior, achievement, and aspirations: Deomgraphic variations across adolescence. Child Development, 75, 1491–1509.

Hill, N. E., & Torres, K. (2010). Negotiating the American dream: The paradox of aspirations and achievement among Latino students and engagement between their families and schools. Journal of Social Issues, 66, 95–112.

Hill, N. E., & Tyson, D. (2009). Parental involvement in middle school: A meta-analytic assessment of the strategies that promote achievement. Developmental Psychology, 45, 740–763.

Hokoda, A., & Fincham, F. D. (1995). Origins of children's helpless and mastery achievement patterns in the family. Journal of Educational Psychology, 87, 375–385.

Hoover-Dempsey, K. V., & Sandler, H. M. (1997). Why do parents become involved in their children's education? Review of Educational Research, 67, 3–42.

Hughes, J., & Kwok, O. (2007). Influence of student–teacher and parent–teacher relationships on lower achieving readers' engagement and achievement in the primary grades. Journal of Educational Psychology, 99, 39–51.

Izzo, C. V., Weissberg, R. P., Kasprow, W. J., & Fendrich, M. (1999). A longitudinal assessment of teacher perceptions of parent involvement in children's education and school performance. American Journal of Community Psychology, 27, 817–839.

Jeynes, W. H. (2003). A meta-analysis: The effects of parental involvement on minority children's academic achievement. Education and Urban Society, 35, 202–218.

Jeynes, W. H. (2005). A meta-analysis of the relation of parental involvement to urban elementary school student academic achievement. Urban Education, 40, 237–269.

Jeynes, W. H. (2007). The relationship between parental involvement and urban secondary school student academic acheivement: A meta-analysis. Urban Education, 42, 82–110.

Jodl, K. M., Michael, A., Malanchuk, O., Eccles, J. S., & Sameroff, A. (2001). Parents' roles in shaping early adolescents' occupational aspirations. Child Development, 72, 1247–1265.

Jose, P. E., & Bcllamy, M. A. (2012). Relationships of parents' theories of intelligence with children's persistence/learned helplessness: A cross-cultural comparison. Journal of Cross-Cultural Psychology, 43, 999–1018.

Kohl, G. O., Lengua, L. J., McMahon, R. J., & Conduct Problems Prevention Research Group. (2000). Parent involvement in school: Conceptualizing multiple dimensions and their relations with family and demographic risk factors. Journal of School Psychology, 38, 501–523.

LeFevre, J., Skwarchuk, S., Smith-Chant, B., Fast, L., Kamawar, D., & Bisanz, J. (2009). Home numeracy experiences and children's math performance in the early school years. Canadian Journal of Behavioural Science, 41, 55–66.

Leone, C. M., & Richards, M. H. (1989). Classwork and homework in early adolescence: The ecology of achievement. Journal of Youth and Adolescence, 18, 531–548.

Maloney, E. A., Ramirez, G., Gunderson, E. A., Levine, S. C., & Beilock, S. L. (2015). Intergenerational effects of low math achievement and high math anxiety. Psychological Science, 26, 1480–1488.

Marinez-Lora, A. M., & Quintana, S. M. (2009). Low-income urban African American and Latino parents' school involvement: Testing a theoretical model. School Mental Health, 1, 212–228.

Mattingly, D. J., Prislin, R., McKenzie, T. L., Rodriguez, J. L., & Kayzar, B. (2002). Evaluating evaluations: The case of parent involvement programs. Review of Educational Research, 72, 549–576.

McKay, M. M., Atkins, M. S., Hawkins, T., Brown, C., & Lynn, C. J. (2003). Inner-city African American parental involvement in children's schooling: Racial socialization and social support from the parent community. American Journal of Community Psychology, 32, 107–114.

Moorman, E. A., & Pomerantz, E. M. (2010). Ability mindsets influence the quality of mothers' involvement in children's learning: An experimental investigation. Developmental Psychology, 46, 1354–1362.

Mueller, C. M., & Dweck, C. S. (1998). Praise for intelligence can undermine children's motivation and performance. Journal of Personality and Social Psychology, 75(1), 33–52.

Muenks, K., Miele, D. B., Ramani, G. B., Stapleton, L. M., & Rowe, M. L. (2015). Parental beliefs about the fixedness of ability. Journal of Applied Developmental Psychology, 41, 78–89.

National Center for Education Statistics. (2015). Parent and family involvement in education from the National Household Education

Surveys Program of 2012 (NCES 2013–028. REV). Washington, DC: Institute of Educational Sciences, U.S. Department of Education.

Ng, F. F., Pomerantz, E. M., & Deng, C. (2014). Why are Chinese mothers more psychologically controlling than American mothers?: "My child is my report card." *Child Development, 85,* 355–369.

Ng, F. F., Pomerantz, E. M., Lam, S.-F., & Deng, C. (2016). *The role of mothers' child-based worth in their affective responses to children's performance.* Manuscript submitted for publication.

Nolen-Hoeksema, S., Wolfson, A., Mumme, D., & Guskin, K. (1995). Helplessness in children of depressed and nondepressed mothers. *Developmental Psychology, 31,* 377–387.

Patall, E. A., Cooper, H., & Robinson, J. C. (2008). Parent involvement in homework: A research synthesis. *Review of Educational Research, 78,* 1039–1101.

Patterson, G. R. (1982). *Coercive family process.* Eugene, OR: Castalia.

Pianta, R. C., Hamre, B. K., & Allen, J. P. (2012). Teacher–student relationships and engagement: Conceptualizing, measuring, and improving the capacity of classroom interactions. In S. L. Christenson, A. L. Reschly, & C. Wylie (Eds.), *Handbook of research on student engagement* (pp. 365–386). New York: Springer.

Pomerantz, E. M., & Dong, W. (2006). The effects of mothers' perceptions of children's competence: The moderating role of mothers' theories of competence. *Developmental Psychology, 42,* 950–961.

Pomerantz, E. M., & Eaton, M. M. (2001). Maternal intrusive support in the academic context: Transactional socialization processes. *Developmental Psychology, 37,* 174–186.

Pomerantz, E. M., Grolnick, W. S., & Price, C. E. (2005). The role of parents in how children approach school: A dynamic process perspective. In A. J. Elliot & C. S. Dweck (Eds.), *Handbook of competence and motivation* (pp. 259–278). New York: Guilford Press.

Pomerantz, E. M., & Kempner, S. (2013). Mothers' daily person and process praise: Implications for children's theory of intelligence and motivation. *Developmental Psychology, 40,* 2040–2046.

Pomerantz, E. M., Kim, E. M., & Cheung, C. S. (2012). Parents' involvement in children's learning. In K. R. Harris, S. Graham, & T. C. Urdan (Eds.), *APA educational psychology handbook: Vol 2. Individual differences and cultural and contextual factors* (pp. 417–440).

Washington, DC: American Psychological Association.

Pomerantz, E. M., & Monti, J. S. (2015). Measuring parents' involvement in children's education. In S. M. Sheridan & E. M. Kim (Eds.), *Research on family–school partnerships: An interdisciplinary examination of state of the science and critical needs: Vol. 1. Foundational aspects of family–school partnerships* (pp. 55–76). New York: Springer.

Pomerantz, E. M., Moorman, E. A., & Litwack, S. D. (2007). The how, whom, and why of parents' involvement in children's schooling: More is not necessarily better. *Review of Educational Research, 77,* 373–410.

Pomerantz, E. M., Ng, F., & Wang, Q. (2006). Mothers' mastery-oriented involvement in children's homework: Implications for the well-being of children with negative perceptions of competence. *Journal of Educational Psychology, 98,* 99–111.

Pomerantz, E. M., Wang, Q., & Ng, F. F. (2005a). Mothers' affect in the homework context: The importance of staying positive. *Developmental Psychology, 42,* 414–427.

Pomerantz, E. M., Wang, Q., & Ng, F. F. (2005b). The role of children's competence experiences in the socialization process: A dynamic process framework for the academic arena. In R. Kail (Ed.), *Advances in child development and behavior* (Vol. 33, pp. 193–227). San Diego, CA: Academic Press.

Program for International Student Assessment (PISA). (2013). PISA 2012 results. Retrieved from *https://nces.ed.gov/surveys/pisa/pisa2012/index.asp.*

Ramani, G. B., & Siegler, R. S. (2014). How informal learning activities can promote children's numerical knowledge. In R. C. Kadosh & A. Dowker (Eds.), *Oxford handbook of mathematical cognition* (pp. 1135–1154). Oxford, UK: Oxford University Press.

Ramirez, A. Y. F. (2003). Dismay and disappointment. *Urban Review, 35,* 93–110.

Rowe, M. L., Ramani, G. B., & Pomerantz, E. M. (in press). Parental involvement and children's motivation and achievement: A domain-specific perspective. In K. Wentzel & D. Miele (Eds.), *Handbook of motivation at school* (2nd ed.). London: Routledge/Taylor & Francis.

Sameroff, A. (1975). Transactional models in early social relations. *Human Development, 18,* 65–79.

Sameroff, A., & Mackenzie, M. J. (2003). Research strategies for capturing transactional models of development: The limits of the possible. *Development and Psychopathology, 15,* 613–640.

Schulting, A. B., Malone, P. S., & Dodge, K. A. (2005). The effect of school-based kindergarten transition policies and practices on child academic outcomes. *Developmental Psychology, 41,* 860–871.

Senechal, M., & LeFevre, J. (2002). Parental involvement in the development of children's reading skill: A five year longitudinal study. *Child Development, 73,* 445–460.

Sheldon, S. B. (2005). Testing a structural equation model of partnership program implementation and parent involvement. *Elementary School Journal, 106,* 171–187.

Silinskas, G., Kiuru, N., Aunola, K., Lerkkanen, M., & Nurmi, J. (2015). The developmental dynamics of children's academic performance and mothers' homework-related affect and practices. *Developmental Psychology, 51,* 419–433.

Simpkins, S. D., Fredricks, J. A., & Eccles, J. S. (2012). Charting the Eccles' expectancy–value model from mothers' beliefs in childhood to youths' activities in adolescence. *Developmental Psychology, 48,* 1019–1032.

Sirin, R. S. (2005). Socioeconomic status and academic achievement: A meta-analytic review of research. *Review of Educational Research, 75,* 417–453.

Skinner, E., Johnson, S., & Snyder, T. (2005). Six dimensions of parenting: A motivational model. *Parenting: Science and Practice, 5,* 175–235.

Steinberg, L., Lamborn, S. D., Dornbusch, S. M., & Darling, N. (1992). Impact of parenting practices on adolescent achievement: Authoritative parenting, school involvement, and encouragement to succeed. *Child Development, 63,* 1266–1281.

Vanneman, A., Hamilton, L., Baldwin Anderson, J., & Rahman, T. (2009). *Achievement gaps: How black and white students in public schools perform in mathematics and reading on the National Assessment of Educational Progress* (NCES 2009–455). Washington, DC: National Center for Education Statistics, Institute of Education Sciences, U.S. Department of Education.

Vasquez, A. C., Patall, E. A., Fong, C. J., Corrigan, A. S., & Pine, L. (2016). Parent autonomy support, academic achievement, and psychosocial functioning: A meta-analysis of research. *Educational Psychology Review, 28*(3), 605–644.

Vickers, H. S., Minke, K. M., & Anderson, K. J. (2002). Best practices in faciliating collaborative family-teacher routine conferences. In A. Thomas & J. Grimes (Eds.), *Best practices in school psychology IV* (Vol. 1, pp. 431–449). Washington, DC: National Association of School Psychologists.

Waanders, C., Mendez, J. L., & Downder, J. T. (2007). Parent characteristics, economic stress and neighbrohood context as predictors of parent involvement in preschool children's education. *Journal of School Psychology, 45,* 619–636.

Walker, J. M. T., Ice, C. L., Hoover-Dempsey, K. V., & Sandler, H. M. (2011). Latino parents' motivations for involvement in their children's schooling: An exploratory study. *Elementary School Journal, 111,* 409–429.

Walker, J. M. T., Wilkins, A. S., Dallaire, J. R., Sandler, H. M., & Hoover-Dempsey, K. V. (2006). Parental involvement: Model revision through scale development. *Elementary School Journal, 106,* 85–104.

Walton, G. M. (2014). The new science of wise psychological interventions. *Current Directions in Psychological Science, 23,* 73–82.

Wang, M.-T., Hill, N. E., & Hofkens, T. (2014). Parental involvement and African American and European American adolescents' academic, behavioral, and emotional development in secondary school. *Child Development, 85,* 2151–2168.

Wang, M.-T., & Sheikh-Khalil, S. (2014). Does parental involvement matter for student achievement and mental health in high school? *Child Development, 85,* 610–625.

Wang, Q., & Pomerantz, E. M. (2009). The motivational landscape of early adolescence in the United States and China: A longitudinal investigation. *Child Development, 80,* 1280–1296.

Wuyts, D., Vansteenkiste, M., Soenens, B., & Assor, A. (2015). An examination of the dynamics involved in parental child-invested contingent self-esteem. *Parenting: Science and Practice, 15,* 55–74.

Yeager, D. S., & Walton, G. M. (2011). Social-psychological interventions in education: They're not magic. *Review of Educational Research, 81,* 267–301.

CHAPTER 31

Peer Relationships, Motivation, and Academic Performance at School

KATHRYN R. WENTZEL

Relationships with peers are of central importance to children throughout childhood and adolescence. They provide a source of companionship and entertainment, help in solving problems, personal validation and emotional support, and a foundation for identity development (Brown, Mory, & Kinney, 1994; Parker & Asher, 1987). In turn, children who enjoy positive relationships with peers appear to experience levels of emotional well-being, beliefs about the self, and values for prosocial forms of behavior and social interaction that are stronger and more adaptive than do children without positive peer relationships (see Rubin, Bukowski, & Parker, 2006). An additional finding is that children who enjoy positive relationships with their peers also tend to be engaged in and even excel at academic tasks more than those who have peer relationship problems. Children's social competence with peers has been related consistently and positively to academic accomplishments throughout the school-age years (see Wentzel, 2013).

In light of evidence that links children's adaptive functioning across social and academic domains, a central issue that is addressed in this chapter is, why do these associations exist? More specifically, what are the mechanisms by which these two domains of functioning might be related? Toward this end, I first provide general criteria for defining social competence and their implications for understanding peer relationships at school, as well as academic motivation and accomplishments. Next, I review the literature on peer relationships and academic outcomes, followed by a discussion of processes and mechanisms that might explain significant relations between peer relationships and positive outcomes in the academic domain. Finally, I offer thoughts about and provocations for future research.

DEFINING SOCIAL COMPETENCE WITH PEERS

Why might students' relationships with peers be related to their academic motivation and accomplishments? One approach to answering this question is to consider the nature of social competence and how students' relationships with each other reflect a critical component of their social adaptation to school that contributes to their academic success. Toward this end, I begin this section by presenting a definition of social competence derived from theoretical perspectives on person–environment fit and personal goal setting. This definition is then applied to the realm of schooling and students' relationships with peers. In this regard, I describe both social and academic correlates of students' competence with peers.

Perspectives on Social Competence

In the social-developmental literature, *social competence* has been described from a variety of perspectives, ranging from the development of individual skills to more general adaptation within a particular setting. In these discussions, social competence frequently is associated with person-level outcomes such as effective behavioral repertoires, social problem-solving skills, positive beliefs about the self, achievement of social goals, and positive interpersonal relationships (Rose-Krasnor, 1997; Rubin et al., 2006). Also central to many definitions of social competence is the notion that contextual affordances and constraints contribute to and mold the development of these individual outcomes in ways that enable them to contribute to the social good (Barker, 1960; Bronfenbrenner, 1989). Social contexts are believed to play an integral role in providing opportunities for healthy social development, as well as defining the appropriate parameters of children's social accomplishments. In this chapter, therefore, social competence is viewed as achieving a balance between the development of positive outcomes for the self (i.e., person-level outcomes) and adherence to context-specific expectations for behavior that contributes to the smooth functioning of social groups (see also Eccles & Midgley, 1989; Ford, 1992).

The application of this perspective to the realm of schooling results in a multifaceted description of children who are socially competent and well adjusted. First, socially competent students achieve goals that are personally valued, as well as those that are sanctioned by others. Second, the goals they pursue result in both social integration and positive developmental outcomes for the student. Socially integrative outcomes are those that promote the smooth functioning of social groups at school (e.g., cooperative, prosocial behavior) and are reflected in levels of social approval and social acceptance;

student-related outcomes reflect healthy development of the self (e.g., perceived social competence, feelings of self-determination) and feelings of emotional security and well-being (Bronfenbrenner, 1989; Ford, 1992; Ryan & Deci, 2000b). From this description, it follows that social competence is achieved to the extent that students accomplish social goals that have both personal and social value, in a manner that supports continued psychological and emotional health. In addition, the ability to be socially competent is contingent on opportunities and affordances of the school context that allow students to pursue multiple social goals.

Goal-directed behavior in social domains historically has been viewed as an aspect of competence rather than a type of motivation to achieve mastery of specific outcomes (see, e.g., Dodge, Asher, & Parkhurst, 1989; Wentzel, 2002). However, a goal-based definition of *social competence* reflects a basic tenet of motivational theories that people set goals for themselves, and that these goals can be powerful motivators of behavior (Austin & Vancouver, 1996; Bandura, 1986; Dweck, 1991). And, as with achievement-related goals, *social goals* are often defined as cognitive representations of desired future outcomes (e.g., Austin & Vancouver, 1996; Dweck, 1991; for a more extensive discussion of social goals, see Wentzel, 2002, 2005). In addition, as with task- or academically related outcomes, the achievement of social goals often is evaluated on the basis of standards. However, social standards are rarely discussed in terms of some sort of social excellence. Rather, evaluations of "success" typically are based on a combined judgment of personal satisfaction with and positive social reactions to specific social outcomes. Achieving an acceptable discrepancy between these two sets of evaluations is the hallmark of social competence, and it is achieved not just by one person's efforts but often as the result of compromise or conflict resolution among two or more individuals.

SOCIAL COMPETENCE WITH PEERS AT SCHOOL

Given this definition of social competence, one strategy for understanding the nature of social competence with peers and its association with academic motivation and achievement is to identify social characteristics and outcomes related to peer approval and acceptance, as well as ways in which peers might contribute to the development of positive outcomes for students themselves. With regard to the former, establishing positive relationships with peers can take many forms, ranging from general acceptance or preference by the peer group to involvement in reciprocated friendships. Therefore, identifying the common correlates of peer acceptance and approval is a first step in understanding the goal pursuits and outcomes that peers demand in exchange for positive regard. In turn, identifying mechanisms of peer influence provides insights into how students provide each other with the necessary resources and create supportive contexts that promote the achievement of both socially and personally desirable outcomes.

Correlates of Peer Approval and Acceptance

Researchers typically have defined children's involvement in peer relationships in three specific ways: degree of peer acceptance or rejection by the larger peer group, peer group membership, and dyadic friendships. Peer acceptance and social (e.g., sociometric) status is typically determined by unilateral assessments of a child's relative standing or reputation within a larger group of peers, such as a classroom or grade mates. Therefore, the social standing of a student is determined by a diverse set of peers who are not necessarily friends with the student and with whom interactions might be infrequent. Based on these assessments, students are assigned to a sociometric status group (i.e., popular, rejected, neglected, controversial, and average status; see Asher & Dodge, 1986), or described in terms of overall acceptance or rejection by peers.

Membership in peer crowds and groups is typically determined by identifying clusters of students who are friends with each other using statistical procedures (e.g., Kindermann & Gest, 2009) or by asking students to identify groups characterized by common activities (e.g., sports) or behavioral

characteristics (e.g., substance use) or, more simply, by those who spend time together (Brown, 1989). Peer crowds and groups have been studied most frequently in adolescent samples (see Brown & Dietz, 2009). Adolescent crowds often include "Populars" (students who engage in positive forms of both academic and social, behavior), "Jocks" (students characterized by their athletic accomplishments), "Druggies" (students engaged in delinquent and other illicit activities), and "Normals" (fairly average students). Research on peer crowds has been mostly descriptive, identifying the central norms and values that uniquely characterize each crowd. A related construct, peer networks, reflects groups of students formed on the basis of mutual friendships.

Finally, peer relationships are studied with respect to dyadic friendships. In this case, students are asked to nominate their best friends at school; often, nominations are then matched to determine reciprocity, or best friendships. Friendships reflect relatively private, egalitarian relationships typically formed on the basis of idiosyncratic criteria, and are enduring aspects of children's peer relationships at all ages.

Each of these relationship "types" has been related to a range of school-based competencies across the school-age years, to include multiple aspects of motivation and achievement (see also Wentzel & Muenks, 2016). With regard to motivation, sociometric status and peer acceptance have been related positively to pursuit of goals to learn, interest in school, and perceived academic competence; moreover, these findings are robust at all ages (see Wentzel, 2013). During middle school, social acceptance and having friends has been related to positive aspects of social (e.g., goals to help, share, cooperate, and follow rules) and academic (e.g., engagement in academic tasks) motivation (see Kindermann & Skinner, 2012; Wentzel, 2005). Peer group membership has been associated with liking and enjoyment of school (Ryan, 2001), and with changes in intrinsic and extrinsic goals over time (Kindermann & Gest, 2009; Kindermann & Skinner, 2012). Finally, peer acceptance and group membership have been related to a range of motivation outcomes during high school (King & Ganotice, 2014; Nichols & White, 2014; Robnett & Leaper, 2013).

Peer relationships have also been related to academic accomplishments. Social status and acceptance have been associated positively with classroom grades, standardized test scores, and IQ in samples ranging from elementary school to high school (see Wentzel, 2013), and these relations tend to be stable over time (e.g., Gest, Demitrovich, & Welsh, 2005; Wentzel & Caldwell, 1997). Simply having friends also has been related positively to grades and test scores (e.g., Jones, Audley-Piotrowski, & Kiefer, 2012; Wentzel, Barry, & Caldwell, 2004). Students who make transitions with their friends, and those who make friends quickly, also tend to make better academic adjustments to new schools than those who do not (e.g., Ladd, 1990; Molloy, Gest, & Rulison, 2011; Wentzel et al., 2004). Finally, adolescent peer groups differ in the degree to which they pressure members to become involved in academic activities, with "Jocks" and "Popular" groups providing significantly more pressure for academic involvement than other groups (Brown & Dietz, 2009). Researchers who identify friendship-based peer groups using statistical procedures also have found relations between group membership and academic performance (e.g., Kindermann & Gest, 2009), and friendship-based groups in middle school have been related to changes in academic performance over time (Wentzel & Caldwell, 1997).

Mechanisms of Peer Influence and Support

How and why might students' relationships with peers contribute to these positive outcomes? Historically, theoretical explanations have focused on the broad notion that positive relationships with peers contribute directly to cognitive development, highlighting fairly structured interactions that take place in formal learning contexts (e.g., Piaget, 1932/1965; Vygotsky, 1978). Additional approaches are based on models of peer socialization that consider how students' interactions and positive relationships with each other, more generally, provide important opportunities for motivating and facilitating positive motivational and academic outcomes (Wentzel, 2005, 2015). In the following sections, I describe each of these perspectives.

Peer Interactions and Cognitive Gains

Theories of cognitive development have a long-standing tradition of relying on social interaction to explain cognitive growth and learning. Piaget (1932/1965) and Vygotsky (1978) both proposed that children are active participants in their own development, and that they acquire knowledge about their world through activity and social interactions. Piaget proposed that mutual discussion, perspective taking, and conflict resolution with peers can motivate the accommodation of new and more sophisticated approaches to intellectual problem solving; development was contingent on the relatively symmetrical nature of same-age peer interactions that allowed conflict resolution within the context of mutual reciprocity. Symmetrical interaction among peers is found most often in collaborative learning contexts. The nature of collaborative problem solving orients children toward discovery and reflection rather than practice and implementation, and requires peers to integrate the multiple perspectives that each student brings to the task. In support of this notion is evidence that problem-solving tasks, which demand the acquisition of basic reasoning skills, have been found to occur best in peer collaborative contexts rather than other forms of peer learning contexts (e.g., tutoring) (Sharan, 1984; Slavin, 1980). Cognitive gains attributed to participation in cooperative learning activities also have been explained with respect to mechanisms associated with symmetrical peer interactions (Slavin, 2011).

Vygotsky (1978) placed primary importance on social activity within small groups or pairs of individuals, in which competent students teach specific strategies and standards for performance to peers who are less skilled. In this manner, asymmetrical interactions contribute to competence development through the process of "scaffolding," which extends the range of the less advanced child by bridging the gap between current and desired skill, thereby allowing him or her to accomplish a task not otherwise possible. From an instructional perspective, scaffolding requires deliberate decision making and choice of peer partners on the part of teachers in order to create the optimal learning environment for participating students.

Peer Interactions and Social Supports

Although the nature of interactions within formal peer learning contexts has the potential to explain the development and refinement of cognitive structures, it is reasonable to expect that additional aspects of peer interactions within these contexts and in less formal settings contribute in positive ways to student competencies. Indeed, most researchers agree that at the core of positive peer relationships and interactions are the benefits they provide in the form of social supports (Bukowski, Motzoi, & Meyer, 2009; Parker & Asher, 1987). These supports serve a range of functions, including maintenance of the peer group by promoting socially valued goals and social cohesion, as well as facilitating the development of individual outcomes such as social skills and psychological well-being. Supports that promote allegiance to the broader group and to engagement in group-valued activities take the form of expectations for the pursuit and achievement of specific outcomes, help to achieve these outcomes, a safe environment, and emotional nurturance (see Wentzel, 2004, for a review). These outcomes reflect essential components of social support in that, if present, (1) information is provided concerning what is expected and valued by the group; (2) attempts to achieve these valued outcomes are met with help and instruction; (3) attempts to achieve outcomes can be made in a safe, nonthreatening environment; and (4) individuals are made to feel like valued members of the group.

Applied specifically to peer activities as they occur in classroom and school settings, this perspective suggests that students will engage in the pursuit of positive social and academic goals, in part, when their peers communicate positive expectations and standards for achieving such goals; provide direct assistance and help in achieving them; and create a climate of emotional support (including protection from physical threats and harm) that facilitates positive engagement in valued classroom activities (see Ford, 1992; Wentzel, 2004). Of relevance for the definition of social competence framing this chapter is that in addition to promoting outcomes valued by peers, these supports also have the potential to facilitate the achievement of students' personal goals by promoting positive perceptions of competence, autonomy, and social relatedness (see Ryan & Deci, 2000a, 2000b; Wentzel, 2004).

In the following sections, I describe specific mechanisms whereby peer supports may influence motivational and academic outcomes. Mechanisms are grouped with respect to informational supports (providing goals, expectations, and assistance) and motivational supports (emotional caring, rewards and reinforcements, and peer pressure).

INFORMATIONAL SUPPORTS

Although teachers play a central role in academic instruction and modeling strategies to learn, students also communicate important information, teach valuable skills, and provide instrumental help to each other. These supports can occur during the course of academic instruction, and they comprise a large part of informal peer interactions at school. As suggested by social-cognitive theory, direct instruction and modeling are powerful mechanisms whereby students learn from peers what is expected of them, along with skills that enable them to go about meeting those expectations (Bandura, 1986). These processes can occur within dyadic or small-group interactions, such as those prescribed by constructivist perspectives. The larger peer group also can be a source of behavioral standards, with direct instruction and modeling serving as means to monitor and enforce group standards and expectations (see Brown, Bakken, Ameringer, & Mahon, 2008; Kindermann, 2007).

Direct Instruction. During the course of interactions with peers, students receive input concerning socially valued goals and expectations for academic performance and social behavior, and standards against which judgments of personal efficacy may be made. From a social-cognitive perspective, peers who convey expectations that academic engagement and positive social interactions are important and enjoyable are likely to lead others to form similar values and goals (Bandura, 1986). Empirical evidence that peers communicate expectations and opinions concerning appropriate behavior and academic outcomes is scant. However, it is clear that these communications do occur, functioning to define, clarify, maintain, and enforce peer norms (Brown et al., 2008). Perceived expectations from peers for social and academic outcomes (Wentzel, 2004; Wentzel, Baker, & Russell, 2012, 2014; Wentzel, Battle, Russell, & Looney, 2010), and peer group norms (e.g., Kindermann, 1993; Kiuru, Aunola, Vuori, & Nurmi, 2007; Sage & Kindermann, 1999) have been related to positive forms of social behavior, motivation, and academic achievement. In addition, advice and feedback from peers following success or failure can lead to adjustments in students' perceived competence and expectations for future academic success (Altermatt, Pomerantz, Ruble, Frey, & Greulich, 2002; see also Gauvain, 2016).

Modeling. Modeling is also a powerful process by which information is communicated (Bandura, 1986). Of interest for this chapter is that modeling effects are especially likely to occur when students are friends (Crockett, Losoff, & Petersen, 1984; Ricciardelli & Mellor, 2012). Findings relating characteristics of friends to changes (positive and negative) in social behavior and academic engagement throughout middle school (Barry & Wentzel, 2006; Berndt, Hawkins, & Jiao, 1999; Wentzel et al., 2004) and high school (Prinstein, Brechwald, & Cohen, 2011) provide indirect evidence for modeling effects. Similarly, changes in younger children's competence perceptions from fall to spring have been associated with the competence perceptions of their very best friends (Altermatt & Pomerantz, 2005; Molloy et al., 2011). Adolescents' perceptions of their friends' academic behavior, engagement, and performance also have predicted students' own achievement-related choices, goal pursuit, engagement, and academic performance (e.g., Jones et al., 2012; Marion, Laursen, Kiuru, Nurmi, & Salmela-Aro, 2014; Nelson & DeBacker, 2008).

MOTIVATIONAL SUPPORTS

Students also exert influence on each other through expressions of emotional caring, dispensing rewards and reinforcements, and engaging in peer pressure. These types of influence are conveyed by way of social acceptance and rejection, intrinsic and extrinsic reinforcements, and group contagion, and are relevant for understanding the nature of social exchanges in both formal and informal instructional settings.

Social Acceptance and Rejection. Students experience varying levels of social belongingness and acceptance with peers within dyadic relationships such as friendships, and within larger peer groups to the extent they are inclusive or exclusive (Bennett, 2014). Models of peer influence posit that students who are rejected by their peers suffer from a lack of opportunities and supports afforded to children accepted by peers, including positive and effective role models, direct instruction concerning normative behavior and skill development, and sources of positive rewards for social and academic behavior (see Parker & Asher, 1987; Patterson & Bank, 1989).

Social acceptance and rejection can also have a powerful impact on students' motivation and emotional well-being. For example, theoretical perspectives suggest that strong affective bonds and perceived support from others serve as buffers from stress and anxiety and contribute to a positive sense of emotional well-being (Sarason, Sarason, & Pierce, 1990). In turn, feelings of emotional security and social connection are believed to facilitate the adoption of goals and interests valued by others (e.g., Ryan & Deci, 2000a). In support of this notion is an extensive literature indicating that experiencing supportive and caring peers is related positively to interest and engagement in classroom life, whereas viewing relationships with peers as negative is related to motivational and academic problems (Juvonen, Nishina, & Graham, 2000). Evidence documents significant relations between psychological distress and depression and a range of achievement-related outcomes, including interest in school, negative attitudes toward academic achievement, actual levels of performance, school avoidance and low levels of class-room participation, and ineffective cognitive functioning (see Wentzel, 2005, 2014).

Theorists also have argued that desires to sustain positive group identity and cohesion can result in exclusionary practices within and between groups (e.g., Abrams & Rutland, 2008; Bennett, 2014), including the formation of stereotypes and discriminating practices (e.g., Dovidio, Gaertner, Hodson, Houlette, & Johnson, 2005; Tajfel & Turner, 1979). As with social acceptance and rejection, these group-level processes can have a profound effect on students' emotional well-being (Brown et al., 2008), their access to opportunities and supports (Haslam, Reicher, & Levine, 2012), and their motivational beliefs, including a sense of group efficacy (Bandura, 1986).

Intrinsic and Extrinsic Reinforcement.

Peers can also exert influence by way of reinforcements and rewards. *Intrinsic rewards* are positive outcomes for the self that are associated with the act of engaging in a task or activity; students might engage in behavior valued by peers because they experience the behavior as enjoyable and of personal value (Boggiano, Klinger, & Main, 1986; Ojanen, Stratman, Card, & Little, 2013). *Extrinsic rewards* are outcomes associated with a task that are externally imposed or viewed as an endpoint, such that the task is viewed as a means to an end. In this case, engaging in positive social interactions and conforming to social expectations is a way to achieve other goals, such as social acceptance or a better grade (see Wentzel, 2002, 2005).

Peer influence has also been studied with respect to negative reinforcements and reward systems, especially peers' use of intimidation, power assertion, and negative reinforcement. These practices have been used to explain the process of peer pressure and how peer groups function to establish normative standards and power hierarchies (e.g., Cairns, Neckerman, & Cairns, 1989). For example, popular children often exert power over others by using social acceptance and status as a reward for compliance and conformity (Cillessen & Rose, 2005; Sandstrom, 2011). An extensive literature has also demonstrated how negative reinforcement in

the form of physical and relational aggression can result in a broad range of negative outcomes related to motivation, emotional functioning, and social behavior (e.g., Crick, Murray-Close, Marks, & Mohajeri-Nelson, 2009). Students can also experience negative reinforcement for doing well academically through labeling and stigmatization (Boehnke, 2008; Fordham & Ogbu, 1986).

Group Contagion.

Group contagion is a mutual influence process that occurs as a function of being a member of a peer group or social network, and of patterns of reinforcement that occur as a product of group functioning (Dishion, 2013). *Peer contagion* is associated most often with children's and adolescent's disinhibition of behavior, the disruption of normative behavior (e.g., Boxer, Guerra, Huesmann, & Morales, 2005; Ehrenreich, Underwood, & Ackerman, 2014), and mood regulation and depressive symptoms (Dishion & Connell, 2006). However, peer group dynamics have also been associated with positive aspects of student motivation, such as pursuit of intrinsic goals (Duriez, Giletta, Kuppens, & Vansteenkiste, 2013) and emotional well-being (Prinstein, 2007; van Workum, Scholte, Cillessen, Lodder, & Giletta, 2013).

Summary

The picture of social competence with peers that emerges from the literature suggests that students' contribution to the "social good" (as indexed by various aspects of peer acceptance and approval) is based in part on positive aspects of motivation and achievement at school. In turn, students have the potential to influence each other's cognitive development and academic accomplishments through a range of mechanisms. The literature on structured peer learning contexts considers "cognitive gains" in fairly narrow terms, that is, as the development of specific cognitive structures and intellectual skills that evolve through certain types of peer interactions. More broadly, peers are believed to influence student motivation and academic accomplishments through provisions of informational and motivational supports.

Although discussion of ways in which these two perspectives on peer learning might be synergistic is rare, it is useful to think about ways in which peer interactions in one type of context might influence interactions in the other. For example, the same supports that are afforded by informal peer contexts also are likely to facilitate the types of positive interactions that are related to cognitive gains within more structured peer learning contexts (see Wentzel & Watkins, 2002). It is also likely that successful peer collaborations can enhance the quality of peer relationships by providing opportunities for students to strengthen interpersonal ties and therefore the likelihood that positive peer supports will become available during other forms of classroom instruction.

The competence perspective that guides this chapter suggests that at the heart of these positive peer interactions and influences are students' desires, or goals, to contribute to the social and academic worlds of the classroom, while maintaining a positive sense of self. Indeed, in order to pay attention to and buy into peer norms and expectations, students must want to be a part of the peer culture, trust that they will be rewarded for doing so, and be assured of safety from emotional and physical harm. Modeling, peer pressure, and other forms of influence are not likely to be effective if these basic conditions are not in place. Similarly, if appropriate goals and supports are not a part of the larger classroom and school culture, students are not likely to offer these basic supports to each other.

Given the critical nature of these contextual supports, it is important to understand the role that adults can play in promoting positive peer relationships and interactions at school, especially as they relate to learning and intellectual growth. Teachers and administrators are the primary architects of the classroom and school contexts in which students interact with each other and, as such, have the potential to facilitate academic achievements by way of positive peer relationships. In the following section, I describe the potential impact that teachers and the broader school context can have on students' ability to provide positive resources and supports to each other, to interact with each other in positive ways, and to encourage the peer group to be socially accepting, cooperative, and welcoming particularly to

students who demonstrate peer problems that interfere with their academic progress (Mikami, Lerner, & Lun, 2010).

LINKING THEORY AND EVIDENCE TO PRACTICE

Given the potentially powerful and positive role that peers can have in student learning and achievement, it becomes important to understand the role of teachers and school administrators in promoting successful interactions and personal relationships among peers. There is evidence that teachers' beliefs and behaviors, classroom organization and instructional practices, and schoolwide structure, composition, and climate affects students' ability to interact successfully in peer learning activities, students' peer choice and general propensity to make friends, and levels of peer acceptance and friendship networks in classrooms. In the following sections, I describe relevant research on teachers and classroom contexts, then research on school-level influences.

Teachers and Peer Learning Activities

The positive effects of peer collaborative and cooperative approaches to learning on cognitive and motivational outcomes is well documented. Although an extensive review of this literature is beyond the scope of this chapter, comprehensive reviews and resources are available on this topic (see, Slavin, 2011; Wentzel & Edelman, 2016). However, it is important to note that in addition to simply implementing these peer learning activities in their classrooms, teachers can play a critical role in their success by ensuring that students have partners who can benefit from the interactions, as well as contribute to the learning of their peer partners. When implementing peer-assisted learning structures, teachers cannot just place students together and hope for the best. These activities require explicit planning and training that will prepare peer partners in academic as well as social skills.

In support of this notion, research on peer learning has confirmed that children do not necessarily develop the constructive interaction patterns or the ability to scaffold that are required for productive engagement to occur without explicit preparation. As Person and Graesser (1999) note, tutoring behaviors tend to be primitive and are often characterized by questioning that is limited in frequency and level of cognitive demand, coupled with infrequent correction of errors, and the giving of positive feedback at inappropriate times. Moreover, students do not necessarily have the ability to engage in positive social interactions that are necessary for successful collaborations with one another (Peterson, Wilkinrson, Spinelli, & Swing, 1984). However, the positive effects of training students to work with peers in collaborative and cooperative learning contexts have been demonstrated. Higher-achieving partners trained to offer positive constructive feedback and guided direction can enhance the quality of social interactions and cognitive functioning of lower-achieving students (e.g., Fuchs, Fuchs, Bentz, Phillips, & Hamlett, 1994).

Teachers and Peer Relationships

Although the nature of causal connections between teacher–student interactions and peer relationships is unclear, it is reasonable to assume that students' positive relationships with peers might be due in large part to teachers' communications of specific expectations for behavior and achievement, and to systematic regulation of student behavior through instruction-related activities. To illustrate, teachers' expectations concerning students' aptitude and performance have been related to levels of peer acceptance and rejection (e.g., Donohue, Perry, & Weinstein, 2003; Farmer, Lines, & Hamm, 2011; Mikami, Griggs, Reuland, & Gregory, 2012). Teachers' verbal and nonverbal behavior toward certain children, especially when critical, also has been related to how these children are treated by their peers (Flanders & Havumaki, 1960; Harper & McCluskey, 2003). In addition, teachers' positive feedback in response to appropriate behavior has been related to students' positive evaluations of and peer preference for students exhibiting that behavior, whereas negative and critical feedback for disruptive and off-task behavior has been related to negative evaluations of and peer dislike

of students exhibiting such behavior (White & Kistner, 1992). Finally, teachers vary in the behaviors they consider to be appropriate and inappropriate when children are interacting with each other, especially with regard to aggression; in turn, teachers' perspectives on the appropriateness of behaviors tend to be adopted by their students (Craig, Henderson & Murphy, 2000; Smith, 2007).

The instructional approach that a teacher adopts also appears to have an impact on students' relationships with peers (Farmer et al., 2011). For example, students enjoy more positive relationships with classmates when teachers use learner-centered practices (e.g., involving students in decision making) as opposed to teacher-centered practices (e.g., focusing on rote learning, norm-referenced evaluation; Donohue et al., 2003) or competitive practices (Mikami et al., 2012). The way in which teachers group students also has been associated with the quality of peer relationships (Gest & Rodkin, 2011) and interactions (Luckner & Pianta, 2011). Finally, middle and high school students in classrooms where students are encouraged to talk to each other about assignments, to work in small groups, and to move about while working on activities also are less likely to be socially isolated or rejected, enjoy greater numbers of friends, and enjoy more diversity and stability in their friendships (e.g., Gest & Rodkin, 2011).

Collectively, this work demonstrates that the quality of teacher–student interpersonal relationships and specific instructional practices has the potential to contribute to positive peer interactions, reputations, academic achievement, and motivation, especially for students with peer problems (Mikami et al., 2012; Pianta & Allen, 2008). Efforts to develop interventions to improve teacher–student relationships have been infrequent. However, several programs appear to be promising and noteworthy. The Responsive Classroom (RC) approach has been associated with improved teacher–student relationships and classroom behavior in addition to academic gains (Rimm-Kaufman & Chiu, 2007; Rimm-Kaufman, Fan, Chiu, & You, 2007). My Teaching Partner–Secondary (MTP-S) intervention was designed to increase teachers' positive interactions with students and promote sensitive instructional practices. RC has demonstrated improvement in positive peer interactions of students high in disruptive behavior (Mikami, Gregory, Allen, Pianta, & Lun, 2011). The Rural Early Adolescent Learning (REAL) program, which includes a focus on teachers' understanding of classroom social dynamics, has demonstrated positive gains in students' motivation and academic outcomes, and changes in peer norms for academic effort and achievement (Hamm, Farmer, Dadisman, Gravelle, & Murray, 2011). The Child Development Project (CDP; *www.devstu.org*) has been successful in increasing levels of positive behavior and academic achievement by focusing in part on improving classroom management practices and interpersonal relationships.

School-Level and Structural Influences

Perhaps the most obvious way that schools can promote positive peer relationships and interactions is by creating cultures and climates that are conducive to positive social and emotional development. Classroom- and school-level programs designed to promote social skills development and positive emotional well-being are relevant to this discussion. As noted earlier, social and emotional competencies can provide a foundation for the types of positive peer interactions in formal settings that are necessary for cognitive gains to occur (e.g., Ladd et al., 2014; Wentzel & Watkins, 2002). Social-emotional skills can also contribute to the development of positive relationships with peers (Fabes, Martin, & Hanish, 2009; Rubin et al., 2006), which in turn provide students with a range of positive supports. In general, schoolwide policies and programs that accentuate the importance of students' prosocial development can also facilitate the development of positive peer relationships (Durlak, Weissberg, Dymnicki, Taylor, & Schellinger, 2011; Gresham, Van, & Cook, 2006). For example, social skills training programs can increase the prevalence of prosocial behaviors (e.g., sharing, cooperating) displayed by students in the classroom by teaching them how to recognize emotions more effectively, negotiate conflict resolutions, and control impulsive behaviors (Gresham et al., 2006). These programs also facilitate a reduction in maladaptive social skills, thus enabling the formation of more functional peer relationships (Wilson & Lipsey, 2007). Programs such as Second Step (Frey, Nolen, Van Schoiack Edstrom, & Hirschstein, 2005), the Fast Track Program (see Bierman et al., 1999; Bierman, Coie, Dodge, Greenberg, Lochman, & McMahon, 2010), and Promoting Alternative Thinking Strategies (PATHS; Bierman et al., 2010) have had documented success in this area.

Of related importance is that although the literature implies that peers might be the primary source of threats to students' physical safety and well-being, teachers and school administrators can play a central role in creating schools that are free of peer harassment and in alleviating the negative effects of harassment once it has occurred (e.g., Espelage & Colbert, 2016; Olweus & Limber, 2009). Interventions designed to offset the often negative influence of peer groups and gangs on behavior and school attendance are especially successful if students have access to adults who provide them with warmth and strong guidance (e.g., Chaskin, 2010). Schools that stress intergenerational bonding also support the development of positive teacher–student relationships that can buffer the potentially negative effects of aggressive peers on behavior (Crosnoe & Needhan, 2004).

From a developmental perspective, improving the quality of peer relationships should be of special concern for teachers and administrators who work with students during transitions to new schools. For example, many young adolescents enter new middle school structures that necessitate interacting with larger numbers of peers on a daily basis. In contrast to the greater predictability of self-contained classroom environments in elementary school, the relative uncertainty and ambiguity of multiple classroom environments, new instructional styles, and more complex class schedules often result in middle school students turning to each other for information, social support, and ways to cope. Students who have access to positive peer supports are likely to adapt to the demands of middle school transition more quickly and in more positive ways than those without such supports (Wentzel et al., 2004). In addition, the value of teacher professional development interventions appears to be particularly important at the secondary school level, where teachers are found to perceive their function as imparting academic content rather than facilitating social relationships with peers (Lynch & Cicchetti, 1997).

Finally, evidence of ways in which school structures and school-level characteristics can influence peer interactions and relationships has been less forthcoming. However, homogenous classroom composition can be deleterious to the formation and maintenance of positive, high-quality peer relationships over time (Barth, Dunlap, Dane, Lochman, & Wells, 2004). Similarly, African American students in classrooms that are ethnically diverse tend to report having more high-quality friendships than those in less diverse classrooms (Jackson, Barth, Powell, & Lochman, 2006). At the school level, greater ethnic diversity tends to result in students who have more friends and more extensive social networks than those in less diverse schools (e.g., Jackson et al., 2006).

CONCLUSIONS AND FUTURE DIRECTIONS

In this chapter, I began by posing the question of how social competence with peers might be related to academic motivation and accomplishments at school. I have argued that social competence with peers reflects the degree to which students are able to meet the social expectations of the peer group, as well as pursue their own personal goals; the achievement of these dual sets of goals is reflected in the psychological and emotional well-being of the student, as well as the smooth functioning of peer relationships and interactions. I also have described pathways whereby students' relationships with peers might be related to academic outcomes.

Much work, however, remains to be done. At the most general level, it is clear that peers can play a powerful role in defining socially valued outcomes at school through direct instruction and modeling, and by rewarding specific behaviors and personal characteristics with social acceptance and approval. Moreover, most students want to be accepted by their peers and are likely to behave in ways that will result in positive relationships with their classmates. However, an understanding of peer influence and determinations of social competence with peers cannot be made without consideration of students' own personal goals. Therefore, researchers need to identify ways in which students learn to coordinate their own social and academic goals with those prompted by others. Issues concerning cause and effect also necessitate continued focus on underlying psychological processes and skills that promote the development and display of competent school-based outcomes.

Lacking direct evidence of causal influence, it is possible that social competence with peers is simply correlated to academic competencies, without any direction of effects. However, a more likely explanation is that a third set of factors contributes to competence in both domains. These factors could reflect specific types of social behavior, as well as psychological or emotional processes that support both positive peer relationships and academic excellence. For example, an extensive body of work has documented associations between peer relationships and social-behavioral outcomes. In general, socially accepted and popular students tend to be more prosocial and sociable, and less aggressive, and rejected students appear to be less compliant, less self-assured, less sociable, and more aggressive and withdrawn. These findings are robust for samples ranging from kindergarten to high school (see Rubin et al., 2006).

Students' friendships and peer groups also are associated with social-behavioral outcomes. Children with friends tend to be more sociable, cooperative, and self-confident when compared to their peers without friends; children with reciprocated friendships also tend to be more independent, emotionally supportive, altruistic and prosocial, and less aggressive than those who do not have such friendships (Newcomb & Bagwell, 1995). As with peer acceptance, these findings appear to be robust for students of all ages. Finally, peer crowds often differ with respect to the reputations for social behavior (see Brown, 1989). Of relevance for this discussion is that these forms of positive social outcomes, to include multiple forms of prosocial and cooperative behavior, have been related consistently and positively to academic outcomes (see Wentzel, 2013), and have been found to mediate relations between sociometric status and academic accomplishments in both early childhood and early adolescence (Buhs & Ladd, 2001; Wentzel, 1991a).

Moreover, teachers report social preference and approval for students who cooperate, share, and follow rules (Wentzel, 1991b, 2003). Therefore, it is possible that students are rewarded by teachers for their positive behavior with high grades. It also is likely that displays of positive behavior and a lack of disruptive behavior in the classroom creates an instructional climate conducive to effective teaching and learning of academic material. In this way, social behavior can contribute directly to learning and task mastery, as well as social approval and acceptance. Finally, metacognitive and self-regulatory processes also are likely to contribute to adaptive outcomes in both social and academic domains. Several theorists have posited a broad range of basic information-processing skills as factors that contribute to the ability to implement planful behavior in both social and academic domains (e.g., Lemerise & Arsenio, 2000).

Assuming that causal connections exist, the contribution of different types of peer involvement to academic outcomes also remains a relatively unexplored area of research. On the one hand, friends are believed to play a central role in providing contexts for self-expression, validation, and affirmation (Hartup & Stevens, 1997). Having friends appears to mediate the negative effects of harsh and punitive home environments on children's relations with the broader peer group (Schwartz, Dodge, Pettit, Bates, & the Conduct Problems Prevention Research Group, 2000), and being without friends predicts less than optimal levels of emotional well-being (e.g., Wenz-Gross, Siperstein, Untch, & Widaman, 1997). In addition, friends appear to elicit behavior that would not necessarily be displayed under other circumstances. For example, when children are with friends, they engage in more positive interactions, resolve more conflicts, and accomplish tasks with greater proficiency than when they are with nonfriends (Newcomb & Bagwell,

1995). Children also typically display more affect and emotional intensity with friends than with nonfriends (Parker & Gottman, 1989), and children are more successful at making transitions when friends accompany them (Ladd, 1990; Ladd & Price, 1987). In contrast, friends tend to play a relatively minor role in socializing each other with respect to larger group norms and expectations (Hartup & Stevens, 1997).

On the other hand, adolescent peer groups and crowds are believed to facilitate the formation of identity and self-concept, and to structure the nature of ongoing social interactions within and across groups (Brown et al., 1994). In both of these roles, peer groups and crowds are likely to provide students with values, norms, and interaction styles that are commonly valued and sanctioned; valued behavior is modeled frequently, so that it can be easily learned and adopted by group members (Brown et al., 1994). Ecological perspectives (Bronfenbrenner, 1989; Cairns et al., 1989) also call attention to the role of peer groups and crowds as intermediaries between the individual and broader peer and adult communities. For these reasons, it is likely that peer groups and crowds can play a central role in contributing to students' academic values and accomplishments. However, the role of other peer relationship "types" in facilitating success at school deserves further attention.

Finally, future research must be conducted within a developmental framework, taking into account the age-related interests and capabilities of the child. From a developmental perspective, the role of peers in motivating academic accomplishments is likely to be especially critical during the middle school and high school years. Although children are interested in and even emotionally attached to their peers at all ages, they exhibit increased interest in their peers, spend more time with them, and exhibit a growing psychological and emotional dependence on them for support and guidance as they make the transition into adolescence (Youniss & Smollar, 1989). Moreover, whereas friendships are enduring aspects of children's peer relationships at all ages, peer groups and crowds emerge primarily in the middle school years, peak at the beginning of high school, then diminish in both prevalence and influence by the end of high school (Brown, 1989). Therefore, efforts to understand the influence of peer relationships on academic motivation and outcomes must be sensitive to not only the qualities and types of relationships that students form with each other but also developmental issues.

In conclusion, we have gained important insights into students' experiences with peers as they relate to academic motivation and achievement. Hopefully, these insights can serve as a foundation to explore further the social antecedents and supports that promote academic accomplishments, and to develop classroom practices that will facilitate positive developmental outcomes in all school-age children.

REFERENCES

Abrams, D., & Rutland, A. (2008). The development of subjective group dynamics. In. S. Levy & M. Killen (Eds.), *Intergroup attitudes and relations in childhood through adulthood* (pp. 47–65). Oxford, UK: Oxford University Press.

Altermatt, E. R., & Pomerantz, E. M. (2005). The implications of having high-achieving versus low-achieving friends: A longitudinal analysis. *Social Development, 14,* 61–81.

Altermatt, E. R., Pomerantz, E. M., Ruble, D. N., Frey, K. S., & Greulich, F. K. (2002). Predicting changes in children's self-perceptions of academic competence: A naturalistic examination of evaluative discourse among classmates. *Developmental Psychology, 38,* 903–917.

Asher, S. R., & Dodge, K. A. (1986). Identifying children who are rejected by their peers. *Developmental Psychology, 22,* 444–449.

Austin, J. T., & Vancouver, J. B. (1996). Goal constructs in psychology: Structure, process, and content. *Psychological Bulletin, 120,* 338–375.

Bandura, A. (1986). *Social foundations of thought and action: A social cognitive theory.* Englewood Cliffs, NJ: Prentice Hall.

Barker, R. G. (1960). Ecology and motivation. In M. R. Jones (Ed.), *Nebraska Symposium on Motivation* (Vol. 8, pp. 1–50). Lincoln: University of Nebraska Press.

Barry, C. M., & Wentzel, K. R. (2006). Friend influence on prosocial behavior: The role of motivational factors and friendship characteristics. *Developmental Psychology, 42,* 153–163.

Barth, J., Dunlap, S., Dane, H., Lochman, J., & Wells, K. (2004). Classroom environment influences on aggression, peer relations, and academic focus. *Journal of School Psychology, 42,* 115–133.

Bennett, M. (2014). Intergroup social exclusion in childhood: Forms, norms, context, and social identity. *Journal of Social Issues, 70,* 183–195.

Berndt, T. J., Hawkins, J. A., & Jiao, Z. (1999). Influences of friends and friendships on adjustment to junior high school. *Merrill–Palmer Quarterly, 45,* 13–41.

Bierman, K., Coie, J., Dodge, K., Greenberg, M., Lochman, J., McMahon, R., et al. (1999). Initial impact of the Fast Track Prevention Trial for conduct problems: II. Classroom effect. *Journal of Consulting and Clinical Psychology, 67,* 648–657.

Bierman, K. L., Coie, J. D., Dodge, K. A., Greenberg, M. T., Lochman, J. E., & McMahon, R. J. (2010). The effects of a multiyear universal social–emotional learning program: The role of student and school characteristics. *Journal of Consulting and Clinical Psychology, 78,* 156–168.

Boehnke, K. (2008). Peer pressure: A cause of scholastic underachievement?: A cross-cultural study of mathematical achievement among German, Canadian, and Israeli middle school students. *Social Psychology of Education, 11,* 149–160.

Boggiano, A., Klinger, C., & Main, D. (1986). Enhancing interest in peer interaction: A developmental analysis. *Child Development, 57,* 852–861.

Boxer, P., Guerra, N., Huesmann, L., & Morales, J. (2005). Proximal peer-level effects of a small-group selected prevention on aggression in elementary school children: An investigation of the peer contagion hypothesis. *Journal of Abnormal Child Psychology, 33,* 325–338.

Bronfenbrenner, U. (1989). Ecological systems theory. In R. Vasta (Ed.), *Annals of child development* (Vol. 6, pp. 187–250). Greenwich, CT: JAI Press.

Brown, B. B. (1989). The role of peer groups in adolescents' adjustment to secondary school. In T. J. Berndt & G. W. Ladd (Eds.), *Peer relationships in child development* (pp. 188–215). New York: Wiley.

Brown, B. B., Bakken, J. P., Ameringer, S. W., & Mahon, S. D. (2008). A comprehensive conceptualization of the peer influence process in adolescence. In M. J. Prinstein & K. A. Dodge (Eds.), *Understanding peer influence in children and adolescents* (pp. 17–44). New York: Guilford Press.

Brown, B. B., & Dietz, E. L. (2009). Informal peer groups in middle childhood and adolescence. In K. H. Rubin, W. M. Bukowski, & B. Laursen (Eds)., *Handbook of peer interactions, relationships, and groups* (pp. 361–376). New York: Guilford Press.

Brown, B. B., Mory, M. S., & Kinney, D. (1994) Casting adolescent crowds in a relational perspective: Caricature, channel, and context. In R. Montemayor, G. R. Adams, & T. P. Gullotta (Eds.), *Personal relationships during adolescence* (pp. 123–167). Newbury Park, CA: Sage.

Buhs, E. S., & Ladd, G. W. (2001). Peer rejection as an antecedent of young children's school adjustment: An examination of mediating processes. *Developmental Psychology, 37,* 550–560.

Bukowski, W. M., Motzoi, C., & Meyer, F. (2009). Friendship as process, function, and outcome. In K. H. Rubin, W. M. Bukowski, & B. Laursen (Eds.), *Handbook of peer interactions, relationships, and groups* (pp. 217–231). New York: Guilford Press.

Cairns, R. B., Neckerman, H. J., & Cairns, B. D. (1989). Social networks and shadows of synchrony. In G. R. Adams, T. P. Gullota, & R. Montemayor (Eds.), *Advances in adolescent development* (pp. 275–305). Beverly Hills, CA: Sage.

Chaskin, R. J. (2010). *Youth gangs and community intervention: Research, practice, and evidence.* New York: Columbia University Press.

Cillessen, A., & Rose, A. (2005). Understanding popularity in the peer system. *Current Directions in Psychological Science, 14,* 102–105.

Craig, W., Henderson, K., & Murphy, J. G. (2000). Prospective teachers' attitudes toward bullying and victimization. *School Psychology International, 21,* 5–21.

Crick, N., Murray-Close, D., Marks, P., & Moharjeri-Nelson, S. (2009). Aggression and peer relationships in school-age children: Relational and physical aggression in group and dyadic contexts. In K. H. Rubin, W. M. Bukowski, & B. Laursen (Eds.), *Handbook of peer interactions, relationships, and groups* (pp. 287–302). New York: Guilford Press.

Crockett, L., Losoff, M., & Petersen, A. C. (1984). Perceptions of the peer group and friendship in early adolescence. *Journal of Early Adolescence, 4,* 155–181.

Crosnoe, R., & Needham, B. (2004). Holism, contextual variability, and the study of friendships in adolescent development. *Child Development, 75,* 264–279.

Dishion, T. (2013). Stochastic agent-based modeling of influence and selection in adolescence: Current status and future directions in understanding the dynamics of peer contagion. *Journal of Research on Adolescence, 23,* 596–603.

Dishion, T. J., & Connell, A. (2006). Adolescents' resilience as a self-regulatory process. *Annals of the New York Academy of Sciences, 1094,* 125–138.

Dodge, K. A., Asher, S. R., & Parkhurst, J. T. (1989). Social life as a goal coordination task. In C. Ames & R. Ames (Eds.), *Research on motivation in education* (Vol. 3, pp. 107–138). New York: Academic Press.

Donohue, K., Perry, K., & Weinstein, R. (2003). Teachers' classroom practices and children's rejection by their peers. *Journal of Applied Developmental Psychology, 24,* 91–118.

Dovidio, J. F., Gaertner, S. L., Hodson, G., Houlette, M. A., & Johnson, K. M. (2005). Social inclusion and exclusion: Recategorization and the perception of intergroup boundaries. In D. Abrams, M. Hogg, & J. Marques (Eds.), *The social psychology of inclusion and exclusion* (pp. 245–264). New York: Psychology Press.

Duriez, B., Giletta, M., Kuppens, P., & Vansteenkiste, M. (2013). Extrinsic relative to intrinsic goal pursuits and peer dynamics: Selection and influence processes among adolescents. *Journal of Adolescence, 36,* 925–933.

Durlak, J. A., Weissberg, R. P., Dymnicki, A. B., Taylor, R. D., & Schellinger, K. B. (2011). The impact of enhancing students' social and emotional learning: A meta-analysis of school-based universal interventions. *Child Development, 82,* 405–432.

Dweck, C. S. (1991). Self-theories and goals: Their role in motivation, personality, and development. In R. Dienstbier (Ed.), *Nebraska Symposium on Motivation* (Vol. 38, pp. 199–236). Lincoln: University of Nebraska Press.

Eccles, J. S., & Midgley, C. (1989). Stage-environment fit: Developmentally appropriate classrooms for young adolescents. In C. Ames & R. Ames (Eds.), *Research on motivation in education* (Vol. 3, pp. 139–186). New York: Academic Press.

Ehrenreich, S., Underwood, M., & Ackerman, R. (2014). Adolescents' text message communication and growth in antisocial behavior across the first year of high school. *Journal of Abnormal Child Psychology, 42,* 251–264.

Espelage, D. L., & Colbert, C. L. (2016). School-based interventions to prevent bullying and promote prosocial behaviors. In K. Wentzel & G. Ramani (Eds.), *Handbook of social influences in school contexts: Social–emotional, motivation, and cognitive outcomes* (pp. 405–422). New York: Taylor & Francis.

Fabes, R. A., Martin, C. L., & Hanish, L. D. (2009). Children's behaviors and interactions with peers. In K. H. Rubin, W. M. Bukowski, & B. Laursen (Eds.), *Handbook of peer interactions, relationships, and groups* (pp. 45–62). New York: Guilford Press.

Farmer, T. W., Lines, M. M., & Hamm, J. (2011). Revealing the invisible hand: The role of teachers in children's peer experiences. *Journal of Applied Developmental Psychology, 32,* 247–256.

Flanders, N. A., & Havumaki, S. (1960). The effect of teacher–pupil contacts involving praise on the sociometric choices of students. *Journal of Educational Psychology, 51,* 65–68.

Ford, M. E. (1992). *Motivating humans: Goals, emotions, and personal agency beliefs.* Newbury Park, CA: Sage.

Fordham, S., & Ogbu, J. U. (1986). Black students' school success: Coping with "the burden of acting white." *Urban Review, 18,* 176–206.

Frey, K. S., Nolen, S. B., Van Schoiack Edstrom, L., & Hirschstein, M. K. (2005). Effects of a school-based social–emotional competence program: Linking children's goals, attributions, and behavior. *Journal of Applied Developmental Psychology, 26*(2), 171–200.

Fuchs, L. S., Fuchs, D., Bentz, J., Phillips, N. B., & Hamlett, C. L. (1994). The nature of student interactions during peer tutoring with and without prior training and experience. *American Educational Research Journal, 31,* 75–103.

Gauvain, M. (2016). Peer contributions to cognitive development. In K. Wentzel & G. Ramani (Eds.), *Handbook of social influences in school contexts: Social–emotional, motivation, and cognitive outcomes* (pp. 80–95). New York: Taylor & Francis.

Gest, S. D., Domitrovich, C. E., & Welsh, J. A. (2005). Peer academic reputation in elementary school: Associations with changes in self-concept and academic skills. *Journal of Educational Psychology, 97,* 337–346.

Gest, S. D., & Rodkin, P. C. (2011). Teaching practices and elementary classroom peer ecologies. *Journal of Applied Developmental Psychology, 32,* 288–296.

Gresham, F., Van, M., & Cook, C. (2006). Social-skills training for teaching replacement behaviors: Remediating acquisition in at-risk students. *Behavioral Disorders, 31,* 363–377.

Hamm, J. V., Farmer, T. W., Dadisman, K., Gravelle, M., & Murray, A. R. (2011). Teachers' attunement to students' peer group affiliations as a source of improved student experiences of the school social–affective context following the middle school transition. *Journal of Applied Developmental Psychology, 32*(5), 267–277.

Harper, L. V., & McCluskey, K. S. (2003). Teacher–child and child–child interactions in inclusive preschool settings: Do adults inhibit peer interactions? *Early Childhood Research Quarterly, 18,* 163–184.

Hartup, W. W., & Stevens, N. (1997). Friendships and adaptation in the life course. *Psychological Bulletin, 121,* 355–370.

Haslam, S., Reicher, S., & Levine, M. (2012). When other people are heaven, when other people are hell: How social identity determines the nature and impact of social support. In J. Jetten, C. Haslam, & S. Haslam (Eds.), *The social cure: Identity, health and well-being* (pp. 157–174). New York: Psychology Press.

Jackson, M., Barth, J., Powell, N., & Lochman, J. (2006). Classroom contextual effects of race on children's peer nominations. *Child Development, 77,* 1325–1337.

Jones, M. H., Audley-Piotrowski, S., & Kiefer, S. M. (2012). Relationships among adolescents' perceptions of friends' behaviors, academic self-concept, and math performance. *Journal of Educational Psychology, 104,* 19–31.

Juvonen, J., Nishina, A., & Graham, S. (2000). Peer harassment, psychological adjustment, and school functioning in early adolescence. *Journal of Educational Psychology, 92,* 349–359.

Kindermann, T. A. (1993). Natural peer groups as contexts for individual development: The case of children's motivation in school. *Developmental Psychology, 29,* 970–977.

Kindermann, T. A. (2007). Effects of naturally existing peer groups on changes in academic engagement in a cohort of sixth graders. *Child Development, 78,* 1186–1203.

Kindermann, T. A., & Gest, S. D. (2009). Assessment of peer group: Identifying naturally occurring social networks and capturing their effects. In K. H. Rubin, W. M. Bukowski, & B. Laursen (Eds.), *Handbook of peer interactions, relationships, and groups* (pp. 100–117). New York: Guilford Press.

Kindermann, T. A., & Skinner, E. A. (2012). Will the real peer group please stand up?: A "tensegrity" approach to examining the synergistic influences of peer groups and friendship networks on academic development. In A. Ryan & G. Ladd (Eds.), *Peer relationships and adjustment at school* (pp. 51–77). Charlotte, NC: Information Age.

King, R. B., & Ganotice, F. A., Jr. (2014). What's happening to our boys?: A personal investment analysis of gender differences in student motivation. *Asia-Pacific Education Researcher, 23,* 151–157.

Kiuru, N., Aunola, K., Vuori, J., & Nurmi, J. E. (2007). The role of peer groups in adolescents' educational expectations and adjustment. *Journal of Youth and Adolescence, 36,* 995–1009.

Ladd, G. W. (1990). Having friends, keeping friends, making friends, and being liked by peers in the classroom: Predictors of children's early school adjustment. *Child Development, 61,* 1081–1100.

Ladd, G. W., Kochenderfer-Ladd, B., Visconti, K. J., Ettekal, I., Sechler, C., & Cortes, K. (2014). Grade-school children's social collaborative skills: Links with partner preference and achievement. *American Educational Research Journal, 51,* 152–183.

Ladd, G. W., & Price, J. M. (1987). Predicting children's social and school adjustment following the transition from preschool to kindergarten. *Child Development, 58,* 1168–1189.

Lemerise, E. A., & Arsenio, W. F. (2000). An integrated model of emotion processes and cognition in social information processing. *Child Development, 71,* 107–118.

Luckner, A. E., & Pianta, R. C. (2011). Teacher–student interactions in fifth-grade classrooms: Relations with children's peer behavior. *Journal of Applied Developmental Psychology, 32,* 257–266.

Lynch, M., & Cicchetti, D. (1997). Children's relationships with adults and peers: An examination of elementary and junior high school students. *Journal of School Psychology, 35,* 81–99.

Marion, D., Laursen, B., Kiuru, N., Nurmi, J., & Salmela-Aro, K. (2014). Maternal affection moderates friend influence on schoolwork engagement. *Developmental Psychology, 50,* 766–771.

Mikami, A. Y., Gregory, A., Allen, J. P., Pianta, R. C., & Lun, J. (2011). Effects of teacher professional development intervention on peer relationships in secondary classrooms. *School Psychology Review, 40*(3), 1–41.

Mikami, A. Y., Griggs, M. S., Reuland, M. M., & Gregory, A. (2012). Teacher practices as predictors of children's classroom social preference. *Journal of School Psychology, 50,* 95–111.

Mikami, A. Y., Lerner, M. D., & Lun, J. (2010). Social context influences on children's rejection by their peers. *Child Development Perspectives, 4,* 123–130.

Molloy, L. E., Gest, S. D., & Rulison, K. L. (2011). Peer influences on academic motivation: Exploring multiple methods of assessing youths' most "influential" peer relationships. *Journal of Early Adolescence, 31,* 13–40.

Nelson, R. M., & DeBacker, T. K. (2008). Achievement motivation in adolescents: The role of peer climate and best friends. *Journal of Experimental Education, 76,* 170–189.

Newcomb, A. F., & Bagwell, C. L. (1995). Children's friendship relations: A meta-analytic review. *Psychological Bulletin, 117,* 306–347.

Nichols, J. D., & White, J. (2014). Friendship cliques: A comparison of the motivational traits of lower/upper track algebra students. *Social Psychology of Education, 17,* 141–159.

Ojanen, T., Stratman, A., Card, N. A., & Little, T. (2013). Motivation and perceived control in early adolescent friendships: Relations with self-, friend-, and peer-reported adjustment. *Journal of Early Adolescence, 33,* 552–577.

Olweus, D., & Limber, S. P. (2009). The Olweus Bullying Prevention Program: Implementation and evaluation over two decades. In S. R. Jimerson, S. M. Swearer, & D. L. Espelage (Eds.), *Handbook of bullying in schools: An international perspective* (pp. 377–402). New York: Routledge.

Parker, J. G., & Asher, S. R. (1987). Peer relations and later personal adjustment: Are low-accepted children at risk? *Psychological Bulletin, 102,* 357–389.

Parker, J. G., & Gottman, J. M. (1989). Social and emotional development in a relational context: Friendship interaction from early childhood to adoelscence. In T. J. Berndt & G. W. Ladd (Eds.), *Peer relationships in child development* (pp. 95–131). Oxford, UK: Wiley.

Patterson, G. R., & Bank, C. L. (1989). Some amplifying mechanisms for pathologic processes in families. In M. R. Gunnar & E. Thelan (Eds.), *Systems and development: The Minnesota Symposia on Child Psychology* (Vol. 22, pp. 167–210). Hillsdale, NJ: Erlbaum.

Person, N. K., & Graesser, A. G. (1999). Evolution of discourse during cross-age tutoring. In A. M. O'Donnell & A. King (Eds.), *Cognitive perspectives on peer learning* (pp. 69–86). Mahwah, NJ: Erlbaum.

Peterson, P. L., Wilkinson, L. C., Spinelli, F., & Swing, S. R. (1984). Merging the process–product and sociolinguistic paradigms: Research on small-group processes. In P. L. Peterson, L. C. Wilkinson, & M. Hallinan (Eds.), *The social context of instruction: Group organization and group processes* (pp. 126–152). New York: Academic Press.

Piaget, J. (1965). *The moral judgment of the child.* New York: Free Press. (Original work published 1932)

Pianta, R. C., & Allen, J. P. (2008). Building capacity for positive youth development in secondary school classrooms: Changing teachers' interactions with students. In M. Shinn & H. Yoshikawa (Eds.), *Toward positive youth development: Transforming schools and community programs* (pp. 21–39). New York: Oxford University Press.

Prinstein, M. (2007). Moderators of peer contagion: A longitudinal examination of depression socialization between adolescents and their best friends. *Journal of Clinical Child and Adolescent Psychology, 36,* 159–170.

Prinstein, M. J., Brechwald, W. A., & Cohen, G. L. (2011). Susceptibility to peer influence: Using a performance-based measure to identify adolescent males at heightened risk for deviant peer socialization. *Developmental Psychology, 47,* 1167–1172.

Ricciardelli, L. A., & Mellor, D. (2012). Influence of peers. In N. Rumsey & D. Harcourt (Eds.), *The Oxford handbook of the psychology of appearance* (pp. 253–272). New York: Oxford University Press.

Rimm-Kaufman, S. E., & Chiu, Y. J. I. (2007). Promoting social and academic competence in the classroom: An intervention study examining the contribution of the Responsive Classroom approach. *Psychology in the Schools, 44*(4), 397–413.

Rimm-Kaufman, S. E., Fan, X., Chiu, Y. J., & You, W. (2007). The contribution of the Responsive Classroom Approach on children's academic achievement: Results from a three year longitudinal study. *Journal of School Psychology, 45*(4), 401–421.

Robnett, R. D., & Leaper, C. (2013). Friendship groups, personal motivation, and gender in relation to high school students' STEM career interest. *Journal of Research on Adolescence, 23,* 652–664.

Rose-Krasnor, L. (1997). The nature of social competence: A theoretical review. *Social Development, 6,* 111–135.

Rubin, K. H., Bukowski, W., & Parker, J. (2006). Peer interactions, relationships, and groups. In N. Eisenberg (Ed.), *Handbook of child psychology: Social, emotional, and personality development* (6th ed., pp. 571–645). New York: Wiley.

Ryan, A. (2001). The peer group as a context for the development of young adolescent motivation and achievement. *Child Development, 72,* 1135–1150.

Ryan, R. M., & Deci, E. (2000a). The darker and brighter sides of human existence: Basic psychological needs as a unifying concept. *Psychological Inquiry, 11,* 319–338.

Ryan, R. M., & Deci, E. L. (2000b). Self-determination theory and the facilitation of intrinsic motivation, social development, and well-being. *American Psychologist, 55,* 68–78.

Sage, N. A., & Kindermann, T. A. (1999). Peer networks, behavior contingencies, and children's engagement in the classroom. *Merrill–Palmer Quarterly, 45,* 143–171.

Sandstrom, M. J. (2011). The power of popularity: Influence processes in childhood and adolescence. In A. H. N. Cillessen, D. Schwartz, & L. Mayeux (Eds.), *Popularity in the peer system* (pp. 219–244). New York: Guilford Press.

Sarason, I. G., Sarason, B. R., & Pierce, G. R. (1990). Social support: The search for theory. *Journal of Social and Clinical Psychology, 9,* 133–147.

Schwartz, D., Dodge, K. A., Pettit, G. S., Bates, J. E., & the Conduct Problems Prevention Research Group. (2000). Friendship as a moderating factor in the pathway between early harsh home environment and later victimization in the peer group. *Developmental Psychology, 36,* 646–662.

Sharan, S. (1984). *Cooperative learning.* Hillsdale, NJ: Erlbaum.

Slavin, R. E. (1980). A review of peer tutoring and cooperative learning projects in twenty-eight schools. *Review of Educational Research, 11,* 315–342.

Slavin, R. E. (2011). Instruction based on cooperative learning. In R. Mayer & P. Alexander (Eds.), *Handbook of research on learning and instruction* (pp. 344–360). New York: Routledge.

Smith, J. (2007). "Ye've got to 'ave balls to play this game sir!"—Boys, peers and fears: The negative influence of school-based "cultural accomplices" in constructing hegemonic masculinities. *Gender and Education, 19,* 179–198.

Tajfel, H., & Turner, J. C. (1979). An integrative theory of intergroup conflict. In W. G. Austin & S. Worchel (Eds.), *The social psychology of intergroup relations* (pp. 33–47). Monterey, CA: Brookes/Cole.

van Workum, N., Scholte, R. H. J., Cillessen, A. H. N., Lodder, G. M. A., & Giletta, M. (2013). Selection, deselection, and socialization processes of happiness in adolescent friendship networks. *Journal of Research on Adolescence, 23,* 563–573.

Vygotsky, L. S. (1978). *Mind in society: The development of higher psychological processes.* Cambridge, MA: Harvard University Press.

Wentzel, K. R. (1991a). Relations between social competence and academic achievement in early adolescence. *Child Development, 62,* 1066–1078.

Wentzel, K. R. (1991b). Social competence at school: Relations between social responsibility and academic achievement. *Review of Educational Research, 61,* 1–24.

Wentzel, K. R. (2002). The contribution of social goal setting to children's school adjustment. In

A. Wigfield & J. Eccles (Eds.), *Development of achievement motivation* (pp. 221–246). New York: Academic Press.

Wentzel, K. R. (2003). Sociometric status and academic adjustment in middle school: A longitudinal study. *Journal of Early Adolescence, 23,* 5–28.

Wentzel, K. R. (2004). Understanding classroom competence: The role of social–motivational and self-processes. In R. Kail (Ed.), *Advances in child development and behavior* (Vol. 32, pp. 213–241). New York: Elsevier.

Wentzel, K. R. (2005). Peer relationships, motivation, and academic performance at school. In A. J. Elliot & C. S. Dweck (Eds.), *Handbook of competence and motivation* (pp. 279–296). New York: Guilford Press.

Wentzel, K. R. (2013). School adjustment. In W. Reynolds & G. Miller (Eds.), *Handbook of psychology: Vol. 7. Educational psychology.* New York: Wiley.

Wentzel, K. R. (2014). Prosocial behavior towards peers and friends. In L. Walker-Padillo & G. Carlo (Eds.), *Prosocial development: A multidimensional approach* (pp. 178–200). New York: Oxford University Press.

Wentzel, K. R. (2015). Competence within context: Implications for the development of positive student identities and motivation at school. In F. Guay, D. M. McInerney, R. Craven, & H. Marsh (Eds.), *Self-concept, motivation and identity: Underpinning success with research and practice* (Vol. 5, pp. 299–336). Charlotte, NC: Information Age.

Wentzel, K. R., & Asher, S. R. (1995). Academic lives of neglected, rejected, popular, and controversial children. *Child Development, 66,* 754–763.

Wentzel, K. R., Baker, S. A., & Russell, S. L. (2012). Young adolescents' perceptions of teachers' and peers' goals as predictors of social and academic goal pursuit. *Applied Psychology, 61,* 605–633.

Wentzel, K. R., Baker, S. A., & Russell, S. (2014). Peer relationships and positive adjustment at school. In R. Gillman, S. Huebner, & M. Furlong (Eds.), *Promoting wellness in children and youth: A handbook of positive psychology in the schools* (pp. 260–277). Mahwah, NJ: Erlbaum.

Wentzel, K. R., Barry, C., & Caldwell, K. (2004). Friendships in middle school: Influences on motivation and school adjustment. *Journal of Educational Psychology, 96,* 195–203.

Wentzel, K. R., Battle, A., Russell, S., & Looney, L. (2010). Teacher and peer contributions to classroom climate in middle school. *Contemporary Educational Psychology, 35,* 193–202.

Wentzel, K. R., & Caldwell, K. (1997). Friendships, peer acceptance, and group membership: Relations to academic achievement in middle school. *Child Development, 68,* 1198–1209.

Wentzel, K. R., & Edelman, D. (2016). Peer relationships and learning: Implications for instruction. In R. Mayer & P. Alexander (Eds.), *Handbook of research on learning and instruction* (2nd ed., pp. 365–387). New York: Routledge.

Wentzel, K. R., & Muenks, K. (2016). Peer influence on students' motivation, academic achievement and social behavior. In K. Wentzel & G. Ramani (Eds.), *Handbook of social influences in school contexts: Social–emotional, motivation, and cognitive outcomes* (pp. 13–30). New York: Taylor & Francis.

Wentzel, K. R., & Watkins, D. E. (2002). Peer relationships and collaborative learning as contexts for academic enablers. *School Psychology Review, 31,* 366–377.

Wenz-Gross, M., Siperstein, G. N., Untch, A. S., & Widaman, K. F. (1997). Stress, social support, and adjustment of adolescents in middle school. *Journal of Early Adolescence, 17,* 129–151.

White, K. J., & Kistner, J. (1992). The influence of teacher feedback on young children's peer preferences and perceptions. *Developmental Psychology, 28,* 933–940.

Wilson, S., & Lipsey, M. W. (2007). School-based interventions for aggressive and disruptive behavior: Update of a meta-analysis. *American Journal of Preventive Medicine, 33*(2, Suppl.), S130–S143.

Youniss, J., & Smollar, J. (1989). Adolescents' interpersonal relationships in social context. In T. J. Berndt & G. Ladd (Eds.), *Peer relationships in child development* (pp. 300–316). New York: Wiley.

CHAPTER 32

The Roles of Schools and Teachers in Fostering Competence Motivation

ERIC M. ANDERMAN
DeLEON L. GRAY

In the first edition of the *Handbook of Competence and Motivation*, Elliot and Dweck (2005) argued that from a motivation perspective, "achievement" can and should be viewed through the lens of "competence." As they noted, the notion of competence is involved in all that humans do on a daily basis. Thus, when one examines schooling, a focus on competence becomes particularly compelling, since schools are designed to foster achievement (i.e., competence) in students. Indeed, students in schools spend time developing competence in not only their academic knowledge and skills but also many other domains (e.g., developing social competence at interacting with peers and teachers and other adults).

As noted by Guskey (2013), *achievement* is an elusive concept that is difficult to define. More specifically, he notes that "student achievement is a multifaceted construct that can address different domains of learning, often measured in many different ways, and for distinctly different purposes" (p. 5). Particularly noteworthy is Guskey's observation that achievement is a construct that serves different purposes for different audiences. For example, achievement can serve as an indicator of learning for student or parents, as an indicator of the quality of a teacher or a school, as an indicator of mastery of content required for entry into an advanced program or university, or as an indicator of national progress for an entire country. Moreover, achievement is influenced by a wide array of variables, including student characteristics, families, schools, teachers, curricula, and instructional strategies, among others (Hattie & Anderman, 2013).

In contrast, *competence* is in many ways a more useful construct than achievement, particularly in discussions of motivation, for a variety of reasons. First, from a psychological and motivational perspective, competence is viewed as a basic human need; moreover, individuals experience greater well-being when they attain competence in various life domains (Deci & Ryan, 2000b; Deci, Vallerand, Pelletier, & Ryan, 1991; Elliot, McGregor, & Thrash, 2002). In addition, *competence* is a construct that is evident across all cultures (Elliot & Dweck, 2005), whereas *achievement* takes on different meanings both within and across cultures. For example, achievement may be defined in terms of attainment of skills in some domains (e.g., in physical education), and as attainment of rote knowledge in other domains (e.g., in a social studies class). However, children, adolescents, and adults in all cultures strive to achieve *competence* in many life domains. These domains, of course, vary greatly, and some are valued more than others (e.g., one adolescent may be interested in developing competence in algebra, whereas another may be interested in developing competence as a hunter); nevertheless, striving for competence is universal.

In this chapter, we examine the roles that schools as organizations, and teachers as individuals, play in the development of competence motivation in children and adults. The connection between school settings and competence motivation can be conceptualized in terms of environmental systems that directly or indirectly regulate students' competence beliefs and behaviors. These environmental systems are the *organizational, instructional,* and *interpersonal* contexts of a school that shape students' daily experiences in these academic spaces (Eccles & Roeser, 1999). Teachers are, of course, the most significant operator in this equation—they are the employees of schools and, by definition, their job is to help students to learn (i.e., to become competent in various subjects and domains). Most teachers feel satisfied with and committed to their jobs when they are helping students to achieve competence (Canrinus, Helms-Lorenz, Beijaard, Buitink, & Hofman, 2012). Thus, teachers' feelings of efficacy (i.e., believing that they are helping students to achieve competence), which have been identified as predictors of beneficial outcomes for both students and teachers, are largely dependent on teachers' daily work in helping students to achieve competence in various academic subjects (Hoy, Hoy, & Davis, 2009; Tschannen-Moran & Hoy, 2001). In this chapter, we focus on how teachers and schools influence competence motivation through the organizational contexts of schools, the instructional strategies employed by educators, and the interpersonal relationships that develop within and outside of the school building.

SCHOOL AS A CONTEXT FOR EXAMINING COMPETENCE MOTIVATION

School is a natural setting in which to study competence motivation. There are many unique features about school environments that dictate the ways motivation scholars approach their research. To date, there are a limited number of peer-reviewed studies that model and describe a truly collaborative, school-centered research partnership aimed at enhancing competence motivation in students. The work of Turner and colleagues (Turner, Christensen, Kackar-Cam, Trucano, Fulmer, 2014; Turner, Warzon, Christensen 2011) represents one such example. Turner and colleagues (2011) conducted an in-depth, 9-month examination of middle school teachers' enactment of motivation-based instructional strategies in the classroom—complete with repeated classroom observations and interviews, and monthly consultations. The authors documented change in teachers' beliefs and practices over time related to competence, belonging, autonomy, and meaning. Results suggested that (1) teachers' consultations with motivation researchers allowed them to think critically about their instructional practices; (2) teacher efficacy explained the extent to which teachers felt accountable for students' motivation; and (3) issues specific to schools that primarily serve ethnic minorities and students from low socioeconomic backgrounds served as barriers to successful implementation of motivation-based instructional strategies (e.g., strong emphasis on test taking).

Whereas the work by Turner and colleagues represents an important step forward in scholarship on teacher and school influences on competence motivation, there are several considerations in conducting this work, and in the everyday pragmatics involved in fostering competence motivation. School-based motivation research is, by nature, complex and contextualized (Kaplan, Katz, & Flum, 2012). We outline facets of schooling (involving both individual teachers and schools as a whole) that affect competence motivation. If not taken into account or discussed explicitly, these features of schooling environments may lead to an oversimplified view of motivational processes in formal education settings. These factors are essential since, as we have argued elsewhere, teachers (e.g., Anderman & Anderman, 2014) and schools (Anderman, 2002) influence academic outcomes in extraordinarily powerful ways.

ORGANIZATIONAL CONTEXTS AND COMPETENCE MOTIVATION

There are many ways to consider the organizational contexts of schools. Schools are generally organized within a hierarchical structure, in which students are nested in classrooms, which in turn are nested in schools that are nested in districts. However, there are other structures that also may impact student motivation. For example, in middle schools and high schools, teachers (classrooms) often are nested within departments (e.g., the math department). In elementary schools, grade level also often is an important organizational structure (e.g., being in the third grade). There are numerous other organizational structures as well (e.g., the presence of unions, school boards). These dimensions are complex but necessary considerations for understanding classroom-based motivational processes.

School organizational contexts can be conceptualized in terms of costs, information flows and networks, and resources (Kilgore & Pendleton, 1993). These factors are discussed less often in the competence motivation literature—presumably because it is difficult to draw direct links between such factors and increments or decrements in student persistence, performance, and choices. Nevertheless, these considerations are important for understanding motivation findings and for distinguishing school-based motivation research from other forms of motivation research (e.g., laboratory-based research).

Enacting Motivation in Students: Potential Drawbacks for Teachers within the Organization

In expectancy–value theory, cost represents the effort, competing demands for time and resources, sacrifices, and the emotional expenses that are required to engage in a task (Flake, Barron, Hulleman, McCoach, & Welsh, 2015). Cost is theorized as being negatively associated with achievement choices (Eccles et al., 1983)—such that the drawbacks of engaging in an achievement task may reduce the likelihood that individuals will choose to engage in such an achievement task. When considering schools

as organizations, cost is relevant to understanding not only student behavior but also the teacher behaviors that can influence student motivation.

The concept of motivation in the practice of education is not always properly understood in the public domain (Maehr & Mayer, 1997). Teachers who recognize the nuances of motivation have an advantage in discussing, identifying, and effectively responding to issues of student motivation. However, in order to fully appreciate the nuances involved in motivating students, teachers must *unpack the concept of motivation* through exposure to the motivation literature, motivation researchers, motivation workshops, or a combination of these. Such exposure may involve (1) learning specific terminology that helps teachers discuss aspects of student motivation with greater precision, (2) understanding why specific pedagogical techniques and methods of assessment support or undermine the development of students' competence motivation, and (3) engaging in trial and error within their classrooms as they work to successfully enact research-based pedagogical principles in their instruction.

Engaging in each of these professional growth activities requires a consideration of costs that are specific to the demands of teaching. Moreover, engagement in these activities must be considered in light of the complex organizational structures previously mentioned. There are several essential prerequisites for such professional development to be effective within this organizational structure. First, teachers must believe that learning about research-based strategies will actually be beneficial for motivating their students or for helping them learn (Urdan & Turner, 2005). Second, the time that teachers are able to invest in learning about strategies for motivating their students is also situated within a number of other competing organizational demands. In particular, teachers today are faced with many responsibilities, and are scrutinized and held accountable for student learning more than in the past. Some teachers may espouse the belief that the strongest curricula, most enthusiastic teachers, and the latest instructional technologies will not be as effective as they can be if students do not care about what they are learning. Even so, the long-term payoff of learning about strategies for motivating students may be eclipsed by more immediate concerns, such as schoolwide initiatives, limited instructional time, preparation for end-of-grade standardized testing, or additional professional learning around new curricular standards (e.g., Common Core State Standards). Third, teachers also may consider cost in terms of personal time investment outside of designated work hours—particularly when they are not regularly afforded protected time to engage in learning about motivation-based instructional strategies during the school day. Finally, it is possible that a trial-and-error process of implementing motivational instructional strategies could lead to frustration, confusion, and even distress, especially if enacting evidence-based practices for motivating students is incompatible with other demands of the organization. For example, teachers who work in schools that consistently recognize high-performing students and afford them special privileges (e.g., making the "Honor Roll" or the "Dean's List") may find it counterintuitive that some goal theorists (e.g., Anderman & Maehr, 1994) caution teachers against universally employing such practices.

Bridging School Information Flow with Competence Motivation

The flow of information within the various structures of the organizational hierarchy of schools also may either facilitate or hinder adaptive motivational outcomes in students. Particularly given the extensive use of technology and social media for communication, it becomes extraordinarily important to consider how policies, practices, and other information are communicated within the various layers of the organization.

School–University Information Flow

Through connections between universities and schools, knowledge of motivation principles may be developed, shared, and utilized by teachers and university researchers alike (e.g, Maehr & Midgley, 1996; Willems & Gonzalez-DeHass, 2012). Even when school–university research networks exist,

the nature of these partnerships can look very different from school to school (Cornelissen et al., 2014). For example, these may be one-way partnerships, in which the research partnership is initiated by one party and requires very little mutual engagement, or they may be reciprocal partnerships, in which the research agenda is collaboratively undertaken, and negotiation of research outcomes and methods is based on input from the project team comprised of practitioners and researchers (Cornelissen, van Swet, Beijaard, & Bergen, 2011).

Another dimension of school–university partnerships is the location in which teacher professional learning occurs (Cornelissen et al., 2013). Opportunities for inservice teacher training also may exist primarily at the university, or primarily in the same school in which teachers are employed. Research on social networks demonstrates that the university–school communication is sustained over a longer period of time when the partnership is embedded within the school, and when research projects are collaboratively designed and undertaken (Cornelissen et al., 2014). Moreover, technology now also is often used to facilitate the professional development of teachers (e.g., Copper & Semich, 2014).

School–Community Information Flow

Models of the causes and consequences of family–school partnerships (Eccles & Harold, 1996) also suggest the importance of school–community information flow for students' competence motivation. In such models, parents form impressions about the roles they should play in their children's academic development based on the school's beliefs about the role of parents; develop perceptions of their abilities to support their children's learning and value systems; and acquire knowledge regarding how to engage in scholastic activities with their children. At the same time, school personnel form impressions about the roles parents should play in their children's academic development based on parents' self-views in each of these areas. Educators and parents also hold beliefs about the motivation, needs, and aptitude of the children, which impact teacher and parent practices regarding family–school collaboration, as well as children's academic self-perceptions, motivation, and ultimately, their performance (e.g., Gonida & Vauras, 2014; Nichols & Zhang, 2011).

Empirical research with parents supports the importance of school–community information flow. For example, when caregivers are provided information about the value of science, technology, engineering, and math (STEM) literacy, the number of mathematics and science courses taken by their adolescents increases on average by nearly one course (Harackiewicz, Rozek, Hulleman, & Hyde, 2012). In addition, parental practices during middle school are linked with higher academic performance among students. These practices include having discussions with their children about high school and next steps after high school (Desimone, 1999), as well as communicating with schools about their child's in-school activities (Sui-Chi & Willms, 1996). These results suggest that consistent messages across in-school and out-of-school organizational structures—facilitated by communication with family members—can further support students' competence motivation in ways that have implications for the beliefs and behaviors they bring with them to formal education settings. Moreover, communication between schools and community members can occur through various means, including greater uses of technology given the prevalence of social media and instantaneous communications (Pollock, 2013).

Information Flow within Districts and Schools

Messages that teachers receive from other teachers and from their schools' leadership can either enhance or reduce their chances of enacting research-based pedagogical principles that facilitate the emergence of competence motivation in students. When school reform researchers refer to *spread*, they mean the extent to which vertical and lateral forms of institutional support lead to the transference of norms, principles, and beliefs across classrooms and schools (Coburn, 2003). Spread at district and school levels occurs when norms and principles serve as a guiding framework for policies, procedures, professional development, and day-to-day operations. Spread at the classroom level occurs when teachers adopt reform-based

norms and principles, and use them as a guiding framework for their instructional practices—even in ways beyond what had been mandated by their school or district level leaders.

In Wake County, North Carolina, school leaders are taking actionable steps to learn about ways of cultivating motivationally supportive learning environments in their schools. Over 170 of Wake County's school principals and approximately 400 of the county's assistant principals are required to read Carol Dweck's *Mindset: The New Psychology of Success* (2006) as part of their training for the Effective Teaching Framework (Wake County Public Schools, 2014). The central purpose of reading this book is to help district and school leaders develop a common understanding of what is meant when they use the term *effective teacher*. When considering that ethnic minorities and students from low-income households may have previously scored below proficiency on tests and received low grades in key academic subject areas (e.g., English and mathematics), the book also serves as a guide for school administrators, who are charged with spreading the belief that all students possess the ability to succeed academically, and to help teachers work through less productive ways of thinking about their students—such as making negative attributions about their scholastic ability in certain subject areas based on demographic information.

School Resources and Competence Motivation

Competence motivation also can be influenced by school resources. Regarding human resources, instructional assistants or paraprofessionals can play a vital role in allowing teachers to develop their capacity to support students' motivation; however, the prevalence of instructional assistants is dependent on local financial resources and community priorities. In addition to fielding students' questions and working with students with special needs during instructional time, these instructional assistants can handle logistical aspects of running the classroom (e.g., materials setup, disciplinary actions)—enabling teachers to focus on employing research-based pedagogical techniques that foster student motivation.

Nevertheless, it is essential to distinguish between instructional assistants who are provided to assist the teacher and all students, and special educators who are placed in classrooms to work with specific students with specific exceptionalities, as required under federal law (Friend & Bursuck, 2012). In the era of digital learning, technology access also allows teachers the choice to engage students in learning tasks that presumably are high in intrinsic appeal and real-world applicability (e.g., robotics kits, smartphone app development, and the construction of heart rate monitors and other devices). Finally, research on teacher professional development indicates that effective professional development programs are typically sustained over a longer span of time, are more intensive, are subject-specific, and are integrated into teachers' daily school activities (Darling-Hammond, Wei, Andree, Richardson, & Orphanos, 2009; Garet, Porter, Desimone, Birman, & Yoon, 2001; Wei, Darling-Hammond, Adamson, & National Staff Development Council, 2010). Schools with an infrastructure that can support teachers' professional learning through these types of motivation-based inservice training and workshops also should be better positioned to support students' motivation in the classroom.

Another significant resource that often is not considered is the school administration. When school administrators (e.g., principals and assistant principals) understand the complexities of human learning and motivation, they can better facilitate the work of teachers. Indeed, the administration represents a level of hierarchy in the school that can facilitate or hinder teachers' efforts to develop student competence and motivation. As noted by Maehr, Midgley, and their colleagues (e.g., Anderman & Urdan, 1994; Maehr & Midgley, 1996; Maehr, Midgley, & Urdan, 1992), the policies that are instituted by school administrators can have either beneficial or detrimental effects on student motivation. For example, a policy that rewards students by allowing them to be on the "honor roll" based on significant improvements in their grades may have different motivational effects on students than a policy that only allows students who earn overall "A" averages/high grade-point averages (GPAs) to be on the honor roll.

Summary

Schools are complex organizations. Organizational structures exist within (e.g., grades, departments), and outside of the school (e.g., districts, regions, states). These organizational structures need to be considered in conversations about student motivation. Whereas often the goals at the various levels of the hierarchy are in sync, at times they conflict and may hinder teachers' efforts to enhance student motivation. Although teachers cannot do much to affect the organizational structures in which they work, they can have a meaningful impact on students via the instructional strategies they use in their classrooms on a daily basis.

INSTRUCTIONAL CONTEXTS AND COMPETENCE MOTIVATION

The instructional context of school environments can be conceptualized as the influence of "teachers, students, content area, and instructional activities on learning, teaching, and motivation" (Turner & Meyer, 2010, p. 70). In an ecological view of schools (Eccles & Roeser, 2009), instructional contexts are seen as having the most immediate impact on competence motivation due to the amount of time students spend in classrooms, and the direct contact that students have with others in these environments.

Instructional contexts are determined by a variety of individuals. The actual course materials (i.e., textbooks) that are used by a particular school often are determined at the district level. Teachers often do not have many opportunities to influence the selection of such materials. Nevertheless, teachers largely determine the instructional practices that are used within the walls of their own individual classrooms. Thus, although two teachers may be using the same textbook or curricular materials, the instructional contexts may be entirely different, depending on the daily instructional techniques and strategies that are used by each teacher. For example, one teacher might present material to students via lectures, wherein students take notes based on what the teacher says daily, whereas another teacher, in a classroom where the same content is being taught, may engage students with the material through cooperative group projects (with virtually no "lecturing" by the teacher) or via technology (e.g., using online tutorials). Thus, these two classes may use the same curriculum but still offer students entirely different instructional contexts. The students' experiences with those contexts affect the development of competence in myriad ways (Urdan & Turner, 2005).

Several theoretical perspectives converge on similar predictions about the role of instructional contexts in fostering competence motivation. From the perspectives of stage–environment fit theory (Eccles et al., 1983), self-determination theory (Deci & Ryan, 1985), and achievement goal theory (Barkoukis & Hagger, 2013; Ciani, Sheldon, Hilpert, & Easter, 2011), autonomy support is a critical driver of students' competence motivation in the classroom. For example, providing students with choices during academic learning activities is associated with increased task and school engagement (Anderman & Maehr, 1994; Reeve & Jang, 2006), less favorable attitudes toward academic cheating (Patall & Leach, 2015), and being oriented toward the development of competence (Midgley, 2002). Achievement goal theory research (Meece, Anderman, & Anderman, 2006) and social-cognitive theory research (Bandura, 1986) also emphasize the important role of instructional activities in fostering student motivation, particularly in terms of offering achievement tasks that are appropriately challenging.

Achievement goal theory in particular provides a specific mechanism to explain the relations of instructional practices to student motivation in the form of perceived goal structures (Kaplan, Middleton, Urdan, & Midgley, 2002; Meece et al., 2006). Goal structures are created by teachers, and are perceived by students; teachers "create" these goal structures via the types of instructional practices they utilize. If a teacher emphasizes mastery, and consistently encourages students to attempt challenging tasks, and to focus on effort and self-improvement, students are likely to perceive a mastery goal structure; in contrast, if a teacher emphasizes testing and assessment, and consistently encourages students to demonstrate their ability and try to outperform others, students are likely to perceive a performance goal structure (Midgley, 2002).

Indeed, research supports the existence of such mastery goal structures, and their relations with competence motivation. For example, results from a longitudinal study of several thousand adolescents indicated that perceptions of a mastery goal structure in high school health classrooms were predictive of value for learning and knowledge about HIV and pregnancy prevention strategies several months after instruction had occurred (Anderman et al., 2011).

In terms of student influences, individual differences between students also interact with other features of instructional contexts to foster competence motivation. In achievement goal theory research, for example, Gray, Chang, and Anderman (2015) found that teachers' emphasis on the development of competence in the classroom was positively associated with the value students placed on academic learning, but only for students with a low or moderate need for cognition (i.e., the extent to which an individual enjoys engaging in effortful cognitive activity). In addition, Yeager and his colleagues (2014) examined the interaction between instructional context and competence when students receive critical feedback. Specifically, in a series of three experiments, they demonstrated that communication of high standards and reassuring students about their potential to be successful is related to increased feelings of trust in school and increased achievement, even when students receive critical feedback from instructors.

Two particular aspects of the instructional context that directly affect competence motivation daily are (1) the nature of the academic tasks that are provided for students and (2) the ways in which assessments are administered. In the next sections, we review each and specifically discuss how these affect competence motivation.

Academic Tasks and Competence Motivation

The selection of academic tasks is a fundamental component of life in schools. Teachers make decisions daily about the types of academic tasks to use with their students. The types of tasks they select have profoundly important effects on the development of competence-based beliefs and the attainment of competence in children and adolescents. In classrooms, competence can be operationalized in terms of students' strivings for mastery (Urdan & Turner, 2005). Thus, the types of tasks that teachers select for their students may either facilitate or hinder the emergence of these strivings for mastery in various academic domains (e.g., Belenky & Nokes-Malach, 2012; Blumenfeld, Mergendoller, & Swarthout, 1987; Guthrie, 2004).

Academic tasks can be classified and selected based on a variety of criteria. As noted by Doyle (1983), classifying academic tasks can be based on the cognitive processes needed to engage successfully with a task. Doyle classified tasks into memory tasks, procedural tasks, comprehension tasks, and opinion tasks. Other categorizations of academic tasks include cooperative versus competitive tasks (e.g., Slavin, 1992), Bloom's taxonomy (both the original and revised taxonomies, which organize tasks according to the cognitive processes needed for success at a task; Anderson & Krathwohl, 2001; Bloom, Engelhart, Furst, Hill, & Krathwohl, 1956), tasks that are matched to students' ability levels, tasks that promote competence more so than control (e.g., Usher, 2016), tasks that convey specific achievement values to students (e.g., attainment value, utility value, intrinsic value, and cost) (Eccles, 2005), and tasks that are presented either partially or completely via technology (Natriello, 2016; Xie, DeBacker, & Ferguson, 2006).

How Do Tasks Affect Competence Motivation?

The selection of tasks can, in many ways, be traced back to school- and district-level policies. The curricula often provided for teachers have been purchased by the school or the district for use in a particular subject domain, for a particular age group. In addition, in the United States, with the growing popularity of highly specific educational standards (e.g., the Common Core State Standards), curricula often are marketed to meet the needs of educators to ensure that their students attain certain academic standards.

Regardless of the factors that ultimately lead to the selection of tasks, the activities in which students engage are pivotal in the development of competence motivation. When students experience success with academic tasks, they are more likely to be motivated to engage in similar tasks, as well as somewhat more challenging tasks, in the future (Wigfield & Eccles, 1992). Studies with special student populations demonstrate how powerful competence beliefs can be. For example, despite the difficulties teachers may face with students with Down syndrome, when children with Down syndrome engage with tasks in which they are engaged and persist, academic competence during adolescence is rated as higher (Gilmore & Cuskelly, 2009). Thus, selection of appropriate tasks is vital.

In a given classroom, variation in students' cognitive abilities, interests, goals, and prior knowledge often is vast. Thus, if a teacher plans a learning activity, some students may experience anxiety before or while engaging in the activity. This anxiety could contribute to the adoption of mastery-avoidance goals (wherein the goal is to avoid misunderstanding) or performance-avoidance goals (wherein the goal is to avoid appearing inferior to others), both of which can have detrimental effects on the development of positive competence beliefs (Hulleman, Schrager, Bodmann, & Harackiewicz, 2010; Van Yperen, Elliot, & Anseel, 2009).

Assessment Practices and Competence Motivation

The area in which teachers and school probably have the strongest influences on the development of competence motivation is assessment of student learning. Assessment occurs throughout the school year and takes on a variety of forms. Moreover, given the prevalence of assessment as a measure of accountability in education, teachers often are compelled to focus their instruction on test preparation rather than other tasks that might facilitate more adaptive motivation (e.g., Ercikan, 2006; Faulkner & Cook, 2006). As noted by Elliot and Dweck (2005) in the introductory chapter of the previous edition of this handbook, one of the most nebulous and ill-defined concepts in the achievement motivation literature is "achievement." Thus, it is important to keep in mind in any examination of assessment the key question: *What exactly is being assessed?*

Moreover, Elliot and Dweck (2005) also note that competence can be assessed in a variety of manners. For example, assessment of competence can be based on meeting standards inherent in the task (i.e., criterion-referenced standards), on demonstrating growth in competence over time, or on normative comparisons. Unfortunately, teachers often are not well trained in either assessment or motivation, and may therefore select assessments that do not foster the development of positive motivational beliefs in their students (e.g., Moore, 1993).

How Do Assessments Affect Competence Motivation?

Consider a high school social studies class that has just completed a 2-week unit on the French Revolution. The teacher quite likely will want and need to assess student learning. He or she may have numerous options regarding how to assess learning, including the following:

- A multiple-choice/fill-in-the-blank exam that assesses knowledge of factual information.
- An essay examination that requires students to analyze aspects of the war on a more conceptual level.
- Participation in an online blog or discussion with fellow students, comparing the French Revolution to another revolution (e.g., the American Revolution).
- An oral presentation about some aspect of the French Revolution.

These are, of course, merely a few examples of assessments; there certainly are numerous other possibilities. Nevertheless, in terms of competence motivation, these choices, which may appear rather inconsequential to teachers, have implications for students' engagement in the classroom (Anderman & Anderman, 2014; Nolen, 2011).

The nature of the student assessment in many ways defines competence for the student. If the assessment focuses on rote memorization of facts, then students may define competence in those terms (at least for the material being covered by that particular assessment); if the assessment involves analysis and synthesis of larger conceptual issues, then students may define competence in those terms. Thus, whereas some students

may come to see the study of the French Revolution (and, more generally, the study of history) as merely memorizing decontextualized facts, others may come to see that the occurrence of the French Revolution led to many of the current governmental, political, and social norms in modern-day France and Europe.

Moreover, characteristics of the assessment also influence students' motivational goals and beliefs. For example, a normatively graded examination may lead students to adopt performance-approach or performance-avoidance goals, whereas a criterion-referenced assessment may lead students to adopt mastery-approach goals. If students are graded on the basis of normative standards, they may begin to define competence in a particular academic domain (e.g., history) in terms of how they compare to others, whereas if students are graded on the basis of having met some specific criterion, they may define competence in terms of task mastery (Anderman & L. Anderman, 2014). The point is not that one of these is better or worse than the other; rather, the type of assessment the teacher decides to use can affect student motivation.

Finally, assessment practices also affect competence beliefs via the ways in which they activate other motivational beliefs. First, when students receive their scores on various assessments, they engage in attributional searches in order to explain their successes or failures (Weiner, 1986). Students may attribute their successes and failures on assessments to factors such as ability (which is largely uncontrollable, stable, and internal) or effort (which is largely controllable, unstable, and internal), among others. These attributions impact students' beliefs about their competence; a student who consistently attributes failures to low ability is unlikely to believe that he or she is highly competent (or able to become highly competent) within a given academic domain. Moreover, as noted by Weiner (2005), the reactions of other individuals (e.g., teachers) to students' academic performance elicit emotions that may be as powerful, if not more powerful, than the attribution experienced by the student.

It is possible for educators to think more broadly about the purposes of assessments (e.g., Baker, 2013). Specifically, the development of positive competence beliefs can be facilitated by assessing facets of motivation, in addition to achievement. As suggested by Urdan and Turner (2005), one way of enhancing competence motivation in classrooms is to assess motivational constructs specifically, including confidence, attributions, and skills, in order to help students to "meet their preferences for challenge and to help students approach tasks with realistic expectations and cope with difficulties adaptively" (p. 307). The use of motivation assessments for improving instructional practices and effectiveness represents a critical area for the future of motivation research for at least two reasons: (1) Such investigations would make practical use of motivation research methodologies, while (2) extending what is known about the use of motivation data by educators. At present, motivation researchers draw from specific theoretical frameworks (e.g., achievement goal theory) to guide their classroom-based research efforts. However, to guide the use of motivation measures in day-to-day instructional practices effectively, motivation researchers may also require more general classroom-based models that guide our thinking about the application of motivation principles in school contexts. Considering that scholars already are proposing (Kaplan et al., 2012) and utilizing (Turner et al., 2014) novel practice-relevant methodologies in motivation research (e.g., collaborative action research; state–space grids), the creation of practice-relevant motivation research models is likely the next frontier of classroom-based motivation research.

THE SPECIAL CASE
OF HIGH-STAKES ASSESSMENTS

Richard Ryan and his colleague noted in the first edition of this handbook that high-stakes testing, in particular, can lead to unintended problematic outcomes for students and teachers (Ryan & Brown, 2005). High-stakes assessments are prevalent in many nations; in general, the results of these examinations often are used as gatekeepers for students (e.g., to allow students to graduate, or to allow them to qualify for certain opportunities). Moreover, results of these

assessments are also often used to judge the quality of schools and teachers. For example, in the United States, value-added assessments, which account for growth in student learning over time, are often used to assess the quality of schools (Lissitz & Jiao, 2014).

Ryan and Brown (2005) note that from a self-determination perspective, individuals are intrinsically motivated to develop competence. However, as the motivation to develop various competencies becomes less autonomous and more controlled, an individual's intrinsic motivation to achieve competence will decline. Most high-stakes assessments are requirements; students seldom choose to engage in high-stakes assessments of their own volition. Thus, the perceived controlling nature of these assessments in particular may be related to decrements in learning and motivation (see also Benware & Deci, 1984; Deci & Ryan, 2000a; Deci, Schwartz, Sheinman, & Ryan, 1981; Ryan & Grolnick, 1986). Importantly, high-stakes testing serves as an example of the interrelated nature of school organizational contexts and instructional contexts.

Summary

We have argued that instructional tasks influence student motivation. The good news is that, unlike organizational structures, teachers often have the ability to make informed decisions about the types of tasks and assessments they use with their students. Whereas teachers may not be able to avoid giving a state-mandated assessment, they can on a daily basis choose instructional tasks and assessments that facilitate the development of competence motivation.

INTERPERSONAL CONTEXTS AND COMPETENCE MOTIVATION

Interactions between teachers and students, and among students, occur daily and continuously. From the moment a student enters the school building until he or she leaves at the end of the day, the student experiences many types of social interactions. In addition, for many students, the interpersonal nature of schooling does not end when school is over, because teachers and students are now able to maintain contact via electronic mail, blogs, online discussions, text messaging, Skype/video conferencing, and many other forms of social media.

The interpersonal context of school environments represents a student's social connections to others; these social connections are facilitated by perceptions of acceptance, respect, inclusion, and support (Goodenow, 1993). Thus, schooling is both an academic *and* a social experience, and school environments are "rich social arenas with constant interaction and affiliation" (Juvonen, 2006, p. 655). Within these social arenas, students engage in various activities and adopt various personal styles to help define themselves in relation to others. Examples of some of these styles include acquiring new speech patterns, participating in afterschool activities, and wearing nontraditional articles of clothing.

Theoretical arguments regarding the role of social bonds in fostering motivation and achievement often acknowledge that students' achievement behaviors occur in the presence of others (Butler, 2011), and are therefore impacted by students' social construals of their achievement settings (e.g., Martin & Dowson, 2009). We do not provide a comprehensive overview of social processes, here because other chapters in this volume are devoted specifically to describing aspects of interpersonal contexts. However, we do wish to emphasize the role that race plays in the development of competence motivation within the school interpersonal context. A consideration of race involves measurement of psychological factors that dictate or modify perceptions of the interpersonal context and, subsequently, competence motivation. Considering that researchers consistently highlight the absence of cultural perspectives in competence motivation research (DeCuir-Gunby & Schutz, 2014; Graham, 1992; Graham & Hudley, 2005; Zusho & Clayton, 2011), we urge motivation researchers to embed the study of race-based constructs into their examinations of interpersonal contexts by examining, for example, the role that institutional diversity practices play in students' social experiences and self-beliefs—and subsequently, their achievement behaviors.

Diversity, Interpersonal Contexts, and Competence

At their best, high schools are structured to cultivate adolescents' productivity and mental health. To clarify their investment in student development, schools often develop mission statements containing buzzwords and terms such as *culture of excellence, engagement, lifelong learning, empowerment,* and the development of leaders. Schools also emphasize their commitment to *diversity*—a word that, in its simplest terms, means contrast, variance, or *difference*. Research on the concept of uniqueness (Snyder & Fromkin, 1980) indicates that seeing oneself as distinct is not only important but also a basic human need. Thus, the ability of schools to accentuate differences in students and to make use of these differences in a productive fashion is practically important—given that learning environments attuned with adolescents' needs produce students with more positive emotions, who are also more motivated to achieve (Eccles & Midgley, 1989; Eccles et al., 1983).

Work by Byrd and Chavous (2011) demonstrates the importance of considering psychological and cultural perspectives in the study of interpersonal contexts and competence motivation. In a study of over 300 African American adolescents, results demonstrated that positive intergroup contact and the valuing of all races at school predicts greater intrinsic motivation among African American adolescents. However, these effects are contingent on racial identity and whether the source of the interpersonal connection is teachers or peers. Specifically, students who take pride in identifying as African American (i.e., private regard) report greater intrinsic motivation when their teachers show equal respect to all races. However, this association is attenuated among African American students with low private regard. A similar pattern is also shown when the school climate variable is positive race relations; students—with high—but not low—private regard show a positive association between peer racial climate and intrinsic motivation.

In addition to examining race-based constructs such as racial identity, we also wish to note that research studies explicitly examining students' uniqueness perceptions remain largely absent within the metanarrative of research on interpersonal school contexts, school connectedness, psychological membership at school, and school belonging. We believe that examining the fulfillment of the basic human desire for uniqueness (Becker et al., 2012) in school settings can yield theoretical insights within the study of interpersonal contexts in general. Moreover, we also believe that explicitly acknowledging uniqueness expands research on the interpersonal contexts of schooling in a way that provides additional considerations of the importance of diversity and culture in motivation theories.

For example, a racial-minority student in a majority white school in the United States might feel that he or she "sticks out" from peers—particularly if the student is denigrated due to his or her race. However, if this very same student is in a school with an identical demographic makeup, but one that welcomes the perspectives of students from all backgrounds and encourages others to learn from different cultures, then he or she might feel that he or she is distinguished and uniquely valued (i.e., he or she "stands out") within the school. In neither example is this student invisible; the student looks different, is different, and is almost guaranteed not to be treated as if he or she were white. Yet the interpersonal experiences of these two hypothetical students differ dramatically.

The construct of race carries meaning and significance in the United States, and it can be difficult to understand fully the influence of teachers and schools on competence motivation without considering how populations with a history of racial denigration and mistreatment perceive and interpret their school's interpersonal context. In future research, the concept of distinctiveness—on a continuum from sticking out (race-based devaluation) to standing out (race-based valuation)—may be a way to provide a race-reimaged view of acceptance, respect, inclusion, and support in schools, thereby providing a window for examining further race-based influences of interpersonal contexts on competence motivation (for an overview of race-focused and -reimaged approaches to research in school settings, see DeCuir-Gunby & Schutz, 2014).

DISCUSSION

The educational contexts in which students spend much of their time are important influences on the development of competence motivation in children and adolescents. Nevertheless, the "school" is a complex system, with many moving parts. Teachers can greatly influence student motivation, but the complexities of schools must be considered from both practice- and research-oriented perspectives.

As we have discussed in this chapter, an examination of competence motivation can be facilitated by considering the organizational, instructional, and interpersonal contexts of school (Eccles & Roeser, 1999). Numerous natural and self-imposed organizational structures exist, and policies, beliefs, and practices at any level of an educational organization can either facilitate or hinder teachers' efforts to motivate their students. Teachers have the ability to make choices about instructional techniques (e.g., academic tasks and assessments), although some of these choices may be affected or thwarted at various levels of the organizational hierarchy. In addition, the interpersonal contexts of schools influence students in many ways. Although we have focused only briefly on specific aspects of these interpersonal relationships (e.g., culture), interpersonal relationships represent complex networks that can impact student motivation.

We conclude by reiterating what Maehr (1976) noted many years ago: Motivation matters, but it often is not considered as a valued outcome in education. Indeed, "achievement" often triumphs over motivation. Many policymakers are proud to claim that students have achieved a certain level of knowledge in a particular domain (e.g., mathematics), but little attention is paid to whether those students subsequently want to continue pursuing mathematics. We believe that the use of "competence," rather than "achievement," as a framework for learning in schools offers more hope that motivation can in fact become more valued, and therefore more easily emphasized by teachers. Moreover, additional classroom-based motivation research that considers and describes protocols for, and findings from, working within organizational, instructional, and interpersonal school contexts will contribute immensely to the next wave of scholarship on teacher and school influences on competence motivation.

REFERENCES

Anderman, E. M. (2002). School effects on psychological outcomes during adolescence. *Journal of Educational Psychology, 94*(4), 795–809.

Anderman, E. M., & Anderman, L. H. (2014). *Classroom motivation* (2nd ed.). Boston: Pearson.

Anderman, E. M., Gray, D. L., O'Connell, A., Cupp, P. K., Lane, D. R., & Zimmerman, R. (2011). Classroom goal structures and HIV and pregnancy prevention education in rural high school health classrooms. *Journal of Research on Adolescence, 21*(4), 904–922.

Anderman, E. M., & Maehr, M. L. (1994). Motivation and schooling in the middle grades. *Review of Educational Research, 64*(2), 287–309.

Anderman, E. M., & Urdan, T. C. (1995). A multilevel approach to middle-level reform. *Principal, 74*(3), 26–28.

Anderson, L. W., & Krathwohl, D. R. (2001). *A taxonomy for learning, teaching, and assessing: A revision of Bloom's taxonomy of educational objectives.* New York: Longman.

Baker, E. L. (2013). Critical moments in research and use of assessment. *Theory Into Practice, 52*, 83–92.

Bandura, A. (1986). *Social foundations of thought and action: A social cognitive theory.* Englewood Cliffs, NJ: Prentice Hall.

Barkoukis, V., & Hagger, M. S. (2013). The trans-contextual model: Perceived learning and performance motivational climates as analogues of perceived autonomy support. *European Journal of Psychology of Education, 28*(2), 353–372.

Becker, M., Vignoles, V. L., Owe, E., Brown, R., Smith, P. B., Easterbrook, M., et al. (2012). Culture and the distinctiveness motive: Constructing identity in individualistic and collectivistic contexts. *Journal of Personality and Social Psychology, 102*(4), 833–855.

Belenky, D. M., & Nokes-Malach, T. J. (2012). Motivation and transfer: The role of mastery-approach goals in preparation for future learning. *Journal of the Learning Sciences, 21*(3), 399–432.

Benware, C., & Deci, E. L. (1984). Quality of learning with an active versus passive motivational set. *American Educational Research Journal, 21*, 755–765.

Bloom, B. S., Engelhart, M. D., Furst, E. J., Hill, W. H., & Krathwohl, D. R. (Eds.). (1956). *Taxonomy of educational objectives: Handbook I. Cognitive domain.* New York: David McKay.

Blumenfeld, P. C., Mergendoller, J. R., & Swartout, D. W. (1987). Task as a heuristic for understanding student learning and motivation. *Journal of Curriculum Studies, 19*(2), 135–148.

Butler, R. (2011, April). *Motivation and development: Some thoughts about the development of achievement motivation and of theories of achievement motivation.* Invited address at the annual meeting of the American Educational Research Association, New Orleans, LA.

Byrd, C. M., & Chavous, T. M. (2011). Racial identity, school racial climate, and school intrinsic motivation among African American youth: The importance of person–context congruence. *Journal of Research on Adolescence, 21*, 849–860.

Canrinus, E. T., Helms-Lorenz, M., Beijaard, D., Buitink, J., & Hofman, A. (2012). Self-efficacy, job satisfaction, motivation and commitment: Exploring the relationships between indicators of teachers' professional identity. *European Journal of Psychology of Education, 27*(1), 115–132.

Ciani, K. D., Sheldon, K. M., Hilpert, J. C., & Easter, M. A. (2011). Antecedents and trajectories of achievement goals: A self-determination theory perspective. *British Journal of Educational Psychology, 81*(2), 223–243.

Coburn, C. E. (2003). Rethinking scale: Moving beyond numbers to deep and lasting change. *Review of Educational Research, 32*, 3–12.

Copper, J., & Semich, G. (2014). YouTube as a teacher training tool: Information and communication technology as a delivery instrument for professional development. *International Journal of Information and Communication Technology Education, 10*(4), 30–40.

Cornelissen, F., Daly, A. J., Liou, Y.-H., van Swet, J., Beijaard, D., & Bergen, T. C. M. (2014). More than a master: Developing, sharing, and using knowledge in school–university research networks. *Cambridge Journal of Education, 44*, 35–57.

Cornelissen, F., van Swet, J., Beijaard, D., & Bergen, T. (2011). Aspects of school–university research networks that play a role in developing, sharing and using knowledge based on teacher research. *Teaching and Teacher Education: An International Journal of Research and Studies, 27*(1), 147–156.

Darling-Hammond, L., Wei, R. C., Andree, A., Richardson, N., & Orphanos, S. (2009). State of the profession: Study measures status of professional development. *Journal of Staff Development, 30*(2), 42–44.

Deci, E. L., & Ryan, R. M. (1985). *Intrinsic motivation and self-determination in human behavior.* New York: Plenum Press.

Deci, E. L., & Ryan, R. M. (2000a). The support of autonomy and the control of behavior. In E. T. Higgins & A. W. Kruglanski (Eds.), *Motivational science: Social and personality perspectives* (pp. 128–145). New York: Psychology Press.

Deci, E. L., & Ryan, R. M. (2000b). The "what" and "why" of goal pursuits: Human needs and the self-determination of behavior. *Psychological Inquiry, 11*(4), 227–268.

Deci, E. L., Schwartz, A. J., Sheinman, L., & Ryan, R. M. (1981). An instrument to assess adults' orientations toward control versus autonomy with children: Reflections on intrinsic motivation and perceived competence. *Journal of Educational Psychology, 73*, 642–650.

Deci, E. L., Vallerand, R. J., Pelletier, L. G., & Ryan, R. M. (1991). Motivation and education: The self-determination perspective. *Educational Psychologist, 26*(3–4), 325–346.

DeCuir-Gunby, J. T., & Schutz, P. A. (2014). Researching race within educational psychology contexts. *Educational Psychologist, 49*, 244–260.

Desimone, L. (1999). Linking parent involvement with student achievement: Do race and income matter? *Journal of Educational Research, 93*, 11–30.

Doyle, W. (1983). Academic work. *Review of Educational Research, 53*, 159–199.

Dweck, C. S. (2006). *Mindset: The new psychology of success.* New York: Random House.

Eccles, J. S. (2005). Subjective task value and the Eccles et al. model of achievement-related choices. In A. J. Elliot & C. S. Dweck (Eds.), *Handbook of competence and motivation* (pp. 105–121). New York: Guilford Press.

Eccles (Parsons), J., Adler, T. F., Futterman, R., Goff, S. B., Kaczala, C. M., Meece, J. L., et al. (1983). Expectancies, values, and academic behaviors. In J. T. Spence (Ed.), *Achievement and achievement motivation* (pp. 75–146). San Francisco: Freeman.

Eccles, J. S., & Harold, R. D. (1996). Family involvement in children's and adolescents' schooling. In A. Booth & J. F. Dunn (Eds.), *Family–school links: How do they affect educational outcomes?* (pp. 3–34). Mahwah, NJ: Erlbaum.

Eccles, J. S., & Midgley, C. (1989). Stage/environment fit: Developmentally appropriate classrooms for young adolescents. In R. Ames & C. Ames (Eds.), *Research on motivation and education: goals and cognitions* (Vol. 3. pp. 139–186). New York: Academic Press.

Eccles, J. S., & Roeser, R. (1999). School and community influences on human development. In M. Bornstein & M. Lamb (Eds.), *Developmental psychology: An advanced textbook* (4th ed., pp. 503–554). Mahwah, NJ: Erlbaum.

Eccles, J. S., & Roeser, R. W. (2009). Schools, academic motivation, and stage–environment fit. In R. M. Lerner & L. Steinber (Eds.), *Handbook of adolescent psychology* (3rd ed., pp. 404–434). Hoboken, NJ: Wiley.

Elliot, A. J., & Dweck, C. S. (Eds.). (2005). *Handbook of competence and motivation.* New York: Guilford Press.

Elliot, A. J., McGregor, H. A., & Thrash, T. M. (2002). The need for competence. In E. L. Deci & R. M. Ryan (Eds.), *Handbook of self-determination research* (pp. 361–387). Rochester, NY: University of Rochester Press.

Ercikan, K. (2006). Development in assessment of student learning. In P. A. Alexander & P. H. Winne (Eds.), *Handbook of educational psychology* (2nd ed., pp. 929–952). Mahwah, NJ: Erlbaum.

Faulkner, S. A., & Cook, C. M. (2006). Testing vs. teaching: The perceived impact of assessment demands on middle grades instructional practices. *RMLE Online: Research in Middle Level Education, 29*(7), 1–13.

Flake, J. K., Barron, K. E., Hulleman, C. S., McCoach, D., & Welsh, M. E. (2015). Measuring cost: The forgotten component of expectancy–value theory. *Contemporary Educational Psychology, 41*, 232–244.

Friend, M., & Bursuck, W. D. (2012). *Including students with special needs: A practical guide for classroom teachers* (6th ed.). Boston: Pearson.

Garet, M. S., Porter, A. C., Desimone, L., Birman, B. F., & Yoon, K. S. (2001). What makes professional development effective?: Results from a national sample of teachers. *American Educational Research Journal, 38*, 915–945.

Gilmore, L., & Cuskelly, M. (2009). A longitudinal study of motivation and competence in children with Down syndrome: Early childhood to early adolescence. *Journal of Intellectual Disability Research, 53*(5), 484–492.

Gonida, E. N., & Vauras, M. (2014). The role of parents in children's school life: Student motivation and socio-emotional functioning. *British Journal of Educational Psychology, 84*(3), 349–351.

Goodenow, C. (1993). The psychological sense of school membership among adolescents: Scale development and educational correlates. *Psychology in the Schools, 30,* 79–90.

Graham, S. (1992). "Most of the subjects were white and middle class": Trends in published research on African Americans in selected APA journals, 1970–1989. *American Psychologist, 47*(5), 629–639.

Graham, S., & Hudley, C. (2005). Race and ethnicity in the study of motivation and competence. In A. J. Elliot & C. S. Dweck (Eds.), *Handbook of competence and motivation* (pp. 392–414). New York: Guilford Press.

Gray, D. L., Chang, Y., & Anderman, E. M. (2015). Conditional effects of mastery goal structure on changes in students' motivational beliefs: need for cognition matters. *Learning and Individual Differences, 40,* 9–21.

Guskey, T. R. (2013). Defining student achievement. In J. Hattie & E. M. Anderman (Eds.), *International guide to student achievement* (pp. 3–6). New York: Routledge/Taylor & Francis Group.

Guthrie, J. T. (2004). Teaching for literacy engagement. *Viewpoint: Journal of Literacy Research, 36*(1), 1–30.

Harackiewicz, J. M., Rozek, C. S., Hulleman, C. S., & Hyde, J. S. (2012). Helping parents to motivate adolescents in mathematics and science an experimental test of a utility–value intervention. *Psychological Science, 23,* 899–906.

Hattie, J., & Anderman, E. M. (2013). *International guide to student achievement*. New York: Routledge.

Hoy, A. W., Hoy, W. K., & Davis, H. A. (2009). Teachers' self-efficacy beliefs. In K. R. Wenzel & A. Wigfield (Eds.), *Handbook of motivation at school* (pp. 627–653). New York: Routledge/Taylor & Francis.

Hulleman, C. S., Schrager, S. M., Bodmann, S. M., & Harackiewicz, J. M. (2010). A meta-analytic review of achievement goal measures: Different labels for the same constructs or different constructs with similar labels? *Psychological Bulletin, 136*(3), 422–449.

Kaplan, A., Katz, I., & Flum, H. (2012). Motivation theory in educational practice: Knowledge claims, challenges, and future directions. In K. R. Harris, S. G. Graham, & T. Urdan (Eds.), *APA educational psychology handbook: Vol. 2. Individual differences, cultural considerations, and contextual factors in educational psychology* (pp. 165–194). Washington, DC: American Psychological Association.

Kaplan, A., Middleton, M. J., Urdan, T., & Midgley, C. (2002). Achievement goals and goal structures. In C. Midgley (Ed.), *Goals, goal structures, and patterns of adaptive learning* (pp. 21–55). Hillsdale, NJ: Erlbaum.

Kilgore, S. B., & Pendleton, W. W. (1993). The organizational context of learning: Framework for understanding the acquisition of knowledge. *Sociology of Education, 66,* 63–87.

Juvonen, J. (2006). Sense of belonging, social relationships, and school functioning. In P. A. Alexander & P. H. Winne (Eds.), *Handbook of educational psychology* (2nd ed., pp. 655–674). Mahwah, NJ: Erlbaum.

Lissitz, R. W., & Jiao, H. (Eds.). (2014). *Value-added modeling and growth modeling with particular application to teacher and school effectiveness*. Charlotte, NC: Information Age.

Maehr, M. L. (1976). Continuing motivation: An analysis of a seldom considered educational outcome. *Review of Educational Research, 46*(3), 443–462.

Maehr, M. L., & Meyer, H. A. (1997). Understanding motivation and schooling: Where we're been, where we are, and where we need to go. *Educational Psychology Review, 9,* 371–409.

Maehr, M. L., & Midgley, C. (1996). *Transforming school cultures*. Boulder, CO: Westview Press.

Maehr, M. L., Midgley, C., & Urdan, T. (1992). School leader as motivator. *Educational Administration Quarterly, 18,* 412–431.

Martin, A., & Dowson, M. (2009). Interpersonal relationships, motivation, engagement, and achievement: Yields for theory, current issues, and educational practice. *Review of Educational Research, 79*(1), 327–365.

Meece, J. L., Anderman, E. M., & Anderman, L. H. (2006). Classroom goal structure, student motivation, and academic achievement. *Annual Review of Psychology, 57,* 487–503.

Midgley, C. (Ed.). (2002). Goals, goal structures, and patterns of adaptive learning. Mahwah, NJ: Erlbaum.

Moore, W. P. (1993, April). *Preparation of students for testing: Teacher differentiation of appropriate and inappropriate practices*. Paper presented at the annual meeting of the National Council on Measurement in Education, Atlanta, GA.

Natriello, G. (2016). Networked learning. In L. Corno & E. M. Anderman (Eds.), *Handbook of educational psychology* (3rd ed., pp. 337–348). New York: Routledge.

Nichols, J. D., & Zhang, G. (2011). Classroom environments and student empowerment: An analysis of elementary and secondary teacher beliefs. *Learning Environments Research, 14*(3), 229–239.

Nolen, S. B. (2011). The role of educational systems in the link between formative assessment and motivation. *Theory Into Practice, 50,* 319–326.

Patall, E. A., & Leach, J. K. (2015). The role of choice provision in academic dishonesty. *Contemporary Educational Psychology, 42,* 97–110.

Pollock, M. (2013). It takes a network to raise a child: Improving the communication infrastructure of public education to enable community cooperation in young people's success. *Teachers College Record, 115*(7), 1–28.

Reeve, J., & Jang, H. (2006). What teachers say and do to support students' autonomy during a learning activity. *Journal of Educational Psychology, 98*(1), 209–218.

Ryan, R. M., & Brown, K. W. (2005). Legislating competence: High-stakes testing policies and their relations with psychological theories and research. In A. J. Elliot & C. S. Dweck (Eds.), *Handbook of competence and motivation* (pp. 354–374). New York: Guilford Press.

Ryan, R. M., & Grolnick, W. S. (1986). Origins and pawns in the classroom: Self-report and projective assessments of individual differences in children's perceptions. *Journal of Personality and Social Psychology, 50*(3), 550–558.

Slavin, R. E. (1992). When and why does cooperative learning increase achievement?: Theoretical and empirical perspectives. In R. Hertz-Lazarowitz & N. Miller (Eds.), *Interaction in cooperative groups: The theoretical anatomy of group learning* (pp. 145–173). Cambridge, UK: Cambridge University Press.

Snyder, C. R., & Fromkin, H. L. (1980). *Uniqueness: The human pursuit of difference.* New York: Plenum Press.

Sui-Chi, H. E., & Willms, D. J. (1996). Effects of parental involvement on eighth-grade achievement. *Sociology of Education, 69,* 126–141.

Tschannen-Moran, M., & Hoy, A. W. (2001). Teacher efficacy: Capturing an elusive construct. *Teaching and Teacher Education, 17*(7), 783–805.

Turner, J. C., Christensen, A., Kackar-Cam, H., Trucano, M., & Fulmer, S. M. (2014). Enhancing students' engagement: Report of a 3-year intervention with middle school teachers. *American Educational Research Journal, 51,* 1195–1226.

Turner, J. C., & Meyer, D. K. (2000). Studying and understanding the instructional contexts of classrooms: Using out past to forge our future. *Educational Psychologist, 35,* 69–85.

Turner, J. C., Warzon, K. B., & Christensen, A. L. (2011). Motivating mathematics learning: Changes in teachers' practices and beliefs during a nine-month collaboration. *American Educational Research Journal, 48,* 718–762.

Urdan, T., & Turner, J. C. (2005). Competence motivation in the classroom. In A. J. Elliot & C. S. Dweck (Eds.), *Handbook of competence and motivation* (pp. 297–317). New York: Guilford Press.

Usher, E. L. (2016). Personal capability beliefs. In L. Corno & E. M. Anderman (Eds.), *Handbook of educational psychology* (3rd ed., pp. 146–159). New York: Routledge/Taylor & Francis.

Van Yperen, N. W., Elliot, A. J., & Anseel, F. (2009). The influence of mastery-avoidance goals on performance improvement. *European Journal of Social Psychology, 39*(6), 932–943.

Wake County Public Schools. (2014, October). Effective teaching framework supports better teaching and learning [Web log comment]. Retrieved from *https://webarchive.wcpss.net/blog/2014/10/effective-teaching-framework-supports-better-teaching-and-learning/.*

Wei, R. C., Darling-Hammond, L., Adamson, F., & National Staff Development Council. (2010). *Professional development in the United States: Trends and challenges: Phase II of a three-phase study* (Executive summary). Oxford, OH: National Staff Development Council.

Weiner, B. (1986). *An attributional theory of motivation and emotion.* New York: Springer-Verlag.

Weiner, B. (2005). Motivation from an attributional perspective and the social psychology of perceived competence. In A. J. Elliot & C. S. Dweck (Eds.), *Handbook of competence and motivation* (pp. 73–84). New York: Guilford Press.

Wigfield, A., & Eccles, J. S. (1992). The development of achievement task values: A theoretical analysis. *Developmental Review, 12*(3), 265–310.

Willems, P. P., & Gonzalez-DeHass, A. R. (2012). School–community partnerships: Using authentic contexts to academically motivate students. *School Community Journal, 22*(2), 9–30.

Xie, K., DeBacker, T. K., & Ferguson, C. (2006). Extending the traditional classroom through online discussion: The role of student motivation. *Journal of Educational Computing Research, 34*(1), 67–89.

Yeager, D. S., Purdie-Vaughns, V., Garcia, J., Apfel, N., Brzustoski, P., Master, A., et al. (2014). Breaking the cycle of mistrust: Wise interventions to provide critical feedback across the racial divide. *Journal of Experimental Psychology: General, 143*(2), 804–824.

Zusho, A., & Clayton, K. (2011). Culturalizing achievement goal theory and research. *Educational Psychologist, 46*(4), 239–260.

CHAPTER 33

Competence and Motivation in the Physical Domain

The Relevance of Self-Theories in Sports and Physical Education

CHRISTOPHER M. SPRAY

Research into competence and motivation in the physical domain has truly burgeoned over the past 40 years. Investigators have adopted various perspectives during this time to understand achievement motivation in contexts in which competence is highly visible, and challenges and threats to the acquisition and demonstration of competence are common. The "physical" domain is taken to comprise sport, structured physical activity (exercise), and physical education (PE) at school and university. Along with theory and research have come evidence-based recommendations for coaches and teachers to adopt behaviors that purportedly optimize motivational processes among individuals participating in these settings. Attempting to synthesize this body of work within a single chapter on competence motivation would likely fail to do justice to the progress that has been made in theory development, knowledge acquisition, and application to professional practice. Consequently, in this chapter I want to focus on self-theories of ability (also referred to as implicit beliefs, mindsets, theories of change, conceptions of ability), with a primary focus on youth

sports and PE (see also Dweck & Molden, Chapter 8, this volume). Following a review of how research in sports and PE has complemented and diverged from research in other domains, I highlight some concerns that require our consideration and proffer a number of avenues for further research. Subsequently, in the spirit of the second edition of the *Handbook of Competence and Motivation,* I turn attention to the application of self-theories research for practitioners, and outline the challenges often faced by coaches and teachers in influencing motivation and competence in physical settings. I hope the chapter serves to inform readers and stimulate continued efforts to learn and apply our knowledge of self-theories in sports and PE.

SELF-THEORIES IN SPORTS AND PE

Beliefs about the nature of human attributes center on an individual's view (or theory) of whether such qualities are fixed and stable, or whether they are malleable and potentially changeable. In the scientific literature, the former belief has been termed an *entity theory*, whereas the latter belief has been labeled an *incremental theory* (Dweck & Leggett, 1988; Dweck, 1999). In more colloquial terms, these theories have often been referred to as *growth (incremental)* and *fixed (entity) mindsets* (Dweck, 2006). As we have seen in Chapter 8 (Dweck & Molden, this volume), these beliefs about competence have received extensive attention from researchers working in diverse contexts such as education, occupations, health, and relationships. Initial work in sports drew heavily on Dweck's research into children's beliefs about intelligence and their links with the adoption of achievement goals and ensuing mastery and helpless responses to challenging tasks (Dweck, 1986; Dweck & Bempechat, 1983; Dweck, Chiu, & Hong, 1995; Dweck & Leggett, 1988). Indeed, over the past 20 years or so, implicit beliefs research in sports, physical activity, and PE has continued to focus predominantly on young people at school and university (Vella, Braithwaite, Gardner, & Spray, 2016). The reason for this attention on formal education contexts is not clear, but most likely it reflects enduring interests of investigators and more significant restrictions encountered in accessing elite sporting populations. In the remainder of this section, I briefly examine the network of motivational variables ("meaning systems") encompassing self-theories. Subsequently, I address measurement and manipulation considerations pertaining to studies of implicit beliefs in the physical domain, drawing comparisons with research in other contexts where possible.

Meaning Systems

Individuals holding an entity perspective are more likely to adopt ego or performance achievement goals in order to demonstrate and validate their ability, whereas those who espouse incremental views tend to adopt task or mastery goals in order to acquire and increase the attribute in question (see Dweck & Molden, 2005, and Chapter 8, this volume). Thus, beliefs and goals combine to influence how individuals interpret competence-based settings, and the perceptual lens adopted leads to important consequences. Early work in youth sports and PE

found support for these propositions with respect to dichotomous (approach) achievement goals (e.g., Biddle, Wang, Chatzisarantis, & Spray, 2003; Ommundsen, 2001a, 2001b, 2003; Wang, Chatzisarantis, Spray, & Biddle, 2002). Following the emergence of the trichotomous and 2×2 approach–avoidance achievement goal frameworks in academic settings (Elliot, 1999; Elliot & Church, 1997; Elliot & McGregor, 2001; Elliot & Hulleman, Chapter 4, this volume), studies in sports and PE have examined the links between self-theories and mastery and performance goals, differentiated by definition (self-task vs. other-related competence) *and* valence (approaching positive vs. avoiding negative outcomes) (e.g., Wang, Liu, Lochbaum, & Stevenson, 2009; Warburton & Spray, 2008). To my knowledge, researchers have yet to examine associations between beliefs and goals in the 3×2 framework (Elliot, Murayama, & Pekrun, 2011) within physical settings. It has yet to be determined, for example, whether incremental beliefs are differentially associated with intrapersonal- and task-based mastery goals. Moreover, little attention has been devoted to how implicit beliefs work in concert with other important intraindividual constructs such as fear of failure and perceived competence, as well as environmental factors in sports and PE, to determine achievement goal adoption and associated outcomes.

Measuring and Manipulating Self-Theories in Sports and PE

The majority of cross-sectional and longitudinal studies measuring athletic ability beliefs have utilized the Conceptions of the Nature of Athletic Ability Questionnaire (CNAAQ; Sarrazin et al., 1996) or its successor, the CNAAQ-2 (Biddle et al., 2003; Wang, Liu, Biddle, & Spray, 2005). This approach to measurement has varied from work in alternative domains that has typically utilized a single scale to label study participants as entity *or* incremental theorists. The CNAAQ-2 (and the CNAAQ) assesses incremental and entity beliefs as distinct higher-order constructs underpinned by more specific beliefs that sports ability can be learned, and therefore is increasable, and that sports ability is a stable and an innate gift. This approach permits the calculation of separate scores for each belief, along with the ability to determine the association of the scores obtained, and the potential to examine within-person permutations of beliefs. The majority of studies have focused on the predictive utility of the higher-order incremental and entity beliefs rather than effects of the more specific beliefs. Moreover, there has been a relative dearth of studies examining change processes, and these longitudinal investigations have focused solely on young people in schools either during a short unit of work in PE, across the primary–secondary school transition, or across 1 year in secondary school (Warburton & Spray, 2008, 2009, 2013).

Few investigators have attempted to temporarily manipulate participants' self-theories in order to examine how the different meaning systems lead to positive or negative outcomes in sports. In our systematic review (Vella et al., 2016), we identified seven experimental studies of self-theories in sports and related contexts, conducted between 1996 and 2010. Searches revealed no published studies since 2010. This state of affairs is somewhat disappointing given the opportunity that these types of investigation afford in designing potentially compelling belief messages to infer causal effects on outcomes of interest. One study, carried out with school students performing a golf-putting task, illustrated the difficulties in creating conditions that reliably produced distinct "high" and "low" incremental groups. While an "entity" message read by participants reliably distinguished groups on entity scores, the "incremental" message failed to distinguish the incremental and control groups on incremental scores (Spray, Wang, Biddle, Chatzisarantis, & Warburton, 2006). Nevertheless, students in the incremental condition were less inclined to make failure attributions to lack of ability than members of the entity group. A second school-based investigation revealed that an incremental beliefs manipulation in PE led to higher levels of intrinsic motivation among students (Moreno, Gonzalez-Cutre, Martin-Albo, & Cervello, 2010). Vella and colleagues (2016) argued for the development and testing of more compelling ways to manipulate beliefs in sports.

Particularly in the education context, investigators have attempted to design longer-term self-theory interventions in school classrooms (e.g., Blackwell, Trzesniewski, & Dweck, 2007). Strategies to induce incremental beliefs have centered on instilling in children the notion of growing connections in the brain to improve intelligence. No studies in sports-related settings have sought to highlight the potential for connections between muscles and the brain to improve motor coordination, or developing fast-twitch muscle fibers to improve speed and power, or stretching muscles to improve ability in activities requiring flexibility. There have been no published investigations with sports coaches and PE teachers that put in place a carefully designed mindset intervention with athletes and students to promote theories of change and to buffer the effects of entity beliefs. Later in this chapter, I address the application of self-theory research to professional practice in physical settings in greater detail.

KEY FINDINGS IN SPORTS AND PE

Following trends in other domains, implicit beliefs research in the physical domain has largely adopted quantitative methods. Very few studies have employed interviews, focus groups, or other forms of qualitative inquiry. Recently, Vella and coworkers (2016) conducted a systematic review and meta-analysis of published research in sports, physical activity, and PE. Studies were eligible for inclusion in the review if a valid and reliable quantitative measure of self-theories was employed. We identified 43 studies conducted between 1991 and 2014 that employed cross-sectional, longitudinal, or experimental designs. Findings showed that incremental beliefs were more strongly associated with theoretically derived correlates than are entity beliefs. Not surprisingly, given the origins of work on implicit theories, the most frequently studied correlates of ability beliefs were achievement goals (conceptualized and measured in either dichotomous or approach–avoidance terms) and motivational climate. Across settings, incremental beliefs about change were positively linked with task orientation, mastery-approach and mastery-avoidance goals, and mastery climate, but negatively correlated with performance climate. On the other hand, entity beliefs about stability positively predicted the adoption of ego orientation, performance-approach and performance-avoidance goals, and performance climate. Moreover, entity beliefs negatively predicted perceptions of mastery climate. These findings are in accordance with theoretical predictions and evidence from other life domains of the meaning systems that individuals adopt (Burnette, O'Boyle, VanEpps, Pollack, & Finkel, 2013). Importantly, incremental beliefs were also linked with more self-determined forms of motivation and perceived competence. In contrast, entity beliefs were negatively associated with autonomous (vs. controlled) motivation and unrelated to perceived competence. More generally, entity beliefs were more weakly associated with outcomes than incremental beliefs.

Notably, the empirical yield of self-theory research in the physical domain is mainly informed by cross-sectional, snapshot studies. There is a need for more, and higher quality, experimental and field-based studies testing a greater range of outcomes (e.g., learning strategies, coping strategies, self-esteem, and achievement). In addition to the outcomes outlined earlier, implicit beliefs have been associated with self-efficacy, beliefs about success, motor learning, skills acquisition, desired future versus present reality focus, and positive and negative affect (e.g., Drews, Chiviacowsky, & Wulf, 2013; Jourden, Bandura, & Banfield, 1991; Kasimatis, Miller, & Marcussen, 1996; Sevincer, Kluge, & Oettingen, 2014). We could begin to look more closely at the influence of key moderators in the beliefs → goals → outcomes sequence, something that our systematic review was unable to reveal because of the disparate nature of empirical endeavors to date. For example, Stenling, Hassmén, and Holmström (2014) have recently identified gender to be an important moderator, but we also need to investigate age, physical context (including elite and recreational sports), motivational climate, need supportive and thwarting coaching styles, as well as intrapersonal variables such as perceived competence and fear of failure.

In addition to quantitative approaches, the utilization of a range of qualitative methods would help to enrich our knowledge of the development and ramifications of self-theories in sports and related settings. Two studies with elite golfers and track-and-field athletes speak to the importance of self-theories in sports. In the first study, eight high-level golfers were interviewed about their self-theories of ability, and a grounded theory approach was adopted to articulate some of the complexities surrounding self-theories in golf (Slater, Spray, & Smith, 2012). Three dimensions emerged: acquirable ability, stable ability, and developing natural attributes, reflecting the coexistence of both types of implicit beliefs. A number of golfing attributes were perceived to be innate and stable, such as coordination and touch, whereas there also emerged the view that natural attributes act as foundations that can be built upon through practice. Interestingly, this study tapped golfers' views of psychological attributes important for success in elite sport. Passion, persistence, and staying in the moment, for example, were considered stable qualities and difficult to develop. Clearly, these findings imply that there is a job to be done by coaches and sports psychologists wishing to cultivate incremental theories of psychological skills among players. More broadly, however, the study revealed the central role played by coaches, other social agents, golf culture, and observations of high-profile professional players in the socialization of self-theories of golf ability. Moreover, the concept of a "ceiling effect" was evident among responses. Some golfers considered that there is always room for improvement, and that certain events (e.g., competitive success) can serve to raise the ceiling, whereas other players endorsed the view that their current level represents the maximum level of competence they will ever attain.

Many of the findings with golfers also emerged in interviews with track-and-field athletes competing in sprinting and throwing events (Jowett & Spray, 2013). At the time of the study, these athletes were hopeful of selection for the 2012 Olympic Games. Again, implicit theories were seen to be intertwined, with participants believing that a combination of innate qualities and sheer hard work and persistence leads to performance improvements and competitive success (building on natural ability). Ceiling effects were observed, although these appeared to be confined to physical attributes; psychological attributes were viewed as more malleable. Also in accordance with Slater and colleagues' (2012) findings were the reported influences on the development of athletes' implicit beliefs: upbringing, career transitions, motivational climate, coaches and fellow athletes, and initial success as a junior. Importantly, and very much in line with theoretical propositions (Dweck, 1999), incremental theories were shown to be essential in overcoming setbacks, taking personal responsibility for successes and failures (controllable attributions), setting approach-focused goals, and overcoming setbacks.

In summary, these two studies show that in elite sports, athletes access both types of self-theories. They recognize that sporting performance is made up of a multitude of specific skills, some of which may be viewed in fixed terms, others in more malleable terms. Performance-enhancing psychological skills, as well as physical attributes, are likely to be considered in both fixed and growth forms. In addition, socialization factors play a key role in individuals' theory development. More qualitative studies would be beneficial, especially with children and adolescents. Results emerging from our recent studies with gymnasts and swimmers are reinforcing many of the points raised by Slater and colleagues (2012) and Jowett and Spray (2013), and attest to the relevance and complexity of self-theories in sports. In the sections that follow, I outline some key conceptual and empirical issues facing researchers in the physical domain (and, no doubt, in other domains), provide suggestions for research questions that appear worthy of our attention, then close the chapter by focusing more closely on the application of research to practice.

CURRENT RESEARCH ISSUES IN SPORTS AND PE

Given the disparate nature of the extant research base in the physical domain, how can investigators bring greater coherence to empirical endeavors and enhance their impact on professional practice?

Measurement of Beliefs

Self-theories of change and stability are conceived as knowledge structures, and individuals have access to both types of beliefs. Individuals' beliefs can differ across and within broad domains such as personality, relationships, health, education, and sports (Dweck, 2005; Dweck & Molden, 2005; Yeager & Dweck, 2012). Research has assumed that people tend chronically to endorse one theory over the other. Early measures tapped only one belief, with the assumption that low scores, or disagreement, denoted the endorsement of the other belief (Dweck, 1999). More recently, in many domains, implicit beliefs have been assessed with a short continuous scale containing both fixed and growth items in which high scores reflect a particular dominant belief. Based on mean scores, participants are classified as entity *or* incremental theorists, reflecting a dominant chronic view. The beliefs are viewed as dichotomous theories (i.e., entity and incremental meaning systems), although measured using one continuous scale (see Leith et al., 2014).

As mentioned earlier, researchers have tended to adopt more comprehensive measurement scales in the physical domain (i.e., the CNAAQ or CNAAQ-2) that permit scores to be derived for both beliefs. Correlations between entity and incremental beliefs (and between the corresponding lower-order beliefs) are typically low to moderate and negative, which suggests that they do not represent opposite ends of the same continuum (Biddle, Soos, & Chatzisarantis, 1999; Lintunen, Valkonen, Leskinen, & Biddle, 1999; Ommundsen, 2001a, 2001b, 2003; Sarrazin et al., 1996; Wang & Biddle, 2003). Using the CNAAQ-2 enables the examination of within-person belief profiles. For example, an individual can believe that certain elements of sports ability are fixed, whereas other contributory qualities (referents; see Nicholls, 1992) are malleable—a high–high or ambivalent profile. Wang and Biddle (2001) demonstrated, with reference to sports, the existence of five motivational profiles among youth, each containing combinations of entity and incremental beliefs.

These clusters were differentially linked with a range of outcomes (see also Biddle & Wang, 2003; Wang, Liu, & Biddle, 2003). Using two short sets of items to measure implicit beliefs about mental toughness, Gucciardi, Jackson, Hodge, Anthony, and Brooke (2015) found two clusters of beliefs among adolescent athletes—an incremental theory (high incremental–low entity scores) and an ambivalent theory (moderate scores on both beliefs). A dominant entity beliefs cluster did not emerge. Our qualitative work with elite athletes has also demonstrated the complexities surrounding implicit beliefs. Athletes conceptualize their sporting attainment as a consequence of many attributes, some that they view as fixed, others that they consider more susceptible to change through sheer hard work (Jowett & Spray, 2013; Slater et al., 2012). In summary, there appears much to be gleaned from analyzing separate scores for the two implicit theories.

Fluidity of Self-Theories

Arguably, too much research in physical settings utilizing the CNAAQ-2 has focused on beliefs about general "sports" ability, either in cross-sectional or longitudinal studies, without identifying the conditions that lead to the adoption or active selection of one belief over the other. Recent work by Leith and colleagues (2014), for instance, has helped to illuminate situational factors that trigger the adoption of one type of implicit belief over the other and has therefore highlighted the potential fluidity of self-theories. Individuals can selectively shift their implicit beliefs to reach desired conclusions about themselves or to protect themselves and liked others. Identifying the circumstances in which athletes regulate their self-theories (i.e., strategically endorse incremental and resist entity views) offers researchers in the physical domain exciting avenues of inquiry.

Manipulation of Beliefs in Experimental Studies

The relatively few experimental studies in the physical domain have either asked participants to read a passage of text espousing one theory or the other, or relevant instructions have been read aloud (e.g., Drews et al., 2013; Jourden et al., 1991; Kasimatis et al., 1996; Spray et al., 2006; Wulf & Lewthwaite, 2009). Typically, "evidence" is presented to provide credibility for the view that ability is either acquired or innate, or a high-profile athlete is described as exemplifying either of the self-theories. Results have generally been supportive of theoretical predictions. Nevertheless, challenges remain, notably, reducing the all-too-appealing nature of incremental belief items to distinguish experimental groups (Dweck, 1999; Spray et al., 2006). We must develop more creative and compelling incremental messages in both laboratory and school settings. These manipulations will likely necessitate inventive use of new technologies and multimedia formats to engage participants. Moreover, researchers and practitioners will need to concurrently deploy powerful and realistic "anti entity" messages.

Urdan and Turner (2005) presented some general arguments for why laboratory-based findings, usually obtained with school or university students, may fail to translate to real-world settings in which numerous situational and cultural factors affect students, coaches, and teachers. These kinds of influences are also likely to operate in physical settings. Thus, we need more varied field-based studies to discover "what works" in PE and sports. Cluster randomized controlled trials are absent from extant research in physical contexts. Moreover, I am unaware of the use of ethnographic techniques or reports of action research studies.

Contextual Nuances

Do the effects of self-theories and their associated meaning systems play out in subtly different ways in elite versus recreational sports, school, and university settings, and in the exercise domain? There is generally a dearth of studies on self-theories in physical activity settings, in which participants are more concerned with maintaining health and fitness than achieving competitive success (see, e.g., Burnette, 2010; Lyons, Kaufman, & Rima, 2015).

Beliefs about What?

Vella, Cliff, Okely, Weintraub, and Robinson (2014) raise the interesting question of whether young people in sports distinguish between relatively general fundamental movement abilities and more specific sports-related skills when responding to implicit belief measures. The development of the CNAAQ was to some extent influenced by such thinking, with the creation of general and specific subscales (Sarrazin et al., 1996). These two variables were later removed in the validation of the CNAAQ-2 (Biddle et al., 2003; Wang et al., 2005). However, we need to know more about individuals' beliefs about the fixed nature of specific skills and fundamental abilities, especially those that underpin a general entity view.

FUTURE RESEARCH DIRECTIONS

Given the current empirical yield, there remains much work to do in physical contexts to assess and manipulate self-theories of ability. Researchers in other domains, notably, education and social psychology, are asking nuanced questions that investigators in the physical domain, where challenging demands, setbacks, threatening transitions, and potential for public displays of incompetence are ubiquitous, would be wise to prioritize (Burnette et al., 2013; Job, Walton, Bernecker, & Dweck, 2015; Leith et al., 2014; Snyder, Malin, Dent, & Linnenbrink-Garcia, 2014; Yeager et al., 2014; Yeager, Trzesniewski, Tirri, Nokelainen, & Dweck, 2011). I offer below a number of avenues of inquiry which I believe would contribute meaningfully to the field.

Socialization of Self-Theories

The development of self-theories of physical ability in young people is understudied. Where do the beliefs come from, and who might be more important in imparting growth and fixed messages across various settings? Some young people may be particularly sensitive to the influence of gender and race stereotypes attached to sporting activities and more readily succumb to entity beliefs following early failure experiences. The role of friendships also deserves our attention. Children and adolescents often identify with a "best friend" in sports and PE (Smith, 2003). Might a desire to be like friends or particular classmates/teammates provide a means by which incremental

messages espoused by adults can be reinforced by such peers?

Resistance to Entity Beliefs in the Face of Failure

Why might some children and adolescents appear to show resistance to endorsing entity beliefs following failure? How are relationships between beliefs and outcomes mediated or moderated by the extant motivational climate, value attached to PE, teacher–student relationship quality, social comparison frames of reference, and motives for comparison in sports and PE?

Triggers that Shift Self-Theories

Considering recent studies pointing toward the potential for individuals to exercise greater self-regulation of beliefs than previously thought (Leith et al., 2014), which circumstances stimulate increased fluidity and susceptibility of implicit beliefs in sports and PE? Candidates for attention include new environments encountered through transitions (new friendships, coaches/teachers) and maturational factors.

Beliefs about Psychological Attributes

To date, research in the physical domain has centered on notions of the fixedness or malleability of athletic (physical) ability. Our qualitative research has nevertheless flagged the existence of implicit beliefs about psychological attributes in sports and alluded to their determinants and consequences (Jowett & Spray, 2013; Slater et al., 2012; see also Gucciardi and colleagues' (2015) study of self-theories of mental toughness operating across occupational, sports, and education achievement contexts). Standout candidates for attention include passion and resilience. My colleagues and I have also begun to examine children and adolescents' implicit beliefs about five characteristics— commitment, confidence, communication, control, and concentration—as they pertain to sports and PE (the 5Cs; Harwood, 2008; Harwood & Anderson, 2015). We are currently considering how to develop ways to promote growth-oriented beliefs about these qualities, particularly around important sports and educational transitions.

Organizational Policies and Practices

Self-theories are particularly important when individuals (teachers, coaches, selectors) are asked to judge the performances and achievements of others and possibly make decisions about their futures (Butler, 2000; Dweck & Molden, 2005). Adults who themselves hold dominant entity beliefs may make rash judgments and selection decisions about young people based on current demonstrated sports competence. Interestingly, in our ongoing studies, we are finding that successful elite athletes report being "rejected" at talent identification events as juniors and that those performers "selected" at the time do not go on to enjoy success in their sport and are no longer competing. We need research into potentially "institutionalized" fixed beliefs about young people's competence in sports and their implications for the policies and practices of National Governing Bodies (e.g., publication of junior rankings, talent identification programs) and professional development opportunities for coaches.

Continued research into coaching and organizational practices will help to reinforce the applied significance and potential impact of self-theories research in sports and education settings. In order to focus more closely on the application of research to practice, in the next section, I discuss several broad recommendations for promoting incremental beliefs in youth sports. Subsequently, I offer some thoughts for sports coaches and teachers as to how the typical practices in which they engage may impact on the accessibility of implicit beliefs among young people.

APPLYING THEORY AND RESEARCH FINDINGS IN SPORTS AND PE

Based on theory and empirical findings, researchers have stressed the importance of promoting incremental beliefs in sport. Chase (2010) documented the benefits to coaches of viewing their leadership abilities in incremental terms, and called on coach education and leadership programs to assist coaches in developing a growth mindset toward their own leadership qualities. Specific coaching behaviors included monitoring communication with individuals and teams, praising effort, providing constructive criticism, and setting and maintaining high expectations. The important point made by Chase is that these behaviors can be learned and improved.

With respect to working in the youth sports context specifically, Vella and colleagues (2014) proposed six interdependent instructional strategies to promote an incremental belief system:

1. *Focusing on effort and persistence.* Focusing on praise for effort and continued engagement, rather than talent, encourages the view that improvement is under personal control, particularly following setbacks.

2. *Facilitating challenge.* The difficulty of tasks and activities should be matched to individuals' current abilities, so that goals for improvement are personally challenging; making mistakes in both training and competition is viewed as an inevitable and necessary part of progressing in sports.

3. *Promoting the value of failure.* Linked with previous strategies, young people's failures in sports can be emphasized to be of value by adults and used to provide specific feedback that otherwise may not have been thought appropriate or relevant. Elements to consider include increased effort at appropriate times, training and competitive strategies, and seeking help (see also Yeager & Dweck, 2012).

4. *Defining success as effort.* Success in sports and other achievement contexts may be perceived from putting forth high effort levels and a sense of personal investment in the activity (Nicholls, 1989). High incremental beliefs promote engagement in the task at hand rather than attention on external outcomes.

5. *Promoting learning.* Incremental beliefs are more likely to flourish within a prevailing mastery-based climate that foregrounds individual and team improvement (Ames, 1992). Learning is placed at the heart of the system.

6. *Providing high expectations.* Coaches should hold high expectations for what young people can control—their cognitive and physical engagement in tasks, drills, games, and activities. Depending on the

context (e.g., long established member of a team, arrival at a new school or club), high expectations will likely have greater impact once professionally caring and sensitive relationships between youth and adults have been forged.

Vella and colleagues (2014) proposed that these strategies facilitate adaptive outcomes for young people in terms of high-quality motivation, positive affect, and behavioral engagement in sports. One can readily see the interdependencies of these six strategies, and it is evident that these broad-based practical recommendations do not stem exclusively from implicit beliefs theory and research. Indeed, components overlap with recommendations emanating from other motivation frameworks (cf. Urdan & Turner's [2005] discussion of common classroom-based recommendations arising from multiple theories).

Despite the appeal of these evidence-based instructional strategies, sports coaches and teachers may not feel sufficiently empowered to put these behaviors into operation, and the reasons may be philosophical and/or efficacy-based. For example, broader organizational and cultural factors may serve to dissuade coaches from deemphasizing winning and facilitating a growth mindset (Vella et al., 2014). Other practitioners may not buy into the principles based on their education and experiences (e.g., "This just won't work in my class/team"). Yet others may want to promote a growth mindset but feel they lack the subject expertise to do so. This situation may typically apply in primary schools in the United Kingdom, for example, where PE is often taught by teachers who are not trained PE specialists and have had little opportunity to undertake relevant development opportunities in their careers.

In an effort to provide further illustration of the relevance of self-theories in sports and school PE, I have summarized in Table 33.1 several pedagogical activities undertaken by coaches and teachers, and have tried to determine how knowledge of self-theories can inform practice. Potential barriers, and suggested ways to overcome them, are also included. This list of behaviors is not intended to be exhaustive, but the practices do represent identifiable components of the

coaching and teaching process. There is a danger that coaching and educating young people is seen as an overly mechanistic process—which it is not. Nevertheless, by breaking down and presenting the following typical tasks, it becomes easier to highlight the relevance of self-theories at a more specific level and consequently facilitate more precise suggestions for behavior change in coaches and teachers:

1. Planning
2. Activities, tasks, drills
3. Demonstrating
4. Grouping
5. Observation
6. Feedback (evaluation and recognition)
7. Recapping the lesson/training session
8. Reporting to parents, head coaches, academy directors

Effective application of theory to practice is not easy. In the first edition of the *Handbook,* Urdan and Turner (2005) eloquently highlighted some of the difficulties encountered by teachers in school classrooms, along with several reasons why recommendations resulting from theory and research may not "work" as effectively as we had hoped. These issues are certainly recognizable in sports and PE settings. Implementation of principles is multifaceted and therefore challenging for practitioners often working with large groups. Concepts such as *competence, meaning, interest, challenge, attributions, achievement emotions, autonomy, control, goals* (and the *reasons* held by individuals for adopting them) present a "heady mix" for the practitioner to take on board. Considered recognition of coaches or teachers' needs and local contexts is called for. We need to help practitioners create and sustain growth motivational systems in their achievement settings in ways that do not engender resistance to, or boredom with, the "message" among young people. How can the sorts of growth-focused messages, carefully composed for participants undertaking discrete tasks in experimental studies, be expanded and infused effectively over a prolonged period of time? Perhaps a starting point is to discuss with teachers and coaches their professional "philosophies." Why did they enter their profession, what do they

TABLE 33.1. Implications of Self-Theories for Teaching and Coaching Behaviors in Sports and PE

Teaching/coaching behaviors	Implications from a self-theories' perspective	Barriers	Overcoming barriers
Planning	• What is the focus of the session and can I infuse an incremental message? • What might competence and success look like in incremental belief terms?	• Lack of knowledge and time to consider carefully and prepare a script or other resources (e.g., YouTube clip, examples of high-profile role models)	• Self-theories workshop (continuous professional development [CPD]) • How can improvement be demonstrated? Faster, farther, longer, smoother, more accurate, more consistent, better understanding
Activities, tasks, drills	• Challenging but not too difficult, varied, fun, appropriate time to move on	• Difficult to be aware of and implement, individually tailored activities and tasks in many school and sports contexts • Operationalizing notions of challenge, meaning, and relevance among diverse learners	• Subject-specific CPD (content-based)
Demonstrating	• Who demonstrates and for what purpose?	• Lack of confidence from the teacher • Lack of knowledge to draw out key points of student demonstration	• Showcase pupils who have improved at different absolute levels • Does not have to be whole class but within groups • How should we utilize social comparison to best effect when watching demonstrators and team/classmates performing skills and activities?
Grouping	• Composition of working groups • When should this be a decision for the adult leader or athletes? • Groupings will often determine social comparison purposes	• Children want to work with their friends, refuse to work with certain teammates/classmates	• Provide a rationale for group selection (e.g., random, friendships, ability, size/weight, gender)
Observation	• Watch, listen for, and challenge attributions to theories of stability from individuals ("I'll never be able to do this") and their peers who may experience initial and easy mastery ("It's so easy!")	• Difficult for teachers to be aware of an individual pupil's psychological characteristics (e.g., attributions, self-efficacy) in a team or class context	• Is the task appropriate? • If it is inappropriate, change it

(continued)

TABLE 33.1. *(continued)*

Teaching/coaching behaviors	Implications from a self-theories' perspective	Barriers	Overcoming barriers
Feedback (evaluation and recognition)	• Present and future focused—related to strategy and effort • Avoid comments such as "You really showed them"; "You nailed that easily"; "You're a quick learner"; "You are a natural/seriously talented"; "What took you so long?"; "You either have it or you don't." • Avoid comforting statements implying "It's OK" not to make progress (low future expectations from the teacher) and "You're just one of those students for whom it doesn't come easy"	• Lack of expertise to identify difficulties and task progressions • Difficult to give individuals equal attention and feedback during activities	• Praise engagement with the task • "How can you make this easier or more difficult?" • Consider space, time, equipment, rules, number of components/opponents • Use "not yet" where possible • "Nothing worth achieving starts off easy" • "Everything is hard before it's easy" • "Be mindful of your mistakes"
Recapping lesson or training session	• Reinforce incremental message of the session • "Who feels they've improved and in what ways? If not, why not?"	• Time to interact with all students, players individually • Some performers may perceive no improvement despite high physical effort and "cognitive investment" in the session	• Value of making mistakes (thoughts of failure as learning opportunities) • Convey high expectations of engagement, persistence, and effort in the next lesson • "Why do you think it's not working at the moment?" • "What do you think you need to work on?" • "How can we change things?"
Reporting to parents, head coaches, academy directors	• Highlight improvements made, referring to both absolute and potential intrapersonal criteria • Avoid "Sports come easily to Jonny as he is a natural who rarely has to exert himself—he will do well at his next school" • Emphasize and reinforce young people's positive approach to overcoming difficulties and learning from mistakes	• Parents often want to know where their child ranks in the class or team • Coaches under pressure to select the current "best" athletes	• Parent education • Examine talent ID programs for implicit entity assumptions underpinning practices • Grading practices on absolute, not normative, outcomes • Employ combination of *current* ability plus effort grades

wish to achieve, and what do they believe are appropriate ways to go about it? Then, we can begin to introduce the psychology of competence and motivation and how it may gel or jar with their personal philosophies and the organizational opportunities and constraints impacting upon them. One example might be: What is their policy for selection to teams—current normative ability? Commitment to training? What is their approach toward giving all players "game time," particularly those youngsters who display a growth mindset and demonstrate personal improvement, yet are not normatively the most talented? How will parents be persuaded of the positives to this approach? These are important yet sensitive issues to address.

CONCLUDING REMARKS

In this chapter, I have articulated the theoretical, empirical, and applied relevance of self-theories of ability in the physical domain, and have discussed some of the issues surrounding definition, measurement, and manipulation of self-theories, followed by an overview of research findings to date. I then addressed key challenges facing researchers, before offering several directions for future work. My attention subsequently was centered on applied implications of the work in this field, including both fairly broad-based and more specific recommendations for practice. A limitation of the review is its primary focus on young people in sports and school-based PE. And self-theories, as central constructs within competence motivation research, by no means stand alone in this respect. We need to extend our reach more fully into the world of elite sports and health/exercise settings. Are the practical recommendations stemming from theory and evidence likely to play out similarly across diverse physical contexts? Or do we need to be a bit more creative and nuanced in how we advise practitioners to utilize their knowledge and skills to develop growth-oriented motivational systems? I suspect that the latter will be more palatable for coaches and teachers, yet more challenging to undertake.

Where does the field go from this point? Undoubtedly, there is a need to bring coherence and more programmatic efforts to the design of our studies (Vella et al., 2016). I would single out the need to design compelling, psychologically precise interventions that sustain growth mindset messages and persistently challenge unproductive fixed mindsets (Yeager & Dweck, 2012). As I mentioned earlier, local factors will need to be considered. That said, self-theories represent an intuitively appealing, elegant, and parsimonious explanatory concept for both the scientist and layperson (Roberts, 2012). Consequently, I look forward to engaging in, and reading about, future studies that have impact on both professional practice and the motivation of countless numbers of athletes and students. These studies, I hope, will feature in the next edition of the *Handbook*.

ACKNOWLEDGMENTS

I wish to thank present and former colleagues and students who have helped conduct studies into this fascinating research area. There are too many individuals to mention, although I would like to say a special thanks to Stuart Biddle for introducing me, as a doctoral student, to the relevance of self-theories in sports and PE.

REFERENCES

Ames, C. (1992). Classrooms: Goals, structures, and student motivation. *Journal of Educational Psychology, 84,* 261–271.

Biddle, S. J. H., Soos, I., & Chatzisarantis, N. (1999). Predicting physical activity intentions using a goal perspectives approach: A study of Hungarian youth. *Scandinavian Journal of Medicine and Science in Sports, 9,* 353–357.

Biddle, S. J. H., & Wang, C. K. J. (2003). Motivation and self-perception profiles and links with physical activity in adolescent girls. *Journal of Adolescence, 26,* 687–701.

Biddle, S. J. H., Wang, C. K. J., Chatzisarantis, N. L. D., & Spray, C. M. (2003). Motivation for physical activity in young people: Entity and incremental beliefs about athletic ability. *Journal of Sports Sciences, 21,* 973–989.

Blackwell, L. S., Trzesniewski, K. H., & Dweck, C. S. (2007). Implicit theories of intelligence predict achievement across an adolescent transition: A longitudinal study and an intervention. *Child Development, 78*, 246–263.

Burnette, J. L. (2010). Implicit theories of body weight: Entity beliefs can weigh you down. *Personality and Social Psychology Bulletin, 36*, 410–422.

Burnette, J. L., O'Boyle, E. H., VanEpps, E. M., Pollack, J. M., & Finkel, E. J. (2013). Mindsets matter: A meta-analytic review of implicit theories and self-regulation. *Psychological Bulletin, 139*, 655–701.

Butler, R. (2000). Making judgments about ability: The role of implicit theories of ability in moderating inferences from temporal and social comparison information. *Journal of Personality and Social Psychology, 78*, 965–978.

Chase, M. A. (2010). Should coaches believe in innate ability?: The importance of a leadership mindset. *Quest, 62*, 296–307.

Drews, R., Chiviacowsky, S., & Wulf, G. (2013). Children's motor skill learning is influenced by their conceptions of ability. *Journal of Motor Learning and Development, 1*, 38–44.

Dweck, C. S. (1986). Motivational processes affecting learning. *American Psychologist, 41*, 1040–1048.

Dweck, C. S. (1999). *Self-theories: Their role in motivation, personality, and development.* Philadelphia: Psychology Press.

Dweck, C. S. (2006). *Mindset: The new psychology of success.* New York: Ballantine.

Dweck, C. S., & Bempechat, J. (1983). Children's theories of intelligence: Consequences for learning. In S. G. Paris, G. M. Olson, & H. W. Stevenson (Eds.), *Learning and motivation in the classroom* (pp. 239–256). Hillsdale, NJ: Erlbaum.

Dweck, C. S., Chiu, C.-Y., & Hong, Y.-Y. (1995). Implicit theories: Elaboration and extension of the model. *Psychological Inquiry, 6*, 322–333.

Dweck, C. S., & Leggett, E. L. (1988). A social-cognitive approach to motivation and personality. *Psychological Review, 95*, 256–273.

Dweck, C. S., & Molden, D. C. (2005). Self-theories: Their impact on competence motivation and acquisition. In A. J. Elliot & C. S. Dweck (Eds.), *Handbook of competence and motivation* (pp. 122–140). New York: Guilford Press.

Elliot, A. J. (1999). Approach and avoidance motivation and achievement goals. *Educational Psychologist, 34*, 169–189.

Elliot, A. J., & Church, M. A. (1997). A hierarchical model of approach and avoidance achievement motivation. *Journal of Personality and Social Psychology, 72*, 218–232.

Elliot, A. J., & McGregor, H. A. (2001). A 2 × 2 achievement goal framework. *Journal of Personality and Social Psychology, 80*, 501–519.

Elliot, A. J., Murayama, K., & Pekrun, R. (2011). A 3 × 2 achievement goal model. *Journal of Educational Psychology, 103*, 632–648.

Gucciardi, D. F., Jackson, B., Hodge, K., Anthony, D. R., & Brooke, L. E. (2015). Implicit theories of mental toughness: Relations with cognitive, motivational, and behavioral correlates. *Sport, Exercise, and Performance Psychology, 4*, 100–112.

Harwood, C. (2008). Developmental consulting in a professional football academy: The 5Cs coaching efficacy program. *The Sport Psychologist, 22*, 109–133.

Harwood, C., & Anderson, R. (2015). Psychosocial development in youth soccer players: Assessing the effectiveness of the 5Cs intervention program. *The Sport Psychologist, 29*, 319–334.

Job, V., Walton, G. M., Bernecker, K., & Dweck, C. S. (2015). Implicit theories about willpower predict self-regulation and grades in everyday life. *Journal of Personality and Social Psychology, 108*, 637–647.

Jourden, F. J., Bandura, A., & Banfield, J. T. (1991). The impact of conceptions of ability on self-regulatory factors and motor skill acquisition. *Journal of Sport and Exercise Psychology, 13*, 213–226.

Jowett, N., & Spray, C. M. (2013). British Olympic hopefuls: The antecedents and consequences of implicit ability beliefs in elite track and field athletes. *Psychology of Sport and Exercise, 14*, 145–153.

Kasimatis, M., Miller, M., & Marcussen, L. (1996). The effects of implicit theories on exercise motivation. *Journal of Research in Personality, 30*, 510–516.

Leith, S. A., Ward, C. L. P., Giacomin, M., Landau, E. S., Ehrlinger, J., & Wilson, A. E. (2014). Changing theories of change: Strategic shifting in implicit theory endorsement. *Journal of Personality and Social Psychology, 107*, 597–620.

Lintunen, T., Valkonen, A., Leskinen, E., & Biddle, S. J. H. (1999). Predicting physical activity intentions using a goal perspectives approach: A study of Finnish youth. *Scandinavian Journal of Medicine and Science in Sports, 9*, 344–352.

Lyons, C., Kaufman, A. R., & Rima, B. (2015). Implicit theories of the body among college women: Implications for physical activity. *Journal of Health Psychology, 20*, 1142–1153.

Moreno, J. A., Gonzalez-Cutre, D., Martin-Albo, J., & Cervello, E. (2010). Motivation and performance in physical education: An experimental test. *Journal of Sports Science and Medicine, 9,* 79–85.

Nicholls, J. G. (1989). *The competitive ethos and democratic education.* Cambridge, MA: Harvard University Press.

Nicholls, J. G. (1992). The general and the specific in the development and expression of achievement motivation. In G. C. Roberts (Ed.), *Motivation in sport and exercise* (pp. 31–56). Champaign, IL: Human Kinetics.

Ommundsen, Y. (2001a). Pupils' affective responses in physical education classes: The association of implicit theories of the nature of ability and achievement goals. *European Physical Education Review, 7,* 219–242.

Ommundsen, Y. (2001b). Self-handicapping strategies in physical education classes: The influence of implicit theories of the nature of ability and achievement goal orientations. *Psychology of Sport and Exercise, 2,* 139–156.

Ommundsen, Y. (2003). Implicit theories of ability and self-regulation strategies in physical education classes. *Educational Psychology, 23,* 141–157.

Roberts, G. C. (2012). Motivation in sport and exercise from an achievement goal theory perspective: After 30 years, where are we? In G. C. Roberts & D. C. Treasure (Eds.), *Advances in motivation in sport and exercise* (pp. 5–58). Champaign, IL: Human Kinetics.

Sarrazin, P., Biddle, S., Famose, J. P., Cury, F., Fox, K., & Durand, M. (1996). Goal orientations and conceptions of the nature of sport ability in children: A social cognitive approach. *British Journal of Social Psychology, 35,* 399–414.

Sevincer, A. T., Kluge, L., & Oettingen, G. (2014). Implicit theories and motivational focus: Desired future versus present reality. *Motivation and Emotion, 38,* 36–46.

Slater, M. J., Spray, C. M., & Smith, B. M. (2012). "You're only as good as your weakest link": Implicit theories of golf ability. *Psychology of Sport and Exercise, 13,* 280–290.

Smith, A. L. (2003). Peer relationships in physical activity contexts: A road less traveled in youth sport and exercise psychology research. *Psychology of Sport and Exercise, 4,* 25–39.

Snyder, K. E., Malin, J. L., Dent, A. L., & Linnenbrink-Garcia, L. (2014). The message matters: The role of implicit beliefs about giftedness and failure experiences in academic self-handicapping. *Journal of Educational Psychology, 106,* 230–241.

Spray, C. M., Wang, C. K. J., Biddle, S. J. H., Chatzisarantis, N. L. D., & Warburton, V. E. (2006). An experimental test of self-theories

of ability in youth sport. *Psychology of Sport and Exercise, 7,* 255–267.

Stenling, A., Hassmén, P., & Holmström, S. (2014). Implicit beliefs of ability, approach–avoidance goals and cognitive anxiety among team sport athletes. *European Journal of Sport Science, 14,* 720–729.

Urdan, T., & Turner, J. C. (2005). Competence motivation in the classroom. In A. J. Elliot & C. S. Dweck (Eds.), *Handbook of competence and motivation* (pp. 297–317). New York: Guilford Press.

Vella, S. A., Braithwaite, R. E., Gardner, L., & Spray, C. M. (2016). A systematic review and meta-analysis of implicit theory research in sport, physical activity, and physical education. *International Review of Sport and Exercise Psychology, 9,* 191–214.

Vella, S. A., Cliff, D. P., Okely, A. D., Weintraub, D. L., & Robinson, T. N. (2014). Instructional strategies to promote incremental beliefs in youth sport. *Quest, 66,* 357–370.

Wang, C. K. J., & Biddle, S. J. H. (2001). Young people's motivational profiles in physical activity: A cluster analysis. *Journal of Sport and Exercise Psychology, 23,* 1–22.

Wang, C. K. J., & Biddle, S. J. H. (2003). Intrinsic motivation towards sports in Singaporean students: The role of sport ability beliefs. *Journal of Health Psychology, 8,* 515–523.

Wang, C. K. J., Chatzisarantis, N. L. D., Spray, C. M., & Biddle, S. J. H. (2002). Achievement goal profiles in school physical education: Differences in self-determination, sport ability beliefs, and physical activity. *British Journal of Educational Psychology, 72,* 433–445.

Wang, C. K. J., Liu, W. C., & Biddle, S. J. H. (2003). Female secondary students' sport ability beliefs and regulatory styles: Relationships with enjoyment, effort and boredom. *Journal of Tianjin Institute of Physical Education, 18,* 13–18.

Wang, C. K. J., Liu, W. C., Biddle, S. J. H., & Spray, C. M. (2005). Cross-cultural validation of the Conceptions of the Nature of Athletic Ability Questionnaire Version 2. *Personality and Individual Differences, 38,* 1245–1256.

Wang, C. K. J., Liu, W. C., Lochbaum, M. R., & Stevenson, S. J. (2009). Sport ability beliefs, 2 × 2 achievement goals, and intrinsic motivation: The moderating role of perceived competence in sport and exercise. *Research Quarterly for Exercise and Sport, 80,* 303–312.

Warburton, V. E., & Spray, C. (2008). Motivation in physical education across the primary–secondary school transition. *European Physical Education Review, 14,* 157–178.

Warburton, V. E., & Spray, C. M. (2009). Antecedents of approach–avoidance achievement goal adoption in physical education: A longitudinal perspective. *Journal of Teaching in Physical Education, 28,* 214–232.

Warburton, V., & Spray, C. (2013). Antecedents of approach–avoidance achievement goal adoption: An analysis of two physical education activities. *European Physical Education Review, 19,* 215–231.

Wulf, G., & Lewthwaite, R. (2009). Conceptions of ability affect motor learning. *Journal of Motor Behavior, 41,* 461–467.

Yeager, D. S., & Dweck, C. S. (2012). Mindsets that promote resilience: When students believe that personal characteristics can be developed. *Educational Psychologist, 47,* 302–314.

Yeager, D. S., Johnson, R., Spitzer, B. J., Trzesniewski, K. H., Powers, J., & Dweck, C. S. (2014). The far-reaching effects of believing people can change: Implicit theories of personality shape stress, health, and achievement during adolescence. *Journal of Personality and Social Psychology, 106,* 867–884.

Yeager, D. S., Trzesniewski, K. H., Tirri, K., Nokelainen, P., & Dweck, C. S. (2011). Adolescents' implicit theories predict desire for vengeance after peer conflicts: Correlational and experimental evidence. *Developmental Psychology, 47,* 1090–1107.

CHAPTER 34

Competence and the Workplace

NICO W. VAN YPEREN

In line with the primary aim of this entire volume, in this chapter, I specifically focus on *competence* as the core concept of achievement motivation (Elliot, 2005; White, 1959; also see Elliot, Dweck, & Yeager, Chapter 1, this volume). *Competence,* or the capacity to perform, is the first factor that Blumberg and Pringle (1982) identified as a critical ingredient for effective job performance in their three-dimensional interactive model. Competence refers to the physical and cognitive capabilities, including knowledge, skills, and abilities that enable workers to perform their tasks effectively. However, even highly competent software engineers cannot perform effectively without a computer. Indeed, the *opportunity to perform,* which refers to the help or hindrance of uncontrollable events and actors in one's environment (e.g., working conditions, equipment, social support, and organizational policies), is Blumberg and Pringle's second determinant of workers' effective performance.

The focus of this chapter is on the third factor in Blumberg and Pringle's (1982) model: workers' *willingness to perform,* which is defined as individuals' psychological characteristics that affect the degree to which they are inclined to perform their tasks. As discussed by Elliot and colleagues (Chapter 1, this volume), people may be motivated by either the positive, appetitive possibility of competence, or the negative, aversive possibility of incompetence. Hence, workers' achievement goals may be directed toward acquiring specific technical knowledge, developing their skills in organizing, or improving their ability to think strategically. Alternatively, they may be motivated to avoid incompetence in these work-related competencies. For example, their goal may be to avoid having their technical knowledge become obsolete. In the following section, first, I discuss this competence-based achievement goal concept more elaborately in the context of the workplace. Second, I review not only the literature on achievement goals in industrial–organizational (I/O) psychology and their impact on job performance, but also that on interpersonal behavior at work, another key organizational outcome. Third, I discuss the implications for effective interventions in the workplace.

ACHIEVEMENT GOALS IN I/O PSYCHOLOGY

Achievement goals are defined as mental representations of the individual's desired level of competence or undesired level of incompetence (see Elliot et al., Chapter 1, this volume). In I/O psychology, the concept of achievement goals was mentioned first by Kanfer (1990) in her chapter on work motivation in the *Handbook of Industrial and Organizational Psychology*. As was common at the time, she discussed the dichotomous conceptualization of achievement goals of Nicholls (1984) and Dweck (1986) by using the labels "task", "mastery" or "learning orientation" versus "ego orientation" or "performance orientation." In today's terms, this dichotomy typically represents mastery-approach goals versus performance goals (i.e., approach and avoidance combined).

Shortly thereafter, in their landmark article, Farr, Hofmann, and Ringenbach (1993) explicitly introduced the achievement goal concept in the I/O domain by first pointing out how achievement goals may influence variables such as goal expectancies, perceived control, task choice, task pursuit, outcome attribution, outcome satisfaction, and task interest. They then discussed the potential implications for I/O psychology in terms of goal setting, performance feedback, training and development, and innovation. More than 20 years after her review in which she introduced the achievement goal concept in I/O psychology, Kanfer (2012) noted that with the development of two adult measures of individuals' goal orientation in the late 1990s (Button, Mathieu, & Zajac, 1996; VandeWalle, 1997; also see the next section), the number of studies on achievement goals in the I/O domain has dramatically increased. Currently, the achievement goal concept is one of the most frequently investigated variables in the literature on work motivation (DeShon & Gillespie, 2005; Elliot, 2005; Van Yperen & Orehek, 2013).

MEASURES OF ACHIEVEMENT GOALS IN I/O PSYCHOLOGY

The first empirical studies on achievement goals in the workplace appeared in the mid-1990s (e.g., Sujan, Weitz, & Kumar, 1994), using achievement goal measures that were based on the measures developed for students in the classroom (Ames & Archer, 1988). Unfortunately, both the (approach-oriented) mastery goal scale and the performance goal scale mixed up achievement goals, affect, error management, effort, impression management, and adherence to supervisors' criteria (see Sujan et al., 1994, Appendix A), which makes it difficult to interpret these early achievement goal findings.

Investigations of achievement goals in the I/O domain grew dramatically with the development of two adult achievement goal measures in the late 1990s (Button et al., 1996; VandeWalle, 1997; also see Kanfer, 2012) that are still used today, despite their conceptual unclarities (Van Yperen, Blaga, & Postmes, 2014). The Button and colleagues (1996) scale represents early achievement goal work in which mastery and performance goals represent mastery-approach goals and performance goals (i.e., approach and avoidance combined), respectively. Across studies, Button and colleagues' undifferentiated performance goal scale appeared to be unrelated to performance attainment (Van Yperen et al., 2014). Recent meta-analyses consistently report positive relationships between performance-approach (PAp) goals and performance, and negative relationships between performance-avoidance (PAv) goals and performance (Hulleman, Schrager, Bodmann, & Harackiewicz, 2010; Van Yperen et al., 2014). These correlation coefficients of opposite valence apparently average to zero when Button and colleagues' measure, which does not differentiate between PAp and PAv goals, is used. This was exactly the reason why the valence dimension was added to the conceptualization of achievement goals in the mid-1990s (Elliot & Church, 1997; VandeWalle, 1997).

Since its introduction, the achievement goal construct has been discussed as having both dispositional and situational components (e.g., Button et al., 1996). From this perspective, one may suspect that a situationally induced achievement goal is particularly effective when it is aligned with a person's dispositional goal orientation (Jagacinski, Madden, & Reider, 2001). Alternatively, goal assignment may be particularly effective among individuals with low trait levels of the corresponding goal orientation (e.g., Bell & Kozlowski, 2008). However, there is *no* strong evidence that trait-like goal orientations moderate the effect of assigned achievement goals on performance. Moreover, the question is whether the achievement goal concept is suited for the dispositional level in the first place. As pointed out by Elliot (2005), the achievement goal approach originated, in part, as a criticism of trait-like constructs, especially the need for achievement. Conceptually, achievement goals are likely to mediate the link between trait-like variables and specific outcomes such as job performance (Elliot & Church, 1997; McCabe, Van Yperen, Elliot, & Verbraak, 2013; Payne, Youngcourt, & Beaubien, 2007). More specifically, as a function of contextual variables, dispositional characteristics may predispose individuals to adopt particular achievement goals, and following this, produce context-specific outcomes. In line with the idea that achievement goals are best suited for the contextual level, Van Yperen, Hamstra, and Van der Klauw (2011) found that individuals tend to hold different dominant achievement goals in different achievement domains (work, education, and sports). Only 21% consistently preferred one particular achievement goal across the three achievement domains.

Acknowledging the context specificity of the achievement goal construct, VandeWalle (1997) developed his widely used trichotomous measure specific to the workplace. Because VandeWalle's definition of *learning goal orientation* exclusively covers mastery-approach goals, that is, "a desire to develop the self by acquiring new skills, mastering new situations, and improving one's competence" (p. 1000), exactly 10 years later, this trichotomous measure was extended by Baranik, Barron, and Finney (2007) with a mastery-avoidance subscale. In contrast to mastery goals, in his original measure, VandeWalle partitioned performance goals into PAp and PAv goals. He referred to these subdimensions as "prove (performance) goal orientation" and "avoid (performance) goal orientation," respectively. Prove goal orientation reflects "the desire to prove one's competence and to gain favorable judgments about it," and avoid goal orientation was defined as "the desire to avoid the disproving of one's competence and to avoid negative judgments about it" (p. 1000). This conceptualization is problematic because the desire to prove and the desire to avoid disproving are not inherent components of performance goals (Elliot, 2005; Vansteenkiste, Lens, Elliot, Soenens, & Mouratidis, 2014). Rather, these *reasons* may underlie any achievement goal, including mastery goals (i.e., "I want to prove that I improved"). The conceptual core of performance goals is other-based striving; that is, performance goal individuals' perceptions of competence are determined by comparisons with others (for a detailed discussion on this issue, see Elliot et al., Chapter 1, this volume).

Quite recently, Van Yperen and Orehek (2013) presented an achievement goal measure specific to the work context that is based on Elliot's (1999) conceptualization of achievement goals (Elliot & McGregor, 2001; also see Pintrich, 2000). In this 2 × 2 framework, achievement goals differ in terms of the standards that individuals use to define competence (a self-referenced standard [mastery] vs. an other-referenced standard [performance], and valence [i.e., approach vs. avoidance]). Individuals who pursue mastery-approach (MAp) goals focus on self-referenced improvement and accomplishments, whereas individuals who pursue performance-approach (PAp) goals focus on performing better than others. Individuals who pursue mastery-avoidance (MAv) goals aim to avoid incompetence on the basis of self-referenced standards, whereas individuals who pursue performance-avoidance (PAv) goals focus on avoiding failure relative to others (Elliot & McGregor, 2001). Note that in their 3 × 2 framework, Elliot, Murayama, and Pekrun (2011) also distinguish between self-referenced and task-referenced mastery goals.

Van Yperen and Orehek's (2013) six-item round-robin measure asks workers to indicate their *dominant* achievement goal in the work context (for an initial, slightly different version, see Van Yperen, 2006). In a sample of 2,158 workers, representing a wide range of professions (e.g., nurses, police officers, teachers, researchers, technicians, physicians, entrepreneurs), businesses (e.g., agriculture, industry, education, health), and private and public organizations, they found that most workers endorsed MAp goals (41.1%), followed by MAv goals (23.0%), PAp goals (13.7%), and PAv goals (9.4%).

Because they also measured the *strength or intensity* of each achievement goal, they were able to present idiographic achievement goal profiles of workers with different dominant achievement goals. As shown in Figure 34.1, these profiles indicate that workers with a dominant achievement goal simultaneously hold other (multiple) achievement goals, but the strength or intensity of a person's own dominant achievement goal is obviously higher relative to the other achievement goals. Among PAp goal workers, goal strength for each achievement goal is relatively high. In contrast, workers with dominant PAv goals or dominant MAv goals tend to focus strongly on either avoidance goal, whereas workers with a dominant MAp goal tend to focus primarily on their dominant MAp goal. The idea that individuals can pursue different achievement goals simultaneously has been referred to as *profiles of goal orientation* (Bouffard, Boisvert, Vezeau, & Larouche, 1995; Somuncuoglu & Yildirim, 1999), *goal configurations* (Schraw, Horn, Thorndikechrist, &

Bruning, 1995), and *multiple-goal perspective* (Barron & Harackiewicz, 2001).

In line with these findings on workers' dominant achievement goals, the extant research in I/O psychology consistently demonstrates that workers score highest on MAp goals and lowest on PAv goals (e.g., Baranik et al., 2007; VandeWalle, 1997). This is good news because across domains, MAp goals are typically related to positive-valenced outcomes, and PAv goals are quite consistently associated with negatively-valenced outcomes, with PAp goals and MAv goals in between these extremes (e.g., Elliot & McGregor, 2001; Van Yperen, 2006). Indeed, the achievement goal approach has been used to understand and predict desirable and undesirable outcomes in the workplace (DeShon & Gillespie, 2005; Farr et al., 1993; Van Yperen & Orehek, 2013). *Performance,* which is discussed below, is arguably a key outcome variable in achievement motivation research because it reveals valuable information about individuals' potential to adapt to the achievement situation.

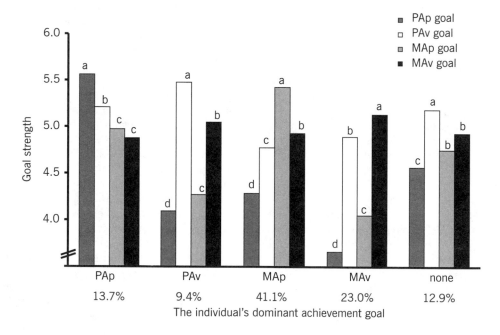

FIGURE 34.1. Idiographic achievement goal profiles of workers with different dominant achievement goals: Differences within each dominant achievement goal. Means adjusted for sex, age, educational level, and number of hours employed (*n* = 2,158). *Within* each dominant achievement goal (i.e., within each cluster), means that differ significantly (*p* < .05) have different letters. From Van Yperen and Orehek (2013). Copyright © 2013 by Elsevier. Adapted with permission.

ACHIEVEMENT GOALS AND JOB PERFORMANCE

Individual Level

Meta-analyses demonstrate that approach goals (either mastery or performance) are positively related to performance, and avoidance goals (either mastery or performance) are negatively related to performance (Baranik, Stanley, Bynum, & Lance, 2010; Hulleman et al., 2010; Payne et al., 2007). In the workplace, the positive link between individuals' MAp goals and job performance appears to be relatively strong (Van Yperen et al., 2014). A possible reason is that, more than performance at school (i.e., exam performance) or on the sports field (i.e., scores), job performance includes extrarole behavior, that is, nonprescribed organizationally beneficial behaviors and gestures (e.g., Podsakoff, MacKenzie, Paine, & Bachrach, 2000). Job performance is a broad and complex construct comprising two fundamentally different aspects: in-role job performance mandated by an organization, and extrarole performance (e.g., providing support to colleagues, creating new ideas for improvement, and searching out new working methods, techniques, or instruments). Because MAp goals (and intrinsic work motivation) are important motivational sources for extrarole behavior in particular, the MAp goal–performance relationship may be particularly strong among workers relative to students and athletes (Van Yperen et al., 2014).

In a study of 170 workers from an energy supply company, for example, Janssen and Van Yperen (2004) found that workers' MAp goals were positively associated with innovative job performance (as rated by their supervisors), including mobilizing support for innovative ideas and generating original solutions to problems. Similarly, in their study of 376 workers from different organizations, Lee, Hui, Tinsley, and Niu (2006) found that workers' MAp goals were positively related to supervisor-rated extrarole behaviors, but only when they felt that the organization emphasized future planning. In addition, workers with stronger MAp goals were more positively rated by their supervisors in terms of in-role job performance, that is, the extent to which they met all the formal performance requirements of the job. Due to their striving to develop and grow, MAp goal workers tend to seek social exchanges with their supervisors in order to discuss and learn how to deal better with emerging problems and opportunities at work. Accordingly, they develop a high-quality exchange relationship with their supervisor, characterized by mutual trust and respect, which enhances their performance on the job (Janssen & Van Yperen, 2004).

Relative to MAp goals, the link between PAp goals and job performance is less strong and less consistent, but across studies, it is positive as well (Van Yperen et al., 2014). In some studies, PAp goals and job performance were not positively, or were even negatively, related (Janssen & Van Yperen, 2004; Lee et al., 2006; Seijts, Latham, Tasa, & Latham, 2004; VandeWalle, Brown, Cron, & Slocum, 1999), but more typically, a positive link was found. For example, in a study of 88 salespeople working from virtual offices for a large multinational computer product and services organization, Porath and Bateman (2006) found a positive relation between salespeople's PAp goals and an objective, lagged measure of in-role job performance (i.e., the percentage of the sales quota met for the subsequent 6 months). In line with their expectations, they showed that salespeople with stronger PAp goals were more likely to seek feedback more actively, using the knowledge gained to outperform others, and to proactively initiate behaviors that would give them a competitive advantage. In other words, PAp goals were positively related to in-role job performance through feedback seeking and proactive behavior.

Team and Unit Level

In the workplace, individuals are typically members of organizational units and teams that work together toward common goals. Therefore, in I/O psychological research, achievement goals are also conceptualized as collective constructs, with a critical impact on collective performance on the job and other team-level outcomes (e.g., Bunderson & Sutcliffe, 2003; Dragoni, 2005). Chadwick and Raver (2015) discuss three mechanisms that may lead individual achievement goals to emerge as a distinct collective construct: (1) Workers' shared exposure to the team or unit environment may create a new collective reality that is distinct from the simple summation of their individual propensities (also see Salancik & Pfeffer, 1978); (2) teams create and maintain a shared reality through social verification processes (i.e., discussions to establish mutually agreed-upon interpretations of the "right" way to behave (also see Hardin & Higgins, 1996); and (3) individuals are attracted to and selected by teams that comprise individuals who are similar to themselves, and team members who nevertheless feel dissimilar tend to either conform or leave (also see Schneider, 1987).

Several studies have provided evidence that units or teams in organizations may be distinguished from each other on the basis of achievement goal preference and strength. For example, in a study of 1,150 members of 230 work units in 230 organizations, Dragoni and Kuenzi (2012) assessed workers' achievement goals at the unit level and at the individual level, and those of unit leaders at the individual level. After it had been demonstrated that more variance existed between units than within units, unit members' responses were aggregated at the unit level (also see Bunderson & Sutcliffe, 2003). Team performance was measured by asking the 230 unit leaders to compare their units' performance with that of other units doing the same kind of work in terms of quality of products, services, or programs. In line with the general pattern observed in the work context (Van Yperen et al., 2014), the best predictors of unit leaders' perceived unit performance were MAp goals. PAp goals were also positively associated with unit performance, and overall, PAv goals were unrelated to job performance (also see Mehta, Feild, Armenakis, & Mehta, 2009). Furthermore, unit leaders' approach goals had an indirect effect on their performance perceptions through the shared corresponding approach goal adopted within the unit, but only in organizations characterized by high levels of autonomy afforded to leaders and employees to perform their jobs.

Similar findings were observed in 485 workers representing 100 research and development teams and 19 Korean companies involved in the telecommunications, electronics, chemical, aerospace, information technology, and pharmaceutical industries. Gong, Kim, Lee, and Zhu (2013) found that, in contrast to team level PAv goals, not only MAp goals but also PAp goals were positively related to team information exchange, which in turn was positively related to team-leader-rated team creativity and individual creativity. Furthermore, as argued and demonstrated by Gong and colleagues, a shared team PAp goal (as well as a shared MAp goal) produces outcome interdependence among team members, motivates them to share task-related information, maintains a collective focus on achieving their goal, and generates a preference for a positive joint outcome, including team effectivity, team cohesion, and team performance.

Bunderson and Sutcliffe (2003) added a cautionary note to the positive MAp goal pattern by pointing out that MAp goals may not be uniformly beneficial. In a study of 438 management team members in 45 business units in a Fortune 100 consumer products company, they showed that team performance in the short term may suffer when teams overemphasize MAp goals, particularly when they have been performing well. In contrast to the effects on individual performance (Gist & Stevens, 1998; Seijts et al., 2004; Winters & Latham, 1996), this may be more pronounced when teams face complex tasks that include large amounts of information and a dynamic environment (Mehta et al., 2009; Nahrgang et al., 2013).

DO ACHIEVEMENT GOALS AFFECT PERFORMANCE, AND WHY?

Particularly for I/O psychologists and other applied scientists and practitioners, an important question is whether performance in the workplace can be improved by achievement goal interventions. The observed positive links between approach goals, and MAp goals in particular, and job performance in survey research are valuable and useful for providing ecologically valid information. However, in order to enhance organizational effectiveness, companies' productivity, and economic success, we need to know the *causal* effects of assigned achievement goals on job performance and other outcomes of interest; that is, only findings from experimental achievement goal research provide a solid basis for the development of effective achievement goal interventions in organizations. Note that in an experimental setting or practical intervention, typically, one particular achievement goal is assigned to the individual, which is assumed to be the individual's *dominant* achievement goal in that particular setting (Van Yperen & Orehek, 2013).

A recent meta-analysis of experimental achievement goal research showed that the observed patterns in the rather small number of experimental studies are generally in line with the overall pattern found in correlational research; that is, relative to avoidance goals (either PAv or MAv), approach goals (either MAp or PAp) *enhance* task performance. Furthermore, in line with the extant survey research in the work domain, MAp goals lead to better performance than PAp goals (Van Yperen, Blaga, & Postmes, 2015). Self-regulation processes related to the positive, appetitive possibility of competence, including mental focus, feedback seeking, and leader–member exchange, may explain the positive effect of approach goals, and MAp goals in particular, on performance (e.g., Anseel, Beatty, Shen, Lievens, & Sackett, 2015; Janssen & Van Yperen, 2004; Lee, Sheldon, & Turban, 2003). For example, in a meta-analysis of the antecedents and outcomes of feedback-seeking behavior in an actual or closely simulated organizational context, Anseel and colleagues (2015) found that approach goals (either MAp or PAp) were positively associated with overall feedback seeking. These results suggest that both MAp and PAp goal workers tend to view feedback seeking as a viable strategy for reaching their goal: to do better than before or to do better than others, respectively, regardless of their tendency to seek different types of feedback information. In a study of 170 medical residents in a hospital, Janssen and Prins (2007) hypothesized and found that MAp goal individuals were particularly interested in information that helped them to improve their competencies, whereas PAp goal individuals found

information that validated the adequacy of their competencies most valuable (also see VandeWalle, 2003).

In contrast, avoidance forms of regulation tend to evoke negative outcomes, including lower levels of self-efficacy and performance (Payne et al., 2007), through increased levels of worry and intrusive negative thoughts (e.g., Elliot & McGregor, 1999; Lee et al., 2003). For example, in two prospective studies, Pekrun, Elliot, and Maier (2006) showed that in contrast to approach goals (either MAp or PAp), PAv goals were positive predictors of anxiety. In a longitudinal study, Lee and colleagues (2003) found a negative link between PAv goals and mental focus, which in turn was positively related to performance. These findings suggest that PAv goals may have undermined individuals' mental focus on the task and, accordingly, their performance on the task, due to worries or intrusive thoughts about potential failure experiences or other cognitive interferences.

MAv goals tend to have a negative impact on performance as well (Van Yperen et al., 2015); this may be particularly true in a multiple-trial context, that is, a context that matches the intrapersonal evaluative focus of MAv goals (Van Yperen, Elliot, & Anseel, 2009). In such a context, an intrapersonal standard is highly diagnostic given that both the dimensions of comparison (the task itself, the conditions, etc.) and the comparison other (the self) are specific, clear, and unambiguous. Accordingly, performing worse than one did before on the same task under identical conditions can yield unequivocal negative feedback that makes it hard to distort the undesired outcome in a self-enhancing manner and to find appropriate excuses for one's poor performance. Hence, negative, interfering thoughts during task performance may even be stronger when pursuing a MAv goal relative to a PAv goal. Indeed, Sideridis (2008) showed that, relative to PAv goals (and approach goals), MAv goals were associated with enhanced negative affect and increases in cognitive and somatic anxiety (as indicated with the use of both self-report and physiological measures). Similarly, Preenen, Van Vianen, and De Pater (2014) found that among individuals ($n = 332$) working for a technical equipment distributor, MAv goals were unrelated to the extent to which workers performed challenging tasks in their work, whereas positive relationships were observed with MAp goals in particular, but also with performance goals (both approach and avoidance). In a study in central Japan of 57 young (average age 22.77 years), newly hired police officers from a middle-size prefecture, Tanaka, Okuno, and Yamauchi (2013) found that MAv goals, particularly, were negatively related to expectations of doing well in one's job. In contrast, among older workers (age 65+), MAv goals may not have such a negative effect on job performance and related variables, since maintenance, loss-prevention, and mastery-avoidance goals are more prevalent in late adulthood (De Lange, Van Yperen, Van der Heijden, & Bal, 2010; Van Yperen & Orehek, 2013). Indeed, among older people, MAv goals appear to be positively associated with positively valenced variables, including well-being, task enjoyment, and work engagement (De Lange et al., 2010; Ebner, Freund, & Baltes, 2006; Senko & Freund, 2015).

Clearly, age is not the only variable that may attenuate or even reverse the effects of a particular achievement goal and performance. For example, performance goal individuals who are inherently focused on external evaluation may be more sensitive to performance contingencies in the achievement context than individuals pursuing MAp goals. Elliot, Shell, Henry, and Maier (2005) showed that, in contrast to MAp goal individuals, PAp goal individuals tended to perform better when they believed that goal attainment was associated with an extra reward on a subsequent task. Such a performance contingency affected PAv goal individuals' performances as well, but in the opposite direction. Among these individuals, performance contingency tends to undermine performance because it enhances their aversive desire to avoid normative failure (also see Raynor, 1969).

The findings of other studies suggest that MAp goals enhance individual performance (relative to PAp goals) when cognitive demands increase (Gist & Stevens, 1998; Seijts et al., 2004; Winters & Latham, 1996). In contrast, external factors such as time pressure and strict adherence to schedules tend to weaken the individual's MAp goals (Beck & Schmidt, 2013), or may undermine the positive effect of MAp goals on performance (Lee et al., 2006; Van Yperen et al., 2015). Thus, particularly when the task is complex and there are no external pressures or constraints, MAp goals may reinforce individuals' feelings of autonomy and self-determination (Deci & Ryan, 1985), and keep their performance efforts channeled toward their intrapersonal standards. Other external factors, including the threat of stereotyping, concern about negative feedback, and praise for being smart rather than praise for effort (Mueller & Dweck, 1998; Steele & Aronson, 1995; Sternberg & Grigorenko, 2001), may also undermine the positive effect of MAp goals on task performance. Similar to *inter*personal standards, these factors may shift the individual's attention away from the task through task-irrelevant interfering thoughts, which undermine performance attainment (e.g., Sarason, Sarason, Keefe, Hayes, & Shearin, 1986).

CAUSAL EFFECTS OF ACHIEVEMENT GOALS ON PERFORMANCE IN THE WORKPLACE

Remarkably, so far, *only one* published experimental study (Van Yperen et al., 2009, Study 2) has examined causal links between achievement goals and performance among workers. In this online experiment, 447 workers (47% female), who had a mean of 14.8 years of work experience in their company, were randomly assigned to one of the four achievement goal conditions from the 2 × 2 framework, or to a no-goal control condition. The dependent variable (as well as the pretest) was workers' performance on an exercise often used in management development programs and procedures for the selection of managers. In line with the extant literature, relative to approach goals (and the no-goal control condition), avoidance goals were detrimental for performance. However, in this particular study, this applied to MAv goals only. This pattern was also observed among undergraduates who completed a verbal skills test (Van Yperen et al., 2009, Study 1).

Thus, there is clearly a lack of (quasi-) experimental or intervention studies of achievement goals and performance in the workplace. However, particularly when an objective, lagged measure of job performance has been used, the findings of longitudinal field tests may suggest that achievement goals affect workers' performance. For example, in a 3-month longitudinal field study among 167 salespeople working for a medical supplies distributor, VandeWalle and colleagues (1999) showed that MAp goal salespersons particularly (i.e., those who valued development of their sales skills) were more likely to set higher goals, to work harder, and to engage in planning activities. This was related to the actual number of units sold, which was obtained from company records. Similarly, Porath and Bateman (2006) demonstrated that salespeople's (n = 88) approach goals (both MAp and PAp) were positively related, and PAv goals were negatively related, to the percentage of the sales quotas met—the company's objective measure of salespeople's performance— for the 6 months (two quarters) after the achievement goals were assessed. Their results also revealed that both approach goals were positively linked to self-reported proactive behavior, a self-regulation tactic that involves actions that effect constructive change rather than passive adaptation to circumstances or compliance with the status quo (Bateman & Crant, 1993). In turn, proactive behavior was positively related to sales performance.

Other field studies were focused on mediators such as self-reported learning and self-efficacy. In a study among 508 workers enrolled in 10 full-time MBA programs and working for over 245 organizations (5.0 years of work experience), participants' achievement goals were assessed about a week before internships started. Self-reported job performance during the 90-day internship was assessed 1–2 weeks after internships ended. Also in line with the typical pattern, Beenen (2014) found that approach goals (both MAp and PAp) were positively related to MBA interns' self-reported job performance, whereas the PAv goals–performance link was negative. Furthermore, relative to performance goal workers, MAp interns reported more improvement in 10 key skills

that employers considered both important and deficient in MBA graduates (e.g., interpersonal skills, leadership skills, negotiation skills, thinking strategically about business problems), which in turn was positively related to job performance. This finding is consistent with research that has shown that undergraduates' MAp goals lead to better task performance through higher levels of self-efficacy (Kozlowski et al., 2001).

In addition, a couple of published field studies have included examination of other potent means of inducing and reinforcing workers' achievement goals, including the framing of errors (Brodbeck, Zapf, Prumper, & Frese, 1993), pay system (Van Yperen, 2003a), and leadership style (Hamstra, Van Yperen, Wisse, & Sassenberg, 2014).

Framing of Errors

Particularly when engaged in learning complex, novel tasks, workers unavoidably make errors. This should be perceived as instrumental for learning and self-improvement (Brodbeck et al., 1993). Hence, in a study in which 350 trainees were engaged in a 3-hour training session, working on a dynamic and complex task that required them to learn a number of basic and strategic skills, Bell and Kozlowski (2008) developed interventions in which errors or mistakes were either accepted as part of the learning process, or as punishment that should be avoided (also see Van Hooft & Noordzij, 2009). Their findings suggest, among other things, that encouraging trainees to make errors and learn from them leads to stronger MAp goals, but only among individuals with low initial MAp goal levels.

Pay System

Another factor that may impact workers' achievement goals through the organization's motivational climate is the organization's pay system. In a job-based pay system, pay is based on the employee's job description; that is, employees who occupy positions with identical job descriptions receive the same salary, irrespective of their actual job performance. In contrast, in a performance-based pay system, in which pay is contingent on job performance, employees receive higher (lower) salaries when they perform better (worse) than their colleagues who occupy positions with identical job descriptions. Hence, relative to job-based pay systems, performance-based pay systems more strongly emphasize norms, interpersonal standards, rankings, and social comparisons. As demonstrated by Van Yperen (2003a), such a policy may strengthen workers' perceptions of a performance goal climate in their firm. Specifically, in this study of 198 workers representing 22 firms, individuals working for successful firms that used performance-based pay systems perceived a relatively strong PAp goal climate within their firm, whereas their counterparts working for unsuccessful firms perceived a relatively strong PAv goal climate. Related to this, in a study of 502 workers from 55 teams, Heidemeier and Bittner (2012) found that workers' individual perceptions of competition within their team was positively related to their tendency to adopt PAp goals.

Leadership Style

Leadership is generally acknowledged to involve influencing followers' motivation and moving followers toward (collective) goal attainment (e.g., Bass, 1990). Two prominent leadership styles that systematically differ in the forms of competence-related encouragement they provide to followers are transformational and transactional leadership. *Transformational leaders* are intellectually stimulating and direct followers to look at things from new perspectives, which may signify to followers that learning is central to competence (Hetland, Skogstad, Hetland, & Mikkelsen, 2011). They treat followers as individuals with their own needs and abilities, and tend to focus followers' attention on improving their own skills rather than comparing themselves with others. In contrast, *transactional leaders* specify that rewards are contingent on achievements. Emphasizing rewards typically signals scarcity of resources or negative interdependence, creating an evaluative context that implies that followers need to demonstrate their competence by outperforming others to receive contingent rewards (e.g., Bolino, Turnley, & Bloodgood, 2002). In a study among 449 followers of 120

leaders, Hamstra and colleagues (2014) demonstrated that transactional leadership, as assessed by other followers of the same leader, was positively related to followers' endorsement of PAp goals and not related to followers' MAp goals. In contrast, transformational leadership was positively related to followers' MAp goals and not related to followers' PAp goals.

In conclusion, an error-encouragement frame, job-based pay, and transformational leadership seem to be instrumental in promoting followers' adoption of mastery goals, whereas an error-avoidance frame, performance-based pay, and transactional leadership may be instrumental in promoting followers' adoption of performance goals. In line with the extant literature, field research further provides some preliminary evidence that whereas approach goals lead to better job performance, avoidance goals lead to worse performance. Most notable, however, is that only one experimental study has been conducted among workers, aimed at testing the effects of achievement goals on performance (Van Yperen et al., 2009, Study 2). Hence, there is a strong need for intervention studies to test the causal effects of assigned, dominant achievement goals on job performance. To develop effective achievement goal interventions in organizations, we may rely on achievement goal manipulations that have been found to be successful in experimental laboratory research, which we discuss next.

DEVELOPING EFFECTIVE ACHIEVEMENT GOAL INTERVENTIONS

As discussed earlier, there are several conceptualizations of achievement goals and, accordingly, several different measures for assessing achievement goals, as well as several procedures that situationally induce individuals' achievement goals. Building on the 2 × 2 framework (Elliot & McGregor, 2001), achievement goal manipulations should differ in terms of the standards that individuals use to define competence (i.e., a self-referenced standard [mastery] vs. an other-referenced standard [performance]) and valence (i.e., approach vs. avoidance). Accordingly, MAp goal interventions direct individuals toward a positive outcome based on a self-referenced (or *intra*personal) standard (e.g., to do better than before) or a task-referenced standard (e.g., master the task, solve the problem), whereas PAp goal interventions focus individuals on a favorable outcome based on an other-referenced (or *inter*personal) standard (e.g., to do better than others, to do well relative to others). MAv goal interventions emphasize an unfavorable outcome based on a self-referenced standard (e.g., not to do worse than before) or a task-referenced standard (e.g., to avoid incorrect answers or solutions). Finally, PAv goal interventions prime individuals to avoid a negative outcome based on an other-referenced standard (e.g., not to do worse than others). A recent meta-analysis of studies that rely on this conceptualization provides evidence for the positive effects of approach goals on performance, and the negative effects of avoidance goals on performance (Van Yperen et al., 2015).

An example of a rigorous, precise, and conceptually clear manipulation is to ask participants to adopt a particular achievement goal from the 2×2 achievement goal framework; that is, in the performance goal conditions, participants' target score is other-referenced, whereas in the mastery goal conditions, participants' target score is self-referenced. In the approach goal conditions, the purpose is to achieve a favorable outcome, and in the avoidance goal conditions, the purpose is to avoid an unfavorable outcome. For example, in the MAp goal condition, Van Yperen (2003b) told the participants that if they reached the target score (e.g., 22 correct answers) on Version 2, they would do better relative to Version 1. In contrast, in the PAv condition, participants were told that if they reached the target score of 22 correct answers on Version 2, they would not do worse than others (also see Van Yperen et al., 2009). This achievement goal manipulation may be strengthened and intensified by asking the participants to elaborate on their assigned achievement goal by describing a situation, including their thoughts and feelings, in which they reached a similar goal. In the case of a MAv goal, for example, participants may recall a situation in which they had not performed worse than they did before, and in the case of a PAp goal, they

may recall a situation in which they did better than others (e.g., Poortvliet, Janssen, Van Yperen, & Van de Vliert, 2007; Van Yperen et al., 2011; Van Yperen & Leander, 2014).

An alternative approach for inducing individuals' achievement goals is to use more complex conceptualizations of achievement goals, that is, to use a combination of cues to induce a dominant achievement goal among individuals (e.g., Bell & Kozlowski, 2008; Cianci, Schaubroeck, & McGill, 2010; Gist & Stevens, 1998; Kozlowski et al., 2001; Steele-Johnson, Heintz, & Miller, 2008). For example, in a study of unemployed job seekers, Van Hooft and Noordzij (2009) encouraged participants in the MAp goal condition to focus on learning different strategies, on viewing errors as learning opportunities, and on searching for challenges and ways to improve their job-search skills. In general, cues used *in mastery goal interventions* include a selected combination of (1) learning instructions in which task mastery is framed as acquirable knowledge and skill; (2) practice presented as an opportunity to improve one's skills or develop one's strategies; (3) encouragement to use errors and diagnostic feedback as learning opportunities; (4) instructions to focus on task mastery rather than outcome achievement; (5) instructions to focus on skills needed to develop proficiency; (6) instruction in self-management as a skills maintenance strategy; (7) instructions to focus on the deep principles and strategies embodied in the task and its performance context; (8) provision of private, self-referenced feedback, whether or not accompanied with rewards based on improvement relative to an intrapersonal standard; and (9) instructions to show another participant how to approach such a task (i.e., a task the participant is going to complete). *In performance goal interventions,* participants are (1) instructed to frame task performance as a demonstration of competence; (2) encouraged to avoid mistakes; (3) instructed to use their score and feedback to gauge their ability; (4) asked to focus on achieving a difficult and specific performance score; (5) informed that their intellectual ability is being tested; (6) focused on comparing their performancee to others' performances; and (7) publicly provided with normative-based feedback, whether or not accompanied by rewards based on an interpersonal standard or ranking.

DeShon and Gillespie (2005) noted, however, that "the lack of consistency in the measurement of goal orientation makes it unclear what the measures of goal orientation actually assess, and the impact of these differences on the comparability of results across research studies is highly uncertain" (p. 1104). Indeed, to optimize conceptual clarity, distinguishing between aim and reason is important. The achievement goal (or *aim*) indicates direction (i.e., standard and valence), whereas *reasons* reflect the type of regulation underlying achievement goal pursuit (Elliot, 2005; Vansteenkiste et al., 2014). From a conceptual point of view, it is preferable if both achievement goal measures and achievement goal interventions are rooted *exclusively* in the two fundamental components of competence: the evaluative standard individuals use to determine their competence (task, self, others) and how it is valenced (approach versus avoidance, Elliot et al., 2011; Van Yperen et al., 2014). For example, as a result of instructing participants to frame task performance as a demonstration of competence, some individuals may prefer to demonstrate competence through self-improvement (MAp), and others by not performing worse than others (PAv; also see Elliot, 2005). Indeed, the strength of the relations between individuals' achievement goals and underlying reasons (< .24; Vansteenkiste et al., 2014) suggests that (1) individuals with the same dominant achievement goal may have different reasons for pursuing this particular goal, and (2) one particular reason may underlie different achievement goals. Vansteenkiste and colleagues (2014) demonstrated that both autonomous and controlled forms of regulation may underlie either achievement goal. Specifically, MAp goal pursuit is related to positive outcomes when individuals indicate that they like pursuing this goal (i.e., autonomous regulation), and it fails to yield desirable outcomes when they feel obliged by others to pursue this goal (i.e., controlled regulation).

Sijbom, Janssen, and Van Yperen (2015a, 2015b) successfully developed MAp and PAp goal manipulations that are rooted exclusively in the two fundamental components of competence and provide cues for practical interventions that are useful owing to their broad scope and emphasis on three coherent aspects of each achievement goal. Note that from an applied perspective, only approach goal interventions are of interest because only approach goals have been found to be positively related to performance (Hulleman et al., 2010; Van Yperen et al., 2014) and, more importantly, appear *to cause* better performance (Van Yperen et al., 2015). In an in-basket setting in which participants had to respond to e-mails from their subordinates, Sijbom and colleagues (2015a, 2015b) assigned participants to a leadership role in which they were responsible for positioning and selling the company's products on the consumer market. In that setting, they were first informed about the *organizational climate*. In the MAp goal condition, the organization was described as having a strong developmental climate, continuously stimulating its leaders to develop their competencies by gaining new knowledge and skills. In the PAp goal condition, it was emphasized that the organization had a strong competitive climate, continuously stimulating its leaders to perform better than others. Second, a *personal leadership motto* imposed on the participants was consistent with the organizational climate described in each condition. In the MAp goal condition, the imposed motto was that leaders are developers and, accordingly, must keep developing their competencies in their executive work. In the PAp goal condition, the personal leadership motto was that leaders are superiors and must therefore demonstrate their superior competencies in their executive work with subordinates. Third, the aligned, specific *achievement goal* was assigned to the participants; that is, it was recommended that participants focus on developing and improving their leadership competences (MAp) or on performing better than others and demonstrating their leadership competencies (PAp). These achievement goal manipulations, which have been found to be successful in experimental laboratory research, may be helpful in developing effective achievement goal interventions in organizations, which may impact not only job performance but also interpersonal behavior at work.

ACHIEVEMENT GOALS AND INTERPERSONAL BEHAVIOR AT WORK

Achievement goal research has predominantly focused on exploring individual cognition, affect, and behavior related to task engagement and task performance in individual task settings (Janssen & Van Yperen, 2004). However, since the early 2000s, more and more attention has been given to the question of how achievement goals influence individuals in the way they interpret and respond to the *interpersonal contexts* of achievement situations. In most work settings, workers interact with colleagues, supervisors, or customers to perform their tasks. Workers with different achievement goals have been found to differ in the way they develop and maintain relationships with other actors in their work context. Although both approach goals (i.e., PAp and MAp) positively affect performance (Van Yperen et al., 2015), PAp goals versus MAp goals are likely to activate different so-called "action plan goals," which are defined as strategies or pathways for achieving desired goals (DeShon & Gillespie, 2005). PAp goal individuals tend to perceive "negative interdependence" with others because their goal can be reached only at the cost of others, that is, by outperforming others (Poortvliet & Darnon, 2010). For example, Janssen and Van Yperen (2004) argued that PAp goal workers may be likely to perceive and approach their supervisor as someone who frustrates their goal of outperforming others, and to feel superior vis-à-vis others, including their supervisor. PAp individuals' tendency to believe that abilities are fixed (e.g., Cury, Elliot, Da Fonseca, & Moller, 2006; Dweck, 1986) may strengthen their perception that their goal of outperforming their superior is unattainable (also see Lockwood & Kunda, 1997). In contrast, MAp goal workers tend to perceive and approach supervisors as valuable sources of work-related knowledge, information, and experience that potentially serve their goal of learning, growth, and development. In turn, supervisors may provide these intrinsically motivated workers with support, decision latitude, and freedom, so that they can initiate, control, and carry out their tasks more

autonomously. Hence, MAp workers and their supervisors are likely to count on each other for support and loyalty, share important resources, and base their exchange relationship on mutual trust, respect, and obligation. Indeed, in a study of 170 workers from a Dutch energy supplier, Janssen and Van Yperen (2004) found that relative to PAp goal individuals, MAp goal individuals reported higher-quality exchange relationships (i.e., more mutual trust and respect) with their supervisors.

Although approach goals, either MAp or PAp, may generally enhance job performance (Van Yperen et al., 2015), such potential additional effects of PAp goals on interpersonal outcomes may be less welcomed by organizations. The pursuit of PAp goals has been found to lead individuals to behave less cooperatively, less honestly, and less constructively in interpersonal conflict, and to be more tactically deceptive. For example, in an experimental study, Poortvliet and colleagues (2007) showed that relative to MAp goal individuals, PAp goal individuals were lower in reciprocity orientation and higher in exploitation orientation, which in turn led to less accurate information giving and more suspicion of exchange partners. Moreover, relative to MAp goal individuals, PAp goal individuals were more willing to hinder their exchange partner's task performance by setting off a loud noise that the other would allegedly hear during task performance, particularly when their exchange partner's competence was high (Poortvliet, Anseel, Janssen, Van Yperen, & de Vliert, 2012). In another experimental study in which disagreement with a cooperation partner and achievement goals were manipulated, Darnon, Butera, and Harackiewicz (2007) observed better learning among MAp goal individuals relative to PAp goal individuals, but only in case of disagreement. Similarly, Darnon, Muller, Schrager, Pannuzzo, and Butera (2006) found that relative to MAp goal individuals, PAp goal individuals were more likely to regulate the conflict situation by asserting and self-affirming their own competence ("relational conflict regulation"). In contrast, MAp goal individuals were more likely to regulate sociocognitive conflict in an epistemic way, that is, by recognizing the other's competence and by attempting to integrate both points of view. Along the same line, Nederveen-Pieterse, Van Knippenberg, and Van Dierendonck (2013) observed that cultural diversity was more positively related to team performance when team members had stronger MAp goals through team members' willingness to exchange and discuss their ideas and viewpoints.

Additional empirical evidence for suboptimal interpersonal behavior in PAp goal individuals (relative to MAp goal individuals) has been found by Sijbom and colleagues (2015a, 2015b). Their quest was to discover why some leaders are motivated to consider and adopt (radical) creative ideas voiced by their subordinates, whereas others oppose this creative input and stick to their own established ideas. Creativity and innovation are critical for the effectiveness and survival of today's organizations, but subordinates' creative ideas often challenge the frameworks of thoughts and routines established by their leaders (Detert & Burris, 2007). In a field study of 128 workers in a supervisory position, Sijbom and colleagues (2015a) demonstrated that leaders' MAp goals were positively related to their tendency to adopt radical creative ideas voiced by their subordinates, whereas leaders' PAp goals were positively associated with their tendency to oppose these radical creative ideas. Indeed, MAp goal leaders may view subordinates' creative ideas as a potentially useful source of diagnostic and new information that can improve their competence and performance as leaders, even though it may challenge the content of the current state of affairs for which they are responsible. In contrast, PAp goal leaders tend to perceive subordinates who voice creative ideas as rivals who challenge and threaten their superior competencies as leader, which strengthens their tendency to stick to the status quo and oppose subordinates' challenging ideas. In follow-up experiments, Sijbom and colleagues (2015a, 2015b) found that this suboptimal tendency among PAp goal leaders was less pronounced, (1) when subordinates voiced their ideas in a considerate mode rather than an aggressive mode (Sijbom et al., 2015a), or (2) when subordinates voiced their creative idea without providing evaluative feedback information that might be perceived by their PAp leaders as a threat to their desired image of being a competent leader (Sijbom et al., 2015b).

CONCLUSION

The provision of a separate chapter called "Competence and the Workplace" might suggest that relative to other achievement domains (e.g., education and sport), achievement goals in the workplace are different in terms of prevalence, strength, determinants, and outcomes. The achievement goal domain is clearly an important moderator, but the similarities across achievement domains appear to be stronger than the differences. Across the achievement domains, approach goals (either MAp or PAp) are associated positively with performance indices, whereas avoidance goals (either MAv or PAv) are associated negatively with performance indices, although the strongest mean correlation between MAp goals and performance is observed in the work domain (Van Yperen et al., 2014).

Hence, with the aim of performance enhancement, achievement goal-based interventions in the workplace (as well as in other achievement contexts) should focus in particular on promoting MAp goals rather than PAp goals. As discussed by Van Yperen and colleagues (2014), there are several reasons for this. First, in achievement settings and contexts, including the workplace, visible and public performance evaluations are typically based on comparisons with others (Klein, 1997; Wheeler & Miyake, 1992; White, Langer, Yariv, & Welch, 2006). Hence, even among mastery goal individuals, there is a consistent reliance on social comparisons over temporal comparisons in their performance self-evaluations (Van Yperen & Leander, 2014). Promoting PAp goals would strengthen individuals' reliance on social comparison even more. Second, in general, the pursuit of MAp goals is considered to be the ideal type of competence-based regulation (Elliot, 2005; Pintrich, 2000). MAp goal individuals have been found to be high in achievement motivation (Elliot & Church, 1997), intrinsic motivation (Rawsthorne & Elliot, 1999), task interest (Harackiewicz, Barron, Pintrich,

Elliot, & Thrash, 2002), and agreeableness and conscientiousness (Day, Radosevich, & Chasteen, 2003; McCabe et al., 2013). Third, MAp goals tend to promote prosocial behavior, such as tolerance for opposing views (Darnon et al., 2006; Nederveen-Pieterse et al., 2013) and sharing resources with others (Levy, Kaplan, & Patrick, 2004; Poortvliet et al., 2007). In contrast, PAp goals show a mixed-valence profile, probably because these hybrid goals contain both a positive component (approach goal) and a negative component (performance goal) (Elliot & McGregor, 2001). On the positive side, individuals who hold PAp goals tend to have high levels of achievement motivation (Elliot & Church, 1997), conscientiousness (Wang & Erdheim, 2007), and positive affectivity (Van Yperen, 2006). However, PAp goals can involve costs in terms of interest (Harackiewicz et al., 2002), anxiety, worry, negative affect (Elliot & McGregor, 2001; Pintrich, 2000), dissatisfaction (Van Yperen & Janssen, 2002), and neuroticism (Hendricks & Payne, 2007; McCabe et al., 2013). Furthermore, PAp goals tend to elicit unethical behaviors such as thwarting behavior and less accurate information giving (Poortvliet et al., 2012) and cheating (Van Yperen et al., 2011). Thus, although PAp goals have consistent positive effects on performance attainment, undesirable social and ethical consequences of these goals might caution practitioners against their promotion.

To enhance job performance and outcomes such as intrinsic work motivation, collaboration, and ethical behavior, practitioners should promote and reinforce the pursuit of MAp goals. Directing workers towards positively valenced task-referenced or intrapersonal standards can be accomplished, for example, by emphasizing evaluation more in terms of progress and effort, by defining success more in terms of improvement, and by creating and maintaining a strong developmental climate in which workers are stimulated to develop their competences (e.g., Ames, 1992; Sijbom et al., 2015a, 2015b). To test the effectiveness of MAp goal-based interventions, repeated measures designs should be applied to MAp workers' self-referenced growth curves (i.e., patterns across time that are independent of others' performances). Remarkably, so far, this has rarely been done in achievement goal research (da Motta Veiga & Turban, 2014; Yeo, Loft, Xiao, & Kiewitz, 2009).

Important to note is that an emphasis on MAp goals does not imply the absence of interpersonal standards, social comparison, or competition. In contrast, in any achievement setting, including the workplace, interpersonal evaluation is apparent (Van Yperen & Leander, 2014), and even necessary (Becker, 1957). As already emphasized by early achievement goal researchers (e.g., Button et al., 1996; Farr et al., 1993), for an organization to be successful, workers must be concerned about meeting normative-based performance standards. In such a performance goal-dominated context, the key is the extent to which managers emphasize other-referenced relative to task-referenced or self-referenced standards, and whether they link task-referenced or self-referenced performance evaluations to (non-) material rewards.

REFERENCES

Ames, C. (1992). Classrooms: Goals, structures, and student motivation. *Journal of Educational Psychology, 84*, 261–271.

Ames, C., & Archer, J. (1988). Achievement goals in the classroom: Students' learning strategies and motivation processes. *Journal of Educational Psychology, 80*, 260–267.

Anseel, F., Beatty, A. S., Shen, W., Lievens, F., & Sackett, P. R. (2015). How are we doing after 30 years?: A meta-analytic review of the antecedents and outcomes of feedback-seeking behavior. *Journal of Management, 41*, 318–348.

Baranik, L. E., Barron, K. E., & Finney, S. J. (2007). Measuring goal orientation in a work domain: Construct validity evidence for the 2 × 2 framework. *Educational and Psychological Measurement, 67*, 697–718.

Baranik, L. E., Stanley, L. J., Bynum, B. H., & Lance, C. E. (2010). Examining the construct validity of mastery-avoidance achievement goals: A meta-analysis. *Human Performance, 23*, 265–282.

Barron, K. E., & Harackiewicz, J. M. (2001). Achievement goals and optimal motivation: Testing multiple goal models. *Journal of Personality and Social Psychology, 80*, 706–722.

Bass, B. M. (1990). *Bass and Stogdill's handbook*

of leadership: Theory, research, and managerial applications (3rd ed.). New York: Free Press.

Bateman, T. S., & Crant, J. M. (1993). The proactive component of organizational behavior: A measure and correlates. *Journal of Organizational Behavior, 14,* 103–118.

Beck, J. W., & Schmidt, A. M. (2013). State-level goal orientations as mediators of the relationship between time pressure and performance: A longitudinal study. *Journal of Applied Psychology, 98,* 354–363.

Becker, G. (1957). *The economics of discrimination.* Chicago: University of Chicago Press.

Beenen, G. (2014). The effects of goal orientations and supervisor concerns on MBA intern learning and performance. *Academy of Management Learning and Education, 13,* 82–101.

Bell, B. S., & Kozlowski, S. W. J. (2008). Active learning: Effects of core training design elements on self-regulatory processes, learning, and adaptability. *Journal of Applied Psychology, 93,* 296–316.

Blumberg, M., & Pringle, C. D. (1982). The missing opportunity in organizational research: Some implications for a theory of work performance. *Academy of Management Review, 7,* 560–569.

Bolino, M. C., Turnley, W. H., & Bloodgood, J. M. (2002). Citizenship behavior and the creation of social capital in organizations. *Academy of Management Review, 27,* 505–522.

Bouffard, T., Boisvert, J., Vezeau, C., & Larouche, C. (1995). The impact of goal orientation on self-regulation and performance among college students. *British Journal of Educational Psychology, 65,* 317–329.

Brodbeck, F. C., Zapf, D., Prumper, J., & Frese, M. (1993). Error handling in office work with computers: A field study. *Journal of Occupational and Organizational Psychology, 66,* 303–317.

Bunderson, J. S., & Sutcliffe, K. M. (2003). Management team learning orientation and business unit performance. *Journal of Applied Psychology, 88,* 552–560.

Button, S. B., Mathieu, J. E., & Zajac, D. M. (1996). Goal orientation in organizational research: A conceptual and empirical foundation. *Organizational Behavior and Human Decision Processes, 67,* 26–48.

Chadwick, I. C., & Raver, J. L. (2015). Motivating organizations to learn: Goal orientation and its influence on organizational learning. *Journal of Management, 41,* 957–986.

Cianci, A. M., Schaubroeck, J. M., & McGill, G. A. (2010). Achievement goals, feedback, and task performance. *Human Performance, 23,* 131–154.

Cury, F., Elliot, A. J., Da Fonseca, D., & Moller, A. C. (2006). The social-cognitive model of achievement motivation and the 2 × 2 achievement goal framework. *Journal of Personality and Social Psychology, 90,* 666–679.

da Motta Veiga, S. P., & Turban, D. B. (2014). Are affect and perceived stress detrimental or beneficial to job seekers?: The role of learning goal orientation in job search self-regulation. *Organizational Behavior and Human Decision Processes, 125,* 193–203.

Darnon, C., Butera, F., & Harackiewicz, J. M. (2007). Achievement goals in social interactions: Learning with mastery vs. performance goals. *Motivation and Emotion, 31,* 61–70.

Darnon, C., Muller, D., Schrager, S. M., Pannuzzo, N., & Butera, F. (2006). Mastery and performance goals predict epistemic and relational conflict regulation. *Journal of Educational Psychology, 98,* 766–776.

Day, E. A., Radosevich, D. J., & Chasteen, C. S. (2003). Construct- and criterion-related validity of four commonly used goal orientation instruments. *Contemporary Educational Psychology, 28,* 434–464.

Deci, E. L., & Ryan, R. M. (1985). *Intrinsic motivation and self-determination in human behavior.* New York: Plenum Press.

De Lange, A. H., Van Yperen, N. W., Van der Heijden, B. I. J. M., & Bal, P. M. (2010). Dominant achievement goals of older workers and their relationship with motivation-related outcomes. *Journal of Vocational Behavior, 77,* 118–125.

DeShon, R. P., & Gillespie, J. Z. (2005). A motivated action theory account of goal orientation. *Journal of Applied Psychology, 90,* 1096–1127.

Detert, J. R., & Burris, E. R. (2007). Leadership behavior and employee voice: Is the door really open? *Academy of Management Journal, 50,* 869–884.

Dragoni, L. (2005). Understanding the emergence of state goal orientation in organizational work groups: The role of leadership and multilevel climate perceptions. *Journal of Applied Psychology, 90,* 1084–1095.

Dragoni, L., & Kuenzi, M. (2012). Better understanding work unit goal orientation: Its emergence and impact under different types of work unit structure. *Journal of Applied Psychology, 97,* 1032–1048.

Dweck, C. S. (1986). Motivational processes affecting learning. *American Psychologist, 41,* 1040–1048.

Ebner, N. C., Freund, A. M., & Baltes, P. B.

(2006). Developmental changes in personal goal orientation from young to late adulthood: From striving for gains to maintenance and prevention of losses. *Psychology and Aging, 21,* 664–678.

Elliot, A. J. (1999). Approach and avoidance motivation and achievement goals. *Educational Psychologist, 34,* 169–189.

Elliot, A. J. (2005). A conceptual history of the achievement goal construct. In A. J. Elliot & C. S. Dweck (Eds.), *Handbook of competence and motivation* (pp. 52–72). New York: Guilford Press.

Elliot, A. J., & Church, M. A. (1997). A hierarchical model of approach and avoidance achievement motivation. *Journal of Personality and Social Psychology, 72,* 218–232.

Elliot, A. J., & McGregor, H. A. (1999). Test anxiety and the hierarchical model of approach and avoidance achievement motivation. *Journal of Personality and Social Psychology, 76,* 628–644.

Elliot, A. J., & McGregor, H. A. (2001). A 2 × 2 achievement goal framework. *Journal of Personality and Social Psychology, 80,* 501–519.

Elliot, A. J., Murayama, K., & Pekrun, R. (2011). A 3 × 2 achievement goal model. *Journal of Educational Psychology, 103,* 632–648.

Elliot, A. J., Shell, M. M., Henry, K. B., & Maier, M. A. (2005). Achievement goals, performance contingencies, and performance attainment: An experimental test. *Journal of Educational Psychology, 97,* 630–640.

Farr, J. L., Hofmann, D. A., & Ringenbach, K. L. (1993). Goal orientation and action control theory: Implications for industrial and organizational psychology. In C. L. Cooper & I. T. Robertson (Eds.), *International Review of Industrial and Organizational Psychology, 8,* 193–232.

Gist, M. E., & Stevens, C. K. (1998). Effects of practice conditions and supplemental training method on cognitive learning and interpersonal skill generalization. *Organizational Behavior and Human Decision Processes, 75,* 142–169.

Gong, Y., Kim, T., Lee, D., & Zhu, J. (2013). A multilevel model of team goal orientation, information exchange, and creativity. *Academy of Management Journal, 56,* 827–851.

Hamstra, M. R. W., Van Yperen, N. W., Wisse, B., & Sassenberg, K. (2014). Transformational and transactional leadership and followers' achievement goals. *Journal of Business and Psychology, 29,* 413–425.

Harackiewicz, J. M., Barron, K. E., Pintrich, P. R., Elliot, A. J., & Thrash, T. M. (2002). Revision of achievement goal theory: Necessary and illuminating. *Journal of Educational Psychology, 94,* 638–645.

Hardin, C. D., & Higgins, E. T. (1996). Shared reality: How social verification makes the subjective objective. In R. M. Sorrentino & E. T. Higgins (Eds.), *Handbook of motivation and cognition: Vol. 3. The interpersonal context* (pp. 28–84). New York: Guilford Press.

Heidemeier, H., & Bittner, J. V. (2012). Competition and achievement goals in work teams. *Human Performance, 25,* 138–158.

Hendricks, J., & Payne, S. (2007). Beyond the Big Five: Leader goal orientation as a predictor of leadership effectiveness. *Human Performance, 20,* 317–343.

Hetland, H., Skogstad, A., Hetland, J., & Mikkelsen, A. (2011). Leadership and learning climate in a work setting. *European Psychologist, 16,* 163–173.

Hulleman, C. S., Schrager, S. M., Bodmann, S. M., & Harackiewicz, J. M. (2010). A meta-analytic review of achievement goal measures: Different labels for the same constructs or different constructs with similar labels? *Psychological Bulletin, 136,* 422–449.

Jagacinski, C. M., Madden, J. L., & Reider, M. H. (2001). The impact of situational and dispositional achievement goals on performance. *Human Performance, 14,* 321–337.

Janssen, O., & Prins, J. (2007). Goal orientations and the seeking of different types of feedback information. *Journal of Occupational and Organizational Psychology, 80,* 235–249.

Janssen, O., & Van Yperen, N. W. (2004). Employees' goal orientations, the quality of leader–member exchange, and the outcomes of job performance and job satisfaction. *Academy of Management Journal, 47,* 368–384.

Kanfer, R. (1990). Motivation theory and industrial and organizational psychology. In M. D. Dunnette (Ed.), *Handbook of industrial and organizational psychology* (2nd ed., Vol. 1, pp. 75–130). Palo Alto, CA: Consulting Psychologists Press.

Kanfer, R. (2012). Work motivation: Theory, practice, and future directions. In S. W. Kozlowski (Ed.), *The Oxford handbook of industrial and organizational psychology* (Vol. 1, pp. 455–495). Oxford, UK: Oxford University Press.

Klein, W. M. (1997). Objective standards are not enough: Affective, self-evaluative, and behavioral responses to social comparison information. *Journal of Personality and Social Psychology, 72,* 763–774.

Kozlowski, S. W. J., Gully, S. M., Brown, K. G., Salas, E., Smith, E. M., & Nason, E. R. (2001). Effects of training goals and goal orientation traits on multidimensional training outcomes and performance adaptability. *Organizational Behavior and Human Decision Processes, 85,* 1–31.

Lee, C., Hui, C., Tinsley, C. H., & Niu, X. Y. (2006). Goal orientations and performance: Role of temporal norms. *Journal of International Business Studies, 37,* 484–498.

Lee, F. K., Sheldon, K. M., & Turban, D. B. (2003). Personality and the goal-striving process: The influence of achievement goal patterns, goal level, and mental focus on performance and enjoyment. *Journal of Applied Psychology, 88,* 256–265.

Levy, I., Kaplan, A., & Patrick, H. (2004). Early adolescents' achievement goals, social status, and attitudes towards cooperation with peers. *Social Psychology of Education, 7,* 127–159.

Lockwood, P., & Kunda, Z. (1997). Superstars and me: Predicting the impact of role models on the self. *Journal of Personality and Social Psychology, 73,* 91–103.

McCabe, K. O., Van Yperen, N. W., Elliot, A. J., & Verbraak, M. (2013). Big Five personality profiles of context-specific achievement goals. *Journal of Research in Personality, 47,* 698–707.

Mehta, A., Feild, H., Armenakis, A., & Mehta, N. (2009). Team goal orientation and team performance: The mediating role of team planning. *Journal of Management, 35,* 1026–1046.

Mueller, C. M., & Dweck, C. S. (1998). Praise for intelligence can undermine children's motivation and performance. *Journal of Personality and Social Psychology, 75,* 33–52.

Nahrgang, J. D., DeRue, D. S., Hollenbeck, J. R., Spitzmuller, M., Jundt, D. K., & Ilgen, D. R. (2013). Goal setting in teams: The impact of learning and performance goals on process and performance. *Organizational Behavior and Human Decision Processes, 122,* 12–21.

Nederveen-Pieterse, A., Van Knippenberg, D., & Van Dierendonck, D. (2013). Cultural diversity and team performance: The role of team member goal orientation. *Academy of Management Journal, 56,* 782–804.

Nicholls, J. G. (1984). Achievement motivation: Conceptions of ability, subjective experience, task choice, and performance. *Psychological Review, 91,* 328–346.

Payne, S. C., Youngcourt, S. S., & Beaubien, J. M. (2007). A meta-analytic examination of the goal orientation nomological net. *Journal of Applied Psychology, 92,* 128–150.

Pekrun, R., Elliot, A. J., & Maier, M. A. (2006). Achievement goals and discrete achievement emotions: A theoretical model and prospective test. *Journal of Educational Psychology, 98,* 583–597.

Pintrich, P. R. (2000). An achievement goal theory perspective on issues in motivation terminology, theory, and research. *Contemporary Educational Psychology, 25,* 92–104.

Podsakoff, P., MacKenzie, S., Paine, J., & Bachrach, D. (2000). Organizational citizenship behaviors: A critical review of the theoretical and empirical literature and suggestions for future research. *Journal of Management, 26,* 513–563.

Poortvliet, P. M., Anseel, F., Janssen, O., Van Yperen, N. W., & de Vliert, E. V. (2012). Perverse effects of other-referenced performance goals in an information exchange context. *Journal of Business Ethics, 106,* 401–414.

Poortvliet, P. M., & Darnon, C. (2010). Toward a more social understanding of achievement goals: The interpersonal effects of mastery and performance goals. *Current Directions in Psychological Science, 19,* 324–328.

Poortvliet, P. M., Janssen, O., Van Yperen, N. W., & Van de Vliert, E. (2007). Achievement goals and interpersonal behavior: How mastery and performance goals shape information exchange. *Personality and Social Psychology Bulletin, 33,* 1435–1447.

Porath, C. L., & Bateman, T. S. (2006). Self-regulation: From goal orientation to job performance. *Journal of Applied Psychology, 91,* 185–192.

Preenen, P., Van Vianen, A., & De Pater, I. E. (2014). Challenging tasks: The role of employees' and supervisors' goal orientations. *European Journal of Work and Organizational Psychology, 23,* 48–61.

Rawsthorne, L. J., & Elliot, A. J. (1999). Achievement goals and intrinsic motivation: A meta-analytic review. *Personality and Social Psychology Review, 3,* 326–344.

Raynor, J. O. (1969). Future orientation and motivation of immediate activity: An elaboration of theory of achievement motivation. *Psychological Review, 76,* 606–610.

Salancik, G. R., & Pfeffer, J. (1978). Social information-processing approach to job attitudes and task design. *Administrative Science Quarterly, 23,* 224–253.

Sarason, I. G., Sarason, B. R., Keefe, D. E., Hayes, B. E., & Shearin, E. N. (1986). Cognitive interference: Situational determinants and traitlike characteristics. *Journal of Personality and Social Psychology, 51,* 215–226.

Schneider, B. (1987). The people make the place. *Personnel Psychology, 40,* 437–453.

Schraw, G., Horn, C., Thorndikechrist, T., & Bruning, R. (1995). Academic goal orientations and student classroom achievement. *Contemporary Educational Psychology, 20,* 359–368.

Seijts, G. H., Latham, G. P., Tasa, K., & Latham, B. W. (2004). Goal setting and goal orientation: An integration of two different yet related literatures. *Academy of Management Journal, 47,* 227–239.

Senko, C., & Freund, A. M. (2015). Are mastery-avoidance achievement goals always detrimental?: An adult development perspective. *Motivation and Emotion, 39,* 477–488.

Sideridis, G. D. (2008). The regulation of affect, anxiety, and stressful arousal from adopting mastery-avoidance goal orientations. *Stress and Health, 24,* 55–69.

Sijbom, R. B. L., Janssen, O., & Van Yperen, N. W. (2015a). How to get radical creative ideas into a leader's mind?: Leader's achievement goals and subordinates' voice of creative ideas. *European Journal of Work and Organizational Psychology, 24,* 279–296.

Sijbom, R. B. L., Janssen, O., & Van Yperen, N. W. (2015b). Leaders' receptivity to subordinates' creative input: The role of achievement goals and composition of creative input. *European Journal of Work and Organizational Psychology, 24,* 462–478.

Somuncuoglu, Y., & Yildirim, A. (1999). Relationship between achievement goal orientations and use of learning strategies. *Journal of Educational Research, 92,* 267–277.

Steele, C. M., & Aronson, J. (1995). Stereotype threat and the intellectual test performance of African Americans. *Journal of Personality and Social Psychology, 69,* 797–811.

Steele-Johnson, D., Heintz, P., Jr., & Miller, C. E. (2008). Examining situationally induced state goal orientation effects on task perceptions, performance, and satisfaction: A two-dimensional conceptualization. *Journal of Applied Social Psychology, 38,* 334–365.

Sternberg, R. J., & Grigorenko, E. L. (2001). *Environmental effects on cognitive abilities.* Mahwah, NJ: Erlbaum.

Sujan, H., Weitz, B. A., & Kumar, N. (1994). Learning orientation, working smart, and effective selling. *Journal of Marketing, 58,* 39–52.

Tanaka, A., Okuno, T., & Yamauchi, H. (2013). Longitudinal tests on the influence of achievement goals on effort and intrinsic interest in the workplace. *Motivation and Emotion, 37,* 457–464.

Van Hooft, E. A. J., & Noordzij, G. (2009). The effects of goal orientation on job search and reemployment: A field experiment among unemployed job seekers. *Journal of Applied Psychology, 94,* 1581–1590.

Van Yperen, N. W. (2003a). The perceived profile of goal orientation within firms: Differences between employees working for successful and unsuccessful firms employing either performance-based pay or job-based pay. *European Journal of Work and Organizational Psychology, 12,* 229–243.

Van Yperen, N. W. (2003b). Task interest and actual performance: The moderating effects of assigned and adopted purpose goals. *Journal of Personality and Social Psychology, 85,* 1006–1015.

Van Yperen, N. W. (2006). A novel approach to assessing achievement goals in the context of the 2 × 2 framework: Identifying distinct profiles of individuals with different dominant achievement goals. *Personality and Social Psychology Bulletin, 32,* 1432–1445.

Van Yperen, N. W., Blaga, M., & Postmes, T. (2014). A meta-analysis of self-reported achievement goals and nonself-report performance across three achievement domains (work, sports, and education). *PLoS ONE, 9,* e93594.

Van Yperen, N. W., Blaga, M., & Postmes, T. (2015). A meta-analysis of the impact of situationally induced achievement goals on task performance. *Human Performance, 28,* 165–182.

Van Yperen, N. W., Elliot, A. J., & Anseel, F. (2009). The influence of mastery-avoidance goals on performance improvement. *European Journal of Social Psychology, 39,* 932–943.

Van Yperen, N. W., Hamstra, M. R. W., & Van der Klauw, M. (2011). To win, or not to lose, at any cost: The impact of achievement goals on cheating. *British Journal of Management, 22,* S5–S15.

Van Yperen, N. W., & Janssen, O. (2002). Fatigued and dissatisfied or fatigued but satisfied?: Goal orientations and responses to high job demands. *Academy of Management Journal, 45,* 1161–1171.

Van Yperen, N. W., & Leander, N. P. (2014). The overpowering effect of social comparison information: On the misalignment between mastery-based goals and self-evaluation criteria. *Personality and Social Psychology Bulletin, 40,* 676–688.

Van Yperen, N. W., & Orehek, E. (2013). Achievement goals in the workplace: Conceptualization, prevalence, profiles, and outcomes. *Journal of Economic Psychology, 38,* 71–79.

VandeWalle, D. (1997). Development and validation of a work domain goal orientation instrument. *Educational and Psychological Measurement, 57,* 995–1015.

VandeWalle, D. (2003). A goal orientation

model of feedback-seeking behavior. *Human Resource Management Review, 13,* 581–604.

VandeWalle, D., Brown, S. P., Cron, W. L., & Slocum, J. W. J. (1999). The influence of goal orientation and self-regulation tactics on sales performance: A longitudinal field test. *Journal of Applied Psychology, 84,* 249–259.

Vansteenkiste, M., Lens, W., Elliot, A. J., Soenens, B., & Mouratidis, A. (2014). Moving the achievement goal approach one step forward: Toward a systematic examination of the autonomous and controlled reasons underlying achievement goals. *Educational Psychologist, 49,* 153–174.

Wang, M., & Erdheim, J. (2007). Does the five-factor model of personality relate to goal orientation? *Personality and Individual Differences, 43,* 1493–1505.

Wheeler, L., & Miyake, K. (1992). Social comparison in everyday life. *Journal of Personality and Social Psychology, 62,* 760–773.

White, J. B., Langer, E. J., Yariv, L., & Welch, J. C. (2006). Frequent social comparisons and destructive emotions and behaviors: The dark side of social comparisons. *Journal of Adult Development, 13,* 36–44.

White, R. (1959). Motivation reconsidered: The concept of competence. *Psychological Review, 66,* 297–333.

Winters, D., & Latham, G. P. (1996). The effect of learning versus outcome goals on a simple versus a complex task. *Group and Organization Management, 21,* 236–250.

Yeo, G., Loft, S., Xiao, T., & Kiewitz, C. (2009). Goal orientations and performance: Differential relationships across levels of analysis and as a function of task demands. *Journal of Applied Psychology, 94,* 710–726.

PART VI

PSYCHOLOGICAL INTERVENTIONS

CHAPTER 35

Turning Point

Targeted, Tailored, and Timely Psychological Intervention

GEOFFREY L. COHEN
JULIO GARCIA
J. PARKER GOYER

In important domains, people create and maintain social systems designed to promote the outcomes they want. Among many of the obvious examples are governments, workplaces, hospitals, and schools. In the last century, Kurt Lewin (1936) pioneered the approach of applying science to social systems. He was convinced that the new discipline of social psychology was the best way to ensure the production of desired social outcomes across a host of human endeavors.

Lewin's conviction was not misplaced. The subsequent decades have provided ample and rigorous evidence that psychologically informed interventions can improve important social outcomes (for reviews, see Cohen & Sherman, 2014; Ross & Gilovich, 2015; Walton, 2014; Wilson, 2011; Yeager & Walton, 2011). In spite of the many seemingly insurmountable obstacles to increasing voter turnout, reducing teenage risky behavior, or closing academic achievement gaps based on race and social class, research shows that it is possible to improve the status quo by changing one key element in a complex system. If, on the night before an election, people are encouraged to label themselves as voters rather than as people who engage in voting, they are more likely to vote (Bryan, Walton, Rogers, & Dweck, 2011). Having the concept of personality presented as something fluid and changeable rather than written in stone led teenagers to be kinder to their peers, earn better grades, and experience less depression (see Yeager, Lee, & Jamieson, 2016). Having a small group of well-connected teenage students generate and then cultivate prosocial norms led to a 30% reduction in disciplinary incidents throughout their school (Paluck, Shepherd, & Aronow, 2016). In a final example, for African American college students, their college grades over four years, participation in extramural activities both before and after graduation, and later career satisfaction increased if as freshmen they had been provided with evidence that difficulty in the transition to college is normal and short-lived (Brady, Walton, Jarvis, & Cohen, 2016; Walton & Cohen, 2007, 2011).

These examples do not speak to the effectiveness of any particular intervention. Rather, they show the power of motivational processes, whether activated intentionally or by chance. The elements of an effective intervention can be characterized as what Jung (1952) termed *synchronicity*. It is a "meaningful coincidence" of two or more apparently unconnected events that alters a process in an important way. Many of us have had the experience of having a bit of advice or encouragement produce positive change in us. Advice or encouragement that we had heard before and that once had no impact, now, because of our readiness, energizes us and moves us to take actions that we had formerly rejected. Interventions aimed to improve motivation work in the same way. They occur at a moment when motivational processes are open, susceptible, and influential. It is not merely the occurrence of an intervention that matters but whether it occurs at the right time, at right place, and for the right person. The confluence of message, moment, and person creates a turning point.

We define *intervention* as any purposeful attempt at change. This chapter classes "psychological intervention" among a large set of motivational and influence practices. These include marketing and political campaigns, social programs, therapy, incentives, praise, and feedback. The chapter thus offers a broad conceptualization of interventions, with a focus on social-psychological interventions. From our perspective, intervention is not merely an exercise in applying knowledge. It is a scientific endeavor. At the heart of this endeavor are two questions. The first, the focus of social psychology, is how to produce a change in the status quo. Social-psychological research shows that people are capable of much more, both good and ill, than our cultural programming would lead many of us to think. Classic studies show that, under certain conditions, ordinary people can be led to kill innocents (Milgram, 1963) or to go to heroic lengths to help (Latané & Darley, 1969). They can sink to the low expectations that others hold for their intelligence and social poise, or they can rise to their high expectations (Rosenthal & Jacobson, 2003; Snyder, Tanke, & Berscheid, 1977). In this respect, social psychology is a science not of human nature but of human potential.

The second question, a new theoretical frontier, is how change is transmitted through time. Although marked change can occur, we do not fully understand when, how, and why it persists. What determines which changes in the status quo are preserved and which decay? In geology, processes such as erosion, deposition, and sedimentation lead to the emergence of complex forms over time. Likewise, the interaction and accumulation of social-psychological processes over time can lead to the emergence of vast inequalities in psychological and material outcomes.

Above all else, our perspective requires going beyond a focus on the behavior one wants to change, the foreground. Rather, it demands a focus on the existing system of forces in the status quo, the background. Though this background regularly operates in plain sight, it often goes unnoticed and may even be invisible. It is where the behavior of interest and our attempts to change it take place. It must inform the timing and placement of any intervention.

OVERVIEW

Our model of intervention is represented in a single formula:

$$B = f(M,C) \times T$$

Behavior (B) is a function of a motivational mechanism (M) unfolding in a specific context (C) through time (T). The first two elements in the equation come from Pawson and Tilley's (1997) insightful model of social change. In general, motivational mechanisms produce a psychological state, often in the form of a motive. Psychological states, like all human experience, are situated in a context and take behavioral form within the constraints of that context. A motive such as self-interest can give rise to different behaviors in different contexts. In a context of abundant and equal opportunity, self-interest would permit and encourage behaviors geared to long-term goals and cooperative enterprises. But in a context where opportunity is highly restricted, self-interest would instead encourage behaviors focused on short-term gains and zero-sum strategies. Time, which captures the changing nature of a given context, creates the possibility for a motive and its behavioral manifestations to alter the context, which in turn alters the person, with the cycle potentially repeating. Cooperative behavior can evoke cooperation from others, establishing a norm. Such feedback loops permit the impact of any intervention to be spread through time rather than limited to the moment of its introduction.

An intervention's success depends on three factors (see Pawson & Tilley, 1997). First, does it activate the targeted motivational mechanism? Second, is the context structured in a way that permits the activated mechanism to express itself in the desired behavior? Third, if the mechanism is activated and allowed to express itself, will its effect be sustained over time? Whether the benefits of an intervention last depends on whether the context contains structures that reinforce the behavioral outputs of the motivational mechanism.

MOTIVATIONAL PROCESSES TRANSFORMING AND TRANSMITTING SOCIAL INFLUENCES THROUGH TIME

The impact of physical mechanisms, at least at the macro level, is fairly direct. It is largely a function of the kinetic and potential energy of one object acting on another. The process is linear and sequential, as when one domino knocks down the next until there are no more dominos standing.

Unlike the more basic laws of physics, psychological processes can act through more dynamic and fluid means. A small influence from the past can come to dominate thought and action in the present. Having homeowners agree to engage in a small act of prosocial behavior, placing a small "Drive Carefully" sign in a window in their home, quadrupled the likelihood that they would agree 2 weeks later to place a large and unsightly sign of the same theme in their front yard (Freedman & Fraser, 1966). Simply asking people about their intentions to buy a new car increased the percentage of those who actually bought a car in the subsequent year (Morwitz, Johnson, & Schmittlein, 1993). People's initial behavior, however fleeting or seemingly trivial, can come to be seen as an indication or telling attribute of their identity, of who they are. The experience then takes on psychological momentum independent of the incident that gave rise to it. A psychological process, in this case the attributional process, transforms a seemingly inconsequential event into an influence that endures.

Because of the dynamic nature of psychological processes, not only can past events influence future thought and action, but present events can alter the influence of past ones. When people write down their deepest thoughts and feelings about a past traumatic experience, they are better able to break free of its influence on them in the present. Having placed it in a meaningful narrative, they experience fewer intrusive thoughts, freeing up working memory and improving health and well-being (Klein & Boales, 2001; Pennebaker & Chung, 2011). Likewise, privately thinking about one's happiest moments, such as a delightful vacation with loved ones, mentally reliving them, pulls their influence into the present, increasing positive emotions for up to a month (Lyubomirsky, Sousa, & Dickerhoof, 2006). Motivational mechanisms can turn even experiences from long ago into powerful causal forces in the present moment.

Insofar as psychological processes stitch past to present, how long a situation lasts is far from clear. A basic tenet in social psychology is the power of the situation, much of which emerges from how people perceive it (Ross & Nisbett, 2011). When a Prisoner's Dilemma game, for instance, was presented as the "Community Game" rather than the "Wall Street Game," more than twice the number of players chose to cooperate rather than pursue their self-interest at the expense of their partner (Liberman, Samuels, & Ross, 2004).

Because the power of a situation lies in large part in how it is perceived, if a situation persists in a person's mind, the situation can also be said to persist. That is, a single experience may last minutes, days, years, or a lifetime. One line of studies showed that a single experience of stereotype threat, where women took a math test that they believed would cast their gender group in a negative light, had effects that persisted a week later. Such women performed worse on a subsequent math test and expressed less confidence in their math ability compared to peers in a control group (Manke & Cohen, 2016). Similarly, college women's likelihood of majoring in a math-intensive discipline, economics, was highly dependent on their grade in the introductory course (Goldin, 2015). Only women who earned an A went onto major in economics at the same rate as men, who, by contrast, majored in economics virtually without regard to their grade in this gateway course. It was as though, for women, only outstanding performance could refute the stereotype that they did not belong. More generally, the effect of positive or negative feedback on people's view of their competence can survive even after its validity has been discredited (Lepper, Ross, & Lau, 1986; Ross, Lepper, & Hubbard, 1975). Although an objective situation may end, as a subjective experience it may be relived repeatedly. Moreover, the objective consequences that follow from a situation and how it is perceived can persist even when the subjective experience fades. The doors of opportunity opened and closed by a student's choice of major is just such a consequence. So is being placed into a remedial track that constrains educational opportunities for years to come (Cohen, Garcia, Purdie-Vaughns, Apfel, & Brzustoski, 2009). How long an event or situation *lasts* is less obvious than it seems.

MOTIVATIONAL PROCESSES IN CONTEXT

People exist in a web of psychological and environmental forces that envelop them in a given moment, what Lewin (1939) called the "life space." There, psychological processes and the proximal environment give rise to behavior. The environment, or context, affects psychological functioning in at least two ways. First, it determines whether a psychological process is activated or not. Second, the context provides constraints and resources that channel the behavioral expression of a process in both the short and the long term.

For example, the demands of an environment might activate the self-affirmation process (Steele, 1988; see also Cohen & Sherman, 2014). A workplace, classroom, or hospital, for instance, can prove stressful and threaten people's sense of personal adequacy. In the face of such threatening circumstances, people engage a self-affirmation process. Its aim is to reaffirm the perceived integrity of the self. Because of the importance of this motivational process, even seemingly minor insults or ambiguous feedback can trigger strong reactions. People often engage in denial and defensiveness that can prove counterproductive. For example, when people are presented with information that their behavior puts them at risk for a serious medical condition, they tend to respond defensively. They challenge the validity of the information and even forego opportunities for medical screening (see Cohen & Sherman, 2014, for a review). However, if the same environment provides them with seemingly minor self-affirming experiences, people can better rise above a threatening event, their default defensive responses curbed. When patients are provided with the opportunity to affirm the self through the chance to write about values they cherish, such as the importance of family, they are more open to threatening health information, more empowered in their interactions with their health care provider, more likely to agree to medical screening, and more likely to take positive behavioral steps in the treatment of their condition (see Cohen & Sherman, 2014, for a review). It is not the act of reflecting on a personal value that is powerful, but the process it triggers (Brady, Reeves, et al., 2016). The act gains causal force from the self-affirmation process it sets in motion.

The context also provides psychological states with constraints and resources that channel their behavioral expression. An institutional goal such as encouraging employees to save for their retirement produces a psychological energy, a motive. People come to think that they must at least consider this as important, and, at the very least, weigh the pros and cons of the options available for reaching the goal. While the environment often presents a fairly fixed array of channels to reach the goal, some channels are easier to access than others. The concept of "nudges," in which access to a contextual channel is facilitated and the link between a motive and a particular course of action strengthened, has proved one of social psychology's most influential exports to social policy (Thaler & Sunstein, 2009). For example, employees are much more likely to sign up for a retirement savings account if they are automatically enrolled and can "opt out" than if initially given the opportunity to opt in to the same account. In another study, when parents of poor children received timely texts on their mobile phones reminding them of concrete ways that they could practice literacy skills with their children, the children earned higher year-end performance on a literary exam (Loeb & York, 2016). Unlike lower animals, people have relatively few preset and fixed behavioral responses to the environment (Geertz, 1973). Their responses often consist of psychological states, with the specific behavioral consequences shaped by context. A parent who wants his or her children to succeed may read to them, praise them, criticize them, or let them fend for themselves. The possible actions are innumerable. Contextual channels guide whether and how people turn general motives into specific actions. They include constraints, resources, rituals, and sources of information such as rules, myths, stories, and norms.

Another way that such nudges, also referred to as *channel factors* (Lewin, 1939; Ross & Nisbett, 2011), can strengthen the link between a motive and action is by explicitly or implicitly normalizing an action. For example, they may imply that enrollment in a retirement account, or practicing literacy skills with one's child, is a common practice and thus lead people to do what they perceive to be normal and expected in their society (Davidai, Gilovich, & Ross, 2012). Such nudges, however, depend on the existence of a motive. Absent a motive, there is nothing to be channeled. For instance, among poor adults filing their federal income tax return, having some of their tax refund defaulted into a savings bond had no impact on savings behavior (Bronchetti, Dee, Huffman, & Magenheim, 2011). The motivation to save for the long term was trumped, it seems, by more pressing short-term motives that could be met by the immediate use of the refund. Motives interacting with context create behavior.

Because of the psychological forces in the life space, there is a fundamental fact about the social context that is hard to appreciate. What appears to be the same situation can in fact be very different for different actors, or for the same actor at different times (Asch, 1952). The psychological experience, the meaning or construal of an environment, can be qualitatively different. Two children presented with an apparently identical academic challenge, insoluble anagrams, may see it differently. For the child who believes that intelligence is fixed, the experience is more likely to be seen as evidence of low ability and thus lead to disengagement (Dweck, 1986). For a child who believes that intelligence is expandable, the experience is more likely to be seen as an opportunity to learn and thus lead to continued engagement. Differences in persistence largely reflect differences not in the children's willpower or character but in the nature of the situation as each perceives it. A visual analogy of this notion is provided by Gestalt bistable figures. Although the visual information provided is the same for everyone, the figures that people perceive may differ. In Figure 35.1, whether the middle character appears to be a B or a 13 depends on whether people perceive the visual information in the context of a line of letters or numbers. Likewise, the meaning of a specific experience in the social world can prove vastly different in light of each actor's unique cognitive context.

The foregoing analysis implies that the effect of any action, including an intervention, depends on the context or life space into which it is introduced. The influence of context is easy to see with interventions that use material rewards or consequences. Although money has no intrinsic causal power, its effectiveness derives from how it interacts with the context. Most obviously, the money must be seen as legitimate and valuable to have purchasing power. More subtly, cash gifts or transfers to the poor have proved an

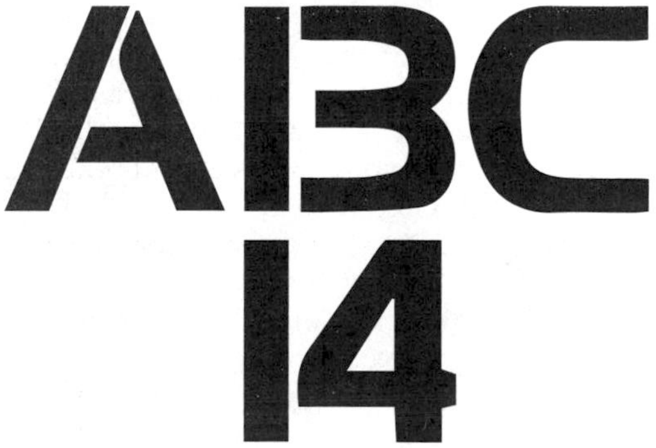

FIGURE 35.1. A Gestalt visual shift. The character in the middle appears to be a B or a 13 as a function of the salient context.

effective and efficient intervention, but only under certain contextual conditions. Money permits people to purchase what they want and what is available to them. People's wants issue out of psychological factors such as goals, desires, and beliefs. What is available to purchase issues out of environmental factors such as what the marketplace offers.

The conditional impact of cash gifts is seen in randomized experiments in developing countries such as Liberia and Uganda. In one study, $200 was given to young men, many of whom were homeless and involved in crime. This cash transfer decreased their engagement in crime and violent behavior over the next several weeks. However, benefits decayed after a year. When the case was delivered with therapy that encouraged the men to see themselves as normal members of society rather than outcasts, and that provided instruction in goal-setting and self-regulation, longer-term reductions in crime and violence were achieved (Blattman, Jamison, & Sheridan, 2015). The rate of drug-selling almost halved. The long-term benefits of the cash gifts arose from the fact that crime in Liberia is driven by young men with few economic opportunities. The recipients now had the psychological tools, such as self-regulatory skills and a positive sense of self, to maintain longer-term positive changes, such as refraining from selling drugs and engaging in theft. Importantly, cash transfers permit recipients to increase their economic opportunity through the paths available in the environment, for instance, by enrolling in vocational training (Blattman & Niehaus, 2014). In contexts where people do not want or do not have access to vocational opportunities or ways to improve their self-control, cash transfers may prove not only ineffective but counterproductive. To paraphrase Pawson and Tilley (1997), the contextual shaping of a mechanism turns its causal potential into a causal outcome.

Although the visible context can shape psychological forces, the life space also contains subtle and even invisible elements that can act as a powerful constraint on motivational processes. Psychological states, unlike everyday physical objects, are not directly observable. In a physical context, it is easy to see how subtle factors, such as moisture, could interfere with the firing of an explosive mechanism in a rocket. But

in a social-psychological context, it can be hard for even a motivated teacher to detect that a student's mistrust is interfering with the "firing" of a motivational mechanism. A teacher may provide feedback on an essay, with the expectation that it will lead a student to improve it. The teacher may not realize that such feedback may be viewed with suspicion if students feel stereotyped as inferior, and thus fail to activate the motivation to act on it (Cohen et al., 2009; Yeager et al., 2014). Because of the subtlety of psychological elements in a context, predicting the effects of psychological interventions can be much harder than for interventions where the key contextual conditions are easily observable. For instance, when jurors deliberate during a legal case, they may appear to be simply discussing the facts of the case as they were presented to them. In reality, however, unseen forces exert a subtle yet powerful influence. Social norms and pressures tend to lead the members of the jury to recommend more extreme punitive damages than any single member would have endorsed independently (Sunstein, 2002). Many of the most influential forces in the social context are not directly observable. They can determine behavior and the effects of our attempts to change it.

MOTIVATIONAL MECHANISMS INTERACT WITH THE CONTEXT OVER TIME

How and when does a social experience such as an intervention have effects that persist? What makes experiences "stick" is a topic that has received scholarly attention (see Heath & Heath, 2008). The question dovetails with both developmental psychology's concern with formative experiences (Worthman, Plotsky, Schechter, & Cummings, 2010) and social psychology's concern with the formation of enduring psychological structures such as attitudes and identity (Aronson, 1968; Steele, 1988). As Lewin (1936) pointed out, situations by definition have a temporal dimension. But when does a situation begin and end? The comments parents make about their teenage daughters' weight can haunt them into adulthood, increasing their dissatisfaction with their bodies many years later (Wansink, Latimer, & Pope, 2016). A single experience of sexual harassment might affect expectations of workplace treatment for an entire career. In short, a situation can be understood at any number of time scales. Contemporary experimental research on motivation uses a time scale of about a half-hour, the time typically required to conduct a laboratory study. Much has been learned using this approach. But the full impact of a process is evident only over a long period of time. An event can have an influence that persists and even grows due to the concatenation of consequences that follows. The line that marks when a situation begins and when it ends depends on the temporal scale of one's analysis.

Widening the temporal lens provides a fuller understanding of psychological processes. The effect of a social interaction between a mentor and a student could be productively examined during the time it takes the utterance of a mentor to be encoded and processed in the student's brain, a matter of microseconds. One could stretch the period of examination to the time it takes for the mentor's utterances to evoke a behavioral response from the student, say a minute or two. One could also examine the interaction for days, observing how multiple interactions, by building a sense of trust, affect the student's ability and willingness to learn. Over years, one could observe how the social interaction, initially focused on building the student's skills, develops into a relationship that takes on a broader range of aims. At such longer time scales, certain moments or events, such as the offer of wisdom or an act of encouragement, may be recalled by the student again and again, fortifying motivation in times of difficulty for years to come. For instance, at-risk students who had engaged in a self-affirming writing activity in the early stages of college—identifying and reflecting on their most important personal values—did not just go on to earn higher grades. When prompted to think about stressors in school 2 years later, they were more likely to spontaneously call to mind self-affirming thoughts like the ones they had written at the start of their college career (Brady, Reeves, et al., 2016). At a long time scale, events that seem to have ended may live on in subjective experience.

How a long-range temporal horizon enriches the understanding of a process can be seen in a number of other studies. The young women who entered Bennington College in the 1930s on the whole were from prosperous and politically conservative families (Alwin, Cohen, & Newcomb, 1991). They may have entered Bennington because of any number of deliberate and random factors. But once there, they began a process of transformation, the effects of which were not limited to college but, for many, lasted the rest of their lives. Most of the students shifted sharply to the left in their political views during their 4 years of being immersed in the liberal college milieu. After graduating, many of these students chose to live in environments that reinforced their political views, befriending and marrying similarly liberal people. Five decades later, the former Bennington students were more likely than women with similar backgrounds to favor Mondale over the more conservative candidate Reagan in the 1984 U.S. presidential election.

In another study, disadvantaged children randomly assigned to participate in the Perry Preschool enrichment programs were more likely to earn higher scores on cognitive tests. Although these cognitive gains tended to fade over time, these children were more likely than their peers in the control condition to graduate from high school 15 years later (see Heckman, Moon, Pinto, Savelyev, & Yavitz, 2009, 2010). Decades later, they had higher earnings and less severe criminal records. Early enrichment seems to have these far-flung consequences when it improves children's relationship to the social environment (Woodhead, 1988). The children tend to project a more positive image to their teachers. They are less likely to be shunted into special education classes and labeled as deficient at a crucial time, when their identities in the academic system are being defined both by themselves and by others. Not only does a wide temporal lens advance an understanding of the process of change, but so does a wide spatial lens. Further data suggest that the mothers of the children who take part in such early enrichment programs also benefit. For instance, they are more likely to be employed when their children become teenagers and more likely to attain education beyond high school (Ramey et al., 2000; see also U.S. Government, 2014).

One can widen the temporal and spatial lens still further. For example, the expansion of educational opportunity to minority students due to the *Brown v. Board of Education* Supreme Court decision benefited not only their academic outcomes but those of their children and their children's children (Johnson, 2012). An assessment of an outcome at a given time provides only a snapshot of an ongoing process.

Even brief experiences can have effects that ripple through both space and time. An experiment with seventh graders revealed that a self-affirmation activity, which guided students to write about important personal values such as relationships and creativity, improved the grades of minority students, the group under the threat of negative stereotypes in school (Cohen, Garcia, Apfel, & Master, 2006). But, in addition, the intervention benefited the classroom as a whole (Powers et al., 2016). Adopting a wide spatial lens revealed that classrooms that, by chance, contained a larger number of minority students who had completed the affirmation writing exercise were higher performing. Regardless of whether they themselves received the intervention, the students in these classrooms earned higher grades. The improvement in performance for the affirmed minority students seems to have triggered a feedback loop, leading to higher achievement norms for the classroom as a whole. Adopting a wide temporal lens on the same study revealed that minority students who had been affirmed as seventh graders were more likely than their nonaffirmed peers to enroll in college years later (Goyer, Garcia, et al., 2016). Success at one transition promotes success at later transitions through a concatenation of consequences (Elder, 1998). The success need not be great. Simply avoiding the remedial track in middle school was a key step that kept affirmed minority students on the path to college (Goyer, Garcia, et al., 2016). As Lewin (1947) asserted, many processes are not simply linear with a discrete beginning and end. Rather, they are circular, with new consequences accumulating with each cycle.

In our model of how outcomes are generated and propagated through time, the "twin engines" of the psychological system and the social system interact with one another to drive the process (Figure 35.2). Our model

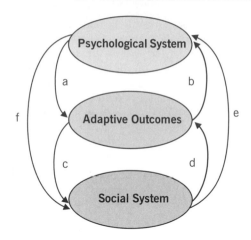

FIGURE 35.2. A field theoretic view of the status quo. Outputs of one system feed back as inputs into the other, producing continuity through time. Adapted from Cohen and Sherman's (2014) cycle of adaptive potential. Examples of paths include Path a: self-affirmed, student performs better; Path b: performing better, student feels more self-affirmed; Path c: because student performs better, teachers and peers treat student differently; Path d: different treatment from teachers and peers elicits higher performance from student; Path e: teachers and peers affirm the student (e.g., through positive feedback, social approval); Path f: the psychology of the student alters the social system through variables other than adaptive outcomes (e.g., by affecting student's mood, speech, nonverbal behavior). From Cohen and Sherman (2014, p. 341). Copyright © 2014 Annual Reviews. Adapted with permission.

draws on Lewin's (1939) field theory (see Cohen & Sherman, 2014). People are enveloped by many contexts making up the social system. These include institutional, cultural, and historical contexts (Bronfenbrenner, 1977). The social and psychological systems each include powerful processes that can transform small inputs into large outputs. The constant interaction of the two systems creates and maintains outcomes through time.

Our model suggests that what it means to scale up an intervention needs to be expanded. It has both a *temporal* and a spatial dimension. Effects should be assessed over an appropriately wide breadth of both time and space. This expanded view requires resources, commitment, and patience to assess the effects of an intervention through time. The goal is to come "to explanatory grips with interactions involving time" (Cronbach, 1975, p. 123): to map the processes that turn early differences in experience and temperament into large differences in life trajectory (Caspi, Elder, & Bem, 1987; Mischel, 2014; Moffitt et al., 2011; Worthman et al., 2010).

Beyond its potential to enrich theory, such a wide-angle lens in the study of motivational processes serves two practical goals. First, it provides a unique vantage point from which to view the connections within systems that produce stable outcomes across time and space. These outcomes can take the form of persistent and wide-ranging inequalities. Second, a wide-angle lens deepens an understanding of how complex systems unfold over time, and through this, permits one to gain a better sense of whether and when to intervene. This is important because there are times and places that can negate the effects of an intervention, as well as times and places that maximize its impact. When aligned to such leverage points, an intervention can have large and long-lasting effects that seem disproportionate to its size or duration.

Our model departs from a common view that ascribes long-term impacts of an intervention or experience primarily to the assets it generates in the person. This view can tempt consumers of research, particularly policymakers and practitioners, to believe that the causal force behind any long-term effects of an intervention must rest in some internal asset it created, such as cognitive aptitude, self-control, or grit. However, there is no necessary reason to think that causality is driven by a force solely within an actor. Causal force emerges from the ongoing dance between person and context. A situation presents itself; the person reacts; the situation reacts back; and the cycle repeats (Cohen & Sherman, 2014).

The literature on self-control yields a result that, while paradoxical in relation to the asset view, resonates with ours. Although adult outcomes such as higher socioeconomic status and fewer criminal convictions are predicted by childhood measures of self-control (Moffitt et al., 2011), self-control has been found to be malleable rather than fixed. Situational interventions,

such as having children take on the role of a favorite superhero, like Superman, can dramatically increase self-control and persistence (Karniol et al., 2011; White & Carlson, 2016; White et al., in press). Moreover, if self-control is acting as a singular causal factor, it should prove highly correlated with itself through time. It appears not to be. Only a modest correlation exists between self-control when measured at age 10 and self-control when measured at age 26 (Moffitt et al., 2011), even though self-control at age 10 correlates at a similar magnitude with larger and more distal criminal outcomes at age 32 (A. Caspi, personal communication, May 18, 2016).

Is it possible for a trait that is both malleable and only modestly stable over time to be the singular cause of an enduring life trajectory? It is unlikely. Causal force issues out of the interactions between the person and the context through time. A brief instance of low self-control, such as an impulsive decision, can be harmless or it can ensnare people in a negative life trajectory, depending on the context in which it occurs (Caspi et al., 1987). A wealthy couple that has an unplanned baby often has sufficient bandwidth and resources to provide for the child, and in many cases can continue on the life trajectory they had been pursuing (see Mullainathan & Shafir, 2013). By contrast, a low-income female adolescent, without such supports, who makes the same impulsive decision will face a constriction of career opportunities (Moffitt et al., 2011), which in turn will tend to reduce the opportunities available to her child as well.

The role of context in modifying the long-range impact of childhood experiences, including interventions, has long been acknowledged in transactional models of social development. Among the most compelling articulations comes from Woodhead (1988). Though he writes about the effects and effectiveness of preschool enrichment programs, his words apply just as aptly to any social intervention.

> The process of long-term effectiveness does not appear to be like a marathon 15-year test of the stamina of a single runner. Rather, it resembles a relay race, in which the burst of superior performance in the first runner (such as cognitive abilities and social adjustment)

soon fades but not before the baton has been passed to later runners on the team (such as parent and teacher expectations, avoidance of referral to special classes, and so on), each of which transmits and even increases that initial superiority. (p. 448)

SOCIAL-PSYCHOLOGICAL INTERVENTIONS: THE PRINCIPLE OF TRIGGER AND CHANNEL

Any timely act, in the right time and place, can create a turning point. In our model, an intervention does not have to be a dedicated program, set of activities, or curriculum. It can be any purposeful attempt to change people. It can range from the everyday mini-interventions we all practice, such as offering advice or feedback, to the large-scale efforts involving many people and resources undertaken by schools, workplaces, and states. Most interventions, regardless of their form, introduce at least one novel element. The new element introduced by social-psychological interventions, if effective, energizes people by triggering a motivational process. The energy is then channeled by the context into new behaviors.

It is because of the intervention's meaning that its initial spark occurs. Like most human behaviors, interventions are symbolic acts. Regardless of their size or duration, their impact depends on the meaning they have. The consequences flowing from a behavior, such as the blink of an eyelid, depend on what it is taken to mean. Is that blink seen as a nervous twitch or a conspiratorial wink (Geertz, 1973; Ryle, 1971/2009)? If the first, it may cause avoidance. If the second, it may kindle a relationship that lasts a lifetime. The same is true of interventions. Their consequences flow from their meaning. For example, the impact of a teacher's constructive criticism depends on how students interpret it. Compliance is more likely if students see the criticism as motivated by the teacher's belief in their ability to reach a higher standard rather than by bias against them (Cohen, Steele, & Ross, 1999; Yeager et al., 2014). Social-psychological interventions often begin by successfully transmitting a meaning. This new meaning, or lens for viewing experiences, is often more important for bringing about change than the intervention's size or duration. Even small acts, when processed by the psychological system, can take on powerful meanings that in turn prompt large change. For example, ethnic-minority teenagers were highly influenced by a one-sentence note from their teacher asserting his belief in their potential to reach a higher standard. Because of it, they not only complied more with their teacher's feedback but also received fewer disciplinary citations in school (Yeager et al., 2014; Yeager, Purdie-Vaughns, Yang, & Cohen, in press).

To return to the notion of synchronicity, it is the confluence of a meaning with an appropriate person, time, and place that is critical: The right message "falls" into a person's life at the moment it matters (Jung, 1952). Because this confluence would seldom occur under the status quo, it can activate assets that were previously inert. For instance, the status quo view in education is that underperformance reflects deficits in students' skill or motivation. The status quo policy that follows is to place underperforming students in remedial programs to address their presumed deficits. However, underperformance can also be a by-product of the school situation. Some students, labeled as "limited," are cut off from positive messages and opportunities. This new view has led to interventions that do virtually the opposite of the approach that predominates under the status quo. They place underperforming students in an honors program. Such programs convey the message that students do not lack skill but rather are seen as capable of reaching a higher standard. Interventions using this high-expectation approach have yielded remarkable gains in the academic achievement of at-risk youth (for reviews, see Cohen et al., 1999; Dweck, Walton, & Cohen, 2011; Steele, 1997). Here, the intervention is an inflection of the standard situation, the effect of which is to activate previously hidden potentials.

In the absence of intervention, the status quo repeatedly regenerates itself. The same forces repeatedly converge in functionally similar situations. Test-taking situations in school provide a glimpse into how this process can play out. Standardized tests are implicitly and sometimes explicitly represented as measures of intellectual aptitude. This representation, which gives legitimacy to the test, is an environmental force. Psychological factors also help to perpetuate the status quo. What is being evaluated is *believed* to be competence on a trait deemed to be fixed and critical to success. A host of psychological processes, ranging from downward social comparison to stereotyping, come to play when people interpret scores from such tests. Indeed, historically, the tests have been misused to provide evidence of the alleged inferiority of different groups. This is not merely distant history but part of the present psychological reality for people being tested. European American students appear to perform better on these tests in part because of stereotype lift, an implicit awareness that these tests favor their racial group (Walton & Cohen, 2003). At the same time, members of negatively stereotyped groups, such as African Americans and Latino Americans, and women in math and science, tend to experience stereotype threat. Aware that their performance could be seen as confirmation of a negative stereotype about their group, they experience extra stress that impedes their performance on difficult tests (Steele, 2010; Steele, Spencer, & Aronson, 2002). Thus, psychology pulls the larger forces of culture and history into the everyday school ritual of the test-taking situation. This configuration of the situation weakens the influence of positive forces for minority students in general, and for women in math and science. It prevents their true academic aptitude from expressing itself. For when placed in a situation that temporarily frees them from stereotype threat, they perform much better, outperforming European Americans and men with similar records of past accomplishment (Walton & Spencer, 2009).

Achievement gaps are persistent because, like many persistent outcomes, a situation repeatedly regenerates them. The test-taking situation repeatedly recurs in school. But if its situational forces are reconfigured, achievement gaps lessen and sometimes vanish. To paraphrase Sapolsky (2010), the status quo can be persistent yet plastic.

Trigger

By introducing a new element into a situation, many social-psychological interventions trigger a motivational process, with its behavioral manifestation shaped by the context. A series of large-scale studies presented incoming college students with one of a variety of social-psychological interventions delivered through a series of online modules (Yeager et al., 2016). The interventions tapped into a process that was expected to sustain students' resilience in the face of difficulty. One intervention conveyed to students that difficulty in school was normal and apt to be short-lived. This permitted them to attribute it to situational factors that were both common to all students and surmountable (see Walton & Cohen, 2011). Another intervention encouraged students to conceptualize intelligence as expandable with effort and practice (see Dweck, 1999). This prompted them to attribute difficulty to the need to expend more effort or find better strategies. Each intervention triggered an attributional process. It lead students to attribute the inevitable challenges of college to a natural adjustment process rather than a deficit in them. When led to this outlook, academically at-risk students, such as negatively stereotyped ethnic-minority students, as well as economically disadvantaged students, e-mailed their professors and joined study groups more, acts that they may have otherwise shunned as evidence of their inadequacy (see Walton & Cohen, 2007).

The germination of the cognitive seeds introduced by the interventions blossomed into a belief structure (see McGuire, 1960). As students acquire firsthand evidence that they can meet the challenges of college, the belief that they belong tends to strengthen. Indeed, this is what appears to have happened both for at-risk minority students and for economically disadvantaged students receiving the interventions (Yeager et al., 2016). The students in one study were more likely to maintain full-enrollment status in their freshman year, an effect driven by the extent to which they used campus resources. Likewise, in an earlier study, at-risk students who had received a similar intervention that protected their sense of belonging in the freshman year of college earned higher grade-point averages (GPAs) throughout their 4 years on campus and, in their final year of college, reported stronger certainty that they belonged in college (Walton &

Cohen, 2011). The dance between the psychological and social systems can alter a trajectory (Figure 35.2). Students' confidence increases as a result of the intervention. They seize opportunities for growth in the environment, which, if well functioning, recognizes and reinforces their efforts. As they see their capacities grow, their confidence strengthens still more in a cycle of adaptive potential (Cohen & Sherman, 2014). The cycle requires both the student and the environment to recognize and act on the assets in each other.

Beyond the attributional process, the self-affirmation process can also be triggered by intervention. This is the process that maintains the perceived integrity or "adequacy" of the self. When that perception is threatened, people try to reaffirm it. Events that appear small can have surprisingly large effects when they serve as inputs into this process. For instance, the act of writing briefly about an important personal value, such as relationships or religion, is an objectively small action that can nevertheless be subjectively large and have a counterintuitively large impact (Steele, 1988; see also Cohen & Sherman, 2014). Signaling one's fidelity to long-held values, the act can convey that one is "moral" and "good" in a way that transcends a threatening situation. After being affirmed in this way, people no longer showed a rise in the stress hormone cortisol when compelled to give an impromptu speech in front of a judgment audience (Creswell et al., 2005). Those under chronic stress maintained higher performance on a creative problem-solving task when being evaluated under time pressure (Creswell, Dutcher, Klein, Harris, & Levine, 2013). From an outsider's perspective, the intervention seems mysteriously powerful, a small act that triggers a large effect. However, from the insider's perspective, the intervention taps into a strong psychological need. The intervention is only a trigger for a powerful process. What influence it has is dependent on the fact that it helps people enact the self-affirmation process already present in their minds.

Beyond attribution and self-affirmation, many other psychological processes can release motivational energy. Interpersonal mechanisms, which involve multiple minds, can also be activated by intervention. An example is the "self-fulfilling prophecy." People's initial beliefs, even if erroneous, can affect their behaviors in ways that turn the belief into a reality. In a classic study, elementary school teachers were told that a subset of their students had been identified as "intellectual bloomers" based on testing (Rosenthal & Jacobson, 2003). In fact, however, they had been selected randomly. Teachers adopted positive expectations for these students, which they then acted on. It appears, for instance, that they invested greater attention and displayed more positive affect toward students labeled as having high potential. The teachers' actions in turn elicited better performance from these students. By year's end, those positively labeled earned higher IQ scores than their peers. The effectiveness of the intervention did not issue out of the causal power of the few sentences given to teachers about the students. Rather, it rested in the psychological and social mechanisms triggered by them.

Channel

Once a motivational mechanism is triggered, the context gives the mechanism its behavioral form and can keep it active through time. Most of the elements in a context exist prior to an intervention's introduction, as in a classroom or workplace. To be effective, an intervention needs to be well placed and well timed in this context. It should be introduced near elements that prevent the interference of inhibiting forces and that channel its effects in the desired direction. Positive behavioral change happens when the mechanism resonates or "gels" with the context (Pawson & Tilley, 1997).

As an analogy, a rocket both triggers and channels the explosive mechanism in liquid hydrogen (Dawson & Bowles, 2004; Pawson & Tilley, 1997). As with many psychological and social systems, liquid hydrogen has many powerful latent assets. For instance, it is both lightweight and burns at extremely high temperatures. Yet for this potential to be actualized as a powerful rocket propellant, it needs to be appropriately channeled and "tamed" by the surrounding context, the rocket. A small change, such as engine exhaust or air friction during flight, could undermine the hydrogen's effectiveness, causing it to evaporate. The rocket is carefully designed to minimize the influence of such external factors on the explosive process. The process is insulated from sources of heat, and its explosive effects are effectively channeled by the rocket nozzle. This phenomenon finds an echo in the realm of psychological interventions. Even relatively subtle forces in a situation, if not checked, can determine an intervention's course and effectiveness.

In contrast to the common view of interventions, a social-psychological intervention is not a remedy unto itself, but a trigger, a catalyst for a process that can then be repeatedly refueled by the context. For example, consider the positive impact on learning and performance of brief "growth mindset" interventions that teach people to see intelligence as an expandable entity rather than a limiting factor (Aronson, Fried, & Good, 2002; Blackwell, Trzesniewski, & Dweck, 2007; Good, Aronson, & Inzlicht, 2003; Yeager et al., 2016). Like all interventions, these do not work in a vacuum but through their interactions with the social context. Examining its impact among first-year college students revealed that it encouraged students to become more involved on campus (Yeager et al., 2016, Study 2). Students who benefited from the intervention most were those who made a relationship with a faculty mentor, joined a campus organization, made friends with students in their building, or availed themselves of services to help them with their studies. A psychological outcome was prompted by the intervention, the belief that one can and will succeed with effort. Students were impelled by this belief to seek out and use the available institutional channels to meet their goals. Using institutional resources and achieving more success can strengthen students' belief in their capacity for further success, leading them to avail themselves of more resources and take on still more challenges. The intervention triggers a psychological process. But its effects on achievement depend on the environmental channels to learn, get help, and advance.

Given this analysis, motivation can be seen less as an internal asset and more as "momentum" (Core, 2014; see also Schwartz, Cheng, Salehi, & Wieman, 2016).

Reciprocal interactions between psychology and situation propel the actor forward. The cycle increases its velocity as psychological assets and environmental opportunity fuel one another. A "motivated" student in this sense is "riding a wave." The intervention helps the student get started. Once high velocity is achieved, minor obstacles have less of a disruptive effect, much as a bicyclist is less likely to be derailed by small bumps at high velocities (Schwartz et al., 2016). Momentum relies as much, if not more, on the structure of the institution as on the psychology of the actor. The institution must offer a channel in the form of a series of opportunities in order for a growth mindset or a sense of belonging to assert an enduring influence on behavior. Absent opportunities to take on new challenges and to acquire necessary support, psychological interventions would act like a flickering flame without kindling. In one study, college students who received an intervention that provided them with a sense of optimism and control over their academic outcomes subsequently performed better on a lecture-based achievement test, but only when the intervention was accompanied with effective teaching (Menec et al., 2006). To keep up motivation or momentum over time, an institution must provide new opportunities for growth and challenge. A channel is not a treadmill. The institution must also keep the intervention's message credible. For example, if opportunities for growth are absent, or if teachers repeatedly praise ability instead of effort, the message that "intelligence can grow" will likely ring hollow. In short, psychological preparation is not enough. People must be able to catch a wave of facilitating processes in an environment rather than fight a tide of countervailing ones. A dearth of positive processes for attaining momentum is one of the reasons why the benefits of an intervention can be short-lived.

Situating an intervention at the right time and place in a given context is critical to the principle of channeling. Seemingly small variations in when or where an intervention is situated can have big effects. For example, in the earlier example of self-affirmation interventions, timing matters. If a values affirmation activity is completed before threatening information is given, it can lessen defensiveness and increase openness. But if the same activity occurs after the threatening information, it may instead strengthen people's confidence in the defensive rationalization they generated to dismiss the information (see Critcher, Dunning, & Armor, 2010). Likewise, in the research on the self-fulfilling prophecy, information about students' academic potential had little effect when given to teachers several weeks into the school year rather than at its beginning (Raudenbusch, 1984). Presumably, teachers' impressions of students, once formed, are hard to change. In each case, a seemingly small variation, like a leak of hydrogen into small holes in the rocket's seams, introduces a factor that negates the intervention's impact.

The trigger and channel approach is illustrated by an experiment in which a random group of seniors in an urban high school received a values affirmation near the time of the deadline to apply for financial aid for college (Fotuhi, Garcia, & Cohen, 2016). This is a threatening and stressful time. The intervention was intended to trigger the self-affirmation mechanism so that feelings of threat would be lessened. Additionally, a treatment designed to open a channel for the desired behavioral response was crossed with the values affirmation. Some of the students received a few reminders, delivered via a mobile application (app), about specific steps they could take to obtain financial aid. Thus, the context was engineered so that the psychological effects of the affirmation—less stress and more bandwidth to focus on long-term goals (Mullainathan & Shafir, 2013)—could be directed to an appropriate behavior. Indeed, it was the combination of affirmation and reminders that produced the highest rate of financial aid awarded, doubling the percentage of those receiving financial aid, from 39 to 78%. Those receiving only the affirmation or only the reminders did not show as strong a benefit.

THE THREE *T*'S OF INTERVENTION: TARGETED, TAILORED, AND TIMELY

The trigger and channel perspective on interventions calls for three necessary actions. An intervention must be targeted, tailored,

and timely. The right person receives the right support at the right time. When this occurs, what would otherwise have been a transient or trivial experience becomes a turning point. An intervention, far from being a product to pack up and scale up to all classrooms, workplaces, or hospitals, has a power that derives from the instant in which it occurs.

Targeted: The Right Person

When an effective intervention is discovered, there is a temptation to "mass vaccinate" and disseminate it as widely as possible. But as with most medical treatments, a psychological treatment should be given to those who need it rather than delivered indiscriminately. A key lesson of research on social-psychological interventions is that their benefits are often moderated, concentrated among a subgroup rather than spread across a population. This is unsurprising given that most of the interventions were designed to meet specific kinds of needs. The benefits of values affirmation interventions, for instance, are confined to people experiencing psychological threat. Those likely to benefit from them include people working in a stressful situation, patients dealing with a medical condition, students contending with threatening negative stereotypes about them, and students with a history of poor performance (Cohen & Sherman, 2014). Moreover, affirmations not only are ineffective in the absence of threat (Hanselman, Bruch, Gamoran, & Borman, 2014) but, like a wrongly prescribed medicine, may also prove counterproductive for some. The act of reflecting on cherished values might lead people to disengage from a task if they feel that their efforts might be better invested elsewhere (see Critcher et al., 2010; Vohs, Park, & Schmeichel, 2013). Online modules that teach a growth mindset, a belief in the malleable nature of intelligence, are another example of moderated interventions. Their benefits tend to be concentrated among the lowest-performing students (Paunesku et al., 2015). Likewise, it is primarily teenagers with low expectations for academic success who benefit from interventions that help them to connect their schoolwork to important issues in their lives (Hulleman,

Godes, Hendricks, & Harackiewicz, 2010; Hulleman & Harackiewicz, 2009). In the pioneering research of Timothy Wilson and colleagues (Wilson, Damiani, & Shelton, 2002; Wilson & Linville, 1982), the benefits of directing attributions for poor performance to unstable rather than stable causes tend to be confined to students who worry about doing well in school. Adding to this complexity, the effect of a moderator can itself be moderated (Cronbach, 1975). In one large-scale study, the positive impact of a values affirmation intervention on middle schoolers' GPA was, consistent with past research, concentrated among stereotyped minority students (Hanselman et al., 2014). However, this was especially true in schools where threatening stereotypes were more salient, that is, schools with fewer minority students and larger achievement gaps between ethnic groups.

Given the complexity of the effects that interventions can have, the best way to maximize their effectiveness and efficiency is to target those people who will most benefit from them. Most of the time, they should be administered not as mass vaccinations but as thoughtfully prescribed treatments. This is for two reasons. First, as a matter of efficiency, it is a waste of time and resources to administer treatments to those who do not benefit from them. Second, as a matter of ethics, the potential benefits of an intervention need to be greater than its potential costs. Because interventions may have foreseeable and unforeseeable side effects, their indiscriminant use should be discouraged.

Tailored: The Right Support

In order for a suit to be comfortable and look good, it should be the right size, style, and color, that is, tailored to the individual wearing it. Like a well-fitting suit, an intervention must be tailored to "fit" in order to be most effective. It must address the motivational mechanism that matters in a given situation. Given that research and lay wisdom suggest that rewards can spark motivation, it is easy to see how they can come to be overused (Skinner, 1969). In fact, people's motivations can be undermined when they are rewarded for doing an activity they already want to do. For instance, when children who enjoyed

drawing with magic markers were offered a "Good Player Certificate" to use them, the amount of time they devoted to that activity 2 weeks later was cut in half (Lepper, 1973). A "one-size-fits-all" assumption is evident in the large and popular scaling up of incentive programs to boost academic achievement (e.g., Fryer, 2011). They assume that what causes underperformance is the same for most students. Perhaps the mixed results of such programs arise from the insistence on widespread dissemination issuing from this assumption. Their effectiveness might be increased if the target were more specific: students lacking intrinsic interest. Our success would be increased, moreover, if we tailored interventions to the diverse array of motivational barriers actually affecting students. In general, poor tailoring of interventions comes from an inaccurate or overgeneralized theory of the underlying psychology at work.

Research on the minority achievement gap in college provides another example of the importance of tailoring interventions. Basic research showed that compared to European American students, African American students tend to see social adversity in school, such as difficulty finding friends, as a sign that others do not want to include them in constructive social relationships due to their race (Walton & Cohen, 2007). For these students, social adversity raises the possibility that they do not belong. When, for instance, African American and European American college students were asked to name eight of their friends in an academic discipline like computer science, most of them had difficulty doing so (Walton & Cohen, 2007). However, the difficulty caused only the African Americans to feel that they lacked belonging and had little potential to succeed there. In another study, college students were asked to record in a daily diary the events that happened to them (Walton & Cohen, 2007). Roughly equal numbers of bad things happened to African American and European American students, such as not being invited to dinner or getting negative feedback in a class. For European American students there was no relationship between these bad events and their sense of social belonging in school. For African Americans, on the other hand, these bad events correlated with a lack of social belonging. African American students appeared to be more likely than European American students to see adversity not as an isolated event but as a global judgment of their fit on campus. They experienced a process of "belonging uncertainty" based on their awareness of prejudice against their racial group.

An intervention that emerged out of this line of basic research was tailored to address the "question of belonging" that African Americans were experiencing in college (Walton & Cohen, 2007, 2011). In a brief laboratory session, students in their freshman year learned that most upperclassmen at their school had also wondered about whether they belonged in college as freshmen. Students read survey statistics and testimonials that conveyed how such concerns were normal and common across racial and gender lines. They also learned that, with time, such concerns tend to fade as students make friends and find their niche on campus. Procedural steps helped students to internalize the message. They were told to make the message "their own" by putting the key themes they learned into their own words (Aronson et al., 2002). They then used their version of the message as the basis of a video they made to help future students adjust to college. This procedure permitted these students to see themselves as agents of change rather than merely candidates for remediation. The results were striking. Relative to a randomized control condition, the intervention improved the GPA of African American students. It reduced the achievement gap over 4 years by more than half. African American students also showed better subjective health at the end of college, and years after graduation they reported being happier and more engaged at work (Brady, Fotuhi, Gomez, Cohen, & Walton, 2016).

In directly addressing a psychological question shown by previous research to be a concern for minority students, the intervention blocked a mechanism that would have undermined their motivation in school. The appropriateness of the message delivered by the intervention was critical, as even an apparently similar message would have failed. For instance, conveying to students that it was normal and transitory to have doubts about one's *ability*, as did another

intervention, had no effect at all on African Americans (Walton & Cohen, 2011). A teacher, parent, or seasoned tutor (Lepper & Woolverton, 2002) providing just the right word of encouragement to a child captures the essence of tailored interventions: Knowledge informs action to maximize effectiveness.

Timely: The Right Time and Place

The timeliness of an intervention can matter as much as its content. A pat on the back before an important game or a bit of advice before a critical health decision can create a turning point. But the same encouragement or advice given days earlier might recede in memory to a mere whisper when the behavioral channel opens, or, if given after, prove to be too little too late. A parent pushing a child on a swing must exert force at the appropriate place, in the appropriate direction, and at the appropriate time. Even a minimal push applied by a parent at the apogee of the child's backward arc will keep the child happily aloft. However, a push applied just moments before may not only interfere with the swing but result in injury to the child (and the parent).

Likewise, a small act of encouragement can have large effects when timed to a moment of need. People regularly ask themselves questions such as "Do I belong?," "Can I do it?," and "Am I valued?" Answering such questions in the affirmative takes on added urgency at moments of high stakes, such as during the transition to college or at the start of a new job. At such gateways are many forces that could propel a person in either a positive or a negative direction (Lewin, 1939). But once one passes through a gateway, often with some timely support, many of the forces in the system serve to propel people forward.

When are the opportune moments to intervene in the social world? One answer is at the time when key cognitions and behaviors arise. Behaviorism, in spite of its flaws, provided a key insight when it asserted that timeliness matters. To produce an effective reinforcement contingency, a reinforcement must occur shortly after the production of the desired behavior. Similarly, to support people through a difficult time, an intervention must occur near the moment when a psychological vulnerability occurs. "Do I belong?," "Why did this happen?," or "Can I do it?" are questions that require a supportive answer the moment that they arise. The importance of timeliness is illustrated in research testing a growth mindset intervention in the context of an educational video (O'Rourke, Haimovitz, Ballwebber, Dweck, & Popović, 2014). A growth mindset message given to children before they played the game had, if anything, a negative impact on their persistence and performance. On the other hand, when the message that intelligence can grow was built into the fabric of the game, timed to the mindset-related actions and cognitions of the learners, persistence and performance improved. The game rewarded new strategies and extra effort, so that children could interpret their entire experience with the game as being "about" growth. Likewise, expert tutors, who consistently produce gains in the learning of at-risk youth in excess of two standard deviations, provide a model of appropriately timed intervention (Bloom, 1984; Lepper & Woolverton, 2002). These tutors use not one strategy but many strategies, each targeted to their students' needs and enacted at the moment it is needed. At the start of a session, a tutor might spend a lot of time getting to know the child through questions about his or her hobbies, thus creating rapport. Then, before a child confronts a challenging problem, the tutor might say, "This next one will be hard." This utterance helps to structure the child's expectations so that he or she attributes the difficulty to the rigor of the work rather than a personal failing. As these examples illustrate, the ultimate aim is for messages of growth, belonging, and affirmation to occur synchronously with their need, something taken for granted as part of the classroom or workplace culture, rather than simply "shots in the arm" (Lewin, 1939).

Beginnings often mark an opportune time to intervene. Transitions into a new environment or role, such as the transition to middle school, college, a new job, and parenthood, mark an important beginning. The outcomes of such a transition, as life-course theorists have suggested, can shape the outcome of later transitions by giving rise to an accumulation of consequences (Elder, 1998). This is especially true when the transition is characterized by a rise in stress and psychological threat, as many transitions throughout the life course are (Crosnoe & Johnson, 2011; Johnson, Crosnoe, & Elder, 2011; Pattwell, Casey, & Lee, 2013). Helping people to cope adaptively with such transitions can yield benefits that compound with time.

In a study touched on earlier, a psychological intervention, a values affirmation writing activity, was given at the beginning of the transition to seventh grade (Cohen et al., 2006, 2009). This is a turbulent time, when many students take a negative turn. Academic motivation and performance tends to decline, while risk behavior rises, especially for negatively stereotyped minority students (Cohen et al., 2006, 2009; Eccles, Lord, & Midgley, 1991; Simmons, Black, & Zhou, 1991). For these students, the intervention led to higher GPAs compared to a control condition. It also bolstered their sense of belonging in school, such that it remained high even when they received a low grade (Cook, Purdie-Vaughns, Garcia, & Cohen, 2012). The benefits persisted through the remaining 2 years of middle school. Moreover, 7 years later, official college enrollment records revealed that affirmation-treated minority students were both more likely to enroll in college and, if they enrolled in a 4-year college, more likely to go to a selective one (Goyer, Garcia, et al., 2016). Interventions that promote college enrollment and persistence like this one deserve special consideration (see also Yeager et al., 2016) because college attendance and graduation are powerful drivers of economic mobility (Douglass, 2009; Haskins, 2008; Reardon, Baker, & Klasik, 2012) and health (Braveman, Egerter, & Williams, 2011; Egerter, Braveman, Sadegh-Nobari, Grossman-Kahn, & Dekker, 2011). Indeed, earning a bachelor's degree is worth $2.8 million in lifetime earnings, 84% more than is earned when one holds only a high school diploma (Carnevale, Rose, & Cheah, 2011).

Longitudinal analysis of how the intervention propagated its influence revealed that it did so through the consequences it set in motion for students at the transition to seventh grade. By earning higher grades at the beginning of middle school, minority students were less likely to be assigned to the remedial track (Cohen et al., 2009) and more likely to be assigned to advanced courses on the college track (Goyer, Garcia, et al., 2016). Indeed, the intervention occurred at a moment when institutional tracking commenced and carried students into increasingly divergent streams of opportunity. As a consequence, affirmed minority students were more likely both to build up a strong academic record and to experience a high sense of belonging in school, especially relative to minority students who had been placed in the remedial track (Goyer, Garcia, et al., 2016). These in turn predicted a greater likelihood of entering college. The consequences of a successful middle school transition seemed to accumulate and stretch into the college transition. Although the start of seventh grade seems to be a brief situation, it can also be seen as the beginning of an institutional situation that lasts for a long time.

Transitions introduce new social systems. Their intricacies can be hard to understand, their consequences still harder to appreciate. These social systems can magnify the consequences of psychological processes. The transition to middle school often marks the beginning of academic tracking, a social reality that is key to understanding the affirmation intervention's long-term effects. Even narrowly avoiding the cutoff for entry into the remedial track can bring about a different academic fate for students, as remediation appears to be among the strongest drivers of unequal opportunity among minority youth (Grubb, 2009; Steele, 1997). The potential for even small performance differences to have dramatic and lasting consequences can be seen in research on institutional cutoffs (Dee, Dobbie, Jacob, & Rockoff, 2016). Students in the state of New York must pass the five core Regents exams in order to graduate from high school, by earning at least a score of 65 on each. Until recently, teachers in students' school could grade their exams. For roughly 40% of students with scores just below the cutoff (scores of 60–64), teachers changed their scores to a passing grade. A series of recent reforms to prohibit both local scoring and the rescoring of scores just below the cutoff appears to have eliminated such flexibility entirely. A quasi-experimental "difference

in differences" analysis indicates that once these reforms were in place, for students with scores in the changeable range, high school graduation rates fell by 3–5%. This happened in spite of the fact that students could retake the exam several times. The strict enforcement of the institutional cutoff turned small variations in test performance into a turning point. Whether a student received a high school diploma, and entered the life channel of opportunities that follow from it, turned on a few exam points. In the context of powerful institutional systems, even minor and psychologically driven differences in performance at key junctures can have life-shaping effects.

Because small initial differences can magnify in a system with feedback loops, even subtle variations in timing can have powerful effects at the beginning of key transitions. In another study, a seemingly minor difference in the timing of the affirmation was experimentally manipulated, again with middle schoolers (Cook et al., 2012). A random subset of students received the intervention in the first week of school in seventh grade rather than 4 weeks later, as had been standard. Strikingly, the positive effect of timing on first-quarter classroom grades was as great as the effect documented in prior research of providing the intervention or not. These findings underscore the importance of the timeliness of an intervention, and how it can matter as much as its occurrence.

Endings, transitioning *out* of an environment, also mark opportune times for intervention. Retirement from a career and graduation from high school or college tend to trigger cognitive consolidation. People focus on larger meanings and prepare for what comes next by thinking about the lessons learned from what occurred before (see Carstensen, Isaacowitz, & Charles, 1999; Hackman, 1998). One study focused on disadvantaged students transitioning out of a high-expectation charter high school. These senior students, on the verge of graduation and about to embark on the path to college, were given a social belonging intervention. It reassured them that it was normal to worry about whether they belonged in college, and that such worries were likely to be short-lived (Yeager et al., 2016). Compared to a randomized control condition, these students proved significantly more likely to stay enrolled in college full-time throughout their freshman year. This study demonstrates that not only are the beginnings of transitions opportune times to intervene, but so are their endings.

Choicepoints are moments when the decisions that people make can launch them onto a new course. These also mark opportune times to intervene. The decision to take the next course in an introductory physics sequence, for example, increases the likelihood that people enter a track toward a physical science degree (Goyer, Stout, et al., 2016). Many factors may be involved in such a choice. In fact, at least for those experiencing a certain amount of ambivalence about the decision, seemingly irrelevant issues, such as whether a friend will also be taking the course, or the posters on the wall, can drive their choice (Cheryan, Plaut, Davies, & Steele, 2009). One study reinforced gender stereotypes of women being bad at math by exposing them to a commercial that depicted them stereotypically. Women seeing such a commercial expressed much lower interest in careers in math and science than women who had not viewed it. Although a choice may seem an act of free will, it can be controlled by gender stereotypes and socialization (Bem & Bem, 1973). This idea gained additional support in a field experiment involving female students enrolled in an introductory physics course at a large state university (Goyer, Stout, et al., 2016; see also Miyake et al., 2010). Students were randomly assigned to complete a values affirmation in their introductory physics class. Women completing the affirmation, relative to their female peers in a control condition, earned better exam scores in the class. Moreover, the intervention was most beneficial over the long term for women with strong preparation, as assessed by their math standardized test scores, and those who expressed relatively more concern with negative gender stereotypes. If affirmed, these women were more likely to take the next physics course in the sequence for physical science majors, and to still bc cnrolled in engineering and physical sciences majors 2 years later. Affirmation had similar positive effects on continued enrollment in a biology track for first-generation college students (Harackiewicz et al., 2014). The long-term effects of many events, experiences, and character traits occur because they launch people onto divergent trajectories through the choices they make.

To target, tailor, and time an intervention appropriately requires that one understand the key elements in the context. In educational and work contexts, these include environmental elements such as institutional tracking systems and psychological elements such as hope and optimism. These can add momentum to a small win or early success. Because of the complexity of social systems, it is impossible to understand all the key elements in a context that help an intervention to "catch fire." Still, the crucial ones, the fuel, can be identified. Among the most important of these are the gateways and pathways to success (Chugh & Brief, 2008).

IMPLICATIONS

Look Beneath Behavior

One key lesson gained from the research reviewed here is the importance of observation. Other people's psychology is not directly accessible, so we must be especially attuned to the first-person perspective of the people we are trying to serve, the actor's perspective (Ross & Nisbett, 2011). We can do this by any number of observational methods such as ethnography and interviews.

The importance of observation was demonstrated in one set of studies conducted in middle school (Yeager et al., in press). Students' level of trust in school was observed for 3 years. Sixth graders reported high levels of trust, and minority and nonminority students did not differ. The seventh grade, however, marked a turning point. In the spring of that year, trust declined sharply. This was especially true for African American students, the predominant minority group at the school. Around this time, children begin to generate general theories about the trustworthiness of institutions based on the events that happen to them (Goyer, Cohen, et al., 2016; Yeager et al., in press). Discipline rates also jumped at this point, again especially for African Americans. This pattern was replicated in a different school with a significant Latino American student population (Yeager et al., in press). It appears that the spring of seventh grade marks the beginning of a process that erodes trust for minority students. Moreover, correlational evidence suggests that once mistrust began, a feedback loop began. Students who initially felt greater mistrust were later more likely to perceive bias at their school, and those who perceived greater bias at this later time felt, still later, more mistrust (Yeager et al., in press). By the time students at both schools graduated middle school, a large race gap in trust had emerged. It had grown out of a slow but steady accumulation of experiences. The striking changes during this time in adolescents' physical maturation are obvious to the eye. The psychological changes can be just as dramatic yet hidden from view.

Because the process that creates the trust gap depends on a feedback loop, interrupting it early could yield benefits that carry forward in time. Such an interruption took the form of a reassuring note from their teacher, called *wise feedback* (Yeager et al., 2014, in press; see also Cohen et al., 1999). It was given to students at the point when mistrust had been found to rise, the spring of seventh grade. The note was handwritten by the teachers and accompanied critical feedback that the teachers gave to students on the first draft of an essay they had written. Students were randomly assigned to receive either the wise feedback note or a neutral note appended to their essay draft (Yeager et al., 2014). The wise feedback note stated, "I'm giving you these comments because I have very high expectations and I know that you can reach them." The note was carefully worded and grounded in previous research (Cohen et al., 1999). It was aimed to reassure negatively stereotyped students that the teacher's feedback reflected the application of high standards rather than bias.

The intervention increased the percentage of African American students who revised their essay from 17% in the neutral feedback condition to 71% in the wise feedback condition, on par with the revision rate of European American students. It also prevented African Americans who had initially expressed low levels of trust in teachers from feeling even less trusting at year's end. Contrary to the easy explanations of lay psychology, African American students in the control condition were not being recalcitrant. Rather, they saw a situation that they could not fully trust and therefore one in which they could not fully invest their efforts. The intervention reassured them that they could trust, releasing their motivation. Consistent with this explanation, in a follow-up study that required all students to submit a revision, minority students who expressed higher levels of mistrust in the control condition wrote weaker revisions, as they used their past experience to make sense of the feedback (Yeager et al., 2014). By contrast, in the wise feedback condition, there was no such correlation between mistrust and the quality of revised essays. The feedback interaction, in other words, helped students to evade the effects of their past experience on their present opportunity. A feedback loop appeared to carry the benefits forward through time. Seven years later, those minority students receiving the wise feedback note in seventh grade were more likely to attend a 4-year college than those who had not (Yeager et al., in press). If the researchers had not taken the time to listen to students' psychology, or to identify the "natural history" of students' trust, they could only have guessed at the message to deliver and the time of delivery required to make a positive difference.

Go with the Flow

Where systemic change is not possible, at least in the short term, attempts to change the status quo should use existing processes rather than attempt to override them. By way of analogy, the Wright brothers realized that they could attain controlled flight by taking advantage of air currents rather than compensating for them through weight-shifting systems. They understood that a wing that could be continually warped when interacting with wind currents would produce both lift and permit control of a plane.

Some of the processes in a social system are not "noise" to be overcome but currents to exploit (see also Paluck, 2009). For example, the effects of an affirmation on later college accomplishment occurred partly because of the institutional tracking system, not in spite of it. In line with the mantra, "The best way to understand something is to try to change it" (Bronfenbrenner, 1977), research on "small" psychological interventions has advanced understanding of the power of "large" structural processes.

Wait for It

Because other people's psychology is difficult to see, large psychological change can take place in the absence of discernible behavioral change. Someone may be in the midst of a turning point, but because the initial shift is psychological, it may go unnoticed. Furthermore, as the effects of many interventions are slow moving rather than abrupt, it may take time for their consequences to become visible.

In one study, even if they earned relatively low grades, minority students who felt that they belonged in middle school as a result of an intervention proved more likely to go to college (Goyer, Garcia, et al., 2016). An invisible state of mind, not just a visible indicator of success, predicted long-term change. Indeed, the teachers who exert the most positive impact on students' psychological development may go unrecognized. This occurs because the predominant metric used to evaluate students' progress, the standardized test, fails to fully capture teachers' effect on students' growth along less visible psychological factors such as belonging and grit (Jackson, 2016). This is especially troubling given that such factors, when measured, predict long-term outcomes, such as college attendance, adult wages, and criminal records, better than standardized tests (Jackson, 2016).

At best, the early returns from the Move to Opportunity program, which provided a random group of poor families with the opportunity to move to somewhat wealthier neighborhoods and schools, were disappointing (Sanbonmatsu, Kling, Duncan, & Brooks-Gunn, 2006). Contrary to expectations, students did not attain higher academic performance. However, in spite of these negative indicators, the seeds of positive change had been laid. Later analyses revealed that the students were, many years later, more likely to attend college and earn higher salaries, especially if they had moved to the wealthier neighborhoods before the teenage years (Chetty, Hendren, & Katz, 2015).

If we judge the efficacy of an intervention only by short-term impacts, we are at risk of abandoning policies and programs with slow-to-emerge or difficult-to-see benefits. Governments and schools may end programs prematurely, either before enough time has elapsed to observe their full impact or before their influence on subtle signs of thriving has a chance to manifest. Indeed, this is what appears to have happened with the small high school movement. It was ended before research revealed, years later, its sizable benefits on high school graduation for disadvantaged students and on college enrollment and persistence for all students (Unterman, 2014). Sometimes change can be vast yet go unnoticed, obscured by the subtlety and gradualness of its unfolding.

Change can also be large and sudden, yet short-lived. This is especially likely if little or no thought is given to how to sustain benefits. In such cases, benefits may decay or even be reversed. For example, a program provided elderly adult residents of a nursing home with a sense of control over a seemingly minor event in their lives by allowing them to schedule visits from a college student (Schulz & Hanusa, 1978). Although residents saw their well-being and health rise in the short term as a result, once the program ended they suffered precipitous declines. To minimize outcomes like this, interventions and the processes they initiate must be viewed through the lens of an "experimental natural history" perspective. This requires that processes be studied over a long time to determine the range of their consequences, as in research on developmental cascades (Masten & Cicchetti, 2010). Moreover, it demands that the trajectory of these processes be compared under natural conditions and under conditions that subject them to experimental alteration. A commitment to studying processes over a long period of time needs to be a higher priority among social scientists, funders, and policymakers.

The Status Quo Is Not Neutral

On the face of it, the fact that a brief affirmation, belonging, or mindset intervention can have large and lasting effects seems a promising and positive message. However, by inverting the lens through which we look at these findings, we can see the background—the context in which the intervention is introduced—as foreground. Doing this reveals a troubling aspect of the status quo in many institutional settings. It is not neutral. If psychological interventions can have large and lasting effects, this implies that students are being underserved psychologically by the current status quo. If, for example, more minority students reach college because, as middle schoolers, they received a series of values affirmation activities (Goyer, Garcia, et al., 2016), a note reassuring them of their potential to reach a high standard (Yeager et al., 2014), or evidence that intelligence is expandable rather than fixed (Blackwell et al., 2007), this suggests that the status quo is failing to communicate these important psychological messages to these students. If merely suggesting to teachers that some of their students are "intellectual bloomers" leads them to draw out higher achievement from them (Rosenthal & Jacobson, 2003), this suggests that many teachers fail to expect as much of their students as they could or should. As a corollary to this logic, a failure to replicate the effects of an intervention in a new context may be a sign that the context is already addressing the psychological need in question (see Yeager et al., 2016, Study 1).

Inequality of opportunity, these data suggest, has not only a material dimension but a psychological one. Under the status quo, there must be many missed opportunities to encourage students, especially those who labor under low expectations. These include sins of omission. Because of stereotypes, people may fail to see potential where it exists. In one experiment, the same job résumés were less likely to receive a callback when the applicant had an African American name rather than a European Amercian name (Bertrand & Mullainathan, 2003). Strikingly, the strength of the résumé mattered little in the decision to call back African Americans. It was as if employers could not see merit where they did not expect it. In another disturbing example, on the exam required for high school graduation, African American and Latino American students were less likely than European American and Asian American students to be bumped above the passing cutoff by their teachers (43% vs. 48%) (Dee et al.,

2016). In still another study, when teachers determined assignment to gifted and talented programs, high-achieving African Americans were less likely than members of ethnic-majority groups to be assigned to them (Grissom & Redding, 2016). This was true even with socioeconomic status, health, and demographic variables controlled. This bias was reduced in one school district when a more objective test was introduced to identify candidates for gifted programs (Card & Giuliano, 2015). The missed opportunities of the status quo to increase equality of opportunity also include sins of commission. These include the documented tendencies of teachers to overpraise and underchallenge minority students (Harber et al., 2012), and their readiness to label misbehaving minority children as troublemakers and subject them to harsher disciplinary sentences (Okonofua & Eberhardt, 2015). Each of these biases has not only a material consequence but also a psychological one. It undercuts for many students the message that they belong, have potential, and are valued. One of the purposes of intervention research is to illuminate the nature of the social system—to shine a light on its inefficiency and injustice.

Consider Subtracting a Force

When we think of sparking change, we often think about adding forces. This is done by crafting new messages, providing new incentives, delivering new information, and so on. However, it is also possible to subtract forces (Lewin, 1939). There may be elements in the status quo that inhibit desired motivational mechanisms. For example, one study looked at college students who were put on academic "probation" because of their unsatisfactory progress (Brady, Fotuhi, et al., 2016). For this student population, conveying that their problems are "normal," as done in previous interventions (Walton & Cohen, 2007; Wilson & Linville, 1982), would miss the mark. Because these students had fallen short of the norms of success in their community, they needed to be alerted to this fact and at the same time assured that they were still respected as capable members of their college. Analyses of the letter notifying these students of their probationary status found it to be based largely on a motivational theory that what students needed was a "wake-up call." In it, "probation" was capitalized and there were dire warnings of the consequences of failing to improve. There was little appreciation of students' need to believe that they belonged in school, that they were members of the college community who could succeed in spite of their poor performance. In response to this, a new letter was devised. It provided the same key information to students but removed the threatening language. Testimonials from previous students who had served on probation reinforced the message that being on probation was not an academic death sentence, and that they belonged in spite of this setback. In a laboratory experiment, this letter produced less shame than the original letter (Brady, Fotuhi, et al., 2016). In a field experiment, it significantly increased the percentage of students who successfully exited probation and remained enrolled at the college. By removing a threatening cue and replacing it with a positive one, the institution better achieved its goals, sending the right message at the right time to the people who needed it.

Be Subtle but Sufficient

Social psychological interventions tend to be subtle but psychologically impactful. One of the barriers to change is that change attempts are often viewed negatively. They can be fragile moments, full of potential and vulnerability (Russell, 2017). A health tip, constructive criticism, a new job, or the start of college can all be experienced in this way. Although such encounters can lead to growth, they can also prove threatening. Persuasion can be seen as high-pressure salesmanship (Lewin, 1939). Reassurances can be seen as insincere, condescending, or stigmatizing (Ross & Nisbett, 2011; Steele, 1997). Constructive criticism can be viewed as biased. Indeed, it is for this reason that agents of change—teachers, managers, doctors, parents—are often viewed with suspicion (see Tyler & Lind, 1996). Many social-psychological interventions strive to convey their message tactfully, helping people to break free of psychological limits with decorum (Russell, 2017). Often a message is conveyed as an invitation to adopt a different outlook, in a manner that respects the diverse circumstances and sensitivities

of individuals in order to preserve their dignity. Defenses assuaged, they can prompt a change in themselves. This tact can be achieved, for example, by having the message conveyed by someone outside of the context of action, such as a scientist rather than a teacher (Walton & Cohen, 2011). Or the message may be conveyed indirectly rather than directly. Expert tutors reassure struggling students less through direct praise than through subtle words and actions that encourage children to generate their own positive meanings (Lepper & Woolverton, 2002). The source of the message can also be what for many is the most credible of sources, the self. In research on self-affirmation, evidence for one's self-integrity is not provided by a teacher, boss, or parent (Steele, 1988; see also Cohen & Sherman, 2014). Rather, it is provided by the threatened student, employee, or child.

Find the Gatekeepers

The "right people" include those individuals whose influence matters most, or as Lewin (1939) called them, "gatekeepers." These are people who channel influence and communication in a social system, for example, teachers, managers, and leaders. Understanding the psychology of the gatekeeper is important because it can affect multitudes. One recent study targeted a small group of middle school teachers, only 15 in number (Okonofua, Paunesku, & Walton, 2016). But combined, the teachers taught hundreds of students across three school districts. The intervention attempted to change the paradigm or lens through which teachers viewed their children. It taught them to have empathy: to see how students sometimes misbehave and act unreasonably when they feel that they do not belong. Rather than label a misbehaving child as a troublemaker, teachers were encouraged to see misbehavior as a product of a larger web of situational processes that could be altered. In short, the intervention helped teachers to unlearn the fundamental attribution error, the tendency to underemphasize the situation, both in its objective and subjective forms, and to overemphasize dispositional factors in the actor (Ross, 1977). Behind misbehavior, teachers learned, there is often a backstory. The intervention encouraged teachers to deal with these situational factors by using their relationships with students as vehicles to build respect rather than primarily to maintain discipline. Although the intervention consisted of only two brief online modules with a handful of teachers, the suspension rate among hundreds of students halved. Viewed from the perspective of the disappointing research on teacher training programs (Harris & Sass, 2007; Jacob & Lefgren, 2002), these results are striking. They show how a leveraged psychological intervention can have large effects when transmitted through key gatekeepers. They also show how the best interventions act not as a behavioral incentive (Lewin, 1939) but as an invitation to see the world in a different way.

Aim for Internalization, Not Compliance

When we focus on the temporal extension of motivational processes, other priorities begin to assert themselves. In the present moment, managers, parents, and teachers often try to achieve compliance. A worker should follow orders, a student complete his or her homework, a child behave. However, the acts that produce short-term compliance may in the long run produce hidden costs. In one study, children severely reprimanded not to play with an attractive toy complied (Freedman, 1965). However, weeks later, they were more likely to play with the toy during free time than were children who complied under mild discouragement, and more likely to cheat on an unrelated game (Freedman, 1965; Lepper, 1973). It was as though children had internalized the self-concept, "I do what's right because of external pressures, not inner scruples." In another study on police arrests, some officers arrested domestic assault suspects in a procedurally unfair way (Paternoster, Brame, Bachman, & Sherman, 1997). They acted in a way that was perceived as disrespectful and coercive. They appeared to have done their job, as they arrested the perpetrator. But there were unforeseen costs that emerged only later and that would have gone unseen had they not been measured and correlated with police treatment. The arrestees who were treated in an unfair manner were more likely to commit assault again when compared to those whose officers had treated them in a more respectful way. Much of the time the impact of our actions on short-term compliance are obvious. However, their psychological and accumulative impacts are not. A single action may create a turning point but we may never know it.

CONCLUSION

Like any attempt at change, a psychological intervention can seem small yet play a decisive role in a larger system. It enters a person's life space and interacts with the forces already there. Its consequences interact with unfolding historical, psychological, social, and cultural processes. Interventions gain their power, when they have any, from the moment when they happen. If there is a synchronicity between the act, actor, and stage—the right support happens to the right person at the right time and place—it can change a destiny. Events that do not happen under the status quo begin to emerge (Cohen & Sherman, 2014; Walton, 2014). More minority teenagers make it to college; fewer disadvantaged children are bullied; and fewer are suspended from school. More patients begin to take their medication, and more citizens go out to vote. Social-psychological research shows how a moment can hold more potential for change than we imagine. A timely and resonant act of support can give rise to more changes in a person's thought and life than prolonged yet poorly aimed intervention.

Interventions can reveal and create turning points in institutions, in relationships, and in other life domains. These are points of latent potential, the importance of which can be hard to grasp without the wide lens of longitudinal research. An intervention's impact on a person, like certain natural phenomena, may be so subtle and gradual as to escape notice if viewed from a short-term perspective. As the research reviewed in this chapter shows, the potential in a person or situation can be tapped and channeled by an everyday practice. In all cases, the full effects of an attempt at change or, indeed, of any act become evident only with both a microscopic perspective that zeroes in on the moment of change and a telescopic perspective that assesses its temporal reach. In summary, this chapter has argued for the adoption of a new wide-angle lens for viewing science-driven attempts at fostering motivation and thriving.

ACKNOWLEDGMENT

We are grateful to Shannon Brady and Roger Cohen for helpful conversations about the subject matter in this chapter.

REFERENCES

Alwin, D. F., Cohen, R. L., & Newcomb, T. M. (1991). *Political attitudes over the life-span: The Bennington women after 50 years*. Madison: University of Wisconsin Press.

Aronson, E. (1968). Dissonance theory: Progress and problems. In R. P. Abelson, E. Aronson, W. J. McGuire, T. M. Newcomb, M. J. Rosenberg, & P. Tannenbaum II (Eds.), *Theories of cognitive consistency: A sourcebook*. Skokie, IL: Rand McNally.

Aronson, J., Fried, C. B., & Good, C. (2002). Reducing the effects of stereotype threat on African American college students by shaping theories of intelligence. *Journal of Experimental Social Psychology, 38*(2), 113–126.

Asch, S. E. (1952). *Social psychology*. Englewood Cliffs, NJ: Prentice Hall.

Bem, S. L., & Bem, D. J. (1973). *Training the woman to know her place: The social antecedents of women in the world of work*. Harrisburg: Pennsylvania State Department of Education.

Bertrand, M., & Mullainathan, S. (2003). *Are Emily and Greg more employable than Lakisha and Jamal?: A field experiment on labor market discrimination* (NBER Working Paper Series 9873). Cambridge, MA: National Bureau of Economic Research.

Blackwell, L. S., Trzesniewski, K. H., & Dweck, C. S. (2007). Implicit theories of intelligence predict achievement across an adolescent transition: A longitudinal study and an intervention. *Child Development, 78*(1), 246–263.

Blattman, C., Jamison, J. C., & Sheridan, M. (2015). *Reducing crime and violence: Experimental evidence on adult noncognitive investments in Liberia* (NBER Working Paper Series 21204). Cambridge, MA: Bureau of Economic Research.

Blattman, C., & Niehaus, P. (2014). Show them the money: Why giving cash helps alleviate poverty. *Foreign Affairs, 93*, 117–126.

Bloom, B. S. (1984). The 2-sigma problem: The search for methods of instruction as effective as one-to-one tutoring. *Educational Researcher, 13*(6), 4–16.

Brady, S. T., Fotuhi, O., Gomez, E., Cohen, G. L., & Walton, G. M. (2016). *Reducing stigma and facilitating student success by reframing institutional messages*. Manuscript in preparation.

Brady, S. T., Reeves, S. L., Garcia, J., Purdie-Vaughns, V., Cook, J. E., Taborsky-Barba, S., et al. (2016). The psychology of the affirmed learner: Spontaneous self-affirmation in the face of stress. *Journal of Educational Psychology, 108*(3), 353–373.

Brady, S. T., Walton, G. M., Jarvis, S. N., & Cohen, G. L. (2016). *Bending the river: Downstream consequences of a social-belonging intervention in the transition to college*. Manuscript in preparation.

Braveman, P., Egerter, S., & Williams, D. R. (2011). The social determinants of health: Coming of age. *Annual Review of Public Health, 32*, 381–398.

Bronchetti, E. T., Dee, T. S., Huffman, D. B., & Magenheim, E. (2011). *When a nudge isn't enough: Defaults and saving among low-income tax filers* (NBER Working Paper Series 16887). Cambridge, MA: National Bureau of Economic Research.

Bronfenbrenner, U. (1977). Toward an experimental ecology of human development. *American Psychologist, 32*(7), 513–531.

Bryan, C. J., Walton, G. M., Rogers, T., & Dweck, C. S. (2011). Motivating voter turnout by invoking the self. *Proceedings of the National Academy of Sciences USA, 108*(31), 12653–12656.

Card, D., & Giuliano, L. (2015). *Can universal screening increase the representation of low income and minority students in gifted education?* (NBER Working Paper Series 21519). Cambridge, MA: National Bureau of Economic Research.

Carnevale, A. P., Rose, S. J., & Cheah, B. (2011). The college payoff: Education, occupations, lifetime earnings. Retrieved from *https://cew.georgetown.edu/wp-content/uploads/2014/11/collegepayoff-complete.pdf*.

Carstensen, L. L., Isaacowitz, D. M., & Charles, S. T. (1999). Taking time seriously: A theory of socioemotional selectivity. *American Psychologist, 54*, 165–181.

Caspi, A., Elder, G. H., Jr., & Bem, D. J. (1987). Moving against the world: Life-course patterns of explosive children. *Developmental Psychology, 23*(2), 308–313.

Cheryan, S., Plaut, V. C., Davies, P., & Steele, C. M. (2009). Ambient belonging: How stereotypical environments impact gender participation in computer science. *Journal of Personality and Social Psychology, 97*(6), 1045–1060.

Chetty, R., Hendren, N., & Katz, L. F. (2015). *The effects of exposure to better neighborhoods on children: New evidence from the*

Moving to Opportunity experiment (NBER Working Paper Series 21156). Cambridge, MA: National Bureau of Economic Research.

Chugh, D., & Brief, A. P. (2008). 1964 was not that long ago: A story of gateways and pathways. In A. P. Brief (Ed.), *Diversity at work* (pp. 318–340). Cambridge, UK: Cambridge University Press.

Cohen, G. L., Garcia, J., Apfel, N., & Master, A. (2006). Reducing the racial achievement gap: A social-psychological intervention. *Science, 313*, 1307–1310.

Cohen, G. L., Garcia, J., Purdie-Vaughns, V., Apfel, N., & Brzustoski, P. (2009). Recursive processes in self-affirmation: Intervening to close the minority achievement gap. *Science, 324*, 400–403.

Cohen, G. L., & Sherman, D. K. (2014). The psychology of change: Self-affirmation and social psychological intervention. *Annual Review of Psychology, 65*(1), 333–371.

Cohen, G. L., Steele, C. M., & Ross, L. D. (1999). The mentor's dilemma: Providing critical feedback across the racial divide. *Personality and Social Psychology Bulletin, 25*(10), 1302–1318.

Cook, J. E., Purdie-Vaughns, V., Garcia, J., & Cohen, G. L. (2012). Chronic threat and contingency belonging: Protective benefits of values affirmation on identity development. *Journal of Personality and Social Psychology, 102*(3), 479–496.

Core, A. (2014). *Change your day, not your life: A realistic guide to sustained motivation, more productivity, and the art of working well.* Hoboken, NJ: Wiley.

Creswell, J. D., Dutcher, J. M., Klein, W. M. P., Harris, P. R., & Levine, J. M. (2013). Self-affirmation improves problem-solving under stress. *PLoS ONE, 8*(5), e62593.

Creswell, J. D., Welch, W. T., Taylor, S. E., Sherman, D. K., Gruenewald, T. L., & Mann, T. (2005). Affirmation of personal values buffers neuroendocrine and psychological stress responses. *Psychological Science, 16*(11), 846–851.

Critcher, C. R., Dunning, D., & Armor, D. A. (2010). When self-affirmations reduce defensiveness: Timing is key. *Personality and Social Psychology Bulletin, 36*(7), 947–959.

Cronbach, L. (1975). Beyond the two disciplines of scientific psychology. *American Psychologist, 30*(2), 116–127.

Crosnoe, R. J., & Johnson, M. K. (2011). Research on adolescence in the twenty-first century. *Annual Review of Sociology, 37*, 439–460.

Davidai, S., Gilovich, T., & Ross, L. D. (2012). The meaning of default options for potential organ donors. *Proceedings of the National Academy of Sciences USA, 109*(38), 15201–15205.

Dawson, V. P., & Bowles, M. D. (2004). Taming liquid hydrogen: The Centaur upper stage rocket, 1958–2002. Retrieved from *http://history.nasa.gov/sp-4230.pdf.*

Dee, T. S., Dobbie, W., Jacob, B. A., & Rockoff, J. (2016). *The causes and consequences of test score manipulation: Evidence from the New York Regents Examinations* (NBER Working Paper Series 22165). Cambridge, MA: National Bureau of Economic Research.

Douglass, J. A. (2009). The race for human capital. In J. A. Douglass, C. J. King, & I. Feller (Eds.), *Globalization's muse: Universities and higher education systems in a changing world* (pp. 45–66). Berkeley, CA: Berkeley Public Policy Press.

Dweck, C. S. (1986). Motivational processes affecting learning. *American Psychologist, 41*(10), 1040–1048.

Dweck, C. S. (1999). *Self-theories: Their role in motivation, personality, and development.* Philadelphia: Psychology Press.

Dweck, C. S., Walton, G. M., & Cohen, G. L. (2011). Academic tenacity: Mindsets and skills that promote long-term learning. Retrieved from *https://ed.stanford.edu/sites/default/files/manual/dweck-walton-cohen-2014.pdf.*

Eccles, J. S., Lord, S., & Midgley, C. (1991). What are we doing to early adolescents?: The impact of educational contexts on early adolescents. *American Journal of Education, 99*(4), 521–542.

Egerter, S., Braveman, P., Sadegh-Nobari, T., Grossman-Kahn, R., & Dekker, M. (2011). *Education and health: Exploring the social determinants of health* (Issue Brief No. 5). Princeton, NJ: Robert Wood Johnson Foundation.

Elder, G. H. (1998). The life course as developmental theory. *Child Development, 69*(1), 1–12.

Fotuhi, O., Garcia, J., & Cohen, G. L. (2016). *Affirmation plus nudges enhance financial aid uptake.* Manuscript in preparation.

Freedman, J. L. (1965). Long-term behavioral effects of cognitive dissonance. *Journal of Experimental Social Psychology, 1*, 145–155.

Freedman, J. L., & Fraser, S. C. (1966). Compliance without pressure: The foot-in-the-door technique. *Journal of Personality and Social Psychology, 4*(2), 195–202.

Fryer, R., Jr. (2011). Financial incentives and student achievement: Evidence from randomized trials. *Quarterly Journal of Economics, 126*(4), 1755–1798.

Geertz, C. (1973). *The interpretation of cultures.* New York: Basic Books.

Goldin, C. (2015). Gender and the undergraduate economics major: Notes on the undergraduate economics major at a highly selective liberal arts college. Retrieved from *http://scholar.harvard.edu/files/goldin/files/claudia_gender_paper.pdf?m=1429198526.*

Good, C., Aronson, J., & Inzlicht, M. (2003). Improving adolescents' standardized test performance: An intervention to reduce the effects of stereotype threat. *Journal of Applied Developmental Psychology, 24*(6), 645–662.

Goyer, J. P., Cohen, G. L., Cook, J. E., Master, A., Okonofua, J. A., Apfel, N., et al. (2016). *A brief social-belonging intervention reduces disciplinary incidents among minority boys over 7 years.* Manuscript submitted for publication.

Goyer, J. P., Garcia, J., Purdie-Vaughns, V., Binning, K. R., Cook, J. E., Reeves, S. L., et al. (2016). *Into swifter currents: Self-affirmation nudges minority middle schoolers onto a college trajectory.* Manuscript submitted for publication.

Goyer, J. P., Stout, J. G., Miyake, A., Finkelstein, N. D., Ito, T. A., & Cohen, G. L. (2016). *Nudging high-potential women to stay in the STEM pipeline: Closing the gender gap in physical sciences with values affirmation.* Manuscript in preparation.

Grissom, J. A., & Redding, C. (2016). Discretion and disproportionality: Explaining the underrepresentation of high-achieving students of color in gifted programs. *AERA Open, 2,* 1–25.

Grubb, W. N. (2009). *The money myth: School resources, outcomes, and equity.* New York: Russell Sage Foundation.

Hackman, J. R. (1998). Why teams don't work. In R. S. Tindale, L. Heath, J. Edwards, E. J. Posavac, F. B. Bryant, Y. Suarez-Balcazar, et al. (Eds.), *Theory and research on small groups* (pp. 245–267). New York: Plenum Press.

Hanselman, P., Bruch, S. K., Gamoran, A., & Borman, G. D. (2014). Threat in context: School moderation of the impact of social identity threat on racial/ethnic achievement gaps. *Sociology of Education, 87*(2), 106–124.

Harackiewicz, J. M., Canning, E. A., Tibbetts, Y., Giffen, C. J., Blair, S. S., Rouse, D. I., et al. (2014). Closing the social class achievement gap for first-generation students in undergraduate biology. *Journal of Educational Psychology, 102*(2), 375–389.

Harber, K. D., Gorman, J. L., Gengaro, F. P., Butisingh, S., Tsang, W., & Ouellette, R. (2012). Students' race and teachers' social support affect the positive feedback bias in public schools. *Journal of Educational Psychology, 104*(4), 1149–1161.

Harris, D. N., & Sass, T. R. (2007). Teacher training, teacher quality and student achievement. Retrieved from *http://files.eric.ed.gov/fulltext/ed509656.pdf.*

Haskins, R. (2008). Education and economic mobility. Retrieved from *www.brookings.edu/~/media/research/files/reports/2008/2/economic-mobility-sawhill/02_economic_mobility_sawhill_ch8.pdf.*

Heath, C., & Heath, D. (2008). *Made to stick: Why some ideas survive and others die.* New York: Random House.

Heckman, J. J., Moon, S. H., Pinto, R., Savelyev, P., & Yavitz, A. (2009). *The rate of return to the High/Scope Perry Preschool Program* (NBER Working Paper Series 15471). Cambridge, MA: National Bureau of Economic Research.

Heckman, J. J., Moon, S. H., Pinto, R., Savelyev, P., & Yavitz, A. (2010). Analyzing social experiments as implemented: A reexamination of the evidence from the HighScope Perry Preschool Program. *Quantitative Economics, 1,* 1–46.

Hulleman, C. S., Godes, O., Hendricks, B. L., & Harackiewicz, J. M. (2010). Enhancing interest and performance with a utility value intervention. *Journal of Educational Psychology, 102*(4), 880–895.

Hulleman, C. S., & Harackiewicz, J. M. (2009). Promoting interest and performance in high school science classes. *Science, 326,* 1410–1412.

Jackson, K. C. (2016). *What do test scores miss?: The importance of teacher effects on non-test score outcomes* (NBER Working Paper Series 22226). Cambridge, MA: National Bureau of Economic Research.

Jacob, B. A., & Lefgren, L. (2002). *The impact of teacher training on student achievement: Quasi-experimental evidence from school reform efforts in Chicago* (NBER Working Paper Series 8916). Cambridge, MA: National Bureau of Economic Research.

Johnson, M. K., Crosnoe, R. J., & Elder, G. H., Jr. (2011). Insights on adolescence from a life course perspective. *Journal of Research on Adolescence, 21*(1), 273–280.

Johnson, R. C. (2012). The grandchildren of Brown: The long legacy of school desegregation (Goldman School of Public Policy Working Paper Series). Retrieved from *http://socrates.berkeley.edu/~ruckerj/rjabstract_browndeseg_grandkids.pdf.*

Jung, C. G. (1952). *Synchronicity: An acausal connecting principle* (2nd ed.). Princeton, NJ: Princeton University Press.

Karniol, R., Galili, L., Shtilerman, D., Naim, R., Stern, K., Manjoch, H., et al. (2011). Why Superman can wait: Cognitive self-transformation in the delay of gratification paradigm. *Journal of Clinical Child and Adolescent Psychology, 40,* 307–317.

Klein, K., & Boals, A. (2001). Expressive writing can increase working memory capacity. *Journal of Experimental Psychology: General, 130*(3), 520–533.

Latane, B., & Darley, J. M. (1969). Bystander "apathy." *American Scientist, 57*(2), 244–268.

Lepper, M. R. (1973). Dissonance, self-perception, and honesty in children. *Journal of Personality and Social Psychology, 25,* 65–74.

Lepper, M. R., Ross, L., & Lau, R. R. (1986). Persistence of inaccurate beliefs about the self: Perseverance effects in the classroom. *Journal of Personality and Social Psychology, 50*(3), 482–491.

Lepper, M. R., & Woolverton, M. (2002). The wisdom of practice: Lessons learned from the study of highly effective tutors. In J. Aronson (Ed.), *Improving academic achievement: Impact of psychological factors on education* (pp. 135–158). San Diego, CA: Academic Press.

Lewin, K. (1936). *Principles of topological psychology.* New York: McGraw Hill.

Lewin, K. (1939). Field theory and experiment in social psychology: Concepts and methods. *American Journal of Sociology, 44*(6), 868–896.

Lewin, K. (1947). Frontiers in group dynamics: Concept, method and reality in social science; social equilibria and social change. *Human Relations, 1*(1), 5–41.

Liberman, V., Samuels, S. M., & Ross, L. (2004). The name of the game: Predictive power of reputations versus situational labels in determining prisoner's dilemma game moves. *Personality and Social Psychology Bulletin, 30*(9), 1175–1185.

Loeb, S., & York, B. (2016). Helping parents help their children. Retrieved from *www.brookings.edu/research/papers/2016/02/18-helping-parents-help-children-loeb-york.*

Lyubomirsky, S., Sousa, L., & Dickerhoof, R. (2006). The costs and benefits of writing, talking, and thinking about life's triumphs and defeats. *Journal of Personality and Social Psychology, 90*(4), 692–708.

Manke, K. J., & Cohen, G. L. (2016). *Stereotype threat perseverance.* Stanford, CA: Stanford University.

Masten, A. S., & Cicchetti, D. (2010). Developmental cascades [Special issue]. *Development and Psychopathology, 22*(3), 491–495.

McGuire, W. J. (1960). A syllogistic analysis of cognitive relationships. In M. J. Rosenberg & C. I. Hoyland (Eds.), *Attitude organization and change* (pp. 140–162). New Haven, CT: Yale University Press.

Menec, V. H., Perry, R. P., Struthers, C. W., Schonwetter, D. J., Hechter, F. J., & Eichholz, B. L. (2006). Assisting at-risk college students with attributional retraining and effective teaching. *Journal of Applied Social Psychology, 24*(8), 675–701.

Milgram, S. (1963). Behavioral study of obedience. *Journal of Abnormal and Social Psychology, 67*(4), 371–378.

Mischel, W. (2014). *The marshmallow test: Why self-control is the engine of success.* New York: Little, Brown.

Miyake, A., Smith-Kost, L., Finkelstein, N. D., Pollock, S., Cohen, G. L., & Ito, T. A. (2010). Reducing the gender achievement gap in college science: A classroom study of values affirmation. *Science, 330,* 1234–1237.

Moffitt, T. E., Arseneault, L., Belsky, D., Dickson, N., Hancox, R. J., Harrington, H., et al. (2011). A gradient of childhood self-control predicts health, wealth, and public safety. *Proceedings of the National Academy of Sciences USA, 108*(7), 2693–2698.

Morwitz, V. M., Johnson, E., & Schmittlein, D. (1993). Does measuring intent change behavior? *Journal of Consumer Research, 20*(1), 46–61.

Mullainathan, S., & Shafir, E. (2013). *Scarcity: Why having too little means so much.* New York: Times Books.

O'Rourke, E., Haimovitz, K., Ballwebber, C., Dweck, C. S., & Popović, Z. (2014, April). *Brain points: A growth mindset incentive structure boosts persistence in an educational game.* Paper presented at the ACM Conference on Human Factors in Computing Systems, Toronto, Ontario, Canada.

Okonofua, J. A., & Eberhardt, J. L. (2015). Two strikes: Race and the disciplining of young students. *Psychological Science, 26*(5), 617–624.

Okonofua, J. A., Paunesku, D., & Walton, G. M. (2016). Brief intervention to encourage empathic discipline cuts suspension rates in half among adolescents. *Proceedings of the National Academy of Sciences USA, 113*(19), 5221–5226.

Paluck, E. L. (2009). Reducing intergroup prejudice and conflict using the media: A field experiment in Rwanda. *Journal of Personality and Social Psychology, 96*(3), 574–587.

Paluck, E. L., Shepherd, H., & Aronow, P. (2016). Changing climates of conflict: A social network driven experiment in 56 schools. *Proceedings of the National Academy of Sciences USA, 113*(3), 566–571.

Paternoster, R., Brame, R., Bachman, R., & Sherman, L. W. (1997). Do fair procedures matter?: The effect of procedural justice on spousal assault. *Law and Society Review, 31*(1), 163–204.

Pattwell, S. S., Casey, B. J., & Lee, F. S. (2013). Altered fear in mice and humans. *Current Directions in Psychological Science, 22*(2), 146–151.

Paunesku, D., Walton, G. M., Romero, C., Smith, E. N., Yeager, D. S., & Dweck, C. S. (2015). Mind-set interventions are a scalable treatment for academic underachievement. *Psychological Science, 26*(6), 784–793.

Pawson, R., & Tilley, N. (1997). *Realistic evaluation*. London: Sage.

Pennebaker, J. W., & Chung, C. K. (2011). Expressive writing: Connections to physical and mental health. In H. S. Friedman (Ed.), *The Oxford handbook of health psychology* (pp. 417–437). New York: Oxford University Press.

Powers, J. T., Cook, J. E., Purdie-Vaughns, V., Garcia, J., Apfel, N., & Cohen, G. L. (2016). Changing environments by changing individuals: The emergent effects of psychological intervention. *Psychological Science, 27*(2), 150–160.

Ramey, C. T., Campbell, F. A., Burchinal, M., Skinner, M. L., Gardner, D. M., & Ramey, S. L. (2000). Persistent effects of early childhood education on high-risk children and their mothers. *Applied Developmental Science, 4*(1), 2–14.

Raudenbush, S. W. (1984). Magnitude of teacher expectancy effects on pupil IQ as a function of the credibility of expectancy induction: A synthesis of findings from 18 experiments. *Journal of Educational Psychology, 76*, 85–97.

Reardon, S. F., Baker, R., & Klasik, D. (2012). Race, income, and enrollment patterns in highly selective colleges, 1982–2004. Retrieved from *http://inequality.stanford.edu/sites/default/files/reardon-baker-klasik_race_income_select_college.pdf*.

Rosenthal, R., & Jacobson, L. F. (2003). *Pygmalion in the classroom: Teacher expectation and pupils' intellectual development* (3rd ed.). Norwalk, CT: Crown House.

Ross, L. (1977). The intuitive psychologist and his shortcomings: Distortions in the attribution process. In L. Berkowitz (Ed.), *Advances in experimental social psychology* (Vol. 10, pp. 173–220). New York: Academic Press.

Ross, L., & Gilovich, T. (2015). *The wisest one in the room: How you can benefit from social psychology's most powerful insights*. New York: Simon & Schuster.

Ross, L., Lepper, M. R., & Hubbard, M. (1975). Perseverance in self-perception and social perception: Biased attributional processes in the debriefing paradigm. *Journal of Personality and Social Psychology, 32*(5), 880–892.

Ross, L., & Nisbett, R. (2011). *The person and the situation: Perspectives of social psychology* (2nd ed.). New York: McGraw-Hill.

Russell, D. (2017). *A literary history of tact: Aesthetic liberalism and the essay form*. Princeton, NJ: Princeton University Press.

Ryle, G. (2009). *Collected essays 1929–1968: Collected papers* (Vol. 2). Oxford, UK: Routledge. (Original work published 1971)

Sanbonmatsu, L., Kling, J. R., Duncan, G. J., & Brooks-Gunn, J. (2006). Neighborhoods and academic achievement: Results from the Moving to Opportunity experiment. *Journal of Human Resources, 41*(4), 649–691.

Sapolsky, R. (2010). Foreword. In C. M. Worthman, P. M. Plotsky, D. S. Schechter, & C. A. Cummings (Eds.), *Formative experiences: The interaction of caregiving, culture, and developmental psychobiology* (pp. xxiii–xxvi). New York: Cambridge University Press.

Schulz, R., & Hanusa, B. H. (1978). Long-term effects of control and predictability-enhancing interventions: Findings and ethical issues. *Journal of Personality and Social Psychology, 36*(11), 1194–1201.

Schwartz, D. L., Cheng, K. M., Salehi, S., & Wieman, C. (2016). The half empty question for socio-cognitive interventions. *Journal of Educational Psychology, 108*(3), 397–404.

Simmons, R. G., Black, A., & Zhou, Y. (1991). African-American versus white children and the transition into junior high school. *American Journal of Education, 99*, 481–520.

Skinner, B. F. (1969). *Contingencies of reinforcement: A theoretical analysis*. New York: Meredith Corporation.

Snyder, M., Tanke, E. D., & Berscheid, E. (1977). Social perception and interpersonal behavior: On the self-fulfilling nature of social stereotypes. *Journal of Personality and Social Psychology, 35*(9), 656–666.

Steele, C. M. (1988). The psychology of self-affirmation: Sustaining the integrity of the self. In L. Berkowitz (Ed.), *Advances in experimental social psychology* (Vol. 21, pp. 261–302). New York: Academic Press.

Steele, C. M. (1997). A threat in the air: How stereotypes shape intellectual identity and performance. *American Psychologist, 52*(6), 613–629.

Steele, C. M. (2010). *Whistling Vivaldi and other clues to how stereotypes affect us*. New York: Norton.

Steele, C. M., Spencer, S. J., & Aronson, J. (2002). Contending with group image: The psychology of stereotype and social identity threat. In M. P. Zanna (Ed.), *Advances in experimental social psychology* (Vol. 34, pp. 379–440). San Diego, CA: Academic Press.

Sunstein, C. R. (2002). The law of group polarization. *Journal of Political Philosophy, 10,* 175–195.

Thaler, R. H., & Sunstein, C. R. (2009). *Nudge: Improving decisions about health, wealth, and happiness.* New York: Penguin Books.

Tyler, T. R., & Lind, E. A. (1996). A relational model of authority in groups. *Advances in Experimental Social Psychology, 25,* 115–191.

Unterman, R. (2014). Headed to college: The effects of New York City's small high schools of choice on postsecondary enrollment. Retrieved from *www.mdrc.org/sites/default/files/headed_to_college_pb.pdf.*

U.S. Government. (2014). The economics of early childhood investments. Retrieved from *www.whitehouse.gov/sites/default/files/docs/early_childhood_report1.pdf.*

Vohs, K. D., Park, J. K., & Schmeichel, B. J. (2013). Self-affirmation can enable goal disengagement. *Journal of Personality and Social Psychology, 104*(1), 14–27.

Walton, G. M. (2014). The new science of wise psychological interventions. *Current Directions in Psychological Science, 23,* 73–82.

Walton, G. M., & Cohen, G. L. (2003). Stereotype lift. *Journal of Experimental Social Psychology, 39,* 456–467.

Walton, G. M., & Cohen, G. L. (2007). A question of belonging: Race, social fit, and achievement. *Journal of Personality and Social Psychology, 92*(1), 82–96.

Walton, G. M., & Cohen, G. L. (2011). A brief social-belonging intervention improves academic and health outcomes of minority students. *Science, 311,* 1447–1451.

Walton, G. M., & Spencer, S. J. (2009). Latent ability: Grades and test scores systematically underestimate the intellectual ability of negatively stereotyped students. *Psychological Science, 20*(9), 1132–1139.

Wansink, B., Latimer, L. A., & Pope, L. (2016). "Don't eat so much": How parent comments relate to female weight satisfaction. *Eating and Weight Disorders.* [Epub ahead of print]

White, R. E., & Carlson, S. M. (2016). What would Batman do?: Self-distancing improves executive function in young children. *Developmental Science, 19*(3), 419–426.

White, R. E., Prager, E. O., Schaefer, C., Kross, E., Duckworth, A. L., & Carlson, S. M. (in press). The "Batman effect": Self-distancing improves perseverance in young children. *Child Development.*

Wilson, T. D. (2011). *Redirect: The surprising new science of psychological change.* New York: Little, Brown.

Wilson, T. D., Damiani, M., & Shelton, N. (2002). Improving the academic performance of college students with brief attributional retraining interventions. In J. Aronson (Ed.), *Improving academic achievement: Impact of psychological factors on education* (pp. 88–108). San Diego, CA: Academic Press.

Wilson, T. D., & Linville, P. W. (1982). Improving the academic performance of college freshmen: Attribution therapy revisited. *Journal of Personality and Social Psychology, 42*(2), 367–376.

Woodhead, M. (1988). When psychology informs public policy: The case of early childhood intervention. *American Psychologist, 43*(6), 443–454.

Worthman, C. M., Plotsky, P. M., Schechter, D. S., & Cummings, C. A. (Eds.). (2010). *Formative experiences: The interaction of caregiving, culture, and developmental psychobiology.* New York: Cambridge University Press.

Yeager, D. S., Lee, H. Y., & Jamieson, J. P. (2016). How to improve adolescent stress responses: Insights from integrating implicit theories of personality and biopsychosocial models. *Psychological Science.* [Epub ahead of print]

Yeager, D. S., Purdie-Vaughns, V., Garcia, J., Apfel, N., Brzustoski, P., Master, A., et al. (2014). Breaking the cycle of mistrust: Wise interventions to provide critical feedback across the racial divide. *Journal of Experimental Psychology: General, 143*(2), 804–824.

Yeager, D. S., Purdie-Vaughns, V., Yang, S., & Cohen, G. L. (in press). Declining institutional trust among racial and ethnic minority adolescents: Consequence of procedural injustice, cause of behavioral disengagement. *Child Development.*

Yeager, D. S., & Walton, G. M. (2011). They're not magic: Social-psychological interventions in education. *Review of Educational Research, 81,* 267–301.

Yeager, D. S., Walton, G. M., Brady, S. T., Akcinarb, E. N., Paunesku, D., Keane, L., et al. (2016). Teaching a lay theory before college narrows achievement gaps at scale. *Proceedings of the National Academy of Sciences USA, 113*(24), E3341–E3348.

Author Index

Subject Index

Page numbers followed by *f* indicate figure; *n*, note; and *t*, table